The GALE ENCYCLOPEDIA of SURGERY AND MEDICAL TESTS

THIRD EDITION

The GALE
ENCYCLOPEDIA *of*
SURGERY AND
MEDICAL TESTS

THIRD EDITION

VOLUME

4

Q–Z

ORGANIZATIONS

GLOSSARY

INDEX

KRISTIN KEY, EDITOR

GALE
CENGAGE Learning®

Farmington Hills, Mich • San Francisco • New York • Waterville, Maine
Meriden, Conn • Mason, Ohio • Chicago

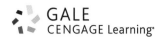

© 2014 Gale, Cengage Learning

WCN: 01-100-101

Gale Encyclopedia of Surgery and Medical Tests, Third Edition

Project Editor: Kristin Key

Editorial: Donna Batten

Product Manager: Rosemary Long

Editorial Support Services: Andrea Lopeman

Indexing Services: Andriot Indexing, LLC

Rights Acquisition and Management: Margaret Chamberlain-Gaston, Moriam Aigoro

Composition: Evi Abou-El-Seoud

Manufacturing: Wendy Blurton

Imaging: John Watkins

Product Design: Kristine Julien

For product information and technology assistance, contact us at
Gale Customer Support, 1-800-877-4253.
For permission to use material from this text or product,
submit all requests online at **www.cengage.com/permissions.**
Further permissions questions can be emailed to
permissionrequest@cengage.com

LIBRARY OF CONGRESS CATALOGING-IN-PUBLICATION DATA

The Gale encyclopedia of surgery and medical tests : a guide for patients and caregivers / Kristin Key, editor. -- 3rd edition.
     p. ; cm
     Encyclopedia of surgery and medical tests
     Includes bibliographical references and index.
     Summary: "Alphabetically arranged encyclopedia that contains approximately 600 entries on medical tests and procedures. Topics include specific surgeries, medical tests, and related concerns, such as postoperative care and anesthesia. Contains images, tables, and illustrations"--Provided by publisher.
     ISBN 978-1-57302-736-6 (set : alk. paper) -- ISBN 978-1-57302-737-3 (vol. 1 : alk. paper) -- ISBN 978-1-57302-738-0 (vol. 2 : alk. paper) -- ISBN 978-1-57302-739-7 (vol. 3 : alk. paper) -- ISBN 978-1-57302-740-3 (vol. 4 : alk. paper) -- ISBN 978-1-57302-741-0 (e-book) -- ISBN 1-57302-741-3 (e-book)
     I. Key, Kristin, editor of compilation.   II. Title: Encyclopedia of surgery and medical tests. [DNLM: 1. Diagnostic Techniques and Procedures--Encyclopedias--English.   2. Diagnostic Techniques and Procedures--Popular Works.   3. Surgical Procedures, Operative--Encyclopedias--English.   4. Surgical Procedures, Operative--Popular Works.   5. Health Services--Encyclopedias--English. 6. Health Services--Popular Works. WO 13]
     RD17
     617.003--dc23
                    2013046369

Gale
27500 Drake Rd.
Farmington Hills, MI, 48331-3535

ISBN-13: 978-1-57302-736-6 (set)   ISBN-13: 978-1-57302-739-7 (vol. 3)
ISBN-13: 978-1-57302-737-3 (vol. 1)   ISBN-13: 978-1-57302-740-3 (vol. 4)
ISBN-13: 978-1-57302-738-0 (vol. 2)

This title is also available as an e-book.
ISBN-13: 978-1-57302-741-0
Contact your Gale, a part of Cengage Learning sales representative for ordering information.

Printed in China
1 2 3 4 5 6 7 18 17 16 15 14

CONTENTS

ALPHABETICAL LIST OF ENTRIES

A

Abdominal ultrasound
Abdominal wall defect repair
Abdominoplasty
Abortion, induced
Abscess drainage
Acetaminophen
Adenoidectomy
Adhesions
Admission to the hospital
Adrenalectomy
Adrenergic drugs
Advance directives
Alanine aminotransferase test
Albumin test
Allergy tests
Alpha-fetoprotein (AFP) test
Ambulatory surgery centers
Amniocentesis
Amputation
Anaerobic bacteria culture
Analgesics
Analgesics, opioid
Anesthesia, general
Anesthesia, local
Anesthesiologist's role
Angiography
Angioplasty
Antianxiety drugs
Antibiotic prophylaxis
Antibiotics
Antibiotics, topical
Antibody tests
Anticoagulant and antiplatelet drugs
Antihypertensive drugs

Antinausea drugs
Antinuclear antibody test
Antiseptics
Antrectomy
Aortic aneurysm repair
Aortic valve replacement
Appendectomy
Arterial blood gas
Arteriovenous fistula creation
Arthrography
Arthroplasty
Arthroscopic surgery
Artificial sphincter insertion
Aseptic technique
Aspartate aminotransferase test
Aspirin
Autologous blood donation
Axillary dissection

B

Balloon valvuloplasty
Bandages and dressings
Bankart procedure
Barium enema
Biliary stenting
Bispectral index
Bladder augmentation
Blast injuries
Blepharoplasty
Blood culture
Blood donation and registry
Blood pressure measurement
Blood salvage
Blood urea nitrogen test

Bloodless surgery
Bone density test
Bone grafting
Bone marrow aspiration and biopsy
Bone marrow transplantation
Bone scan
Bone x-rays
Bowel preparation
Bowel resection
Bowel resection, small intestine
Breast biopsy
Breast implants
Breast reconstruction
Breast reduction
Bronchoscopy
BUN-creatinine ratio
Bunionectomy

C

Cardiac catheterization
Cardiac event monitor
Cardiac marker tests
Cardiac monitor
Cardiopulmonary resuscitation
Cardioversion
Carotid endarterectomy
Carpal tunnel release
Cephalosporins
Cerebral aneurysm repair
Cerebrospinal fluid (CSF) analysis
Cervical cerclage
Cervical cryotherapy
Cesarean section
Chemistry screen

Heart surgery for congenital defects
Heart transplantation
Heart-lung machines
Heart-lung transplantation
Heller myotomy
Hemangioma excision
Hematocrit
Hemispherectomy
Hemoglobin test
Hemoperfusion
Hemorrhoidectomy
Hepatectomy
Hepatitis virus tests
Hernia repair, femoral
Hernia repair, incisional
Hernia repair, inguinal
Hernia repair, umbilical
HIDA scan
Hip osteotomy
Hip replacement
Hip revision surgery
HIV and AIDS tests
Home care
Hospice
Hospital services
Hospital-acquired infections
Hospitalist
Human chorionic gonadotropin
    (hCG) pregnancy test
Human leukocyte antigen (HLA) test
Hydrocelectomy
Hypophysectomy
Hypospadias repair
Hysterectomy
Hysteroscopy

 I

Ileal conduit surgery
Ileoanal anastomosis
Ileostomy
Immunoassay tests
Immunologic therapies
Immunosuppressant drugs
Immunosuppression
Implantable cardioverter defibrillator
In vitro fertilization
Incentive spirometry

Incision care
Informed consent
Intensive care unit
Intensive care unit equipment
Intestinal obstruction repair
Intraoperative parathyroid hormone
    measurement
Intrauterine device (IUD) insertion
    and removal
Intravenous rehydration
Intussusception reduction
Iridectomy
Iron tests
Islet cell transplantation

 J

Joint fluid analysis

 K

Kidney dialysis
Kidney function tests
Kidney transplantation
Knee arthroscopic surgery
Knee osteotomy
Knee replacement
Knee revision surgery
Kneecap removal

 L

Laceration repair
Laminectomy
Laparoscopy
Laparoscopy for endometriosis
Laparotomy, exploratory
Laryngectomy
Laser iridotomy
Laser posterior capsulotomy
Laser skin resurfacing
Laser surgery
Laser-assisted in situ keratomileusis
    (LASIK)
Latex allergy
Laxatives
LDL cholesterol test

Leg lengthening or shortening
Length of hospital stay
Limb salvage
Lipid profile
Liposuction
Lithotripsy
Liver biopsy
Liver function tests
Liver transplantation
Living will
Lobectomy, cerebral
Lobectomy, pulmonary
Long-term care insurance
Lumpectomy
Lung biopsy
Lung transplantation
Lymph node biopsy
Lymphadenectomy

M

Magnetic resonance angiogram
Magnetic resonance imaging
Magnetic resonance venogram
Mammography
Managed care plans
Mantoux test
Mastectomy
Mastoidectomy
Maze procedure for atrial fibrillation
Mechanical circulatory support
Mechanical ventilation
Meckel's diverticulectomy
Mediastinoscopy
Medicaid
Medical charts
Medical comorbidities
Medical errors
Medicare
Medication monitoring
Meningocele repair
Mental health assessment
Mentoplasty
Microsurgery
Migraine surgery
Minimally invasive heart surgery
Mitral valve repair
Mitral valve replacement

Modified radical mastectomy
Mohs surgery
Multiple-gated acquisition (MUGA) scan
Myelography
Myocardial resection
Myomectomy
Myringotomy and ear tubes

N

Necessary surgery
Needle bladder neck suspension
Negative pressure rooms
Nephrectomy
Nephrolithotomy, percutaneous
Nephrostomy
Nerve conduction study
Neurosurgery
Nonsteroidal anti-inflammatory drugs
Nuclear medicine scans
Nursing homes

O

Obesity and surgery
Obstetric and gynecologic surgery
Omphalocele repair
Oophorectomy
Operating room
Ophthalmologic surgery
Ophthalmoscopy
Oral and maxillofacial surgery
Oral glucose tolerance test
Orchiectomy
Orchiopexy
Orthopedic surgery
Otoplasty
Outpatient surgery
Oxygen therapy

P

Pacemakers
Pain and pain management
Pallidotomy

Pancreas transplantation
Pancreatectomy
Pap test
Paracentesis
Parathyroid hormone test
Parathyroid scan
Parathyroidectomy
Parentage testing
Parotidectomy
Partial thromboplastin time
Patent urachus repair
Patient confidentiality
Patient Protection and Affordable Care Act
Patient rights
Patient-controlled analgesia
Pectus excavatum repair
Pediatric concerns
Pediatric surgery
Pelvic ultrasound
Penile prostheses
Pericardiocentesis
Peripheral endarterectomy
Peripheral vascular bypass surgery
Peritoneovenous shunt
pH monitoring
Phacoemulsification for cataracts
Pharyngectomy
Phlebography
Phlebotomy
Photocoagulation therapy
Photorefractive keratectomy (PRK)
Physical examination
Planning a hospital stay
Plastic, reconstructive, and cosmetic surgery
Pneumonectomy
Polypectomy
Portal vein bypass
Positron emission tomography
Post-anesthesia care unit
Postoperative antiemetics
Postoperative care
Postoperative infections
Postoperative pain
Power of attorney
Preanesthesia evaluation
Prenatal surgery
Prenatal testing

Preoperative care
Preparing for surgery
Pressure ulcers
Presurgical testing
Private insurance plans
Prostate biopsy
Prostatectomy
Protein components test
Prothrombin time
Proton pump inhibitors
Pulmonary function tests
Pulse oximeter
Pyloroplasty

Q

Quadrantectomy

R

Radical neck dissection
Recovery at home
Rectal prolapse repair
Rectal resection
Red blood cell indices
Red reflex testing
Reoperation
Retinal cryopexy
Retropubic suspension
Rh blood typing
Rheumatoid factor testing
Rhinoplasty
Rhizotomy
Robot-assisted surgery
Root canal treatment
Rotator cuff repair

S

Sacral nerve stimulation
Salpingo-oophorectomy
Salpingostomy
Scar revision surgery
Scleral buckling
Sclerostomy
Sclerotherapy for esophageal varices
Sclerotherapy for varicose veins

LIST OF ENTRIES BY BODY SYSTEM

▌Cardiovascular

Angiography

Angioplasty

Aortic aneurysm repair

Aortic valve replacement

Arteriovenous fistula creation

Balloon valvuloplasty

Cardiac catheterization

Cardiac event monitor

Cardiac marker tests

Cardiac monitor

Cardiopulmonary resuscitation

Cardioversion

Carotid endarterectomy

Coronary artery bypass graft surgery

Coronary stenting

Defibrillation

Echocardiography

Electrocardiography

Electrophysiology study of the heart

Endovascular stent surgery

Heart surgery for congenital defects

Heart transplantation

Heart-lung machines

Heart-lung transplantation

Hemangioma excision

Hernia repair, femoral

Implantable cardioverter defibrillator

Magnetic resonance angiogram

Magnetic resonance venogram

Maze procedure for atrial fibrillation

Mechanical circulatory support

Minimally invasive heart surgery

Mitral valve repair

Mitral valve replacement

Multiple-gated acquisition (MUGA) scan

Myocardial resection

Pacemakers

Pericardiocentesis

Peripheral endarterectomy

Peripheral vascular bypass surgery

Portal vein bypass

Sclerotherapy for varicose veins

Stress test

Vascular access devices

Vascular surgery

Vein ligation and stripping

Venous thrombosis prevention

Ventricular assist device

Ventricular shunt

▌Endocrine

Adenoidectomy

Adrenalectomy

Endoscopic retrograde cholangiopancreatography

Hypophysectomy

Intraoperative parathyroid hormone measurement

Islet cell transplantation

Oral glucose tolerance test

Pancreas transplantation

Pancreatectomy

Parathyroid hormone test

Parathyroid scan

Parathyroidectomy

Sestamibi scan

Thyroid function tests

Thyroidectomy

Whipple procedure

▌Gastrointestinal

Antrectomy

Appendectomy

Artificial sphincter insertion

Barium enema

Biliary stenting

Bowel preparation

Bowel resection

Bowel resection, small intestine

Cholecystectomy

Colonic stent

Colonoscopy

Colorectal surgery

Colostomy

Defecography

Endoscopic ultrasound

Esophageal atresia repair

Esophageal function tests

Esophageal resection

Esophagogastrectomy

Esophagogastroduodenoscopy

Gastrectomy

Gastric acid inhibitors

Gastric bypass

Gastroduodenostomy

Gastroenterologic surgery

Gastroesophageal reflux scan

Gastroesophageal reflux surgery

Gastrostomy

Glossectomy

Heller myotomy

Hemorrhoidectomy

Hepatectomy

HIDA scan

Ileoanal anastomosis

Ileostomy

Intestinal obstruction repair

Intussusception reduction

Laxatives

Liver biopsy

Liver transplantation

Parotidectomy

Pyloroplasty

Rectal prolapse repair

Rectal resection

Sclerotherapy for esophageal
  varices

Sigmoidoscopy

Total parenteral nutrition

Tube enterostomy

Upper gastrointestinal exam

Vagotomy

Vertical banded gastroplasty

▌Hematological

Alanine aminotransferase test

Albumin test

Allergy tests

Alpha-fetoprotein (AFP) test

Antinuclear antibody test

Arterial blood gas

Aspartate aminotransferase test

Autologous blood donation

Blood culture

Blood donation and registry

Blood pressure measurement

Blood salvage

Blood urea nitrogen test

Bloodless surgery

Bone marrow aspiration and biopsy

Bone marrow transplantation

BUN-creatinine ratio

Chemistry screen

Cholesterol and triglyceride tests

Coagulation and clotting tests

Complete blood count

Creatine phosphokinase (CPK)

Electrolyte tests

Enhanced external counterpulsation

Enzyme-linked immunosorbent
  assay (ELISA)

Epstein-Barr virus test

HDL cholesterol test

Hematocrit

Hemoglobin test

Hemoperfusion

Hepatitis virus tests

HIV and AIDS tests

Human chorionic gonadotropin
  (hCG) pregnancy test

Human leukocyte antigen (HLA)
  test

Iron tests

LDL cholesterol test

Lipid profile

Liver function tests

Meckel's diverticulectomy

Partial thromboplastin time

Phlebography

Phlebotomy

Photocoagulation therapy

Protein components test

Prothrombin time

Pulse oximeter

Red blood cell indices

Rh blood typing

Rheumatoid factor testing

Sedimentation rate

Serum calcium level

Serum carbon dioxide level

Serum chloride level

Serum creatinine level

Serum glucose level

Serum lead level

Serum phosphate level

Serum potassium level

Serum sodium level

Sphygmomanometer

Stem cell transplantation

Thrombectomy

Thrombolytic therapy

Toxicology screen

Transfusion

Type and screen

White blood cell count and
  differential

▌Integumentary

Allergy tests

Blepharoplasty

Cleft lip and palate repair

Debridement

Dermabrasion

Face lift

Face transplantation

Fasciotomy

Forehead lift

Laceration repair

Laser skin resurfacing

Mohs surgery

Pressure ulcers

Skin biopsy

Skin culture

Skin grafting

Tattoo removal

Webbed finger or toe repair

▌Musculoskeletal

Abdominal wall defect repair

Abdominoplasty

Amputation

Arthrography

Arthroplasty

Arthroscopic surgery

Bankart procedure

Bone density test

Bone grafting

Bone scan

Bone x-rays

Bunionectomy

Club foot repair

Craniofacial reconstruction

Disk removal

Elbow surgery

Electromyography

Eye muscle surgery

Finger reattachment

Fracture repair

Ganglion cyst removal
Hammer, claw, and mallet toe
    surgery
Hand surgery
Hernia repair, incisional
Hernia repair, inguinal
Hernia repair, umbilical
Hip osteotomy
Hip replacement
Hip revision surgery
Joint fluid analysis
Knee arthroscopic surgery
Knee osteotomy
Knee replacement
Knee revision surgery
Kneecap removal
Laminectomy
Leg lengthening or shortening
Limb salvage
Mastoidectomy
Mentoplasty
Orthopedic surgery
Pectus excavatum repair
Rotator cuff repair
Shoulder joint replacement
Shoulder resection arthroplasty
Skull x-rays
Spinal fusion
Spinal instrumentation
Tendon repair
Tenotomy
Traction
Wrist replacement

Neurological

Bispectral index
Carpal tunnel release
Cerebral aneurysm repair
Cerebrospinal fluid (CSF) analysis
Corpus callosotomy
Craniotomy
Deep brain stimulation
Electroencephalography
Hemispherectomy
Lobectomy, cerebral
Meningocele repair
Migraine surgery

Myelography
Nerve conduction study
Neurosurgery
Pallidotomy
Rhizotomy
Stereotactic radiosurgery
Sympathectomy
Vagus nerve stimulation

Reproductive, Female

Abortion, induced
Amniocentesis
Breast biopsy
Breast implants
Breast reconstruction
Breast reduction
Cervical cerclage
Cervical cryotherapy
Cesarean section
Colporrhaphy
Colposcopy
Colpotomy
Cone biopsy
Dilatation and curettage
Episiotomy
Fetoscopy
Hysterectomy
Hysteroscopy
In vitro fertilization
Intrauterine device (IUD) insertion
    and removal
Laparoscopy for endometriosis
Lumpectomy
Mammography
Mastectomy
Modified radical mastectomy
Myomectomy
Obstetric and gynecologic surgery
Oophorectomy
Pap test
Prenatal surgery
Prenatal testing
Quadrantectomy
Salpingo-oophorectomy
Salpingostomy

Sexually transmitted disease
    cultures
Simple mastectomy
Tubal ligation

Reproductive, Male

Circumcision
Hydrocelectomy
Hypospadias repair
Orchiectomy
Orchiopexy
Penile prostheses
Prostate biopsy
Prostatectomy
Sexually transmitted disease
    cultures
Transurethral resection of the
    prostate
Vasectomy
Vasovasostomy

Respiratory

Bronchoscopy
Chest tube insertion
Cricothyroidotomy
Endotracheal intubation
Functional endoscopic sinus
    surgery
Incentive spirometry
Laryngectomy
Lobectomy, pulmonary
Lung biopsy
Lung transplantation
Mantoux test
Mechanical ventilation
Mediastinoscopy
Pharyngectomy
Pneumonectomy
Pulmonary function tests
Septoplasty
Snoring surgery
Spirometry
Thoracentesis
Thoracoscopy
Tracheotomy

Sensory

Cochlear implants
Corneal transplantation
Cryotherapy
Cyclocryotherapy
Electronystagmography
Endolymphatic shunt
Enucleation, eye
Extracapsular cataract extraction
Goniotomy
Iridectomy
Laser iridotomy
Laser posterior capsulotomy
Laser-assisted in situ keratomileusis (LASIK)
Myringotomy and ear tubes
Ophthalmologic surgery
Ophthalmoscopy
Otoplasty
Phacoemulsification for cataracts
Photorefractive keratectomy (PRK)
Red reflex testing
Retinal cryopexy
Scleral buckling
Sclerostomy
Stapedectomy
Tarsorrhaphy
Tonometry
Trabeculectomy
Tube-shunt surgery
Tympanoplasty

Urinary

Bladder augmentation
Collagen periurethral injection
Cystectomy
Cystocele repair
Cystoscopy
Gallstone removal
Human chorionic gonadotropin (hCG) pregnancy test
Ileal conduit surgery
Kidney dialysis
Kidney function tests
Kidney transplantation
Lithotripsy
Needle bladder neck suspension
Nephrectomy
Nephrolithotomy, percutaneous
Nephrostomy
Patent urachus repair
Retropubic suspension
Sacral nerve stimulation
Sexually transmitted disease cultures
Sling procedure
Transurethral bladder resection
Ureteral stenting
Ureterosigmoidostomy
Ureterostomy, cutaneous
Urinalysis
Urinary anti-infectives
Urinary catheterization
Urine culture
Urologic surgery

Other Surgeries

Abscess drainage
Axillary dissection
Curettage and electrosurgery
Debulking surgery
Ear, nose, and throat surgery
Elective surgery
Emergency surgery
Essential surgery
Exenteration
General surgery
Gingivectomy
Laparoscopy
Laparotomy, exploratory
Laser surgery
Lymph node biopsy
Lymphadenectomy
Microsurgery
Necessary surgery
Omphalocele repair
Oral and maxillofacial surgery
Outpatient surgery
Pediatric surgery
Plastic, reconstructive, and cosmetic surgery
Polypectomy
Radical neck dissection
Rhinoplasty
Robot-assisted surgery
Root canal treatment
Scar revision surgery
Second-look surgery
Segmentectomy
Sex reassignment surgery
Splenectomy
Telesurgery
Thoracic surgery
Thoracotomy
Tonsillectomy
Tooth extraction
Tooth replantation
Trabeculectomy
Transplant surgery
Trauma surgery
Tumor removal

Other Tests & Procedures

Abdominal ultrasound
Anaerobic bacteria culture
Antibody tests
Chest x-ray
Computed tomography
Cryotherapy for cataracts
Cytology
Dental implants and restoration
Dental x-rays
Epidural therapy
Fecal occult blood test
Genetic testing
Glucose tests
Hair transplantation
Immunoassay tests
Immunologic therapies
Intravenous rehydration
Liposuction
Magnetic resonance imaging
Medication monitoring
Mental health assessment
Nuclear medicine scans
Oxygen therapy
Paracentesis
Parentage testing

Pelvic ultrasound
Peritoneovenous shunt
pH monitoring
Physical examination
Positron emission tomography
Sentinel lymph node biopsy
Sexually transmitted disease cultures
Single photon emission computed
    tomography
Stoma
Stool culture
Stool fat test
Stool O and P test
Temperature measurement
Tumor grading
Tumor marker tests
Tumor staging
Ultrasound
Weight management

Drugs

Acetaminophen
Adrenergic drugs
Analgesics
Analgesics, opioid
Anesthesia, general
Anesthesia, local
Antianxiety drugs
Antibiotic prophylaxis
Antibiotics
Antibiotics, topical
Anticoagulant and antiplatelet drugs
Antihypertensive drugs
Antinausea drugs
Antiseptics
Aspirin
Cephalosporins
Corticosteroids
Diuretics
Erythromycins
Fluoroquinolones
Immunosuppressant drugs
Nonsteroidal anti-inflammatory
    drugs
Postoperative antiemetics
Preanesthesia evaluation
Proton pump inhibitors

Scopolamine patch
Sedation, conscious
Sulfonamides
Tetracyclines

Related Issues & Topics

Adhesions
Admission to the hospital
Advance directives
Ambulatory surgery centers
Anesthesiologist's role
Aseptic technique
Bandages and dressings
Blast injuries
Choosing a hospital
Closures
Complementary/alternative
    medicine (CAM) and surgery
Crush injuries
Death and dying
Diabetes and surgery
Discharge from the hospital
Do not resuscitate (DNR) order
Drug-resistant organisms
Exercise
Fibrin sealants
Finding a surgeon
Health care proxy
Health history
Home care
Hospice
Hospital services
Hospital-acquired infections
Hospitalist
Immunosuppression
Incision care
Informed consent
Intensive care unit
Intensive care unit equipment
Latex allergy
Length of hospital stay
Living will
Long-term care insurance
Managed care plans
Medicaid
Medical charts

Medical comorbidities
Medical errors
Medicare
Medication monitoring
Mental health assessment
Negative pressure rooms
Nursing homes
Obesity and surgery
Operating room
Pain and pain management
Patient confidentiality
Patient Protection and Affordable
    Care Act
Patient rights
Patient-controlled analgesia
Pediatric concerns
Planning a hospital stay
Post-anesthesia care unit
Postoperative care
Postoperative infections
Postoperative pain
Power of attorney
Preoperative care
Preparing for surgery
Presurgical testing
Private insurance plans
Recovery at home
Reoperation
Second opinion
Smoking cessation
Stethoscope
Surgeons
Surgery and the elderly
Surgical instruments
Surgical mesh
Surgical oncology
Surgical risk
Surgical team
Surgical training
Surgical triage
Syringe and needle
Talking to the health care provider
Thermometer
Treatment refusal
Trocars
Vital signs
Wound care
Wound culture

PLEASE READ—IMPORTANT INFORMATION

The *Gale Encyclopedia of Surgery and Medical Tests, 3rd Edition* is a health reference product designed to inform and educate readers about a wide variety of surgeries, tests, diseases and conditions, treatments and drugs, equipment, and other issues associated with surgical and medical practice. Cengage Learning believes the product to be comprehensive, but not necessarily definitive. It is intended to supplement, not replace, consultation with physicians or other healthcare practitioners. While Cengage Learning has made substantial efforts to provide information that is accurate, comprehensive, and up-to-date, Cengage Learning makes no representations or warranties of any kind, including without limitation, warranties of merchantability or fitness for a particular purpose, nor does it guarantee the accuracy, comprehensiveness, or timeliness of the information contained in this product. Readers should be aware that the universe of medical knowledge is constantly growing and changing, and that differences of opinion exist among authorities. Readers are also advised to seek professional diagnosis and treatment for any medical condition, and to discuss information obtained from this book with their healthcare provider.

INTRODUCTION

The *Gale Encyclopedia of Surgery and Medical Tests, 3rd Edition* is a unique and invaluable source of information. This collection of approximately 600 entries provides in-depth coverage of various surgeries, medical tests, diseases and conditions, medications, and other issues related to hospitalization. Topics related to general health care round out the set, including entries on death and dying, discharge from the hospital, do not resuscitate (DNR) orders, exercise, finding a surgeon, hospice, hospital services, informed consent, living wills, long-term care insurance, managed care plans, Medicaid, Medicare, patient rights, planning a hospital stay, power of attorney, private insurance plans, second opinions, talking to the health care provider, and others.

SCOPE

The *Gale Encyclopedia of Surgery and Medical Tests, 3rd Edition* covers a wide variety of topics, but entries follow a standardized format to help users find information at a glance. Rubrics include the following headings (as applicable):

- Definition
- Purpose
- Demographics
- Description
- Precautions
- Diagnosis
- Preparation
- Aftercare
- Recommended dosage
- Risks
- Side effects
- Interactions
- Complications
- Morbidity and mortality rates
- Alternatives
- Results

- Health care team roles
- Questions to Ask Your Doctor (sidebar)
- Key Terms (sidebar)
- Resources

INCLUSION CRITERIA

A preliminary list of topics was compiled from a wide variety of sources, including health reference books, general medical encyclopedias, and consumer health guides. The advisory board evaluated the topics and made suggestions for inclusion. Final selection of topics was made by the advisory board in conjunction with the editor.

ABOUT THE CONTRIBUTORS

The essays were compiled by experienced medical writers, including doctors, pharmacists, and registered nurses. Medical advisors reviewed the completed essays to ensure that they are appropriate, up to date, and accurate.

HOW TO USE THIS BOOK

The *Gale Encyclopedia of Surgery and Medical Tests, 3rd Edition* has been designed with ready reference in mind.

- Straight **alphabetical arrangement** of topics allows users to locate information quickly.
- **Bold-faced terms** within entries inform readers of related articles.
- **Cross-references** placed throughout the encyclopedia direct readers from alternate names and related topics to specific entries.
- A list of **key terms** is included in most entries to define terms or concepts that may be unfamiliar to the user. A **glossary** of key terms in the back matter contains a complete list of all terms, arranged alphabetically.

• **Questions to Ask Your Doctor** sidebars provide users with questions to help facilitate discussions with physicians and other health care providers.

• **Resources** sections in all entries present readers with additional sources of information on a topic.

• Valuable **contact information** for health organizations is included with most entries. An appendix of organizations in the back matter contains an extensive list of organizations, arranged alphabetically.

• A comprehensive **general index** guides readers to significant topics mentioned in the text.

GRAPHICS

The *Gale Encyclopedia of Surgery and Medical Tests, 3rd Edition* is enhanced by more than 300 color photographs, illustrations, and tables.

ADVISORY BOARD

A number of experts in the medical community provided invaluable assistance in the formulation of this encyclopedia, and the editor would like to express her appreciation. The advisory board performed a myriad of duties, from defining the scope of coverage to reviewing individual entries for accuracy and accessibility.

CONTRIBUTORS

Margaret Alic
Medical and Science Writer
Eastsound, WA

Tammy Allhoff, CST, CSFA, AAS
Program Director, Surgical Technology
Pearl River Community College
Hattiesburg, MS

William Atkins
Science Writer
Pekin, IL

Laurie Barclay, MD
Neurological Consulting Services
Tampa, FL

Jeanine Barone
Nutritionist, Exercise Physiologist
New York, NY

Julia Barrett
Science Writer
Madison, WI

Donald G. Barstow, RN
Clinical Nurse Specialist
Oklahoma City, OK

Maria Basile, PhD
Medical Writer
Roselle, NJ

Mary Bekker
Medical Writer
Willow Grove, PA

Mark A. Best, MD, MPH, MBA
Associate Professor of Pathology
St. Matthew's University
Grand Cayman, BWI

Randall J. Blazic, MD, DDS
Oral and Maxillofacial Surgeon
Goodyear, AZ

Robert Bockstiegel
Medical Writer
Portland, OR

Maggie Boleyn, RN, BSN
Medical Writer
Oak Park, MN

Susan Joanne Cadwallader
Medical Writer
Cedarburg, WI

Diane M. Calabrese
Medical Sciences and Technology Writer
Silver Spring, MD

Richard H. Camer
Editor
International Medical News Group
Silver Spring, MD

Rosalyn Carson-DeWitt, MD
Medical Writer
Durham, NC

Laura Jean Cataldo, RN, EdD
Nurse
Myersville, MD

Lisa Christenson, PhD
Science Writer
Hamden, CT

Rhonda Cloos, RN
Medical Writer
Austin, TX

Constance Clyde
Medical Writer
Dana Point, CA

Angela M. Costello
Medical Writer
Cleveland, OH

L. Lee Culvert, PhD
Medical Writer
Portland, ME

Tish Davidson, AM
Medical Writer
Fremont, CA

Lori De Milto
Medical Writer
Sicklerville, NJ

Victoria E. DeMoranville
Medical Writer
Lakeville, MA

Altha Roberts Edgren
Medical Writer
Medical Ink
St. Paul, MN

Lorraine K. Ehresman
Medical Writer
Northfield, Quebec, Canada

Abraham F. Ettaher, MD

L. Fleming Fallon, Jr, MD, DrPH
Professor of Public Health
Bowling Green State University
Bowling Green, OH

Paula Ford-Martin
Medical Writer
Warwick, RI

Janie F. Franz
Journalist
Grand Forks, ND

Rebecca J. Frey, PhD
Medical Writer
New Haven, CT

Debra Gordon
Medical Writer
Nazareth, PA

Jill Granger, MS
Sr. Research Associate
Department of Pathology
University of Michigan Medical Center
Ann Arbor, MI

Peter Gregutt
Medical Writer
Asheville, NC

Laith Farid Gulli, MD, MS
*Consultant Psychotherapist in
    Private Practice*
Lathrup Village, MI

**Stephen John Hage, AAAS,
    RT(R), FAHRA**
Medical Writer
Chatsworth, CA

Maureen Haggerty
Medical Writer
Ambler, PA

Robert Harr
Associate Professor and Chair
Department of Public and Allied
    Health
Bowling Green State University
Bowling Green, OH

Dan Harvey
Medical Writer
Wilmington, DE

Katherine Hauswirth, APRN
Medical Writer
Deep River, CT

Caroline A. Helwick
Medical Writer
New Orleans, LA

Lisette Hilton
Medical Writer
Boca Raton, FL

Fran Hodgkins
Medical Writer

René A. Jackson, RN
Medical Writer
Port Charlotte, FL

Nadine M. Jacobson, RN
Medical Writer
Takoma Park, MD

Michelle L. Johnson, MS, JD
Patent Attorney
ZymoGenetics, Inc.
Seattle, WA

Paul Johnson
Medical Writer
San Diego, CA

Cindy L. A. Jones, PhD
Biomedical Writer
Sagescript Communications
Lakewood, CO

Linda D. Jones, BA, PBT (ASCP)
Medical Writer
Asheboro, NY

Crystal H. Kaczkowski, MSc
Medical Writer
Chicago, IL

Beth A. Kapes
Medical Writer
Bay Village, OH

Mary Jeanne Krob, MD, FACS
Medical Writer
Pittsburgh, PA

Monique Laberge, PhD

Richard H. Lampert
Medical Editor
W.B. Saunders Co.
Philadelphia, PA

Renee Laux, MS
Medical Writer
Manlius, NY

Victor Leipzig, PhD
Biological Consultant
Huntington Beach, CA

Lorraine Lica, PhD
Medical Writer
San Diego, CA

John T. Lohr, PhD
Assistant Director, Biotechnology Center
Utah State University
Logan, UT

Jennifer Lee Losey, RN
Medical Writer
Madison Heights, MI

Nicole Mallory, MS, PA-C
Medical Student
Wayne State University
Detroit, MI

Jacqueline N. Martin, MS
Medical Writer
Albrightsville, PA

Nancy McKenzie, PhD
Public Health Consultant
Brooklyn, NY

Mercedes McLaughlin
Medical Writer
Phoenixville, CA

Miguel A. Melgar, MD, PhD
Neurosurgeon
New Orleans, LA

**Christine Miner Minderovic,
    BS, RT, RDMS**
Medical Writer
Ann Arbor, MI

Mark Mitchell, MD, MPH, MBA
Medical Writer
Bothell, WA

**Alfredo Mori, MD, FACEM,
    FFAEM**
Emergency Physician
The Alfred Hospital
Victoria, Australia

Bilal Nasser, MD, MS
*Senior Medical Student, Wayne
    State University*
Detroit, MI

Erika J. Norris
Medical Writer
Oak Harbor, WA

Teresa Norris, RN
Medical Writer
Ute Park, NM

Debra Novograd, BS, RT(R)(M)
Medical Writer
Royal Oak, MI

Jane E. Phillips, PhD
Medical Writer
Chapel Hill, NC

J. Ricker Polsdorfer, MD
Medical Writer
Phoenix, AZ

**Elaine R. Proseus, MBA/TM,
    BSRT, RT(R)**
Medical Writer
Farmington Hills, MI

Robert Ramirez, BS
Medical Student
University of Medicine & Dentistry
    of New Jersey
Stratford, NJ

Esther Csapo Rastegari, RN, BSN, EdM
Medical Writer
Holbrook, MA

Martha Reilly, OD
Clinical Optometrist, Medical Writer
Madison, WI

Toni Rizzo
Medical Writer
Salt Lake City, UT

Richard Robinson
Medical Writer
Sherborn, MA

Nancy Ross-Flanigan
Science Writer
Belleville, MI

Belinda Rowland, PhD
Medical Writer
Voorheesville, NY

Laura Ruth, PhD
Medical, Science, & Technology Writer
Los Angeles, CA

Uchechukwu Sampson, MD, MPH, MBA

Kausalya Santhanam, PhD
Technical Writer
Branford, CT

Joan M. Schonbeck
Medical Writer

Nursing
Massachusetts Department of Mental Health
Marlborough, MA

Stephanie Dionne Sherk
Medical Writer
University of Michigan
Ann Arbor, MI

Lee A. Shratter, MD
Consulting Radiologist
Kentfield, CA

Jennifer E. Sisk, MA
Medical Writer
Havertown, PA

Allison Joan Spiwak, MSBME
Circulation Technologist
Ohio State University
Columbus, OH

Kurt Richard Sternlof
Science Writer
New Rochelle, NY

Margaret A Stockley, RGN
Medical Writer
Boxborough, MA

Dorothy Elinor Stonely
Medical Writer
Los Gatos, CA

Bethany Thivierge
Biotechnical Writer and Editor
Technicality Resources
Rockland, ME

Carol A. Turkington
Medical Writer
Lancaster, PA

Samuel D. Uretsky, PharmD
Medical Writer
Wantagh, NY

Chitra Venkatasubramanian, MD
Clinical Associate Professor, Neurology and Neurological Sciences
Stanford University School of Medicine
Palo Alto, CA

Ellen S. Weber, MSN
Medical Writer
Fort Wayne, IN

Barbara Wexler
Medical Writer
Chatsworth, CA

Abby Wojahn, RN, BSN, CCRN
Medical Writer
Milwaukee, WI

Kathleen D. Wright, RN
Medical Writer
Delmar, DE

Mary Zoll, PhD
Science Writer
Newton Center, MA

Michael Zuck, PhD
Medical Writer
Boulder, CO

Contributors

Quadrantectomy

Definition

Quadrantectomy is a surgical procedure in which a quadrant (approximately one-fourth) of the breast, including tissue surrounding a cancerous tumor, is removed. It is also called a partial or segmental **mastectomy**.

Purpose

Quadrantectomy is a type of breast-conserving surgery used as a treatment for breast cancer. Prior to the advent of breast-conserving surgeries, total mastectomy (complete removal of the breast) was considered the standard surgical treatment for breast cancer. Procedures such as quadrantectomy and **lumpectomy** (removing the tissue directly surrounding the tumor) have allowed doctors to treat cancer without sacrificing the entire affected breast.

Demographics

The American Cancer Society estimates that approximately 232,600 new cases of breast cancer are diagnosed annually in the United States, and 39,600 women die as a result of the disease. Approximately one in eight women will develop breast cancer at some point in her life. The risk of developing breast cancer increases with age: women ages 30–40 have a one in 252 chance; ages 40–50 have a one in 68 chance; ages 50–60 have a one in 35 chance; and ages 60–70 have a one in 27 chance.

In the 1990s, the incidence of breast cancer was higher among white women (113.1 cases per 100,000 women) than African American women (100.3 per 100,000). The death rate associated with breast cancer, however, was higher among African American women (29.6 per 100,000) than Caucasian women (22.2 per 100,000). Rates were lower among Hispanic women (14.2 per 100,000), Native American women (12.0 per 100,000), and Asian women (11.2 per 100,000).

Description

The patient is usually placed under **general anesthesia** for the duration of the procedure. In some instances, a local anesthetic may be administered with sedation to help the patient relax.

During quadrantectomy, a margin of normal breast tissue, skin, and muscle lining is removed around the periphery of the tumor. This decreases the risk of any abnormal cells being left behind and spreading locally or to other parts of the body (a process called metastasis). The amount removed is generally about one-fourth of the size of the breast (hence, the "quadrant" in quadrantectomy). The remaining tissue is then reconstructed to minimize any cosmetic defects, and then sutured closed. Temporary drains may be placed through the skin to remove excess fluid from the surgical site.

Some patients may have the lymph nodes removed from under the arm (called the axillary lymph nodes) on the same side as the tumor. Lymph nodes are small oval- or bean-shaped masses found throughout the body that act as filters against foreign materials and cancer cells. If cancer cells break away from their primary site of growth, they can travel to and begin to grow in the lymph nodes first, before traveling to other parts of the body. Removal of the lymph nodes is therefore a method of determining whether a cancer has begun to spread. To remove the nodes, a second incision is made in the area of the armpit and the fat pad that contains the lymph nodes is removed. The tissue is then sent to a pathologist, who extracts the lymph nodes from the fatty tissue and examines them for the presence of cancer cells.

Diagnosis

Breast tumors may be found during self-examination or an examination by a health care professional. In other cases, they are visualized during a routine mammogram.

Symptoms such as breast pain, changes in breast size or shape, redness, dimpling, or irritation may be an indication that medical attention is warranted.

Preparation

Prior to surgery, the patient is instructed to refrain from eating or drinking after midnight on the night before the operation. The physician will tell the patient what will take place during and after surgery, as well as expected outcomes and potential complications of the procedure.

Aftercare

The patient may return home the same day or remain in the hospital for one to two days after the procedure. Discharge instructions will include how to care for the incision and drains, which activities to restrict (e.g., driving and heavy lifting), and how to manage **postoperative pain**. Patients are often instructed to wear a well-fitting support bra for at least a week following surgery. A follow-up appointment to remove stitches and drains is usually scheduled 10–14 days after surgery.

If lymph nodes are removed, specific steps should be taken to minimize the risk of developing lymphedema of the arm, a condition in which excess fluid is not properly drained from body tissues, resulting in chronic swelling. This swelling can sometimes become severe enough to interfere with daily activity. Prior to being discharged, the patient will learn how to care for the arm, and how to avoid infection. She will also be told to avoid sunburn, refrain from heavy lifting, and to be careful not to wear tight jewelry and elastic bands.

Most patients undergo radiation therapy as part of their complete treatment plan. The radiation usually begins immediately or soon after quadrantectomy, and involves a schedule of five days of treatment a week for five to six weeks. Other treatments, such as chemotherapy or hormone therapy, may also be prescribed depending on the size and stage of the patient's cancer.

Risks

Risks associated with the surgical removal of breast tissue include bleeding, infection, breast asymmetry, changes in sensation, reaction to the anesthesia, and unexpected scarring.

Some of the risks associated with removal of the lymph nodes include excessive bleeding, infection, pain, excessive swelling, and damage to nerves during surgery. Nerve damage may be temporary or permanent, and may result in weakness, numbness, tingling, and drooping. Lymphedema is also a risk whenever lymph nodes have

been removed; it may occur immediately following surgery or months to years later.

Results

Most patients will not experience recurrences of the cancer following a treatment plan of quadrantectomy and radiation therapy. One study followed patients for a period of 20 years after breast-conserving surgery, and found that only 9% experienced recurrence of the cancer.

Morbidity and mortality rates

Following removal of the axillary lymph nodes, there is approximately a 10% risk of lymphedema and a 20% risk of abnormal skin sensations. Approximately 17% of women undergoing breast-conserving surgery have a poor cosmetic result (e.g., asymmetry or distortion of shape). The risk of complications associated with general anesthesia is less than 1%.

Alternatives

A full mastectomy, in which the entire affected breast is removed, is one alternative to quadrantectomy. A **simple mastectomy** removes the entire breast, while a radical mastectomy removes the entire breast plus parts of the chest muscle wall and the lymph nodes. In terms of recurrence and survival rates, breast-conserving surgery has been shown to be equally effective as mastectomy in treating breast cancer.

A new technique that may eliminate the need for removing many axillary lymph nodes is called sentinel node biopsy. When lymph fluid moves out of a region, the sentinel lymph node is the first node it reaches. The theory behind **sentinel lymph node biopsy** is that if cancer is not present in the sentinel node, it is unlikely to have spread to other nearby nodes. This procedure may allow individuals with early stage cancers to avoid the complications associated with partial or radical removal of lymph nodes if there is little or no chance that cancer has spread to them.

QUESTIONS TO ASK YOUR DOCTOR

- Why is quadrantectomy recommended?
- What methods of anesthesia and pain relief will be used?
- Where will the incision be located, and how much tissue will be removed?
- Will a lymph node dissection be performed?
- Is sentinel node biopsy appropriate in this case?
- Is postsurgical radiation therapy recommended?

Health care team roles

Quadrantectomy is usually performed by a general surgeon, breast surgeon, or surgical oncologist. Radiation therapy is administered by a radiation oncologist, and chemotherapy by a medical oncologist. The surgical procedure is frequently done in a hospital setting (especially when lymph nodes are to be removed at the same time), but specialized outpatient facilities are sometimes preferred.

Resources

BOOKS

Townsend, Courtney M., et al. *Sabiston Textbook of Surgery.* 19th ed. Philadelphia: Saunders/Elsevier, 2012.

PERIODICALS

Magno, Stefano, et al. "Accessory Nipple Reconstruction following a Central Quadrantectomy: A Case Report." *Cases Journal* 2, no. 1 (2009): 32. http://dx.doi.org/10.1186/1757-1626-2-32 (accessed October 2, 2013).

Pusiol, T., et al. "Middle Ear Metastasis from Dormant Breast Cancer as the Initial Sign of Disseminated Disease 20 Years after Quadrantectomy." *Ear, Nose & Throat Journal* 92, no. 3 (2013): 121–24.

WEBSITES

American Cancer Society. "Surgery for Breast Cancer." http://www.cancer.org/cancer/breastcancer/detailedguide/breast-cancer-treating-surgery (accessed October 2, 2013).

ORGANIZATIONS

American Cancer Society, 250 Williams St. NW, Atlanta, GA 30303, (800) 227-2345, http://www.cancer.org.

Society of Surgical Oncology, 9525 W. Bryn Mawr Ave., Ste. 870, Rosemont, IL 60018, (847) 427-1400, info@surgonc.org, http://surgonc.org.

Stephanie Dionne Sherk

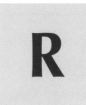

R

Radical neck dissection

Definition

Radical neck dissection is a surgical operation used to remove cancerous tissue in the head and neck.

Purpose

The purpose of radical neck dissection is to remove lymph nodes and other structures in the head and neck that are likely or known to be malignant. Variations on neck dissections exist, depending on the extent of the cancer. A radical neck dissection removes the most tissue. It is performed when the cancer has spread widely in the neck. A modified neck dissection removes less tissue, and a selective neck dissection even less.

Demographics

Experts estimate that there are approximately 5,000–10,000 radical neck dissections in the United States each year. Men and women undergo radical neck dissections at about the same rate.

Description

Cancers of the head and neck often spread to nearby tissues and into the lymph nodes. Removing these structures is one way of controlling the cancer.

Of the 600 lymph nodes in the body, approximately 200 are in the neck. Only a small number of these are removed during a neck dissection. In addition, other structures such as muscles, veins, and nerves may be removed during a radical neck dissection. These include the sternocleidomastoid muscle (one of the muscles that functions to flex the head), internal jugular (neck) vein, submandibular gland (one of the salivary glands), and the spinal accessory nerve (a nerve that helps control speech, swallowing, and certain movements of the head and neck). The goal is always to remove all the cancer, but

also to save as many components surrounding the nodes as possible.

An incision is made in the neck, and the skin is pulled back (retracted) to reveal the muscles and lymph nodes. The surgeon is guided in what to remove by tests performed prior to surgery and by examination of the size and texture of the lymph nodes.

Precautions

This operation should not be performed if the cancer has metastasized (spread) beyond the head and neck, or if the cancer has invaded the bones of the cervical vertebrae

---

KEY TERMS

Barium swallow—Barium is used to coat the throat to highlight the tissues lining the throat, allowing them to be visualized using x-ray pictures.

Computed tomography (CT or CAT) scan—Using x-rays taken from many angles and computer modeling, CT scans help locate and estimate the size of tumors and provide information on whether they can be surgically removed.

Lymph nodes—Small, bean-shaped collections of tissue found in lymph vessels. They produce cells and proteins that fight infection and filter lymph. Nodes are sometimes called lymph glands.

Magnetic resonance imaging (MRI)—Uses magnetic fields and computers to create detailed cross-sectional pictures of the interior of the body.

Malignant—Cancerous. Cells tend to reproduce without normal controls on growth and form tumors or invade other tissues.

Metastasize—Spread of cells from the original site of a cancer to other parts of the body where secondary tumors are formed.

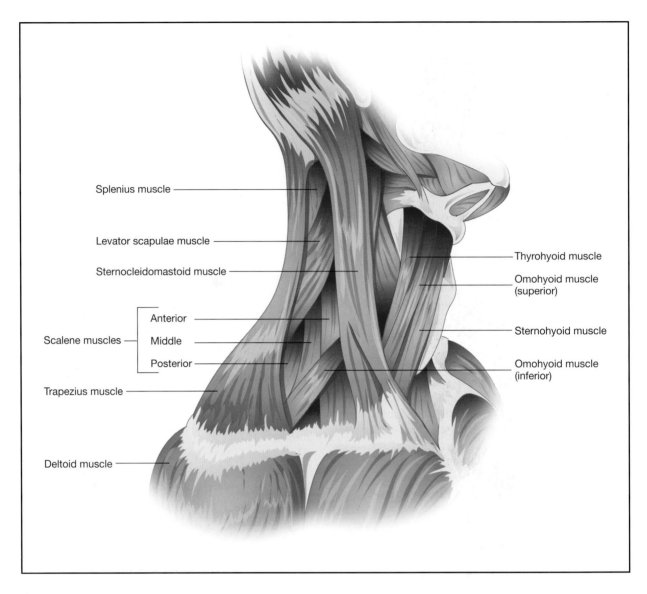

Splenius muscle

Levator scapulae muscle

Sternocleidomastoid muscle

Scalene muscles — Anterior

Middle

Posterior

Trapezius muscle

Deltoid muscle

Thyrohyoid muscle

Omohyoid muscle (superior)

Sternohyoid muscle

Omohyoid muscle (inferior)

Major muscles of the neck. *(Illustration by Electronic Illustrators Group. Copyright © 2014 Cengage Learning®.)*

(the first seven bones of the spinal column) or the skull. In these cases, the surgery will not effectively contain the cancer.

Preparation

Radical neck dissection is a major operation. Extensive tests are performed before the operation to try to determine where and how far the cancer has spread. These may include lymph node biopsies, **computed tomography** (CT) scans, **magnetic resonance imaging** (MRI) scans, and barium swallows, as well as standard preoperative blood and **liver function tests**. The candidate may meet with various health care professionals, including an anesthesiologist, nutritionist, and speech therapist, before or shortly after the operation.

The candidate should tell the anesthesiologist about any drug allergies and all medications (including over-the-counter drugs, vitamins, and supplements) that are presently being taken.

Aftercare

A person who has had a radical neck dissection will stay in the hospital for up to one week after the operation. Drains are inserted under the skin to remove fluid that accumulates in the neck area. The patient may need to keep at least one drain in for a short period of time after being discharged from the hospital. After the surgery, the patient will find it painful to swallow and may need to follow a liquid or soft-food diet while the neck heals. Follow-up doctor visits are required. Depending on how

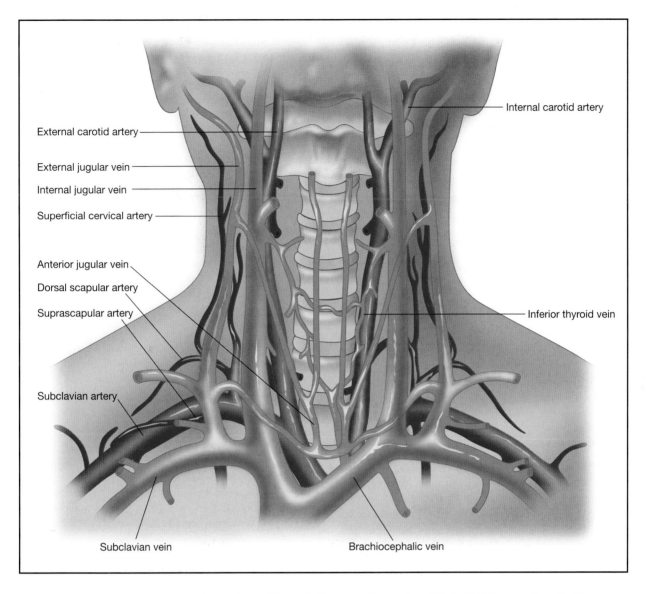

External carotid artery

External jugular vein

Internal jugular vein

Superficial cervical artery

Anterior jugular vein

Dorsal scapular artery

Suprascapular artery

Subclavian artery

Internal carotid artery

Inferior thyroid vein

Subclavian vein

Brachiocephalic vein

Major veins and arteries in the neck. *(Illustration by Electronic Illustrators Group. Copyright © 2014 Cengage Learning®.)*

many structures are removed, a person who has had a radical neck dissection may require physical therapy to regain use of the arm and shoulder.

Risks

The greatest risk in a radical neck dissection is damage to the nerves, muscles, and veins in the neck. Nerve damage can result in numbness (either temporary or permanent) to different regions on the neck and loss of function (temporary or permanent) to parts of the neck, throat, and shoulder. The more extensive the neck dissection, the more function a person is likely to lose. It is common following radical neck dissection for people to have stooped shoulders, limited ability to lift one or both arms, and limited head and neck rotation and flexion

due to the removal of nerves and muscles. Other risks are the same as for all major surgery: potential bleeding, infection, and allergic reaction to anesthesia.

Results

Normal lymph nodes are small and show no cancerous cells under a microscope. Abnormal lymph nodes may be enlarged and show malignant cells when examined under a microscope.

Morbidity and mortality rates

The mortality rate for radical neck dissection can be as high as 14%. Morbidity rates are somewhat higher and are due to bleeding, postsurgical infections, and medicine errors.

QUESTIONS TO ASK YOUR DOCTOR

- What tests will be performed to determine if the cancer has spread?

- Which parts of the neck will be removed?

- How will a radical neck dissection affect my daily activities after recovery?

- What is the likelihood that all of the cancer can be removed with a radical neck dissection?

- Are the involved lymph nodes on one or both sides of the neck?

- What will be my resulting appearance after the surgery?

- How will my speech and breathing be affected?

- Is my surgeon board-certified in otolaryngology head and neck surgery?

- How many radical neck procedures has my surgeon performed?

- What is my surgeon's complication rate?

Alternatives

Alternatives to radical neck dissection depend on the reason for the proposed surgery. Most alternatives are far less acceptable. Radiation and chemotherapy may be used instead of or in addition to a radical neck dissection in the case of cancer. Alternatives for some surgical procedures may reduce scarring but are not as effective in the removal of all pathological tissue. Chemotherapy and radiation or altered fractionated radiotherapy are reasonable alternatives.

Health care team roles

A radical neck dissection is usually performed by a surgeon with specialized training in otolaryngology head and neck surgery. Occasionally, a general surgeon will perform a radical neck dissection. The procedure is performed in a hospital under **general anesthesia**.

Resources

BOOKS

Goldman, Lee, and Andrew I. Schafer. *Goldman's Cecil Medicine.* 24th ed. Philadelphia: Saunders/Elsevier, 2012.

Lucioni, Marco. *Practical Guide to Neck Dissection: Focusing on the Larynx.* 2nd ed. New York: Springer, 2013.

Townsend, Courtney M., et al. *Sabiston Textbook of Surgery.* 19th ed. Philadelphia: Saunders/Elsevier, 2012.

PERIODICALS

Dautremont, J. F., et al. "Planned Neck Dissection Following Radiation Treatment for Head and Neck Malignancy." *International Journal of Otolaryngology*, art. ID no. 954203 (September 24, 2012). http://dx.doi.org/10.1155/2012/954203 (accessed August 2, 2013).

Ferlito, A., et al. "Is the Standard Radical Neck Dissection No Longer Standard?" *Acta Otolaryngolica* 122, no. 7 (2002): 792–95.

Lango, Miriam N., et al. "Impact of Neck Dissection on Long-Term Feeding Tube Dependence in Head and Neck Cancer Patients Treated with Primary Radiation or Chemoradiation." *Head & Neck* 32, no. 3 (2010): 341–47. http://dx.doi.org/10.1002/hed.21188 (accessed August 2, 2013).

Nobis, J. F., et al. "Head and Neck Salivary Gland Carcinomas—Elective Neck Dissection, Yes or No?" *Journal of Oral and Maxillofacial Surgery* (July 25, 2013): e-pub ahead of print. http://dx.doi.org/10.1016/j.joms.2013.05.024 (accessed August 2, 2013).

Popescu, B., et al. "Functional Implications of Radical Neck Dissection and the Impact on the Quality of Life for Patients with Head and Neck Neoplasia." *Journal of Medicine and Life* 5, no. 4 (2012): 410–13.

Seethala, Raja R. "Current State of Neck Dissection in the United States." *Head and Neck Pathology* 3, no. 3 (2009): 238–45. http://dx.doi.org/10.1007/s12105-009-0129-y (accessed August 2, 2013).

WEBSITES

A.D.A.M. Medical Encyclopedia. "Neck Dissection." MedlinePlus. http://www.nlm.nih.gov/medlineplus/ency/article/007573.htm (accessed August 5, 2013).

MedStar Georgetown University Hospital. "Neck Dissection Patient Information." http://www.georgetownuniversityhospital.org/body_dept.cfm?id=1016 (accessed August 5, 2013).

National Cancer Institute. "Metastatic Squamous Neck Cancer with Occult Primary Treatment (PDQ)." http://www.cancer.gov/cancertopics/pdq/treatment/metastatic-squamous-neck/Patient (accessed August 5, 2013).

ORGANIZATIONS

American Academy of Otolaryngology—Head and Neck Surgery, 1650 Diagonal Rd., Alexandria, VA 22314-2857, (703) 836-4444, http://www.entnet.org.

American Cancer Society, 250 Williams St. NW, Atlanta, GA 30303, (800) 227-2345, http://www.cancer.org.

American College of Surgeons, 633 N. Saint Clair St., Chicago, IL 60611-3211, (312) 202-5000, (800) 621-4111, Fax: (312) 202-5001, postmaster@facs.org, http://www.facs.org.

American Osteopathic Colleges of Otolaryngology—Head and Neck Surgery, 4764 Fishburg Rd., Ste. F, Huber Heights, OH 45424, (800) 455-9404, info@aocoohns.org, http://www.aocoohns.org.

National Cancer Institute, 6116 Executive Blvd., Ste. 300, Bethesda, MD 20892-8322, (800) 4-CANCER (422-6237), http://cancer.gov.

L. Fleming Fallon, Jr, MD, DrPH

Radical prostatectomy *see* **Prostatectomy**

Radioimmunoassay *see* **Immunoassay tests**

Reconstructive surgery *see* **Plastic, reconstructive, and cosmetic surgery**

Recovery at home

Definition

Recovery at home after surgery may require certain dietary and environmental restrictions, recommended rest and limitations to physical activities, and other required or restricted activities as recommended by a physician or surgeon.

Purpose

Postoperative recovery at home should promote physical healing and rest and recovery from the stress of surgery. For patients who undergo **orthopedic surgery**, the home recovery period will also involve rehabilitation to regain diminished musculoskeletal functioning. Emotional and psychological recovery from life-altering surgeries may also begin during the home recovery period.

Description

When patients are discharged from either an ambulatory surgical facility or a hospital, they will receive written instructions from their physician containing restrictions, requirements, and recommendations for their postoperative recovery at home. A nurse will usually review these instructions verbally with the patient and answer any questions and concerns. They may also call one or up to several days after a surgical discharge to follow up on how the patient is feeling and answer any questions about home recovery.

Restrictions and recommendations outlined in home recovery instructions may include:

- Driving restrictions. A patient may be prohibited from driving for a period of time due to functional limitations or to medication that impairs driving ability.

- Work restrictions. Depending on the nature of the patient's job, he or she may be required to stay home from work or request alternate duties until recovery is complete.

- Social restrictions. Patients at high risk of complications from infection, such as an organ transplant patient, may be advised to avoid anyone with a cold or flu and to stay away from crowds or social gatherings during the initial recovery period.

- Medication recommendations. Prescription and/or over the counter drugs may be recommended on an as-needed basis for pain and nausea. Other drugs may also be required.

- Dietary limitations. Certain types of gastrointestinal procedures and other surgeries may require a restricted diet during the recovery period. Alcohol may also be prohibited, particularly if pain medication has been prescribed.

- Ambulation recommendations. The doctor will note if the patient should refrain from lifting heavy objects, climbing stairs, having sex, or participating in other potentially strenuous activities.

- Exercise recommendations. If movement, stretches, or exercise is encouraged as part of recovery, that fact will also be noted.

- Incision care. Patients are instructed on how to care for their incision and educated on signs of infection (e.g., redness, warmth, swelling, fever, odor).

- Home care needs. Some patients may require a visiting nurse or live-in health aide for a period of time as they recover from surgery.

- Adaptive equipment. Assistive or adaptive devices such as crutches, a walker, prosthetics, or bed or bathroom hand rails may be necessary.

- Follow-up with physician. A patient may be instructed to call the doctor's office to schedule a follow-up appointment. The patient should also be given criteria for warning signs and symptoms that may occur with the procedure, and when to call the physician if the symptoms appear.

- Other required medical appointments. If a patient has undergone orthopedic surgery or another procedure that requires rehabilitation, he or she may need to see a physical or occupational therapist to regain range of motion, strength, and mobility. Depending on the type of surgery performed, the expertise of other medical professionals may also be required.

The postoperative period is also a time of emotional healing. Patients who face a long recovery and rehabilitation may feel depressed or anxious about their situation. Providing a patient with realistic goals and expectations for recovery both before and after the surgery can help avoid feelings of failure or let down when things do not progress as quickly as the patient had hoped. Realistic recovery expectations can also prevent a patient from doing too much too early and potentially hindering the healing process.

Certain life-altering surgeries, such as an **amputation** or a **mastectomy**, carry their own set of emotional issues. Counseling, therapy, or participation in a patient support group may be an important part of postoperative recovery as a patient adjusts to the new postsurgical life.

Preparation

Discharge recommendations for home recovery are typically explained to the patient before he or she is allowed to leave the hospital or ambulatory care facility. In some cases, the patient may be required to sign paperwork indicating that he or she has both received and understood home care instructions.

Depending on the surgical procedure undergone, a patient may be taught some home care techniques while still in the hospital. Physical therapy exercises, **incision care**, and use of assistive devices such as crutches or splints are a few self-care skills that may be demonstrated and practiced in an inpatient environment.

A physical and emotional support system is a crucial part of a successful home recovery. Faced with restrictions to movement, driving, and possibly more, a patient needs someone at home to help with the daily tasks of independent living. If family or friends are not nearby or available, a visiting nurse or home healthcare aide should be hired before the patient is discharged to home recovery.

Results

Following home care instructions can help to speed a patient's recovery time and ensure the safe resumption of normal activities. In some cases, the familiar, comforting home environment may even speed the healing process or improve the degree of recovery. One study of patients 64 and older undergoing hip surgery found that patients who were allowed to undergo rehabilitation at home had significantly better outcomes than those who underwent rehabilitation as hospital inpatients. On average, the former had better physical capacity and independent living skills when assessed six months after surgery.

Some studies have also indicated that gender may have an impact on the success and speed of postoperative home recovery. Some studies have found that women recover more rapidly than men. However, animal and laboratory studies have found that progesterone and estrogen may be involved in the period immediately after surgery or injury. This would indicate that women may have a natural advantage in recovery. Scientists continue to study the recovery process to try to understand it and help patient recovery as quickly and completely as possible.

Resources

BOOKS

Brunicardi, F. Charles, et al. *Schwartz's Principles of Surgery.* 10th ed. New York: McGraw-Hill, 2014.

Hatfield, Anthea and Michael Tronson. *The Complete Recovery Room Book.* 4th ed. New York: Oxford University Press, 2009.

PERIODICALS

Evenson, Mallorie, Daniel Payne, and Ingrid Nygaard. "Recovery at Home after Major Gynecologic Surgery: How Do Our Patients Fare?" *Obstetrics & Gynecology* 119, no. 4 (2012): 780–84. http://dx.doi.org/10.1097/AOG.0b013e31824bb15e (accessed October 17, 2013).

OTHER

Johns Hopkins Medicine. *The Road To Recovery after Lumbar Spine Surgery.* http://www.hopkinsortho.org/JHULumbSpineSurgeryGuide.pdf (accessed October 17, 2013).

WEBSITES

American Cancer Society. "Going Home after Cancer Surgery." http://www.cancer.org/treatment/treatmentsandsideeffects/treatmenttypes/surgery/surgery-going-home (accessed October 17, 2013).

Beth Israel Deaconess Medical Center. "Home After Heart Surgery: The Journey Back to Normal." http://www.bidmc.org/YourHealth/HealthNotes/KeepingYourHeartHealthy/DidYouKnow/HomeAfterHeartSurgery.aspx (accessed October 17, 2013).

Cleveland Clinic. "Heart Surgery Recovery." http://my.clevelandclinic.org/heart/disorders/recovery_ohs.aspx (accessed October 17, 2013).

Dunkin, Mary Anne. "Prepare for Your Post-Surgery Homecoming." *Arthritis Today.* http://www.arthritistoday.org/arthritis-treatment/surgery/recovery-and-rehab/post-surgery-recovery.php (accessed October 17, 2013).

"Helping Seniors with Post Surgical Recovery: Advice for Families and Caregivers." Care.com. http://my.clevelandclinic.org/

heart/disorders/recovery_ohs.aspx (accessed October 17, 2013).

MedlinePlus. "After Surgery." U.S. National Library of Medicine, National Institutes of Health. http://www.nlm.nih.gov/medlineplus/aftersurgery.html (accessed October 17, 2013).

NHS (UK National Health Service). "Having an Operation (Surgery)—Getting Back to Normal." http://www.nhs.uk/Conditions/surgery/Pages/getting-back-to-normal.aspx (accessed October 17, 2013).

Sutter Health. "Abdominal Surgery: Caring for Yourself at Home." http://www.cpmc.org/learning/documents/rg-abdom-home.html (accessed October 17, 2013).

University of California, San Francisco. "Recovering from Hip Replacement Surgery." http://www.ucsfhealth.org/education/recovering_from_hip_replacement_surgery (accessed October 17, 2013).

ORGANIZATIONS

National Association for Home Care & Hospice, 228 Seventh St. SE, Washington, DC 20003, (202) 547-7424, Fax: (202) 547-3540, http://www.nahc.org.

VNAA (Visiting Nurse Associations of America), 601 Thirteenth St. NW, Ste. 610N, Washington, DC 20005, (202) 384-1420, (888) 866-8773, vnaa@vnaa.org, http://vnaa.org.

Paula Ford-Martin
Robert Bockstiegel

Recovery room *see* **Post-anesthesia care unit**

Rectal artificial sphincter *see* **Artificial sphincter insertion**

Rectal prolapse repair

Definition

Rectal prolapse repair surgery treats a condition in which the rectum falls, or prolapses, from its normal anatomical position because of a weakening in the surrounding supporting tissues.

Purpose

A prolapse occurs when an organ falls or sinks out of its normal anatomical place. The pelvic organs normally have tissue (muscle, ligaments, etc.) holding them in place. Certain factors, however, may cause those tissues to weaken, leading to prolapse of the organs. The rectum is the last out of six divisions of the large intestine; the anus is the opening from the rectum through which stool exits the body. A complete rectal prolapse occurs when the rectum protrudes through the anus. If rectal prolapse is present, but the rectum does not protrude through the anus, it is called occult rectal prolapse, or rectal intussusception. In females, a rectocele occurs when the rectum protrudes into the posterior (back) wall of the vagina.

Factors that are linked to the development of rectal prolapse include age, repeated childbirth, constipation, ongoing physical activity, heavy lifting, prolapse of other pelvic organs, and prior **hysterectomy**. Symptoms of rectal prolapse include protrusion of the rectum during and after defecation, fecal incontinence (inadvertent leakage of feces with physical activity), constipation, and rectal bleeding. Women may experience a vaginal bulge, vaginal pressure or pain, painful sexual intercourse, and lower back pain.

Demographics

The overall incidence of rectal prolapse in the United States is approximately 4.2 per 1,000 people. The incidence of the disorder increases to 10 per 1,000 among patients older than 65. Most patients with rectal prolapse are women; the ratio of male-to-female patients is one to six.

Description

Surgery is generally not performed unless the symptoms of the prolapse have begun to interfere with daily life. Because of the numerous defects that can cause rectal prolapse, there are more than 50 operations that may be used to treat the condition. A perineal or abdominal approach may be used. While abdominal surgery is associated with a higher rate of complications and a longer recovery time, the results are generally longer lasting. Perineal surgery is generally used for older patients who are unlikely to tolerate the abdominal procedure well.

Abdominal and laparoscopic approach

Rectopexy and anterior resection are the two most common abdominal surgeries used to treat rectal prolapse. The patient is usually placed under **general anesthesia** for the duration of surgery. During rectopexy, an incision into the abdomen is made, the rectum isolated from surrounding tissues, and the sides of the rectum lifted and fixed to the sacrum (lower backbone) with stitches or with a nonabsorbable mesh. Anterior resection removes the S-shaped sigmoid colon (the portion of the large intestine just before the rectum); the two cut ends are then reattached. This straightens the lower portion of the colon and makes it easier for stool to pass. Rectopexy and anterior resection may also be performed in combination and may lead to a lower rate of prolapse recurrence.

As an alternative to the traditional laparotomy (large incision into the abdomen), laparoscopic surgery may be

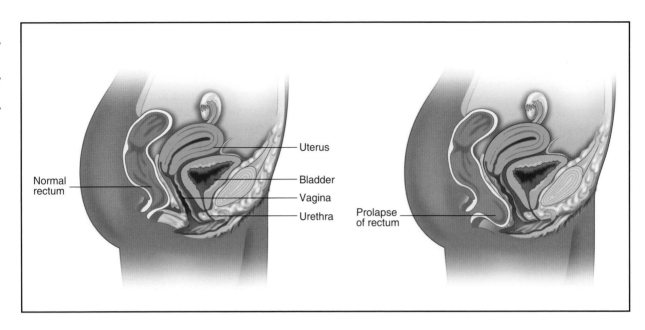

Normal rectum

Uterus
Bladder
Vagina
Urethra

Prolapse of rectum

Rectale prolapse occurs when the rectum slides down into the anus. The normal location of the rectum is shown on the left; the prolapsed rectum is shown on the right. *(Illustration by Electronic Illustrators Group. Copyright © 2014 Cengage Learning®.)*

performed. **Laparoscopy** is a surgical procedure in which a laparoscope (a thin, lighted tube) and various instruments are inserted into the abdomen through small incisions. Rectopexy and anterior resection have been performed laparoscopically with good results. A patient's recovery time following laparoscopic surgery is shorter and less painful than following traditional abdominal surgery.

Perineal approach

Perineal repair of rectal prolapse involves a surgical approach around the anus and perineum. The patient may be placed under general or regional anesthesia for the duration of surgery.

The most common perineal repair procedures are the Altemeier and Delorme procedures. During the Altemeier procedure (also called a proctosigmoidectomy), the prolapsed portion of the rectum is resected (removed) and the cut ends reattached. The weakened structures supporting the rectum may be stitched into their anatomical position. The Delorme procedure involves the resection of only the mucosa (inner lining) of the prolapsed rectum. The exposed muscular layer is then folded and stitched up and the cut edges of mucosa stitched together.

A rarely used procedure is anal encirclement. Also called the Thiersch procedure, anal encirclement involves the insertion of a thin circular band of non-absorbable material under the skin of the anus. This narrows the anal opening and prevents the protrusion of the rectum

through the opening. This procedure, however, does not address the underlying condition and therefore is generally reserved for patients who are not good candidates for more invasive surgery.

Diagnosis

Physical examination is most often used to diagnose rectal prolapse. The patient is asked to strain as if defecating; this increase in intra-abdominal pressure will maximize the degree of prolapse and aid in diagnosis. In some instances, imaging studies such as **defecography** (x-rays taken during the process of defecation) may be administered to determine the extent of prolapse.

Preparation

Before surgery, an intravenous (IV) line is placed so that fluid and/or medications may be easily administered to the patient. A Foley catheter will be placed to drain urine. **Antibiotics** are usually given to help prevent infection. The patient will be given a bowel prep to cleanse the colon and prepare it for surgery.

Aftercare

A Foley catheter may remain for one to two days after surgery. The patient will be given a liquid diet until normal bowel function returns. The recovery time following perineal repair is faster than recovery after abdominal surgery and usually involves a shorter hospital stay (one to three days following perineal surgery, three to seven days following abdominal surgery). The patient will be instructed to avoid activities for several weeks that will cause strain on the surgical site; these include lifting, coughing, long periods of standing, sneezing, straining with bowel movements, and sexual intercourse. High-fiber foods should be gradually added to the diet to avoid constipation and straining that could lead to prolapse recurrence.

Risks

Risks associated with rectal prolapse surgery include potential complications associated with anesthesia, infection, bleeding, injury to other pelvic structures, recurrent prolapse, and failure to correct the defect. Following a resection procedure, a leak may occur at the site where two cut ends of colon are reattached, requiring surgical repair.

Results

Most patients undergoing rectal prolapse repair will be able to return to normal activities, including work, within four to six weeks after surgery. The majority of patients will experience a significant improvement in symptoms and have a low chance of prolapse recurrence if heavy lifting and straining is avoided.

Morbidity and mortality rates

The approximate recurrence rates for the most commonly performed surgeries as reported by several studies are as follows:

- Altemeier procedure: 5%–54%
- Delorme procedure: 5%–26%
- anal encirclement: 25%
- rectopexy: 2%–10%
- anterior resection: 7%–9%
- rectopexy with anterior resection: 0%–4%

Abdominal surgeries are associated with a higher rate of complications than perineal repairs; rectopexy, for example, has a morbidity rate of 3%–29%, and anterior resection a rate of 15%–29%. The complication rate for combined rectopexy and anterior resection is slightly lower at 4%–23%. Approximately 25% of patients undergoing anal encirclement will eventually require surgery to treat complications associated with the procedure.

Alternatives

There are currently no medical therapies available to treat rectal prolapse. In cases of mild prolapse where the rectum does not protrude through the anus, a high-fiber diet, stool softeners, enemas, or **laxatives** may help to avoid constipation, which may make the prolapse worse.

Health care team roles

Rectal prolapse repair is usually performed in a hospital **operating room**. The surgery may be performed by a general surgeon, a colon and rectal surgeon (who focuses on diseases of the colon, rectum, and anus), or a gastrointestinal surgeon (who focuses on diseases of the gastrointestinal system).

Resources

BOOKS

Feldman, M., et al. *Sleisenger & Fordtran's Gastrointestinal and Liver Disease.* 9th ed. Philadelphia: Saunders/Elsevier, 2010.

Wein, Alan J., et al. *Campbell-Walsh Urology.* 10th ed. Philadelphia: Saunders/Elsevier, 2012.

PERIODICALS

Brown, S. "The Evidence Base for Rectal Prolapse Surgery: Is Resection Rectopexy Worth the Risk?" *Diseases of the Colon & Rectum* (October 1, 2013): e-pub ahead of print. http://dx.doi.org/10.1007/s10151-013-1077-9 (accessed October 2, 2013).

Mustain, W. C., et al. "Abdominal versus Perineal Approach for Treatment of Rectal Prolapse: Comparable Safety in a Propensity-Matched Cohort." *American Surgeon* 79, no. 7 (2013): 686–92.

Perrenot, Cyril, et al. "Long-Term Outcomes of Robot-Assisted Laparoscopic Rectopexy for Rectal Prolapse." *Diseases of the *Colon & Rectum* 56, no. 7 (2013): 909–14. http://dx.doi.org/10.1097/DCR.0b013e318289366e (accessed October 2, 2013).

WEBSITES

A.D.A.M. Medical Encyclopedia. "Rectal Prolapse Repair." MedlinePlus. http://www.nlm.nih.gov/medlineplus/ency/article/002932.htm (accessed October 2, 2013).

American Society of Colon and Rectal Surgeons. "Rectal Prolapse." http://www.fascrs.org/patients/conditions/rectal_prolapse (accessed October 2, 2013).

Mayo Clinic staff. "Rectal Prolapse Surgery." MayoClinic.com. http://www.mayoclinic.com/health/rectal-prolapse-surgery/MY00312/DSECTION=what-you-can-expect (accessed October 2, 2013).

ORGANIZATIONS

American Society of Colon and Rectal Surgeons, 85 W. Algonquin Rd., Ste. 550, Arlington Heights, IL 60005, (847) 290-9184, Fax: (847) 290-9203, ascrs@fascrs.org, http://www.fascrs.org.

Stephanie Dionne Sherk

Rectal resection

Definition

A rectal resection is the surgical removal of a portion of the rectum.

Purpose

Rectal resections repair damage to the rectum caused by diseases of the lower digestive tract, such as cancer, diverticulitis, and inflammatory bowel disease (ulcerative colitis and Crohn's disease). Injury, obstruction, and ischemia (compromised blood supply) may require rectal resection. Masses and scar tissue can grow within the rectum, causing blockages that prevent normal elimination of feces. Other diseases, such as diverticulitis and ulcerative colitis, can cause perforations in the rectum. Surgical removal of the damaged area can return normal rectal function.

Demographics

The American Cancer Society estimated 142,820 new colorectal cancer diagnoses in the United States for 2013, with 50,830 deaths. Rectal cancer incidence is approximately 28% of the total colorectal incidence rate. Surgery is the optimal treatment for rectal cancer, resulting in cure for 45% of patients. Recurrence due to surgical failure is low, from 4%–8%, when the procedure is meticulously performed.

Crohn's disease and ulcerative colitis, both chronic inflammatory diseases of the colon, each affect approximately 500,000 young adults. Surgery is recommended when medication fails patients with ulcerative colitis. Nearly three-fourths of all Crohn's patients will require surgery to remove a diseased section of the intestine or rectum.

Description

During a rectal resection, the surgeon removes the diseased or perforated portion of the rectum. If the diseased or damaged section is not very large, the separated ends are reattached. Such a procedure is called rectal anastomosis.

Diagnosis

A number of tests identify masses and perforations within the intestinal tract:

• A lower GI (gastrointestinal) series is a series of x-rays of the colon and rectum that can help identify ulcers, cysts, polyps, diverticuli (pouches in the intestine), and cancer. The patient is given a barium enema to coat the intestinal tract, making disease easier to see on the x-rays.

• Flexible sigmoidoscopy involves insertion of a sigmoidoscope, a flexible tube with a miniature camera, into the rectum to examine the lining of the rectum and the sigmoid colon, the last third of the intestinal tract. The sigmoidoscope can also remove polyps or tissue for biopsy.

• A colonoscopy is similar to the flexible sigmoidoscopy, except the flexible tube examines the entire intestinal tract.

• Magnetic resonance imaging (MRI), used both prior to and during surgery, allows physicians to determine the precise margins for the resection, so that all of the diseased tissue can be removed. This also identifies patients who could most benefit from adjuvant therapy such as chemotherapy or radiation.

Preparation

To cleanse the bowel, the patient may be placed on a restricted diet for several days before surgery, then placed on a liquid diet the day before, with nothing by mouth after midnight. A series of enemas and/or oral preparations (GoLytely, Colyte, or senna) may be ordered to empty the bowel. Oral anti-infectives (neomycin, erythromycin, or kanamycin sulfate) may be ordered to decrease bacteria in the intestine and help prevent postoperative infection. The operation can be done with an abdominal incision (laparotomy) or using minimally

Rectal resection

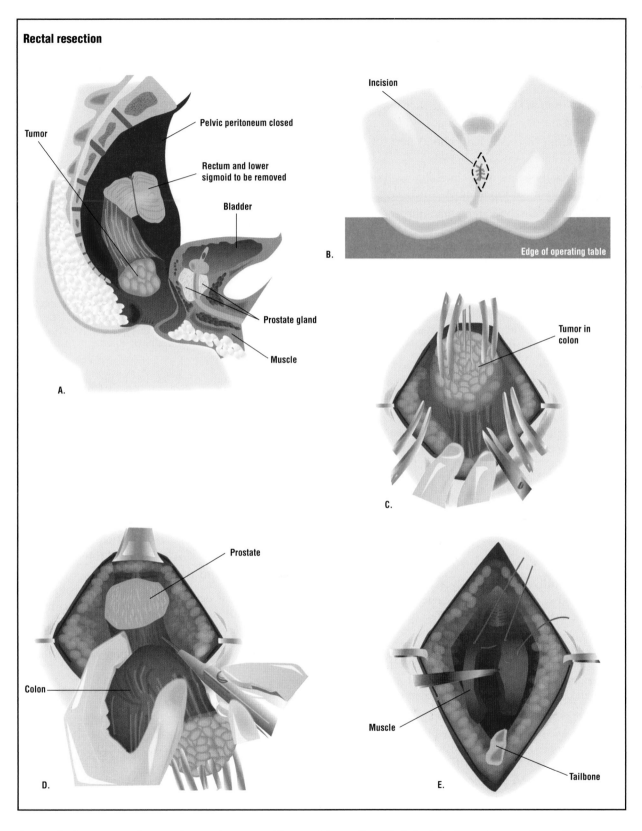

A. **Tumor** / **Pelvic peritoneum closed** / **Rectum and lower sigmoid to be removed** / **Bladder** / **Prostate gland** / **Muscle**

B. **Incision** / **Edge of operating table**

C. **Tumor in colon**

D. **Prostate** / **Colon**

E. **Muscle** / **Tailbone**

A tumor in the rectum or lower colon can be removed by a rectal resection (A). An incision is made around the patient's anus (B). The tumor is pulled down through the incision (C). An attached area of the colon is also removed (D). The area is repaired, leaving an opening for bowel functioning (E). *(Illustration by GGS Information Services. Copyright © Cengage Learning®.)*

invasive techniques with small tubes to allow insertion of the operating instruments (**laparoscopy**).

Aftercare

Postoperative care involves monitoring blood pressure, pulse, respiration, and temperature. Breathing tends to be shallow because of the effect of the anesthesia and the patient's reluctance to breathe deeply due to discomfort around the surgical incision. The patient is taught how to support the incision during deep breathing and coughing, and given pain medication as necessary. Fluid intake and output is measured, and the wound is observed for color and drainage.

Fluids and electrolytes are given intravenously until the patient's diet can be resumed, starting with liquids, then adding solids. The patient is helped out of bed the evening of the surgery and allowed to sit in a chair. Most patients are discharged in two to four days.

Risks

Rectal resection has potential risks similar those of other major surgeries. Complications usually occur while the patient is in the hospital and the patient's general health prior to surgery will be an indication of the risk potential. Patients with heart problems and stressed immune systems are of special concern. Both during and following the procedure, the physician and nursing staff will monitor the patient for:

- excessive bleeding
- wound infection
- thrombophlebitis (inflammation and blood clot in the veins in the legs
- pneumonia
- pulmonary embolism (blood clot or air bubble in the lungs' blood supply)
- cardiac stress due to allergic reaction to the general anaesthetic

Symptoms that the patient should report, especially after discharge, include:

- increased pain, swelling, redness, drainage, or bleeding in the surgical area
- flu-like symptoms such as headache, muscle aches, dizziness, or fever
- increased abdominal pain or swelling, constipation, nausea or vomiting, or black, tarry stools

Results

Complete healing is expected without complications. The recovery rate varies, depending on the patient's overall health prior to surgery. Typically, full recovery takes six to eight weeks.

Morbidity and mortality rates

Mortality has decreased from nearly 28% to under 6%, through the use of prophylactic **antibiotics** before and after surgery.

Alternatives

If the section of the rectum to be removed is very large, the rectum may not be able to be reattached. Under those circumstances, a **colostomy** would be preformed. The distal end of the rectum would be closed and left to atrophy. The proximal end would be brought through an opening in the abdomen to create an opening, a **stoma**, for feces to be removed from the body.

Health care team roles

Rectal resections are performed by general **surgeons** and colorectal surgeons as in-patient surgeries under **general anesthesia**.

Resources

BOOKS

American Cancer Society. *QuickFACTS Colorectal Cancer*. Chicago: American Cancer Society, 2012.

Johnston, Lorraine. *Colon & Rectal Cancer: A Comprehensive Guide for Patients and Families*. Sebastopol, CA: O'Reilly, 2000.

Levin, Bernard, et al. *American Cancer Society's Complete Guide to Colorectal Cancer*. Atlanta: American Cancer Society, 2006.

PERIODICALS

Fernandez, Ramiro, et al. "Laparoscopic versus Robotic Rectal Resection for Rectal Cancer in a Veteran Population." *American Journal of Surgery* 206, no. 4 (2013): 509–17. http://dx.doi.org/10.1016/j.amjsurg.2013.01.036 (accessed October 2, 2013).

Turina, Matthias, et al. "Quantification of Risk for Early Unplanned Readmission after Rectal Resection: A Single-Center Study." *Journal of the American College of Surgeons* 217, no. 2 (2013): 200–208. http://dx.doi.org/10.1016/j.jamcollsurg.2013.05.016 (accessed October 2, 2013).

WEBSITES

American Cancer Society. "Surgery for Colorectal Cancer." http://www.cancer.org/cancer/colonandrectumcancer/detailedguide/colorectal-cancer-treating-surgery (accessed October 2, 2013).

Society of American Gastrointestinal Endoscopic Surgeons. "Guidelines for Laparoscopic Resection of Curable Colon and Rectal Cancer." http://www.sages.org/publications/guidelines/guidelines-for-laparoscopic-resection-of-curable-colon-and-rectal-cancer (accessed October 2, 2013).

ORGANIZATIONS

American Board of Colon and Rectal Surgery, 20600 Eureka Rd., Ste. 600, Taylor, MI 48180, (734) 282-9400, Fax: (734) 282-9402, admin@abcrs.org, http://www.abcrs.org.

Society of American Gastrointestinal Endoscopic Surgeons (SAGES), 11300 W. Olympic Blvd., Ste. 600, Los Angeles, CA 90064, (310) 437-0544, Fax: (310) 437-0585, webmaster@sages.org, http://www.sages.org.

Janie Franz

Red blood cell indices

Definition

Red blood cell (RBC) indices are calculations derived from the **complete blood count** that aid in the diagnosis and classification of anemia.

Purpose

Red blood cell indices help classify types of anemia, a decrease in the oxygen carrying capacity of the blood. Healthy people have an adequate number of correctly sized red blood cells containing enough hemoglobin to carry sufficient oxygen to all the body's tissues. Anemia is diagnosed when either the hemoglobin or **hematocrit** of a blood sample is too low.

Description

Measurements needed to calculate RBC indices are the red blood cell count, hemoglobin, and hematocrit. The hematocrit is the percentage of blood by volume that is occupied by the red cells. The three main RBC indices are:

- Mean corpuscular volume (MCV). The average size of the red blood cells expressed in femtoliters (fL). MCV is calculated by dividing the hematocrit (as percent) by the RBC count in millions per microliter of blood, then multiplying by 10.

- Mean corpuscular hemoglobin (MCH). The average amount of hemoglobin inside an RBC expressed in picograms (pg). The MCH is calculated by dividing the hemoglobin concentration in grams per deciliter by the RBC count in millions per microliter, then multiplying by 10.

- Mean corpuscular hemoglobin concentration (MCHC). The average concentration of hemoglobin in the RBCs expressed as a percent. It is calculated by dividing the hemoglobin in grams per deciliter by the hematocrit, then multiplying by 100.

The mechanisms by which anemia occurs will alter the RBC indices in a predictable manner. Therefore, the RBC indices permit the physician to narrow down the possible causes of an anemia. The MCV is an index of the size of the RBCs. When the MCV is below normal, the RBCs will be smaller than normal and are described as microcytic. When the MCV is elevated, the RBCs will be larger than normal and are termed macrocytic. RBCs of normal size are termed normocytic.

Failure to produce hemoglobin results in smaller than normal cells. This occurs in many diseases, including iron deficiency anemia, thalassemia (an inherited disease in

KEY TERMS

Anemia—A variety of conditions in which a person's blood cannot carry as much oxygen as is needed by the tissues.

Hypochromic—A descriptive term applied to a red blood cell with a decreased concentration of hemoglobin.

Macrocytic—A descriptive term applied to a larger than normal red blood cell.

Mean corpuscular hemoglobin (MCH)—A calculation of the average weight of hemoglobin in a red blood cell.

Mean corpuscular hemoglobin concentration (MCHC)—A calculation of the average concentration of hemoglobin in a red blood cell.

Mean corpuscular volume (MCV)—A measure of the average volume of a red blood cell.

Microcytic—A descriptive term applied to a smaller than normal red blood cell.

Normochromic—A descriptive term applied to a red blood cell with a normal concentration of hemoglobin.

Normocytic—A descriptive term applied to a red blood cell of normal size.

Red cell distribution width (RDW)—A measure of the variation in the size of red blood cells.

which globin chain production is deficient), and anemias associated with chronic infection or disease. Macrocytic cells occur when division of RBC precursor cells in the bone marrow is impaired. The most common causes of macrocytic anemia are vitamin B_{12} deficiency, folate deficiency, and liver disease. Normocytic anemia may be caused by decreased production (e.g., malignancy and other causes of bone marrow failure), increased destruction (hemolytic anemia), or blood loss. The RBC count is low, but the size and amount of hemoglobin in the cells are normal.

A low MCH indicates that cells have too little hemoglobin. This is caused by deficient hemoglobin production. Such cells will be pale when examined under the microscope and are termed hypochromic. Iron deficiency is the most common cause of a hypochromic anemia. The MCH is usually elevated in macrocytic anemias associated with vitamin B_{12} and folate deficiency.

The MCHC is the ratio of hemoglobin mass in the RBC to cell volume. Cells with too little hemoglobin are lighter in color and have a low MCHC. The MCHC is low in microcytic, hypochromic anemias such as iron deficiency, but is usually normal in macrocytic anemias. The MCHC is elevated in hereditary spherocytosis, a condition with decreased RBC survival caused by a structural protein defect in the RBC membrane.

Cell indices are usually calculated from tests performed on an automated electronic cell counter. However, these counters measure the MCV, which is directly proportional to the voltage pulse produced as each cell passes through the counting aperture. Electronic cell counters calculate the MCH, MCHC, hematocrit, and an additional parameter called the red cell distribution width (RDW).

The RDW is a measure of the variance in red blood cell size. It is calculated by dividing the standard deviation (a measure of variation) of RBC volume by the MCV and multiplying by 100. A large RDW indicates abnormal variation in cell size, termed anisocytosis. The RDW aids in differentiating anemias that have similar indices. For example, thalassemia minor and iron deficiency anemia are both microcytic and hypochromic anemias, and overlap in MCV and MCH. However, iron deficiency anemia has an abnormally wide RDW, but thalassemia minor does not.

Preparation

RBC indices require 3–5 mL of blood collected by vein puncture with a needle. A nurse or phlebotomist usually collects the sample.

Aftercare

Discomfort or bruising may occur at the puncture site. Pressure to the puncture site until the bleeding stops reduces bruising; warm packs relieve discomfort. Some people feel dizzy or faint after blood has been drawn and should be allowed to lie down and relax until they are stable.

Risks

Other than potential bruising at the puncture site, and/or dizziness, there are no complications associated with this test. However, certain prescription medications may affect the test results. These drugs include zidovudine (Retrovir), phenytoin (Dilantin), and azathioprine (Imuran). When the hematocrit is determined by centrifugation, the MCV and MCHC may differ from those derived by an electronic cell counter, especially in anemia. Plasma trapped between the RBCs tends to cause an increase in the hematocrit, giving rise to a somewhat higher MCV and lower MCHC.

Results

Normal results for red blood cell indices are as follows:

• MCV: 80–96 fL

• MCH: 27–33 pg

• MCHC: 33%–36%

• RDW: 12%–15%

Resources

BOOKS

Hoffman, Ronald, et al. *Hematology: Basic Principles and Practice.* 6th ed. Philadelphia: Saunders/Elsevier, 2013.

McPherson, Richard A., and Matthew R. Pincus, eds. *Henry's Clinical Diagnosis and Management by Laboratory Methods.* 22nd ed. Philadelphia: Saunders/Elsevier, 2011.

WEBSITES

A.D.A.M. Medical Encyclopedia. "RBC Indices." MedlinePlus. http://www.nlm.nih.gov/medlineplus/ency/article/003648.htm (accessed October 17, 2013).

American Association for Clinical Chemistry. "Red Blood Cell Count." Lab Tests Online. http://labtestsonline.org/understanding/analytes/rbc (accessed October 17, 2013).

ORGANIZATIONS

American Association for Clinical Chemistry, 1850 K St. NW, Ste. 625, Washington, DC 20006, (800) 892-1400, Fax: (202) 887-5093, custserv@aacc.org, http://www.aacc.org.

Victoria E. DeMoranville
Robert Harr
Mark A. Best
Rosalyn Carson-DeWitt, MD

Red blood cell test *see* **Hemoglobin test**

Red reflex testing

Definition

Red reflex (RR) testing is an examination of the red reflex—light reflected back from the retina at the rear of the eye, which causes the pupil of the eye to appear red, as in flash photographs. RR testing is used to screen for abnormalities or obstructions of the retina—such as a cataract or tumor—that distort or eliminate the red reflex. The red reflex test is also called a light reaction test.

Purpose

Red reflex testing is considered to be an essential component of all healthcare visits for newborns, infants, and children through five years of age or until they are old enough to read an eye chart. Basic eye examinations in newborns, including RR testing, have become even more important as the number of premature and medically fragile infants born in the United States continues to increase. Although many more of these children are surviving, they often suffer visual impairment.

The primary purpose of RR testing is to screen for vision- and life-threatening conditions, especially retinoblastoma and congenital, infantile, or juvenile cataracts. Retinoblastoma is an inherited malignant (cancerous) tumor of the retina that can grow to fill much of the eye and spread to other parts of the body. A cataract is a clouding of the lens of the eye or its surrounding transparent membrane that prevents the passage of light into the eye. Although these conditions are rare, they are much more likely to be successfully treated with early detection. However, it is estimated that 75% of U.S. children under age five have never had a comprehensive eye exam, and only about 22% of preschoolers have had any type of vision screening.

Other abnormalities that can be detected by RR testing include:

• other opacities—areas of the eye that are not transparent to light—and abnormalities of the retina

• white spots in the eye

• strabismus—misalignment of the eyes caused by an imbalance in the muscles of the eyeball, resulting in an eye that turns in toward the nose (crosseyed) or outward away from the nose (walleyed)

• high refractive error, or the inability of an eye to focus light properly due to an irregularly shaped cornea, causing blurry vision—includes nearsightedness, farsightedness, or astigmatism

• asymmetric refractive error—significant differences in refractive error between the two eyes

• congenital glaucoma—a disease characterized by increased pressure within the eyeball

• lenticonus—a rare, usually congenital condition, in which the lens of the eye has a conical surface

• certain systemic diseases that affect the eyes

Demographics

About 60% of children who develop retinoblastoma have no known family history that would cause them to be screened. As many as 80% of retinoblastomas are initially detected by the child's family or friends, often by noticing that the child has one red eye and one white eye in a flash photograph. However, by the time the condition is this obvious, it is often too late to save the affected eye.

The American Academy of Pediatrics (AAP) recommends RR testing with an ophthalmoscope for all infants within the first two months of life, in a darkened room to maximize pupil dilation. Pediatricians often fail to diagnose retinoblastoma early because the exams are conducted in well-lit rooms in which the pupils are very small. For this reason, some states have considered legislation that would mandate RR testing of eye drop–dilated pupils for all newborns, and possibly at all six-week to eight-week and six-month to nine-month well-baby exams.

Description

In red reflex testing, a bright light is transmitted from an ophthalmoscope through all of the parts of the eye that are normally transparent, including the tear film, cornea, aqueous humor (the transparent fluid in the space between the cornea and lens), crystalline lens, and vitreous body (the transparent jelly that fills the eyeball behind the lens). The light reflects off the ocular fundus—the part of the eye opposite the pupil—and is transmitted back through the eye and the aperture of the ophthalmoscope. Any obstruction of this optical pathway results in an abnormal red reflex.

A direct ophthalmoscope or retinoscope is used to detect the red reflex in each eye individually and then in both eyes simultaneously to compare the red light reflection from each pupil. The ophthalmoscope is held close to the examiner's eye, about 12–18 inches (30–46 cm) from the child's eye. Sometimes RR testing is performed at two different distances and lens settings. If the baby's eyelids do not open adequately, a lid speculum may be used to hold them open.

A Bruckner test is RR testing combined with a simultaneous corneal light reflex test. The latter involves observing the location of a shined light on each cornea with respect to the pupil to check for ocular misalignment or other abnormalities. With a Bruckner test, the direct ophthalmoscope is held 2–3 feet (60–90 cm) from the child, and the red reflexes and corneal light reflexes of both eyes are viewed simultaneously.

Photoscreening is a newer type of RR testing in which a photograph of a child's eyes are analyzed for anomalies. It is especially useful for children who have trouble keeping still during an exam. RR testing for leukocoria—a white pupil reflex—is also sometimes performed by taking a flash photograph of the eyes after the child has been in a dark room for three to five minutes. Leukocoria may be more apparent in flash photographs because the pupil is exposed to a large amount of light only briefly, so that it does not have time to contract.

Infants and children who are at high risk due to a family history of retinoblastoma; congenital, infantile, or juvenile cataracts; congenital retinal dysplasia (abnormal growth in the retina); glaucoma; or other congenital disorders of the lens or retina should have initial RR testing performed with eye-drop dilation of the pupils. These children should be examined by an experienced pediatric ophthalmologist, even when their RR test results are normal.

Preparation

Sometimes, particularly with high-risk infants and children or when an abnormality is suspected, the pupils are artificially dilated with ophthalmic eye drops or sprays called mydriatic agents prior to RR testing. This ensures that the pupils remain dilated when exposed to bright light. Mydriatic agents are administered about 15 minutes prior to RR testing. In infants younger than nine months, a combination medication containing 0.2% or 0.25% cyclopentolate and 1% or 2.5% phenylephrine (Cyclomydril) is used. Lower concentrations are used for preterm infants. In babies older than nine months, one drop of 1% or less tropicamide and/or 2.5% phenylephrine are used.

Aftercare

There is no necessary aftercare for red reflex testing.

Risks

The use of mydriatic agents to dilate infants' pupils for RR testing is somewhat controversial. Some experts contend that infant pupils are so small that there is only a 30% chance of detecting retinoblastoma and other abnormal conditions inside the eye unless the pupil is dilated. Pediatric ophthalmologists routinely use mydriatic agents on infants older than two weeks, and they are often used on premature infants in neonatal intensive care units. However, rare but significant medical complications have been reported in infants with all commercially available dilating agents, and preterm infants may be particularly sensitive. Some practitioners believe that these side effects occur more often than the retinoblastomas detected by RR testing. The AAP recommends dilation with mydriatic agents only if there is evidence of an abnormality.

Reported complications of mydriatic agents include:

• increased blood pressure
• slowed or increased heart rate
• heart arrhythmias
• respiratory depression
• behavioral disturbances

KEY TERMS

Amblyopia—Lazy eye; poor vision in one eye with no apparent structural cause.

Aqueous humor—The clear, watery fluid between the cornea and the crystalline lens of the eye.

Astigmatism—A refractive error caused by an irregular-shaped cornea.

Cataract—Opacity or cloudiness of the eye lens, which can prevent a clear image from forming on the retina.

Cornea—The transparent covering of the iris and pupil that admits light to the interior of the eye.

Glaucoma—Damage to the optic nerve resulting in vision loss and usually accompanied by inflammation and increased pressure in the eye (intraocular pressure).

Iris—Pigmented tissue behind the cornea that gives color to the eye and varies the size of the pupil to control the amount of light entering the eye.

Lens—The transparent biconvex crystalline tissue that focuses light rays on the retina of the eye.

Lenticonus—A rare, usually congenital, condition in which the surface of the lens of the eye is conical.

Leukocoria—A pupil reflex that is white instead of red or that has white spots.

Mydriatic—Causing dilation or widening of the pupil of the eye.

Ocular fundus—The part of the eye opposite the pupil.

Opacity—An opaque spot in a normally transparent structure, such as the lens of the eye.

Ophthalmoscope—An instrument for examining the inner structure of the eye.

Pupil—The black circular opening at the center of the iris that regulates the amount of light that enters the eye.

Refractive error—The inability of the eye to properly focus light due to an irregularly shaped cornea, resulting in blurry vision, nearsightedness, farsightedness, or astigmatism.

Retina—The light-sensitive tissue at the back of the eye.

Retinoblastoma—A hereditary malignant tumor of the retina that develops during childhood.

Retinoscope—An instrument for determining the state of refraction of the eye by illuminating the retina with a mirror.

Strabismus—An imbalance of the eyeball muscles that prevents one eye from attaining binocular vision with the other.

Vitreous body—The transparent jelly that fills the eyeball behind the lens.

- hives (urticaria)

- contact dermatitis

- discomfort or pain

Results

Results of red reflex testing are considered to be negative or normal if the reflections from the two eyes, viewed both individually and simultaneously, are symmetrical—equivalent in color, brightness or intensity, size, and clarity—and without opacities or leukocoria (white spots). The reflected color is usually a bright reddish yellow. However, the red reflex can vary significantly depending on the child's racial or ethnic background, due to differing levels of pigmentation of the ocular fundus. The reflex may be light gray in dark pigmented, brown-eyed children.

Normal red reflexes indicate that the ocular media are free of opacities, that there are no large refractive errors, and that the eyes are aligned.

Abnormal results

Positive or abnormal RR testing results that require referral to an ophthalmologist include:

- dark spots in the red reflex

- a diminished or blunted red reflex

- opacities or dark spots or white spots in one area of the red reflex

- a white reflex (leukocoria)

- absence of a red reflex

- any differences in red reflex between the two eyes

Abnormalities in red reflexes or asymmetries between the two eyes can be due to:

- mucus or other foreign bodies in the tear film, which move and disappear upon blinking

- unequal or high refractive errors that indicate the need for glasses

- strabismus (eye misalignment)

- opacities in the cornea or aqueous or vitreous media

Reoperation

- abnormalities of the iris that affect the pupil
- cataracts
- glaucoma
- retinoblastoma
- other retinal abnormalities

Specific abnormalities in red reflexes may suggest certain conditions:

- A brighter red reflex in one eye may suggest that the eye is misaligned or strabismic.
- A difference in red reflex color between the two eyes may indicate unequal refractive power in the eyes (anisometropia) and a risk for amblyopia.
- Leukocoria, or a white pupil reflex, is the most common symptom of retinoblastoma.
- Strabismus is the second most common sign of retinoblastoma.
- Leukocoria can also be due to coloboma—a congenital cleft, fissure, or slit in the eye.
- An absent, dull, or patchy red reflex may suggest a cataract. Cataracts can also cause the pupil to appear white or yellow.
- Although lenticonus is usually detected by a slit-lamp examination, it may also appear as a dimple or oil droplet that moves with eye movement in the red reflex.

An abnormal RR testing result is usually followed by RR testing after pupil dilation of each eye and/or referral to a pediatric ophthalmologist. The ophthalmologist will conduct a complete eye exam, including an ocular fundus examination by indirect **ophthalmoscopy** with pupil dilation.

All infants and children with a positive family history of retinoblastoma; congenital, infantile, or juvenile cataracts; glaucoma; or retinal abnormalities should be referred to a pediatric ophthalmologist, regardless of the results of RR testing. The age at which the child should be referred depends on the specific risk factor. However, any infant with consistently white pupils requires examination for retinoblastoma. Any infant with large eyes, excessive tearing, and cloudy corneas should be tested for congenital glaucoma, which can also lead to blindness.

Health care team roles

RR testing is quick and is usually performed by a pediatrician or other primary care provider who has been trained in the technique. It should be performed in a dim or darkened room so that the baby's pupils dilate or widen to increase the retinal reflection and provide the examiner with a better view.

Resources

PERIODICALS

American Academy Of Pediatrics Section on Ophthalmology, American Association for Pediatric Ophthalmology and Strabismus, American Academy of Ophthalmology, and American Association of Certified Orthoptists. "Red Reflex Examination in Neonates, Infants, and Children." *Pediatrics* 122, no. 6 (2008): 1401–4. http://dx.doi.org/10.1542/peds.2008-2624 (accessed October 7, 2013).

WEBSITES

American Academy for Pediatric Ophthalmology and Strabismus. "Vision Screening." http://www.aapos.org/terms/conditions/107 (accessed October 7, 2013).

ORGANIZATIONS

American Academy of Ophthalmology, 655 Beach St., San Francisco, CA 94109, (415) 561-8500, Fax: (415) 561-8533, http://www.aao.org.

American Academy for Pediatric Ophthalmology and Strabismus (AAPOS), PO Box 193832, San Francisco, CA 94119-3832, (415) 561-8505, Fax: (415) 561-8531, aapos@aao.org, http://www.aapos.org.

American Academy of Pediatrics, 141 Northwest Point Blvd., Elk Grove Village, IL 60007-1098, (847) 434-4000, (800) 433-9016, Fax: (847) 434-8000, http://www.aap.org.

National Eye Institute, NEI Information Office, 31 Center Dr., MSC 2510, Bethesda, MD 20892-2510, (301) 496-5248, 2020@nei.nih.gov, http://www.nei.nih.gov.

Margaret Alic, PhD

Regional anesthetic *see* **Anesthesia, local**
Remote surgery *see* **Telesurgery**
Renal transplant *see* **Kidney transplantation**

Reoperation

Definition

Reoperation is a term used by **surgeons** for the duplication of a surgical procedure.

Purpose

A variety of reasons may necessitate reoperation. The repeated surgery may be done at the same site, at another site for the same condition, or to repair a structure that was treated in a previous surgery.

Description

Success for most surgical procedures depends upon the lack of a need to repeat the surgery. However, failure

1556 GALE ENCYCLOPEDIA OF SURGERY AND MEDICAL TESTS, 3ᴿᴰ EDITION of some feature of a procedure may be only one of many reasons that reoperation is necessary. Reasons for repeat surgery depend upon surgical skills, as well as the reason for the primary surgery. Some diseases and conditions necessitate or make probable repeating the operation.

Cancer

Surgeries for cancer are sometimes repeated because a new tumor or more surrounding tissue has been affected by the original malignancy. This is often the case with breast surgery for cancer that involves breast conservation management. Often it is necessary to re-excise the site of the previously biopsied primary cancer. In the case of breast cancer, only 50% of re-excision specimens show residual tumor. If cancer cells are found with the re-excision, this may change the treatment protocol. Colon cancer sometimes involves more surgeries to resect newly affected areas beyond the previous primary site.

Coronary artery surgery

Currently, about 10% of coronary artery procedures are reoperations due to the progression of the disease into native vessels between operations, as well as to treat diseased vein grafts. The mortality associated with reoperation is significantly higher than that of the original bypass procedures. In one study, patients undergoing their first coronary artery bypass graft (CABG) had a mortality rate of 1.7% versus 5.2% for elective reoperation.

Orthopedic surgeries

Arthroplasty—the operative restoration of a joint like the elbow, knee, hip, or shoulder, often involves components that need repair. Infections of the joint may also require reoperation with the complete removal of all prostheses and cement. Re-implantation is repeated after a six-week course of **antibiotics**. Other bone surgeries that have a high reoperation rate are back surgeries, including spinal surgeries involving discectomy in which discs are fused together to reduce pain. Due to scarring or infection, there may be a need for reoperation. As the frequency of repeat back surgeries increases, the chance of a satisfactory result drops precipitously.

Gastrointestinal surgeries

Crohn's disease surgeries are often repeated. Operations that cut and stitch only the area of obstruction, called strictureplasty, often have repeat operations if the affected area is the small intestine. Another gastrointestinal surgery that often requires reoperation is fundoplication or flap wrapping of the lower part of the esophagus

KEY TERMS

Reoperation—The repeat of a surgical procedure required for a variety of reasons, from surgical failure, replacement of failed component parts, or treatment of progressive disease.

Surgical revision—The failure of a procedure, which requires surgery be performed to improve the result.

to prevent the reflux of acid from the stomach back into the esophagus. Folding the loose valve above the stomach in such a way as to tighten its ability to close treats the condition known as gastroesophageal reflux disease (GERD). The surgery has a high failure rate of between 30% after five years and 63% after 10 years. Reoperation may be required because of surgical failure, breakdown of tissue, injury to nearby organs, or an excessively wrapped fundus that leads to trouble swallowing.

Vasectomy and penile prostheses

These surgeries often have complications that lead to reoperation, largely due to surgical failure.

Risks

In general, reoperation is more difficult and involves more risks than the original procedure. It requires more operative time, more blood is lost, and the incidences of infection and clots are higher. Advancements in design and improvements in cementing techniques for component failure in **arthroplasty** have improved the results of reoperation.

Resources

BOOKS

Khatri, V. P., and J. A. Asensio. *Operative Surgery Manual.* Philadelphia: Saunders, 2003.

Townsend, Courtney M., et al. *Sabiston Textbook of Surgery.* 19th ed. Philadelphia: Saunders/Elsevier, 2012.

PERIODICALS

Burns, E., et al. "Variation in Reoperation after Colorectal Surgery in England as an Indicator of Surgical Performance: Retrospective Analysis of Hospital Episode Statistics." *BMJ* 343 (August 16, 2011): d4836. http://dx.doi.org/10.1136/bmj.d4836 (accessed October 17, 2013).

Chen, Michelle M., et al. "Postdischarge Complications Predict Reoperation and Mortality after Otolaryngologic Surgery." *Otolaryngology—Head and Neck Surgery* (September 18,

2013): e-pub ahead of print. http://dx.doi.org/10.1177/0194599813505078 (accessed October 17, 2013).

Groh, Gordon I, and Griffin M. Groh. "Complications Rates, Reoperation Rates, and the Learning Curve in Reverse Shoulder Arthroplasty." *Journal of Shoulder and Elbow Surgery* (September 9, 2013): e-pub ahead of print. http://dx.doi.org/10.1016/j.jse.2013.06.002 (accessed October 17, 2013).

Murphy, D. K., et al. "Treatment and Displacement Affect the Reoperation Rate for Femoral Neck Fracture." *Clinical Orthopaedics and Related Research*® 471, no. 8 (2013): 2691–702. http://dx.doi.org/10.1007/s11999-013-3020-9 (accessed October 17, 2013).

WEBSITES

American Association of Endocrine Surgeons. "Re-Operative (Re-Do) Parathyroid Surgery." http://endocrinediseases.org/parathyroid/re-operative.shtml (accessed October 17, 2013).

Conley, Mikaela. "Re-Operation Rates Vary Among Breast Cancer Surgery Patients." ABC News, January 31, 2012. http://abcnews.go.com/Health/high-variability-rate-breast-tumor-excision-rates/story?id=15480739#.TyllqePLyRk (accessed October 17, 2013).

University of Texas MD Anderson Cancer Center. "Surgery and Reoperation Options for Brain Tumors." Video, 68:08. http://endocrinediseases.org/parathyroid/re-operative.shtml (accessed October 17, 2013).

ORGANIZATIONS

American College of Surgeons, 633 N. Saint Clair St., Chicago, IL 60611-3211, (312) 202-5000, (800) 621-4111, Fax: (312) 202-5001, postmaster@facs.org, http://www.facs.org.

Nancy McKenzie, PhD

Replantation of digits *see* **Finger reattachment**

Retinal cryopexy

Definition

Retinal cryopexy, also called retinal **cryotherapy**, is a procedure that uses intense cold to induce a chorioretinal scar and to destroy retinal or choroidal tissue.

Purpose

The retina is the very thin membrane in the back of the eye that acts like the "film" in a camera. It is held against the inside back portion of the eye by pressure from fluid within the eye. In the front part of the eye, the retina is firmly attached at a ring just behind the lens called the pars plana. In the back part of the eye, the retina is continuous with the optic nerve. In between the pars plana and the optic nerve the retina has no fixed attachments. The retina collects information from the images projected on it from the eye lens and sends it along the optic nerve to the brain, where the information is interpreted and experienced as sight.

Several disorders can affect the retina and retinal cryopexy is used to treat the following conditions:

• retinal breaks or detachments

• retinal ischemia (retinal tissue that lacks oxygen)

• neovascularization (proliferation of blood vessels in the retina)

• Coats' disease (abnormal retinal blood vessels that cause loss of vision)

• retinoblastoma (intraocular tumors)

Demographics

Disease and disorders affecting the retina cause the majority of the visual disability and blindness in the United States. Retinal detachment occurs in one in 10,000 Americans each year, with middle-aged and older individuals being at higher risk than the younger population. Coats' disease usually affects children, especially boys, in the first 10 years of life, but it can also affect young adults. The condition affects central vision, typically in only one eye. Severity can range from mild vision loss to total retinal detachment and blindness. No cause has yet been identified for Coats' disease. According to the National Cancer Institute, retinoblastoma accounts for approximately 11% of cancers developing in the first year of life, and for 3% of the cancers developing among children younger than 15 years. In the United States, approximately 300 children and adolescents below the age of 20 are diagnosed with retinoblastoma each year. The majority of cases occur among young children, with 63% of all retinoblastoma occurring before the age of two years.

Description

Usually, retinal cryopexy is administered under **local anesthesia**. The procedure involves placing a metal probe against the eye. When a foot pedal is depressed, the tip of the cryopexy probe becomes very cold as a result of the rapid expansion of very cold gases (usually nitrous oxide) within the probe tip. When the probe is placed on the eye, the formation of water crystals followed by rapid thawing results in tissue destruction. This is followed by healing and scar tissue formation.

KEY TERMS

Chorioretinal—Relating to the choroid coat of the eye and retina.

Choroid—Middle layer of the eye, between the retina and sclera.

Coats' disease—Also called exudative retinitis, a chronic abnormality characterized by the deposition of cholesterol on the outer retinal layers.

Ophthalmoscope—An instrument for viewing the interior of the eye, particularly the retina. Light is thrown into the eye by a mirror (usually concave) and the interior is then examined with or without the aid of a lens.

Retina—Light-sensitive layer of the eye.

Retinoblastoma—Malignant tumor of the retina.

Sclera—The tough white outer coat of the eyeball.

In the case of retinal detachment, treatment calls for irritating the tissue around each of the retinal tears. Cryopexy stimulates scar formation, sealing the edges of the tear. This is typically done by looking into the eye using the indirect ophthalmoscope while pushing gently on the outside of the eye using the cryopexy probe, producing a small area of freezing that involves the retina and the tissues immediately underneath it. Using multiple small freezes like this, each of the tears is surrounded. Irritated tissue forms a scar, which brings the retina back into contact with the tissue underneath it.

Diagnosis

The earlier the retinal disorder diagnosis is confirmed, the greater the chance of successful outcome. Diagnosis is based on symptoms and a thorough examination of the retina. An ophthalmoscope is used to examine the retina. This is a small, hand-held instrument consisting of a battery-powered light and a series of lenses that is held up to the eye. The ophthalmologist is able to see the retina and check for abnormalities by shining the light into the eye and looking through the lens. Eye drops are placed in the eyes to dilate the pupils and help visualization. Afterward, an indirect ophthalmoscope is used. This instrument is worn on the specialist's head, and a lens is held in front of the patient's eye. It allows a better view of the retina. Examination with a slit lamp microscope may also be done. This microscope enables the ophthalmologist to examine the different parts of the eye under magnification. After instilling drops to dilate the pupil, the slit lamp

is used to detect retinal tears and detachment. A visual acuity test is also usually performed to assess vision loss. This test involves reading letters from a standard eye chart.

Additional diagnostic procedures are used in the case of Coats' disease and retinoblastoma. Ultrasonography helps in differentiating Coats' disease from retinoblastoma. CT scan may be used to characterize the intraocular features of Coats' disease. MRI is another very useful diagnostic tool used to distinguish retinoblastoma from Coats' disease.

Aftercare

After the procedure, patients are taken to a recovery room, and observed for 30–60 minutes. Tylenol or pain medication is usually given. Healing typically takes 10–14 days. Vision may be blurred briefly, and the operated eye is usually red and swollen for some time following cryopexy. Cold compresses applied to the eyelids relieve some of the discomfort. Most patients are able to walk the day after surgery and are discharged from the hospital within a week. After discharge, patients are advised to gently cleanse their eyelids every morning, and as necessary, using warm tap water and cotton balls or tissues. Day surgery patients are usually allowed to go home two hours after the surgery is complete.

Risks

Risks involved in retinal cryopexy include infection, perforation of the eye with the anesthetic needle, bleeding, double vision, and glaucoma. All of these complications, however, are quite uncommon.

Results

If treated early, the outcome of cryopexy for Coats' disease may be successful in preventing progression and in some cases can improve vision, but this is less effective if the retina has completely detached. For retinal reattachments, the retina can be repaired in about 90% of cases. Early treatment almost always improves the vision of most patients with retinal detachment. Some patients, however, require more than one cryopexy procedure to repair the damage.

Morbidity and mortality rates

Survival rates for children with retinoblastoma are favorable, with more than 93% alive five years after diagnosis. Males and females had similar five-year survival rates for the period 1976–1994, namely 93% and 94% respectively. African American children had slightly lower survival rates (86%) than Caucasian children (94%).

Alternatives

Several alternatives to retinal cryopexy are available, depending on the condition being treated. A few examples include:

- Laser photocoagulation. This type of surgery induces a therapeutic effect by destroying outer retinal tissue, thus reducing the oxygen requirements of the retina, and increasing oxygen delivery to the remaining retina through alterations in oxygen diffusion from the choroid. It is used for repairing retinal tears.
- Pneumatic retinopexy. This procedure is used to reattach retinas. After numbing the eye with a local anesthesia, the surgeon injects a small gas bubble into the inside of the eye. The bubble presses against the retina, flattening it against the back wall of the eye. Since the gas rises, this treatment is most effective for detachments located in the upper portion of the eye.
- Scleral buckle. With this technique, a tiny sponge or silicone band is attached to the outside of the eye, pressing inward and holding the retina in position. After removing the vitreous gel from the eye (vitrectomy), the surgeon seals a few areas of the retina into position with laser or cryotherapy.
- Radiation therapy. For neuroblastomas, this treatment uses high-energy radiation to kill or shrink cancer cells.
- Chemotherapy. Another alternative for neuroblastoma. Chemotherapy uses drugs to kill cancer cells. The drugs are delivered through the bloodstream, and spread throughout the body to the cancer site.

Health care team roles

Retinal cryopexy is performed in the treating physician's office or in a hospital setting depending on the condition motivating the surgery. The physician is usually an ophthalmologist, specialized in the treatment of retinal disorders. An ophthalmologist is a physician who specializes in the medical and surgical care of the eyes and visual system and in the prevention of eye disease and injury. Ophthalmologists must complete four or more years of college premedical education, four or more years of medical school, one year of internship, and three or more years of specialized medical and surgical and refractive training and experience in eye care.

Resources

BOOKS

Packer, A. J., ed. *Manual of Retinal Surgery.* Boston: Butterworth-Heinemann, 2001.

Schepens, C. L., M. E. Hartnett, and T. Hirose, eds. *Schepens's Retinal Detachment and Allied Diseases.* Boston: Butterworth-Heinemann, 2000.

Yanoff, Myron, and Jay S. Duker. *Ophthalmology.* St. Louis, MO: Mosby/Elsevier, 2009.

PERIODICALS

Uno, T., et al. "Accommodative Loss After Retinal Cryotherapy." *American Journal of Ophthalmology* 147, no. 1 (June 2009): 116–20. http://dx.doi.org/10.1016/j.ajo.2008.07.031 (accessed October 2, 2013).

WEBSITES

Mayo Clinic staff. "Retinal Detachment: Treatments and Drugs." MayoClinic.com. http://www.mayoclinic.com/health/retinal-detachment/DS00254/DSECTION=treatments-and-drugs (accessed October 2, 2013).

National Eye Institute. "Facts about Retinal Detachment." http://www.nei.nih.gov/health/retinaldetach/retinaldetach.asp (accessed October 2, 2013).

ORGANIZATIONS

American Academy of Ophthalmology, 655 Beach St., San Francisco, CA 94109, (415) 561-8500, Fax: (415) 561-8533, http://www.aao.org.

National Eye Institute, NEI Information Office, 31 Center Dr., MSC 2510, Bethesda, MD 20892-2510, (301) 496-5248, 2020@nei.nih.gov, http://www.nei.nih.gov.

Monique Laberge, PhD

Retinal detachment surgery *see* **Scleral buckling**

Retropubic suspension

Definition

Retropubic suspension refers to the surgical procedures used to correct incontinence by supporting and stabilizing the bladder and urethra.

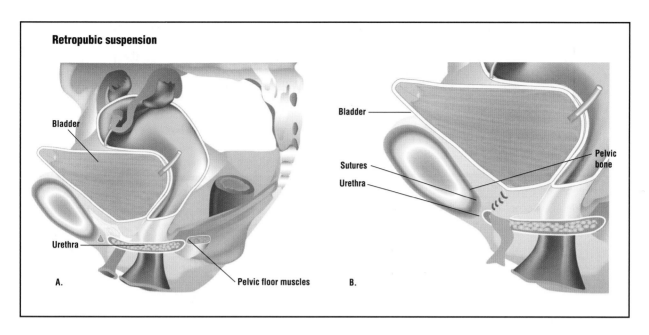

Retropubic suspension

Bladder

Urethra

A.

Pelvic floor muscles

Bladder

Sutures

Urethra

Pelvic bone

B.

Weak pelvic floor muscles (A) can cause stress incontinence. In a retropubic suspension, the neck of the bladder is elevated and stitched to the pubic bone to hold it in place (B). *(Illustration by GGS Information Services. Copyright © Cengage Learning®.)*

Purpose

The primary purpose of retropubic suspension is to treat incontinence. The Burch procedure, also known as retropubic urethropexy procedure or Burch colposuspension, and Marshall-Marchetti-Krantz procedure (MMK) are the two primary surgeries for treating stress incontinence. The major difference between these procedures is the method for supporting the bladder. The Burch procedure uses sutures to attach the urethra and bladder to muscle tissue in the pelvic area. MMK uses sutures to attach these organs to the pelvic cartilage. Laparoscopic retropubic surgery can be performed with a video laparoscope through small incisions in the belly button and above the pubic hairline.

Demographics

Over 15 million Americans have urinary incontinence and women comprise 85% of all cases. It affects 25% of women of reproductive age and 50% of women past menopause. Due to the female anatomy, women have twice the risk for stress incontinence compared to men. In addition, childbirth places pressure and burden on the pelvic muscles that often weaken with age, thereby weakening urethra stability. Women are more prone to surgeries for urological changes than men and severe urinary incontinence is often associated with these surgeries as well as hysterectomies. The majority of women with incontinence have stress incontinence or mixed incontinence. Male incontinence occurs primarily in response to blockage in the prostate or after prostate

surgery. It is usually treated with implants and/or an artificial sphincter insert.

Description

The urinary system expels a quart and a half of urine per day. The amount of urine produced depends upon diet and medications taken, as well as **exercise** and loss of water due to sweating. The ureters, two tubes connecting the kidneys and the bladder, pass urine almost continually and when the bladder is full the brain sends a signal to the bladder to relax and let urine pass from the bladder to the urethra. People who are continent control the release of urine from the urethra via the sphincter muscles. These two sets of muscles act like rubber bands to keep the bladder closed until a conscious decision is made to urinate. The intrinsic sphincter or urethral sphincter muscles keep the bladder closed and the extrinsic sphincter muscles surround the urethra and prevent leakage. Incontinence is common when either the urethra lacks tautness and stability (genuine stress urine incontinence, SUI) and/or the sphincter muscles are unable to keep the bladder closed (intrinsic sphincter deficiency [ISD]).

Types of incontinence

Incontinence occurs in many forms with four primary types related to disease and injury or anatomic, neurological, or dietary causes.

STRESS INCONTINENCE. The most frequent form of incontinence is stress incontinence. This relates to leakage of the urethra with activity that puts stress on the abdominal muscles. The primary sign of stress incontinence is this leakage at sneezing, coughing, exercise, or other straining activities, which indicates a lack of support for the urethra due to weakened muscles, fascia, or ligaments. Pressure from the abdomen with movement, like exercising, uncompensated by tautness or stability in the urethra, causes the urethra to be displaced or mobile leading to leakage. Essentially, this hypermobility of the urethra is an indication that it is moving down or herniating through weakened pelvic structures.

To diagnose incontinence and determine treatment, three grades of severity for stress incontinence are used:

• Type I. Moderate movement of the urethra, with no hernia or cystocele.

• Type II. Severe or hypermobility in the urethra of more than 0.8 in. (2 cm), with or without decent of the urethra into pelvic structures.

• Type III. Hypermobility of the urethra where the primary source of incontinence is the inability of the sphincter muscles to keep the bladder closed. This is due to weakness or deficiency in the intrinsic sphincter muscles.

URGE INCONTINENCE. Urge incontinence relates to the frequent need to urinate and may involve going to the bathroom every two hours. Accidents are common when not reaching a bathroom in time. Urge incontinence is not due to general changes in the urethra or supporting muscles. It is often linked to other disorders that produce muscle spasms in the bladder, such as infections. Urge incontinence can also be due to underlying illnesses like stroke, spinal cord injury, multiple sclerosis and Alzheimer's disease, which cause detrusor hyperreflexia—the contracting of the bladder muscle responsible for sending urine from the bladder to the urethra. Urge incontinence is very common in the elderly, especially those in long term care facilities.

MIXED INCONTINENCE. Mixed incontinence is a combination of stress incontinence and urge incontinence, especially in older women. Since each form of incontinence pertains to different functions or anatomy, it is very important to distinguish which part of the incontinence is to be treated by surgery.

OVERFLOW INCONTINENCE. Overflow incontinence results in leakage from a bladder that never completely empties due to weakened bladder muscles. Overflow incontinence is involuntary and not accompanied by the urge to urinate. Many causes exist for overflow incontinence, including weak bladder muscles due to diabetes, nerve damage, or a blocked urethra. Men are more frequently affected than women.

Types of surgery

There are a variety of retropubic suspension surgeries available to treat stress incontinence. The variations differ by the types of structures used to support the urethra and bladder. In all procedures, parts of the pelvic anatomy (pubic bone, ligaments) serve as an anchor or wall upon which the urethra is tacked for stability. The surgery is called a suspension surgery because it stabilizes the urethra from tilting by suspending it against a part of the pelvic anatomy. The Burch procedure is often performed when other surgery is needed such as repair of the urethra for cystoceles and urethral reconstruction. However, this procedure is the most difficult of the anti-incontinent surgeries and is more common in mild forms of stress incontinence where intrinsic sphincter deficiency is not present.

The Burch procedure can be done through open abdominal surgery, which requires a long incision at the bikini line, or surgery performed through the vagina. The patient, in stirrups, receives **general anesthesia**. Within the retropubic area, the anterior vaginal wall is separated from the bladder manually. The bladder neck is identified and old **adhesions** or fatty tissues are removed. The neck of the bladder is sutured to pubic ligaments where it will form adhesions and thereby gain stability. The surgeon examines for bladder injury and the surgery is completed. Urethral position is tested by placing a cotton-tipped swab in the urethra and measuring the angle. With abdominal surgery or vaginal surgery a catheter may be put in place by the surgeon for postoperative voiding and to decrease the risks of infection. A suction drain may be placed in the retropubic space for bleeding. The drain is removed one to three days after surgery.

Recently, laparoscopic surgery has been used to perform retropubic suspensions. Laparoscopic surgery requires only three or four 0.25 in. (0.6 cm) incisions in the belly button, pubic hairline, or groin area and uses small instruments without opening the abdominal cavity. A shorter healing time is seen with this procedure. The hospital stay is usually not more than 24 hours and recovery to normal activities takes about 7 to 14 days. However, the Burch procedure performed using laparoscopic techniques requires great skill on the part of the surgeon and research indicates that the results may not be as long lasting as those developed with abdominal or vaginal surgery.

Diagnosis

A patient with incontinence may have multiple factors that induce transient or chronic incontinence. It is crucial that the physician obtain a complete history, physical, clinical, neurological and medication evaluation of the patient, as well as a radiographic assessment before continuing urological tests aimed at a surgical solution. The specific indications for the Burch colposuspension procedure or its variants is the correction of stress urinary incontinence. This can be a patient who also requires abdominal surgery that cannot be performed vaginally, like **hysterectomy** or sigmoid surgery, as well as patients who have SUI without ISD.

A urodynamic study with a point pressure leak test will allow a diagnosis to be made that can distinguish the patient who has a hypermobile urethra from the patient who also has ISD. The point pressure leak test, also known as the Valsalva leak test, measures the amount of abdominal pressure required to induce leakage. The patient is asked to cough or strain in order to encourage leakage. The point at which the patient leaks helps determine if stress incontinence with ISD contribution is present. Obese patients and patients that engage in high impact exercise regimens are not considered good candidates for retropubic suspension.

Aftercare

Patients with open retropubic procedures are given pain medication postoperatively that is tapered down over the next two days. A suprapubic catheter stays in place for approximately five days with voiding difficulties encountered initially in many patients. Patients with laparoscopic suspensions are reported to have less blood loss during surgery, less postoperative narcotic requirements, and shorter hospital stays. Patients are expected to refrain from strenuous activity for three months and to have a follow-up visit within three weeks after surgery.

Risks

As with any major abdominal or pelvic surgical procedures, complications that may occur after a retropubic suspension include bleeding; injury to the bladder, urethra, and ureters; wound infection; and blood clots. Specific to the Burch procedure are complications that involve urethral obstruction because of urethral kinking due to elevation of the vagina or bladder base. Postoperative voiding difficulties are common and depend upon the suture tension of the urethral axis. Corrective surgery and the release of the urethra to a more anatomic position resolves voiding issues with a very high rate of success. Vaginal prolapse is also a risk of this procedure.

Results

The patient can expect more than 80%–90% cure or great improvement in their incontinence. There is a large body of literature documenting the success of the Burch

KEY TERMS

Genuine urinary stress incontinence (USI)—Stress incontinence due to hypermobility of the urethra.

Intrinsic sphincter deficiency (ISD)—A factor in severe stress incontinence due to the inadequacy of the sphincter muscles to keep the bladder closed.

Retropubic urethropexy—A generic term for the Burch procedure and its variants that treat mild stress incontinence by stabilizing the urethra with retropubic surgery.

Stress incontinence—Leakage of urine upon movements that put pressure on the abdominal muscles such as coughing, sneezing, laughing, or exercise. One of four types of incontinence.

Urethra hypermobility—Main factor in stress urinary incontinence, with severity based upon how far the urethra has descended into the pelvic floor through herniation or cystocele.

procedure. Published research shows a cure rate ranging from 63% to 93%, according to the actual version of colposuspension used. Laparoscopic surgery has not produced the long term results that open surgery has and there is the possibility that the fibrosis (adhesion) necessary for a successful outcome does not occur as easily with the laparoscopic procedure. Patients not carefully screened out for ISD will not have a high level of success with the Burch procedure since the source of the incontinence will not have been treated. Sling procedures are recommended for patients with ISD instead of colosuspension surgery.

Morbidity and mortality rates

The Burch procedure may aggravate vaginal wall weakness or vaginal prolapse. This incident varies between 3% and 17%. Research on the Marshall-Marchetti-Krantz procedure pertaining to 2,712 patients found a complication rate of 21%, with wound complications and infections making up the majority, 5.5% and 3.9% respectively. Direct wound injury occurred in 1.6% and obstructions in 0.3% overall.

Alternatives

General or simple severe stress incontinence related primarily to weakening of the urethral support can be remedied with changes in diet, weight loss, and certain behavioral and rehabilitative measures. These include:

- regular, daily exercising of the pelvic muscles called Kegel exercises, requiring 30–200 contractions a day for eight weeks

- biofeedback to gain awareness and control of pelvic muscles

- vaginal weight training in which small weights are inserted in the vagina to tighten vaginal muscles

- mild electrical stimulation to increase contractions in pelvic muscles

- bladder retraining in which the patient is taught how to resist the urge to urinate and expand the intervals between urinations

There are also medications that can facilitate continence for those experiencing stress or urge incontinence. These include some kinds of antidepressants, although the mechanism of action is not quite understood, as well as antispasmodic medication and estrogen therapy. Finally, should behavioral, rehabilitative, and surgical procedures fail, there remain alternatives through the use of vaginal cones and urethral plugs that can be inserted and removed by the patient.

Health care team roles

Retropubic suspension procedures are performed by a urological surgeon specially trained in incontinence surgeries. Surgery is performed in a general hospital.

Resources

BOOKS

Wein, Alan J., et al. *Campbell-Walsh Urology.* 10th ed. Philadelphia: Saunders/Elsevier, 2012.

WEBSITES

A.D.A.M. Medical Encyclopedia. "Urinary Incontinence—Retropubic Suspension." MedlinePlus. http://www.nlm.nih.gov/medlineplus/ency/article/007374.htm (accessed October 2, 2013).

National Kidney and Urologic Diseases Information Clearing-house. "Urinary Incontinence in Women." http://kidney.niddk.nih.gov/kudiseases/pubs/uiwomen/index.aspx (accessed October 2, 2013).

University of Minnesota Medical Center. "Laparoscopic Retropubic Suspension." http://www.uofmmedicalcenter.org/healthlibrary/Article/88464 (accessed October 2, 2013).

ORGANIZATIONS

National Kidney and Urologic Diseases Information Clearing-house, 3 Information Way, Bethesda, MD 20892-3580, (800) 891-5390, (866) 569-1162, Fax: (703) 738-4929, nkudic@info.niddk.nih.gov, http://kidney.niddk.nih.gov.

Simon Foundation for Continence, PO Box 835, Wilmette, IL 60091, (847) 864-3913, (800) 23-SIMON (237-4666), info@simonfoundation.org, http://simonfoundation.org.

Nancy McKenzie, PhD

Rh blood typing

Definition

Rh blood typing is performed in order to determine the Rh factor of an individual's blood. The term "Rh factor" refers to an antigen on the surface of the red blood cells. All red blood cells have certain substances on their surfaces. These substances are called "antigens," and may be molecules of protein, carbohydrate, glycolipid, or glycoprotein. Blood typing categorizes blood by identifying the presence or absence of these antigens on the surface of the red blood cell.

The Rh system identifies the presence (denoted as positive) or absence (denoted as negative) of a particular antigen termed the Rhesus antigen. Its name stems from the fact that the Rh factor was first identified on the red blood cell surfaces of Rhesus monkeys. When the Rh factor is present on the surface of the red blood cell, the blood is said to be Rh-positive; when the Rh factor is absent from the surface of the red blood cell, the blood is said to be Rh-negative.

The Rh factor status is reported in conjunction with identification of the major ABO blood group of the individual. The ABO blood group system identifies a type of protein antigen on the red blood cell surface as Type A, Type B, Type AB, or Type O. An individual's blood type, then, is reported as a combination of information obtained about the ABO and RH blood group systems; for example, A-positive, or A-negative, etc.

Blood typing is particularly important when an individual needs to receive a blood **transfusion**. If the wrong blood type is given, there is a high risk of an adverse transfusion reaction. For example, the first time an Rh-negative individual is given blood from an Rh-positive donor, there will probably not be any problem. However, if the Rh-negative individual receives future transfusions of Rh-positive blood, the recipient's immune system will recognize the Rh antigen on the donor blood as foreign, and will begin to produce antibodies directed against that antigen. The antibodies will attack the donor blood, damaging and bursting the donor red blood cells. This results in high serum levels of hemoglobin spilling from the burst red blood cells (called hemoglobinemia), disseminated intravascular coagulation or DIC (a condition in which clotting factors are used up very rapidly, resulting in the potential for severe, uncontrollable bleeding), kidney failure, and eventually complete cardiovascular collapse (a combination of heart attack, shock, and lack of blood flow to all major organs and tissues).

Knowing a pregnant woman's Rh-factor is crucial because there is always a chance during pregnancy, labor, and delivery, that some of the baby's blood will get into the mother's bloodstream. If this happens in an Rh-negative mother with an Rh-positive baby, the mother's body will identify the baby's Rh-negative blood as foreign and begin producing antibodies against the Rh-factor. This is called Rh-sensitization. The first time this sensitization occurs between a mother and her baby, the baby usually doesn't suffer any ill-effects. But in subsequent pregnancies, if the mother is again carrying an Rh-positive baby, having already been exposed to the Rh-antigen previously, her body will begin to produce Rh-antibodies more quickly and in greater numbers. If these cross over into the baby's bloodstream, they can begin destroying the baby's red blood cells, resulting in severe illness. This problem is referred to as Rh disease, hemolytic disease of the newborn, or erythroblastosis fetalis. In order to avoid this problem, Rh testing is done prior to pregnancy or early in pregnancy. Rh-negative women can be given a special shot called Rh-immune globulin that can prevent Rh-sensitization.

Purpose

Blood typing is ordered prior to a blood transfusion, to make sure that the donor blood type is appropriately compatible with the recipient's blood type. It is also done on donor blood, on a donor who is giving an organ to be used for transplantation, as well as prior to surgery (so that the patient's blood type is known, should the individual needs an unexpected, emergency blood transfusion). Rh-typing is also important in pregnant women. When

the mother and the baby have different Rh-types, there is a risk to the baby of illness caused by the mother's antibodies; if the mother is identified as having Rh-negative blood, a shot called Rh-immune globulin can prevent the problem from developing.

Description

This test requires blood to be drawn from a vein (usually one in the forearm), generally by a nurse or phlebotomist (an individual who has been trained to draw blood). A tourniquet is applied to the arm above the area where the needle stick will be performed. The site of the needle stick is cleaned with antiseptic, and the needle is inserted. The blood is collected in vacuum tubes. After collection, the needle is withdrawn, and pressure is kept on the blood draw site to stop any bleeding and decrease bruising. A bandage is then applied.

Precautions

Some situations may confuse the results of blood typing, including recent x-ray test using contrast or use of medications such as methyldopa, levodopa, and certain **antibiotics** (including cephalexin). Other factors that may confuse test results include having received a blood transfusion in the previous three months, having had a bone marrow transplant in the past, or having a history of cancer or leukemia.

Preparation

There are no restrictions on diet or physical activity, either before or after the blood test.

Aftercare

As with any blood test, discomfort, bruising, and/or a very small amount of bleeding is common at the puncture site. Immediately after the needle is withdrawn, it is helpful to put pressure on the puncture site until the bleeding has stopped. This decreases the chance of significant bruising. Warm packs may relieve minor discomfort. Some individuals may feel briefly woozy after a blood test, and they should be encouraged to lie down and rest until they feel better.

Risks

Basic blood tests, such as Rh blood typing, do not carry any significant risks, other than slight bruising and the chance of brief dizziness.

Results

Rh blood typing reports back whether the individual's red blood cells have the Rh antigen present on their surface (Rh-positive) or absent from their surface (Rh-negative). About 84% of all people are Rh-positive; about 16% are Rh-negative.

Resources

BOOKS

Goldman, Lee, and Andrew I. Schafer. *Goldman's Cecil Medicine*. 24th ed. Philadelphia: Saunders/Elsevier, 2012.

Hoffman, Ronald, et al. *Hematology: Basic Principles and Practice*. 6th ed. Philadelphia: Saunders/Elsevier, 2013.

McPherson, Richard A., and Matthew R. Pincus, eds. *Henry's Clinical Diagnosis and Management by Laboratory Methods*. 22nd ed. Philadelphia: Saunders/Elsevier, 2011.

PERIODICALS

Sandler, S. Gerald. "New Laboratory Procedures and Rh Blood Type Changes in a Pregnant Woman." *Obstetrics & Gynecology* 119, no. 2 pt. 2 (2012): 426–28. http://dx.doi.org/10.1097/AOG.0b013e31823f6f76 (accessed October 17, 2013).

WEBSITES

American Red Cross. "Blood Types." http://www.redcross blood.org/learn-about-blood/blood-types (accessed October 17, 2013).

American Pregnancy Association. "Rh Factor." http://american pregnancy.org/pregnancycomplications/rhfactor-2.html (accessed October 17, 2013).

Nemours Foundation. "Rh Incompatibility." KidsHealth.org. http://kidshealth.org/parent/pregnancy_center/your_ pregnancy/rh.html (accessed October 17, 2013).

ORGANIZATIONS

American Association for Clinical Chemistry, 1850 K St. NW, Ste. 625, Washington, DC 20006, (800) 892-1400, Fax: (202) 887-5093, custserv@aacc.org, http://www.aacc.org.

American Red Cross, 2025 E St., Washington, DC 20006, (800) RED CROSS (733-2767), http://www.redcross.org.

Rosalyn Carson-DeWitt, MD

■ Rheumatoid factor testing

Definition

Rheumatoid factor is a type of antibody. A rheumatoid factor test checks the amount of rheumatoid factor in the bloodstream.

Purpose

Rheumatoid factor testing is usually done when an individual is having symptoms compatible with an autoimmune disorder, particularly rheumatoid arthritis or Sjögren's syndrome. Suspicious symptoms include joint stiffness, pain and swelling (especially in the morning), bumps (nodules) under the skin, and/or dry eyes, mouth, and skin.

Description

Antibodies, also called immunoglobulins, are proteins produced by the body. Antibodies work to clear the body of potentially threatening infections or substances, fighting off various invaders, such as viruses, bacteria, toxins, mold spores, etc.

The body's immune system is made up of lymphoid organs, including lymph nodes, the bone marrow (located within the center of long bones) and the thymus (located in the chest). These lymphoid organs produce lymphocytes, including T cells and B cells. These lymphocytes circulate within the bloodstream, within the lymph system, and are also positioned in clumps within organs and on mucosal surfaces of the body. When a B cell encounters a foreign invader, it recognized it as foreign by virtue of a chemical identifier on its surface (called an antigen). Once the B cell recognizes an antigen, the B cell gives rise to a large number of plasma cells. These plasma cells are capable of producing antibodies.

Antibodies are made up of units called "chains." All antibodies are composed of two larger chains (called heavy chains) and two smaller chains (called light chains). The tip of the antibody is referred to as the hypervariable region. This hypervariable region is responsible for unique chemical properties possessed by each antibody that allow a specific antibody to "recognize" and match up to a particular antigen. The combination of an antibody with a specific antigen, creates an antibody-antigen complex, marking the invader as foreign and in need of inactivation or destruction by other immune cells in the body.

The first time an antigen is encountered by the immune system, the body's response is slow. Time is required in order to activate the machinery necessary to produce the very specific type of antibody necessary to combat that antigen. However, if that particular antigen is encountered in the future, the needed machinery is already available, and antibody production in response to a "familiar" antigen is quite rapid.

One of the important attributes of a healthy, well-functioning immune system rests on its ability to distinguish between "self" and "other." This means that it's crucial that the antibodies don't mistakenly identify parts of the body itself as foreign invaders. When this does happen, the body's immune system attacks the body, damaging and destroying it. Conditions in which this occurs are referred to as autoimmune disorders. One example of an autoimmune disorder is the condition called rheumatoid arthritis or RA. In RA, the lining of the joints (synovium) is misrecognized by the immune system as foreign, resulting in the immune system creating specific antibodies that repeatedly attack, damage, and destroy the joints' lining, resulting in the cluster of symptoms that accompany this disease.

Rheumatoid factor belongs to the class of antibodies known as IgM antibodies. IgM antibodies are primarily found in the blood, and comprise about 13% of all antibodies. IgM functions to kill bacteria, and is found in the earlier phases of immune response to bacterial invasion of the bloodstream (bacteremia).

In rheumatoid arthritis, rheumatoid factor is directed against IgG antibodies. IgG antibodies are very common circulating antibodies; in fact, about 80% of all circulating antibodies are IgG. IgG is found in blood and tissue fluids. IgG functions to coat invading particles, marking them so that they can more easily and rapidly be taken up by other types of immune cells. IgG is the predominant antibody cell in the later or secondary phase of the immune response.

When rheumatoid factor encounters IgG, it attaches itself to the IgG, forming an immune complex. This immune complex kicks off a complicated immune cascade, prompting the production and release of a variety of chemicals that ultimately misidentify the synovium as "non-self," attack the lining, and over time cause tremendous destruction.

Blood draw

This test requires blood to be drawn from a vein (usually one in the forearm), generally by a nurse or phlebotomist (an individual who has been trained to draw blood). A tourniquet is applied to the arm above the area where the needle stick will be performed. The site of the needle stick is cleaned with antiseptic, and the needle is inserted. The blood is collected in vacuum tubes. After collection, the needle is withdrawn, and pressure is kept

---

KEY TERMS

Antibody—A protein that the body produces in response to exposure to a foreign invader such as a virus, bacteria, fungus, or allergen.

Antigen—The protein marker that prompts the body's immune system to produce antibodies.

Autoimmune disorder—A condition in which the body produces antibodies that serve to attack organs or tissues of the body itself.

Immune system—The collection of organs, tissues, and cells that serve to protect the body against foreign invaders, such as bacteria, viruses, and fungi.

Lymphocyte—A white blood cell; part of the immune system responsible for the production of antibodies.

Plasma cell—The specific type of white blood cell that produces antibodies.

Rheumatoid arthritis—A condition in which the immune system damages and destroys the synovial lining of the joints. Red, warm, swollen, stiff joints are a common symptom. Over time, other organ systems may also be affected, including the heart, eyes, lungs, and kidneys.

Sjögren's syndrome—A disease in which the immune system damages and destroys exocrine glands, such as those that produce tears and saliva. Dry eyes and mouth are the usual initial symptoms of this disorder, but other organ systems can also be severely affected over time, including the skin, pancreas, liver, lungs, brain, and kidneys.

---

on the blood draw site to stop any bleeding and decrease bruising. A bandage is then applied.

Precautions

Rheumatoid factor testing is not diagnostic. This means that getting a specific result does not definitively confirm the presence of any particular disease. Instead, the test is used to correlate with the clinical picture, meaning the history and the symptoms that an individual is experiencing.

Some situations may confuse the results of testing for rheumatoid factor, including very high blood levels of triglycerides or other fats, or advanced age (people over 65 years of age have a higher chance of having a higher-than-normal rheumatoid factor that is not associated with disease).

Preparation

There are no restrictions on diet or physical activity, either before or after the blood test.

Aftercare

As with any blood test, discomfort, bruising, and/or a very small amount of bleeding is common at the puncture site. Immediately after the needle is withdrawn, it is helpful to put pressure on the puncture site until the bleeding has stopped. This decreases the chance of significant bruising. Warm packs may relieve minor discomfort. Some individuals may feel briefly woozy after a blood test, and they should be encouraged to lie down and rest until they feel better.

Risks

Basic blood tests, such as rheumatoid factor testing, do not carry any significant risks, other than slight bruising and the chance of brief dizziness.

Results

Normal rheumatoid factor results would demonstrate a rheumatoid factor titer less than 1:20–1:40, or a rheumatoid factor of less than 43 nephelometry units.

The patient's, history, symptoms, and rheumatoid factor results are used together in order to arrive at a diagnosis. An elevated rheumatoid factor may indicate the possibility of rheumatoid arthritis or Sjögren's syndrome. However, some patients (about 20%) with these diseases do not have an elevated rheumatoid factor, or have the condition for several years before their rheumatoid factor becomes abnormally elevated.

Rheumatoid factor may also be elevated in a number of other autoimmune conditions, such as systemic lupus erythematosus, vasculitis, or scleroderma; in severe infections such as syphilis or tuberculosis, mononucleosis, malaria, hepatitis, or endocarditis; in certain types of cancer, including leukemia; and in a number of other conditions, such as cirrhosis of the liver, and lung or kidney disease.

Resources

BOOKS

Firestein, Gary S., et al. *Kelley's Textbook of Rheumatology.* 9th ed. Philadelphia: Saunders/Elsevier, 2013.

Goldman, Lee, and Andrew I. Schafer. *Goldman's Cecil Medicine.* 24th ed. Philadelphia: Saunders/Elsevier, 2012.

Hoffman, Ronald, et al. *Hematology: Basic Principles and Practice.* 6th ed. Philadelphia: Saunders/Elsevier, 2013.

McPherson, Richard A., and Matthew R. Pincus, eds. "Meta-Analysis: Diagnostic Accuracy of Anti—Cyclic Citrullinated Peptide Antibody and Rheumatoid Factor for Rheumatoid Arthritis." *Annals of Internal Medicine* 146, no. 11.

PERIODICALS

WEBSITES

A.D.A.M. Medical Encyclopedia. "Rheumatoid Factor (RF)." MedlinePlus. http://www.nlm.nih.gov/medlineplus/ency/article/003548.htm (accessed October 2, 2013).

American Association for Clinical Chemistry. "Rheumatoid Factor." Lab Tests Online. http://labtestsonline.org/understanding/analytes/rheumatoid (accessed October 2, 2013).

ORGANIZATIONS

American Association for Clinical Chemistry, 1850 K St. NW, Ste. 625, Washington, DC 20006, (800) 892-1400, Fax: (202) 887-5093, custserv@aacc.org, http://www.aacc.org.

Rosalyn Carson-DeWitt, MD

Rhinoplasty

Definition

The term rhinoplasty means "nose molding" or "nose forming." It refers to a procedure in **plastic surgery** in which the structure of the nose is changed. The change can be made by adding or removing bone or cartilage, grafting tissue from another part of the body, or implanting synthetic material to alter the shape of the nose.

Purpose

Rhinoplasty is most often performed for cosmetic reasons. A nose that is too large, crooked, misshapen, malformed at birth, or deformed by an injury can be given a more pleasing appearance. If breathing is impaired due to the form of the nose or to an injury, it can often be improved with rhinoplasty.

Demographics

Rhinoplasty is the most common cosmetic procedure performed in men and the second most common in women. The total number of rhinoplasty procedures performed in the United States in 2012 was 242,684, according to the American Society of Plastic Surgeons, with 25% performed on men.

Description

The external nose is composed of a series of interrelated parts that include the skin, the bony pyramid, cartilage, and the tip of the nose, which is composed of

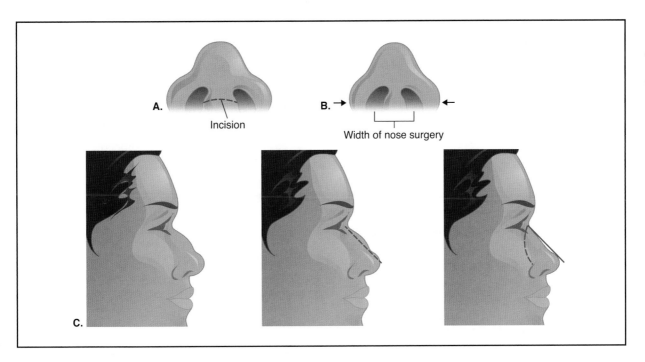

During an open rhinoplasty, an incision is made in the skin between the nostrils (A). Closed rhinoplasty involves only incisions inside the nose. Rhinoplasty may involve a change in nostril width (B) or removal of a hump on the nose (C) using bone sculpting. *(Illustration by Electronic Illustrators Group. Copyright © 2014 Cengage Learning®.)*

cartilage and skin. The strip of skin separating the nostrils is called the columella.

Surgical approaches to nasal reconstruction are varied. Internal rhinoplasty involves making all incisions from inside the nasal cavity. The external, or "open," technique involves a skin incision across the base of the nasal columella. An external incision allows the surgeon to expose the bone and cartilage more fully and is most often used for complicated procedures. During surgery, the surgeon will separate the skin from the bone and cartilage support. The framework of the nose is then reshaped in the desired form. Shape can be altered by removing or adding bone, cartilage, or skin. The remaining skin is then replaced over the new framework. If the procedure requires adding to the structure of the nose, the donated bone, cartilage, or skin can come from another location on the patient's body or from a synthetic source.

When the operation is completed, the surgeon will apply a splint to help the bones maintain their new shape. The nose may also be packed, or stuffed with a dressing, to help stabilize the septum.

When a local anesthetic is used, light sedation is usually given first, after which the operative area is numbed. It will remain insensitive to pain for the length of the surgery. A general anesthetic is used for lengthy or complex procedures, or if the doctor and patient agree that it is the best option.

Precautions

The quality of the skin plays a major role in the outcome of rhinoplasty. Persons with extremely thick skin may not see a significant change in the underlying bone structure after surgery. On the other hand, thin skin provides almost no cushion to hide many minor bone irregularities or imperfections.

Rhinoplasty should not be performed until the pubertal growth spurt is complete, age 14–15 for girls and older for boys.

Preparation

During the initial consultation, the candidate and surgeon will determine what changes can be made in the shape of the nose. Most doctors take photographs during that consult. The surgeon will also explain the techniques and anesthesia options available to the candidate.

The candidate and surgeon should also discuss guidelines for eating, drinking, smoking, taking or avoiding certain medications, and washing the face for the weeks immediately following surgery.

Aftercare

Patients usually feel fine immediately after surgery. As a precaution, most surgery centers do not allow patients to drive themselves home after an operation.

KEY TERMS

Cartilage—Firm supporting tissue that does not contain blood vessels.

Columella—The strip of skin running from the tip of the nose to the upper lip, which separates the nostrils.

Septum—The dividing barrier in the center of the nose.

QUESTIONS TO ASK YOUR DOCTOR

- What will be the resulting appearance?
- Is the surgeon board certified in plastic and reconstructive surgery?
- How many rhinoplasty procedures has the surgeon performed?
- What is the surgeon's complication rate?

The first day after surgery, there will be some swelling of the face. Persons should stay in bed with their heads elevated for at least a day. The nose may hurt and a headache is common. The surgeon will prescribe medication to relieve these conditions. Swelling and bruising around the eyes will increase for a few days, but will begin to diminish after about the third day. Slight bleeding and stuffiness are normal, and vary according to the extent of the surgery performed. Most people are walking in two days, and back to work or school in a week. No strenuous activities are allowed for two to three weeks.

Patients are given a list of postoperative instructions, which include requirements for hygiene, **exercise**, eating, and follow-up visits to the doctor. Patients should not blow their noses for the first week to avoid disruption of healing. It is extremely important to keep the surgical dressing dry. **Dressings**, splints, and stitches are removed in one to two weeks. Patients should avoid excessive sun or sunburn.

Risks

Any type of surgery carries a degree of risk. There is always the possibility of unexpected events such as an infection or a reaction to the anesthesia.

When the nose is reshaped or repaired from inside, the scars are not visible. If the surgeon needs to make the incision on the outside of the nose, there will be some slight scarring. In addition, tiny blood vessels may burst, leaving small red spots on the skin. These spots are barely visible, but may be permanent.

Results

The best candidates for rhinoplasty are those persons with relatively minor deformities. Nasal anatomy and proportions are quite varied and the final look of any rhinoplasty operation depends on a person's anatomy, as well as the surgeon's skill.

A cosmetic change of the nose will change a person's appearance, but it will not change self-image.

A person who expects a different lifestyle after rhinoplasty is likely to be disappointed.

The cost of rhinoplasty depends on the difficulty of the work required and on the specialist chosen. If the problem was caused by an injury, insurance will usually cover the cost. A rhinoplasty done only to change a person's appearance is not usually covered by insurance.

Morbidity and mortality rates

Death from a rhinoplasty procedure is exceedingly rare. When it occurs, the cause is often due to an adverse reaction to anesthesia or postoperative medications or to an infection. About 10% of persons receiving rhinoplasty require a second procedure.

Alternatives

Persons contemplating rhinoplasty may wish to seek alternative measures, such as counseling or therapy, to address any body image issues before undergoing rhinoplasty.

Health care team roles

Simple rhinoplasty is usually performed in an **outpatient surgery** center or in the surgeon's office. Most procedures take only an hour or two, and patients go home right away. Complex procedures may be performed in a hospital and require a short stay.

Rhinoplasty is usually performed by a surgeon with advanced training in plastic and **reconstructive surgery**.

Resources

BOOKS

Flint, Paul F., et al. *Cumming's Otolaryngology: Head and Neck Surgery.* 5th ed. rev. Philadelphia: Mosby/Elsevier, 2010.

PERIODICALS

Sklar, Michael, Jerod Golant, and Philip Solomon. "Rhinoplasty with Intravenous and Local Anesthesia." *Clinics in*

Plastic Surgery 40, no. 4 (2013): 627–29. http://dx.doi.org/10.1016/j.cps.2013.08.002 (accessed October 14, 2013).

OTHER

American Society of Plastic Surgeons. *2012 Plastic Surgery Statistics Reports.* 2013. http://www.plasticsurgery.org/Documents/news-resources/statistics/2012-Plastic-Surgery-Statistics/full-plastic-surgery-statistics-report.pdf (accessed October 1, 2013).

WEBSITES

American Academy of Facial Plastic and Reconstructive Surgery. "Nasal Surgery." http://www.aafprs.org/patient/procedures/rhinoplasty.html (accessed October 14, 2013).

American Society for Aesthetic Plastic Surgery. "Nose Reshaping (Rhinoplasty)." http://www.surgery.org/consumers/procedures/head/nose-reshaping (accessed October 14, 2013).

American Society of Plastic Surgeons. "Nose Surgery." http://www.plasticsurgery.org/cosmetic-procedures/nose-surgery-.html (accessed October 14, 2013).

ORGANIZATIONS

American Academy of Facial Plastic and Reconstructive Surgery, 310 S. Henry St., Alexandria, VA 22314, (703) 299-9291, info@aafprs.org, http://www.aafprs.org.

American Board of Plastic Surgery, 7 Penn Ctr., Ste. 400, 1635 Market St., Philadelphia, PA 19103-2204, (215) 587-9322, info@abplsurg.org, https://www.abplsurg.org.

American Society for Aesthetic Plastic Surgery (ASAPS), 11262 Monarch St., Garden Grove, CA 92841, (562) 799-2356, (800) 364-2147, Fax: (562) 799-1098, asaps@surgery.org, http://www.surgery.org.

American Society for Dermatologic Surgery, 5550 Meadowbrook Dr., Ste. 120, Rolling Meadows, IL 60008, (847) 956-0900, Fax: (847) 956-0999, http://www.asds.net.

American Society of Plastic Surgeons, 444 E. Algonquin Rd., Arlington Heights, IL 60005, http://www.plasticsurgery.org.

L. Fleming Fallon, Jr., MD, DrPH

Rhizotomy

Definition

Rhizotomy is the cutting of nerve roots as they enter the spinal cord.

Purpose

Rhizotomy (also called dorsal rhizotomy, selective dorsal rhizotomy, and selective posterior rhizotomy) is a treatment for spasticity that is unresponsive to less invasive procedures.

Demographics

Spasticity (involuntary muscle contractions) affects many thousands of Americans, but very few are affected seriously enough to require surgery for its treatment.

Description

Rhizotomy is performed on patients with spasticity that is insufficiently responsive to oral medications or injectable therapies (botulinum toxin, phenol, or alcohol). It is most commonly performed for those patients with lower extremity spasticity that interferes with walking or severe spasticity that prevents hygiene or positioning of the legs. It is most commonly performed on children with cerebral palsy.

Rhizotomy is performed under **general anesthesia**. The patient lies face down. An incision is made along the lower spine, exposing the sensory nerve roots at the center the spinal cord. Individual nerve rootlets are electrically stimulated. Since these are sensory nerves, they should not stimulate muscle movement. Those that do (and therefore cause spasticity) are cut. Typically, one-quarter to one-half of nerve rootlets tested are cut.

Preparation

Patients undergoing rhizotomy receive a large battery of tests before the procedure, in order to document the functional effects of spasticity, and the patient's medical health and likely response to anesthesia and other operative stresses. Rhizotomy is performed as an in-patient procedure, and the patient is likely to require an overnight hospital stay before the operation.

Aftercare

After surgery, the patient will spend one to several days in the hospital. Physical therapy and strength training usually begin the next day, in order to maximize the gains expected from surgery, and to keep the limbs mobile. Medication may be given for pain.

Risks

Rhizotomy carries small but significant risks of nerve damage, permanent loss of sensation or altered sensation, weakness of the lower extremities, bowel and bladder dysfunction, increased likelihood of hip dislocation, and scoliosis progression. Anesthesia carries its own risks.

QUESTIONS TO ASK YOUR DOCTOR

- How many rhizotomies has the surgeon performed?
- What is the complication rate?
- Is orthopedic surgery still likely to be necessary later on?

Results

Rhizotomy reduces spasticity, which should allow more normal gait and improve mobility. Patients may require fewer walking aids, such as walkers or crutches.

Morbidity and mortality rates

Other than the risks from anesthesia, rhizotomy does not carry a risk of death during surgery. Morbidity rates vary among centers performing the surgery. Persistent and significant adverse effects may occur in 1%–5% of patients, including bowel or bladder changes and low back pain.

Alternatives

Other spasticity treatments include oral medications and an implanted pump delivering baclofen to the space around the spinal cord (intrathecal baclofen). These may be appropriate alternatives for some patients. **Orthopedic surgery** can correct deformities that occur from untreated spasticity. Some controversy exists whether rhizotomy can delay or prevent the need for other spasticity procedures, especially orthopedic surgery such as **tenotomy**, with some evidence suggesting it can, and other evidence suggesting it may not.

Health care team roles

Rhizotomy is performed by a neurosurgeon in a hospital. The patient's neurologist and physical therapist may also be in attendance to help with the evaluation during surgery.

Resources

BOOKS

Sindou, Marc, ed. *Practical Handbook of Neurosurgery: From Leading Neurosurgeons*. Wein; New York: Springer-Verlag, 2009.

PERIODICALS

Bakir, Mustafa Sinan, et al. "Temporal but Not Spatial Variability during Gait Is Reduced after Selective Dorsal Rhizotomy in Children with Cerebral Palsy." *PLoS ONE* 8, no. 7 (July 26, 2013): e69500. http://dx.doi.org/10.1371/journal.pone.0069500 (accessed October 2, 2013).

Dudley, Roy W. R., et al. "Long-Term Functional Benefits of Selective Dorsal Rhizotomy for Spastic Cerebral Palsy." *Journal of Neurosurgery: Pediatrics* 12, no. 2 (2013): 142–50. http://dx.doi.org/10.3171/2013.4.PEDS12539 (accessed October 2, 2013).

Landau, William M. "Rootless Century: Posterior Rhizotomy for Spastic Cerebral Palsy." *Journal of Child Neurology* 28, no. 1 (2013): 7–12. http://dx.doi.org/10.1177/0883073812442588 (accessed October 2, 2013).

WEBSITES

Cleveland Clinic. "Selective Dorsal Rhizotomy." http://my.clevelandclinic.org/services/selective_dorsal_rhizotomy/ns_overview.aspx (accessed October 2, 2013).

ORGANIZATIONS

United Cerebral Palsy (UCP), 1825 K St. NW, Ste. 600, Washington, DC 20006, (202) 776-0406, (800) 872-5827, http://www.ucp.org.

WE MOVE (Worldwide Education and Awareness for Movement Disorders), 5731 Mosholu Ave., Bronx, NY 10471, wemove@wemove.org, http://www.wemove.org.

Richard Robinson

Rhytidoplasty *see* **Face lift**

Robot-assisted surgery

Definition

Robot-assisted surgery involves the use of a robot under the direction and guidance of a surgeon.

Purpose

Robot-assisted surgery provides many benefits in the surgical care of patients. Computer-assisted robots provide exact motion and trajectories to minimize the side effects of surgical intervention. Robot-assisted surgeries can use three-dimensional imaging and smaller surgical tools to operate in a closed environment through smaller incisions. For example, traditional methods of cardiac surgery usually require a 6–8 inch incision in the sternum and the use of a heart-lung machine to maintain the functions of the heart and lungs while they are stopped for the surgery. Robot-assisted surgery has furthered the use of the keyhole approach, in which multiple small incisions are made between the ribs instead of one large incision. With robot-assisted surgery, the surgeon is also able to make more precise movements using motion scaling. In this practice, an image is enlarged on a monitor, and the movements of the surgeon's hands are translated by the computer into smaller movements. This allows **surgeons** to perform more

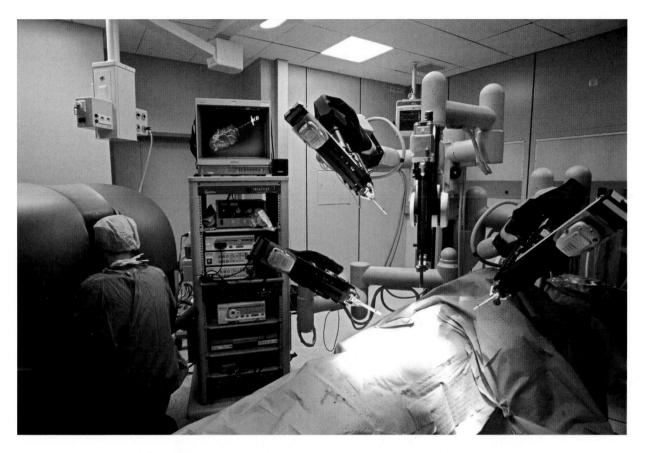

Surgery being performed using the da Vinci robot surgical system. *(Patrick Landmann)*

precisely, which can be especially important when the surgery is performed on small parts of the body.

Description

Robot-assisted surgical techniques are used in the fields of **neurosurgery**, **gynecologic surgery**, **general surgery**, **orthopedic surgery**, radio surgery and radiotherapy, **prostatectomy**, endoscopy, **laparoscopy**, cardiac surgery, and craniofacial surgery.

Neurosurgery

A high level of accuracy is required when operating on the brain to avoid damage to the sensitive brain tissue. Biopsies and minor interventions are best assisted by a robotic device. Interventions include drilling into the skull and making an incision through the dura mater—the outermost layer of the membranes that sheathe the spinal cord and brain—to gain brain tissue samples, drain cysts, or eliminate hemorrhage.

Gynecoloic surgery

Hysterectomies and other gynecologic surgeries can be performed using robotic-assisted techniques. Multiple

gynecologic procedures are performed through use of a laparoscope. The addition of the robotic-assisted technique allows the surgeon to perform more difficult procedures such as removal of larger fibroids, cysts, or the uterus through the same smaller incisions. This technique benefits patients by providing reduced recovery time and less **postoperative pain**.

General surgery

Laparoscopic methods have led to a significant expansion of minimally invasive techniques in recent years, and robotic-assisted laparoscopy is addressing some of the limitations of laparoscopic surgery. This includes significant improvements in instrument dexterity, diminishing natural hand tremors, three-dimensional visualization, ergonomics, and camera stability. Robotic-assisted procedures in general surgery include laparoscopic **cholecystectomy**, Nissen fundoplication, **Heller myotomy**, gastric banding procedures, colectomy, **splenectomy**, **adrenalectomy**, pancreatic surgery, and **gastric bypass**.

Orthopedic surgery

Applications such as cementless **hip replacement**, total knee **arthroplasty**, and pedicle screw placement can benefit from the more accurate cutting and drilling provided by a robot. Femur bone-cutting devices provide improved drilling to carve a cavity in the bone for prosthesis implant. Pins inserted into the bone before surgery are used as landmarks for **computed tomography** (CT) imaging. The CT image provides the surgeon with the necessary information for choosing an implant. The surgeon removes the head from the femur bone, eliminating the joint. The leg is then secured and the robot is brought into position. A high-speed cutter is applied to create the cavity, followed by a smoothing tool. The surgeon manually inserts the implant into the femur and completes the cap implant into the pelvic bone.

Radiosurgery and radiotherapy

Radiation treatment is provided by a robot. A CT or **magnetic resonance imaging** (MRI) scan is used to determine where the radiation treatment should be delivered. The robot aligns with patient anatomy, delivering specific doses of radiation to the intended location.

Prostatectomy

Removal of all or part of the prostate is another robot-assisted procedure. The robot controls instruments inserted through the urethra to the prostate gland. A diathermic hot wire cutting loop is guided to remove tissue in an appropriate pattern around the urethra. Fastening the guiding frame to the upper legs of the patient secures the device for accurate guidance.

Endoscopy

Endoscopy is used to examine patient cavities for the presence of polyps, tumors, and other diseases. The endoscope can be better passed through cavities such as the colon or trachea. Three-dimensional images of the cavity are obtained and used to dictate the path taken by the endoscope. Sedation and heavy analgesia can be avoided.

Laparoscopy

In laparoscopic surgeries, three to four small incisions are made in the abdominal or thoracic cavity to insert the **surgical instruments** and video equipment. The surgeon performs the operation from a remote console that provides the human-machine interface. The console provides video monitoring images that are three-dimensional. Joysticks are used to manipulate the tools within the chest cavity to complete the surgical procedure.

Cardiac surgery

Robots can be used in coronary artery bypass grafting surgeries and cardiac valve replacement and

---

KEY TERMS

Cardiac surgery—Surgery performed on the heart.

Craniofacial surgery—Surgery of the facial tissue and skull.

Endoscopy—Used to visualize internal structures of the body, such as the trachea, esophagus or intestines.

General surgery—General surgery includes procedures on the abdominal cavity organs and other body areas such as breast and thyroid. It also includes procedures on various other body regions that may be associated with multiple specialties.

Gynecologic surgery—Gynecologic procedures include surgeries on the female reproductive system.

Laparoscopy—Surgery on internal structures through small incisions and visualized with the laparoscope.

Neurosurgery—Surgery performed on the brain.

Orthopedic surgery—Surgery performed on the bones. May include joint replacements and surgery of the vertebrae.

Prostatectomy—Performed for the treatment of prostate disease including prostate cancer.

Radio surgery and radiotherapy—Used in the treatment of cancerous growths or kidney stones.

---

repair surgeries. The harvesting of artery and vein grafts can also be accomplished with the aid of laparoscopic techniques.

Craniofacial surgery

Difficult bone cuts and bone tumor removals can be successfully accomplished using robotic instruments. Preplanned trajectories are programmed into the machine. Precision cuts are made in the manner desired to achieve an aesthetically satisfactory result. As the surgeon manipulates the saw, he or she is guided along the path by a predetermined trajectory determined during an initial run on a model of the surgical site.

Da Vinci Surgical System

Approved by the U.S. Food and Drug Administration in 2000, the da Vinci surgical system is the most popular surgical robotic system. According to the company that manufactures the system, Intuitive Surgical, more than 2,000 systems are used in hospitals throughout the world. The system has four robotic arms that move cameras and tools that a surgeon controls from a console. Although the da Vinci is very expensive, many surgeons who use the system say that is has become an indispensable aid to complicated surgical procedures. Moreover, it has been estimated that hospitals save money overall because the length of postsurgical hospitalization is cut in half.

Preparation

Preparation for robot-assisted surgery follows the same guidelines as traditional surgery and depends on the specific procedure.

Aftercare

Patients typically experience shorter recovery times with robotic surgery than with traditional surgical procedures.

Risks

Although the use of robotic tools often shortens the length of surgery, some procedures may require more time to achieve the same desired outcome as the traditional surgical approach. There is an increased risk of anesthesia-related complications as surgical times increase. Additionally, if the robotic procedure is not successful, the surgeon may need to complete the procedure with a traditional technique.

Results

Results for robot-assisted procedures are usually comparable to or even better than their standard surgical counterparts. Numerous studies have shown equivalent or improved patient outcomes when robotic-assisted devices are used.

Morbidity and mortality rates

Complications are comparable to standard surgical procedures and are often reduced. Some complications may only be associated with the robot-assisted procedure.

Alternatives

The alternative to using robot-assisted surgery is for the surgeon to employ a traditional surgical approach.

Resources

BOOKS

DiGioia, Anthony, et al., eds. *Computer and Robotic Assisted Hip and Knee Surgery.* New York: Oxford University Press, 2004.

Faust, Russel A., ed. *Robotics in Surgery: History, Current and Future Applications.* New York: Nova Science Publishers, 2007.

Stiehl, James B., Werner H. Konermann and Rolf G. Haaker, eds. *Navigation and Robotics in Total Joint and Spine Surgery.* New York: Springer, 2004.

PERIODICALS

Aly, E. H. "Robotic Colorectal Surgery: Summary of the Current Evidence." *International Journal of Colorectal Disease* (September 1, 2013): e-pub ahead of print. http://dx.doi.org/10.1007/s00384-013-1764-z (accessed September 6, 2013).

Blanco, Ray Gervacio F., and Kofi Boahene. "Robotic-Assisted Skull Base Surgery: Preclinical Study." *Journal of Laparoendoscopic & Advanced Surgical Techniques* 23, no. 9 (2013): 776–82. http://dx.doi.org/10.1089/lap.2012.0573 (accessed September 6, 2013).

Cirocchi, Roberto, et al. "Current Status of Robotic Distal Pancreatectomy: A Systematic Review." *Surgical Oncology* 22, no. 3 (2013): 201–7. http://dx.doi.org/10.1016/j.suronc.2013.07.002 (accessed September 6, 2013).

Cooper, Michol A., et al. "Underreporting of Robotic Surgery Complications." *Journal for Healthcare Quality* (August 27, 2013): e-pub ahead of print. http://dx.doi.org/10.1111/jhq.12036 (accessed September 6, 2013).

Phillips, Carmen. "Tracking the Rise of Robotic Surgery for Prostate Cancer." *NCI [National Cancer Institute] Cancer Bulletin* 8, no. 16 (August 9, 2011). http://www.cancer.gov/ncicancerbulletin/080911/page4 (accessed September 6, 2013).

Seder, Christopher W., and Stephen D. Cassivi. "Navigating the Pathway to Robotic Competency in General Thoracic Surgery." *Innovations: Technology & Techniques in Cardiothoracic & Vascular Surgery* 8, no. 3 (2013): 184–89. http://dx.doi.org/10.1097/IMI.0b013e3182a05788 (accessed September 6, 2013).

Seror, Julien, et al. "Laparoscopy versus Robotics in the Surgical Management of Endometrial Cancer: Comparison of Intra-Operative and Post-Operative Complications." *Journal of Minimally Invasive Gynecology* (August 29, 2013): e-pub ahead of print. http://dx.doi.org/10.1016/j.jmig.2013.07.015 (accessed September 6, 2013).

WEBSITES

A.D.A.M. Medical Encyclopedia. "Robotic Surgery." Medline Plus. http://www.nlm.nih.gov/medlineplus/ency/article/007339.htm (accessed September 6, 2013).

Intuitive Surgical. "Frequently Asked Questions." http://www.intuitivesurgical.com/products/products_faq.html (accessed September 6, 2013).

"Surgical Robots: The Kindness of Strangers." *Babbage* (blog), *The Economist*, January 18, 2012. http://www.economist.com/blogs/babbage/2012/01/surgical-robots (accessed September 6, 2013).

ORGANIZATIONS

American College of Surgeons, 633 N. Saint Clair St., Chicago, IL 60611-3211, (312) 202-5000, (800) 621-4111, Fax: (312) 202-5001, postmaster@facs.org, http://www.facs.org.

Society of Robotic Surgery, 1100 E. Woodfield Rd., Ste. 350, Schaumburg, IL 60173, (847) 517-7225, srs@wjweiser.com, http://www.srobotics.org.

Allison Joan Spiwak, MSBME
Robert Bockstiegel
Tammy Allhoff, CST/CSFA, AAS

Root canal treatment

Definition

Root canal treatment, also known as endodontic treatment, is a dental procedure in which the diseased or damaged pulp (central core) of a tooth is removed and the inside areas (the pulp chamber and root canals) are filled and sealed.

Purpose

An inflamed or infected pulp is called pulpitis. It is the most common cause of a toothache. To relieve the pain and prevent further complications, the tooth may be extracted (surgically removed) or saved by root canal treatment.

Demographics

Root canal treatment has become a common dental procedure. According to the American Association of Endodontists, more than 14 million root canal treatments are performed every year, with a 95% success rate.

Description

Inside the tooth, the pulp of a tooth is comprised of soft tissue that contains the blood supply, by which the tooth receives its nutrients; and the nerve, by which the tooth senses hot and cold. This tissue is vulnerable to damage from deep dental decay, accidental injury, tooth fracture, or trauma from repeated dental procedures such as multiple fillings or restorations over time. If a tooth becomes diseased or injured, bacteria may build up inside the pulp, spreading infection from the natural crown of the tooth to the root tips in the jawbone. Pus accumulating at the ends of the roots can form a painful abscess that can damage the bone supporting the teeth. Such an infection may produce pain that is severe, constant, or throbbing. It can also result in prolonged sensitivity to heat or cold, swelling, and tenderness in the surrounding gums, facial swelling, or discoloration of the tooth. In some cases, however, the pulp may die so gradually that there is little noticeable pain.

Root canal treatment is performed under **local anesthesia**. A thin sheet of rubber, called a rubber dam, is placed in the mouth and around the base of the tooth to isolate the tooth and help to keep the operative field dry. The dentist removes any tooth decay and makes an opening through the natural crown of the tooth into the pulp chamber. Creating this access also relieves the pressure inside the tooth and can dramatically ease pain.

The dentist determines the length of the root canals, usually with a series of x-rays. Small wire-like files are then used to clean the entire canal space of diseased pulp tissue and bacteria. The debris is flushed out with large amounts of water (irrigation). The canals are also slightly enlarged and shaped to receive an inert (non-reactive) filling material called gutta percha. However, the tooth is not filled and permanently sealed until it is completely free of active infection. The dentist may place a temporary seal, or leave the tooth open to drain, and prescribe an antibiotic to counter any spread of infection from the tooth. This is why root canal treatment may require several visits to the dentist.

Once the canals are completely clean, they are filled with gutta percha and a sealer cement to prevent bacteria from entering the tooth in the future. A metal post may be placed in the pulp chamber for added structural support and better retention of the crown restoration. The tooth is protected by a temporary filling or crown until a permanent restoration may be made. This restoration is usually a gold or porcelain crown, although it may be a gold inlay, or an amalgam or composite filling (paste fillings that harden).

Diagnosis

Signs that a root canal treatment is necessary include severe pain while chewing, prolonged sensitivity to heat or cold, or a darkening of the tooth. Swelling and tenderness of the gums or pimples appearing on the gums are also common symptoms. However, it is also possible that no symptoms will be noticed. The dentist will take

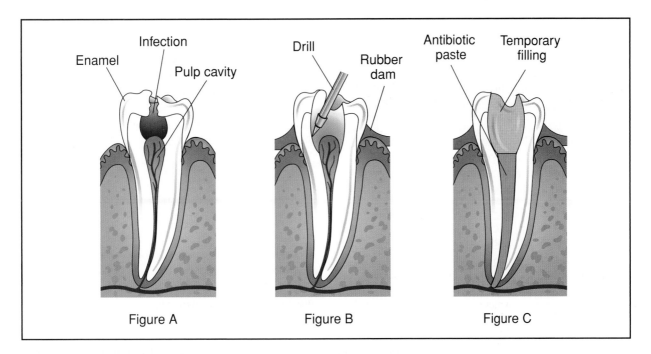

Root canal treatment is a dental procedure in which the diseased pulp of a tooth (A) is removed and the inside areas are filled and sealed. The dentist drills into the enamel and extracts the diseased area (B). The dentist then fills the pulp cavity with antibiotic paste and a temporary filling (C). *(Illustration by Electronic Illustrators Group. Copyright © Cengage Learning®.)*

an x-ray of the tooth to determine if there is any sign of infection in the surrounding bone.

Aftercare

Once a root canal treatment is performed, the recipient must have a crown placed over the tooth to protect it. The cost of the treatment and the crown may be expensive. However, replacing an extracted tooth with a fixed bridge, a removable partial denture, or an implant to maintain the space and restore the chewing function is typically even more expensive.

During the time when **antibiotics** are being used, care should be taken to avoid using the tooth to chew food. The tooth has been structurally weakened and may break, or there is a possibility of the interior of the tooth becoming reinfected.

If the tooth feels sensitive following the procedure, a standard over-the-counter pain medication such as ibuprofen or naproxen may be taken. This sensitivity will fade after a few days. In most cases the patient can resume regular activity the following day.

Risks

There is a possibility that a root canal treatment will not be successful the first time. If infection and inflammation recur and an x-ray indicates a repeat treatment is feasible, the old filling material is removed

and the canals are thoroughly cleaned out. The dentist will try to identify and correct problems with the first root canal treatment before filling and sealing the tooth a second time.

In cases where an x-ray indicates that another root canal treatment cannot correct the problem, endodontic surgery may be performed. In a procedure called an apicoectomy, or root resectioning, the root end of the tooth is accessed in the bone, and a small amount is shaved away. The area is cleaned of diseased tissue and a filling is placed to reseal the canal.

Results

With successful root canal treatment, the tooth will no longer cause pain. However, because it does not contain an internal nerve, it no longer has sensitivity to hot, cold, or sweets. Because these are signs of dental decay, the root canal recipient must receive regular dental check-ups with periodic x-rays to avoid further disease in the tooth. The restored tooth may last a lifetime. However, with routine wear, the filling or crown may eventually need to be replaced.

Morbidity and mortality rates

In some cases, despite proper root canal treatment and endodontic surgery, the tooth dies and must be extracted. This is relatively uncommon.

Abscess—A cavity or space in tooth or gum tissue filled with pus as the result of infection. Its swelling exerts pressure on the surrounding tissues, causing pain.

Apicoectomy—Also called root resectioning. The root tip of a tooth is accessed in the bone and a small amount is shaved away. The diseased tissue is removed and a filling is placed to reseal the canal.

Crown—The natural crown of a tooth is that part of the tooth covered by enamel. Also, a restorative crown is a protective shell that fits over a tooth.

Endodontic—Pertaining to the inside structures of the tooth, including the dental pulp and tooth root, and the periapical tissue surrounding the root.

Endodontist—A dentist who specializes in the diagnosis and treatment of disorders affecting the inside structures of teeth.

Extraction—The surgical removal of a tooth from its socket in a bone.

Gutta percha—An inert, latex-like substance used for filling root canals.

Pulp—The soft innermost layer of a tooth, containing blood vessels and nerves.

Pulp chamber—The area within the tooth occupied by dental pulp.

Pulpitis—Inflammation of the pulp of a tooth involving the blood vessels and nerves.

Root canal—The space within a tooth that runs from the pulp chamber to the tip of the root.

Root canal treatment—The process of removing diseased or damaged pulp from a tooth, then filling and sealing the pulp chamber and root canals.

Alternatives

The only alternative to performing a root canal procedure is to extract the diseased tooth. After restoration or extraction, the two main goals are to allow normal chewing and to maintain proper alignment and spacing between teeth. A fixed bridge, a removable partial denture or an implant will accomplish both goals. However, these are usually more expensive than a root canal treatment.

Health care team roles

A root canal treatment may be performed by a general dentist or by an endodontist. An endodontist is a

- What will be the resulting functional capacity of the tooth?
- Is the oral surgeon board certified in endodontic surgery?
- How many root canal procedures has the oral surgeon performed?
- What is the oral surgeon's complication rate?

dentist who specializes in endodontic (literally "inside of the tooth") procedures. The procedure is usually performed in a professional dental office. In rare situations, it may be performed in a hospital outpatient facility.

Resources

BOOKS

Hupp, James R., Edward Ellis, and Myron R Tucker. *Contemporary Oral and Maxillofacial Surgery.* 6th ed. St. Louis, MO: Elsevier/Mosby, 2014.

Walton, Richard E., and Mahmoud Torabinejad. *Endodontics: Principles and Practice.* St. Louis, MO: Elsevier/Mosby, 2009.

PERIODICALS

Arias, A., et al. "Predictive Models of Pain following Root Canal Treatment: A Prospective Clinical Study." *International Endodontic Journal* 46, no. 8 (2013): 784–93. http://dx.doi.org/10.1111/iej.12059 (accessed October 2, 2013).

Cousson, Pierre-Yves, Emmanuel Nicolas, and Martine Hennequin. "A Follow-Up Study of Pulpotomies and Root Canal Treatments Performed Under General Anaesthesia." *Clinical Oral Investigations* (September 1, 2013): e-pub ahead of print. http://dx.doi.org/10.1007/s00784-013-1090-4 (accessed October 2, 2013).

Gilbert, G. H., et al. "Outcomes of Root Canal Treatment in Dental PBRN Practices." *Texas Dental Journal* 130, no. 4 (2013): 351–59.

Xavier, Ana Claudia C., et al. "One-Visit Versus Two-Visit Root Canal Treatment: Effectiveness in the Removal of Endotoxins and Cultivable Bacteria." *Journal of Endodontics* 39, no. 8 (2013): 959–64. http://dx.doi.org/10.1016/j.joen.2013.04.027 (accessed October 2, 2013).

WEBSITES

American Association of Endodontists. "Root Canals." http://www.aae.org/patients/treatments-and-procedures/root-canals/root-canals.aspx (accessed October 2, 2013).

American Dental Association. "Root Canals." http://www.mouthhealthy.org/en/az-topics/r/root-canals (accessed October 2, 2013).

ORGANIZATIONS

Academy of General Dentistry, 211 E. Chicago Ave., Ste. 900, Chicago, IL 60611-1999, (888) AGD-DENT (243-3368), membership@agd.org, http://www.agd.org.

American Academy of Pediatric Dentistry, 211 E. Chicago Ave., Ste. 1700, Chicago, IL 60611-2637, (312) 337-2169, http://www.aapd.org.

American Association of Endodontists, 211 E. Chicago Ave., Ste. 1100, Chicago, IL 60611-2691, (312) 266-7255, (800) 872-3636, info@aae.org, http://aae.org.

American Dental Association, 211 E. Chicago Ave., Chicago, IL 60611, (312) 440-2500, http://www.ada.org.

L. Fleming Fallon, Jr., MD, DrPH

Rotator cuff repair

Definition

Rotator cuff surgery is the repair of inflammation or tears of the rotator cuff tendons in the shoulder. There are four tendons in the rotator cuff, and these tendons are attached individually to the following muscles: teres minor, subscapularis, infraspinatus, and the supraspinatus. The tears and inflammation associated with rotator cuff injury occur in the region near where these tendon/muscle complexes attach to the humerus (upper arm) bone.

Purpose

Rotator cuff surgery is necessary when chronic shoulder pain associated with rotator cuff injury does not respond to conservative therapy such as rest, heat/ice application, or the use of **nonsteroidal anti-inflammatory drugs** (NSAIDs). Rotator cuff injuries are often lumped into the category referred to as rotator cuff syndrome. Rotator cuff syndrome describes a range of symptoms from basic sprains and tendon swelling (tendinitis) to total rupture or tearing of the tendon.

Demographics

Approximately 5%–10% of the general population is believed to have rotator cuff syndrome at a given time. It is not commonly found in individuals under the age of 20 years, even though many in this population are athletically active. In general, males are more likely than females to develop rotator cuff syndrome and require surgery. Most rotator cuff injuries are associated with athletic activities such as baseball, tennis, weight lifting, and swimming, where the arms are repeatedly lifted over the head. Rotator cuff injuries can also occur in accidents involving falling to the ground or when the humerus is pushed into the shoulder socket. Rotator cuff injuries can also occur in older, active individuals because the rotator cuff tendons begin to deteriorate after age 40. Occupations that have been associated with rotator cuff injuries include nursing, painting, carpentry, tree pruning, fruit picking, and grocery clerking.

Description

For most patients, if the pain begins to subside, they are encouraged to undergo a period of physical therapy. If the pain does not subside after a few weeks, then the physician may suggest the use of cortisone injections into the shoulder region. Rotator cuff repair is then considered if the more conservative methods are not successful.

The primary aim of rotator cuff repair is to repair the connection between the damaged tendon and the bone. Once this bridge is re-established and the connection between the tendon and the bone has thoroughly healed, the corresponding muscles can once again move the arm in a normal fashion. The goal of the surgery is to ensure the smooth movement of the rotator cuff tendons and bursa under the upper part of the shoulder blade. The surgery is also performed to improve the comfort of the patient and to normalize the function of the shoulder and arm. There are a variety of surgical approaches that can be used to accomplish rotator cuff repair. The most common approach is called the anterior acromioplasty approach. This approach allows for excellent access to the most common sites of tears—the biceps groove, anterior cuff, and the undersurface of the joint.

Three types of rotator cuff repair surgeries are performed: open incision, mini-open incision, and arthroscopic. Most rotator cuff repairs are accomplished using incisions that minimize cosmetic changes in the skin following healing. If possible, the surgery is performed with an arthroscope to minimize cosmetic damage to the skin. Typically, the incision made is about the size of a buttonhole. The arthroscope, a pencil-sized instrument, is then inserted into the joint. The surgeon usually accesses the rotator cuff by opening part of the deltoid muscle. If bone spurs, **adhesions**, and damaged bursa are present in the rotator cuff region, then the surgeon will generally remove these damaged structures to improve function in the joint. In cases where the arthroscopic technique is not advised or when it fails to achieve the desired results, a conversion to open surgery is made. This involves a larger incision and usually requires more extensive anesthesia and a longer recovery period.

The success of the rotator cuff repair is dependent on the following factors:

• age of the patient

• type of surgical technique employed

Rotator cuff repair

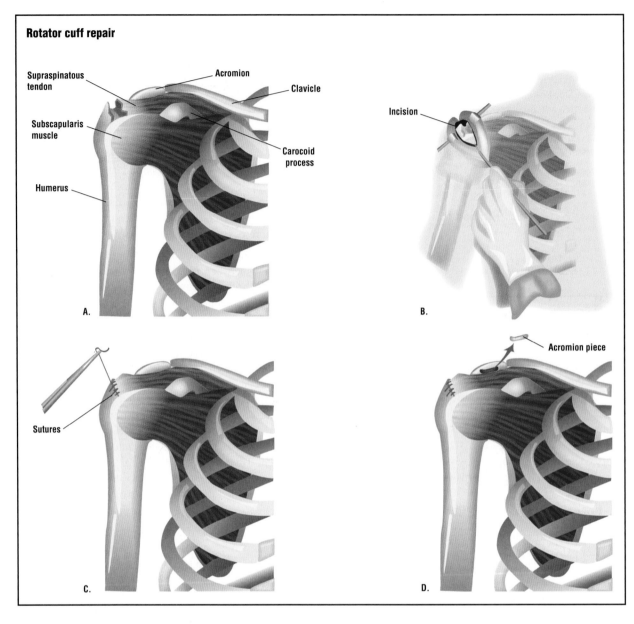

Supraspinatous tendon

Acromion

Clavicle

Subscapularis muscle

Carocoid process

Humerus

A.

Incision

B.

Sutures

C.

Acromion piece

D.

A rotator cuff injury results in a torn tendon at the top of the shoulder (A). To repair it, an incision is made over the site of the tear (B). The tendon's attachment to the bone is repaired with sutures (C), and a small piece of bone from the acromion may be removed (D) to ensure smoother movement of the tendons. *(Illustration by GGS Information Services. Copyright © Cengage Learning®.)*

- degree of damage present
- patient's recovery goals
- patient's ability to follow a physical therapy program following surgery
- smoking status
- number of previous cortisone injections

Diagnosis

The diagnosis of rotator cuff injury is based on a combination of clinical signs and symptoms, coupled with diagnostic testing. The most common clinical signs and symptoms include:

- tenderness in the rotator cuff
- pain associated with the movement of the arm above the head
- pain that is fairly constant but more intense at night
- weakness or pain with the forward movement of the arm
- muscle atrophy (wasting) in long-term injuries that involve a complete tendon tear

KEY TERMS

Adhesions—A fibrous band that holds together tissue that are usually separated and that are associated with wound healing.

Arthrography—Visualization of a joint by radiographic means following injection of a contrast dye into the joint space.

Arthroscope—An endoscope, or a tube containing an optical system, that is used to examine the interior of a joint.

Bone spurs—A sharp or pointed calcified projection.

Bursa—A sac found in connective tissue that acts to reduce friction between tendon and bone.

Deltoid muscle—Muscle that covers the prominence of the shoulder.

X-rays are used to rule out other types of injuries or abnormalities present in the shoulder region. While x-rays are often used to help solidify the diagnosis, **arthrography**, ultrasonography, **computed tomography** (CT), and **magnetic resonance imaging** (MRI) are the definitive tests in the diagnosis of rotator cuff injury. Arthrography and ultrasonography of the shoulder can help determine whether or not there is a full tear in the rotator cuff. An MRI can help determine whether there is a full tear, partial tear, chronic tendinitis, or other cause of the shoulder pain. The final decision to repair the tear ultimately rests on the amount of pain and restriction suffered by the patient.

Aftercare

Following the procedure, the patient will typically spend several hours in the recovery room. Generally, an ice pack will be applied to the affected shoulder joint for a period up to 48 hours. The patient will usually be given either prescription or non-prescription pain medication. The dressing is usually removed the day after surgery and is replaced by adhesive strips. The patient should contact a physician if there are any significant changes in the affected area once the patient goes home. These changes can include increased swelling, pain, bleeding, drainage in the affected area, nausea, vomiting, or signs of infection. Signs of infection include fever, dizziness, headache, and muscle aches.

It often takes several days for the arthroscopic puncture wounds to heal, and the joint usually takes several weeks to recover. Most patients can resume normal

daily activities, with the permission of a physician, within a few days following the procedure. Most patients are advised to undergo a rehabilitation program that includes physical therapy. Such a program can facilitate recovery and improve the functioning of the joint in the future.

Risks

Complications following arthroscopic rotator cuff surgery are very rare. Such complications occur in less than 1% of cases. These complications include instrument breakage, blood vessel or nerve damage, blood vessel clots, infection, and inflammation. Complications, though still rare, are more common following open surgery. This is due to the larger incisions and more complicated anesthesia that is often necessary.

Results

The prognosis for the long-term relief from rotator cuff syndrome is good, especially when both conservative and surgical therapeutic approaches are used. In those patients who do require surgery, six weeks of physical therapy is typically instituted following surgery. Complete recovery following surgery may take several months. In rare cases, the rotator cuff injury is so severe that the patient may require muscle transfers and tendon grafts. Even more rarely, the injury can be so severe that the tendons are not repairable. This typically occurs when a severe rotator cuff injury is neglected for a long period of time.

Morbidity and mortality rates

Morbidity is rare in both the arthroscopic and open procedures. Mortality is exceedingly rare in patients undergoing rotator cuff repair.

Alternatives

Conservative approaches are typically used before surgery is considered in patients with rotator cuff injury. This is true even in cases where there is evidence of a full tendon tear. Some patients with a full or partial tear do not suffer a significant amount of pain and retain normal or nearly normal range of motion in shoulder movement. A majority of those with rotator cuff syndrome respond to conservative nonsurgical approaches. Conservative therapies include the following:

• heat or ice to reduce pain and swelling
• cessation or reduction of activities that involve the movement of the arms overhead
• medication such as nonsteroidal anti-inflammatory agents to reduce pain and inflammation
• cortisone injections to reduce pain and inflammation
• rest

QUESTIONS TO ASK YOUR DOCTOR

- What are my alternatives?
- Is surgery the answer for me?
- Can you recommend a surgeon who performs rotator cuff repairs?
- If surgery is appropriate for me, what are the next steps?
- How many times have you performed rotator cuff repair?
- Are you a board-certified surgeon?
- What type of outcomes have you had?
- What are the most common side effects or complications?
- What should I do to prepare for surgery?
- What should I expect following the surgery?
- Can you refer me to one of your patients who has had this procedure?
- What type of diagnostic procedures are performed to determine if patients require surgery?
- Will I need to see another specialist for the diagnostic procedures?

Once the pain begins to subside, the patient usually is encouraged to begin a program of physical therapy to help re-institute normal motion and function to the shoulder.

Health care team roles

Rotator cuff repair is generally performed by a specialist known as an orthopedic surgeon, who has received specialized training in the diseases and injuries of the musculoskeletal system. Orthopedic **surgeons** who perform rotator cuff repair receive extensive training in **general surgery** and in the specific techniques involving the musculoskeletal system. Rotator cuff repairs are often performed in the specialized department of a general hospital, but they are also performed in specialized **orthopedic surgery** clinics or institutes for orthopedic conditions.

Resources

BOOKS

Browner, Bruce D., et al. *Skeletal Trauma: Basic Science, Management, and Reconstruction.* 4th ed. Philadelphia: Saunders/Elsevier, 2009.

Canale, S. T., ed. *Campbell's Operative Orthopaedics.* 12th ed. St. Louis, MO: Mosby, 2012.

DeLee, Jesse, David Drez, and Mark D. Miller. *DeLee and Drez's Orthopaedic Sports Medicine: Principles and Practice.* 3rd ed. Philadelphia: Saunders/Elsevier, 2010.

PERIODICALS

Karas, V., et al. "Comparison of Subjective and Objective Outcomes After Rotator Cuff Repair." *Arthroscopy* (September 25, 2013): e-pub ahead of print. http://dx.doi.org/10.1016/j.arthro.2013.08.001 (accessed October 14, 2013).

WEBSITES

American Academy of Orthopaedic Surgeons. "Rotator Cuff Tears: Surgical Treatment Options." OrthoInfo. http://orthoinfo.aaos.org/topic.cfm?topic=A00406 (accessed October 14, 2013).

MedlinePlus. "Rotator Cuff Injuries." U.S. National Library of Medicine, National Institutes of Health. http://www.nlm.nih.gov/medlineplus/rotatorcuffinjuries.html (accessed October 14, 2013).

Sutter Health. "Rotator Cuff Tear and Repair." http://www.sutterhealth.org/orthopedics/shoulder/rotator-cuff-injuries-repair.html (accessed October 14, 2013).

University of Washington, Department of Orthopaedics and Sports Medicine. "Repair of Rotator Cuff Tears." http://www.orthop.washington.edu/?q=patient-care/articles/shoulder/repair-of-rotator-cuff-tears.html (accessed October 14, 2013).

ORGANIZATIONS

American Academy of Orthopaedic Surgeons (AAOS), 6300 N. River Rd., Rosemont, IL 60018-4262, (847) 823-7186, Fax: (847) 823-8125, pemr@aaos.org, http://www.aaos.org.

Mark Mitchell

Routine urinalysis *see* **Urinalysis**

S

Sacral nerve stimulation

Definition

Sacral nerve stimulation, also known as sacral neuromodulation, is a procedure in which the sacral nerve at the base of the spine is stimulated by a mild electrical current from an implanted device. It is done to improve functioning of the urinary tract, to relieve pain related to urination, and to control fecal incontinence.

Purpose

As a proven treatment for urinary incontinence, sacral nerve stimulation (SNS) has recently been found effective in the treatment of interstitial cystitis, a disorder that involves hyperreflexia of the urinary sphincter. SNS is also used to treat pelvic or urinary pain as well as fecal incontinence.

A person's ability to hold urine or feces depends on three body functions:

- a reservoir function represented by the urethra/bladder or colon
- a gatekeeping function represented by the urethral or anal sphincter
- the brain's ability to control urination, defecation, and nerve sensitivity

A dysfunction or deficiency in any of these components can result in incontinence. The most common forms of incontinence are stress urinary incontinence and urge incontinence. Stress incontinence is related to an unstable detrusor muscle that controls the urinary sphincter. When the detrusor muscle is weak, urine can leak out of the bladder from pressure on the abdomen caused by sneezing, coughing, and other movements. Urge incontinence is characterized by a sudden strong need to urinate and inability to hold urine until an appropriate time; it is also associated with hyperactivity of the urinary sphincter. Both conditions can be treated by SNS. SNS requires an implanted device that sends continuous stimulation to the sacral nerve that controls the urinary sphincter. This treatment has been used with over 1,500 patients with a high rate of success. It was approved in Europe in 1994. The U.S. Food and Drug Administration (FDA) approved SNS for the treatment of urinary urge incontinence in 1997 and for urinary frequency in 1999.

Interstitial cystitis (IC) is a chronic condition of unknown origin that causes pain in the bladder and lower abdomen, urinary urgency, a frequent need to urinate at night, and pain during intercourse. IC has no known cause; it is diagnosed by the level of reported discomfort and by excluding other sources of urinary pain, frequency, and urgency. SNS has only recently been used to treat IC. According to three studies presented to the American Urological Association in 2001, SNS significantly reduced urinary urgency and frequency, with some relief of pain, in patients who had not responded to other treatments. The use of SNS in treating IC is still considered experimental, however.

Treatment of fecal incontinence with SNS is very recent; it is also considered experimental. Newer research from Italy, however, indicates that patients with anorectal disturbances that are usually treated by augmentation of the sphincter muscle or implanting an artificial sphincter can benefit from electrical stimulation of the sacral nerve. Although the mechanism of SNS is not completely clear, researchers believe that the patient's control of the pelvic region is restored by the stimulation or activation of afferent fibers in the muscles of the pelvic floor.

Demographics

Urinary incontinence affects between 15% and 30% of American adults living in the community, and as many as 50% of people confined to **nursing homes**. It is a disorder that affects women far more frequently than men; 85% of people suffering from urinary incontinence are women. According to the chief of geriatrics at a Boston hospital, 25 million Americans suffer each year from occasional episodes of urinary or fecal incontinence.

Interstitial cystitis is less common than urinary or fecal incontinence but still affects about 12% of women in the United States each year. The average age of IC patients is 40; 25% of patients are younger than 30. Although 90% of patients diagnosed with IC are women, it is thought that the disorder may be underdiagnosed in men.

Description

Sacral nerve stimulation (SNS) is conducted through an implanted device that includes a thin insulated wire called a lead and a neurostimulator much like a cardiac pacemaker. The device is inserted in a pocket in the patient's lower abdomen. SNS is first tried on an outpatient basis in the doctor's office with the implantation of a test lead. If the trial treatment is successful, the patient is scheduled for inpatient surgery.

Permanent surgical implantation is done under **general anesthesia** and requires a one-night stay in the hospital. After the patient has been anesthetized, the surgeon implants the neurostimulator, which is about the size of a pocket stopwatch, under the skin of the patient's abdomen. Thin wires, or leads, running from the

stimulator carry electrical pulses from the stimulator to the sacral nerves located in the lower back. After the stimulator and leads have been implanted, the surgeon closes the incision in the abdomen.

Diagnosis

Incontinence significantly affects a patient's quality of life; thus patients usually consult a doctor when their urinary problems begin to cause difficulties in the workplace or on social occasions. A family care practitioner will usually refer the patient to a urologist for diagnosis of the cause(s) of the incontinence. Patients with urinary and fecal incontinence are evaluated carefully through the taking of a complete patient history and a **physical examination**. The doctor will use special techniques to assess the capacity of the bladder or rectum as well as the functioning of the urethral or anal sphincter in order to determine the cause or location of the incontinence. **Cystoscopy**, which is the examination of the full bladder with a scope attached to a small tube, allows the physician to rule out certain disorders as well as plan the most effective treatment. These extensive tests are especially important in diagnosing interstitial cystitis because all other causes of urinary urgency, frequency, and pain must be ruled out before surgery can be suggested. Cystoscopy is done under anesthesia and often works as a treatment for IC. Once the doctor has made the diagnosis of urinary incontinence due to sphincter insufficiency, he or she will explain and discuss the surgical implant with the patient. SNS may be tried out on a temporary basis. The same pattern of diagnosis and treatment is used for patients with IC and fecal incontinence. Temporary implants can help eliminate those patients who will not benefit from a permanent implant.

Aftercare

Following surgery, the patient remains overnight in the hospital. **Antibiotics** may be given to reduce the risk of infection and pain medications to relieve discomfort. The patient will be given instructions on **incision care** and follow-up appointments before he or she leaves the hospital.

Aftercare includes fine-tuning of the SNS stimulator. The doctor can adjust the strength of the electrical impulses in his or her office with a handheld programmer. The stimulator runs for about five to ten years and can be replaced during an outpatient procedure. About a third of patients require a second operation to adjust or replace various elements of the stimulator device.

Risks

In addition to the risks of bleeding and infection that are common to surgical procedures, implanting an SNS device carries the risks of pain at the insertion site, discomfort when urinating, mild electrical shocks, and displacement or dislocation of the leads.

Results

Patients report improvement in the number of urinations, the volume of urine produced, lessened urgency, and higher overall quality of life after treatment with SNS. Twenty-two patients undergoing a three- to seven-day test of sacral nerve stimulation on an outpatient basis reported significant reduction in urgency and frequency, according to the American Urological Association. Studies have indicated complete success in about 50% of patients. Sacral nerve stimulation is being used to treat fecal incontinence in the United States and Europe, with promising early reports. SNS is the least invasive of the recognized surgical treatments for fecal incontinence.

Morbidity and mortality rates

Sacral nerve stimulation has been shown to be a safe and effective procedure for the treatment of both urinary and fecal incontinence. Two groups of researchers, in Spain and the United Kingdom respectively, have reported that "the effects of neuromodulation are long-lasting and associated morbidity is low." The most commonly reported complications of SNS are pain at the site of the implant (15.3% of patients); pain on urination (9%); and displacement of the leads (8.4%).

Alternatives

There are three types of nonsurgical treatments that benefit some patients with IC:

• Behavioral approaches include biofeedback, diet modifications, bladder retraining, and pelvic muscle exercises.

• Medications include antispasmodic drugs; tricyclic antidepressants; and pentosan polysulfate sodium, which is sold under the trade name Elmiron. Elmiron appears to work by protecting the lining of the bladder from bacteria and other irritating substances in urine.

• Intravesical medications are medications that affect the muscular tissues of the bladder. Oxybutynin is a drug that is prescribed for patients who are incontinent because their bladders fail to store urine properly. Capsaicin and resiniferatoxin are used to treat hyperreflexia of the detrusor muscle.

Surgical alternatives to SNS are considered treatments of last resort for IC because they are invasive, irreversible, and benefit only 30%–40% of patients. In addition, some studies indicate that these surgeries can

QUESTIONS TO ASK YOUR DOCTOR

• Am I likely to benefit from SNS?

• How many stimulators have you implanted?

• How many of your patients consider SNS a successful treatment?

• What side effects have your patients reported?

lead to long-term kidney damage. They include the following procedures:

• Augmentation cystoplasty. In this procedure, the surgeon removes the patient's bladder and replaces it with a section of the bowel—in effect creating a new bladder. The patient passes urine through the urethra in the normal fashion.

• Urinary diversion. The surgeon creates a tube from a section of the patient's bowel and places the ureters (tubes that carry urine from the kidneys to the bladder) in this tube. The tube is then attached to a stoma, or opening in the abdomen. Urine is carried into an external collection bag that the patient must empty several times daily.

• Internal pouch. The surgeon creates a new bladder from a section of the bowel and attaches it inside the abdomen. The patient empties the pouch by self-catheterization four to six times daily.

Health care team roles

SNS devices are implanted under general anesthesia by urologists, who are physicians specializing in treating disorders of the urinary tract. The procedure is usually performed in a hospital.

Resources

BOOKS

Feldman, M., et al. *Sleisenger & Fordtran's Gastrointestinal and Liver Disease.* 9th ed. Philadelphia: Saunders/Elsevier, 2010.

Lentz, Gretchen, et al. *Comprehensive Gynecology.* 5th ed. St. Louis: Mosby/Elsevier, 2012.

Wein, Alan J., et al. *Campbell-Walsh Urology.* 10th ed. Philadelphia: Saunders/Elsevier, 2012.

PERIODICALS

Altomare, D. F., et al. "The Effects of Sacral Nerve Stimulation on Continence Are Temporarily Maintained after Turning the Stimulator Off." *Colorectal Disease* (September 14, 2013): e-pub ahead of print. http://dx.doi.org/10.1111/codi.12418 (accessed October 17, 2013).

Maeda, Y., et al. "Outcome of Sacral Nerve Stimulation for Fecal Incontinence at 5 Years." *Annals of Surgery* (June

28, 2013): e-pub ahead of print. http://dx.doi.org/10.1097/SLA.0b013e31829d3969 (accessed October 17, 2013).

Thomas, G., et al. "A Pilot Study of Transcutaneous Sacral Nerve Stimulation for Faecal Incontinence." *Colorectal Disease* (August 3, 2013): e-pub ahead of print. http://dx.doi.org/10.1111/codi.12371 (accessed October 17, 2013).

OTHER

Addenbrooke's Hospital. "Sacral Nerve Stimulation (Permanent Implant): Frequently-Asked Questions." http://www.camurology.org.uk/wp-content/uploads/sns-permanent-implant-35.pdf (accessed October 17, 2013).

WEBSITES

Bladder & Bowel Foundation. "Sacral Nerve Stimulation." http://www.bladderandbowelfoundation.org/bladder/bladder-problems/sacral-nerve-stimulation.asp (accessed October 17, 2013).

National Institute for Health and Care Excellence. "Sacral Nerve Stimulation for Urge Incontinence and Urgency-Frequency." http://publications.nice.org.uk/sacral-nerve-stimulation-for-urge-incontinence-and-urgency-frequency-ipg64/the-procedure (accessed October 17, 2013).

ORGANIZATIONS

Bladder & Bowel Foundation, SATRA Innovation Park, Rockingham Rd., Kettering, Northants NN16 9JH, United Kingdom, +44 01536 533255, info@bladderandbowelfoundation.org, http://www.bladderandbowelfoundation.org.

National Association for Continence (NAFC), PO Box 1019, Charleston, SC 29402-1019, (843) 377-0900, (800) BLADDER (252-3337), Fax: (843) 377-0905, member-services@nafc.org, http://www.nafc.org.

National Kidney and Urologic Diseases Information Clearinghouse, 3 Information Way, Bethesda, MD 20892-3580, (800) 891-5390, (866) 569-1162, Fax: (703) 738–4929, nkudic@info.niddk.nih.gov, http://kidney.niddk.nih.gov.

National Kidney Foundation, 30 E. 33rd St., New York, NY 10016, (212) 889-2210, (800) 622-9010, Fax: (212) 689-9261, http://www.kidney.org.

Urology Care Foundation, 1000 Corporate Blvd., Linthicum, MD 21090, (410) 689-3700, (800) 828-7866, Fax: (410) 689-3998, info@urologycarefoundation.org, http://auafoundation.org.

Nancy McKenzie, PhD

Salpingo-oophorectomy

Definition

Unilateral salpingo-oophorectomy is the surgical removal of a fallopian tube and an ovary. If both sets of fallopian tubes and ovaries are removed, the procedure is called a bilateral salpingo-oophorectomy.

Purpose

This surgery is performed to treat ovarian or other gynecological cancers, or infections caused by pelvic inflammatory disease. Occasionally, removal of one or both ovaries may be done to treat endometriosis, a condition in which the lining of the uterus (the endometrium) grows outside of the uterus (usually on and around the pelvic organs). The procedure may also be performed if a woman has been diagnosed with an ectopic pregnancy in a fallopian tube and a **salpingostomy** (an incision into the fallopian tube to remove the pregnancy) cannot be done. If only one fallopian tube and ovary are removed, the woman may still be able to conceive and carry a pregnancy to term. If both are removed, however, the woman is rendered permanently infertile. This procedure is commonly combined with a **hysterectomy** (surgical removal of the uterus); the ovaries and fallopian tubes are removed in about one-third of hysterectomies.

Until the 1980s, women over age 40 having hysterectomies routinely had healthy ovaries and fallopian tubes removed at the same time. Many physicians reasoned that a woman over 40 was approaching menopause and soon her ovaries would stop secreting estrogen and releasing eggs. Removing the ovaries would eliminate the risk of ovarian cancer and only accelerate menopause by a few years.

In the 1990s, the thinking about routine salpingo-oophorectomy began to change. The risk of ovarian cancer in women who have no family history of the disease is less than 1%. Moreover, removing the ovaries increases the risk of cardiovascular disease and accelerates osteoporosis unless a woman takes prescribed hormone replacements.

Demographics

Overall, ovarian cancer accounts for only 4% of all cancers in women. For women at increased risk, **oophorectomy** may be considered after the age of 35 if childbearing is complete. Factors that increase a woman's risk of developing ovarian cancer include age (most ovarian cancers occur after menopause), the presence of a mutation in the BRCA1 or BRCA2 gene, the number of menstrual periods a woman has had (affected by age of onset, pregnancy, breast-feeding, and oral contraceptive use), history of breast cancer, diet, and family history. The incidence of ovarian cancer is highest among Native American (17.5 cases per 100,000 population), Caucasian (15.8 per 100,000), Vietnamese (13.8 per 100,000), Hispanic (12.1 per 100,000), and Hawaiian (11.8 per 100,000) women; it is lowest among Korean (7.0 per 100,000) and Chinese (9.3 per 100,000)

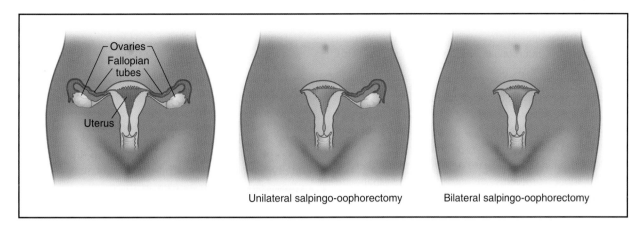

Unilateral salpingo-oophorectomy   Bilateral salpingo-oophorectomy

During a salpingo-oophorectomy, one (unilateral) or both (bilateral) sets of a woman's ovaries and fallopian tubes are removed. *(Illustration by Electronic Illustrators Group. Copyright © 2014 Cengage Learning®.)*

women. African American women have an ovarian cancer incidence of 10.2 per 100,000 population.

Endometriosis, another reason why salpingo-oophorectomy may be performed, has been estimated to affect up to 10% of women. Approximately four out of every 1,000 women are hospitalized as a result of endometriosis each year. Women 25–35 years of age are affected most, with 27 being the average age of diagnosis.

Description

General or regional anesthesia will be given to the patient before the procedure begins. If the procedure is performed through a laparoscope, the surgeon can avoid a large abdominal incision and can shorten recovery. With this technique, the surgeon makes a small cut through the abdominal wall just below the navel. A tube containing a tiny lens and light source (a laparoscope) is then inserted through the incision. A camera can be attached that allows the surgeon to see the abdominal cavity on a video monitor. When the ovaries and fallopian tubes are detached, they are removed though a small incision at the top of the vagina. The organs can also be cut into smaller sections and removed. When the laparoscope is used, the patient can be given either regional or **general anesthesia**; if there are no complications, the patient can leave the hospital in a day or two.

If a laparoscope is not used, the surgery involves an incision 4–6 in. (10–15 cm) long into the abdomen extending either vertically up from the pubic bone toward the navel, or horizontally (the "bikini incision") across the pubic hairline. The scar from a bikini incision is less noticeable, but some **surgeons** prefer the vertical incision because it provides greater visibility while operating. A disadvantage to abdominal salpingo-oophorectomy is

that bleeding is more likely to be a complication of this type of operation. The procedure is more painful than a laparoscopic operation and the recovery period is longer. A woman can expect to be in the hospital two to five days and will need three to six weeks to return to normal activities.

Preparation

Before surgery, the doctor will order blood and urine tests, and any additional tests such as **ultrasound** or x-rays to help the surgeon visualize the woman's condition. The woman may also meet with the anesthesiologist to evaluate any special conditions that might affect the administration of anesthesia. A colon preparation may be done if extensive surgery is anticipated.

On the evening before the operation, the woman should eat a light dinner, then take nothing by mouth, including water or other liquids, after midnight.

Aftercare

If performed through an abdominal incision, salpingo-oophorectomy is major surgery that requires three to six weeks for full recovery. However, if performed laparoscopically, the recovery time can be much shorter. There may be some discomfort around the incision for the first few days after surgery, but most women are walking around by the third day. Within a month or so, patients can gradually resume normal activities such as driving, exercising, and working.

Immediately following the operation, the patient should avoid sharply flexing the thighs or the knees. Persistent back pain or bloody or scanty urine indicates that a ureter may have been injured during surgery.

If both ovaries are removed in a premenopausal woman as part of the operation, the sudden loss of estrogen will trigger an abrupt premature menopause that may involve severe symptoms of hot flashes, vaginal dryness, painful intercourse, and loss of sex drive. (This is also called "surgical menopause.") In addition to these symptoms, women who lose both ovaries also lose the protection these hormones provide against heart disease and osteoporosis many years earlier than if they had experienced natural menopause. Women who have had their ovaries removed are seven times more likely to develop coronary heart disease and much more likely to develop bone problems at an early age than are premenopausal women whose ovaries are intact. For these reasons, some form of hormone replacement therapy (HRT) may be prescribed to relieve the symptoms of surgical menopause and to help prevent heart and bone disease.

Reaction to the removal of fallopian tubes and ovaries depends on a wide variety of factors, including the woman's age, the condition that required the surgery, her reproductive history, how much social support she has, and any previous history of depression. Women who have had many gynecological surgeries or chronic pelvic pain seem to have a higher tendency to develop psychological problems after the surgery.

Risks

Major surgery always involves some risk, including infection, reactions to the anesthesia, hemorrhage, and scars at the incision site. Almost all pelvic surgery causes some internal scars, which in some cases can cause discomfort years after surgery.

Potential complications after a salpingo-oophorectomy include changes in sex drive, hot flashes, and other symptoms of menopause if both ovaries are removed. Women who have both ovaries removed and who do not take estrogen replacement therapy run an increased risk for cardiovascular disease and osteoporosis. Women with a history of psychological and emotional problems before an oophorectomy are more likely to experience psychological difficulties after the operation.

Results

If the surgery is successful, the fallopian tubes and ovaries will be removed without complication, and the underlying problem resolved. In the case of cancer, all the cancer will be removed. A woman will become infertile following a bilateral salpingo-oophorectomy.

Morbidity and mortality rates

Studies have shown that the complication rate following salpingo-oophorectomy is essentially the same as that following hysterectomy. The rate of complications

KEY TERMS

BRCA1 or BRCA2 genetic mutation—A genetic mutation that predisposes otherwise healthy women to breast cancer.

Endometriosis—A painful disease in which cells from the lining of the uterus (endometrium) become attached to other organs in the pelvic cavity. The condition is hard to diagnose and often causes severe pain as well as infertility.

Fallopian tubes—Tubes that extend from either end of the uterus that convey the egg from the ovary to the uterus during each monthly cycle.

Hysterectomy—The surgical removal of the uterus.

Ureter—The tube that carries urine from the bladder to the kidneys.

differs by the type of hysterectomy performed. Abdominal hysterectomy is associated with a higher rate of complications (9.3%), while the overall complication rate for vaginal hysterectomy is 5.3%, and 3.6% for laparoscopic vaginal hysterectomy. The risk of death is about one in every 1,000 women having a hysterectomy. The rates of some of the more commonly reported complications are:

- excessive bleeding (hemorrhaging): 1.8%–3.4%
- fever or infection: 0.8%–4.0%
- accidental injury to another organ or structure: 1.5%–1.8%

Because of the cessation of hormone production that occurs with a bilateral oophorectomy, women who lose both ovaries also prematurely lose the protection these hormones provide against heart disease and osteoporosis. Women who have undergone bilateral oophorectomy are seven times more likely to develop coronary heart disease and much more likely to develop bone problems at an early age than are premenopausal women whose ovaries are intact.

Alternatives

Depending on the specific condition that warrants an oophorectomy, it may be possible to modify the surgery so at least a portion of one ovary remains, allowing the woman to avoid early menopause. In the case of endometriosis, there are a number of alternative treatments that are usually pursued before a salpingo-oophorectomy (with or without hysterectomy) is performed. These include excising the growths without removing any organs, blocking or destroying the nerves that provide sensation to some of the pelvic structures, or prescribing drugs that decrease estrogen levels.

Health care team roles

Salpingo-oophorectomies are usually performed in a hospital **operating room** by a gynecologist, a medical doctor who has completed specialized training in the areas of women's general health, pregnancy, labor and childbirth, **prenatal testing**, and genetics.

Resources

PERIODICALS

Dongwon, Kim, et al. "Factors Affecting the Decision to Undergo Risk-Reducing Salpingo-oophorectomy among Women with BRCA Gene Mutation." *Familial Cancer* (March 16, 2013): e-pub ahead of print. http://dx.doi.org/10.1007/s10689-013-9625-z (accessed October 2, 2013).

Mannis, Gabriel N., et al. "Risk-Reducing Salpingo-oophorectomy and Ovarian Cancer Screening in 1077 Women after BRCA Testing." *JAMA Internal Medicine* 173, no. 2 (2013): 96–103. http://dx.doi.org/10.1001/2013.jamainternmed.962 (accessed October 2, 2013).

Tan, Bee K., et al. "A Retrospective Review of Patient-Reported Outcomes on the Impact on Quality of Life in Patients Undergoing Total Abdominal Hysterectomy and Bilateral Salpingo-oophorectomy for Endometriosis." *European Journal of Obstetrics & Gynecology and Reproductive Biology* 170, no. 2 (2013): 533–38. http://dx.doi.org/10.1016/j.ejogrb.2013.07.030 (accessed October 2, 2013).

WEBSITES

National Cancer Institute. "Ovarian Cancer." http://www.cancer.gov/cancertopics/types/ovarian (accessed October 2, 2013).

NYU Langone Medical Center. "Ovarian Cancer." http://robotic-surgery.med.nyu.edu/for-patients/our-departments/gynecology/procedures/salpingo-oopherectomy-for-malignant-conditions (accessed October 2, 2013).

ORGANIZATIONS

American Cancer Society, 250 Williams St. NW, Atlanta, GA 30303, (800) 227-2345, http://www.cancer.org.

American Congress of Obstetricians and Gynecologists, 409 12th St. SW, Washington, DC 20024-2188, (202) 638-5577, (800) 673-8444, resources@acog.org, http://www.acog.org.

Carol A. Turkington
Stephanie Dionne Sherk

Salpingostomy

Definition

A salpingostomy is a surgical incision into a fallopian tube. This procedure may be done to repair a damaged tube or to remove an ectopic pregnancy (one that occurs outside of the uterus).

Purpose

The fallopian tubes are the structures that carry a mature egg from the ovaries to the uterus. These tubes, which are about 4 inches (10 cm) long and 0.2 inches (0.5 cm) in diameter, are found on the upper outer sides of the uterus, and open into the uterus through small channels. It is within the fallopian tubes that fertilization, the joining of an egg and a sperm, takes place.

During a normal pregnancy, the fertilized egg passes from the fallopian tubes into the uterus and then implants into the lining of the uterus. If the fertilized egg implants anywhere outside of the uterus, it is called an ectopic (or tubal) pregnancy. The majority of ectopic pregnancies occur in the fallopian tubes (95%); they may also occur in the uterine muscle (1%–2%), the abdomen (1%–2%), the ovaries (less than 1%), and the cervix (less than 1%).

As an ectopic pregnancy progresses, the fallopian tubes are unable to contain the growing embryo and may rupture. A ruptured ectopic pregnancy is considered a medical emergency as it can cause significant hemorrhaging (excessive bleeding). If an ectopic pregnancy is diagnosed early (i.e., before rupture has occurred), it may be possible to manage medicinally; the drug methotrexate targets rapidly dividing fetal cells, preventing the fetus from developing further. If medicinal management is not possible or has failed, surgical intervention may be necessary. A salpingostomy may then be performed to remove the pregnancy.

Salpingostomy may also be performed in an effort to restore fertility to a woman whose fallopian tubes have

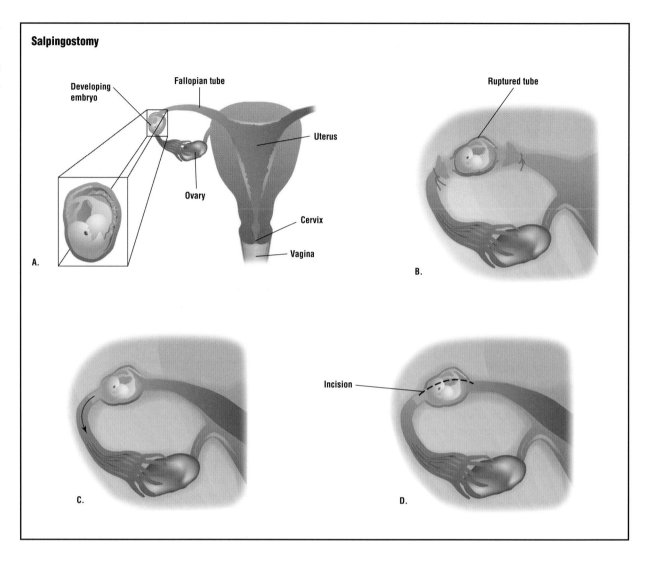

Salpingostomy

Developing embryo

Fallopian tube

Uterus

Ovary

Cervix

Vagina

A.

Ruptured tube

B.

C.

Incision

D.

A tubal or ectopic pregnancy can be removed in several ways. If the fallopian tube is ruptured (A), the tube is tied off on both sides and the embryo is removed. If the tube is intact, the embryo can be pulled out the end of the tube (C) or the tube can be cut open (D). *(Illustration by GGS Information Services. Copyright © Cengage Learning®.)*

been damaged, such as by **adhesions** (bands of scar tissue that may form after surgery or trauma). In the case of hydrosalpinx, a condition in which a tube becomes blocked and filled with fluid, a salpingostomy may be performed to create a new tubal ostium (opening).

Demographics

Ectopic pregnancy occurs in approximately 2% of all pregnancies. Once a woman has an ectopic pregnancy, she has an increased chance (10%–25%) of having another. Women between the ages of 25 and 34 have a higher incidence of ectopic pregnancy, although the mortality rate among women over the age of 35 is 2.5–5.9 times higher. Minority women are also at an increased risk of ectopic pregnancy-related death.

Description

Salpingostomy may be performed via laparotomy or **laparoscopy**, under general or regional anesthesia. A laparotomy is an incision made in the abdominal wall through which the fallopian tubes are visualized. If the tube has already ruptured as a result of an ectopic pregnancy, a salpingectomy will be performed to remove the damaged fallopian tube. If rupture has not occurred, a drug called vasopressin is injected into the fallopian tube to minimize the amount of bleeding. An incision (called a linear salpingostomy) is made through the wall of the tube in the area of the ectopic pregnancy. The products of conception are then flushed out of the tube with an instrument called a suction-irrigator. Any bleeding sites are treated by suturing or by applying pressure with forceps. The incision is not sutured but instead left to heal on its own (called closure by secondary intent). The abdominal wall is then closed.

A neosalpingostomy is similar to a linear salpingostomy but is performed to treat a tubal blockage (e.g., hydrosalpinx). An incision is made to create a new opening in the fallopian tube; the tissue is folded over and stitched into place. The new hole, or ostium, replaces the normal opening of the fallopian tube through which the egg released by an ovary each menstrual cycle is collected.

Salpingostomy may also be performed laparoscopically. With this surgery, a tube (called a laparoscope) containing a tiny lens and light source is inserted through a small incision in the navel. A camera can be attached that allows the surgeon to see the abdominal cavity on a video monitor. The salpingostomy is then performed with instruments inserted through **trocars**, small incisions of 0.2–0.8 in. (0.5–2 cm) made through the abdominal wall.

An advantage of laparoscopic salpingostomy is that the operation is less invasive, thus recovery time is quicker and less painful as compared to a laparotomy; the average duration of recovery following laparoscopy is 2.4 weeks, compared to 4.6 weeks for laparotomy. An abdominal incision, on the other hand, allows the surgeon a better view of and easier access to the pelvic organs. Several studies have indicated a reduced rate of normal pregnancy after salpingostomy by laparoscopy versus laparotomy.

Diagnosis

It has been estimated that 40%–50% of ectopic pregnancies are incorrectly diagnosed when first presenting to emergency room medical personnel. Often the symptoms of ectopic pregnancy are confused with other conditions such as miscarriage or pelvic inflammatory disease. Diagnosis is usually based on presentation of symptoms, a positive pregnancy test, and detection of a pregnancy outside of the uterus by means of ultrasonography (using a machine that transmits high frequency sound waves to visualize structures in the body).

Diagnosis of hydrosalpinx or other defects of the fallopian tubes may be done surgically, using a laparoscope to visualize the fallopian tubes. Alternatively, a hysterosalpingogram may be performed, in which the uterus is filled with a dye and an x-ray is taken to see if the dye flows through the fallopian tubes.

Aftercare

If performed through an abdominal incision, a salpingostomy requires three to six weeks for full recovery. If salpingostomy is performed laparoscopically, the recovery time can be much shorter (an average

QUESTIONS TO ASK YOUR DOCTOR

- Why is a salpingostomy being recommended?
- How will the procedure be performed?
- If an ectopic pregnancy is suspected, how will the diagnosis be confirmed?
- What alternatives to salpingostomy are available to me?

of 2.4 weeks). There may be some discomfort around the incision for the first few days after surgery, but most women are walking by the third day. Within a month or so, patients can gradually resume normal activities such as driving, exercising, and working.

Risks

Complications associated with the surgical procedure include reaction to anesthesia, excessive bleeding, injury to other organs, and infection. With an ectopic pregnancy, there is a chance that not all of the products of conception will be removed and that the persistent tissue will continue growing. If this is the case, further treatment will be necessary.

Results

In the case of ectopic pregnancy, the products of conception will be removed without significantly impairing fertility. If salpingostomy is being performed to restore fertility, the procedure will increase a woman's chance of conceiving without resorting to artificial reproductive techniques.

Morbidity and mortality rates

Abdominal pain occurs in 97% of women with an ectopic pregnancy, vaginal bleeding in 79%, abdominal tenderness in 91%, and infertility in 15%. Persistent ectopic pregnancy after surgical treatment occurs in 5%–10% of cases. Ectopic pregnancy accounts for 10%–15% of all maternal deaths; the mortality rate for ectopic pregnancy is approximately one in 2,500 cases.

Alternatives

Some ectopic pregnancies may be managed expectantly (allowing the pregnancy to progress to see if it will resolve on its own). This may occur in up to 25% of ectopic pregnancies. There is, of course, a chance that the fallopian tube will rupture during the period of observation. Treatment with methotrexate is gaining popularity and has been shown to have success rates similar to laparoscopic salpingostomy if multiple doses are given and the patient is in stable condition. Salpingectomy is another surgical option and is indicated if a tube has ruptured or is seriously damaged.

Health care team roles

Salpingostomies are usually performed in a hospital **operating room** by a surgeon or gynecologist, a medical doctor who has completed specialized training in the areas of women's general health, pregnancy, labor and childbirth, **prenatal testing**, and genetics.

Resources

PERIODICALS

Beall, Stephanie, and Alan H. DeCherney. "Management of Tubal Ectopic Pregnancy: Methotrexate and Salpingostomy Are Preferred to Preserve Fertility." *Fertility and Sterility* 98, no. 5 (2012): 1118–20. http://dx.doi.org/10.1016/j.fertnstert.2012.07.1115 (accessed October 4, 2013).

Rabischong, Benoit, et al. "Predicting Success of Laparoscopic Salpingostomy for Ectopic Pregnancy." *Obstetrics & Gynecology* 116, no. 3 (2010): 701–7. http://dx.doi.org/10.1097/AOG.0b013e3181eeb80f (accessed October 4, 2013).

WEBSITES

American Pregnancy Association. "Ectopic Pregnancy." http://americanpregnancy.org/pregnancycomplications/ectopic-pregnancy.html (accessed October 4, 2013).

Harvard Medical School. "Hysterosalpingogram." http://www.health.harvard.edu/diagnostic-tests/hysterosalpingogram.htm (accessed October 4, 2013).

ORGANIZATIONS

American Congress of Obstetricians and Gynecologists, 409 12th St. SW, Washington, DC 20024-2188, (202) 638-5577, (800) 673-8444, resources@acog.org, http://www.acog.org.

American Pregnancy Association, 1425 Greenway Dr., Ste. 440, Irving, TX 75038, questions@americanpregnancy.org, http://americanpregnancy.org.

Stephanie Dionne Sherk

Saphenous vein bypass *see* **Peripheral vascular bypass surgery**

Scar revision surgery

Definition

Scar revision surgery refers to a group of procedures that are done to partially remove scar tissue following surgery or injury, or to make the scar(s) less noticeable. The specific procedure that is performed depends on the type of scar; its cause, location, and size; and the characteristics of the patient's skin.

Purpose

Scar revision surgery is performed to improve the appearance of the patient's face or other body part, but it is also done to restore or improve functioning when the formation of a scar interferes with the movement of muscles and joints. The shortening or tightening of the skin and underlying muscles that may accompany scar formation is known as contracture. Contractures may interfere with range of motion and other aspects of joint functioning, as well as deform the shape of the hand or other body part. Contractures in the face often affect the muscles that control facial expressions.

Scar revision surgery may be considered as either a cosmetic procedure or a **reconstructive surgery**, depending on whether the patient's concern is primarily related to appearance or whether contractures have also affected functioning. Some insurance companies will cover the cost of scar revision surgery if the scarring resulted from injury. Patients who are considering scar revision surgery should consult their insurance carriers to learn whether their condition may be covered. According to the American Academy of Facial Plastic and Reconstructive Surgery (AAFPRS), the average cost for scar revision surgery on the face is $1,135, compared to $1,376 for **dermabrasion**, $149 for microdermabrasion, and $2,484 for **laser skin resurfacing**.

Demographics

The demographics of scar revision are difficult to establish precisely because of the number of different procedures that are grouped under this heading and the different types of scars that they are intended to treat. In addition, although dermabrasion and laser resurfacing of the skin are often described as surgical methods of scar treatment to distinguish them from medical modalities, they are usually listed separately in statistical tables. According to the American Society of Plastic Surgeons, in 2012 the number of procedures, by type, were as follows: 171,000 for scar revision, 72,805 for dermabrasion, 509,055 for laser skin resurfacing, and 973,556 for microdermabrasion.

The female to male ratio for scar revision surgery is about four to three, whereas women are almost five times as likely as men to have laser skin resurfacing and almost 13 times as likely to have a microdermabrasion procedure. Most patients who have scar revision surgery are between 15 and 39, although a significant number choose to undergo this type of surgery in their 40s and 50s.

It is difficult to compare scar revision surgery with other treatments across ethnic and racial groups because skin color is a factor in the effectiveness of some forms of therapy. In addition, some types of scars—particularly keloids—are more likely to form in darker skin. On the whole, it is estimated that between 4.5% and 16% of the United States population is affected by keloids and hypertrophic scars. These are the most difficult scars to treat, and are discussed in further detail below.

Description

Scar formation

A description of the process of scar formation may be helpful in understanding scar revision surgery and other procedures intended to improve the appearance of scarred skin. There are three phases in the formation of a scar:

• Inflammation. This phase begins right after the injury and lasts until the wound is closed. It is the body's way of preventing infection, because a wound is not sterile until it is covered by a new outer layer of skin.

• Transitional repair. Scar tissue is formed during this phase to hold the wound together. The length of this phase depends on the severity of the injury.

• Maturation. This phase usually begins about 7 to 12 weeks after the injury occurs. It is also the phase in which problem scars appear. Under normal conditions, a repair process takes place in which the development of new skin is combined with breaking down the scar tissue that was formed in the second phase of healing. A problem scar is likely to develop when the repair process is interrupted or disturbed.

Causes and types of problem scars

Problem scars may result from inflammatory diseases, particularly acne; trauma, including cuts and burns; previous surgery; and a genetic predisposition for the skin to overreact to injury. Tension on the skin around the wound, foreign material in the wound, infection, or anything that delays closure of the wound may also contribute to scar formation.

The most difficult types of scars to treat are characterized by overproduction of collagen, which is the extracellular protein found in connective tissue that gives it strength and flexibility. The two types of scars that are most often considered for treatment are keloids and hypertrophic scars. Keloids are shiny, smooth benign tumors that arise in areas of damaged skin and look like irregular growths in the wound area. Hypertrophic scars, on the other hand, are thick, ropy-textured scars that are often associated with contractures.

Keloids can be distinguished from hypertrophic scars by the following characteristics:

• Timing. Hypertrophic scars usually begin to form within weeks of the injury, whereas keloids may not appear until a year later.

• Growth pattern. Hypertrophic scars do not continue to grow after they form, and remain within the original area of injury. Keloids continue to grow and spread outward into normal tissue.

• Role of genetic factors. Keloids tend to run in families, whereas hypertrophic scars do not.

• Racial and age distribution. Keloids occur more frequently in persons with darker skin than in fair-skinned persons. They are also more likely to develop during adolescence and pregnancy, which are periods of high hormone production.

• Recurrence. Hypertrophic scars may fade with time and do not recur. Keloids, on the other hand, may recur even after surgical removal.

• Collagen structure. The collagen fibers in a hypertrophic scar are shorter and generally arranged in a wavelike pattern, whereas the collagen fibers in keloids tend to be randomly arranged.

Surgical approaches to scar revision

The treatment of scars is highly individualized. Most plastic surgeons use a variety of nonsurgical and surgical approaches to improve the appearance of scars. In addition, patients might need several different surgical procedures if their scar revisions require a series of operations at different stages of the healing process.

SURGICAL EXCISION. Surgical excision is a procedure in which the surgeon shaves down and cuts out scar tissue to reduce the size of the scar. This technique is most commonly used on large scars that cannot be treated adequately with medications or other nonsurgical means. When excision is done in stages, it is referred to as "serial excision." This is performed if the area of the scar is too large to remove at one time without distorting nearby skin.

FLAPS, GRAFTS, AND ARTIFICIAL SKIN. Flaps, grafts, and artificial skin are used to treat contractures and large areas of scarring resulting from burns and other traumatic injuries. When there is not enough skin at the site of the injury to cover an incision made to remove scar tissue, the surgeon implants a skin graft or flap after cutting out the scar tissue itself. Skin grafts are thin layers of skin that are removed from another part of the patient's body and carefully matched to the color and texture of the face or other area where the graft is to be placed. A skin flap is a full-thickness piece of tissue with its own blood supply that is taken from a site as close as possible to the scarred area.

Dermal regeneration templates, often called "artificial skin," are used to treat people with contracture scars or severe burns. These devices were approved by the U.S. Food and Drug Administration (FDA) in April 2002. The templates are made of two layers of material, a bottom layer composed of collagen derived from cows and a top layer made of silicone. To use the artificial skin, the surgeon first removes all the burned skin or scar tissue from the patient's wound. The collagen layer, which is eventually absorbed, allows the patient's body to start growing new skin while the silicone layer closes and protects the wound. After 14–21 days, the silicone layer can be removed and a very thin graft of the patient's own skin is applied to the surface of the wound. The advantages of using a dermal regeneration template are that it lowers the risk of infection and minimizes the amount of tissue that must be removed from the patient's other body sites.

Z-PLASTY AND W-PLASTY. Z-plasty and W-plasty are surgical techniques used to treat contractures and to minimize the visibility of scars by repositioning them along the natural lines and creases in the patient's skin. They are not usually used to treat keloids or hypertrophic scars. In Z-plasty, the surgeon makes a Z-shaped incision with the middle line of the Z running along the scar tissue. The flaps of skin formed by the other lines of the Z are rotated and sewn into a new position that reorients the scar about 90 degrees. In effect, the Z-plasty minimizes the appearance of the scar by breaking up the straight line of the scar into smaller units.

A W-plasty is similar to a Z-plasty in that the goal of the procedure is to minimize the visibility of a scar by turning a straight line into an irregular one. The surgeon makes a series of short incisions to form a zigzag pattern to replace the straight line of the scar. The primary difference between a Z-plasty and a W-plasty is that a W-plasty does not involve the formation and repositioning of skin flaps. A variation on the W-plasty is known as the geometric broken line closure, or GBLC.

LASER SKIN RESURFACING AND DERMABRASION. Skin resurfacing and dermabrasion are techniques used to treat acne scars or to smooth down scars with raised or uneven surfaces. They are known as ablative skin treatments because they remove the top layer of skin, or the epidermis. In dermabrasion, the surgeon moves an instrument with a high-speed rotating wheel over the scar tissue and surrounding skin several times in order to smooth the skin surface down to the lowest level of scarring. Laser skin resurfacing involves the use of a carbon dioxide or Er:YAG laser to evaporate the top layer of skin and tighten the underlying layer. Keloid or hypertrophic scars are treated with a pulsed dye laser. Dermabrasion or laser resurfacing can be used about five weeks after a scar excision to make the remaining scar less noticeable.

Laser skin resurfacing, however, is less popular than it was in the late 1990s because of increasing awareness of its potential complications. The skin of patients who have undergone laser skin resurfacing takes several months to heal, often with considerable discomfort as well as swelling and reddish discoloration of the skin. In addition, there is a 33%–85% chance that changes in the color of the skin will be permanent; the risk of permanent discoloration is higher for patients with darker skin. Some plastic surgeons are recommending laser resurfacing only for patients with deep wrinkles or extensive sun damage who are willing to accept the pain and permanent change in skin color.

Preparation

Preparation for scar revision surgery includes the surgeon's assessment of the patient's psychological stability as well as the type and extent of potential scar tissue. Many patients respond to scarring following trauma with intense anger, particularly if the face is disfigured or their livelihood is related to their appearance. Some people are impatient to have the scars treated as quickly as possible, and may have the idea that revision surgery will restore their skin to its original condition. During the initial interview, the surgeon must explain that scar revision may take months or years to complete; that some techniques essentially replace one scar with another, rather than remove all scar tissue; and that it is difficult to predict the final results in advance. Most plastic surgeons recommend waiting at least six months, preferably a full year, for a new scar to complete the maturation phase of development. Many scars will begin to fade during this period of time, and others may respond to more conservative forms of treatment.

Good candidates for scar revision surgery are people who have a realistic understanding of its risks as well as its benefits, and equally realistic expectations of its potential outcomes. On the other hand, the following are considered psychological warning signs:

• The patient is considering scar revision surgery to please someone else—most often a spouse or partner.

• The patient has a history of multiple cosmetic procedures and/or complaints about previous surgeons.

• The patient has an unrealistic notion of what scar revision surgery will accomplish.

• The patient seems otherwise emotionally unstable.

In addition to discussing the timing and nature of treatments, the surgeon will take a careful medical history, noting whether the patient is a heavy smoker or has a family history of keloids, as well as other disorders that may influence the healing of scar tissue. These disorders include diabetes, lupus, scleroderma, and other disorders that compromise the body's immune system.

Aftercare

Aftercare following Z-plasty or surgical removal of a scar is relatively uncomplicated. The patient is given pain medication, told to rest for a day or two at home, and advised to avoid any activities that might put tension or pressure on the new incision(s). Most patients can return to work on the third day after surgery. The most important aspect of long-term aftercare is protecting the affected area from the sun because the surgical scar will take about a year to mature and is only about 80% as strong as undamaged skin. Sunlight can cause burns, permanent redness, loss of pigment in the skin, and breakdown of the collagen that maintains the elasticity of the skin.

Aftercare following the use of skin grafts, flaps, or dermal regeneration templates begins in the hospital with standard postoperative patient care. If sutures have been used, they are usually removed three to four days after surgery on the face and five to seven days after surgery for incisions elsewhere on the body. Patients are usually asked to return to the hospital at regular intervals so that the graft sites can be monitored. If artificial skin has been used, the patients must keep the site absolutely dry, which may require special precautions or restrictions on bathing or showering.

Aftercare for some patients includes going to psychotherapy or joining a support group to deal with emotions related to disfigurement and scar treatment.

Risks

Scar revision surgery carries the same risks as other surgical procedures under anesthesia, such as bleeding, infection at the incision site, and an adverse reaction to the anesthetic. The chief risk specific to this type of surgery is that the scar may grow, change color, or otherwise become more noticeable. Some plastic surgeons use the "90–10 rule," which means that there is a 90% chance that the scar will look better after surgery; a 9% chance that it will look about the same; and a 1% chance that it will look significantly worse.

Results

Normal results of scar revision surgery and associated nonsurgical treatments are a less noticeable scar.

Morbidity and mortality rates

Mortality rates for scar revision surgery are very low. Rates of complications depend on the specific technique that was used, the condition of the patient's general health, and genetic factors affecting the condition of the patient's skin.

Alternatives

There are a number of nonsurgical treatments that can be used before, after, or in place of scar revision surgery.

Drugs

Medications may be used during the initial inflammatory phase of scar formation, as well as during therapy for such specific skin disorders as acne. Keloids are often treated by direct injections of **corticosteroids** to reduce itching, redness, and burning; steroid treatment may also cause the keloid to shrink. Corticosteroid injections, gels, or tapes impregnated with medication are also used after scar excisions and Z-plasty to prevent recurrence or formation of hypertrophic scars. Acne scars are treated with oral **antibiotics** or isotretinoin.

Massage, wraps, radiation, and nonablative treatments

The most conservative treatments of scar tissue include several techniques that help to minimize scar formation and improve the appearance of scars that exist already. The simplest approach is repeated massage of the scarred area with cocoa butter or vitamin E preparations. Burn scars are treated typically with the application of pressure **dressings**, which restrict movement of the affected area and provide insulation. Another technique that is often used is silicone gel sheeting. The

QUESTIONS TO ASK YOUR DOCTOR

- Am I a candidate for treatment by a nonsurgical method of scar revision?
- What treatment technique(s) would be best for my scar?
- How long should I wait before scar revision surgery?
- What are the risks of the specific procedures you are recommending in my case?

sheeting is applied to the scarred area, and remains for a minimum of 12 hours a day over a period of three to six months. It is effective in improving the appearance of keloids in about 85% of cases.

Keloids that do not respond to any other form of treatment may be treated with low-dose radiation therapy.

Nonablative treatments, which do not remove the epidermal layer of skin, include microdermabrasion and superficial chemical peels. Microdermabrasion, the use of which has increased widely since 2000, is a technique for smoothing the skin. During this procedure, the physician uses a handheld instrument that buffs the skin with aluminum oxide crystals; skin flakes are removed through a vacuum tube. Microdermabrasion does not remove deep wrinkles or extensive scar tissue, but can make scars somewhat less noticeable without the risk of serious side effects. Mild chemical peels, such as those made with alpha-hydroxy acid (AHA), are used sometimes to treat acne scars or uneven skin pigmentation resulting from other types of scar revision treatment.

Camouflage

Scars on the face and legs can often be covered with specially formulated cosmetics that even out the color of the surrounding skin and help to make the scar less noticeable. Some of these preparations are available in waterproof formulations for use during swimming and other athletic activities that cause perspiration.

Health care team roles

Scar revision surgery is a specialized procedure performed only by a qualified plastic surgeon. Plastic surgeons are physicians (with MD or DO [doctors of osteopathy]) who have completed three years of general **surgical training**, followed by two to three years of specialized training in **plastic surgery**.

Scar revision may be conducted either in a hospital or in an outpatient clinic that specializes in plastic surgery. Scar revision surgery that involves skin grafts and flaps, however, is usually done in a hospital as an inpatient procedure. Microdermabrasion, chemical peels, steroid injections, pressure wraps, and silicone treatments may be performed in the surgeon's office.

Resources

BOOKS

Canale, S. T., ed. *Campbell's Operative Orthopaedics*. 12th ed. St. Louis, MO: Mosby, 2012.

Flint, Paul F., et al. *Cumming's Otolaryngology: Head and Neck Surgery*. 5th ed. rev. Philadelphia: Mosby/Elsevier, 2010.

Wein, Alan J., et al. *Campbell-Walsh Urology*. 10th ed. Philadelphia: Saunders/Elsevier, 2012.

PERIODICALS

Watson, Deborah, and Marsha Sonia Reuther. "Scar Revision Techniques—Pearls and Pitfalls." *Facial Plastic Surgery* 28, no. 5 (2012): 487–91. http://dx.doi.org/10.1055/s-0032-1325642 (accessed October 1, 2013).

OTHER

American Society of Plastic Surgeons. *2012 Plastic Surgery Statistics Reports*. 2013. http://www.plasticsurgery.org/Documents/news-resources/statistics/2012-Plastic-Surgery-Statistics/full-plastic-surgery-statistics-report.pdf (accessed October 1, 2013).

WEBSITES

A.D.A.M. Medical Encyclopedia. "CO2 blood test." MedlinePlus. http://www.nlm.nih.gov/medlineplus/ency/article/002991.htm (accessed October 17, 2013).

American Academy of Facial Plastic and Reconstructive Surgery. "Facial Scar Revision." http://www.aafprs.org/patient/procedures/facial_scar.html (accessed October 17, 2013).

American Society of Plastic Surgeons. "Scar Revision." http://www.plasticsurgery.org/reconstructive-procedures/scar-revision.html (accessed October 17, 2013).

ORGANIZATIONS

American Academy of Facial Plastic and Reconstructive Surgery, 310 S. Henry St., Alexandria, VA 22314, (703) 299-9291, info@aafprs.org, http://www.aafprs.org.

American Burn Association, 311 S. Wacker Dr., Ste. 4150, Chicago, IL 60606, (312) 642-9260, Fax: (312) 642-9130, info@ameriburn.org, http://www.ameriburn.org.

American Society of Plastic Surgeons, 444 E. Algonquin Rd., Arlington Heights, IL 60005, http://www.plasticsurgery.org.

FACES: The National Craniofacial Association, PO Box 11082, Chattanooga, TN 37401, (800) 3-FACES-3 (332-2373), faces@faces-cranio.org, http://www.faces-cranio.org.

Rebecca Frey, PhD

Scleral buckling

Definition

Scleral buckling is a surgical procedure in which a piece of silicone plastic or sponge is sewn onto the sclera at the site of a retinal tear to push the sclera toward the retinal tear. The buckle holds the retina against the sclera until scarring seals the tear. It also prevents fluid leakage, which could cause further retinal detachment.

Purpose

Scleral buckling is used to reattach the retina if the break is very large or if the tear is in one location. It is also used to seal breaks in the retina.

Demographics

Retinal detachment occurs in 25,000 Americans each year. Patients suffering from retinal detachments are commonly nearsighted, have had eye surgery, experienced ocular trauma, or have a family history of retinal detachments. Retinal detachments also are common after cataract removal. White males are at a higher risk, as are people who are middle-aged or older. Patients who already have had a retinal detachment also have a greater chance for another detachment.

Some conditions, such as diabetes or Coats' disease in children, make people more susceptible to retinal detachments.

Description

Scleral buckling is performed in an **operating room** under general or local anesthetic. Immediately before the procedure, patients are given eye drops to dilate the pupil to allow better access to the eye. After the eye is numbed, the surgeon cuts the eye membrane, exposing the sclera. If bleeding or inflammation blocks the surgeon's view of the retinal detachment or hole, he or she may perform a vitrectomy before scleral buckling.

Vitrectomy is necessary only in cases in which the surgeon's view of the damage is hindered. The surgeon makes two incisions into the sclera, one for a light probe and the other for instruments to cut and aspirate. The surgeon uses a tiny, guillotine-like device to remove the vitreous, which he or she then replaces with saline. After the removal, the surgeon may inject air or gas to hold the retina in place.

After the surgeon is able to see the retina, he or she will perform one of two companion procedures:

• Laser photocoagulation is used when the retinal tear is small or the detachment is slight. The surgeon points the laser beam through a contact lens to burn the area around the retinal tear. The laser creates scar tissue that will seal the hole and prevent leakage. It requires no incision.

• Cryopexy involves the use of a freezing probe to freeze the outer surface of the eye over the tear or detachment. The inflammation caused by the freezing leads to scar formation that seals the hole and prevents leakage. Cryopexy is used for larger holes or detachments, and for areas that may be hard to reach with a laser.

After the surgeon has performed laser photocoagulation or cryopexy, he or she indents the affected area of the sclera with silicone. The silicone, either in the form of a sponge or buckle, closes the tear and reduces the eyeball's circumference. This reduction prevents further pulling and separation of the vitreous. Depending on the severity of the detachment or hole, a buckle may be placed around the entire eyeball.

When the buckle is in place, the surgeon may drain subretinal fluid that might interfere with the retina's reattachment. After the fluid is drained, the surgeon will suture the buckle into place and then cover it with the conjunctiva. The surgeon then inserts an antibiotic (drops or ointment) into the affected eye and patches it.

For less severe detachments, the surgeon may choose a temporary buckle that will be removed later. Usually, however, the buckle remains in place for the patient's lifetime. It does not interfere with vision. Scleral buckles in infants, however, will need to be removed as the eyeball grows.

Preparation

Retinal detachment is considered an emergency situation. In the case of acute onset detachment, the longer it takes to repair the detachment, the less chance of successful reattachment. Usually the patient sees floating spots and experiences peripheral visual field loss. Patients commonly describe the vision loss as having someone pull a shade over their eyes. In extreme cases, patients may lose vision completely.

An ophthalmologist or optometrist will take a complete medical history, including family history of retinal detachment and any recent ocular trauma. In addition to performing a general eye exam, which includes a slit lamp examination, examination of the macula, and lens evaluation, physicians may perform the following tests to determine the extent of retinal detachment:

• echography

• three-mirror contact lens/panfunduscopic

• scleral indentation

Scleral buckling

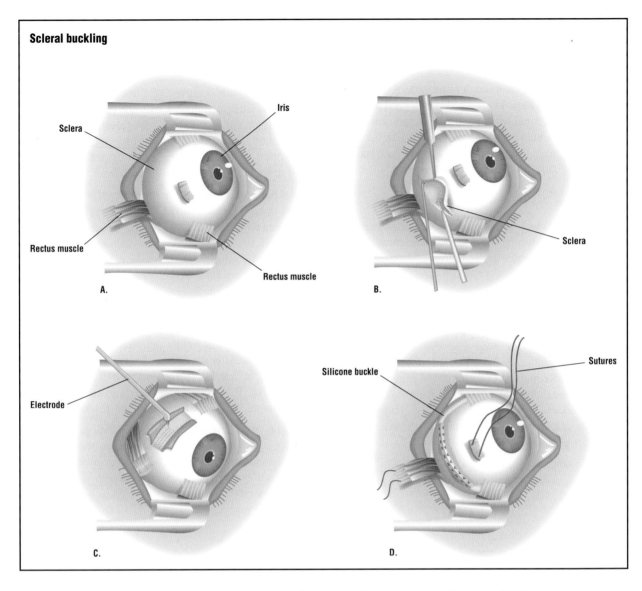

In a scleral buckling procedure, one of the eye's rectus muscles is severed to gain access to the sclera (A). The sclera is cut open (B), and an electrode is applied to the area of retinal detachment (C). A silicone buckle is threaded into place beneath the rectus muscles (D), and the severed muscle is repaired. *(Illustration by GGS Information Services. Copyright © Cengage Learning®.)*

Small breaks in the retina will not require surgery, but patients with acute onset detachment require reattachment in 24–48 hours. Chronic retinal detachments should be repaired within one week.

Because this is usually an emergency procedure, there is no long-term preparation. Patients are required to fast for at least six hours before surgery.

Aftercare

Immediately following the surgery, patients will need help with meals and walking. Some patients must remain hospitalized for several days. However, many scleral buckling procedures are performed on an outpatient basis.

After release from the hospital, patients should avoid heavy lifting or strenuous **exercise** that could increase intraocular pressure. Rapid eye movements should also be avoided; reading may be prohibited until the surgeon gives permission. Sunglasses should be worn during the day and an eye patch at night. Pain, redness, and a scratchy sensation in the eyes may also occur after surgery. Ice packs may be applied if the conjunctiva swells. Patients may take pain medication, but should check with their physician before taking any over-the-counter medication.

Excessive pain, swelling, bleeding, discharge from the eye, or decreased vision is not normal, and should immediately be reported to the physician.

If a vitrectomy was performed in conjunction with the scleral buckling, patients must sleep with their heads elevated. They also must avoid air travel until the air bubble is absorbed.

After scleral buckling, patients will use dilating, antibiotic, or corticosteroid eye drops for up to six weeks to decrease inflammation and the chance of infection. Best visual acuity cannot be determined for at least six to eight weeks after surgery. Driving may be prohibited or restricted while vision stabilizes. At the six-to-eight week postoperative visit, physicians determine if the patient needs corrective lenses or stronger prescription lenses. Full vision restoration depends on the location and severity of the detachment.

Risks

Complications are rare but may be severe. In some instances, patients lose sight in the affected eye or lose the entire eye.

Scar tissue, even pre-existing scar tissue, may interfere with the retina's reattachment and the scleral buckling procedure may have to be repeated. Scarring, along with infection, is the most common complication.

Other possible but infrequent complications include:

- bleeding under the retina
- cataract formation
- double vision
- glaucoma
- vitreous hemorrhage

Patients may also become more nearsighted after the procedure. In some instances, although the retina reattaches, vision is not restored.

Results

The National Institutes of Health reports that scleral buckling has a success rate of 85%–90%. Restored vision depends largely on the location and extent of the detachment, and the length of time before the detachment was repaired. Patients with a peripheral detachment have a quicker recovery then those patients whose detachment was located in the macula. The longer the patient waits to have the detachment repaired, the worse the prognosis.

Morbidity and mortality rates

The danger of mortality and loss of vision depends on the cause of the retinal detachment. Patients with Marfan syndrome, preeclampsia, and diabetes, for example, are more at risk during the scleral buckling procedure than a patient in relatively good health. The risk of surgery also rises with the use of **general anesthesia**. Scleral buckling, however, is considered a safe, successful procedure.

Severe infections that are left untreated can cause vision loss, but following the prescribed regimen of eye drops and follow-up treatment greatly minimizes this risk.

Alternatives

Vitrectomy is sometimes performed alone to treat retinal detachments. Laser photocoagulation and cryopexy also may be used to treat less serious tears. The more common alternative, however, is pneumatic retinopexy, which is used when the tear is located in the upper portion of the eye. The surgeon uses cryopexy to freeze the area around the tear, then removes a small amount of fluid. When the fluid is drained and the eye softened, the surgeon injects a gas bubble into the vitreous cavity. As the gas bubble expands, it seals the retinal tear by pushing the retina against the choroid. Eventually, the bubble will be absorbed.

The patient is required to remain in a certain position for at least a few days after surgery while the bubble helps seal the hole. Pneumatic retinopexy also is not as successful as scleral buckling. Complications include recurrent retinal detachments and the chance of gas getting under the retina.

Health care team roles

Scleral buckling can be performed by a general ophthalmologist, an MD who specializes in treatment of

Sclerostomy

QUESTIONS TO ASK YOUR
DOCTOR

- How many scleral buckling procedures have you performed?
- Could other treatments be an option?
- Will I have to stay in the hospital?
- Will my sight be completely restored?
- What is the probability of having another retinal detachment in the same eye?
- Am I likely to have a retinal detachment in my unaffected eye?

the eye. Even more specialized ophthalmologists, vitreoretinal **surgeons** who specialize in diseases of the retina, may be called upon for serious cases.

The surgery is usually performed in a hospital setting. Because of the delicacy of the procedure, sometimes an overnight hospital stay is required. Less severe retinal detachments can be treated on an outpatient basis at surgery centers.

Resources

BOOKS

Bhavsar, Abdhish R. *Retina and Vitreous Surgery*. Philadelphia: Saunders/Elsevier, 2009.

Brinton, Daniel A., and C. P. Wilkinson. *Retinal Detachment: Principles and Practices*. 3rd ed. New York: Oxford University, 2009.

PERIODICALS

Codenotti, Marco, et al. "Scleral Buckling Dislocation Mimicking Glaucoma Progression." *European Journal of Ophthalmology* 23, no. 2 (2013): 271–74. http://dx.doi.org/10.5301/ejo.5000165 (accessed October 4, 2013).

Dehghani, A., et al. "The Comparison of Retinal Blood Flow after Scleral Buckling Surgery with or without Encircling Procedure." *Journal of Research in Medical Sciences* 18, no. 3 (2013): 222–24.

Miura, Masahiro, et al. "Choroidal Thickness after Scleral Buckling." *Ophthalmology* 119, no. 7 (2012): 1497–98. http://dx.doi.org/10.1016/j.ophtha.2012.02.038 (accessed October 4, 2013).

WEBSITES

Golonka, Debby. "Scleral Buckling Surgery for Retinal Detachment." Bon Secours St. Francis Health System. http://www.stfrancishealth.org/health-library.html?documentID=hw187645 (accessed October 4, 2013).

National Eye Institute. "Facts About Retinal Detachment." http://www.nei.nih.gov/health/retinaldetach/retinaldetach.asp (accessed October 4, 2013).

ORGANIZATIONS

American Academy of Ophthalmology, 655 Beach St., San Francisco, CA 94109, (415) 561-8500, Fax: (415) 561-8533, http://www.aao.org.

American Board of Ophthalmology, 111 Presidential Blvd., Ste. 241, Bala Cynwyd, PA 19004-1075, (610) 664-1175, info@abop.org, http://abop.org.

National Eye Institute, NEI Information Office, 31 Center Dr., MSC 2510, Bethesda, MD 20892-2510, (301) 496-5248, 2020@nei.nih.gov, http://www.nei.nih.gov.

Mary Bekker

Sclerostomy

Definition

A sclerostomy is a procedure in which the surgeon makes a small opening in the outer covering of the eyeball to reduce intraocular pressure (IOP) in patients with open-angle glaucoma. It is classified as a type of glaucoma filtering surgery. The name of the surgery comes from the Greek word for "hard," which describes the tough white outer coat of the eyeball, and the Greek word for "cutting" or "incision."

Purpose

Sclerostomies are usually performed to reduce IOP in open-angle glaucoma patients who have not been helped by less invasive forms of treatment, specifically medications and **laser surgery**. In some cases—most commonly patients who are rapidly losing their vision or who cannot tolerate glaucoma medications—an ophthalmologist (eye specialist) may recommend a sclerostomy without trying other forms of treatment first.

Glaucoma is not considered a single disease but rather a group of diseases characterized by three major characteristics: elevated intraocular pressure (IOP) caused by an overproduction of aqueous humor in the eye or by resistance to the normal outflow of fluid; atrophy of the optic nerve; and a resultant loss of visual field. A sclerostomy works to reduce the IOP by improving the outflow of aqueous humor. Between 80% and 90% of aqueous humor leaves the eye through the trabecular meshwork while the remaining 10%–20% passes through the ciliary muscle bundles. A sclerostomy allows the fluid to collect under the conjunctiva, which is the thin membrane lining the eyelids, to form a filtration bleb.

1600

GALE ENCYCLOPEDIA OF SURGERY AND MEDICAL TESTS, 3ʳᴰ EDITION

Demographics

According to the National Eye Institute, approximately 2.7 million people in the United States have glaucoma. Primary open-angle glaucoma (POAG) accounts for the majority of cases. "Primary" means that the glaucoma is not associated with a tumor, injury to the eye, or other eye disorder.

Although glaucoma can occur at any age, it is most common in adults over 40 and in people with a familial history of the disease. People of African, Latino, or Asian descent are at higher risk for developing POAG.

With regard to race, African Americans are four times as likely to develop glaucoma as Caucasians, and six to eight times more likely to lose their sight to the disease. African Americans also develop glaucoma at earlier ages; while everyone over age 60 is at increased risk for POAG, the risk for African Americans rises sharply after age 40. A 2001 study reported that the rate for Mexican Americans lies between the rate of POAG in African Americans and that in Caucasians. Mexican Americans, however, are more likely to suffer from undiagnosed glaucoma—62% as compared to 50% for other races and ethnic groups in the United States. In addition, the rate of POAG in Mexican Americans was found to rise rapidly after age 65; in the older age groups, it approaches the rates reported for African Americans. Among Caucasians, people of Scandinavian, Irish, or Russian ancestry are at higher risk of glaucoma than people from other ethnic groups.

The question of a sex ratio in open-angle glaucoma is debated. Three studies done in the United States between 1991 and 1996 reported that the male to female ratio for open-angle glaucoma is about one to one. Three other studies carried out in the United States, Barbados, and the Netherlands, however, found that the male to female ratio was almost two to one. A 2002 study from western Africa reported a male to female ratio of 2.26 to one. It appears that further research is needed in this area.

Description

Most sclerostomies are performed as outpatient procedures under **local anesthesia**. In some cases the patient may be given an intravenous sedative to help him or her relax before the procedure.

Conventional sclerostomy

After the patient has been sedated, the surgeon injects a local anesthetic into the area around the eye as well as a medication to prevent eye movement. Using very small instruments with the help of a microscope, the surgeon makes a tiny hole in the sclera as a passageway for aqueous humor. Some **surgeons** use an Erbium YAG laser to create the hole. Most surgeons apply an antimetabolite drug during the procedure to minimize the risk that the new drainage channel will be closed by tissue regrowth. The most common antimetabolites that are used are mitomycin and 5-fluorouracil.

After the surgery, the aqueous humor begins to flow through the sclerostomy hole and forms a small blister-like structure on the upper surface of the eye. This structure is known as a bleb or filtration bleb, and is covered by the eyelid. The bleb allows the aqueous humor to leave the eye in a controlled fashion.

Enzymatic sclerostomy

A newer technique that was first described in 2002 is enzymatic sclerostomy, which was developed at the Weizmann Institute of Science in Israel. In enzymatic sclerostomy, the surgeon applies an enzyme called collagenase to the eye to increase the release of aqueous humor. The collagenase is applied through an applicator that is attached to the eye with tissue glue for 22–24 hours and then removed. According to the researchers, the procedure reduced the intraocular pressure in all patients immediately following the procedure and in 80% of the subjects at one-year follow-up. None of the patients developed systemic complications. However, enzymatic sclerostomy is still considered experimental.

Diagnosis

Open-angle glaucoma is not always diagnosed promptly because it is insidious in onset, which means that it develops slowly and gradually. Unlike closed-angle glaucoma, open-angle glaucoma rarely has early symptoms. It is usually diagnosed either in the course of an eye examination or because the patient has noticed that they are having problems with their peripheral vision—that is, they are having trouble seeing objects at the side or out of the corner of the eye. In some cases the patient notices that he or she is missing words while reading; having trouble seeing stairs or other objects at the bottom of the visual field; or having trouble seeing clearly when driving. Other symptoms of open-angle glaucoma may include headaches, seeing haloes around lights, or difficulty adjusting to darkness. It is important to diagnose open-angle glaucoma as soon as possible because the vision that has been already lost cannot be recovered. Although open-angle glaucoma cannot be cured, it can be stabilized and controlled in almost all patients. Because of the importance of catching open-angle glaucoma as early as possible, adults should have their eyes examined every two years at least.

KEY TERMS

Angle—The open point in the anterior chamber of the eye at which the iris meets the cornea.

Aqueous humor—The watery fluid produced in the eye that ordinarily leaves the eye through the angle of the anterior chamber and Schlemm's canal.

Atrophy—Wasting away or degeneration. Atrophy of the optic nerve is one of the defining characteristics of glaucoma.

Bleb—A thin-walled auxiliary drain created on the outside of the eyeball during filtering surgery for glaucoma. It is sometimes called a filtering bleb.

Conjunctiva—The thin membrane that lines the eyelids and covers the visible surface of the sclera.

Cornea—The transparent front portion of the exterior cover of the eye.

Endophthalmitis—An infection on the inside of the eye, which may result from an infected bleb. Endophthalmitis can result in vision loss.

Glaucoma—A group of eye disorders characterized by increased fluid pressure inside the eye that eventually damages the optic nerve. As the cells in the optic nerve die, the patient gradually loses vision.

Gonioscopy—A technique for examining the angle between the iris and the cornea with the use of a special mirrored lens applied to the cornea.

Hyphema—Blood inside the anterior chamber of the eye. Hyphema is one of the risks associated with sclerostomies.

Hypotony—Intraocular fluid pressure that is too low.

Insidious—Developing in a stealthy and inconspicuous way. Open-angle glaucoma is an insidious disorder.

Ocular hypertension—A condition in which fluid pressure inside the eye is higher than normal but the optic nerve and visual fields are normal.

Open-angle glaucoma—A form of glaucoma in which fluid pressure builds up inside the eye even though the angle of the anterior chamber is open and looks normal when the eye is examined with a gonioscope. Most cases of glaucoma are open-angle.

Ophthalmology—The branch of medicine that deals with the diagnosis and treatment of eye disorders.

Peripheral vision—The outer portion of the visual field.

Schlemm's canal—A circular channel located at the point where the sclera of the eye meets the cornea. Schlemm's canal is the primary pathway for aqueous humor to leave the eye.

Sclera—The tough white fibrous membrane that forms the outermost covering of the eyeball.

Tonometry—Measurement of the fluid pressure inside the eye.

Trabecular meshwork—The main drainage passageway for fluid to leave the anterior chamber of the eye.

Visual field—The total area in which a person can see objects within his or her peripheral vision while the eyes are focused on a central point.

High-risk groups

Not everyone is at equal risk for glaucoma. People with any of the risk factors listed below should consult their doctor for advice about the frequency of eye checkups:

• Age over 40 (African Americans) or over 60 (other races and ethnic groups).

• Ocular hypertension. The normal level of IOP is between 11 mm Hg and 21 mm Hg. It is possible for people to have an IOP above 21 mm Hg without signs of damage to the optic nerve or loss of visual field; this condition is referred to as ocular hypertension. Conversely, about one out of six of patients diagnosed with open-angle glaucoma have so-called normal-tension glaucoma, which means that their optic nerve

is being damaged even though their IOP is within the "normal" range. Ocular hypertension does, however, increase a person's risk of developing glaucoma in the future.

• Family history of glaucoma in a first-degree relative.

• An unusually thin cornea (the clear front portion of the outer cover of the eye). A recent National Eye Institute (NEI) study found that patients whose corneas are thinner than 555 microns are three times as likely to develop glaucoma as those whose corneas are thicker than 588 microns.

• Extreme nearsightedness. People who are very near-sighted are two to three times more likely to develop glaucoma than those who are not nearsighted.

• Diabetes.

• History of traumatic injury to the eye or surgery for other eye disorders.

• Use of steroid medications.

• Migraine headaches or sleep-related breathing disorder.

• Male sex.

Some patients should not be treated with filtration surgery. Contraindications for a sclerostomy include cardiovascular disorders and other severe systemic medical problems, eyes that are already blind, or the presence of an intraocular tumor or bleeding in the eye.

Diagnostic tests

Ophthalmologists use the following tests to screen patients for open-angle glaucoma:

• Tonometry. Tonometry is a painless procedure for measuring IOP. One type of tonometer blows a puff of pressurized air toward the patient's eye as the patient sits near a lamp; it measures the changes in the light reflections on the patient's corneas. Another method of tonometry involves the application of a local anesthetic to the outside of the eye and touching the cornea briefly with an instrument that measures the fluid pressure directly.

• Visual field test. This test measures loss of peripheral vision. In the simplest version of this test, the patient sits directly in front of the examiner with one eye covered. The patient looks at the examiner's eye and indicates when he or she can see the examiner's hand. In the automated version, the patient sits in front of a hollow dome and looks at a central target inside the dome. A computer program flashes lights at intervals at different locations inside the dome, and the patient presses a button whenever he or she sees a light. At the end of the test, the computer prints an assessment of the patient's responses.

• Gonioscopy. Gonioscopy measures the size of the angle in the anterior chamber of the eye with the use of a special mirrored contact lens. The examiner numbs the outside of the eye with a local anesthetic and touches the outside of the cornea with the gonioscopic lens. He or she can use a slit lamp to magnify what appears on the lens. Gonioscopy is necessary in order to distinguish between open- and closed-angle glaucoma; it can also distinguish between primary and many secondary glaucomas.

• Ophthalmoscopic examination of the optic nerve. An ophthalmoscope is an instrument that contains a perforated mirror as well as magnifying lenses. It allows the examiner to view the interior of the eye. If the patient has open-angle glaucoma, the examiner can see a cup-shaped depression in the optic disk.

Newer diagnostic devices include a laser-scanning microscope known as the Heidelberg retinal tomograph (HRT) and **ultrasound** biomicroscopy (UBM). UBM has proved to be a useful method of long-term follow-up of sclerostomies.

Preparation

Preparation for a sclerostomy begins with the patient's decision to undergo incisional surgery rather than continuing to take medications or having repeated laser procedures. Three factors commonly influence the decision: the present extent of the patient's visual loss, the speed of visual deterioration, and the patient's life expectancy.

With regard to the procedure itself, patients may be asked to take oral antibiotic and anti-inflammatory medications for several days prior to surgery.

Aftercare

Patients can use their eyes after filtering surgery, although they should have a friend or relative to drive them home after the procedure. They can go to work the next day, although they will probably notice some blurring of vision in the operated eye for about a month. Patients can carry out their normal activities with the exception of heavy lifting, although they should not drive until their vision has completely cleared. Most ophthalmologists recommend that patients wear their eyeglasses during the day and tape an eye shield over the operated eye at night. They should apply eye drops prescribed by the ophthalmologist to prevent infection, manage pain, and reduce swelling. They should also avoid rubbing, bumping, or getting water into the operated eye. Complete recovery after filtering surgery usually takes about six weeks. Long-term aftercare includes avoiding damage to or infection of the bleb.

It is important for patients recovering from filtering surgery to see their doctor for frequent checkups in the first few weeks following surgery. In most cases the ophthalmologist will check the patient's eye the day after surgery and about once a week for the next several weeks.

Risks

The risks of a sclerostomy include the following:

• Infection. Infections may develop in the bleb (blebitis), but may spread to the interior of the eye (endophthalmitis). The symptoms of an infection include pain and redness in the eye, blurred vision, teariness, and a discharge. Infections must be treated promptly, as they can lead to loss of vision.

- Hyphema. Hyphema refers to the presence of blood inside the anterior chamber of the eye. Hyphemas are most common within the first two to three days after surgery and are usually treated with corticosteroid medications to reduce inflammation.

- Suprachoroidal hemorrhage. A suprachoroidal hemorrhage, or massive bleeding behind the retina, is a serious complication that can occur during as well as after eye surgery.

- Cataract formation.

- Hypotony (low IOP). If hypotony is not corrected, it can lead to failure of the bleb and eventual cataract formation.

- Loss of central vision. This is a very rare complication.

- Bleb leak or failure. Blebs can develop leaks at any time, from several days after surgery to years later. Bleb failure usually results from inadequate control of the intraocular pressure and a new obstruction of aqueous humor outflow.

- Closing of the opening in the sclera by new tissue growth. A sclerostomy can be repeated if necessary.

Results

According to the National Eye Institute, sclerostomy is 80%–90% effective in lowering intraocular pressure. The success rate is highest in patients who have not had previous eye surgery.

Morbidity and mortality rates

Mortality following a sclerostomy is very low because the majority of procedures are performed under local anesthesia. The most common complications of filtering surgery are cataract formation (30% of patients develop cataracts within five years of a sclerostomy) and closure of the drainage opening requiring additional surgery (10%–15% of patients). Bleeding or infection occur in less than 1% of patients.

Alternatives

There are two surgical alternatives to sclerostomy that are called nonpenetrating deep sclerectomies because they do not involve entering the anterior chamber of the eye. The first alternative, viscocanalostomy, is a procedure that involves creating a window in Descemet's membrane (a layer of tissue in the cornea) to allow aqueous humor to leave the anterior chamber and injecting a viscoelastic substance into Schlemm's canal, which is the main pathway for aqueous humor to leave the eye. The viscoelastic helps to keep the canal from scarring shut following surgery.

The second type of nonpenetrating surgery involves implanting a device called the Aquaflow® collagen wick about 0.8 in. (2 cm) long under the sclera. The wick keeps open a space created by the surgeon to allow drainage of the aqueous humor. The wick is made of a material that is absorbed by the body within six to nine months, but the drainage pathway remains open after the wick is absorbed. The Aquaflow® wick was approved by the U.S. Food and Drug Administration (FDA) in July 2001.

Both types of nonpenetrating deep sclerectomies allow patients to recover faster, with fewer complications than traditional sclerostomies. Their drawbacks include a lower success rate and the need for additional procedures to control the patient's IOP. Viscocanalostomy in particular is not as effective in reducing IOP levels as traditional filtering surgery.

Complementary and alternative (CAM) approaches

Bilberry (European blueberry) extract has been recommended for improving night vision; it was given to pilots during World War II for this reason. There is evidence that 80–160 mg of bilberry extract taken three times a day does improve night vision temporarily. The plant does not have any serious side effects, but it should not be used in place of regular eye examinations or other treatments for glaucoma.

People who support the medicinal use of marijuana have argued that cannabinoids, the active chemical compounds found in the plant, lower intraocular pressure in patients with glaucoma. According to the Glaucoma Research Foundation, however, very high doses of marijuana are required to produce any significant effect on IOP. A Canadian researcher has concluded that the effects of cannabinoids on IOP "are not sufficiently strong, long lasting, or reliable to provide a valid basis for therapeutic use [of marijuana]."

Health care team roles

Sclerostomies are performed by ophthalmologists, who are physicians who have completed four to five years of specialized training following medical school in the medical and surgical treatment of eye disorders. Ophthalmology is one of 24 specialties recognized by the American Board of Medical Specialties.

Sclerostomies are usually done as outpatient procedures, either in the ophthalmologist's office or in an ambulatory surgery center; however, they may also be performed in a hospital with sedation as well as local anesthesia.

QUESTIONS TO ASK YOUR DOCTOR

- How many sclerostomies have you performed?
- Do you prefer using miniature instruments or a laser, and why?
- What are my chances of developing a cataract if I have this procedure?
- Would you recommend nonpenetrating surgery? Why or why not?

Resources

BOOKS

Yanoff, Myron, and Jay S. Duker. *Ophthalmology*. St. Louis, MO: Mosby/Elsevier, 2009.

PERIODICALS

Tse, Kwong Ming, et al. "Do Shapes and Dimensions of Scleral Flap and Sclerostomy Influence Aqueous Outflow in Trabeculectomy? A Finite Element Simulation Approach." *British Journal of Ophthalmology* 96, no. 3 (2012): 432–37. http://dx.doi.org/10.1136/bjophthalmol-2011-300228 (accessed October 4, 2013).

OTHER

John M. Eisenberg Center for Clinical Decisions and Communications Science, Baylor College of Medicine. *Treatments for Open-Angle Glaucoma: A Review of the Research for Adults.* Pub. No. 12(13)-EHC038-A. Rockville, MD: Agency for Healthcare Research and Quality, 2013. http://www.ncbi.nlm.nih.gov/pubmedhealth/PMH0054461/pdf/consglau.pdf (accessed October 4, 2013).

WEBSITES

A.D.A.M. Medical Encyclopedia. "Glaucoma." MedlinePlus. http://www.nlm.nih.gov/medlineplus/ency/article/001620.htm (accessed October 4, 2013).
The Glaucoma Foundation. "Primary Open-Angle Glaucoma (POAG)." http://glaucomafoundation.org/Primary_Open-Angle_Glaucoma.htm (accessed October 4, 2013).
The Glaucoma Foundation. "Who's at Risk?" http://glaucomafoundation.org/Risk.htm (accessed October 4, 2013).
Glaucoma Research Foundation. "Symptoms of Open-Angle Glaucoma." http://glaucoma.org/glaucoma/symptoms-of-primary-open-angle-glaucoma.php (accessed October 4, 2013).
National Eye Institute. "Facts About Glaucoma." http://glaucoma.org/glaucoma/symptoms-of-primary-open-angle-glaucoma.php (accessed October 4, 2013).
National Eye Institute. "Statistics and Data: Glaucoma, Open-Angle." http://www.nei.nih.gov/eyedata/glaucoma.asp (accessed October 4, 2013).

ORGANIZATIONS

American Academy of Ophthalmology, 655 Beach St., San Francisco, CA 94109, (415) 561-8500, Fax: (415) 561-8533, http://www.aao.org.
American Optometric Association, 243 N. Lindbergh Blvd., St. Louis, MO 63141, (800) 365-2219, http://www.aoa.org.
Canadian Ophthalmological Society, 610-1525 Carling Ave., Ottawa, Ontario, Canada K1Z 8R9, (613) 729-6779, cos@eyesite.ca, http://www.eyesite.ca.
The Glaucoma Foundation, 80 Maiden Ln., Ste. 700, New York, NY 10038, (212) 285-0080, info@glaucomafoundation.org, http://www.glaucomafoundation.org.
Glaucoma Research Foundation, 251 Post St., Ste. 600, San Francisco, CA 94108, (415) 986-3162, grf@glaucoma.org, http://glaucoma.org.
National Eye Institute, NEI Information Office, 31 Center Dr., MSC 2510, Bethesda, MD 20892-2510, (301) 496-5248, 2020@nei.nih.gov, http://www.nei.nih.gov.
Prevent Blindness America, 211 West Wacker Dr., Ste. 1700, Chicago, IL 60606, (800) 331-2020, http://www.preventblindness.org.
Wills Eye Institute, 840 Walnut St., Philadelphia, PA 19107, (877) AT-WILLS (289-4557), http://www.willseye.org.

Rebecca Frey, PhD

Sclerotherapy for esophageal varices

Definition

Sclerotherapy for esophageal varices, also called endoscopic sclerotherapy, is a treatment for esophageal bleeding that involves the use of an endoscope and the injection of a sclerosing solution into veins.

Purpose

Esophageal varices are enlarged or swollen veins on the lining of the esophagus that are prone to bleeding. They are life-threatening; each episode of bleeding carries a 20%–30% risk of death. 70% of patients who do not receive treatment for their varices die of bleeding within a year of their first episode of bleeding. Esophageal varices are a complication of portal hypertension, a condition characterized by increased blood pressure in the portal vein resulting from liver disease, such as cirrhosis. Increased pressure causes the veins to balloon outward. The vessels may rupture, causing vomiting of blood and bloody stools.

In most hospitals, sclerotherapy for esophageal varices is the treatment of choice to stop esophageal

KEY TERMS

Cirrhosis—A chronic degenerative liver disease causing irreversible scarring of the liver.

Endoscope—An instrument used to examine the inside of a canal or hollow organ. Endoscopic surgery is less invasive than traditional surgery.

Esophagus—The part of the digestive canal located between the pharynx (part of the digestive tube) and the stomach. Also called the food pipe.

Portal hypertension—Abnormally high pressure within the veins draining into the liver.

Sclerosant—An irritating solution that stops bleeding by hardening the blood or vein it is injected into.

Varices—Swollen or enlarged veins, in this case on the lining of the esophagus.

bleeding during acute episodes, and to prevent further incidences of bleeding. Emergency sclerotherapy is often followed by preventive treatments to eradicate distended esophageal veins.

Demographics

Bleeding esophageal varices are a serious complication of liver disease. In the United States, at least 50% of people who survive bleeding esophageal varices are at risk of recurrent bleeding during the next one to two years.

Description

Sclerotherapy for esophageal varices involves injecting a strong and irritating solution (a sclerosant) into the veins and/or the area beside the distended vein. Sclerosant injected directly into the vein causes blood clots to form and stops the bleeding, while sclerosant injected into the area beside the distended vein stops the bleeding by thickening and swelling the vein to compress the blood vessel. Most physicians inject the sclerosant directly into the vein, although injections into the vein and the surrounding area are both effective. Once bleeding has been stopped, the treatment can be used to significantly reduce or destroy the varices.

Sclerotherapy for esophageal varices is performed with the patient awake but sedated. Hyoscine butylbromide (Buscopan) may be administered to freeze the esophagus, making injection of the sclerosant easier. During the procedure, an endoscope is passed through the patient's mouth to the esophagus to allow the surgeon to view the inside. The branches of the blood vessels at or just above where the stomach and esophagus come together, the usual site of variceal bleeding, are located. After the bleeding vein is identified, a long, flexible sclerotherapy needle is passed through the endoscope. When the tip of the needle's sheath is in place, the needle is advanced, and the sclerosant is injected into the vein or the surrounding area. The most commonly used sclerosants are ethanolamine and sodium tetradecyl sulfate. The needle is withdrawn. The procedure is repeated as many times as necessary to eradicate all distended veins.

Preparation

A radiologist assesses patients for sclerotherapy based on blood work and liver imaging studies performed using CT scans, **ultrasound**, or MRI scans, and in consultation with the treating gastroenterologist, hepatologist, or surgeon. Tests to localize bleeding and detect active bleeding are also performed.

Before a sclerotherapy procedure, the patient's **vital signs** and other pertinent data are recorded, an intravenous line is inserted to administer fluid or blood, and a sedative is prescribed.

Aftercare

After sclerotherapy for esophageal varices, the patient will be observed for signs of blood loss, lung complications, fever, a perforated esophagus, or other complications. Vital signs are monitored, and the intravenous line maintained. Pain medication is usually prescribed. After leaving the hospital, the patient follows a diet prescribed by the physician, and, if appropriate, can take mild pain relievers.

Risks

Risks associated with sclerotherapy include complications that can arise from use of the sclerosant or from the endoscopic procedure. Minor complications, which cause discomfort but do not require active treatment or prolonged hospitalization, include transient chest pain, difficulty swallowing, and fever, which usually go away after a few days. Some patients may have allergic reactions to the sclerosant solution. Infection occurs in up to 50% of cases. In 2%–10% of patients, the esophagus tightens, but this can usually be treated with dilatation. More serious complications may occur in 10%–15% of patients. These include perforation or bleeding of the esophagus and lung problems, such as aspiration pneumonia. Long-term sclerotherapy can also damage the esophagus, and increase the patient's risk of developing cancer.

Patients with advanced liver disease complicated by bleeding are at very high risk for experiencing complications with this procedure. The surgery, premedications, and anesthesia may be sufficient to tip the patient into protein intoxication and hepatic coma. The blood in the bowels acts like a high-protein meal and may induce protein intoxication.

Results

Normal sclerotherapy results include the control of acute bleeding if present and the shrinking of the esophageal varices.

Morbidity and mortality rates

Sclerotherapy for esophageal varices has a 20%–40% incidence of complications and a 1%–2% mortality rate. The procedure controls acute bleeding in about 90% of patients, but it may have to be repeated within the first 48 hours to achieve this success rate. During the initial hospitalization, sclerotherapy is usually performed two or three times. Preventive treatments are scheduled every few weeks or so, depending on the patient's risk level and healing rate. Several studies have shown that the risk of recurrent bleeding is much lower in patients treated with sclerotherapy: 30%–50% as opposed to 70%–80% for patients not treated with sclerotherapy.

Alternatives

Pharmacological agents are also used in the treatment of esophageal varices. Drugs such as vasopressin and somatostatin are administered to actively bleeding patients on admission, while propranolol, nadolol, or subcutaneous octreotide are used to prevent subsequent bleeding after successful endoscopic variceal eradication. Vasopressin or vasopressin with nitroglycerin has been proven effective in the acute control of variceal hemorrhage. Somatostatin is more effective in the control of active bleeding when compared to vasopressin, glypressin, endoscopic sclerotherapy, or balloon tamponade. Octreotide has comparable outcomes to vasopressin, terlipressin, or endoscopic sclerotherapy. **Liver transplantation** should be considered as an alternative for patients with bleeding varices from liver disease.

Another alternative treatment is provided by transjugular intrahepatic porto-systemic shunting (TIPS). In TIPS, a catheter fitted with a stent, a wire mesh tube used to prop open a vein or artery, is inserted through a vein in the neck into the liver. Under x-ray guidance, the stent is placed in an optimal position within the liver so as to

---

QUESTIONS TO ASK YOUR DOCTOR

- What are esophageal varices?
- Are there alternatives to sclerotherapy?
- How do I prepare for surgery?
- What type of anesthesia will be used?
- How is the surgery performed?
- How long will I be in the hospital?
- How many sclerotherapy procedures do you perform in a year?

---

allow blood to flow more easily through the portal vein. This treatment reduces the excess pressure in the esophageal varices, and thus decreases the risk of recurrent bleeding.

Sclerotherapy for esophageal varices is performed by a surgeon specialized in gastroenterology or hepatology in a hospital setting, very often as an emergency procedure.

Resources

BOOKS

Feldman, M., et al. *Sleisenger & Fordtran's Gastrointestinal and Liver Disease.* 9th ed. Philadelphia: Saunders/Elsevier, 2010.

Townsend, Courtney M., et al. *Sabiston Textbook of Surgery.* 19th ed. Philadelphia: Saunders/Elsevier, 2012.

PERIODICALS

Croffie, J., et al. "Sclerosing Agents for Use in GI Endoscopy." *Gastrointestinal Endoscopy* 66, no. 1 (2007): 1–6. http://dx.doi.org/10.1016/j.gie.2007.02.014 (accessed October 17, 2013).

WEBSITES

A.D.A.M. Medical Encyclopedia. "Bleeding Esophageal Varices." MedlinePlus. http://www.nlm.nih.gov/medlineplus/ency/article/000268.htm (accessed October 17, 2013).

Mount Sinai Hospital. "Esophageal Variceal Injection." http://www.mountsinai.org/patient-care/health-library/treatments-and-procedures/esophageal-variceal-injection (accessed October 17, 2013).

ORGANIZATIONS

Society of American Gastrointestinal Endoscopic Surgeons (SAGES), 11300 West Olympic Blvd., Ste. 600, Los Angeles, CA 90064, (310) 437-0544, Fax: (310) 437-0585, webmaster@sages.org, http://www.sages.org.

Lori De Milto
Monique Laberge, PhD

Sclerotherapy for varicose veins

Definition

Sclerotherapy, which takes its name from a Greek word meaning "hardening," is a method of treating enlarged veins by injecting an irritating chemical called a sclerosing agent into the vein. The chemical causes the vein to become inflamed, which leads to the formation of fibrous tissue and closing of the lumen, or central channel of the vein.

Purpose

Sclerotherapy in the legs is performed for several reasons. It is most often done to improve the appearance of the legs, and is accomplished by closing down spider veins—small veins in the legs that have dilated under increased venous blood pressure. A spider vein is one type of telangiectasia, which is the medical term for a reddish-colored lesion produced by the permanent enlargement of the capillaries and other small blood vessels. The word telangiectasia comes from three Greek words that mean "end," "blood vessel," and "stretch out."

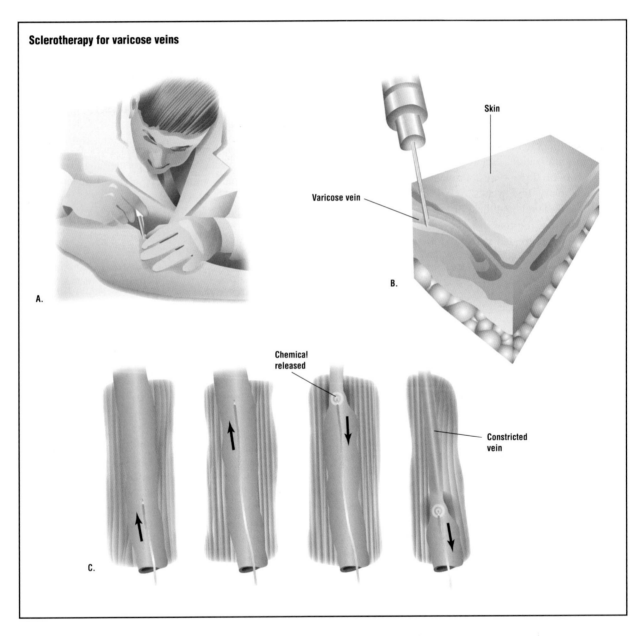

Sclerotherapy for varicose veins

Skin

Varicose vein

B.

Chemical released

Constricted vein

A.

C.

During sclerotherapy for the treatment of varicose veins, the doctor injects a chemical solution directly into the vein (A, B). The needle travels up the vein, and as it is pulled back, the chemical is released, causing the vein to form fibrous tissue that collapses the inside of it (C). *(Illustration by GGS Information Services. Copyright © Cengage Learning®.)*

In a spider vein, also called a "sunburst varicosity," there is a central reddish area that is visible to the eye because it lies close to the surface of the skin; smaller veins spread outward from it in the shape of a spider's legs. Spider veins may also appear in two other common patterns—they may look like tiny tree branches or like extra-fine separate lines.

In addition to the cosmetic purposes sclerotherapy serves, it is also performed to treat the soreness, aching, muscle fatigue, and leg cramps that often accompany small- or middle-sized varicose veins in the legs. It is not, however, used by itself to treat large varicose veins.

Because sclerotherapy is usually considered a cosmetic procedure, it is usually not covered by health insurance. People who are being treated for cramps and discomfort in their legs, however, should ask their insurance companies whether they are covered for sclerotherapy. Sclerotherapy costs usually reflect the number of syringes of sclerosant required; the average cost of each syringe is $225. Many procedures will require the use of two syringes of sclerosant. The average cost is $326.

Sclerotherapy as a general treatment modality is also performed to treat hemorrhoids (swollen veins) in the esophagus.

Demographics

The American College of Phlebology (ACP), a group of dermatologists, plastic **surgeons**, gynecologists, and general surgeons with special training in the treatment of venous disorders, comments that about 60% of all people in the United States suffer from spider veins or varicose veins. Women are more commonly affected than men, with about half of all women experiencing some type of vein disorder. The American Society of Plastic Surgeons (ASPS) estimates that more than 40% of women over 50 in the United States have spider veins.

Women are more likely to develop spider veins than men, but the incidence among both sexes increases with age. The results of a recent survey of middle-aged and elderly people in San Diego, California, show that 80% of the women and 50% of the men had spider veins. Men are less likely to seek treatment for spider veins for cosmetic reasons, however, because the discoloration caused by spider veins is often covered by leg hair. On the other hand, men who are bothered by aching, burning sensations or leg cramps can benefit from sclerotherapy.

According to the ASPS, there were 358,152 sclerotherapy procedures performed in the United States in 2012. Most people who are treated with sclerotherapy are between the ages of 30 and 60.

Spider veins are most noticeable and common in Caucasians. Hispanics are less likely than Caucasians but more likely than either African or Asian Americans to develop spider veins.

Description

Causes of spider veins

To understand how sclerotherapy works, it is helpful to begin with a brief description of the venous system in the human body. The venous part of the circulatory system returns blood to the heart to be pumped to the lungs for oxygenation. This is in contrast to the arterial system, which carries oxygenated blood away from the heart to be distributed throughout the body. The smallest parts of the venous system are the capillaries, which feed into larger superficial veins. All superficial veins lie between the skin and a layer of fibrous connective tissue called fascia, which covers and supports the muscles and the internal organs. The deeper veins of the body lie within the muscle fascia. This distinction helps to explain why superficial veins can be treated by sclerotherapy without damage to the larger veins.

Veins contain one-way valves that push blood inward and upward toward the heart when they are functioning normally. The blood pressure in the superficial veins is usually low, but if it rises and remains at a higher level over a period of time, the valves in the veins begin to fail and the veins dilate, or expand. Veins that are not functioning properly are said to be "incompetent." As the veins expand, they become more noticeable because they lie closer to the surface of the skin, forming the typical patterns seen in spider veins.

Some people are at greater risk for developing spider veins. These risk factors include:

• Sex. Females in any age group are more likely than males to develop spider veins.

• Genetic factors. Some people have veins with abnormally weak walls or valves. They may develop spider veins even without a rise in blood pressure in the superficial veins.

• Pregnancy. A woman's total blood volume increases during pregnancy, which increases the blood pressure in the venous system. In addition, the hormonal changes of pregnancy cause the walls and valves in the veins to soften.

• Using birth control pills.

• Obesity. Excess body weight increases pressure on the veins.

• Occupational factors. People whose jobs require standing or sitting for long periods of time without the opportunity to walk or move around are more likely

KEY TERMS

Arteriole—A very small branch of an artery, usually close to a capillary network.

Edema—The presence of abnormally large amounts of fluid in the soft tissues of the body.

Electrodesiccation—A method of treating spider veins or drying up tissue by passing a small electric current through a fine needle into the affected area.

Hemosiderin—A form of iron that is stored inside tissue cells. The brownish discoloration of skin that sometimes occurs after sclerotherapy is caused by hemosiderin.

Hirsutism—Abnormal hair growth on the part of the body treated by sclerotherapy. It is also called hypertrichosis.

Incompetent—In a medical context, insufficient. An incompetent vein is one that is not performing its function of carrying blood back to the heart.

Lumen—The channel or cavity inside a tube or hollow organ of the body.

Palpation—Examining by touch as part of the process of physical diagnosis.

Percussion—Thumping or tapping a part of the body with the fingers for diagnostic purposes.

Phlebology—The study of veins, their disorders, and their treatments. A phlebologist is a doctor who specializes in treating spider veins, varicose veins, and associated disorders.

Sclerose—To harden or undergo hardening. Sclerosing agents are chemicals that are used in sclerotherapy to cause swollen veins to fill with fibrous tissue and close down.

Spider nevus (plural, nevi)—A reddish lesion that consists of a central arteriole with smaller branches radiating outward from it. Spider nevi are also called spider angiomas; they are most common in small children and pregnant women.

Spider veins—Telangiectasias that appear on the surface of the legs, characterized by a reddish central point with smaller veins branching out from it like the legs of a spider.

Telangiectasia—The medical term for the visible discolorations produced by permanently swollen capillaries and smaller veins.

Varicose—Abnormally enlarged and distended.

to develop spider veins than people whose jobs allow more movement.

• Trauma. Falls, deep bruises, cuts, or surgical incisions may lead to the formation of spider veins in or near the affected area.

There is no known method to prevent the formation of spider veins.

Sclerotherapy procedures

In typical outpatient sclerotherapy treatment, the patient changes into a pair of shorts at the doctor's office and lies on an examination table. After cleansing the skin surface with an antiseptic, the doctor injects a sclerosing agent into the veins. This agent is eliminated when the skin is stretched tightly over the area with the other hand. The doctor first injects the larger veins in each area of the leg, then the smaller ones. In most cases, one injection is needed for every inch of spider vein; a typical treatment session will require 5 to 40 separate injections. No anesthetic is needed for sclerotherapy, although the patient may feel a mild stinging or burning sensation at the injection site.

The liquid sclerosing agents that are used most often to treat spider veins are polidocanol (Aethoxysklerol), sodium tetradecyl sulfate, and saline solution at 11.7% concentration. Some practitioners prefer to use saline because it does not cause allergic reactions. The usual practice is to use the lowest concentration of the chemical that is still effective in closing the veins.

A newer type of sclerosing agent is a foam instead of a liquid chemical that is injected into the veins. The foam has several advantages: It makes better contact with the wall of the vein than a liquid sclerosing agent; it allows the use of smaller amounts of chemical; and its movement in the vein can be monitored on an **ultrasound** screen. Sclerosing foam has been shown to have a high success rate with a lower cost, and causes fewer major complications.

After all the veins in a specific area of the leg have been injected, the doctor covers the area with a cotton ball or pad and compression tape. The patient may be asked to wait in the office for 20–30 minutes after the first treatment session to ensure that there is no hypersensitivity to the sclerosing chemicals. Most sclerotherapy treatment sessions are short, lasting from 15 to 45 minutes.

It is not unusual for patients to need a second treatment to completely eliminate the spider veins; however, it is necessary to wait four to six weeks between procedures.

Diagnosis

The most important aspect of diagnosis prior to undergoing sclerotherapy is distinguishing between telangiectasias and large varicose veins, and telangiectasias and spider nevi. Because sclerotherapy is intended to treat only small superficial veins, the doctor must confirm that the patient does not have a more serious venous disorder.

Spider nevi, which are also called "spider angiomas," are small, benign reddish lesions that consist of a central arteriole, which is a very small branch of an artery with smaller vessels radiating from it. Although the names are similar, spider nevi occur in the part of the circulatory system that carries blood away from the heart, whereas spider veins occur in the venous system that returns blood to the heart. To distinguish between the two, the doctor will press gently on the spot in the center of the network. A spider nevus will blanch, or lose its reddish color, when the central arteriole is compressed. When the doctor releases the pressure, the color will return. Spider veins are not affected by compression in this way. In addition, spider nevi occur most frequently in children and pregnant women, rather than in older adults. They are treated by laser therapy or electrodesiccation, rather than by sclerotherapy.

After taking the patient's medical history, the doctor examines the patient from the waist down, both to note the location of spider veins and to palpate (touch with gentle pressure) them for signs of other venous disorders. Ideally, the examiner will have a small, raised platform for the patient to stand on during the examination. The doctor will ask the patient to turn slowly while standing, and will be looking for scars or other signs of trauma, bulges in the skin, areas of discolored skin, or other indications of chronic venous insufficiency. While palpating the legs, the doctor will note areas of unusual warmth or soreness, cysts, and edema (swelling of the soft tissues due to fluid retention). Next, the doctor will percuss certain parts of the legs where the larger veins lie closer to the surface. By gently tapping or thumping on the skin over these areas, the doctor can feel fluid waves in the veins and determine whether further testing for venous insufficiency is required. If the patient has problems related to large varicose veins, these must be treated before sclerotherapy can be performed to eliminate spider veins.

Some conditions and disorders are considered contraindications for sclerotherapy:

• Pregnancy and lactation. Pregnant women are advised to postpone sclerotherapy until at least three months after the baby is born, because some spider veins will fade by themselves after delivery. Nursing mothers should postpone sclerotherapy until the baby is weaned because it is not yet known whether the chemicals used in sclerotherapy may affect the mother's milk.

• Diabetes.

• A history of AIDS, hepatitis, syphilis, or other diseases that are carried in the blood.

• Heart conditions.

• High blood pressure, blood clotting disorders, and other disorders of the circulatory system.

Preparation

Patients are asked to discontinue **aspirin** or aspirin-related products for a week before sclerotherapy. Further, they are told not to apply any moisturizers, creams, tanning lotions, or sunblock to the legs on the day of the procedure. Patients should bring a pair of shorts to wear during the procedure, as well as compression stockings and a pair of slacks or a long skirt to cover the legs afterwards.

Most practitioners will take photographs of the patient's legs before sclerotherapy to evaluate the effectiveness of treatment. In addition, some insurance companies request pretreatment photographs for documentation purposes.

Aftercare

Aftercare following sclerotherapy includes wearing medical compression stockings that apply either 20–30 mm Hg or 30–40 mm Hg of pressure for at least seven to ten days (preferably four to six weeks) after the procedure. Wearing compression stockings minimizes the risk of edema, discoloration, and pain. Fashion support stockings are a less acceptable alternative because they do not apply enough pressure to the legs.

The surgical tape and cotton balls used during the procedure should be left in place for 48 hours after the patient returns home.

Patients are encouraged to walk, ride a bicycle, or participate in other low-impact forms of **exercise** (examples: yoga and tai chi) to prevent the formation of blood clots in the deep veins of the legs. They should, however, avoid prolonged periods of standing or sitting, and high-impact activities, such as jogging.

Risks

Cosmetically, the chief risk of sclerotherapy is that new spider veins may develop after the procedure. New spider veins are dilated blood vessels that can form when some of the venous blood forms new pathways back to the larger veins; they are not the original blood vessels that were sclerosed. Some patients may develop telangiectatic matting, which is a network of new spider veins that surface around the treated area. Telangiectatic matting usually clears up by itself within 3 to 12 months after sclerotherapy, but it can also be treated with further sclerosing injections.

Other risks of sclerotherapy include:

- Venous thrombosis. A potentially serious complication, thrombosis refers to the formation of blood clots in the veins.
- Severe inflammation.
- Pain after the procedure lasting several hours or days. This discomfort can be eased by wearing medical compression stockings and by walking briskly.
- Allergic reactions to the sclerosing solution or foam.
- Permanent scarring.
- Loss of feeling resulting from damage to the nerves in the treated area.
- Edema (swelling) of the foot or ankle. This problem is most likely to occur when the foot or ankle is treated for spider veins. The edema usually resolves within a few days or weeks.
- Brownish spots or discoloration in the skin around the treated area. These changes in skin color are caused by deposits of hemosiderin, which is a form of iron that is stored within tissue cells. The spots usually fade after several months.
- Ulceration of the skin. This complication may result from reactive spasms of the blood vessels, the use of overly strong sclerosing solutions, or poor technique in administering sclerotherapy. It can be treated by diluting the sclerosing chemical with normal saline solution.
- Hirsutism. Hirsutism is the abnormal growth of hair on the area treated by sclerotherapy. It usually develops several months after treatment and goes away on its own. It is also known as hypertrichosis.

Results

Normal results of sclerotherapy include improvement in the external appearance of the legs and relief of aching or cramping sensations associated with spider veins. It is common for complete elimination of spider veins to require three to four sclerotherapy treatments.

Morbidity and mortality rates

Mortality associated with sclerotherapy for spider veins is almost 0% when the procedure is performed by a competent doctor. The rates of other complications vary somewhat, but have been reported as falling within the following ranges:

- Hemosiderin discoloration: 10%–80% of patients, with fewer than 1% of cases lasting longer than a year.
- Telangiectatic matting: 5%–75% of patients.
- Deep venous thrombosis: Fewer than 1%.
- Mild aching or pain: 35%–55%.
- Skin ulceration: About 4%.

Alternatives

Conservative treatments

Patients who are experiencing some discomfort from spider veins may be helped by any or several of the following approaches:

- Exercise. Walking or other forms of exercise that activate the muscles in the lower legs can relieve aching and cramping because these muscles keep the blood moving through the leg veins. One exercise that is often recommended is repeated flexing of the ankle joint. By flexing the ankles five to ten times every few minutes and walking around for one to two minutes every half hour throughout the day, the patient can prevent the venous congestion that results from sitting or standing in one position for hours at a time.
- Avoiding high-heeled shoes. Shoes with high heels do not allow the ankle to flex fully when the patient is walking. This limitation of the range of motion of the ankle joint makes it more difficult for the leg muscles to contract and force venous blood upward toward the heart.
- Elevating the legs for 15–30 minutes once or twice a day. This change of position is frequently recommended for reducing edema of the feet and ankles.
- Wearing compression hosiery. Compression benefits the leg veins by reducing inflammation as well as improving venous outflow. Most manufacturers of medical compression stockings now offer some relatively sheer hosiery that is both attractive and that offers support.
- Medications. Drugs that have been used to treat the discomfort associated with spider veins include nonsteroidal anti-inflammatory drugs (NSAIDs) and preparations of vitamins C and E. One prescription medication that is sometimes given to treat circulatory problems in the legs and feet is pentoxifylline, which improves

blood flow in the smaller capillaries. Pentoxifylline is sold under the brand name Trendar.

If appearance is the patient's primary concern, spider veins on the legs can often be covered with specially formulated cosmetics that come in a wide variety of skin tones. Some of these preparations are available in waterproof formulations for use during swimming and other athletic activities.

Electrodesiccation, laser therapy, and pulsed light therapy

Electrodesiccation is a treatment modality whereby the doctor seals off the small blood vessels that cause spider veins by passing a weak electric current through a fine needle to the walls of the veins. Electrodesiccation seems to be more effective in treating spider veins in the face than in treating those in the legs; it tends to leave pitted white scars when used to treat spider veins in the legs or feet.

Laser therapy, like electrodesiccation, works better in treating facial spider veins. The sharply focused beam of intense light emitted by the laser heats the blood vessel, causing the blood in it to coagulate and close the vein. Various lasers have been used to treat spider veins, including argon, KTP 532nm, and alexandrite lasers. The choice of light wavelength and pulse duration are based on the size of the vein to be treated. Argon lasers, however, have been found to increase the patient's risk of developing hemosiderin discoloration when used on the legs. The KTP 532nm laser gives better results in treating leg spider veins, but is still not as effective as sclerotherapy.

Intense pulsed light (IPL) systems differ from lasers because the light emitted is noncoherent and not monochromatic. The IPL systems enable doctors to use a wider range of light wavelengths and pulse frequencies when treating spider veins and other skin problems, such as pigmented birthmarks. This flexibility, however, requires considerable skill and experience on the part of the doctor to remove spider veins without damaging the surrounding skin.

Complementary and alternative (CAM) treatments

According to Dr. Kenneth Pelletier, the former director of the program in complementary and alternative treatments at Stanford University School of Medicine, California, horse chestnut extract is as safe and effective as compression stockings when used as a conservative treatment for spider veins. Horse chestnut (*Aesculus hippocastanum*) has been used in Europe for some years to treat circulatory problems in the legs; the most recent research has been conducted in Great Britain and

QUESTIONS TO ASK YOUR DOCTOR

- How likely am I to develop new spider veins in the treated areas?
- Do you use the newer sclerosing foams when you administer sclerotherapy?
- What technique(s) do you prefer to use for sclerotherapy and why?

Germany. The usual dosage is 75 mg twice a day at meals. The most common side effect of oral preparations of horse chestnut is occasional indigestion in some patients.

Health care team roles

Sclerotherapy is usually performed by general surgeons, dermatologists, or plastic surgeons, but it can also be done by family physicians or naturopaths who have been trained to do it. The American College of Phlebology holds workshops and intensive practical courses for interested practitioners. The ACP can be contacted for a list of members in each state.

Sclerotherapy is done as an outpatient procedure, most often in the doctor's office or in a **plastic surgery** clinic.

Resources

BOOKS

Townsend, Courtney M., et al. *Sabiston Textbook of Surgery.* 19th ed. Philadelphia: Saunders/Elsevier, 2012.

OTHER

American Society of Plastic Surgeons. *2012 Plastic Surgery Statistics Reports.* 2013. http://www.plasticsurgery.org/ Documents/news-resources/statistics/2012-Plastic-Surgery-Statistics/full-plastic-surgery-statistics-report.pdf (accessed October 1, 2013).

WEBSITES

American Society of Plastic Surgeons. "Spider Vein Treatment." http://www.plasticsurgery.org/cosmetic-procedures/spider-veins.html (accessed October 17, 2013).
MedlinePlus. "Varicose Veins." U.S. National Library of Medicine, National Institutes of Health. http://www.nlm. nih.gov/medlineplus/varicoseveins.html (accessed October 17, 2013).

ORGANIZATIONS

American Academy of Dermatology, 930 E. Woodfield Rd., Schaumburg, IL 60173, (847) 240-1280, (866) 503-SKIN (7546), http://www.aad.org.

American College of Phlebology, 101 Callan Ave., Ste. 210, San Leandro, CA 94577, (510) 346-6800, http://www.phlebology.org.

American Society of Plastic Surgeons, 444 E. Algonquin Rd., Arlington Heights, IL 60005, http://www.plasticsurgery.org.

Peripheral Vascular Surgery Society (PVSS), 100 Cummings Ctr., Ste. 124A, Beverly, MA 01915, (978) 927-7800, Fax: (978) 927-7872, pvss@administrare.com, http://www.pvss.org.

Society for Vascular Surgery, 633 N. Saint Clair St., 22nd Fl., Chicago, IL 60611, (312) 334-2300, (800) 258-7188, vascular@vascularsociety.org, http://www.vascularweb.org.

Rebecca Frey, PhD

Scoliosis surgery, arthrodesis *see* **Spinal fusion**

Scopolamine patch

Definition

A scopolamine patch (Transderm Scōp® or Transderm-V®) is an adhesive medication patch that is applied to the skin behind the ear the night before surgery or a caesarean section. The patch is treated with the belladonna alkaloid scopolamine, an anticholinergic drug that is a central nervous system depressant and an antiemetic.

Purpose

Scopolamine patches are prescribed to reduce postoperative nausea and vomiting (PONV) associated with anesthesia and surgery. Scopolamine also has a mild analgesic and sedative effect, which adds to its therapeutic value for some surgical patients. In addition to PONV, scopolamine patches are also used for the treatment of motion sickness.

Demographics

Elderly patients may be more sensitive to scopolamine treatment and its use should be prescribed with caution in this group. The safety of scopolamine patches has not been determined in children; according to the U.S. Food and Drug Administration (FDA), the patch should not be used in children.

Description

A potent drug derived from an alkaloid of belladonna (*Atropa belladonna*; common name deadly

nightshade), scopolamine works by depressing the action of the nerve fibers near the ear and the vomiting center of the brain and central nervous system (CNS). The patch itself is designed with special layered materials that slowly release a small dose of the drug transdermally (through the skin) over a period of several days.

Patients who are instructed to apply their patch at home should wash their hands thoroughly both before and after the procedure. Scopolamine can be spread to the eyes by hand, which can cause blurred vision and pupil dilation. Patches should never be cut into pieces, as cutting destroys the time-release mechanism of the drug. The directions for use for the patch should be read thoroughly before application, and specific physician instructions should also be followed. The drug will start to work approximately four hours after the patch is applied.

Precautions

Patients with a history of glaucoma, prostate enlargement, kidney or liver problems, bladder obstruction, gastrointestinal obstruction, or contact dermatitis (allergic skin rash) in response to topical drugs may not be suitable candidates for scopolamine patch therapy. A physician or anesthesiologist should take a full medical history before prescribing scopolamine to determine if the medication is appropriate.

Preparation

The dime-sized scopolamine patch is applied just behind either the left or right ear. The area should be clean and hairless prior to the application, which should occur the evening before a scheduled surgery. For women who are prescribed a scopolamine patch to reduce nausea and vomiting related to a **cesarean section**, the patch should be applied just one hour before the procedure to minimize the baby's exposure to the drug. Scopolamine does cross the placental barrier, but there are not enough studies in humans to show whether the drug has any negative effects on newborn babies of mothers who used scopolamine during caesarean delivery.

Aftercare

Patients who receive a scopolamine patch should not drive or operate heavy machinery until the therapy is complete. Patch therapy generally lasts about three days. Patches should be disposed of according to the manufacturer's directions in a secure place to ensure that small children or pets do not get access to them. If PONV has not resolved after patch therapy has ended, patients should talk to their doctor about their treatment options.

Risks

Possible complications or side effects from transdermal scopolamine include but are not limited to: short-term memory loss, fatigue, confusion, hallucinations, difficulty urinating, and changes in heart rate. The drug can trigger seizures and psychotic delusions in patients with a history of these problems. Dizziness, nausea, headache, and hypotension (low blood pressure) have also been reported in some patients upon discontinuation of scopolamine patch therapy.

Patients who experience eye pain with redness and possible blurred vision should remove the patch immediately and call their doctor, since the symptoms could be signs of a rare but possible side effect of scopolamine called narrow-angle glaucoma. Blurriness with or without pupil dilation is also a potential but generally harmless side effect of the drug.

The FDA recommends that patients who are scheduled for a **magnetic resonance imaging** (MRI) scan remove the patch before the scan, as the patch's backing contains aluminum. The aluminum absorbs energy and heats up during the scan, which may cause a mild burn of the skin beneath the patch.

Results

When scopolamine patch therapy works, it reduces or eliminates postsurgical nausea and vomiting. Two-thirds of patients experience dry mouth, the most common side effect of the drug.

Alternatives

Intravenous or intramuscular injection of scopolamine may be used as alternatives to patch therapy for some patients. Other antiemetics that may be prescribed for PONV include anticholinergic drugs, dopaminergic drugs (e.g., promethazine, droperidol), antihistamines (e.

g., diphenhydramine), and the serotonin receptor antagonists (e.g., ondansetron, granisetron, tropisetron, dolasetron). **Corticosteroids** may also be recommended for PONV in some patients.

Health care team roles

When used for surgical implications, a scopolamine patch may be ordered by a physician, surgeon, or anesthesiologist, typically in a hospital setting or an ambulatory surgery center. The patch may be applied at home by the patient, or by a nurse or physician's assistant as part of preoperative preparation.

Resources

BOOKS

Deglin, Judith Hopfer, and April Hazard Vallerand. *Davis's Drug Guide for Nurses.* 10th ed. Philadelphia: F. A. Davis, 2007.

PERIODICALS

Seo, S. W., et al. "Mental Confusion Associated with Scopolamine Patch in Elderly with Mild Cognitive Impairment (MCI)." *Archives of Gerontology and Geriatrics* 49, no. 2 (2009): 204–7. http://dx.doi.org/10.1016/j.archger.2008.07.011 (accessed October 17, 2013).

WEBSITES

AHFS Consumer Medication Information. "Scopolamine Transdermal Patch." American Society of Health-System Pharmacists. Available from: http://www.nlm.nih.gov/medlineplus/druginfo/meds/a682509.html (accessed October 17, 2013).
Micromedex. "Scopolamine (Transdermal Route)." MayoClinic.com. http://www.mayoclinic.com/health/drug-information/DR602935 (accessed October 17, 2013).

ORGANIZATIONS

U.S. Food and Drug Administration, 10903 New Hampshire Ave., Silver Spring, MD 20993, (888) INFO-FDA (463-6332), http://www.fda.gov.

Paula Ford-Martin
Rebecca Frey, PhD

> ## QUESTIONS TO ASK YOUR DOCTOR
>
> - When and how do I apply the patch?
> - What should I do if the patch becomes loose or falls off?
> - When can I remove or replace the patch?
> - Are there any warning symptoms that should signal me to remove the patch?

Second opinion

Definition

A second opinion is the result of seeking an evaluation by another doctor or surgeon to confirm the diagnosis and treatment plan of a primary physician, or to offer an alternative diagnosis and/or treatment approach.

Purpose

Getting a second surgical opinion can fill an important emotional need as well as establish medical needs and treatment goals. When a second opinion confirms initial findings, it can provide reassurance and feelings of acceptance for the patient, and may reduce anxiety and uncertainty.

From a cost-effectiveness point of view, second opinions can save health insurance providers money by establishing the certainty of a clinical need (or lack of need) for surgery, particularly when the diagnosis is life-threatening.

Patients with a diagnosis of cancer may also benefit from a second-opinion pathology review of their biopsy material. A Johns Hopkins study reported that 1.4% of patients scheduled for cancer-related surgery at their facility were found to have been misdiagnosed when their tissue samples were reevaluated by a second pathologist. Similarly, a study published in the *Annals of Surgical Oncology* in 2002 found that a pathological second opinion of breast cancers changed the initial diagnosis, prognosis, or treatment approach in 80% of the 340 study subjects.

Several clinical research studies, however, have found that patients often seek second opinions not necessarily because they doubt the diagnosis or recommendations of their first provider, but because they were dissatisfied with either the amount of information given to them or the style of communication of their doctor. A 2002 Northwestern University study found that only 46% of patients coming into a breast cancer treatment center for a second opinion had been offered a complete discussion of treatment options during their initial consultation.

Description

Doctors often have differing viewpoints as to how a particular medical problem should be managed, whether through surgery or less-invasive treatment means. One surgeon may prefer to take a "watchful waiting" approach before recommending surgery, while another may believe in performing surgery as soon as possible to avoid later complications. In some cases, several surgical

KEY TERMS

Informed consent—Providing a patient with complete, objective information on the risks, benefits, and potential and probable outcomes of different surgical or therapeutic options so that they may make an informed decision or consent to treatment.

Pathologist—A physician with specialized training in recognizing and identifying diseases through the analysis of abnormal bodily tissues.

Postoperative care—Medical care and support required after surgery to promote healing and recovery.

Watchful waiting—Monitoring a patient's disease state carefully to see if the condition worsens before trying surgery or another therapy. This term is often associated with prostate cancer.

techniques may be viable options for a patient. Medicine is not as black-and-white as many patients are led to believe, and physicians are not infallible. For these reasons, and because surgery is a major procedure with associated risks that should not be taken lightly, second opinions are an important part of the process of **informed consent** and decision-making.

Although a physician may strive to be objective, personal views and subjective experiences can influence their treatment recommendations. In addition, both the education and experience of a doctor in a given medical area can also influence the advice they offer a patient. For these reasons, seeking a second opinion from another physician and/or surgeon can be invaluable in making a decision on a course of treatment.

Second opinions are most frequently sought in cases of elective (nonemergency) surgery, when the patient has time to consider options and make a more informed choice about his or her course of treatment. While a second surgical opinion may be requested in some cases of **emergency surgery**, they are not as common, simply because of the logistical limitations involved with getting a qualified second opinion if a patient requires immediate care.

In some cases, a doctor or surgeon may encourage seeking a second opinion, particularly when the preferred course of treatment is not clear-cut or another surgeon with advanced training or expertise may provide more insights into surgical options. A doctor or surgeon may also recommend seeking a second opinion when the patient is suffering from multiple medical disorders.

Patients should remember that it is their right to seek a second opinion before committing to surgery or another treatment plan. Embarrassment or fear of disapproval from a primary care provider should not be a barrier to getting a second opinion. A competent physician will not consider the decision to seek a second opinion an insult to their ability or experience. Instead, they will consider the patient an informed individual who is proactive and responsible for his or her own health care.

Patients seeking a second-opinion consultation may ask the provider questions similar to those they asked their primary provider. Questions may include:

• Are there other options besides surgery?
• What are the risks and benefits of each treatment option?
• How might each possible treatment impact quality-of-life for the patient?
• What kind of success rate is associated with surgery and other potential therapies?
• How is the surgery performed?
• Is surgery a permanent, long-term, or temporary solution to the condition?
• What type of anesthesia will be used?
• If surgery is chosen by the patient, how soon must it be done?
• What type of aftercare and recovery time is required once the surgery is complete?
• How much pain is to be expected postoperatively, and how is it typically treated?
• What are the costs involved with surgery and other treatment options, including postoperative care?

Providing the second surgeon with appropriate background information is important, but so is refraining from detailed descriptions of what the first provider did or did not recommend before the consultation begins. Patients should allow the surgeon to draw objective conclusions based on the medical history and diagnostic data before them. If the second opinion differs from the first provider's opinion, and the patient feels comfortable doing so, he or she might then offer information on the first provider's recommendations to get further feedback and input for a final decision.

Preparation

Before seeking a second opinion, patients should contact their health insurance provider to find out if the service is covered. Some insurance companies may request that a second opinion be sought before major **elective surgery**, and may reserve the right to designate a physician or surgeon to provide the patient evaluation.

Medicare Part B covers 80% of costs for surgical second opinions after deductible, and 80% for a third opinion if the first two opinions are contradictory. Other Medicare programs may cover second opinions as well; patients should check with their Medicare carrier for details.

There are several ways to find an appropriate health care professional to provide a second opinion. Patients can:

• ask friends and family for references
• ask their primary care physician or another trusted health care provider
• contact an appropriate specialty medical organization (e.g., American College of Surgeons)
• call their local medical licensing board
• check with their insurance provider or Medicare carrier

Cancer patients can also consult a list of multidisciplinary institutions that will provide a second opinion on request. The list is available at http://www.blochcancer.org.

When seeking a second surgical opinion, patients should find a surgeon who is board certified in the appropriate specialty by an organization that is part of the American Board of Medical Specialties (ABMS). For example, surgery of the urinary tract may be performed by a provider who is board certified by the American Board of Urology and/or the American Board of Surgery (ABS), two member organizations of the ABMS. Diplomates of ABMS member boards are **surgeons** who have passed rigorous written and oral testing on these specialties and have met specific accredited educational and residency requirements. In some cases, surgeons may also be certified in subspecialties within a discipline (for example, a vascular surgeon may be board certified by the **vascular surgery** board of the ABS). The ABMS provides a verification service for patients to check on the certification status of their provider.

In addition, the surgeon may also be a Fellow of the American College of Surgery (ACS), as indicated by the designation FACS after their name. This indicates that he or she has met standards of clinical experience, education, ethical conduct, and professional expertise as prescribed by the ACS.

Once a second health care provider is selected, patients should speak with their primary doctor about providing the appropriate medical history, test results, and other pertinent information to the physician who will give the second opinion. The patient may have to sign an information release form to allow the files to be sent. If x-rays, **magnetic resonance imaging** (MRI), or other radiological testing was performed, the second physician may request to see the original films, rather than the radiologist's report of the results, in order to interpret them objectively. In some cases, the office of the surgeon giving the second opinion can arrange to have these materials transferred with a patient's written approval. Patients should call ahead to ensure that all needed materials arrive at the second provider's office before the appointment, to give that physician adequate time to review them and to avoid potentially costly repeat testing.

Results

Second opinions that agree with the first provider's conclusions may help ease the patient's mind and provide a clearer picture of the necessary course of treatment or surgery. However, if a patient still feels uncomfortable with the treatment plan outlined by the first and second physicians, or strongly disagrees with their conclusions, a third opinion from another provider is an option.

In cases in which the second provider disagrees with the first provider on diagnosis and/or treatment, the patient has harder choices to face. Again, a third evaluation may be in order from yet another physician, and some insurance companies may actually require this step in cases of conflicting opinions. If a patient is very comfortable with and confident in their primary care provider, they may wish to revisit them to review the second opinion.

In all cases, a patient should remember that their personal preferences, beliefs, and lifestyle considerations must also be considered in their final decision on surgery or treatment, as they are the ones who will live with the results.

Resources

BOOKS

Horton, Richard C. *Second Opinion: Doctors, Diseases, and Decisions in Modern Medicine.* London: Granta Books, 2003.

OTHER

Center for Medicare & Medicaid Services (CMS). *Getting a Second Opinion Before Surgery.* June 2010. http://www.medicare.gov/Publications/Pubs/pdf/02173.pdf (accessed October 17, 2013).

WEBSITES

Breastcancer.org. "When to Get a Second Opinion." http://www.breastcancer.org/treatment/second_opinion/when (accessed October 17, 2013).
Center for Medicare & Medicaid Services (CMS). "Second Surgical Opinions." http://www.medicare.gov/coverage/second-surgical-opinions.html (accessed October 22, 2013).
Johns Hopkins Medicine. "Questions to Ask Before Surgery." http://www.hopkinsmedicine.org/healthlibrary/conditions/ surgical_care/questions_to_ask_before_surgery_85, P01409 (accessed October 17, 2013).
Pompa, Frank, and Peter Eisler. "Why You Should Get a Second Opinion before Getting Surgery." *USA Today,* June 19, 2013. http://www.usatoday.com/story/news/ nation/2013/06/19/surgery-second-opinion-interactive/ 2439275 (accessed October 17, 2013).

ORGANIZATIONS

American Board of Medical Specialties, 222 N. LaSalle St., Ste. 1500, Chicago, IL 60601, (312) 436-2600, http://www.abms.org.
American College of Surgeons, 633 N. Saint Clair St., Chicago, IL 60611-3211, (312) 202-5000, (800) 621-4111, Fax: (312) 202-5001, postmaster@facs.org, http://www.facs.org.

Paula Ford-Martin
Rebecca Frey, PhD

Second-look surgery

Definition

Second-look surgery is performed after a procedure or course of treatment to determine if the patient is free of disease. If disease is found, additional procedures may or may not be performed at the time of second-look surgery.

Purpose

Second-look surgery may be performed under numerous circumstances on patients with various medical conditions.

Cancer

A second-look procedure is sometimes performed to determine if a cancer patient has responded successfully to a particular treatment. Examples of cancers that are assessed during second-look surgery are ovarian cancer and colorectal cancer. In many cases, before a round of chemotherapy and/or radiation therapy is started, a patient will undergo a surgical procedure called cytoreduction to reduce the size of a tumor. This debulking increases the sensitivity of the tumor and decreases the number of necessary treatment cycles. Following cytoreduction and chemotherapy, a second-look procedure may be necessary to determine if the area is cancer-free.

An advantage to second-look surgery following cancer treatment is that if cancer is found, it may be removed during the procedure in some patients. In other cases, if a tumor cannot be entirely removed, the surgeon can debulk the tumor and improve the patient's chances of responding to another cycle of chemotherapy. However, second-look surgery cannot definitively prove that a patient is free of cancer; some microscopic cancer cells can persist and begin to grow in other areas of the body. Even if no cancer is found during second-look surgery, the rate of cancer relapse is approximately 25%.

Pelvic disease

Second-look surgery may benefit patients suffering from a number of different conditions that affect the pelvic organs. Endometriosis is a condition in which the tissue that lines the uterus grows elsewhere in the body, usually in the abdominal cavity, leading to pain and scarring. Endometrial growths may be surgically removed or treated with medications. A second-look procedure may be performed following the initial surgery or course of medication to determine if treatment was successful in reducing the number of growths. Additional growths may be removed at this time.

Second-look surgery may also be performed following the surgical removal of **adhesions** (bands of scar tissue that form in the abdomen following surgery or injury) or uterine fibroids (noncancerous growths of the uterus). If the results are positive, an additional procedure may be performed to remove the adhesions or growths. Patients undergoing treatment for infertility may benefit from a second-look procedure to determine if the cause of infertility has been cured before ceasing therapy.

Abdominal disease

In patients suffering from bleeding from the gastrointestinal (GI) tract, recurrence of bleeding after attempted treatment remains a significant risk; approximately 10%–25% of cases do not respond to initial treatment. Second-look surgery following treatment for GI bleeding may be beneficial in determining if bleeding has recurred and, if necessary, in treating the cause of the bleeding before it becomes more extensive.

Patients suffering from a partial or complete blockage of the intestine are at risk of developing bowel ischemia (death of intestinal tissue due to a lack of oxygen). Initial surgery is most often done to remove the diseased segment of bowel; a second-look procedure is commonly performed to ensure that only healthy tissue remains and that the new intestinal connection (called an anastomosis) is healing properly.

Other conditions

A variety of other conditions can be assessed with second-look surgery. Patients who have undergone surgical repair of torn muscles in the knee might undergo a procedure called second-look arthroscopy to assess whether the repair is healing. A physician may use second-look mastoidoscopy to visualize the middle ear after removal of a cholesteatoma (a benign but destructive growth in the middle ear). A second endoscopic procedure may be performed on a patient who underwent endoscopic treatment for sinusitis (chronic infection of the sinuses) to evaluate the surgical site and remove debris.

Description

Second-look surgery may be performed within hours, days, weeks, or months of the initial procedure or treatment. This time interval depends on the patient's condition and the type of procedure.

Laparotomy

A laparotomy is a large incision through the abdominal wall to visualize and explore the structures inside the abdominal cavity. After placing the patient under **general anesthesia**, the surgeon first makes a large incision through the skin, then through each layer under the skin in the region that the surgeon wishes to explore. This may include the muscle, fascia, and subcutaneous layers. The area will then be assessed for evidence of remaining disease. For example, in the case of second-look laparotomy following treatment for endometriosis, the abdominal organs will be examined for evidence of endometrial growths. In the case of cancer, a "washing" of the abdominal cavity may be performed; sterile fluid is instilled into the abdominal cavity and washed around the organs, then extracted with a syringe. The fluid is then analyzed for the presence of cancerous cells. Biopsies may also be taken of various abdominal tissues and analyzed.

If the surgeon discovers evidence of disease or a failed surgical repair, additional procedures may be performed to remove the disease or repair the dysfunction. For example, if adhesions are encountered during a second-look procedure on an infertile female patient, the surgeon may remove the adhesions at that time. Upon completion of the procedure, the incision is closed.

Laparoscopy

Laparoscopy is a surgical technique that permits a view of the internal abdominal organs without an extensive surgical incision. During laparoscopy, a thin lighted tube called a laparoscope is inserted into the abdominal cavity through a tiny incision. Images taken by the laparoscope are seen on a video monitor connected to the scope. The surgeon may then examine the abdominal cavity, albeit with a more limited operative

KEY TERMS

Adhesion—A band of internal scar tissue that develops after injury or surgery.

Anastomosis (plural, anastomoses)—The surgical connection of two structures, such as blood vessels or sections of the intestine.

Cholesteatoma—A destructive and expanding sac that develops in the middle ear or mastoid process.

Debulking—The removal of part of a malignant tumor in order to make the remainder more sensitive to radiation or chemotherapy.

Endometriosis—The growth of tissue like the lining of a woman's uterus (endometrium) outside the uterus in other parts of the body.

Endoscopy—A surgical technique that uses an endoscope (a thin, lighted, telescope-like instrument) to visualize structures inside the human body.

Infertility—The inability to become pregnant or carry a pregnancy to term.

Ischemia—Inadequate blood supply to an organ or area of tissue due to obstruction of a blood vessel.

Kidney stones—Small solid masses that form in the kidney.

view than with laparotomy. Procedures such as the removal of growths or repair of deformities can be performed by instruments inserted through other small incisions or **trocars** in the abdominal wall. After the procedure is completed, any incisions are closed with stitches or surgical glue products. Surgical glues are also known as wound adhesives or sealants.

Other procedures

Depending on the area of the body in question, other procedures may be used to perform second-look surgery:

- Arthroscopy uses a thin endoscope to visualize the inner space of a joint such as the knee or elbow. Second-look arthroscopy may be used to determine if previous surgery on the joint is healing properly.

- Percutaneous nephrolithotomy (PNL) is a minimally invasive procedure used to remove kidney stones. Second-look PNL may be used to remove fragments of stones that could not be removed during the initial procedure.

- A hysteroscope is an instrument used to visualize and perform procedures on the inner cavity of the uterus.

Second-look hysteroscopy may be used after surgery or medical treatment to treat adhesions or benign growths in the uterus to determine if they have been effectively removed.

- Mastoidectomy is a surgical procedure used to treat cholesteatoma; a second-look procedure is generally performed to ensure that the entire cholesteatoma was removed during the initial procedure.

Resources

BOOKS

Cushner, Fred D., W. Norman Scott, and Giles R. Scuderi, eds. *Surgical Techniques for the Knee.* New York: Thieme, 2005.

Hatch, Kenneth D. *Laparoscopy for Gynecology and Oncology.* Philadelphia: Wolters Kluwer/Lippincott Williams & Wilkins Health, 2008.

Sabel, Michael S., Vernon K. Sondak, and Jeffrey J. Sussman, eds. *Surgical Foundations: Essentials of Surgical Oncology.* Philadelphia: Mosby/Elsevier, 2007.

PERIODICALS

Ahn, J. H., et al. "Second-Look Arthroscopic Findings of 208 Patients after ACL Reconstruction." *Knee Surgery, Sports Traumatology, Arthroscopy* 15 (March 2007): 242–48.

Dell Anna, T., et al. "Systematic Lymphadenectomy in Ovarian Cancer at Second-Look Surgery: A Randomised Clinical Trial." *British Journal of Cancer* 107 (August 21, 2012): 785–92. http://dx.doi.org/10.1038/bjc.2012.336 (accessed September 12 2013).

Marmo, Riccardo, et al. "Outcome of Endoscopic Treatment for Peptic Ulcer Bleeding: Is a Second Look Necessary?" *Gastrointestinal Endoscopy* 57, no. 1 (January 2003): 62–67.

Shenoy, Ashok M., et al. "The Utility of Second Look Microlaryngoscopy after Trans Oral Laser Resection of Laryngeal Cancer." *Indian Journal of Otolaryngology and Head & Neck Surgery* 64, no. 2 (2012): 137–41. http://dx.doi.org/10.1007/s12070-012-0496-7 (accessed September 12, 2013).

Sood, A. K. "Second-Look Laparotomy for Ovarian Germ Cell Tumors: To Do or Not to Do?" *Journal of Postgraduate Medicine* 52 (October–December 2006): 246–47.

Yanar, H., et al. "Planned Second-Look Laparoscopy in the Management of Acute Mesenteric Ischemia." *World Journal of Gastroenterology* 13 (June 28, 2007): 3350–353.

WEBSITES

Horlbeck, Drew. "Middle Ear Endoscopy." Medscape Reference. http://emedicine.medscape.com/article/860570-overview (accessed September 12, 2013).

Murphy, Kate. "Second Look Surgery for Peritoneal Carcinomatosis." FightColorectalCancer.org. http://fightcolorectalcancer.org/uncategorized/2011/05/second_look_surgery_for_peritoneal_carcinomatosis (accessed September 12, 2013).

ORGANIZATIONS

American College of Surgeons, 633 N. Saint Clair St., Chicago, IL 60611-3211, (312) 202-5000, (800) 621-4111, Fax: (312) 202-5001, postmaster@facs.org, http://www.facs.org.

Society of Surgical Oncology, 9525 W. Bryn Mawr Ave., Ste. 870, Rosemont, IL 60018, (847) 427-1400, info@surgonc.org, http://surgonc.org.

Stephanie Dionne Sherk
Rebecca Frey, PhD

Sedation, conscious

Definition

Conscious sedation, produced by the administration of certain medications, is an altered level of consciousness that still allows a patient to respond to physical stimulation and verbal commands, and to maintain an unassisted airway.

Purpose

The purpose of conscious sedation is to produce a state of relaxation and/or pain relief by using benzodiazepine-type and narcotic medications to facilitate a procedure such as a biopsy, radiologic imaging study, endoscopic procedure, radiation therapy, or **bone marrow aspiration**.

Description

Sedation is used inside or outside the **operating room**. Outside the operating suite, medical specialists use sedation to calm and relax their patients.

If the patient is to undergo a minor surgical procedure, screening and assessment of medical conditions that may interfere with conscious sedation must be explored. These potential risk factors include advanced age, history of adverse reactions to the proposed medications, and a past medical history of severe cardiopulmonary (heart/lung) disease. Other than those risk factors, contraindications for conscious sedation include recent ingestion of large food or fluid volumes or a physical class IV or greater.

Once it has been established that the patient would be a good candidate for conscious sedation, just prior to the surgery or procedure, the patient will receive the sedating drug intravenously. A clip-like apparatus will be placed on the patient's finger to monitor oxygen intake during the sedation. This oxygen monitoring is called pulse oximetry and is a valuable, continuous monitor of patient oxygenation.

Dosing of medications that produce conscious sedation is individualized, and the medication is administered slowly to gauge a patient's response to the sedative. The two most common medications used to sedate patients for medical procedures are midazolam and fentanyl.

Fentanyl is a medication classified as an opioid narcotic analgesic (pain reliever) that is 50 to 100 times more potent than morphine. Given intravenously, the onset of action of fentanyl is almost immediate, and peak analgesia occurs within 10 to 15 minutes. A single dose of fentanyl given intravenously can produce good analgesia for only 20 to 45 minutes for most patients because the drug's distribution shifts from the brain (central nervous system) to peripheral tissues. The key to correct dosage is titration, or giving the medication in small amounts until the desired patient response is achieved.

Midazolam is a medication classified as a short-acting benzodiazepine (sedative) that depresses the central nervous system. Midazolam is ineffective for pain and has no analgesic effect during conscious sedation. The drug is a primary choice for conscious sedation because midazolam causes patients to have no recollection of the medical procedure. In general, midazolam has a fast-acting, short-lived sedative effect when given intravenously, achieving sedation within one to five minutes and peaking within 30 minutes. The effects of midazolam typically last one hour but may persist for six hours (including the amnestic effect). Patients who receive midazolam for conscious sedation should not be allowed to drive home after the procedure.

Monitoring

Patient monitoring during conscious sedation must be performed by a trained and licensed health care professional. This clinician must not be involved in the procedure, but should have primary responsibility of monitoring and attending to the patient. Equipment must be in place and organized for monitoring the patient's blood pressure, pulse, respiratory rate, level of consciousness, and, most important, the oxygen saturation (the measure of oxygen perfusion inside the body) with a **pulse oximeter** (a machine that provides a continuous real-time recording of oxygenation). The oxygen saturation is the most sensitive parameter affected during increased levels of conscious sedation. **Vital signs** and other pertinent recordings must be monitored before the start of the administration of medications, and then at a minimum of every five minutes thereafter until the procedure is completed. After the procedure has been completed, monitoring should continue every 15 minutes for the first hour after the last dose of medication(s) was administered. After the first hour, monitoring can continue as needed. Children who receive sedative medication with a long half-life may require extended observation.

Risks

The American Academy of Pediatrics (AAP) has established safe practice guidelines to manage conscious sedation without an anesthesiologist for minor procedures. These AAP criteria include (1) a full-time licensed clinician (nurse, physician, physician assistant, surgeon assistant, respiratory therapist) who is strictly and exclusively monitoring the patient's breathing, level of consciousness, vital signs, and airway; (2) standard procedures for monitoring vital signs; and (3) immediate availability (on site) of airway equipment, resuscitative medications, suction apparatus, and supplemental oxygen delivery systems.

If adverse reactions occur while using fentanyl, the antidote is a drug called naloxone. It provides rapid reversal of fentanyl's narcotic effect. The incidence of oversedation or decreased respiration is low using fentanyl if the medication is carefully titrated.

Health care team roles

Conscious sedation is administered by medical or pediatric specialists performing a procedure that may be diagnostic and/or therapeutic. It may be used in a hospital, outpatient care facility, or doctor's office.

Resources

BOOKS

Kliegman, Robert M., et al. *Nelson Textbook of Pediatrics.* 19th ed. Philadelphia: Saunders/Elsevier, 2011.

PERIODICALS

Jones, Dean R., Peter Salgo, and Joseph Meltzer. "Conscious Sedation for Minor Procedures in Adults." *New England Journal of Medicine* 364 (June 23, 2011): e54. http://dx.doi.org/10.1056/NEJMvcm0800732 (accessed October 17, 2013).

OTHER

American Academy of Pediatrics and the American Academy of Pediatric Dentistry. "Guidelines for Monitoring and Management of Pediatric Patients during and after Sedation for Diagnostic and Therapeutic Procedures." *Clinical Guidelines Reference Manual* 35, no. 6 (2011). http://www.aapd.org/media/Policies_Guidelines/G_Sedation.pdf (accessed October 17, 2013).

Council for Public Interest in Anesthesia. *Conscious Sedation: What Patients Should Expect.* American Association of Nurse Anesthetists. http://www.aana.com/forpatients/Documents/sedation_brochure03.pdf (accessed October 17, 2013).

WEBSITES

A.D.A.M. Medical Encyclopedia. "Conscious Sedation for Surgical Procedures." MedlinePlus. http://www.nlm.nih.gov/medlineplus/ency/article/007409.htm (accessed October 17, 2013).

Society of Gastroenterology Nurses and Associates. "Sedation Levels & Definitions." http://www.sgna.org/issues/sedationfactsorg/sedationadministration/sedationlevels.aspx (accessed October 17, 2013).

ORGANIZATIONS

American Association of Nurse Anesthetists (AANA), 222 S. Prospect Ave., Park Ridge, IL 60068-4001, (847) 692-7050, (855) 526-2262, Fax: (847) 692-6968, info@aana.com, http://www.aana.com.

Laith Farid Gulli, MD, MS
Alfredo Mori, MBBS
Renee Laux, MS

Sedimentation rate

Definition

The sedimentation rate (or erythrocyte sedimentation rate) is a test that measures the degree of inflammation occurring in the body. Inflammation is the sum total of the body's reaction to infection, allergy, irritation, malignancy (cancer), or injury. The test is neither specific to a particular type of disease or condition, nor does it identify what tissues or organs are inflamed. In other words, while the sedimentation rate is a useful test to verify an impression of the possible presence of a particular illness, it cannot stand alone as a definitive diagnostic tool. The patient's history and symptoms must be correlated with the sedimentation rate and other laboratory tests in order for physicians to arrive at a clinical diagnosis.

The sedimentation rate is literally a measure of the distance that red blood cells (erythrocytes) fall through a test tube filled with blood in an hour's time. This process leaves clear plasma, devoid of red blood cells, at the top of the tube. When there is an inflammatory process occurring in the body, the body produces a variety of proteins that stick to red blood cells. These protein-red blood cell complexes are heavier than unaffected red blood cells, allowing them to fall more quickly and farther through the blood in the test tube. As a result, when inflammation is present in the body, the red blood cells drop through the test tube more quickly, and more of them accumulate at a lower part of the test tube, resulting in a higher sedimentation rate.

Purpose

A sedimentation rate test is usually done when an individual is having symptoms compatible with an inflammatory disorder, particularly polymyalgia rheumatica and temporal arteritis. Symptoms that might prompt a practitioner to order a sedimentation rate include unexplained headache, joint pain or stiffness, anemia, unintentional weight loss, fevers, and severe fatigue. The sedimentation rate is also frequently used to monitor a disease process that has already been diagnosed, such as Hodgkin's lymphoma, or autoimmune disorders such as rheumatoid arthritis or systemic lupus erythematosus. It is also performed to see how well a treatment is working.

Precautions

The sedimentation rate is not diagnostic, which means getting a specific result does not definitively confirm the presence of a particular disease. Instead, the test is used to correlate with the clinical picture, meaning the history and the symptoms that an individual is experiencing.

Description

This test requires blood to be drawn from a vein (usually one in the forearm), generally by a nurse or phlebotomist (an individual who has been trained to draw blood). A tourniquet is applied to the arm above the area where the needle stick will be performed. The site of the needle stick is cleaned with antiseptic, and the needle is inserted. The blood is collected in vacuum tubes. After collection, the needle is withdrawn, and pressure is kept

---

KEY TERMS

Autoimmune disorder—A condition in which the body's immune system is accidentally attacking tissues or organs of the body, causing injury and disease.

Inflammation—Pain, swelling, redness, and heat that often occur when tissues of the body are injured, infected, or irritated in some way.

Lupus—A chronic inflammatory disease that is caused by autoimmunity. Patients with lupus have antibodies that target their own body tissues. Lupus can cause disease of the skin, heart, lungs, kidneys, joints, and nervous system. The cause of lupus is unknown but is hereditary.

Malignancy—Conditions that are cancerous, meaning that they produce abnormal cells capable of invading and destroying other local and distant tissues.

Polymyalgia rheumatica—A condition with symptoms of achiness and stiffness, primarily striking older adults.

Red blood cells (erythrocytes)—The blood cells that carry oxygen. Red cells contain hemoglobin, which permits them to transport oxygen (and carbon dioxide). Hemoglobin, aside from being a transport molecule, is a pigment. It gives the cells their red color (and their name).

Temporal arteritis—A condition in which inflammation of the blood vessels that supply the head and neck result in severe, chronic headache, particularly over one temple, as well as fever, weight loss, and severe fatigue.

---

on the blood draw site to stop any bleeding and decrease bruising. A bandage is then applied.

Preparation

There are no restrictions on diet or physical activity, either before or after the blood test.

Aftercare

As with any blood test, discomfort, bruising, and/or a very small amount of bleeding is common at the puncture site. Immediately after the needle is withdrawn, it is helpful to put pressure on the puncture site until the bleeding has stopped. This decreases the chance of significant bruising. Warm packs may relieve minor discomfort. Some individuals may feel briefly woozy after a blood test, and they should be encouraged to lie down and rest until they feel better.

Risks

Basic blood tests, such as sedimentation testing, do not carry any significant risks, other than slight bruising and the chance of brief dizziness.

Results

The normal sedimentation rate range in men is 0-15 mm/hr. The normal sedimentation rate range in women is 0-20 mm/hr. The normal sedimentation rate range in children is 0-10 mm/hr. The normal sedimentation rate range in newborn babies is 0-2 mm/hr. Women normally have higher sedimentation rates than men. People over the age of 50 years also have higher normal sedimentation rates than do younger individuals. Other factors that may increase the sedimentation rate without suggesting the presence of disease include obesity and pregnancy.

An elevated sedimentation rate can be caused by a number of conditions, including an episode of crisis in sickle cell disease, osteomyelitis, stroke, prostate cancer, coronary artery disease, rheumatoid arthritis, chronic infections, certain cancers (including Hodgkin's disease and renal cell carcinoma), ankylosing spondylitis, thyroid disease, temporal arteritis, scleroderma, polyarteritis nodosa, systemic lupus erythematosus, infections (appendicitis, osteomyelitis, pelvic inflammatory disease, pneumonia), and Kawasaki disease in children.

An extremely elevated sedimentation rate can be caused by multiple myeloma and polymyalgia rheumatica.

An abnormally low sedimentation rate can be caused by sickle cell anemia (not during painful crisis), use of steroid medications, polycythemia, or high serum glucose.

Resources

BOOKS

Fischbach, Francis, and Marshall B. Dunning III, eds. *A Manual of Laboratory and Diagnostic Tests.* 8th ed. Philadelphia: Lippincott Williams and Wilkins, 2009.

Goldman, Lee, and Andrew I. Schafer, eds. *Goldman's Cecil Medicine.* 24th ed. Philadelphia: Saunders, 2011.

Kushner, I., and S. P. Ballou. "Acute-Phase Reactants and the Concept of Inflammation." In *Kelley's Textbook of Rheumatology,* 8th ed. Edited by G. S. Firestein, et al. Philadelphia: Saunders/Elsevier, 2009.

Warner, E. A., et al. "Common Laboratory Tests." In *Textbook of Family Medicine,* edited by R. A. Rakel. 8th ed. Philadelphia: Saunders/Elsevier 2011.

WEBSITES

A.D.A.M. Medical Encyclopedia. "ESR." MedlinePlus. http://www.nlm.nih.gov/medlineplus/ency/article/003638.htm (accessed October 2, 2013).

ORGANIZATIONS

American Association of Clinical Chemistry, 1850 K St. NW, Ste. 625, Washington, DC 20006, http://www.aacc.org.

Rosalyn Carson-DeWitt, MD
Karl Finley

Segmentectomy

Definition

Segmentectomy is the excision (removal) of a portion of any organ or gland. The procedure has several variations and many names, including segmental resection, wide excision, **lumpectomy**, tumorectomy, **quadrantectomy**, and partial **mastectomy**.

Purpose

Segmentectomy is the surgical removal of a defined segment or portion of an organ or gland performed as a treatment. In this case, the purpose is the removal of a cancerous tumor. Common organs that have segments are the breasts, lungs, and liver.

Demographics

Segmentectomies are usually performed on patients with lung, liver, or breast cancer.

Lung cancer is the second most common cancer among both men and women, and is the leading cause of cancer death for both genders. Lung cancer kills more people (approximately 157,000 per year) than cancers of the breast, prostate, colon, and pancreas combined. Almost 90% of all lung cancers are caused by cigarette smoking. Other causes include secondhand smoke and exposure to asbestos and other occupation-related substances.

In each of the racial and ethnic groups, the rates among men are about two to three times greater than the rates among women. Among men, age-adjusted lung cancer incidence rates (per 100,000) range from a low of about 14 among Native Americans to a high of 117 among African Americans, an eight-fold difference. For women, the rates range from approximately 15 per 100,000 among Japanese to nearly 51 among Alaska Natives, approximately a three-fold difference.

Excluding cancers of the skin, breast cancer is the most common form of cancer among women in the United States. The increase in incidence is primarily due to increased screening by **physical examination** and **mammography**. Although breast cancer occurs among both women and men, it is quite rare among men. Caucasian non-Hispanic women have the highest rates of breast cancer, over twice the rate for Hispanic women. There are a low number of cases for Alaska Native, Native American, Korean, and Vietnamese women.

Primary cancers of the liver account for approximately 1.5% of all cancer cases in the United States. About two-thirds of liver cancers are clearly associated with hepatitis B and hepatitis C viral infections and cirrhosis. This type of liver cancer occurs more frequently in men than in women by a ratio of two to one.

Description

When cancer is confined to a segment of an organ, removal of that portion may offer cancer-control results equivalent to those of more extensive operations. This is especially true for breast and liver cancers. For breast and lung cancers, a segmentectomy is often combined with removal of some or all regional lymph nodes.

Treatment options for lung cancer depend on the stage of the cancer (whether it is in the lung only or has spread to other places in the body); tumor size; the type of lung cancer; presence (or lack) of symptoms; and the patient's general health.

A disease in which malignant (cancer) cells form in the tissues of the lung is called non-small cell lung cancer (NSCLC). There are five types of NSCLC; each consists of different types of cancer cells, which grow and spread in different ways. The types of NSCLC are named for the kinds of cells found in the cancer, and how the cells appear when viewed under a microscope.

Segmentectomy may be the treatment of choice for cancerous tumors in the occult, or hidden stage, as well as in stage 0, stage I, or stage II NSCLC. When the site and nature of the primary tumor is defined in occult stage lung cancer, it is generally removed by segmentectomy.

Segmentectomy is the usual treatment for stage 0 cancers of the lung, as they are limited to the layer of tissue that lines air passages, and have not invaded the nearby lung tissue. Chemotherapy or radiation therapy is not normally required.

Segmentectomy is recommended only for treating the smallest stage I cancers and for patients with other medical conditions that make removing part or the entire lobe of the lung (lobectomy) dangerous. If the patient does not have sufficient pulmonary function to tolerate this more extensive operation, a segmentectomy will be performed. Additional chemotherapy after surgery for stage I NSCLC is not routinely recommended. If a patient has serious medical problems, radiation therapy may be the primary treatment.

A cancerous tumor will be surgically removed by segmentectomy or lobectomy in cases of stage II NSCLC. A wedge resection might be done if the patient cannot withstand lobectomy. Sometimes **pneumonectomy** (removal of the entire lung) is needed. Radiation therapy may be used to destroy cancer cells left behind after surgery, especially if malignant cells are present at the edge of the tissue removed by surgery. Some doctors may recommend additional radiation therapy even if the edges of the sample have no detectable cancer cells.

Segmentectomy is under investigation for the treatment of small-cell lung cancers.

Precautions

Because of the need for radiotherapy after segmentectomy, some patients, such as pregnant women and those with syndromes not compatible with radiation treatment, may not be candidates for segmentectomy. As in any surgery, patients should alert their physician about all allergies and any medications they are taking.

Diagnosis

The following methods may be used to help diagnose breast cancer:

- complete physical exam and family medical history
- clinical breast exam
- mammography
- biopsy (incisional, excisional, or needle)
- ultrasonography
- fine-needle aspiration

Tests help to determine whether cancer cells have spread within the lungs or to other parts of the body after a diagnosis of lung cancer. The following tests and procedures may be used in the staging process to diagnose lung cancer:

- complete physical exam, including personal and family medical history
- chest x-ray
- computed tomography (CT) scan
- positron emission tomography (PET) scan
- other radiologic exams
- laboratory tests (tissue, blood, urine, or other substances in the body)
- bronchoscopy

KEY TERMS

Angiogram—An examination of a part of the body by injecting dye into an artery so that the blood vessels show up on an x-ray.

Anterior mediastinotomy—A surgical procedure to look at the organs and tissues between the lungs and between the breastbone and spine for abnormal areas. An incision (cut) is made next to the breastbone and a thin, lighted tube is inserted into the chest. Tissue and lymph node samples may be taken for biopsy.

Biopsy—Removal and examination of tissue, cells, or fluids from the living body.

Bronchoscope—A tubular illuminated instrument used for inspecting or passing instruments into the bronchi.

Chemoprevention—The use of drugs, vitamins, or other substances to reduce the risk of developing cancer or of the cancer returning.

Chemotherapy—Cancer treatment that uses drugs to stop the growth of cancer cells, either by killing the cells or by stopping them from dividing.

Clinical breast exam—An examination of the breast and surrounding tissue by a physician, who is feeling for lumps and looking for other signs of abnormality.

Computed tomography—An x-ray machine linked to a computer that takes a series of detailed

pictures of the organs and blood vessels in the body.

Conservation surgery—Surgery that preserves the aesthetics of the area undergoing an operation.

Excision—To surgically remove.

Excisional biopsy—Procedure in which a surgeon removes all of a lump or suspicious area and an area of healthy tissue around the edges. The tissue is then examined under a microscope to check for cancer cells.

Fine-needle aspiration—A procedure in which a thin needle removes fluid and cells from a breast lump to be examined.

Incisional biopsy—A procedure in which a surgeon cuts out a sample of a lump or suspicious area.

Laser therapy—A cancer treatment that uses a laser beam (a narrow beam of intense light) to kill cancer cells.

Lobectomy—Removal of a section of the lung.

Lymph node biopsy—The removal of all or part of a lymph node to view under a microscope for cancer cells.

Lymph nodes—Small, bean-shaped organs located throughout the lymphatic system. Lymph nodes

---

- mediastinoscopy
- anterior mediastinotomy
- lymph node biopsy

Treatment is determined when the stage of the tumor is known.

Preparation

Routine preoperative preparations, such as not eating or drinking after midnight on the night before surgery, are typically ordered for a segmentectomy. Information about expected outcomes and potential complications is also part of the preparation for this surgery.

Aftercare

After a segmentectomy, patients are usually cautioned against doing moderate lifting for several days. Other activities may be restricted (especially if lymph nodes were removed) according to individual needs. Pain is often enough to limit inappropriate motion, and is generally controlled with medication. If pain medications

are ineffective, the patient should contact the physician, as severe pain may be a sign of a complication requiring medical attention. Women who undergo segmentectomy of the breast are often instructed to wear a well-fitting support bra both day and night for approximately one week after surgery.

The length of the hospital stay depends on the specific surgery performed and the extent of organ or tissue removed, as well as other factors.

Radiation therapy usually begins four to six weeks after surgery, and continues for four to five weeks. The timing of additional therapy is specific to each patient.

Risks

The risks for any surgical procedure requiring anesthesia include reactions to the medications and breathing problems. Bleeding and infection are risks for any surgical procedure. Infection in the area affecting a segmentectomy occurs in only 3%–4% of patients. Pneumonia is also a risk.

store special cells that can trap cancer cells and bacteria traveling through the body.

Magnetic resonance imaging (MRI)—A powerful magnet linked to a computer used to make detailed images of areas inside the body. These pictures are viewed on a monitor and can also be printed.

Mammography—An x-ray of the breast.

Mediastinoscopy—A surgical procedure to look at the organs, tissues, and lymph nodes between the lungs for abnormal areas. An incision (cut) is made at the top of the breastbone and a thin, lighted tube is inserted into the chest. Tissue and lymph node samples may be taken for biopsy.

Needle biopsy—The use of a needle to remove tissue from an area that looks suspicious on a mammogram but cannot be felt. Tissue removed in a needle biopsy goes to a lab to be checked for cancer cells.

Photodynamic therapy—A cancer treatment that uses a drug that is activated by exposure to light. When the drug is exposed to light, the cancer cells are killed.

Positron emission tomography (PET) scan—A procedure to find malignant tumor cells in the body. A

small amount of radionuclide glucose (sugar) is injected into a vein. The PET scanner rotates around the body and makes a picture of where the glucose is being used in the body. Malignant tumor cells show up brighter in the picture because they are more active and take up more glucose than normal cells.

Radiation therapy—A cancer treatment that uses high-energy x-rays or other types of radiation to kill cancer cells.

Radiologic exams—The use of radiation or other imaging methods to find signs of cancer.

Radiosurgery—A method of delivering radiation directly to the tumor. This method does not involve surgery and causes little damage to healthy tissue.

Radiotherapy—The treatment of disease with high-energy radiation, such as x-rays or gamma rays.

Ultrasonography—A procedure using high-frequency sound waves to show whether a lump is a fluid-filled cyst (not cancer) or a solid mass (which may or may not be cancer).

Ultrasound test—A device using sound waves that produce a pattern of echoes as they bounce off internal organs. The echoes create a picture of the organs.

Results

Successful removal of the tumor with no major bleeding or infection at the wound site after surgery is considered a normal outcome.

Morbidity and mortality rates

Although the incidence of breast cancer has been rising in the United States for the past two decades, the mortality rate has remained relatively stable since the 1950s. Mortality rates range from 15% of the incidence rate for Japanese women to 33% of the incidence rate for African American women. The highest age-adjusted mortality occurs among African American women, followed by Caucasian and Hawaiian women.

African American women have the highest mortality rates in the age groups 30–54 years and 55–69 years, followed by Hawaiian and Caucasian non-Hispanic women. The mortality rate for Caucasian women exceeds

that for African American women in the 70 year and older age group.

Five-year survival rates for liver cancer patients are usually less than 10% in the United States. The reported statistics for these cancers often include mortality rates that exceed the incidence rates. The discrepancy occurs when the cause of death is misclassified as "liver cancer" for patients whose cancer originated as a primary tumor in another organ and spread to the liver, becoming a secondary cancer.

For primary liver cancer, non-Hispanic Caucasian men and women have the lowest age-adjusted mortality rates in the United States, roughly one-half that of the African American and Hispanic populations.

Liver cancer mortality rates for Asian American groups are several times higher than that of the Caucasian population. The highest age-adjusted mortality rates for all groups are among the Chinese population. Alaska Native and Native American populations have a very low incidence of liver cancer.

Factors that affect the prognosis (chance of recovery) for lung cancer include:

- stage of the cancer (whether it is in the lung only or has spread to other places in the body)
- tumor size
- type of lung cancer
- presence of symptoms
- shortness of breath during activities
- shortness of breath with less and less activity
- the patient's general health

Current treatments are not a cure for most patients with non-small cell lung cancer. If it returns after treatment, it is called recurrent non-small cell lung cancer. The cancer may reappear in the brain, lung, or other parts of the body. Further treatment is then required.

Alternatives

Other cancer treatments include:

- chemotherapy
- radiation therapy
- radiosurgery
- laser therapy
- photodynamic therapy
- chemoprevention

Using a segmentectomy to remove breast cancers (as a technique that conserves the aesthetic appearance of a breast) is being investigated for large tumors after several cycles of preoperative chemotherapy.

Cancers in some locations (such as where the windpipe divides into the left and right main bronchi) are difficult to remove completely by surgery without also removing an entire lung.

Health care team roles

Segmentectomies are performed in a hospital by a general surgeon, a medical doctor who specializes in surgery. If there are complicating factors, a specialized surgeon may perform the surgery.

Resources

BOOKS

Clavien, Pierre-Alain, et al. *Malignant Liver Tumors: Current and Emerging Therapies.* 3rd ed. Oxford, UK: Wiley-Blackwell, 2010.

Dixon, J. M. *Breast Surgery.* Edinburgh, UK; New York: Saunders/Elsevier, 2014.

PERIODICALS

Rothenberg, Steven S., et al. "Thoracoscopic Segmentectomy for Congenital and Acquired Pulmonary Disease: A Case for Lung-Sparing Surgery." *Journal of Laparoendoscopic & Advanced Surgical Techniques* (September 28, 2013): e-pub ahead of print. http://dx.doi.org/10.1089/lap.2013.0337 (accessed October 4, 2013).

Sawabata, Noriyoshi. "Is Segmentectomy Suitable for Solid-Type Lung Cancer?" *Journal of American Medical Association* 146, no. 3 (2013): 728–29. http://dx.doi.org/10.1016/j.jtcvs.2013.04.019 (accessed October 4, 2013).

Xu, Meiqing, et al. "VATS Left Upper Lobe Posterior Segmentectomy." *Journal of Thoracic Disease* 5, suppl. 3 (2013): S317–18. http://dx.doi.org/10.3978/j.issn.2072-1439.2013.08.54 (accessed October 4, 2013).

WEBSITES

American Cancer Society. "Liver Cancer." http://www.cancer.org/cancer/livercancer (accessed October 4, 2013).

MedlinePlus. "Breast Cancer." U.S. National Library of Medicine, National Institutes of Health. http://www.nlm.nih.gov/medlineplus/breastcancer.html (accessed October 4, 2013).

National Cancer Institute. "Lung Cancer." http://www.cancer.gov/cancertopics/types/lung (accessed October 4, 2013).

ORGANIZATIONS

ABCD (After Breast Cancer Diagnosis), 5775 N. Glen Park Rd., Ste. 201, Glendale, WI 53209, (414) 977-1780, (800) 977-4121, abcdinc@abcdmentor.org, helpline@abcdmentor.org, http://www.abcdbreastcancersupport.org.

American Cancer Society, 250 Williams St. NW, Atlanta, GA 30303, (800) 227-2345, http://www.cancer.org.

National Cancer Institute, 6116 Executive Blvd., Ste. 300, Bethesda, MD 20892-8322, (800) 4-CANCER (422-6237), http://cancer.gov.

National Comprehensive Cancer Network (NCCN), 275 Commerce Dr., Ste. 300, Fort Washington, PA 19034, (215) 690-0300, Fax: (215) 690-0280, http://www.nccn.org.

Laura Ruth, PhD
Crystal H. Kaczkowski, MSc

Selective dorsal rhizotomy *see* **Rhizotomy**
Senna *see* **Laxatives**

Sentinel lymph node biopsy

Definition

Sentinel **lymph node biopsy** (SLNB) is a minimally invasive procedure in which a lymph node near the site of a cancerous tumor is first identified as a sentinel node and then removed for microscopic analysis. SLNB was developed by researchers in several different cancer centers following the discovery that the human lymphatic system can be mapped with radioactive dyes, and that the lymph node(s) closest to a tumor serve to filter and trap cancer cells. These nodes are known as sentinel nodes because they act like sentries to warn doctors that a patient's cancer is spreading.

The first descriptions of sentinel nodes come from studies of penile and testicular cancers done in the 1970s. A technique that uses blue dye to map the lymphatic system was developed in the 1980s and applied to the treatment of melanoma in 1989. The extension of sentinel lymph node biopsy to the treatment of breast cancer began at the John Wayne Cancer Institute in Santa Monica, California, in 1991. Today, SLNB is used in the diagnosis and treatment of many other cancers, including cancers of the head and neck, anus, bladder, lung, and male breast.

Purpose

Sentinel lymph node biopsy has several purposes, including to:

- improve the accuracy of cancer staging, a system used to classify malignant tumors according to the extent of their spread in the body and guide decisions about treatment

- catch the spread of cancer to nearby lymph nodes as early as possible

- define homogeneous patient populations for clinical trials of new cancer treatments

Description

A sentinel lymph node biopsy is done in two stages. In the first part of the procedure, which takes one to two hours, the patient goes to the nuclear medicine department of the hospital for an injection of a radioactive tracer known as technetium-99. A doctor who specializes in nuclear medicine first numbs the area around the tumor with a local anesthetic and then injects the radioactive technetium. He or she usually injects a blue dye as well. The doctor will then use a gamma camera to take pictures of the lymph nodes before surgery. This type of imaging study is called lymphoscintigraphy.

After the lymphoscintigraphy, the patient must wait several hours for the dye and the radioactive material to travel from the tissues around the tumor to the sentinel lymph node. He or she is then taken to the **operating room** and put under **general anesthesia**. Next, the surgeon injects more blue dye into the area around the tumor. The surgeon then uses a hand-held probe connected to a gamma ray counter to scan the area for the radioactive technetium. The sentinel lymph node can be pinpointed by the sound made by the gamma ray counter. The surgeon makes an incision about 0.5 in. long to remove the sentinel node. The blue dye that has been injected helps to verify that the surgeon is removing the right node. The incision is then closed and the tissue is sent to the hospital laboratory for examination.

Precautions

Some cancer patients should not be given an SLNB. They include women with cancer in more than one part of the breast; women who have had previous breast surgery, including **plastic surgery**; women with breast cancer in advanced stages; and women who have had radiation therapy. Melanoma patients who have undergone wide excision (removal of surrounding skin as well as the tumor) of the original skin cancer are also not candidates for an SLNB.

Preparation

Apart from evaluating the patient's fitness for an SLNB, no additional preparation is necessary.

Aftercare

A sentinel lymph node biopsy does not require extensive aftercare. In most cases, the patient goes home after the procedure or after an overnight stay in the hospital.

The surgeon will discuss the laboratory findings with the patient. If the sentinel node was found to contain cancer cells, the surgeon will usually recommend a full axillary lymph node dissection (ALND). This is a more invasive procedure in which a larger number of lymph nodes—usually 12–15—is surgically removed. A drainage tube is placed for two to three weeks, and the patient must undergo physical therapy at home.

Risks

Risks associated with an SLNB include the following:

- mild discomfort after the procedure

- lymphedema (swelling of the arm due to disruption of the lymphatic system after surgery)

Sentinel lymph node biopsy

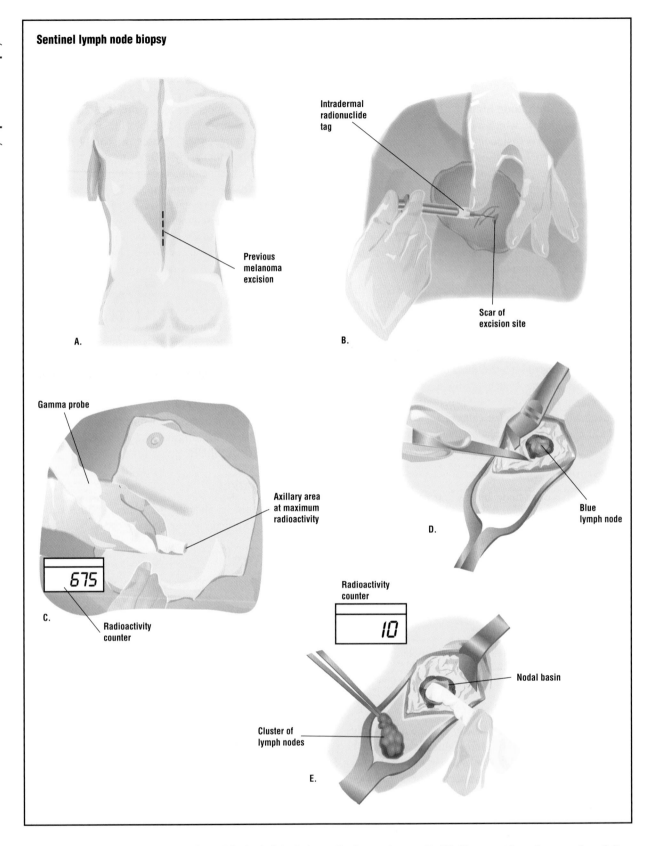

A.

Previous
melanoma
excision

B.

Intradermal
radionuclide
tag

Scar of
excision site

C.

Gamma probe

Axillary area
at maximum
radioactivity

675

Radioactivity
counter

D.

Blue
lymph node

E.

Radioactivity
counter

10

Nodal basin

Cluster of
lymph nodes

In a sentinel lymph node biopsy, radionuclide dye is injected near the known tumor site (B). The area of maximum radioactivity is traced to the sentinel lymph node (C). The area is cut open, and the lymph node is identified by its blue dye (D). After the lymph node is removed, the area is checked for further radioactivity (E). *(Illustration by GGS Information Services. Copyright © Cengage Learning®.)*

KEY TERMS

Biopsy—The removal of a piece of living tissue from the body for diagnostic purposes.

Lymph—A clear yellowish fluid derived from tissue fluid. It is returned to the blood via the lymphatic system.

Lymph nodes—Small masses of tissue located at various points along the course of the lymphatic vessels.

Lymphedema—Swelling of the arm as a result of removal of lymphatic tissue.

Lymphoscintigraphy—A technique for detecting the presence of cancer cells in lymph nodes by using a radioactive tracer.

Prophylactic—Intended to prevent or protect against disease.

Sentinel lymph node—The lymph node(s) closest to a cancerous tumor. They are the first nodes that receive lymphatic drainage from the tissues surrounding the tumor.

Staging—The classification of cancers according to the extent of the tumor.

• damage to the nerves in the area of the biopsy
• temporary discoloration of the skin in the area of the dye injection
• false negative laboratory report

A false negative means that there is cancer in other lymph nodes in spite of the absence of cancer in the sentinel node. False negatives usually result from either poor timing of the dye injection, the way in which the pathologist prepared the tissue for examination, or the existence of previously undiscovered sentinel nodes.

Results

Sentinel lymph node biopsies have a high degree of accuracy, with relatively few false negatives. A negative laboratory report means that there is a greater than 95% chance that the other nearby lymph nodes are also free of cancer.

Morbidity and mortality rates

Compared to axillary lymph node dissection, sentinel lymph node biopsy has a significantly lower rate of complications, including a lower rate of postoperative pain and infection, as well as a lower long-term risk of lymphedema.

QUESTIONS TO ASK YOUR DOCTOR

• Am I a candidate for sentinel lymph node biopsy?
• How many SLNBs have you performed?
• Do you perform this procedure on a regular basis?
• What is your false negative rate?

Alternatives

Breast cancer patients who should not have a sentinel lymph node biopsy usually undergo an axillary lymph node dissection to determine whether their cancer has spread. Melanoma patients who have already had a wide excision of the original melanoma may have nearby lymph nodes removed to prevent the cancer from spreading. This procedure is called a prophylactic lymph node dissection.

Health care team roles

An SLNB is usually performed in a hospital that has a department of nuclear medicine, although it is sometimes done as an outpatient procedure. The radioactive material or dye is injected by a physician who specializes in nuclear medicine. The sentinel lymph node is removed by a surgeon with experience in the technique. It is then analyzed in the hospital laboratory by a pathologist, who is a doctor with special training in studying the effects of disease on body organs and tissues.

The accuracy of a sentinel lymph node biopsy depends greatly on the skill of the surgeon who removes the node. Recent studies indicate that most doctors need to perform 20–30 SLNBs before they achieve an 85% success rate in identifying the sentinel node(s) and 5% or fewer false negatives. They can gain the necessary experience through special residency programs, fellowships, or training protocols. It is vital for patients to ask their surgeon how many SLNBs he or she has performed, as those who do these biopsies on a regular basis generally have a higher degree of accuracy.

Resources

BOOKS

Lentz, Gretchen, et al. *Comprehensive Gynecology*. 5th ed. St. Louis: Mosby/Elsevier, 2012.

Niederhuber, John E., et al. *Abeloff's Clinical Oncology*. 5th ed. Philadelphia: Saunders/Elsevier, 2013.

Pagana, Kathleen Deska, and Timothy J. Pagana. *Mosby's Diagnostic and Laboratory Test Reference*. 11th ed. St. Louis, MO: Mosby/Elsevier, 2013.

PERIODICALS

Yamada, K., et al. "Accuracy and Validity of Sentinel Lymph Node Biopsy for Breast Cancer Using a Photosensitizer: 8-Year Follow-Up." *Lasers in Surgery and Medicine* 45, no. 9 (2013): 558–63. http://dx.doi.org/10.1002/lsm.22183 (accessed October 18, 2013).

WEBSITES

National Cancer Institute. "Sentinel Lymph Node Biopsy." http://www.cancer.gov/cancertopics/factsheet/detection/sentinel-node-biopsy (accessed October 18, 2013).

Whaley, J. Taylor. "Sentinel Node Biopsy." OncoLink. http://www.oncolink.org/treatment/article.cfm?c=249&id=508 (accessed October 18, 2013).

ORGANIZATIONS

American Cancer Society, 250 Williams St. NW, Atlanta, GA 30303, (800) 227-2345, http://www.cancer.org.

National Cancer Institute, 6116 Executive Blvd., Ste. 300, Bethesda, MD 20892-8322, (800) 4-CANCER (422-6237), http://cancer.gov.

Society of Nuclear Medicine and Molecular Imaging, 1850 Samuel Morse Dr., Reston, VA 20190, (703) 708-9000, http://www.snm.org.

Rebecca Frey, PhD

Septoplasty

Definition

Septoplasty is a surgical procedure to correct the shape of the septum of the nose. The goal of this procedure is to correct defects or deformities of the septum.

Purpose

Septoplasty is performed to correct a crooked (deviated) or dislocated septum, often as part of **plastic surgery** of the nose (**rhinoplasty**). The nasal septum has three functions: to support the nose, to regulate air flow, and to support the mucous membranes (mucosa) of the nose. Septoplasty is done to correct the shape of the nose caused by a deformed septum or correct deregulated airflow caused by a deviated septum. Septoplasty is often needed when the patient is having an operation to reduce the size of the nose (reductive rhinoplasty), because this operation usually reduces the amount of breathing space in the nose.

Demographics

About one-third of the population may have some degree of nasal obstruction. Among those with nasal obstruction, about one-fourth have deviated septa.

Description

The nasal septum is the separation between the two nostrils. In adults, the septum is composed partly of cartilage and partly of bone. Septal deviations are either congenital (present from birth) or develop as a result of an injury. Most people with deviated septa do not develop symptoms. It is typically only the most severely deformed septa that produce significant symptoms and require surgical intervention. However, many septoplasties are performed during rhinoplasty procedures, which are most often performed for cosmetic purposes.

Septal deformities can cause nasal airway obstruction. Such airway obstruction can lead to mouth breathing, chronic nasal infections, or obstructive sleep apnea. Septal spurs can produce headaches when these growths lead to increased pressure on the nasal septum. **Polypectomy**, ethmoidectomy, **tumor removal**, and turbinate surgical procedures often include septoplasty. Individuals who have used significant quantities of cocaine over a long period of time often require septoplasty because of alterations in the nasal passage structures.

During surgery, the patient's own cartilage that has been removed can be reused to provide support for the nose if needed. External septum supports are not usually needed. Splints may be needed occasionally to support cartilage when extensive cutting has been done. External splints can be used to support the cartilage for the first few days of healing. Tefla gauze is inserted in the nostril to support the flaps and cartilage and to absorb any bleeding or mucus.

Diagnosis

The primary conditions that may suggest a need for septoplasty include:

- nasal air passage obstruction
- nasal septal deformity
- headaches caused by septal spurs
- chronic and uncontrolled nosebleeds
- chronic sinusitis associated with a deviated septum
- obstructive sleep apnea
- polypectomy (polyp removal)
- tumor excision
- turbinate surgery
- ethmoidectomy (removal of all or part of a small bone on the upper part of the nasal cavity)

Septoplasty

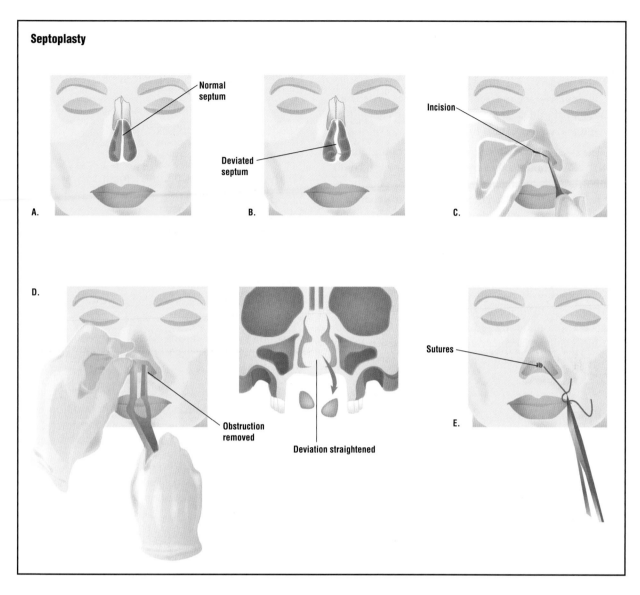

A. Normal septum

B. Deviated septum

C. Incision

D. Obstruction removed

Deviation straightened

E. Sutures

Septoplasty is used to correct a deviated septum (B). First, an incision is made to expose the nasal septum (C). Pieces of septum that are obstructing air flow are removed (D), and the incision is then closed (E). *(Illustration by GGS Information Services. Copyright © Cengage Learning®.)*

Septal deviation is usually diagnosed by direct observation of the nasal passages. In addition, a **computed tomography** (CT) scan of the entire nasal passage is often performed. This scan allows the physician to fully assess the structures and functioning of the area. Additional tests that evaluate the movement of air through the nasal passages may also be performed.

Preparation

Before performing a septoplasty, the surgeon will evaluate the difference in airflow between the two nostrils. In children, this assessment can be done very simply by asking the patient to breathe out slowly on a small mirror held in front of the nose.

As with any other operation under **general anesthesia**, patients are evaluated for any physical conditions that might complicate surgery and for any medications that might affect blood clotting time. If a general anesthetic is used, then the patient is advised not to drink or eat after midnight the night before the surgery. In many cases, septoplasty can be performed on an outpatient basis using **local anesthesia**. Conditions that might preclude a patient from receiving a septoplasty include excessive cocaine abuse, Wegener's granulomatosis, malignant lymphomas, and an excessively large septal perforation.

Aftercare

Patients who receive septoplasty are usually sent home from the hospital later the same day or the morning after the surgery. All **dressings** inside the nose are usually removed before the patient leaves. Aftercare includes a list of detailed instructions for the patient that focus on preventing trauma to the nose.

The head needs to be elevated while resting during the first 24-48 hours after surgery. Patients will have to breathe through the mouth while the nasal packing is still in place. A small amount of bloody discharge is normal, but excessive bleeding should be reported to the physician immediately. **Antibiotics** are usually not prescribed unless the packing is left in place more than 24 hours. Most patients do not suffer significant amounts of pain, but those who do have severe pain are sometimes given narcotic pain relievers. Patients are often advised to place an ice pack on the nose to enhance comfort during the recovery period. Patients who have splint placement usually return seven to ten days after the surgery for examination and splint removal.

Risks

The risks from septoplasty are similar to those from other operations on the face: **postoperative pain** with some bleeding, swelling, bruising, or discoloration. A few patients may have allergic reactions to the anesthetics. The operation in itself, however, is relatively low-risk in that it does not involve major blood vessels or vital organs. Infection is unlikely if proper surgical technique is observed. One of the extremely rare but serious complications of septoplasty is cerebrospinal fluid leak. This complication can be treated with proper nasal packing, bed rest, and antibiotic use. Follow-up surgery may be necessary if the nasal obstruction relapses.

Results

Normal results include improved breathing and airflow through the nostrils, and an acceptable outward shape of the nose. Most patients have significant improvements in symptoms following surgery.

Morbidity and mortality rates

Significant morbidity associated with septoplasty is rare. Mortality is extremely rare and associated with the risks involving anesthesia. This procedure can be performed using local anesthesia on an outpatient basis or under general anesthesia during a short hospital stay.

Cartilage—A tough, elastic connective tissue found in the joints, outer ear, nose, larynx, and other parts of the body.

Obstructive sleep apnea—A temporary cessation of breathing that occurs during sleep and is associated with poor sleep quality.

Polyp—A tumor commonly found in vascular organs such as the nose that is often benign but can become malignant.

Rhinoplasty—Plastic surgery of the nose.

Septum (plural, septa)—The dividing partition in the nose that separates the two nostrils. It is composed of bone and cartilage.

Sinusitis—Inflammation of the sinuses.

Splint—A thin piece of rigid material that is sometimes used during nasal surgery to hold certain structures in place until healing is underway.

Spurs—A sharp horny outgrowth of the skin.

Wegener's granulomatosis—A rare condition that consists of lesions within the respiratory tract.

General anesthesia is associated with a greater mortality rate, but this risk is minimal.

Alternatives

In cases of sinusitis or allergic rhinitis, nasal airway breathing can be improved by using nasal sprays, such as phenylephrine (Neo-Synephrine). Patients with a history of chronic, uncontrolled nasal bleeding should receive conservative therapy that includes nasal packing to identify the source of the bleeding before surgery is contemplated. Those who have been diagnosed with obstructive sleep apnea have a variety of conservative alternatives before surgery is seriously considered. These alternatives include weight loss, changes in sleep posture, and the use of appliances during sleep that enlarge the upper airway.

Health care team roles

Septoplasty is performed by a medical doctor (MD) who has received additional training in surgery. Typically, septoplasty is performed by a board-certified plastic surgeon, a specialist called an otolaryngologist, or a head and neck surgeon. The procedure can be performed in a hospital or in a specialized surgical clinic.

Resources

BOOKS

Brunicardi, F. Charles, et al. *Schwartz's Principles of Surgery.* 10th ed. New York: McGraw-Hill, 2014.

PERIODICALS

Karatas, Duran, et al. "The Contribution of Computed Tomography to Nasal Septoplasty." *Journal of Craniofacial Surgery* 24, no. 5 (2013): 1549–51. http://dx.doi.org/10.1097/SCS.0b013e3182902729 (accessed October 4, 2013).

Steele, T., et al. "Correction of the Severely Deviated Septum: Extracorporeal Septoplasty." *Ear, Nose & Throat Journal* 92, no. 9 (2013): 421–24. http://dx.doi.org/10.1097/SCS.0b013e3182902729 (accessed October 4, 2013).

WEBSITES

A.D.A.M. Medical Encyclopedia. "Septoplasty." MedlinePlus. http://www.nlm.nih.gov/medlineplus/ency/article/003012.htm (accessed October 4, 2013).

Mark Mitchell

▌Serum calcium level

Definition

Calcium is the most prevalent mineral in the body. It is a major component of bones and teeth and is also important in the functioning of the muscles, nervous system, heart, and the blood clotting system. A blood calcium test assesses the total amount of calcium present in the bloodstream.

Purpose

A blood calcium level may be drawn as part of a general metabolic panel during a routine **physical examination**. It may also be ordered if there are concerns regarding arrhythmias of the heart, problems with the muscles or nervous system, kidney stones, pancreatitis, infection, evidence of kidney disease, concerns about intestinal absorption, or problems with blood clotting. The test may also be useful if the patient has signs of too much blood calcium (hypercalcemia) or low blood calcium (hypocalcemia). Signs of hypercalcemia include abnormal tiredness, weakness, decreased appetite, nausea and vomiting, constipation, excessive thirstiness, and increased urination; signs of hypocalcemia include muscle spasms, numbness or a tingling sensation in the hands and feet and around the mouth, and abdominal cramps. Blood calcium levels may also be monitored regularly in patients who have conditions that may cause abnormal calcium levels, such as cancers of the breast, lung, head and neck, kidney, and multiple myeloma; malnutrition (including due to anorexia or other eating disorders); thyroid disease; intestinal disorders; kidney disease; or a history of kidney transplant, as well as patients undergoing treatment with calcium or vitamin D supplements.

Description

The bones are the body's major storage compartment for calcium. About 99% of the body's total calcium is located in bone. In the blood, calcium is either free or bound to the protein albumin. The bound calcium is essentially inactive, whereas the free calcium is considered biologically active. Calcium is obtained through the diet, and requires the presence of a normal quantity of vitamin D for efficient absorption from the intestine into the bloodstream.

Hormones involved in calcium metabolism include parathyroid hormone and calcitonin. Parathyroid hormone is released by the parathyroid glands, which are located behind the thyroid gland in the mid-neck. When blood calcium levels are low, the parathyroid glands are stimulated to produce and release parathyroid hormone. Parathyroid hormone acts to induce the release of calcium from bone. Parathyroid hormone is also active in the kidney, and is involved in keeping calcium from being excreted out of the body. Parathyroid hormone also stimulates the kidney to convert vitamin D into its active form, calcitriol, which is paramount to the intestinal absorption of calcium. Calcitonin is produced by special cells (parafollicular cells) in the thyroid gland. Calcitonin is involved in prompting bone to resorb calcium from the bloodstream.

The calcium test requires blood to be drawn from a vein (usually one in the forearm), generally by a nurse or phlebotomist (an individual who has been trained to draw blood). A tourniquet is applied to the arm above the area where the needle stick will be performed. The site of the needle stick is cleaned with antiseptic, and the needle is inserted. The blood is collected in vacuum tubes. After collection, the needle is withdrawn, and pressure is kept on the blood draw site to stop any bleeding and decrease bruising. A bandage is then applied.

Preparation

Patients who use calcium or vitamin D supplements should stop taking them for the 24 hours prior to their blood test.

Aftercare

As with any blood test, discomfort, bruising, and/or a very small amount of bleeding are common at the puncture site. Immediately after the needle is withdrawn, it is helpful to put pressure on the puncture site until the bleeding has stopped. This decreases the chance of significant bruising. Warm packs may relieve minor discomfort. Some individuals may briefly feel woozy after a blood test, and they should be encouraged to lie down and rest until they feel better.

Risks

Basic blood tests, such as blood calcium levels, do not carry any significant risks, other than slight bruising and the chance of brief dizziness.

Results

The blood calcium level can be determined by measuring the total blood calcium (the calcium that is bound to the protein albumin and the calcium that is free in the blood serum), or by measuring the free (ionized) calcium. Although measuring the total blood calcium is generally easier and usually sufficient in most patients, some patients have conditions that will affect these results; in these patients, it is important to measure the free calcium. Such patients include those who are extremely, critically ill; patients who are getting blood transfusions or large quantities of intravenous fluids or nutrition; patients who will undergo or have recently undergone major surgery; and patients who do not have normal levels of blood protein (albumin).

Normal results for a total blood calcium level in adults range from 0.0–103.5 milligrams per deciliter (mg/dL) or 2.25–2.75 millimoles per liter (mmol/L). Children have higher calcium levels because their bones are in such a high-growth phase. Normal total blood calcium levels in children range from 7.6–10.8 mg/dL or 1.9–2.7 mmol/L. A normal free or ionized calcium level in adults is 4.65–5.28 mg/dL.

High levels

High blood calcium levels may be due to:

• prolonged bed rest

• hyperparathyroidism (overactive parathyroid glands)

KEY TERMS

Calcitonin—A hormone made by the thyroid gland. Calcitonin is involved in regulating levels of calcium and phosphorus in the blood.

Hypercalcemia—High levels of blood calcium.

Hypocalcemia—Low levels of blood calcium.

Pancreatitis—Inflammation of the pancreas.

Parathyroid hormone—A hormone that is secreted by the parathyroid glands. Parathyroid hormone is involved in the regulation of calcium levels in the blood.

• kidney disease

• tuberculosis

• cancer in the bones

• too much calcium, vitamin D, or vitamin A in the diet (e.g., from excessive intake of dairy products, antacids, or supplements)

• dehydration

• sarcoidosis

• Paget's disease

• Addison's disease

• chronic kidney or liver diseases

Low levels

Low blood calcium levels may be due to:

• hypoparathyroidism (underactive parathyroid glands)

• intestinal problems that interfere with appropriate absorption of nutrients

• bone disorders

• kidney disease

• pancreatitis

• low serum albumin (hypoalbuminemia)

• low magnesium

• pregnancy

• advanced age in men

Resources

BOOKS

Brenner, B. M., and F. C. Rector, eds. *Brenner & Rector's The Kidney.* 9th ed. Philadelphia: Saunders/Elsevier, 2012.

Goldman, Lee, and Andrew I. Schafer. *Goldman's Cecil Medicine.* 24th ed. Philadelphia: Saunders/Elsevier, 2012.

McPherson, Richard A., and Matthew R. Pincus, eds. *Henry's Clinical Diagnosis and Management by Laboratory Methods.* 22nd ed. Philadelphia: Saunders/Elsevier, 2011.

PERIODICALS

Hazari, Mohammed Abdul Hannan, et al. "Serum Calcium Level in Hypertension." *North American Journal of Medical Sciences* 4, no. 11 (2012): 569–72. http://dx.doi.org/10.4103/1947-2714.103316 (accessed May 22, 2013).

Uusi-Rasi, Kirsti, Merja U.M. Kärkkäinen, and Christel J.E. Lamberg-Allardt. "Calcium Intake in Health Maintenance— A Systematic Review." *Food and Nutrition Research* 57, article no. 21082 (May 2013). http://dx.doi.org/10.3402/fnr.v57i0.21082 (accessed May 22, 2013).

WEBSITES

A.D.A.M. Medical Encyclopedia. "Calcium—Blood Test." MedlinePlus. http://www.nlm.nih.gov/medlineplus/ency/article/003477.htm (accessed May 22, 2013).

American Association for Clinical Chemistry. "Calcium." Lab Tests Online. http://labtestsonline.org/understanding/analytes/calcium (accessed May 22, 2013).

ORGANIZATIONS

American Association for Clinical Chemistry, 1850 K St. NW, Ste. 625, Washington, DC 20006, (800) 892-1400, Fax: (202) 887-5093, custserv@aacc.org, http://www.aacc.org.

Rosalyn Carson-DeWitt, MD

Serum carbon dioxide level

Definition

Carbon dioxide (CO_2) is the waste product of the respiratory system. It is a gas that is exchanged for oxygen in the body's tissues, transported to the lungs, and then excreted during exhalation. A blood carbon dioxide test assesses the amount of CO_2 in the bloodstream.

Purpose

A blood carbon dioxide level is usually drawn as part of a larger panel of electrolytes. Other measurements in the electrolyte panel include chloride, potassium, and sodium. Sometimes the blood carbon dioxide level is drawn along with an **arterial blood gas**, and the results are correlated to help determine whether the acid-base imbalance is due to respiratory causes or metabolic causes. Respiratory acid-base imbalances are due to an imbalance in the intake of oxygen relative to the output of carbon dioxide. Metabolic acid-base imbalances are due to inappropriate amounts of bicarbonate in the blood. Excess bicarbonate results in metabolic alkalosis; a shortage of bicarbonate results in metabolic acidosis.

Description

Carbon dioxide travels throughout the body in the form of bicarbonate, or HCO_3-. Bicarbonate levels are involved in keeping the body in appropriate acid-base balance (pH level). When the kidneys sense that the body's acid-base balance is shifting toward the acidic, they secrete extra bicarbonate to neutralize the acid. When the kidneys sense that the body's acid-base balance is leaning more toward the alkaline, they reabsorb bicarbonate from the bloodstream to decrease the body's alkalinity.

On a cellular level, bicarbonate works in concert with sodium, chloride, and potassium to attain and maintain appropriate pH balance within cells.

A blood carbon dioxide level reflects the presence of all three forms of carbon dioxide in the blood, including bicarbonate (HCO_3-), carbonic acid (H_2CO_3), and dissolved CO_2. The level of bicarbonate present, therefore, is extrapolated from the overall blood carbon dioxide level; it is not an exact measurement, but rather an estimate based on the total blood carbon dioxide level measured.

The CO_2 test requires blood to be drawn from a vein (usually one in the forearm), generally by a nurse or phlebotomist (an individual who has been trained to draw blood). A tourniquet is applied to the arm above the area where the needle stick will be performed. The site of the needle stick is cleaned with antiseptic, and the needle is inserted. The blood is collected in vacuum tubes. After collection, the needle is withdrawn, and pressure is kept on the blood draw site to stop any bleeding and decrease bruising. A bandage is then applied.

Precautions

Patients who are taking anticoagulant medications should inform their healthcare practitioner, since this may increase their chance of bleeding or bruising after a blood test.

Preparation

There are no restrictions on diet or physical activity, either before or after the blood test.

Aftercare

As with any blood test, discomfort, bruising, and/or a very small amount of bleeding are common at the puncture site. Immediately after the needle is withdrawn, it is helpful to put pressure on the puncture site until the bleeding has stopped. This decreases the chance of significant bruising. Warm packs may relieve minor discomfort. Some individuals may feel slightly woozy after a blood test, and they should be encouraged to lie down and rest until they feel better.

Risks

Basic blood tests, such as blood carbon dioxide levels, do not carry any significant risks, other than slight bruising and the chance of brief dizziness.

Results

In adults, a normal blood carbon dioxide level is 23–29 millimoles per liter (mmol/L). In children, a normal blood carbon dioxide level is 20–28 mmol/L. In infants, a normal blood carbon dioxide level is 13–22 mmol/L.

A number of drugs may affect the results of the test. Blood carbon dioxide levels may be elevated in patients who are using steroid medications, barbiturates, bicarbonates, and loop **diuretics**. Blood carbon dioxide levels may be lower in patients who are using methicillin, nitrofurantoin, tetracycline, thiazide diuretics, and triamterene. It is important that the healthcare provider takes into consideration the effects that these drugs may have on the blood carbon dioxide level.

High levels

High blood carbon dioxide levels may be due to:

- chronic obstructive pulmonary disease
- emphysema
- pneumonia
- Cushing's syndrome
- Conn's syndrome
- alcoholism
- vomiting

Low levels

Low blood carbon dioxide levels may be due to:

- pneumonia
- cirrhosis of the liver
- liver failure
- hyperventilation (fast, shallow breathing)
- diabetes
- kidney failure
- liver failure
- salicylate (aspirin) overdose
- shock states
- chronic diarrhea
- dehydration
- chronic severe malnutrition
- ingestion of toxins such as antifreeze (ethylene glycol) or wood alcohol (methanol)

KEY TERMS

Acid—Any chemical or compound that lowers the pH of a solution below 7.0, meaning that there is a surplus of hydrogen ions dissociated within that solution.

Alkaline—Any chemical or compound that raises the pH of a solution above 7.0, meaning that there is a relative shortage of hydrogen ions dissociated within that solution.

Metabolic—Pertaining to metabolism, the physical and chemical processes of living things that produce energy.

Neutralize—The way the body addresses acidity or alkalinity: adding acid to an alkaline environment to arrive at a neutral pH value, or adding bicarbonate to an acidic environment to arrive at a neutral pH value.

pH—A measure of the acidity or alkalinity of a solution, relative to a standard solution. A neutral pH value is 7.0. An acidic pH value is below 7.0. An alkaline pH value is above 7.0.

Resources

BOOKS

Brenner, B. M., and F. C. Rector, eds. *Brenner & Rector's The Kidney.* 9th ed. Philadelphia: Saunders/Elsevier, 2012.

Goldman, Lee, and Andrew I. Schafer. *Goldman's Cecil Medicine.* 24th ed. Philadelphia: Saunders/Elsevier, 2012.

Mason, Robert J., et al., eds. *Murray & Nadel's Textbook of Respiratory Medicine.* 5th ed. Philadelphia: Saunders/Elsevier, 2010.

McPherson, Richard A., and Matthew R. Pincus, eds. *Henry's Clinical Diagnosis and Management by Laboratory Methods.* 22nd ed. Philadelphia: Saunders/Elsevier, 2011.

WEBSITES

A.D.A.M. Medical Encyclopedia. "CO2 Blood Test." MedlinePlus. http://www.nlm.nih.gov/medlineplus/ency/article/003469.htm (accessed May 22, 2013).

American Association for Clinical Chemistry. "Bicarbonate." Lab Tests Online. http://labtestsonline.org/understanding/analytes/co2 (accessed May 22, 2013).

Lewis, James L. "Overview of Acid-Base Balance." *The Merck Manual Home Health Handbook* (online). http://www.merckmanuals.com/home/hormonal_and_metabolic_disorders/acid-base_balance/overview_of_acid-base_balance.html (accessed May 22, 2013).

ORGANIZATIONS

American Association for Clinical Chemistry, 1850 K St. NW, Ste. 625, Washington, DC 20006, (800) 892-1400, Fax: (202) 887-5093, custserv@aacc.org, http://www.aacc.org.

Rosalyn Carson-DeWitt, MD

Serum chloride level

Definition

Chloride is a mineral that is found throughout the body. Along with other electrolytes (such as sodium, potassium, and carbon dioxide), chloride is involved in maintaining an appropriate fluid balance throughout the body, including an appropriate blood volume; maintaining an stable blood pressure; and equilibrating the pH of the body fluids. For the body to function normally, serum chloride levels have to be maintained at a very narrow range; when chloride levels are too high or too low, it can have serious health consequences. The body keeps its chloride levels in equilibrium by prompting the kidneys to resorb more (when the body needs chloride) or excrete more (when there is excess chloride). When serum chloride levels get too high, the condition is called hyperchloremia. When serum chloride levels get too low, the condition is called hypochloremia.

Purpose

A serum chloride level is usually drawn as part of a larger panel of electrolytes. Other measurements in the electrolyte panel include sodium, potassium, and carbon dioxide. A serum chloride level is usually checked during a routine **physical examination**, as well as to evaluate patients who are experiencing prolonged or severe vomiting and/or diarrhea, fatigue, weakness, confusion, muscle spasms, or respiratory distress. Electrolyte panels are frequently used to diagnose, monitor, or otherwise evaluate patients with kidney disease, liver disease, high blood pressure, heart failure, and other chronic conditions.

Description

This test requires blood to be drawn from a vein (usually one in the forearm), generally by a nurse or phlebotomist (an individual who has been trained to draw blood). A tourniquet is applied to the arm above the area where the needle stick will be performed. The site of the needle stick is cleaned with antiseptic, and the needle is inserted. The blood is collected in vacuum tubes. After collection, the needle is withdrawn, and pressure is kept on the blood draw site to stop any bleeding and decrease bruising. A bandage is then applied.

Precautions

Serum chloride levels can be affected by a number of medications. Patients who are on these medications should inform their doctor, so that test results can be interpreted

KEY TERMS

Addison's disease—A disease involving decreased functioning of the adrenal glands.

Antidiuretic hormone (ADH)—Also called vasopressin. A hormone produced by the hypothalamus and stored in and excreted by the pituitary gland. ADH acts on the kidneys to reduce the flow of urine, increasing total body fluid. When too much ADH is produced, resulting in the body retaining fluid, the sodium concentration becomes abnormally low.

Cushing's syndrome—A disorder affecting the adrenal glands and their secretion of cortisol.

Diuretic—A medication that increases the flow of urine through the kidneys and out of the body.

Hyperchloremia—Elevated serum chloride levels.

Hypochloremia—Low serum chloride levels.

Metabolic acidosis—A condition in which either too much acid or too little bicarbonate in the body results in a drop in the blood pH (toward acidity).

Metabolic alkalosis—A condition in which either too little acid or too much bicarbonate in the body results in an elevation in the blood pH (toward alkalinity).

Respiratory acidosis—A condition in which abnormal exchange of oxygen and carbon dioxide in the lungs results in too much carbon dioxide being accumulated, and a resultant drop in the blood pH (toward acidity).

Respiratory alkalosis—A condition in which abnormal exchange of oxygen and carbon dioxide in the lungs results in the exhalation of too much carbon dioxide, and a resultant rise in the blood pH (toward alkalinity).

appropriately. Medications that may affect serum chloride levels include steroid medications, **nonsteroidal anti-inflammatory drugs** (such as ibuprofen), estrogen-containing medications, male hormones (androgens), some blood pressure medications, cholesterol-lowering agents (such as cholestyramine), and diuretic medications. Another factor that may skew the results of a serum chloride level involves the patient's level of hydration. When a patient is dehydrated, the serum chloride level will be elevated; when a patient is over-hydrated, the serum chloride level will be artificially lowered.

Patients who are taking anticoagulant medications should inform their healthcare practitioner, since this may increase their chance of bleeding or bruising after a blood test.

Preparation

There are no restrictions on diet or physical activity, either before or after the blood test.

Aftercare

As with any blood test, discomfort, bruising, and/or a very small amount of bleeding is common at the puncture site. Immediately after the needle is withdrawn, it is helpful to put pressure on the puncture site until the bleeding has stopped. This decreases the chance of significant bruising. Warm packs may relieve minor discomfort. Some individuals may feel briefly woozy after a blood test, and they should be encouraged to lie down and rest until they feel better.

Risks

Basic blood tests, such as serum chloride levels, do not carry any significant risks, other than slight bruising and the chance of brief dizziness.

Results

In adults, a normal serum chloride level is 98-106 milliequivalents per liter (mEq/L), or 98-106 millimoles per liter (mmol/L). In children, a normal serum chloride level is 90-110 milliequivalents per liter (mEq/L), or 90-110 millimoles per liter (mmol/L). In newborns, a normal serum chloride level is 96-106 milliequivalents per liter (mEq/L), or 96-106 millimoles per liter (mmol/L). In premature infants, a normal serum chloride level is 95-110 milliequivalents per liter (mEq/L), or 95-110 millimoles per liter (mmol/L).

High levels

High serum chloride levels occur whenever there is low blood sodium (hyponatremia), or may also be due to:

• dehydration (increased loss of body fluid without sufficient replacement)
• hyperventilation
• kidney disease
• excessive consumption of salt
• anemia
• use of carbonic anhydrase inhibitors (glaucoma medications)
• hyperparathyroidism (an overactive parathyroid gland)
• metabolic acidosis
• respiratory alkalosis
• excess bromide

Low levels

Low serum chloride levels may be due to any disorder that causes low blood sodium (hyponatremia), or may be due to:

• Cushing's syndrome
• Addison's disease
• syndrome of inappropriate ADH secretion (SIADH)
• repeated vomiting, or prolonged gastric suction
• chronic diarrhea
• serious burns
• excess sweating
• chronic lung diseases, including emphysema and chronic obstructive pulmonary disorder
• congestive heart failure
• kidney disease
• cystic fibrosis
• respiratory acidosis
• metabolic alkalosis
• overhydration

Resources

BOOKS

Goldman, Lee, and Andrew I. Schafer. *Goldman's Cecil Medicine.* 24th ed. Philadelphia: Saunders/Elsevier, 2012.
McPherson, Richard A., and Matthew R. Pincus, eds. *Henry's Clinical Diagnosis and Management by Laboratory Methods.* 22nd ed. Philadelphia: Saunders/Elsevier, 2011.

WEBSITES

American Association for Clinical Chemistry. "Chloride." Lab Tests Online. http://labtestsonline.org/understanding/analytes/chloride (accessed October 17, 2013).

ORGANIZATIONS

American Association for Clinical Chemistry, 1850 K St. NW, Ste. 625, Washington, DC 20006, (800) 892-1400, Fax: (202) 887-5093, custserv@aacc.org, http://www.aacc.org.

Rosalyn Carson-DeWitt, MD

Serum creatinine level

Definition

Creatinine is actually a chemical waste product that is produced by the muscles. The chemical "creatine" is an important chemical involved in the production of energy needed for muscle contraction. During the course of every day, about 2% of the body's creatine becomes creatinine. Creatinine enters the bloodstream and goes to the kidneys. Healthy kidneys filter out this waste material from the blood. It passes into the urine and out of the body. Unhealthy kidneys are unable to filter out the creatinine from the blood. The creatinine remains circulating in the bloodstream, and levels rise as the muscles continue to produce more and more.

The serum creatinine level is used to predict how the kidneys are functioning. In many cases, the serum creatinine level will begin to rise before a patient is even aware of any symptoms of kidney malfunction. High creatinine levels indicate the need for further investigation into the possibility of kidney failure. If a creatinine level is elevated, then other tests such as blood urea nitrogen (BUN) or urine creatinine will be performed. Calculations involving serum and urine creatinine levels will give the creatinine clearance, a figure that reflects the capacity of the kidneys to filter small molecules out of the bloodstream. Calculations involving the serum creatinine level and the individual's gender, height, weight, and age will allow estimation of the glomerular filtration rate, which can screen for kidney damage and disease.

Serum creatinine level is tied to muscle contraction, therefore, the normal value of an individual's serum creatinine level will be dependent on the individual's size and their overall muscle mass. In general, the normal serum creatinine level for men is higher than the normal serum creatinine level in either women or children. Because athletes tend to have greater muscle mass, their normal creatinine level may be higher than that of non-athletes.

Purpose

A serum creatinine level is usually drawn as part of a larger metabolic panel or screen. Other tests performed in this panel include electrolytes (sodium, potassium, chloride, and carbon dioxide), as well as calcium, glucose, and BUN. A serum creatinine level is usually checked during a routine **physical examination**, as well as to evaluate patients for the presence of kidney disease, to monitor patients who have illnesses or who are taking medications that might affect the functioning of their kidneys, or to make sure that treatment for kidney disease is effective.

Description

This test requires serum to be drawn from a vein (usually one in the forearm), generally by a nurse or phlebotomist (an individual who has been trained to draw serum). A tourniquet is applied to the arm above the area where the needle stick will be performed. The site of the

---

KEY TERMS

Blood urea nitrogen (BUN)—Blood urea nitrogen is a chemical waste product of protein metabolism that circulates in the bloodstream. Healthy kidneys remove urea from the bloodstream and it leaves the body in the urine. When the kidneys are not functioning properly, they are unable to filter the urea out of the blood, and blood urea nitrogen levels become elevated.

Creatine—Creatine is a substance produced by proteins and stored in the muscles. Creatine is a source for energy, allowing muscle contraction to take place. Some creatine is converted to creatinine, and enters the bloodstream, where it is filtered out by healthy kidneys and leaves the body in the urine. When the kidneys are not functioning properly, creatinine levels in the blood become abnormally elevated.

Diabetic nephropathy—Kidney damage or disease brought on by the long-term effects of diabetes.

Glomerulonephritis—A condition in which the filtering structures within the kidneys become damaged, limiting the kidneys' ability to filter waste products from the blood.

Preeclampsia—A condition occurring in pregnancy in which high blood pressure leads to a number of complications, including a decreased ability of the kidneys to appropriately filter wastes from the blood.

Urine creatinine level—A value obtained by testing a 24–hour collection of urine for the amount of creatinine present.

---

needle stick is cleaned with antiseptic, and the needle is inserted. The serum is collected in vacuum tubes. After collection, the needle is withdrawn, and pressure is kept on the serum draw site to stop any bleeding and decrease bruising. A bandage is then applied.

Precautions

Serum creatinine levels can be affected by a number of medications. Patients who are on these medications should inform their doctor, so that test results can be interpreted appropriately. Medications that may affect serum creatinine levels include methyldopa, trimethoprim, vitamin C, cimetidine, certain **diuretics**, and cephalosporin **antibiotics**. Additionally, if the serum creatinine level is going to be used in calculations with the urine creatinine or the BUN levels to evaluate kidney

---

functioning, results may be skewed by the following medications: vitamin C, phenytoin, cephalosporin antibiotics, captopril, aminoglycosides, trimethoprim, cimetidine, quinine, quinidine, procainamide, amphotericin B, steroid medications, and tetracycline antibiotics.

Patients who are taking anticoagulant medications should inform their healthcare practitioner, since this may increase their chance of bleeding or bruising after a blood test.

Preparation

In the 24–48 hours prior to a serum creatinine level, patients should be advised to avoid strenuous **exercise** and to limit the amount of protein they ingest. Creatinine is a waste product of muscle contraction and, therefore, vigorous exercise in the 48 hours prior to a serum creatinine level could alter the results of the test. Similarly, ingesting more than eight ounces of meat (particularly beef) or other protein sources in the 24 hours prior to the serum creatinine level may affect the results.

Aftercare

As with any blood test, discomfort, bruising, and/or a very small amount of bleeding is common at the puncture site. Immediately after the needle is withdrawn, it is helpful to put pressure on the puncture site until the bleeding has stopped. This decreases the chance of significant bruising. Warm packs may relieve minor discomfort. Some individuals may feel briefly woozy after a serum test, and they should be encouraged to lie down and rest until they feel better.

Risks

Basic serum tests, such as serum creatinine levels, do not carry any significant risks, other than slight bruising and the chance of brief dizziness.

Results

In adult men, a normal serum creatinine level is 0.6–1.2 milligrams per deciliter (mg/dL) or 53–106 micromoles/L (mcmol/L). In adult women, a normal serum creatinine level is 0.5–1.1 mg/dL or 44–97 mcmol/L. In teenagers, a normal serum creatinine level is 0.5–1.0 mg/dL. In children, a normal serum creatinine level is 0.3–0.7 mg/dL. In newborn babies, a normal serum creatinine level is 0.3–1.2 mg/dL.

High levels

High serum creatinine levels suggest that the kidneys are suffering from damage or disease. Kidneys can be damaged by severe infections, shock, cancer, or conditions that limit the blood flow reaching the kidneys. High serum creatinine levels can also occur when the urinary tract is blocked, or due to:

• obstruction of the urinary tract from a kidney stone or tumor
• acute tubular necrosis
• diabetic nephropathy
• preeclampsia
• glomerulonephritis
• dehydration
• heart failure
• extreme blood loss
• gout
• muscular dystrophy
• rhabdomyolysis (conditions resulting in the abnormal breakdown of muscle tissue)
• myasthenia gravis
• acromegaly
• gigantism

Low levels

Low serum creatinine levels may be due to:

• abnormally low muscle mass, as may occur from aging or muscle-wasting diseases like muscular dystrophy
• liver disease
• extreme low-protein diets
• pregnancy

Resources

BOOKS

Brenner, B. M., and F. C. Rector, eds. *Brenner & Rector's The Kidney.* 9th ed. Philadelphia: Saunders/Elsevier, 2012.
Goldman, Lee, and Andrew I. Schafer. *Goldman's Cecil Medicine.* 24th ed. Philadelphia: Saunders/Elsevier, 2012.
McPherson, Richard A., and Matthew R. Pincus, eds. *Henry's Clinical Diagnosis and Management by Laboratory Methods.* 22nd ed. Philadelphia: Saunders/Elsevier, 2011.

WEBSITES

American Association for Clinical Chemistry. "Creatinine." Lab Tests Online. http://labtestsonline.org/understanding/analytes/creatinine (accessed October 17, 2013).

ORGANIZATIONS

American Association for Clinical Chemistry, 1850 K St. NW, Ste. 625, Washington, DC 20006, (800) 892-1400, Fax: (202) 887-5093, custserv@aacc.org, http://www.aacc.org.

Rosalyn Carson-DeWitt, MD

Serum electrolyte tests *see* **Electrolyte tests**

Serum glucose level

Definition

The serum glucose or blood sugar level is a measurement of the amount of a particular form of simple sugar in the blood. When carbohydrates are ingested, they are broken down in the intestines into component parts, including sugars such as glucose. Glucose is absorbed from the small intestine into the bloodstream. It circulates throughout the body and is used by all of the body's tissues and organs to generate the energy necessary for their normal functioning. In order for glucose to enter the body's cells, insulin must be present. Insulin is a hormone produced in and excreted by the pancreas. Insulin functions to allow the transport of glucose into the cells of the body and is involved in the body's storage of excess glucose in the form of glycogen or triglycerides.

The blood levels of glucose and insulin are intimately related. When carbohydrates are metabolized after a meal, the blood glucose begins to rise. Under normal circumstances, the pancreas then secretes insulin, in an amount relative to the blood glucose elevation. Between meals, or after heavy exertion, glucose levels may begin to drop below a safe threshold for the body's cells (particular cells of the brain and nervous system). In response to this lowering of blood glucose, the pancreas secretes a different hormone, called glucagon. Glucagon prompts the liver to convert glycogen into glucose, thereby elevating the blood glucose back into a safe range.

Abnormal levels of blood glucose can be life-threatening. High blood glucose is termed hyperglycemia; low blood glucose is termed hypoglycemia. Either of these conditions can result in organ failure, severe brain damage, coma, or death. Diabetes occurs when the pancreas fails to produce normal amounts of insulin, or when it completely stops producing any insulin at all (this is often referred to as insulin-dependent or type I diabetes). Diabetes can also occur when cells of the body become less responsive to the effects of insulin (this is often referred to as insulin-resistant, or type II diabetes). Diabetes causes abnormal perturbations of the serum glucose level. Chronic high levels of serum glucose (which may occur in poorly controlled diabetes) can result in severe damage over time to the heart, the eyes, the kidneys, the circulatory system, and the nervous system. In diabetics, sudden, acute increases in the serum glucose level can result in the condition called diabetic ketoacidosis, in which the extremely high levels of blood glucose lead to a life-threatening illness. Diabetics can also suffer from sudden drops in serum glucose levels; if untreated, glucose deprivation can affect the organs and tissues of the body and may also be life-threatening.

Purpose

A serum glucose level is usually drawn as part of a larger metabolic panel or screen. Other tests performed in this panel include electrolytes (sodium, potassium, chloride, and carbon dioxide), as well as calcium, creatinine, and BUN (blood urea nitrogen). A serum glucose level is usually checked during a routine **physical examination** or may be performed specifically to screen for diabetes, especially when there is a strong family history of diabetes or when an individual has other specific risk factors, such as being overweight.

Serum glucose levels are also an important part of monitoring the health of pregnant women since some women develop gestational diabetes during pregnancy. Untreated, this can result in problems with the baby as well as the mother. Gestational diabetes in early pregnancy can cause birth defects (particularly of the brain and/or heart) and increase the chance of miscarriage. Gestational diabetes in the second and third trimesters can cause the baby to grow very large. The baby's size can result in problems for the mother during labor and delivery. Additionally, once the baby is born, it can suffer sudden hypoglycemia. In utero, the baby will have acclimated to its mother's high serum glucose levels by producing high levels of insulin. After birth, suddenly deprived of that glucose, the baby's relatively high insulin levels can result in severe hypoglycemia.

A serum glucose level may be ordered when there are symptoms suspicious of diabetes, such as excessive thirst and/or hunger, urinary frequency, unintentional weight loss, severe fatigue and weakness, and poor healing. The diagnosis of diabetes requires that a random high serum glucose level be confirmed by a high fasting serum glucose level or by abnormal results of an **oral glucose tolerance test**. Patients who are diabetic may also be required to check their own blood glucose one or more times a day, to make sure that their condition is under good control.

A serum glucose level may be ordered when there are symptoms suspicious of low blood sugar (hypoglycemia), such as shakiness, sweating, anxiety, confusion, dizziness, or fainting.

Description

This test requires serum to be drawn from a vein (usually one in the forearm), generally by a nurse or phlebotomist (an individual who has been trained to draw serum). A tourniquet is applied to the arm above the area where the needle stick will be performed. The site of the needle stick is cleaned with antiseptic, and the needle is inserted. The serum is collected in vacuum tubes. After collection, the needle is withdrawn, and pressure is kept on the serum draw site to stop any bleeding and decrease bruising. A bandage is then applied.

Self-glucose testing is often performed one or more times per day by diabetics themselves. This involves using a special sharp instrument, called a lancet, to prick a finger. Frequently, these lancets are placed in a spring-loaded mechanism to make it easier to accomplish the finger prick. A drop of blood from this finger prick is then put onto a special strip of paper and slipped into a machine called a blood glucose meter. The meter gives a digital readout of the serum glucose level. Alternatively, the drop of blood can be put onto a special strip of test paper that changes color based on the glucose level; this is less accurate than the blood glucose meter.

Precautions

The serum glucose level is highly affected by when an individual has last eaten, therefore, appropriate interpretation of the test results must take this into consideration. Serum glucose levels may be examined under random conditions, after an eight to ten hour fast (referred to as a fasting serum glucose level); two hours after a meal has been completed (referred to as a two-hour post-prandial serum glucose level); or after an individual has been given a standardized amount of a glucose-containing beverage (referred to as an oral glucose tolerance test or OGTT).

Serum glucose levels can be affected by a number of medications. Patients who are on these medications should inform their doctor, so that test results can be interpreted appropriately. Medications that may affect serum glucose levels include birth control pills, high blood pressure medications, phenytoin, furosemide, triamterene, hydrochlorothiazide, niacin, propranolol, and steroid medications. Additionally, the use of alcohol, the use of caffeine, recent illness, infection, or emotional distress may affect test results.

Patients who are taking anticoagulant medications should inform their healthcare practitioner, since this may increase their chance of bleeding or bruising after a blood test.

Preparation

There are no special preparations necessary prior to a random serum glucose level. For a two-hour post-prandial serum glucose level, the individual should be instructed to eat a meal exactly two hours before the blood draw. For a fasting serum glucose level, the individual should ingest nothing other than water for a

---

KEY TERMS

Gestational diabetes—A type of diabetes that occurs during pregnancy. Untreated, it can cause severe complications for the mother and the baby; however, it usually does not lead to long-term diabetes in either the mother or the child.

Glucagon—A hormone produced in the pancreas that is responsible for elevating blood glucose when it falls below a safe level for the body's organs and tissues.

Glucose—A simple sugar that is the product of carbohydrate metabolism. It is the major source of energy for all of the organs and tissues of the body.

Glycogen—The form in which glucose is stored in the body.

Hyperglycemia—Elevated blood glucose levels.

Hypoglycemia—Low blood glucose levels.

Insulin—A hormone produced by the pancreas that is responsible for allowing the body's cells to utilize glucose. The deficiency or absence of insulin is one of the causes of the disease diabetes.

Insulinoma—A tumor within the pancreas that produces insulin, potentially causing the serum glucose level to drop to dangerously low levels.

Ketoacidosis—A potentially life-threatening condition in which abnormally high blood glucose levels result in the blood becoming too acidic.

Pancreas—An organ located near the liver and stomach, responsible for various digestive functions. The pancreas produces insulin and glucagon, hormones that are responsible for maintaining safe blood levels of glucose.

---

minimum of eight hours prior to the blood draw. Diabetics may be asked to delay their morning dose of insulin or oral diabetes medication (oral hypoglycemic agents) prior to the blood draw.

Aftercare

As with any blood test, discomfort, bruising, and/or a very small amount of bleeding is common at the puncture site. Immediately after the needle is withdrawn, it is helpful to put pressure on the puncture site until the bleeding has stopped. This decreases the chance of significant bruising. Warm packs may relieve minor discomfort. Some individuals may feel briefly woozy after a serum test, and they should be encouraged to lie down and rest until they feel better.

Risks

Basic blood tests, such as serum glucose levels, do not carry any significant risks, other than slight bruising and the chance of brief dizziness.

Results

Normal results of a random serum glucose test range from 70–125 milligrams per deciliter (mg/dL). Normal results of a two-hour post-prandial serum glucose level range from 70–145 mg/dL. Normal results of a fasting serum glucose level range from 70–99 mg/dL.

High levels

High serum glucose levels suggest the possibility of diabetes; however, a single high, random serum glucose level is not sufficient for definitively diagnosing diabetes. The American Diabetes Association has specific criteria that must be met in order to diagnose diabetes. They require that results are verified through testing on a minimum of two different days. Levels indicative of diabetes are as follows:

• random serum glucose level of 200 mg/dL in the presence of actual symptoms of diabetes (such as increased thirst and/or hunger, urinary frequency, unintentional weight loss, weakness and fatigue, numbness/tingling in hands and feet, blurred vision, or erection problems)

• fasting serum glucose level of at least 126 mg/dL

• two-hour oral glucose tolerance test of at least 200 mg/dL

Individuals who don't meet the criteria for an actual diagnosis of diabetes but who have a higher-than-normal fasting serum glucose level, also known as an impaired fasting glucose (ranging from 100 mg/dL to 125 mg/dL), have an increased risk of eventually developing diabetes, and should be followed closely. These individuals are considered to have "prediabetes."

Other causes of high serum glucose levels include:

• severe stress

• heart attack

• stroke

• Cushing's syndrome

• steroid medications

• acromegaly (elevated growth hormone)

Low levels

Low serum glucose levels may be due to:

• the presence of an insulinoma (a tumor that secretes insulin)

• Addison's disease

• hypothyroidism (underactive thyroid)

• pituitary gland tumor

• liver disease, including cirrhosis

• kidney disease

• malnutrition

• eating disorders, including anorexia nervosa

• inappropriate doses of medicines used to treat diabetes, such as insulin or oral hypoglycemic agents

Resources

BOOKS

Goldman, Lee, and Andrew I. Schafer. *Goldman's Cecil Medicine.* 24th ed. Philadelphia: Saunders/Elsevier, 2012.

McPherson, Richard A., and Matthew R. Pincus, eds. *Henry's Clinical Diagnosis and Management by Laboratory Methods.* 22nd ed. Philadelphia: Saunders/Elsevier, 2011.

Melmed, Shlomo, et al. *Williams Textbook of Endocrinology.* 12th ed. Philadelphia: Saunders/Elsevier, 2011.

WEBSITES

American Association for Clinical Chemistry. "Glucose." Lab Tests Online. http://labtestsonline.org/understanding/analytes/glucose (accessed October 17, 2013).

American Diabetes Association. "Checking Your Blood Glucose." http://www.diabetes.org/living-with-diabetes/treatment-and-care/blood-glucose-control/checking-your-blood-glucose.html (accessed October 17, 2013).

MedlinePlus. "Blood Sugar." U.S. National Library of Medicine, National Institutes of Health. http://www.nlm.nih.gov/medlineplus/bloodsugar.html (accessed October 17, 2013).

ORGANIZATIONS

American Association for Clinical Chemistry, 1850 K St. NW, Ste. 625, Washington, DC 20006, (800) 892-1400, Fax: (202) 887-5093, custserv@aacc.org, http://www.aacc.org.

American Diabetes Association, 1701 North Beauregard St., Alexandria, VA 22311, (800) DIABETES (342-2383), AskADA@diabetes.org, http://www.diabetes.org.

Rosalyn Carson-DeWitt, MD

Serum lead level

Definition

A blood lead test (BLL) is a test done on a sample of a child or adult's blood to test for exposure to lead in the home or work environment.

Purpose

Screening

A blood lead test is done most often for screening: to see whether a person has been exposed to dangerous levels of lead in their home or workplace. Lead is a soft element classified as a heavy metal. It is plentiful in the earth's crust and has been used by humans since the late Stone Age (around 6500 B.C.) for making jewelry. Later, it was used—most heavily by the ancient Romans—in construction, pottery and other crafts, cosmetics, and metalwork. Lead was favored for such purposes because it has a relatively low melting point and is easy to cast into a desired shape. Unfortunately, none of the ancient civilizations known to have used lead were aware that it is poisonous to humans; there is documented evidence of lead poisoning from ancient China and the Greek city-states as well as the Roman Empire.

Unlike some metallic elements like copper or zinc, which serve as dietary trace minerals, lead serves no known purpose in the human body. In fact, there is no known level of lead that can be considered safe for humans. Although most people's bodies contain low levels of lead simply because it is so widespread in the natural as well as the human-built environment, higher levels of lead are dangerous because this metal is a neurotoxin. Lead is, however, still widely used in the modern world; in the early twentieth century it was a common additive to gasoline to reduce engine knocking; it was used as an alloy in hot metal typesetting; and it was added to house paints to speed up drying, preserve the fresh appearance of the pigments, and increase the paint's resistance to weathering. It was not until 1978 that the United States banned the use of lead-based paints in housing, and not until 1996 that it banned the use of lead as a gasoline additive. Lead is still used to make ceramic glazes, batteries, bullets, stained glass, costume jewelry, some types of artists' oil paints, the plastic that coats electrical cords, some forms of vinyl, some of the components of solar energy panels, the x-ray shields used in dentists' offices and hospitals, and infrared detectors.

Lead enters the human body most often through the mouth or the respiratory tract, when people touch a surface coated with lead dust or soil contaminated by lead and then carry their hands to the mouth; drink water conveyed through lead pipes; or breathe in lead dust during a home or workplace renovation. Parents who work in occupations that involve the use of lead may carry lead dust on their clothes when they leave the workplace and bring it into the home. Less common ways for people to ingest lead include the use of folk medicines made outside the United States that are contaminated with lead; swallowing lead shot, curtain weights, or other small lead objects; drinking fluids stored in pottery made with lead glazes; or inhaling fumes from burning lead-painted wood or battery casings. People are not harmed, however, by simply holding or touching an object made of or containing lead, because lead is not absorbed through the skin.

Once inside the human body, lead rapidly enters the bloodstream and is carried to other organs, but it eventually accumulates in the bones and teeth. Lead remains in blood for several weeks, in soft tissues for several months, and in bone for years. The estimated half-life of lead in human bone is 20–30 years; moreover, bone can reintroduce lead into the bloodstream long after the initial exposure period. Without therapy, lead is removed from the body very slowly, primarily through urine. A smaller amount is excreted through the feces; only very small amounts of lead are removed through sweat, hair, or fingernails.

It is important to keep in mind that a blood lead test measures only the amount of lead in the person's bloodstream at the time the test is performed; it does not measure the total amount of lead in the person's body. The danger that a particular level of lead in the body represents depends on the age and health of the person being tested; the amount of lead he or she is exposed to; and the length of time he or she has been exposed to elevated lead levels. In cases of suspected plumbism (lead poisoning), the doctor must order additional tests, usually microscopic study of the patient's red blood cells and dense lines in the bones visible on x-ray. These lines are called lead lines; in children, they are most visible in the long bones of the legs near the knees.

Diagnosis

A BLL may be performed to diagnose actual cases of plumbism. First, it is possible for people to be harmed by lead in their bodies long before they develop noticeable symptoms. Second, the initial symptoms of lead poisoning are often vague and nonspecific, particularly when people are exposed to low or moderate levels of lead over long periods of time. This type of lead poisoning is called chronic lead poisoning. In adults, early symptoms may include loss of fertility in men; miscarriages or smaller infants in women; depression; difficulties with anger management; abdominal pain, nausea, and diarrhea; insomnia; gradual loss of kidney function; headaches; fatigue; and a strange taste in the mouth. Acute lead poisoning, which is rare in the developed world due to the phasing out of organic lead compounds as gasoline additives, results from short-term exposure to very high levels of lead; it is characterized by muscle pain and weakness, tingling sensations in the extremities, blood in the urine resulting from the rupture of red blood cells, and a metallic taste in the mouth, in addition to the gastrointestinal symptoms of chronic lead poisoning.

Children exposed to lead have a somewhat different symptom profile from adults because their nervous systems are still developing; in addition, their bodies absorb lead more rapidly than adults' bodies. To begin with, children can be exposed to lead before birth, because lead can cross from the mother's circulatory system to the child's bloodstream through the placenta. Children are most likely to develop lead poisoning as toddlers, however, when they begin to actively explore their environments and take in lead by breathing in or tasting lead-contaminated dust or soil. Signs and symptoms of lead poisoning in children include loss of appetite, abdominal pain, vomiting, weight loss, constipation, anemia, kidney failure, irritability, lethargy, learning disabilities, and behavioral problems. These children are also slow to develop such normal childhood behaviors as language skills, and they may suffer permanent intellectual disability.

Monitoring

In addition to screening children or adults for exposure to lead, blood lead testing may also be done to monitor the effectiveness of treatment for lead poisoning or to confirm that a person's blood lead levels are decreasing over time.

Description

Who should be tested for blood lead levels

It is very important to screen children at risk for lead poisoning because they are at greater risk of lifelong damage to health than adults, as their nervous systems are still developing. The American Academy of Pediatrics (AAP) and the Centers for Disease Control and Prevention (CDC) have drawn up the following guidelines for screening infants and children for high blood lead levels:

- Every child eligible for Medicaid, at age 1 and again at 2 years of age.
- Other children at age 2, unless lead contamination of the child's home can be confidently excluded.
- Other children as recommended by the local public health department or the child's pediatrician.
- Children whose parents work with lead as part of their jobs.
- Immigrant, refugee, or foreign-born children of any age entering the United States.

Adults should have their blood tested for lead if they show symptoms of lead poisoning, work in industries where they are exposed to lead, or pursue hobbies that involve the use of lead.

- Industries that involve exposure to high levels of lead include smelting; auto repair; battery manufacturing; construction; bridge reconstruction; cable splicing; mining; steel welding; plumbing; printing; lead plating; firing range instruction or maintenance; and the manufacture of plastics, rubber, jet engines, radiation shields, ammunition, certain types of surgical equipment, fetal heart monitors, and paints and pigments.
- Hobbies that involve the use of lead include ceramics, painting with oil-based pigments containing lead, using solder to make jewelry or stained-glass objects; casting fishing lures or homemade bullets; remodeling older homes; and target shooting on firing ranges.

How the test is performed

There are three ways to obtain a blood sample for testing for lead levels: venipuncture, fingerstick, or heelstick. Venipuncture is the most common way of obtaining a blood sample from adults and older children. In venipuncture, the blood is drawn from a vein on the inside of the arm near the elbow by a phlebotomist or other trained professional through a needle into a vacuum tube. In a fingerstick, the nurse or other health care professional uses a small sharp double-edged needle called a lancet to break through the skin on the patient's fingertip to produce a small quantity of venous blood. The blood is drawn up through a capillary tube in order to be sent to a laboratory for analysis.

The heelstick method is usually used to obtain blood samples from infants because their fingers are too small for the fingerstick method. To perform a heelstick, the infant's skin in the heel area is first cleansed with alcohol. The nurse then uses a lancet in the same way as for a fingerstick, and the blood is withdrawn into a capillary tube. A small bandage may be applied afterward.

Some doctors prefer venipuncture as the most reliable method for obtaining an accurate test result. The reason for this preference is that the patient's skin may be contaminated by lead dust or soil containing lead. If test results from a fingerstick or heelstick test indicate a suspicious level of lead, the doctor will order a second test, with the blood collected by venipuncture.

After the blood sample is collected, it is sent to a laboratory for analysis; results are usually ready within a week.

Preparation

Adults and older children do not require any special preparation for a blood lead test. Younger children may require a simple explanation as to why the test is necessary and some reassurance from the parents that it can be completed quickly. Some health professionals recommend having the child wear a short-sleeved shirt to the doctor's office or clinic to make the blood withdrawal as quick and easy as possible.

Aftercare

Aftercare following venipuncture for an adult blood test consists of the application of pressure, a gauze pad, and adhesive tape to the puncture site. The phlebotomist or other health care professional will instruct the patient to hold the arm straight and upward for a few seconds, continue to apply pressure, and keep the bandage on the site for a few hours after the test.

No special aftercare is needed if the blood is withdrawn by fingerstick or heelstick, although parents may find it necessary to comfort or reassure a child who is upset by the test.

Risks

Risks associated with venipuncture in adults include pain or a stinging sensation when the needle is inserted in the vein, a feeling of lightheadedness or dizziness, a swelling or bruise (hematoma) at the site of the venipuncture, excessive bleeding, and infection.

There is very little risk with a heelstick, although some infants may develop a small bruise at the location where the lancet penetrated the skin.

Results

The interpretation of blood lead level test results is different for adults and children, again because the potential consequences of lead poisoning are much more severe for children than for adults. It is also important to note that the CDC has changed its standards over the years in regard to the blood lead levels considered a reason for concern. The most recent change occurred in 2012, when the CDC lowered the acceptable BLL for children from 10 mcg/dL (micrograms per deciliter) to 5 mcg/dL. The AAP currently defines lead poisoning in children as any level above 10 mcg/dL. The current reference range for an acceptable blood lead level in adults is 25 mcg/dL or lower; the upper acceptable limit for workers exposed to lead is 30 mcg/dL, according to the Occupational Safety and Health Administration (OSHA).

The current CDC recommendations for children with BLLs at or above 10 mcg/dL are as follows:

- 10–14 mcg/dL: Educate the child's parents about the significance of the test results and screen the child again.

KEY TERMS

Chelation therapy—A method for removing lead from the body by administering an agent that binds lead ions in the body, allowing the body to excrete the lead through the urine. The agent most often used is dimercaptosuccinic acid (DMSA), also known as succimer.

Heme—The nonprotein iron-containing pigment that is part of the hemoglobin molecule in red blood cells.

Neurotoxin—Any substance that affects the functioning of the human nervous system, whether mature or developing. In addition to lead, neurotoxins include ethanol (beverage alcohol), nitric oxide, tetanus toxin, and botulinum toxin.

Phlebotomist—A person specially trained to withdraw blood from a vein for testing, research, or transfusion.

Plumbism—Another word for lead poisoning; it is derived from *plumbum*, the Latin word for lead.

Venipuncture—The withdrawal of blood from a patient's vein for purposes of testing or research. The most common procedure used in adults involves the withdrawal of blood from the medial cubital vein near the elbow using a hypodermic needle and a vacuum tube.

Zinc protoporphyrin (ZPP) test—A blood test that can be performed to screen for high blood lead levels by measuring the levels of a compound called zinc protoporphyrin.

- 15–19 mcg/dL: Repeat the screening test and place the child under case management to evaluate the child's environment for lead contamination.
- 20–44 mcg/dL: Place the child under case management and evaluate him or her for signs of lead poisoning.
- 45–69 mcg/dL: Place the child under case management; evaluate him or her for signs of lead poisoning; and begin chelation therapy.
- 70 mcg/dL or higher: A BLL this high in a child is considered a medical emergency; hospitalize the child at once and begin immediate chelation therapy.

There are no nationwide standards for BLLs in adults similar to the CDC's 2012 standards for children. In general, adults should be treated with chelation therapy if they have BLLs above 60 mcg/dL or have developed symptoms of lead poisoning. One of the difficulties with establishing national standards for adults is that some show

QUESTIONS TO ASK YOUR DOCTOR

- Should I have a blood lead test, given that I do not work in an occupation that exposes me to lead?

- I live in an older house. Should I have it tested for lead-based paint? Should my children be screened for exposure to lead?

- How can I tell whether I have early symptoms of lead poisoning?

- Have you ever treated a child or adult for lead poisoning?

signs of lead poisoning at much lower BLLs than others. Some adults show evidence of lead poisoning when the BLL reaches 25 mcg/dL, but most adults are more likely to show symptoms only above 50–60 mcg/dL. Above 80 mcg/dL, adults will typically develop anemia and severe abdominal cramping; above 100 mcg/dL, most adults will develop brain swelling, severe headaches, delirium, coma, and seizures. It is extremely rare for an adult to have a BLL above 100 mcg/dL and be asymptomatic.

Alternatives

As noted above, x-rays of the long bones and microscopic examination of the patient's red blood cells may be used to confirm the results of a blood lead level test.

Another blood test that can be used to screen adults for elevated blood lead levels is the zinc protoporphyrin or ZPP test. Zinc protoporphyrin is a compound formed in red blood cells when the production of heme is hindered either by the presence of lead in the blood or by a lack of iron. Instead of incorporating a ferrous ion to form heme, the precursor compound of heme incorporates a zinc ion to form ZPP. A high level of ZPP in the blood, therefore, indicates either lead poisoning or low iron levels.

Health care team roles

A blood sample for testing may be taken in a doctor's office, outpatient clinic, or diagnostic testing facility. The blood may be taken by a doctor, nurse, physician assistant, or phlebotomist.

Resources

BOOKS

Chernecky, Cynthia C., and Barbara J. Berger. *Laboratory Tests and Diagnostic Procedures*, 6th ed. St. Louis, MO: Elsevier, 2013.

Lieseke, Constance L., and Elizabeth A. Zeibig. *Essentials of Medical Laboratory Practice*. Philadelphia: F.A. Davis Co., 2012.

Reddy, Vishnu, Marisa B. Marques, and George A. Fritsma. *Quick Guide to Hematology Testing*, 2nd ed. Washington, DC: American Association for Clinical Chemistry, Inc., 2013.

PERIODICALS

Centers for Disease Control and Prevention (CDC). "Blood Lead Levels in Children Aged 1–5 Years—United States, 1999–2010." *Morbidity and Mortality Weekly Report* 62 (April 5, 2013): 245–248.

Centers for Disease Control and Prevention (CDC). "Take-home Lead Exposure among Children with Relatives Employed at a Battery Recycling Facility—Puerto Rico, 2011." *Morbidity and Mortality Weekly Report* 61 (November 30, 2012): 967–970.

McCloskey, L.J., et al. "Decreasing the Cutoff for Elevated Blood Lead (EBL) Can Decrease the Screening Sensitivity for EBL." *American Journal of Clinical Pathology* 139 (March 2013): 360–367.

McLaine, P., et al. "Elevated Blood Lead Levels and Reading Readiness at the Start of Kindergarten." *Pediatrics* 131 (June 2013): 1081–1089.

Schmidt, C.W. "Unsafe Harbor? Elevated Blood Lead Levels in Refugee Children." *Environmental Health Perspectives* 121 (June 2013): a190–a195.

Taylor, M.P., et al. "Environmental Lead Exposure Risks Associated with Children's Outdoor Playgrounds." *Environmental Pollution* 178 (July 2013): 447–454.

Zhang, N., et al. "Early Childhood Lead Exposure and Academic Achievement: Evidence from Detroit Public Schools, 2008–2010." *American Journal of Public Health* 103 (March 2013): e72–e77.

WEBSITES

American Academy of Pediatrics (AAP). "Blood Lead Levels in Children: What Parents Need to Know." http://www.healthychildren.org/English/safety-prevention/all-around/Pages/Blood-Lead-Levels-in-Children-What-Parents-Need-to-Know.aspx (accessed July 1, 2013).

American Association for Clinical Chemistry (AACC) Lab Tests Online. "Lead." http://labtestsonline.org/understanding/analytes/lead/tab/glance (accessed July 1, 2013).

Centers for Disease Control and Prevention (CDC). "New Blood Lead Level Information." http://www.cdc.gov/nceh/lead/ACCLPP/blood_lead_levels.htm (accessed July 1, 2013).

MedlinePlus. "Lead Levels—Blood." http://www.nlm.nih.gov/medlineplus/ency/article/003360.htm (accessed July 1, 2013).

Medscape Reference. "Lead Toxicity." http://emedicine.medscape.com/article/1174752-overview (accessed July 1, 2013).

National Institute of Environmental Health Sciences (NIEHS). "Lead and Your Health." http://www.niehs.nih.gov/health/materials/niehs_lead_and_your_health_508.pdf (accessed July 1, 2013).

Nemours Foundation. "Blood Test: Lead." http://kidshealth.org/parent/system/medical/test_lead.html (accessed July 1, 2013).

Occupational Safety and Health Administration (OSHA). "Lead." http://www.osha.gov/SLTC/lead (accessed July 1, 2013).

WebMD Children's Health. "Lead." http://children.webmd.com/lead-test (accessed July 1, 2013).

ORGANIZATIONS

American Academy of Pediatrics (AAP), 141 Northwest Point Boulevard, Elk Grove Village, IL 60007-1098, (847) 434-4000, Fax: (847) 434-8000, (800) 433-9016, http://www.aap.org/en-us/Pages/Default.aspx.

American Association for Clinical Chemistry (AACC), 1850 K St. NW, Ste. 625, Washington, DC United States 20006, (800) 892-1400, Fax: (202) 887-5093, http://www.aacc.org/Pages/default.aspx.

Centers for Disease Control and Prevention (CDC), 1600 Clifton Rd., Atlanta, GA 30333, (800) CDC-INFO (232-4636), http://www.cdc.gov/cdc-info/requestform.html, http://www.cdc.gov.

National Institute of Environmental Health Sciences (NIEHS), PO Box 12233, MD K3-16, Research Triangle Park, NC 27709, (919) 541-3345, Fax: (301) 480-2978, webcenter@niehs.nih.gov, http://www.niehs.nih.gov.

Occupational Safety and Health Administration (OSHA), 200 Constitution Avenue, Washington, DC 20210, (800) 321-OSHA (6742), http://www.osha.gov/ecor_form.html, http://www.osha.gov/index.html.

Rebecca J. Frey, PhD

Serum phosphate level

Definition

Phosphate is a mineral that is found in abundance in the body. About 85% of the body's phosphate is in bone. Phosphate is also a major component of teeth. Phosphate is involved in producing and repairing bone, as well as in the functioning of both nerves and muscles. It is used to help produce energy for the cell and in the production of DNA.

A blood phosphate test assesses the total amount of phosphate in the blood.

Purpose

A blood phosphate level is usually drawn as part of a larger panel of electrolytes. Other measurements in the electrolyte panel include calcium, chloride, potassium, and sodium. Blood phosphate level is usually checked when there are concerns about the functioning of a patient's kidneys, to monitor patients who are on renal dialysis, in the presence of bone disease, to diagnose disorders of the parathyroid glands, to monitor intestinal disorders that affect nutrient absorption, and as part of the monitoring process for diabetic ketoacidosis.

Description

Calcium and phosphate are both present in the blood, but in inverse proportions. In other words, higher blood calcium levels result in lower blood phosphate levels; lower blood calcium levels result in higher blood phosphate levels. Excess phosphate in the blood, beyond what is needed for proper functioning, is processed by the kidneys and excreted in the urine.

Phosphate is acquired through the diet, in foods such as yeast, beans, lentils, grains, peanuts, and almonds. As with calcium, vitamin D is required for the proper absorption of phosphate. Excess phosphate in the body is excreted through the urine and the stool.

The phosphate test requires blood to be drawn from a vein (usually one in the forearm), generally by a nurse or phlebotomist (an individual who has been trained to draw blood). A tourniquet is applied to the arm above the area where the needle stick will be performed. The site of the needle stick is cleaned with antiseptic, and the needle is inserted. The blood is collected in vacuum tubes. After collection, the needle is withdrawn, and pressure is kept on the blood draw site to stop any bleeding and decrease bruising. A bandage is then applied.

Precautions

The test results can be affected by alcohol and by some medications, such as steroids, androgen hormones, vitamin D supplements, enemas containing phosphate, antacids containing aluminum, insulin, acetazolamide, epinephrine, or large quantities of glucose. Patients who are taking anticoagulant medications should inform their healthcare practitioner, since this may increase their chance of bleeding or bruising after a blood test.

Preparation

There are no restrictions on diet or physical activity either before or after the blood test.

Aftercare

As with any blood test, discomfort, bruising, and/or a very small amount of bleeding are common at the puncture site. Immediately after the needle is withdrawn, it is helpful to put pressure on the puncture site until the bleeding has stopped. This decreases the chance of significant bruising. Warm packs may relieve minor discomfort. Some individuals may feel briefly woozy after a blood test, and they should be encouraged to lie down and rest until they feel better.

Risks

The test does not carry any significant risks, other than slight bruising and the chance of brief dizziness.

Results

In adults, a normal blood phosphate level is 3.0–4.5 milligrams per deciliter (mg/dL) or 0.97–1.45 millimoles per liter (mmol/L). Children and infants normally have higher blood phosphate levels because their bodies are in a phase involving rapid bone growth. In children, a normal blood phosphate level is 4.5–6.5 mg/dL or 1.45–2.10 mmol/L. In infants, a normal blood phosphate level is 4.3–9.3 mg/dL or 1.4–3.0 mmol/L.

High levels (hyperphosphatemia)

High blood phosphate levels may be due to:

- kidney disease
- poorly functioning parathyroid glands (hypoparathyroidism)
- acromegaly (a condition in which the pituitary is overactive, and secretes too much growth hormone)
- rhabdomyolysis (a condition in which muscle is broken down, releasing phosphate, among other substances)
- bone diseases, including recently fractured bones
- diabetic ketoacidosis (a condition in which the blood glucose becomes extremely elevated)
- excess vitamin D
- shortage of magnesium
- pregnancy

Low levels (hypophosphatemia)

Low blood phosphate levels may be due to:

- overactive parathyroid glands (hyperparathyroidism)
- kidney disease
- liver disease
- malnutrition or outright starvation
- burns
- severe alcoholism
- excess blood calcium (hypercalcemia)
- vitamin D deficiency
- bone disorders, such as osteomalacia (an adult type of rickets in which the bones become softer due to a vitamin D deficiency)
- intestinal disorders that result in poor absorption of nutrients

KEY TERMS

Dialysis—A blood filtration therapy that replaces the function of the kidneys, filtering fluids and waste products out of the bloodstream. There are two types of dialysis treatment: hemodialysis, which uses an artificial kidney, or dialyzer, as a blood filter; and peritoneal dialysis, which uses the patient's abdominal cavity (peritoneum) as a blood filter.

Hyperphosphatemia—Elevated blood phosphate levels.

Hypophosphatemia—Low blood phosphate levels.

Parathyroid—Several small glands located behind the thyroid glands in the mid-neck. The parathyroid glands secrete parathyroid hormone, which is highly involved in the chemical equilibrium of calcium and phosphate throughout the body.

Resources

BOOKS

Brenner, B. M., and F. C. Rector, eds. *Brenner & Rector's The Kidney*. 9th ed. Philadelphia: Saunders/Elsevier, 2012.

Goldman, Lee, and Andrew I. Schafer. *Goldman's Cecil Medicine*. 24th ed. Philadelphia: Saunders/Elsevier, 2012.

McPherson, Richard A., and Matthew R. Pincus, eds. *Henry's Clinical Diagnosis and Management by Laboratory Methods*. 22nd ed. Philadelphia: Saunders/Elsevier, 2011.

WEBSITES

A.D.A.M. Medical Encyclopedia. "Phosphorus—Blood." MedlinePlus. http://www.nlm.nih.gov/medlineplus/ency/article/003478.htm (accessed May 22, 2013).

American Association for Clinical Chemistry. "Phosphorus." Lab Tests Online. http://labtestsonline.org/understanding/analytes/phosphorus (accessed May 22, 2013).

ORGANIZATIONS

American Association for Clinical Chemistry, 1850 K St. NW, Ste. 625, Washington, DC 20006, (800) 892-1400, Fax: (202) 887-5093, custserv@aacc.org, http://www.aacc.org.

Rosalyn Carson-DeWitt, MD

Serum potassium level

Definition

Potassium is a mineral that is found in abundance in the body, primarily within its cells. Only about 2% of the body's total potassium is located outside of the cells. Potassium levels are crucial to the appropriate functioning of all cells, especially nerve and muscle cells. For the body to function normally, blood potassium levels have to be maintained at a very narrow range; when potassium levels are too high or too low, there can be serious health consequences. The body keeps its potassium levels in equilibrium by prompting the kidneys to resorb more (when the body needs potassium) or excrete more (when there is excess potassium). The hormone responsible for stimulating the processing of potassium in the kidneys is called aldosterone. Aldosterone is secreted by the adrenal glands. When blood potassium levels get too high, the condition is called hyperkalemia. When blood potassium levels get too low, the condition is called hypokalemia.

Purpose

A blood potassium level is usually drawn as part of a larger panel of electrolytes. Other measurements in the electrolyte panel include sodium, chloride, and carbon dioxide. A blood potassium level is usually checked during a regular **physical examination**. It may also be performed when there are concerns about the functioning of a patient's kidneys, on patients with high blood pressure (hypertension), to monitor the potassium levels of patients taking medications that affect its equilibrium (such as certain **diuretics**, which cause potassium to be lost in the urine), on patients undergoing dialysis, on patients receiving intravenous fluids or parenteral nutrition, or on patients experiencing symptoms such as unexplained weakness or abnormal heart rhythm (cardiac arrhythmia).

Description

This test requires blood to be drawn from a vein (usually one in the forearm), usually by a nurse or phlebotomist (an individual who has been trained to draw blood). A tourniquet is applied to the arm above the area where the needle stick will be performed. The site of the needle stick is cleaned with antiseptic, and the needle is inserted. The blood is collected in vacuum tubes. After collection, the needle is withdrawn, and pressure is kept on the blood draw site to stop any bleeding and decrease bruising. A bandage is then applied.

Precautions

Blood potassium levels can be affected by a number of medications. Patients who are on these medications should inform their doctor, so that test results can be interpreted appropriately. Medications that increase blood potassium levels include some chemotherapy agents, aminocaproic acid, high blood pressure medications (specifically angiotensin-converting enzyme or ACE inhibitors), certain diuretics (referred to as potassium-sparing or potassium-conserving diuretics), epinephrine, heparin, histamine, isoniazid, mannitol, and succinylcholine. Medications that decrease blood potassium levels include acetazolamide, aminosalicylic acid, amphotericin B, carbenicillin, cisplatin, potassium-wasting diuretics (such as thiazide diuretics and furosemide), insulin, **laxatives**, penicillin G, phenothiazines, salicylates, and sodium polystyrene sulfonate. Other factors that may skew the results of blood potassium level tests include intravenous infusion of fluids containing potassium, as well as intravenous infusion of either glucose-containing solutions or insulin.

Patients who are taking anticoagulant medications should inform their healthcare practitioner since this may increase their chance of bleeding or bruising after a blood test.

Proper technique in drawing the potassium blood level and in handling the sample is crucial to an accurate result. If the patient is clenching and relaxing arm muscles in the arm from which the blood is being drawn, the potassium blood level may be falsely elevated. If the flow of blood into the vacuum tubes is not carefully regulated and the blood flows too quickly or too slowly into the tubes, the blood cells may be damaged due to turbulence. This will cause the blood cells to leak potassium into the sample, falsely elevating the result. Delay in testing the blood at the laboratory will also result in an artificially elevated blood potassium level being reported.

Preparation

There are no restrictions on diet or physical activity, either before or after the blood test.

Aftercare

As with any blood test, discomfort, bruising, and/or a very small amount of bleeding are common at the puncture site. Immediately after the needle is withdrawn, it is helpful to put pressure on the puncture site until the bleeding has stopped. This decreases the chance of significant bruising. Warm packs may relieve minor discomfort. Some individuals may feel woozy after a blood test, and they should be encouraged to lie down and rest until they feel better.

Risks

Basic blood tests, such as blood potassium levels, do not carry any significant risks other than slight bruising and the chance of brief dizziness.

Results

In adults, a normal blood potassium level is 3.5–5.0 milliequivalents per liter (mEq/L) or 3.5–5.0 millimoles per liter (mmol/L). In children, a normal blood potassium level is 3.4–4.7 mEq/L or 3.4–4.7 mmol/L. In infants, a normal blood potassium level is 4.13–5.3 mEq/L or 4.1–5.3 mmol/L. In newborns, a normal blood potassium level is 3.9–5.9 mEq/L or 3.9–5.9 mmol/L.

High levels

High blood potassium levels may be due to:

• kidney disease, either acute or chronic kidney failure
• Addison's disease (a disease in which the adrenal gland is underfunctioning)
• low blood levels of the hormone aldosterone (hypoaldosteronism)
• tissue injury, resulting in the release of potassium into the bloodstream, including trauma, heart attack, and severe burns
• infection
• dehydration
• diabetes
• excess intake of foods containing potassium (in particular, fruits and fruit juices are often high in potassium)
• excess intake of potassium supplements
• medications that elevate potassium, including NSAIDS (ibuprofen); beta blockers (propranolol and atenolol); ACE inhibitors (captopril, enalapril, lisinopril); and diuretics such as triamterene, amiloride, and spironolactone

Low levels

Low blood potassium levels may be due to:

• dehydration
• severe vomiting
• severe diarrhea
• insulin use
• Cushing's syndrome
• cystic fibrosis
• poor nutritional status due to alcoholism, an eating disorder, or other causes of malnutrition
• Bartter syndrome
• too much aldosterone in the blood (hyperaldosteronism)
• diuretic use (thiazide diuretics and furosemide, in particular)
• poor dietary intake of potassium

KEY TERMS

Addison's disease—A condition in which the adrenal glands are not functioning properly. Addison's disease can be caused by a problem in the adrenal glands themselves, or in the pituitary gland (which secretes a hormone that affects the adrenal glands).

Bartter syndrome—An inherited disorder that affects a number of body processes, including the functioning of the part of the kidney that regulates potassium excretion and absorption. People with Bartter's syndrome have abnormally low blood potassium levels (hypokalemia).

Diuretic—A medication that increases the flow of urine through the kidneys and out of the body.

Hyperkalemia—Elevated blood potassium levels.

Hypokalemia—Low blood potassium levels.

NSAIDs—Nonsteroidal anti-inflammatory drugs.

Resources

BOOKS

Goldman, Lee, and Andrew I. Schafer. *Goldman's Cecil Medicine.* 24th ed. Philadelphia: Saunders/Elsevier, 2012.

McPherson, Richard A., and Matthew R. Pincus, eds. *Henry's Clinical Diagnosis and Management by Laboratory Methods.* 22nd ed. Philadelphia: Saunders/Elsevier, 2011.

PERIODICALS

Weaver, Connie M. "Potassium and Health." *Advances in Nutrition* 4, no. 3 (May 2013): 368S–77S. http://dx.doi.org/10.3945/an.112.003533 (accessed May 22, 2013).

WEBSITES

A.D.A.M. Medical Encyclopedia. "Potassium Test." MedlinePlus. http://www.nlm.nih.gov/medlineplus/ency/article/003484.htm (accessed May 22, 2013).

American Association for Clinical Chemistry. "Potassium." Lab Tests Online. http://labtestsonline.org/understanding/analytes/potassium (accessed May 22, 2013).

ORGANIZATIONS

American Association for Clinical Chemistry, 1850 K St. NW, Ste. 625, Washington, DC 20006, (800) 892-1400, Fax: (202) 887-5093, custserv@aacc.org, http://www.aacc.org.

Rosalyn Carson-DeWitt, MD

Serum protein level *see* **Protein components test**

Serum sodium level

Definition

Sodium is a mineral that is found throughout the body and is crucial (along with other electrolytes) to the appropriate balance of fluid in the body. Sodium is primarily found in bodily fluids and blood. For the body to function normally, blood sodium levels have to be maintained at a very narrow range; when sodium levels are too high or too low, serious health consequences can result. The body keeps its sodium levels in equilibrium by prompting the kidneys to resorb more (when the body needs sodium) or excrete more (when there is excess sodium). The hormones responsible for stimulating the processing of sodium in the kidneys include natriuretic peptides, which prompt the kidneys to excrete sodium into the urine and out of the body; aldosterone, which prompts the kidneys to hold onto or resorb sodium; and antidiuretic hormone (ADH), which prompts the retention of fluids in the bloodstream, thus increasing the amount of water in the bloodstream and diluting the blood sodium level. The mechanism of thirst is another important way that blood sodium levels are controlled; as small as a 1% increase in blood sodium level will prompt thirst, which initiates drinking behavior and serves to drop the elevated blood sodium level. When blood sodium levels get too high, the condition is called hypernatremia. When blood sodium levels get too low, the condition is called hyponatremia.

Purpose

A blood sodium level is usually drawn as part of a larger panel of electrolytes. Other measurements in the electrolyte panel include chloride, potassium, and carbon dioxide. Blood sodium level is usually checked during a routine **physical examination**, as well as when there are concerns about the functioning of the patient's kidneys; when the patient has high blood pressure (hypertension); to monitor sodium levels during the use of intravenous fluid therapy; to monitor patients on dialysis; in patients who have symptoms of heart failure or who are known to have heart failure; in patients with liver disease; in patients with lower leg swelling or other fluid accumulation; and in patients with symptoms that could possibly be due to electrolyte imbalance, specifically low blood sodium levels or hyponatremia. These symptoms can include confusion, severe fatigue and weakness, extreme thirst, low urine output, muscle twitching, irritability, or agitation.

Description

The test requires blood to be drawn from a vein (usually one in the forearm), generally by a nurse or phlebotomist (an individual who has been trained to draw blood). A tourniquet is applied to the arm above the area where the needle stick will be performed. The site of the needle stick is cleaned with antiseptic and the needle is inserted. The blood is collected in vacuum tubes. After collection, the needle is withdrawn and pressure is kept on the blood draw site to stop any bleeding and decrease bruising. A bandage is then applied.

Precautions

Blood sodium levels can be affected by a number of medications. Patients who are on these medications should inform their doctor, so that test results can be interpreted appropriately. Medications that increase blood sodium levels include birth control pills, some **antibiotics**, clonidine, steroid medications, anabolic steroid use, cough preparations, **laxatives**, methyldopa, and nonsteroidal anti-inflammatory agents (including ibuprofen). Medications that decrease blood sodium levels include carbamazepine, **diuretics**, sulfonylureas, triamterene, and vasopressin. Other factors that may skew the results include intravenous infusion of fluids containing sodium; excess ingestion of food or beverages containing salt; excess consumption of fluids; use of the hormone aldosterone; and recent severe injury, surgery, or shock.

Patients who are taking anticoagulant medications should inform their healthcare practitioner, since this may increase their chance of bleeding or bruising after a blood test.

Preparation

There are no restrictions on diet or physical activity before or after the blood test.

Aftercare

As with any blood test, discomfort, bruising, and/or a very small amount of bleeding are common at the puncture site. Immediately after the needle is withdrawn, it is helpful to put pressure on the puncture site until the bleeding has stopped. This decreases the chance of significant bruising. Warm packs may relieve minor discomfort. Some individuals may feel woozy for a short time after the blood test, and they should be encouraged to lie down and rest until they feel better.

Risks

Basic blood tests, such as blood sodium levels, do not carry any significant risks other than slight bruising and the chance of brief dizziness.

Results

A normal blood sodium level is 136–145 milli-equivalents per liter (mEq/L), or 136–145 millimoles per liter (mmol/L).

High levels

High blood sodium levels may be due to:

- dehydration (increased loss of body water without sufficient replacement by drinking, which often occurs in febrile illnesses; with severe diarrhea and/or vomiting; or in situations involving heavy exercise in hot weather, resulting in fluid loss through sweating)
- high blood levels of the hormone aldosterone (hyperaldosteronism)
- Cushing's syndrome
- diabetes insipidus (caused by a shortage of antidiuretic hormone)
- diabetic ketoacidosis
- diuretic use
- head injury or brain surgery, particularly if the pituitary gland is affected
- sickle cell anemia
- kidney disease
- medications including lithium, demeclocycline, or diuretics
- ingestion of an extremely high-sodium diet

Low levels

Low blood sodium levels may be due to:

- Addison's disease
- thyroid insufficiency
- severe diarrhea
- diuretic use
- excess sweating
- serious burns
- kidney disease, including those resulting in the loss of protein from the body (nephrotic syndrome)
- cirrhosis of the liver
- cystic fibrosis
- increased retention of water in the body, due to excess consumption of water, heart failure, or cirrhosis of the liver
- poor nutritional status due to alcoholism, an eating disorder, or other causes of malnutrition
- disorders involving the pituitary gland
- certain medications, including chlorpropamide, carbamazepine, vincristine, clofibrate, antipsychotic

medications, aspirin, ibuprofen, synthetic vasopressin, and oxytocin

- too much antidiuretic hormone (also called vasopressin) in the blood (referred to as syndrome of inappropriate antidiuretic hormone or SIADH) can occur due to a wide variety of conditions involving the lung and brain, including brain injury, infections such as meningitis and encephalitis, pneumonia, acute respiratory failure, brain tumors, lung cancer, and psychosis
- any of a number of conditions that stimulate release of ADH from the pituitary, such as pain, stress, exercise, dehydration, increased levels of other blood electrolytes, or low blood sugar levels
- poor dietary intake of sodium (this is extremely rare)

Resources

BOOKS

Goldman, Lee, and Andrew I. Schafer. *Goldman's Cecil Medicine.* 24th ed. Philadelphia: Saunders/Elsevier, 2012.

McPherson, Richard A., and Matthew R. Pincus, eds. *Henry's Clinical Diagnosis and Management by Laboratory Methods.* 22nd ed. Philadelphia: Saunders/Elsevier, 2011.

> **KEY TERMS**
>
> **Addison's disease**—A condition in which the adrenal glands are not functioning properly. Addison's disease can be caused by a problem in the adrenal glands themselves, or in the pituitary gland, which secretes a hormone that affects the adrenal glands.
>
> **Aldosterone**—A hormone secreted by the adrenal glands that prompts the kidneys to hold onto sodium.
>
> **Antidiuretic hormone (ADH)**—Also called vasopressin; a hormone produced by the hypothalamus and stored in and excreted by the pituitary gland. ADH acts on the kidneys to reduce the flow of urine, increasing total body fluid.
>
> **Cushing's syndrome**—A disorder affecting the adrenal glands and their secretion of cortisol.
>
> **Diuretic**—A medication that increases the flow of urine through the kidneys and out of the body.
>
> **Hypernatremia**—Elevated blood sodium levels.
>
> **Hyponatremia**—Low blood sodium levels.
>
> **Natriuretic peptides**—Peptides that prompt the kidneys to excrete sodium into the urine and out of the body.

WEBSITES

A.D.A.M. Medical Encyclopedia. "Sodium—Blood." MedlinePlus. http://www.nlm.nih.gov/medlineplus/ency/article/003481.htm (accessed May 22, 2013).

American Association for Clinical Chemistry. "Sodium." Lab Tests Online. http://labtestsonline.org/understanding/analytes/sodium (accessed May 22, 2013).

ORGANIZATIONS

American Association for Clinical Chemistry, 1850 K St. NW, Ste. 625, Washington, DC 20006, (800) 892-1400, Fax: (202) 887-5093, custserv@aacc.org, http://www.aacc.org.

Rosalyn Carson-DeWitt, MD

Sestamibi scan

Definition

A sestamibi scan is a highly sensitive and highly specific nuclear medicine test used to locate and image an overactive parathyroid gland in a patient with known hyperparathyroidism. Information from the test can help with planning for surgery to remove the overactive gland.

Located in the neck behind the thyroid gland, the four parathyroid glands are pea-sized endocrine glands that are responsible for the production of parathyroid hormone or PTH. PTH is important in the balance of calcium and phosphate throughout the body.

Under normal conditions, low calcium concentrations in the bloodstream prompt the parathyroid gland to put out increased amounts of PTH. PTH acts on several areas of the body. It directs the kidneys to absorb calcium back into the body, rather than flushing it out of the body in the urine. It activates osteoclasts in bone to degrade bone material, releasing calcium for use in the body. It increases the activity of vitamin D, which allows more calcium to be absorbed in the intestine.

Hyperparathyroidism is usually due to the presence of an adenoma, a benign (not cancerous) growth on one or more of the parathyroid glands. A sestamibi scan is used to generate images of the parathyroid glands prior to surgery so that the surgeon knows which of the four glands will require removal. Surgery to remove a parathyroid gland is called a **parathyroidectomy**.

During a sestamibi scan, the patient is given an injection of the radioactive material technetium-99, bound to a tiny protein called sestamibi. Unlike normal parathyroid glands, adenomatous parathyroid glands absorb the radioactive material, permitting visualization and localization of the tumor or tumors on the scan images. This test can be performed in preparation for an operation to remove the parathyroid adenoma, or during the course of such an operation (intraoperatively).

Purpose

Hyperparathyroidism is a condition in which one or more of the parathyroid glands become overactive. Too much bone is broken down, and too much calcium circulates in the bloodstream (termed hypercalcemia). The consequences of this excess bone breakdown and excess circulating calcium include:

- weakness
- fatigue
- depression
- achiness
- decreased appetite
- heartburn
- nausea and vomiting
- constipation
- high blood pressure
- confusion
- difficulty thinking
- poor memory
- excess thirst
- frequent urination
- thinner, weaker bones
- increased risk of bone fracture
- kidney stones

Hyperparathyroidism is often considered idiopathic, which means that there is no known underlying cause of the disorder. In about 5% of people with parathyroidism, there is a family tendency for the disorder, such as familial multiple endocrine neoplasia type 1 or familial hypocalciuric hypercalcemia.

About 100,000 people in the United States are diagnosed with hyperparathyroidism annually. Women are twice as likely to get the disorder than men, and it is more common in people over the age of 60.

Description

Prior to starting the scanner for a sestamibi scan, radioactive contrast is injected through an IV in the patient's arm. The radionuclide (the technetium-99 bound to sestamibi molecules) circulates in the blood stream, concentrating in diseased parathyroid glands. The patient lies on an examination table, and a gamma camera is positioned over the patient's neck. The camera consists of a crystal detector that detects emitted radiation from the radioactive contrast.

KEY TERMS

Adenoma—A benign tumor of an endocrine gland.

Hypercalcemia—Excess concentration of calcium in the blood.

Hyperparathyroidism—A condition in which the parathyroid gland is overactive; usually caused by the presence of an adenoma on one or more of the glands.

Parathyroidectomy—An operation performed in order to remove one or more parathyroid gland.

Thyroid gland—An endocrine organ in the neck that produces thyroid hormone. Thyroid hormone is involved in important growth and metabolic processes throughout the body.

A computer converts the signal into a digital image of the parathyroid glands. Scanning is done immediately after injection of the radionuclide, and again 90–120 minutes after injection. Each scan takes about 10 minutes.

Preparation

There is nothing patients need to do in preparation for a sestamibi scan. To avoid confusing results, patients who have recently had another type of nuclear scan may need to wait several days to allow that radioactive tracer to leave their bodies, prior to undergoing a sestamibi scan.

Women who are pregnant or who think they may be pregnant are advised against undergoing a sestamibi scan. Women who are breast-feeding and who require a sestamibi scan should feed their baby with formula for two days following the procedure, and should pump and discard their breast milk, since it will be contaminated with the radioactive dye.

Aftercare

There is no aftercare necessary following a sestamibi scan. The patient can return immediately to a normal diet and normal activities.

Risks

A sestamibi scan poses very little risk to the patient. Rarely, a patient may have an allergy to the radioactive contrast utilized.

Results

Normal results of a sestamibi scan would reveal no uptake of the radionuclide tracer in the neck, suggesting that no parathyroid adenoma is present.

Abnormal results

An abnormal sestamibi scan will reveal an area where the radionuclide has been absorbed by a parathyroid adenoma. Even small, single adenomas on a parathyroid gland will "light up," due to their tendency to absorb the radionuclide. This allows highly accurate localization of the exact area requiring operation. In some cases, a falsely positive sestamibi scan may occur in patients with thyroid disease.

Resources

BOOKS

Adam, A., and A. K. Dixon, eds. *Grainger & Allison's Diagnostic Radiology.* 5th ed. Philadelphia: Churchill Livingstone/Elsevier, 2008.

Melmed, Shlomo, et al. *Williams Textbook of Endocrinology.* 12th ed. Philadelphia: Saunders/Elsevier, 2011.

Mettler, Fred A. Jr. *Essentials of Radiology.* 3rd ed. Philadelphia: Saunders/Elsevier, 2014.

PERIODICALS

Opoku-Boateng, A., et al. "Use of a Sestamibi-Only Approach to Routine Minimally Invasive Parathyroidectomy." *The American Surgeon* 79, no. 8 (2013): 797–801.

WEBSITES

University of Michigan Health System. "Primary Hyperparathyroidism." http://surgery.med.umich.edu/general/endocrine/patient/conditions/parathyroid/primary_hyperparathyroidism.shtml (accessed October 4, 2013).

Rosalyn Carson-DeWitt, MD

Seton glaucoma surgery *see* **Tube-shunt surgery**

Sex reassignment surgery

Definition

Also known as sex change or gender reassignment surgery, sex reassignment surgery is a procedure that changes genital organs from one gender to another.

Purpose

There are two main reasons to alter the genital organs from one sex to another:

• Newborns with intersex deformities must be assigned to one sex or the other. These deformities represent intermediate stages between the primordial female genitals and the change into male genitals caused by male hormone stimulation.

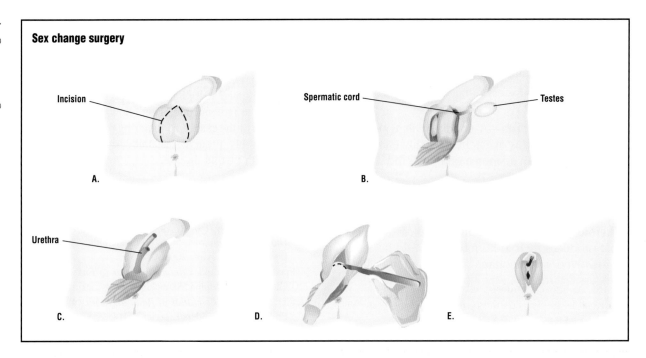

Sex change surgery

Incision

A.

Spermatic cord   Testes

B.

Urethra

C.   D.   E.

To change male genitalia to female genitalia, an incision is made into the scrotum (A). The flap of skin is pulled back, and the testes are removed (B). The skin is stripped from the penis but left attached, and a shorter urethra is cut (C). All but a stump of the penis is removed (D). The excess skin is used to create the labia (external genitalia) and vagina (E). *(Illustration by GGS Information Services. Copyright © Cengage Learning®.)*

• Both men and women occasionally believe they are physically a different sex than they are mentally and emotionally. This dissonance is so profound that they are willing to be surgically altered.

In both cases, technical considerations favor successful conversion to a female rather than a male. Newborns with ambiguous organs will almost always be assigned to the female gender unless the penis is at least an inch (2.5 cm) long. Whatever their chromosomes, they are much more likely to be socially well-adjusted as females, even if they cannot have children.

Demographics

Reliable statistics are extremely difficult to obtain. Many sexual reassignment procedures are conducted in private facilities that are not subject to reporting requirements. Sexual reassignment surgery is often conducted outside of the United States. The number of gender reassignment procedures conducted in the United States each year is estimated at between 100 and 500. The number worldwide is estimated to be two to five times larger.

Description

Converting male to female anatomy requires removal of the penis, reshaping genital tissue to appear

more female, and constructing a vagina. A vagina can be successfully formed from a skin graft or an isolated loop of intestine. Following the surgery, female hormones (estrogen) will reshape the body's contours and stimulate the growth of satisfactory breasts.

Female-to-male surgery has achieved lesser success due to the difficulty of creating a functioning penis from the much smaller clitoral tissue available in the female genitals. Penis construction is not attempted less than a year after the preliminary surgery to remove the female organs. One study in Singapore found that a third of the persons would not undergo the surgery again. Nevertheless, they were all pleased with the change of sex. Besides the genital organs, the breasts need to be surgically altered for a more male appearance. This can be successfully accomplished.

The capacity to experience an orgasm, or at least "a reasonable degree of erogenous sensitivity," can be expected by almost all persons after gender reassignment surgery.

Preparation

Gender identity is an extremely important characteristic for human beings. Assigning sex must take place immediately after birth for the mental health of both children and their parents. Changing sexual identity is

KEY TERMS

Androgens—A class of chemical compounds (hormones) that stimulates the development of male secondary sexual characteristics.

Chromosomes—The carriers of genes that determine gender and other characteristics.

Estrogens—A class of chemical compounds (hormones) that stimulates the development of female secondary sexual characteristics.

Hysterectomy—Surgical removal of the uterus.

Oophorectomy—Surgical removal of the ovaries.

among the most significant changes that a human can experience. It should therefore be undertaken with extreme care and caution. By the time most adults come to surgery, they have lived for many years with a dissonant identity. The average in one study was 29 years. Nevertheless, even then they may not be fully aware of the implications of becoming a member of the opposite gender.

In-depth psychological counseling should precede and follow any gender reassignment surgical procedure.

Sex reassignment surgery is expensive. The cost for male-to-female reassignment is $10,000 to $20,000. The cost for female-to-male reassignment can exceed $50,000.

Aftercare

Social support, particularly from the person's family, is important for readjustment as a member of the opposite gender. If surgical candidates are socially or emotionally unstable before the operation, over the age of 30, or have an unsuitable body build for the new gender, they tend not to fare well after gender reassignment surgery; however, in no case studied did the gender reassignment procedure diminish the ability to work.

Risks

All surgery carries the risks of infection, bleeding, and a need to return for repairs. Gender reassignment surgery is irreversible, so a candidate must have no doubts about accepting the results and outcome.

Results

Persons undergoing gender reassignment surgery can expect to acquire the external genitalia of a member of the opposite gender. Persons having male-to-female

gender reassignment surgery retain a prostate. Individuals undergoing female-to-male gender reassignment surgery undergo a **hysterectomy** to remove the uterus and **oophorectomy** to remove their ovaries. Developing the habits and mannerisms characteristic of the patient's new gender requires many months or years.

Morbidity and mortality rates

The risks that are associated with any surgical procedure are present in gender reassignment surgery. These include infection, **postoperative pain**, and dissatisfaction with anticipated results. Accurate statistics are extremely difficult to find. Intraoperative death has not been reported.

The most common complication of male-to-female surgery is narrowing of the new vagina. This can be corrected by dilation or using a portion of colon to form a vagina.

A relatively common complication of female-to-male surgery is dysfunction of the penis. Implanting a penile prosthesis is technically difficult and does not have uniformly acceptable results.

Psychiatric care may be required for many years after sex-reassignment surgery.

The number of deaths in male-to-female transsexuals was five times the number expected, due to increased numbers of suicide and death from an unknown cause.

Alternatives

There is no alternative to surgical reassignment to alter the external genitalia. The majority of persons who experience gender disorder problems never surgically alter their appearance. They dress as members of the desired gender, rather than gender of birth. Many use creams or pills that contain hormones appropriate to the desired gender to alter their bodily appearance. Estrogens (female hormones) will stimulate breast development, widening of the hips, loss of facial hair, and a slight increase in voice pitch. Androgens (male hormones) will stimulate the development of facial and chest hair and cause the voice to deepen. Most individuals who undergo gender reassignment surgery lead happy and productive lives.

Health care team roles

Gender reassignment surgery is performed by **surgeons** with specialized training in urology, gynecology, or plastic and **reconstructive surgery**. The surgery is performed in a hospital setting, although many procedures are completed in private clinics.

QUESTIONS TO ASK YOUR DOCTOR

- What will my body look like afterward?
- Is the surgeon board certified in urology, gynecology, or plastic and reconstructive surgery?
- How many gender reassignment procedures has the surgeon performed?
- How many surgeries of the type similar to the one being contemplated (i.e., male-to-female or female-to-male) has the surgeon performed?
- What is the surgeon's complication rate?

Resources

BOOKS

Wein, Alan J., et al. *Campbell-Walsh Urology.* 10th ed. Philadelphia: Saunders/Elsevier, 2012.

PERIODICALS

Monstrey, Stan J., Peter Ceulemans, Piet Hoebeke. "Sex Reassignment Surgery in the Female-to-Male Transsexual." *Seminars in Plastic Surgery* 25, no. 3 (2011): 229–44. http://dx.doi.org/10.1055/s-0031-1281493 (accessed October 14, 2013).

WEBSITES

Gender Matters. "Female to Male (FtM)." http://gender-matters.org.uk/links/female-to-male-%28ftm%29 (accessed October 14, 2013).

Gender Matters. "Male to Female (MtF)." http://gender-matters.org.uk/links/male-to-female-%28mtf%29 (accessed October 14, 2013).

University of California Santa Cruz. "Sexual Reassignment Surgery." http://queer.ucsc.edu/resources/trans/srs.html (accessed October 14, 2013).

University of Michigan Health System. "Gender Affirming Surgery." http://www.uofmhealth.org/medical-services/gender-affirming-surgery (accessed October 14, 2013).

ORGANIZATIONS

American Medical Association, 515 N. State St., Chicago, IL 60654, (800) 621-8335, http://www.ama-assn.org.

American Psychiatric Association, 1000 Wilson Blvd., Ste. 1825, Arlington, VA 22209, (703) 907-7300, (888) 35-PSYCH (357-7924), apa@psych.org, http://www.psychiatry.org.

American Psychological Association, 750 First St. NE, Washington, DC 20002-4242, (202) 336-5500, (800) 374-2721, (202) 336-6123, http://www.apa.org.

Gender Matters, The Mill House, 5b Bridgnorth Rd., Wolverhampton, West Midlands WV6 8AB, United Kingdom, +44 (0) 1902 744424, info@gender-matters.org.uk, http://gender-matters.org.uk.

The Philadelphia Center for Transgender Surgery, 19 Montgomery Ave., Bala Cynwyd, PA 19004, (610) 667-1888, DrShermanLeis@DrShermanLeis.com, http://www.thetransgendercenter.com.

Urology Care Foundation, 1000 Corporate Blvd., Linthicum, MD 21090, (410) 689-3700, (800) 828-7866, Fax: (410) 689-3998, info@urologycarefoundation.org, http://auafoundation.org.

World Professional Association for Transgender Health, wpath@wpath.org, http://www.wpath.org.

L. Fleming Fallon Jr., MD, DrPH

Sexually transmitted disease cultures

Definition

Sexually transmitted diseases are infections spread from person to person through sexual contact. A culture is a test in which a laboratory attempts to grow and identify the microorganism causing an infection.

Purpose

Sexually transmitted diseases (STDs) produce symptoms such as genital discharge, pain during urination, bleeding, pelvic pain, skin ulcers, or urethritis. Often, however, they produce no immediate symptoms. Therefore, the decision to test for these diseases must be based not only on the presence of symptoms, but on whether or not a person is at risk of having one or more of the diseases. Activities such as drug use and sex with more than one partner place a person at high risk for these diseases.

STD cultures are necessary to diagnose certain types of STDs. Only after the infection is diagnosed can it be treated and further spread of the infection prevented. Left untreated, the consequences of these diseases range from discomfort to infertility and even to death. In addition, these diseases, if present in a pregnant woman, can be passed from mother to fetus.

Description

Gonorrhea, syphilis, chlamydia, chancroid, herpes, human papillomavirus, human immunodeficiency virus (HIV), and mycoplasma are common sexually transmitted diseases. Not all are diagnosed with a culture. For those that are, a sample of material is taken from the infection site, placed in a sterile container, and sent to the laboratory.

Bacterial cultures

In the laboratory, a portion of material from the infection site is spread over the surface of several different types of culture plates and placed in an incubator at body temperature for one to two days. Bacteria present in the sample will multiply and appear on the plates as visible colonies. They are identified by the appearance of their colonies and by the results of biochemical tests and a Gram stain. The Gram stain is performed by smearing part of a colony onto a microscope slide. After it dries, the slide is stained with purple and red and is examined under a microscope. The color of stain picked up by the bacteria (purple or red), the shape (such as round or rectangle), and the size provide valuable clues as to the identity and which **antibiotics** might work best. Bacteria that stain purple are called gram-positive; those that stain red are called gram-negative.

The result of the gram stain is available the same day or in less than an hour if requested by the physician. An early report, known as a preliminary report, is usually available after one day. This report will tell if any microorganisms have been found and, if so, their Gram stain appearance—for example, a gram-negative rod or a gram-positive cocci. The final report, usually available in one to seven days, includes complete identification and an estimate of the quantity of the microorganisms isolated.

A sensitivity test, also called an antibiotic susceptibility test and commonly performed on bacteria isolated from an infection site, is not always done on bacteria isolated from a sexually transmitted disease. These bacteria often are treated using antibiotics that are part of a standard treatment protocol.

GONORRHEA. *Neisseria gonorrhoeae*, also called gonococcus or GC, causes gonorrhea. It infects the surfaces of the genitourinary tract, primarily the urethra in males and the cervix in females. On a Gram stain done on material taken from an infection site, the bacteria appear as small gram-negative diplococci (pairs of round bacteria) inside white blood cells. *Neisseria gonorrhoeae* grows on a special culture plate called Thayer-Martin (TM) media in an environment with low levels of oxygen and high levels of carbon dioxide.

The best specimen from which to culture *Neisseria gonorrhoeae* is a swab of the urethra in a male or the cervix in a female. Other possible specimens include vagina, body fluid discharge, swab of genital lesion, or the first urine of the day. Results are usually available after two days. Rapid nonculture tests are available to test for GC and provide results on the same or following day.

CHANCROID. Chancroid is caused by *Haemophilus ducreyi*. It is characterized by genital ulcers with nearby swollen lymph nodes. The specimen is collected by swabbing one of these pus-filled ulcers. The Gram stain may not be helpful as this bacteria looks just like other *Haemophilus* bacteria. This bacterium only grows on special culture plates, so the physician must request a specific culture for a person who has symptoms of chancroid. Even using special culture plates, *Haemophilus ducreyi* is isolated from less than 80% of the ulcers it infects. If a culture is negative, the physician must diagnose chancroid based on the person's symptoms and by ruling out other possible causes of these symptoms, such as syphilis.

MYCOPLASMA. Three types of mycoplasma organisms cause sexually transmitted urethritis in males and pelvic inflammatory disease and cervicitis in females: *Mycoplasma hominis*, *Mycoplasma gentialium*, and *Ureaplasma urealyticum*. These organisms require special culture plates and may take up to six days to grow. Samples are collected from the cervix in a female, the urethra or semen in a male, or urine.

SYPHILIS. Syphilis is caused by *Treponema pallidum*, one in a group of bacteria called spirochetes. It causes ulcers or chancres at the site of infection. The organism does not grow in culture. Using special techniques and stains, it is identified by looking at a sample of the ulcer or chancre under the microscope. Various blood tests also may be performed to detect the treponema organism.

CHLAMYDIA. Chlamydia is caused by the gram-negative bacterium *Chlamydia trachomatis*. It is one of the most common STDs in the United States and generally appears in sexually active adolescents and young adults. While chlamydia often does not have any initial symptoms, it can, if left untreated, lead to pelvic inflammatory disease and sterility. Samples are collected from one or more of these infection sites: cervix in a female, urethra in a male, or the rectum. A portion of specimen is combined with a specific type of cell and allowed to incubate. Special stains are performed on the cultured cells, looking for evidence of the chlamydia organism within the cells. A swab can also be taken from the woman's vulva. Men and women can now be screened for chlamydia with a urine sample. Urine-based screening has increased screening significantly, especially among men.

Viral cultures

To culture or grow a virus in the laboratory, a portion of specimen is mixed with commercially prepared animal cells in a test tube. Characteristic changes to the cells caused by the growing virus help identify the virus. The time to complete a viral culture varies with the type of virus. It may take several days or up to several weeks.

HERPES VIRUS. Herpes simplex virus type 2 is the cause of genital herpes. Diagnosis is usually made based on the person's symptoms. If a diagnosis needs confirmation, a viral culture is performed using material taken from an ulcer. A Tzanck smear is a microscope test that can rapidly detect signs of herpes infection in cells taken from an ulcer. The cell culture test takes up to 14 days to complete. In addition, the polymerase chain reaction (PCR) blood test is able to diagnosis genital herpes even when symptoms are not present. The test does this by looking for pieces of deoxyribonucleic acid (DNA) within the virus. The PCR blood test, which is very accurate in its results, is considered the most commonly used test for diagnosing genital herpes.

HUMAN PAPILLOMAVIRUS. Human papillomavirus causes genital warts. This virus will not grow in culture; the diagnosis is based on the appearance of the warts and the person's symptoms. A human papillomavirus (HPV) DNA test with a Pap smear is performed to diagnosis HPV in women age 30 years and older. (The test is rarely given to women under 30 years of age because most of these younger women can rid themselves of the HPV without medical treatment.) Older women are usually given the test after a regular Pap smear comes back with an abnormal result. The combined test also helps physicians determine which women are at extremely low risk for cervical cancer and which should be more closely monitored.

The Hybrid Capture II (HC II) is a test for human papillomavirus that is used to show the presence or absence of genetic material (DNA) from HPV in cells from a woman's cervix. The test is able to detect the virus in a very accurate manner when compared with the previous tests of Hybrid Capture I (HC I) and PCR. HPV detection with the HC II test is also a much more convenient and easier test than the PCR test. In 2013, the HC II was the most commonly used HPV test in the United States.

HIV. Human immunodeficiency virus (HIV) is usually diagnosed with a blood test. Cultures for HIV are possible, but rarely needed for diagnosis. The HIV test detects antibodies to the human immunodeficiency virus, along with detecting the genetic material, either DNA or ribonucleic acid (RNA) of HIV in the blood. Thus, this test determines whether an HIV infection is present (HIV-positive) or not present (HIV-negative). Others tests are also used to find genetic material or antibodies of HIV. The **enzyme-linked immunosorbent assay (ELISA)** test will determine if HIV antibodies are present (HIV-positive). A positive result on a test will usually mean that another test should be performed to confirm the initial finding. If the test is negative, then other tests are not normally needed.

The Western blot test is usually performed when confirmation is needed with two positive ELISA tests. The test is more difficult to perform than the ELISA test, which is why it is not the first test to be used for detection of HIV. The PCR test determines either RNA or DNA of HIV within white blood cells. The PCR test is also very difficult to perform and requires expensive equipment.

Preparation

Generally, the type of specimen collected depends on the type of infection. Cultures always should be collected before the person begins taking antibiotics. After collection of these specimens, each is placed into a sterile tube containing a liquid in which the organism can survive while en route to the laboratory. The new rapid **HIV tests** rely on blood samples collected from a finger stick or vein or on saliva collected from the mouth. Initial results are not sent to a laboratory but are processed on site.

Urethral specimen

Men should not urinate one hour before collection of a urethral specimen. The physician inserts a sterile, cotton-tipped swab into the urethra.

Cervical specimen

Women should not douche or take a bath within 24 hours of collection of a cervical or vaginal culture. The physician inserts a moistened, nonlubricated vaginal speculum. After the cervix is exposed, the physician

QUESTIONS TO ASK YOUR DOCTOR

- What does STD testing involve?
- If my symptoms for STD come and go, should I still be tested?
- Should I be tested for HIV/AIDS?
- When will the results of the tests be available?
- Should I avoid sexual activity until the test results are available? If not, what types of precautions should I take to reduce the risk for infecting my partner?
- Should my partner also be tested for STDs?
- Is the STD that I have been diagnosed with treatable? Curable?
- Does having this diagnosed STD increase my risk for other health problems, including other STDs?
- Are there long-term risks or complications associated with the STD that I have been diagnosed with? If so, what are these long-term risks?
- What is the treatment that you recommend for this STD? Which medication(s) will be used to treat this STD? What are the benefits, risks, side effects, and possible complications associated with this STD treatment?

removes the cervical mucus using a cotton ball. Next, he or she inserts a sterile cotton-tipped swab into the endocervical canal and rotates the swab with firm pressure for about 30 seconds.

Vaginal specimen

Women should not douche or take a bath within 24 hours of collection of a cervical or vaginal culture. The physician inserts a sterile, cotton-tipped swab into the vagina.

Anal specimen

The physician inserts a sterile, cotton-tipped swab about 1 inch (2.5 centimeters) into the anus and rotates the swab for 30 seconds. Stool must not contaminate the swab.

Oropharynx (throat) specimen

The person's tongue is held down with a tongue depressor, as a healthcare worker moves a sterile, cotton-

tipped swab across the back of the throat and tonsil region.

Urine specimen

To collect a "clean-catch" urine sample, the person first washes the perineum, and the penis or labia and vulva. He or she begins urinating, letting the first portion pass into the toilet, then collecting the remainder into a sterile container.

Results

These microorganisms are not found in a normal culture. Many types of microorganisms, normally found on a person's skin and in the genitourinary tract, may contaminate the culture. If a mixture of these microorganisms grow in the culture, they are reported as normal flora.

Abnormal results

If a person has a positive culture for one or more of these microorganisms, treatment is started and his or her sexual partners should be notified and tested. Certain laws govern reporting and partner notification of various STDs. After treatment is completed, the person's physician may want a follow-up culture to confirm the infection is gone.

Resources

BOOKS

Aral, Sevgi O., Kevin A. Fenton, and Judith A. Lipshutz, eds. *The New Public Health and STD/HIV Prevention: Personal, Public and Health Systems Approaches.* New York: Springer, 2013.

Papadakis, Maxine A., and Stephen J. McPhee, eds. *Current Medical Diagnosis and Treatment 2013.* New York: McGraw-Hill Medical, 2013.

Stanberry, Lawrence R., and Susan L. Rosenthal, eds. *Sexually Transmitted Diseases: Vaccines, Prevention, and Control.* Amsterdam and Boston: Elsevier Academic Press, 2013.

Sutton, Amy L., ed. *Sexually Transmitted Diseases Sourcebook.* Detroit: Omnigraphics, 2013.

Wecker, Lynn, et al. *Brody's Human Pharmacology: Molecular to Clinical.* Philadelphia: Mosby/Elsevier, 2010.

White, Lois, Gena Duncan, and Wendy Baumle, ed. *Medical-surgical Nursing: An Integrated Approach.* Clifton Park, NY: Delmar Cengage Learning, 2013.

WEBSITES

Mayo Clinic staff. "STD Testing: What's Right for You?" MayoClinic.com. http://www.mayoclinic.com/health/std-testing/ID00047 (accessed September 5, 2013).

MedlinePlus. "Sexually Transmitted Diseases." U.S. National Library of Medicine, National Institutes of Health. http://www.nlm.nih.gov/medlineplus/sexuallytransmitteddiseases.html (accessed September 17, 2013).

Planned Parenthood. "STD Testing." http://www.planned parenthood.org/health-topics/stds-hiv-safer-sex/std-testing-21695.asp (accessed September 17, 2013).

ORGANIZATIONS

American Social Health Association, PO Box 13827, Research Triangle Pk., NC 27709, (919) 361-8400, Fax: (919) 361-8425, http://www.ashastd.org.

Centers for Disease Control and Prevention, National Center for HIV, STD, and TB Prevention, 1600 Clifton Rd., Atlanta, GA 30333, (800) 232-4636, cdcinfo@cdc.gov, http://www.cdc.gov/nchhstp.

Nancy J. Nordenson
Teresa G. Odle
William A. Atkins, BB, BS, MBA

Shoulder arthroscopic surgery *see* **Bankart procedure; Rotator cuff repair**

Shoulder joint replacement

Definition

Shoulder joint replacement surgery is performed to replace a shoulder joint with artificial components (prostheses) when the joint is severely damaged by degenerative joint diseases such as arthritis, or in complex cases of upper arm bone fracture.

Purpose

The shoulder is a ball-and-socket joint that allows the arms to be raised; twisted; bent; and moved forward, to the side, and backward. The head of the upper arm bone (humerus) is the ball, and a circular cavity (glenoid) in the shoulder blade (scapula) is the socket. A soft-tissue rim (labrum) surrounds and deepens the socket. The head of the humerus is also covered with a smooth, tough tissue (articular cartilage), and the joint, also called the acromioclavicular (AC) joint, has a thin inner lining (synovium) that facilitates movement, while surrounding muscles and tendons provide stability and support.

The AC joint can be damaged by the following conditions to such an extent as to require replacement by artificial components:

• Osteoarthritis. This is a degenerative joint disease characterized by degeneration of the articular cartilage. When nonsurgical treatment is no longer effective and shoulder resection not possible, joint replacement surgery is usually indicated.

• Rheumatoid arthritis. Shoulder replacement surgery is the most commonly performed procedure for the arthritic shoulder with severe inflammatory or rheumatoid arthritis.

• Severe fracture of the humerus. A fracture of the upper arm bone can be so severe as to require replacement of the AC joint.

• Osteonecrosis. This condition usually follows a three- or four-part fracture of the humeral head that disrupts the blood supply, resulting in bone death and disruption of the AC joint.

• Charcot's arthropathy. Also called neuropathic arthropathy or arthritis, Charcot's arthropathy is a condition in which the shoulder joint is destroyed following loss of its nerve supply.

Demographics

Shoulder arthritis is among the most prevalent causes of shoulder pain and loss of function. In the United States, arthritis of the shoulder joint is less common than arthritis of the hip or knee. Individuals with arthritis in one joint are more likely to get it in another joint. Overall, arthritis is quite common in the United States, affecting about 21% of adult Americans, and 50% of Americans over the age of 65. Projections suggest that, by the year 2030, there will be 67 million Americans who have received the diagnosis of arthritis from their doctor. Osteoarthritis is also the most common joint disorder, extremely common by age 70. Men and women are equally affected, but onset is earlier in men.

Description

Shoulder joint replacement surgery can either replace the entire AC joint, in which case it is referred to as total shoulder joint replacement or total shoulder **arthroplasty**; or replace only the head of the humerus, in which case the procedure is called a hemiarthroplasty.

Implants

The two artificial components that can be implanted in the shoulder during shoulder joint replacement surgery are:

• The humeral component. This part replaces the head of the humerus. It is usually made of cobalt or chromium-based alloys and has a rounded ball attached to a stem that can be inserted into the bone. It comes in various sizes and may consist of a single piece or a modular unit.

• The glenoid component. This component replaces the glenoid cavity. It is made of very high-density

Shoulder joint replacement

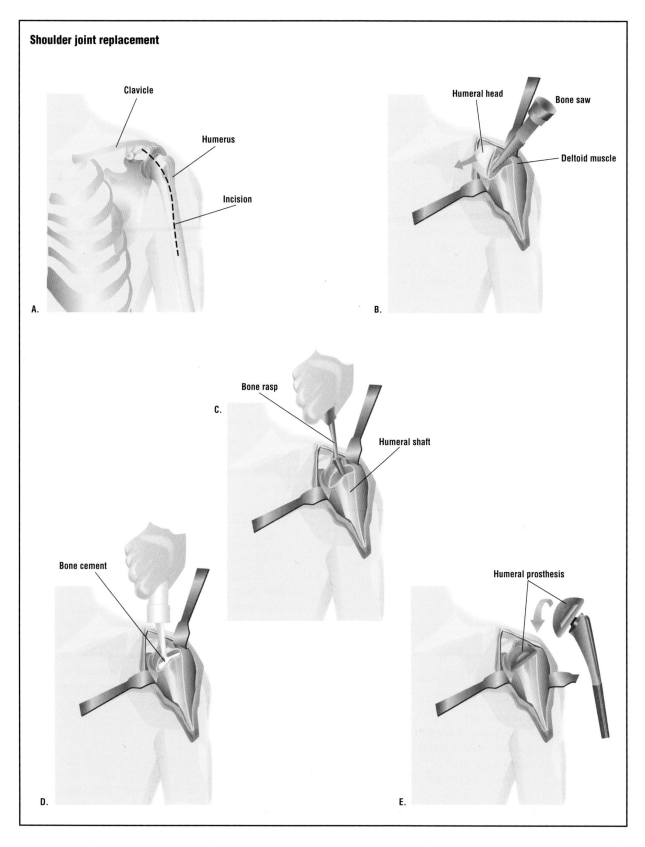

During a total shoulder joint replacement, an incision is first made in the shoulder and upper arm (A). The head of humerus is removed with a bone saw (B). The shaft of the humerus is shaped with a bone rasp to ready it for the prosthesis (C). After the shoulder joint, or glenoid cavity, is similarly prepared, bone cement is applied to the areas that will receive prostheses (D). The ball and socket prostheses are put in place, and the incision is closed (E). *(Illustration by GGS Information Services. Copyright © Cengage Learning®.)*

polyethylene. Some models feature a metal tray, but the 100% polyethylene type is more common.

Shoulder joint replacement surgery is performed under either regional or **general anesthesia**, depending on the specifics of the case. The surgeon makes a 3–4 in. (7.6–10.2 cm) incision on the front of the shoulder from the collarbone to the point where the shoulder muscle (deltoid) attaches to the humerus. The surgeon also inspects the muscles to see if any are damaged. He or she then proceeds to dislocate the humerus from the socket-like glenoid cavity to expose the head of the humerus. Only the portion of the head covered with articular cartilage is removed. The center cavity of the humerus (humeral shaft) is then cleaned and enlarged with reamers of gradually increasing size to create a cavity matching

the shape of the implant stem. The top end of the bone is smoothed so that the stem can be inserted flush with the bone surface.

If the glenoid cavity of the AC joint is not damaged and the surrounding muscles are intact, the surgeon does not replace it, thus performing a simple hemiarthroplasty; however, if the glenoid cavity is damaged or diseased, the surgeon moves the humerus to the back and implants the artificial glenoid component as well. The surgeon prepares the surface by removing the cartilage and equalizes the glenoid bone to match the implant. Protrusions on the polyethylene glenoid implant are then fitted into holes drilled in the bone surface. Once a precise fit is achieved, the implant is cemented into position. The humerus, with its new implanted artificial head, is replaced in the glenoid socket. The surgeon reattaches the supporting tendons and closes the incision.

Diagnosis

Damage to the AC joint is usually assessed using x-rays of the joint and humerus. They provide information on the state of the joint space, the position of the humeral head in relation to the glenoid, the presence of bony defects or deformity, and the quality of the bone. If glenoid wear is observed, a **computed tomography (CT) scan** is usually performed to evaluate the degree of bone loss.

Preparation

The treating physician usually performs a general medical evaluation several weeks before shoulder joint replacement surgery to assess the patient's general health condition and risk for anesthesia. The results of this examination are forwarded to the orthopedic surgeon, along with a surgical clearance. Patients are advised to eat properly and take a daily iron supplement some weeks before surgery. Several types of tests are usually required, including blood tests, a cardiogram, a urine sample, and a **chest x-ray**. Patients may be required to stop taking certain medications until surgery is over.

Aftercare

Following surgery, the operated arm is placed in a sling, and a support pillow is placed under the elbow to protect the repair. A drainage tube is used to remove excess fluid and is usually removed on the day after surgery.

A careful and well-planned rehabilitation program is very important for the successful outcome of a shoulder joint replacement. It should start no later than the first postoperative day. A physical therapist usually starts the patient with gentle, passive-assisted range of motion exercises. Before the patient leaves the hospital (usually two or three days after surgery), the therapist provides instruction on using a pulley device to help bend and extend the operated arm.

Risks

Complications after shoulder replacement surgery occur less frequently than with other joint replacement surgeries; however, there are risks associated with the surgery, including infection, intraoperative fracture of the humerus or postoperative fractures, biceps tendon rupture, and postoperative instability and loosening of the glenoid implant. Advances in surgical techniques and prosthetic innovations are helping to significantly lower the occurrence of complications.

Results

Pain relief is expected after shoulder joint replacement because the diseased joint surfaces have been replaced with smooth gliding surfaces. Improved motion, however, is variable and depends on the following:

• the surgeon's ability to reconstruct the shoulder's supporting tissues, namely the shoulder ligaments, capsule, and muscle attachments

• the patient's preoperative muscle strength

• the patient's motivation and compliance in participating in postoperative rehabilitation therapy

Morbidity and mortality rates

Good to excellent outcomes usually follow shoulder joint replacement surgery, including pain relief and a functional range of motion that provides the ability to dress and perform the normal activities of daily living. In the hands of experienced orthopedic **surgeons**, such outcomes occur 90% of the time. Shoulders with artificial joints are reported to function well for more than 20 years. No death has ever been reported for shoulder joint replacement procedures.

Alternatives

Arthritis treatment is very complex, as it depends on the type of arthritis and the severity of symptoms. Alternatives to joint replacement may include medications and therapy. It is known that arthritis is characterized by an increased rate of cartilage degradation and a decreased rate of cartilage production. An experimental therapy featuring the use of joint supplements such as glucosamine and chondroitin is being investigated for its effectiveness to repair cartilage. The pain and inflammation resulting from arthritis are also commonly treated

---

QUESTIONS TO ASK YOUR DOCTOR

• What type of joint replacement surgery does my shoulder require?

• What are the risks associated with the surgery?

• How long will it take for my shoulder to recover from the surgery?

• How long will the artificial components last?

• Is there a risk of implant infection?

• How many shoulder joint replacement surgeries do you perform in a year?

---

with nonsteroidal anti-inflammatory pain medication (NSAIDs) or cortisone injections (steroidal).

Health care team roles

Shoulder replacement surgery is performed in a hospital by orthopedic surgeons with specialized training in shoulder joint replacement surgery.

Resources

BOOKS

Browner, Bruce D., et al. *Skeletal Trauma: Basic Science, Management, and Reconstruction*. 4th ed. Philadelphia: Saunders/Elsevier, 2009.

Canale, S. T., ed. *Campbell's Operative Orthopaedics*. 12th ed. St. Louis, MO: Mosby, 2012.

DeLee, Jesse, David Drez, and Mark D. Miller. *DeLee and Drez's Orthopaedic Sports Medicine: Principles and Practice*. 3rd ed. Philadelphia: Saunders/Elsevier, 2010.

PERIODICALS

Rasmussen, J. V., et al. "A Review of National Shoulder and Elbow Joint Replacement Registries." *Journal of Shoulder and Elbow Surgery* 21, no. 10 (2012): 1328–35. http://dx.doi.org/10.1016/j.jse.2012.03.004 (accessed October 14, 2013).

Sandow, Michael J., Huw David, and Steven J. Bentall. "Hemiarthroplasty vs Total Shoulder Replacement for Rotator Cuff Intact Osteoarthritis: How Do They Fare after a Decade?" *Journal of Shoulder and Elbow Surgery* 22, no. 7 (2013): 877–85. http://dx.doi.org/10.1016/j.jse.2012.10.023 (accessed October 14, 2013).

WEBSITES

American Academy of Orthopaedic Surgeons. "Shoulder Joint Replacement." OrthoInfo. http://orthoinfo.aaos.org/topic.cfm?topic=A00094 (accessed October 14, 2013).

Cleveland Clinic. "Joint Replacement—Shoulder." http://my.clevelandclinic.org/services/shoulder_replacement/

hic_total_shoulder_joint_replacement.aspx (accessed October 14, 2013).

Craig, Edward V. "Shoulder Replacement Surgery: Diagnosis, Treatment, and Recovery." Hospital for Special Surgery. http://orthoinfo.aaos.org/topic.cfm?topic=A00094 (accessed October 14, 2013).

MedlinePlus. "Shoulder Injuries and Disorders." U.S. National Library of Medicine, National Institutes of Health. http://www.nlm.nih.gov/medlineplus/shoulderinjuriesanddisorders.html (accessed October 14, 2013).

University of California, San Francisco Medical Center. "Recovering from Shoulder Replacement Surgery." http://www.ucsfhealth.org/education/recovering_from_shoulder_replacement_surgery (accessed October 14, 2013).

University of Maryland Medical Center. "Reverse Shoulder Replacement Surgery." http://umm.edu/programs/orthopaedics/services/shoulder-and-elbow/reverse-shoulder-prosthesis (accessed October 14, 2013).

ORGANIZATIONS

American Academy of Orthopaedic Surgeons (AAOS), 6300 N. River Rd., Rosemont, IL 60018-4262, (847) 823-7186, Fax: (847) 823-8125, pemr@aaos.org, http://www.aaos.org.

American Shoulder and Elbow Surgeons, 6300 N. River Rd., Ste. 727, Rosemont, IL 60018, (847) 698-1629, ases@aaos.org, http://www.ases-assn.org.

Monique Laberge, PhD

Shoulder resection arthroplasty

Definition

Shoulder resection **arthroplasty** is surgery performed to repair a shoulder acromioclavicular (AC) joint. The procedure is most commonly recommended for AC joint problems resulting from osteoarthritis or injury.

Purpose

The shoulder consists of three bones: the shoulder blade, the upper arm bone (humerus), and the collarbone (clavicle). The part of the shoulder blade that makes up the roof of the shoulder is called the acromion and the joint where the acromion and the collarbone join is called the acromioclavicular (AC) joint.

Some joints in the body are more likely to develop problems due to normal wear and tear, or degeneration resulting from osteoarthritis, a progressive and degenerative joint disease. The AC joint is a common target for developing osteoarthritis in middle age. This condition can

lead to pain and difficulty using the shoulder for everyday activities. Besides osteoarthritis, AC joint disease (arthrosis) may develop from an old injury to the joint such as an acromioclavicular dislocation, which is the disruption of the normal articulation between the acromion and the collarbone. This type of injury is quite common in competitive sports, but can also result from a simple fall on the shoulder.

The goal of shoulder resection arthroplasty is to restore function to an impaired shoulder, with its required motion range, stability, strength, and smoothness.

Demographics

According to the National Ambulatory Medical Care Survey, osteoarthritis is one of the most common confirmed diagnoses in individuals over the age of 65, with the condition starting to develop in middle age.

As for AC joint injuries, they are seen especially in high-level athletes such as football or hockey players, and occur most frequently in the second decade of life. Males are more commonly affected than females, with a male-to-female ratio of approximately five to one.

Description

A resection arthroplasty involves the surgical removal of the last 0.5 in. (1.3 cm) of the collarbone.

This removal leaves a space between the acromion and the cut end of the collarbone where the AC joint used to be. The joint is replaced by scar tissue, which allows movement to occur, but prevents the rubbing of the bone ends. The end result of the surgery is that the flexible connection between the acromion and the collarbone is restored. The procedure is usually performed by making a small 2 in. (5 cm) incision in the skin over the AC joint. In some cases, the surgery can be done arthroscopically. In this approach, the surgeon uses an endoscope to look through a small hole into the shoulder joint. The endoscope is an instrument the size of a pen, consisting of a tube fitted with a light and a miniature video camera, which transmits an image of the joint interior to a television monitor. The surgeon proceeds to remove the segment of collarbone through a small incision with little disruption of the other shoulder structures.

Diagnosis

The diagnosis is made by physical exam. Tenderness over the AC joint is usually present, with pain upon compression of the joint. X-rays of the AC joint may show narrowing of the joint and bone spurs around the joint. A **magnetic resonance imaging** (MRI) scan may also be performed. An MRI scan is a special imaging test that uses magnetic waves to create pictures that show the tissues of the shoulder in slices and has the advantage of showing tendons as well as bones. In some cases, an **ultrasound** test may be also be performed to inspect the soft tissues of the joint.

Preparation

Prior to arthroplasty surgery, all the standard preoperative blood and urine tests are performed. The patient also meets with the anesthesiologist to discuss any special conditions that may affect the administration of anesthesia.

Aftercare

The rehabilitation following surgery for a simple resection arthroplasty is usually fairly rapid. Patients should expect the soreness to last for three to six weeks. Postoperatively, patients usually have the affected arm in a sling for two weeks. Thereafter, a progressive passive shoulder range-of-motion **exercise** program is started, usually with range-of-motion exercises that gradually evolve into active stretching and strengthening. The patient's arm remains in the sling between sessions. At six weeks, healing is sufficient to encourage progressive functional use. Physiotherapy usually continues until range of motion and strength are maximized. The therapist may also use massage and other types of hands-on treatments to ease muscle spasm and pain. Heavy physical use of the shoulder is prohibited for an additional six weeks.

Risks

Patients who undergo shoulder resection arthroplasty are susceptible to the same complications associated with any such surgery. These include wound infection, osteomyelitis, soft tissue ossification, and failure of fixation (remaining in place), with recurrent deformity. Symptomatic AC joint arthritis may develop in patients who undergo the surgery as a result of injury.

Specific risks associated with shoulder resection arthroplasty include:

- Fractures. Fractures of the humerus may occur after surgery, although the risk is considered low.
- Shoulder instability. Shoulder dislocations may occur during the early postoperative period due to soft tissue imbalance or to inadequate postoperative protection; late dislocation may result from glenoid cavity wear.
- Degenerative changes. Progressive degeneration of the AC joint is a common late complication.

Results

Shoulder resection arthroplasty is generally very effective in reducing pain and restoring motion of the shoulder.

Morbidity and mortality rates

In a four-year follow-up study on shoulder arthroplasty patients, all patients experienced pain relief. Functional improvement was good in 77% of patients. Average shoulder abduction improved from 37–79° and forward flexion from 52–93°. No deaths resulting from shoulder resection arthroplasty have ever been reported.

Alternatives

Nonsurgical treatments

Doctors commonly attempt to treat AC joint problems using conservative treatments. Patients may be prescribed anti-inflammatory medications such as **aspirin** or ibuprofen. Treatment also may include disease-modifying drugs such as methotrexate and sulfasalazine, as well as gold injections. Researchers are also working on biologic agents that can interrupt the progress of osteoarthritis. These agents target specific chemicals in the body to prevent them from acting on the joints. Resting the sore joint and applying ice to it can also ease pain and inflammation. Injections of cortisone into the joint may also be prescribed. Cortisone is a

QUESTIONS TO ASK YOUR DOCTOR

- How can I regain the use of my shoulder?
- What will it take to make my shoulder healthy again?
- Why do I have problems with my shoulder?
- What surgical procedures do you follow?
- How many shoulder resection arthroplasties do you perform each year?
- Will surgery on my shoulder condition allow me to resume my activities?

strong steroidal medication that decreases inflammation and reduces pain. The effects of the drug are temporary, but it provides effective relief in the short term. Physicians may also prescribe sessions with a physical or occupational therapist, who may use various treatments to relieve inflammation of the AC joint, including heat and ice.

Surgical alternatives

Alternative surgical approaches include replacing the entire shoulder joint with a prosthesis (total shoulder arthroplasty) or replacing the head of the humerus (hemiarthroplasty).

Health care team roles

Shoulder resection arthroplasty is performed in a hospital. It is performed by experienced orthopedic **surgeons** who are specialists in AC joint problems. Some medical centers specialize in joint surgery and tend to have higher success rates than less specialized centers.

Resources

BOOKS

Browner, Bruce D., et al. *Skeletal Trauma: Basic Science, Management, and Reconstruction.* 4th ed. Philadelphia: Saunders/Elsevier, 2009.

Canale, S. T., ed. *Campbell's Operative Orthopaedics.* 12th ed. St. Louis, MO: Mosby, 2012.

DeLee, Jesse, David Drez, and Mark D. Miller. *DeLee and Drez's Orthopaedic Sports Medicine: Principles and Practice.* 3rd ed. Philadelphia: Saunders/Elsevier, 2010.

PERIODICALS

Boileau, P., et al. "Revision Surgery of Reverse Shoulder Arthroplasty." *Journal of Shoulder and Elbow Surgery* 22, no. 10 (2013): 1359–70. http://dx.doi.org/10.1016/j.jse.2013.02.004 (accessed October 17, 2013).

WEBSITES

American Academy of Orthopaedic Surgeons. "Arthritis of the Shoulder." OrthoInfo. http://orthoinfo.aaos.org/topic.cfm?topic=A00222 (accessed October 17, 2013).

Hospital for Special Surgery. "Distal Clavicle Resection." http://www.hss.edu/animation-distal-clavicle-resection.htm (accessed October 17, 2013).

ORGANIZATIONS

American Academy of Orthopaedic Surgeons (AAOS), 6300 N. River Rd., Rosemont, IL 60018-4262, (847) 823-7186, Fax: (847) 823-8125, pemr@aaos.org, http://www.aaos.org.

American Shoulder and Elbow Surgeons, 6300 N. River Rd., Ste. 727, Rosemont, IL 60018, (847) 698-1629, ases@aaos.org, http://www.ases-assn.org.

Monique Laberge, PhD

Sigmoidoscopy

Definition

Sigmoidoscopy is a diagnostic and screening procedure in which a rigid or flexible tube with a camera on the end (a sigmoidoscope) is inserted into the anus to examine the rectum and lower colon (bowel) for bowel disease, cancer, precancerous conditions, or causes of bleeding or pain.

Purpose

Sigmoidoscopy is used most often in screening for colorectal cancer or to determine the cause of rectal bleeding. It is also used in diagnosis of inflammatory bowel disease, microscopic and ulcerative colitis, and Crohn's disease.

Cancer of the rectum and colon is the second most common cancer in the United States. About 148,300 new cases are diagnosed annually. Between 55,000 and 60,000 Americans die each year of cancer in the colon or rectum.

After reviewing a number of studies, experts recommend that people over 50 be screened for colorectal cancer using sigmoidoscopy every three to five years. Individuals with inflammatory bowel conditions such as Crohn's disease or ulcerative colitis, and thus at increased risk for colorectal cancer, may begin their screenings at a younger age, depending on when their disease was diagnosed. Many physicians screen such persons more often than every three to five years. Screening should also be performed in people who have a family history of colon or rectal cancer, or small growths in the colon (polyps).

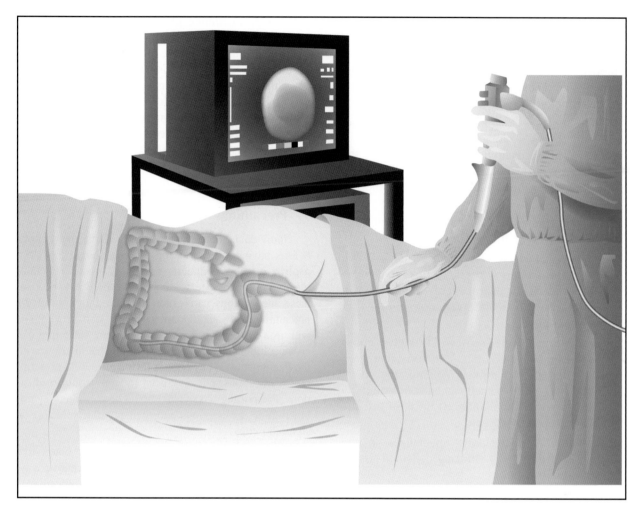

Sigmoidoscopy is a procedure most often used in screening for colorectal cancer and as a test in diagnosis of possible inflammatory bowel disease. The physician can view the rectum and colon through a sigmoidoscope, a flexible fiber-optic tube that contains a light source and a lens. *(Illustration by GGS Information Services. Copyright © Cengage Learning®.)*

Some physicians do this screening with a colonoscope, which allows them to see the entire colon. Most physicians prefer sigmoidoscopy, which is less time-consuming, less uncomfortable, and less costly.

Studies have shown that one-quarter to one-third of all precancerous or small cancerous growths can be seen with a sigmoidoscope. About one-half are found with a 1 ft. (30 cm) scope, and two-thirds to three-quarters can be seen using a 2 ft. (60 cm) scope.

In some cases, the sigmoidoscope can be used therapeutically in conjunction with other equipment such as electrosurgical devices to remove polyps and other lesions found during the sigmoidoscopy.

Demographics

Experts estimate that in excess of 525,000 sigmoidoscopy procedures are performed each year. This number includes most of the persons who are diagnosed with colon cancer each year, a greater number who are screened and receive negative results, persons who have been treated for colon conditions and receive a sigmoidoscopy as a follow-up procedure, and individuals who are diagnosed with other diseases of the large colon.

Description

Sigmoidoscopy may be performed using either a rigid or flexible sigmoidoscope. A sigmoidoscope is a thin tube with fiberoptics, electronics, a light source, and camera. A physician inserts the sigmoidoscope into the anus to examine the rectum (the first 1 ft [30 cm] of the colon) and its interior walls. If a 2 ft (60 cm) scope is used, the next portion of the colon can also be examined for any irregularities. The camera of the sigmoidoscope is connected to a viewing monitor, allowing the interior of the rectum and colon to be enlarged and viewed on the

KEY TERMS

Biopsy—The removal of a small portion of tissue during sigmoidoscopy to perform laboratory tests to determine if the tissue is cancerous.

Colonoscopy—A diagnostic endoscopic procedure that uses a long flexible tube called a colonoscope to examine the inner lining of the entire colon; may be used for colorectal cancer screening or for a more thorough examination of the colon.

Colorectal cancer—Cancer of the large intestine, or colon, including the rectum.

Electrosurgical device—A medical device that uses electrical current to cauterize or coagulate tissue during surgical procedures, often used in conjunction with laparoscopy, colonoscopy, or sigmoidoscopy.

Inflammatory bowel diseases—Ulcerative colitis or Crohn's disease: chronic conditions characterized by periods of diarrhea, bloating, abdominal cramps, and pain, sometimes accompanied by weight loss and malnutrition because of the inability to absorb nutrients.

Pathologist—A doctor who specializes in the diagnosis of disease by studying cells and tissues under a microscope.

Polyp—A small growth, usually not cancerous, but often precancerous when it appears in the colon.

monitor. Images can then be recorded as still pictures or the entire procedure can be videotaped. The still pictures are useful for comparison purposes with the results of future sigmoidoscopic examinations.

If polyps, lesions, or other suspicious areas are found, the physician biopsies them for analysis. During the sigmoidoscopy, the physician may also use forceps, graspers, snares, or electrosurgical devices to remove polyps, lesions, or tumors.

A typical sigmoidoscopy procedure requires 15 to 20 minutes to perform. Preparation begins one day before the procedure. There is some discomfort when the scope is inserted and throughout the procedure, similar to that experienced when a physician performs a rectal exam using a finger to test for occult blood in the stool (another important screening test for colorectal cancer). Individuals may also feel some minor cramping pain. There is rarely severe pain, except for persons with active inflammatory bowel disease.

Private insurance plans almost always cover the cost of sigmoidoscopy examinations for screening in healthy individuals over 50, or for diagnostic purposes. **Medicare** covers the cost for diagnostic exams, and may cover the costs for screening exams. **Medicaid** benefits vary by state, but sigmoidoscopy is not a covered procedure in many states. Some community health clinics offer the procedure at reduced cost, but this can only be done if a local gastroenterologist (a physician who specializes in treating stomach and intestinal disorders) is willing to donate personal time to perform the procedure.

Precautions

Individuals need to be careful about medications before having sigmoidoscopy. They should not take **aspirin**, products containing aspirin, or products containing ibuprofen for one week prior to the exam, because these medications can exacerbate bleeding during the procedure. They should not take any iron or vitamins with iron for one week prior to the exam, since iron can cause color changes in the bowel lining that interfere with the examination. They should take any routine prescription medications, but may need to stop certain medications. Prescribing physicians should be consulted regarding routine prescriptions and their possible effect(s) on sigmoidoscopy.

Individuals with renal insufficiency or congestive heart failure need to be prepared in an alternative way, and must be carefully monitored during the procedure.

Preparation

The purpose of preparation for sigmoidoscopy is to cleanse the lower bowel of fecal material or stool so the physician can see the lining. Preparation begins 24 hours before the procedure, when an individual must begin a clear liquid diet. Preparation kits are available in drug stores. In normal preparation, about 20 hours before the exam, a person begins taking a series of **laxatives**, which may be oral tablets or liquid. The individual must stop drinking any liquid four hours before the exam. An hour or two prior to the examination, the person uses an enema or laxative suppository to finish cleansing the lower bowel.

Aftercare

There is no specific aftercare necessary following sigmoidoscopy. If a biopsy was taken, a small amount of blood may appear in the next stool. Persons should be encouraged to pass gas following the procedure to relieve any bloating or cramping that may occur after the procedure. In addition, an infection may develop following sigmoidoscopy. Persons should be instructed to call their physician if a fever or pain in the abdomen develops over the few days after the procedure.

Risks

There is a slight risk of bleeding from the procedure. This risk is heightened in individuals whose blood does not clot well, either due to disease or medication, and in those with active inflammatory bowel disease. Rarely, trauma to the bowel or other organs can occur, resulting in an injury (perforation) that must be repaired, or peritonitis, which must be treated with medication.

Sigmoidoscopy may be contraindicated in persons with severe active colitis or toxic megacolon (an extremely dilated colon). In general, people experiencing continuous ambulatory peritoneal dialysis are not candidates due to a high risk of developing intraperitoneal bleeding.

Results

The results of a normal examination reveal a smooth colon wall, with sufficient blood vessels for good blood flow.

Morbidity and mortality rates

For a cancer screening sigmoidoscopy, an abnormal result is one or more noncancerous or precancerous polyps, or clearly cancerous polyps. People with polyps have an increased risk of developing colorectal cancer in the future and may be required to undergo additional procedures such as **colonoscopy** or more frequent sigmoidoscopic examinations.

Small polyps can be completely removed. Larger polyps may require the physician to remove a portion of the growth for laboratory biopsy. Depending on the laboratory results, a person is then scheduled to have the polyp removed surgically, either as an urgent matter if it is cancerous, or as an elective procedure within a few months if it is noncancerous.

In a diagnostic sigmoidoscopy, an abnormal result shows signs of active inflammatory bowel disease, either a thickening of the intestinal lining consistent with ulcerative colitis, or ulcerations or fissures consistent with Crohn's disease.

Mortality from a sigmoidoscopy examination is rare and is usually due to uncontrolled bleeding or perforation of the colon.

Alternatives

A screening examination for colorectal cancer is a test for fecal occult blood. A dab of fecal material from toilet tissue is smeared onto a card. The card is treated in

QUESTIONS TO ASK YOUR DOCTOR

- Is the supervising physician appropriately certified to conduct a sigmoidoscopy?
- How many sigmoidoscopy procedures has the doctor performed?
- What other steps will be taken as a result of my test findings?

a laboratory to reveal the presence of bleeding. This test is normally performed prior to a sigmoidoscopic examination.

A less invasive alternative to a sigmoidoscopic examination is an x-ray of the colon and rectum. Barium is used to coat the inner walls of the colon. This lower GI (gastrointestinal) x-ray may reveal the outlines of suspicious or abnormal structures. It has the disadvantage of not allowing direct visualization of the colon. It is less costly than a sigmoidoscopic examination.

A more invasive procedure is direct visualization of the colon during surgery. This procedure is rarely performed in the United States.

Health care team roles

A colonoscopy procedure is usually performed by a gastroenterologist, a physician with specialized training in diseases of the colon. Alternatively, general **surgeons** or experienced family physicians perform sigmoidoscopic examinations. In the United States, the procedure is usually performed in an outpatient facility of a hospital or in a physician's professional office.

Persons with rectal bleeding may need full colonoscopy in a hospital setting. Individuals whose blood does not clot well (possibly as a result of blood-thinning medications) may require the procedure to be performed in a hospital setting.

Resources

BOOKS

Balakrishnan, V., ed. *Practical Gastroenterology*. 3rd ed. Tunbridge Wells, Kent, UK: Anshan Ltd., 2007.

Gillison, W., and H. Buchwald. *Pioneers in Surgical Gastroenterology*. Shrewsbury, Shropshire, UK: TFM Publishing, 2006.

PERIODICALS

Carter, Xiaolu Wu, et al. "Role of Anxiety in the Comfort of Nonsedated Average-Risk Screening Sigmoidoscopy."

Southern Medical Journal 106, no. 4 (2013): 280–84. http://dx.doi.org/10.1097/SMJ.0b013e31828de613 (accessed October 14, 2013).

Holme, Ø., et al. "Flexible Sigmoidoscopy versus Faecal Occult Blood Testing for Colorectal Cancer Screening in Asymptomatic Individuals." *Cochrane Database of Systematic Reviews* 9, art. no. CD009259 (September 30, 2013). http://dx.doi.org/10.1002/14651858.CD009259. pub2 (accessed October 14, 2013).

van Dam, L., et al. "What Influences the Decision to Participate in Colorectal Cancer Screening with Faecal Occult Blood Testing and Sigmoidoscopy?" *European Journal of Cancer* 49, no. 10 (2013): 2321–30. http://dx. doi.org/10.1016/j.ejca.2013.03.007 (accessed October 14, 2013).

WEBSITES

American Cancer Society. "Frequently Asked Questions about Colonoscopy and Sigmoidoscopy." http://www.cancer. org/healthy/findcancerearly/examandtestdescriptions/faq-colonoscopy-and-sigmoidoscopy (accessed October 14, 2013).

American Society for Gastrointestinal Endoscopy. "Six Questions That Could Save Your Life (Or the Life of Someone You Love): What Women Need to Know about Colon Cancer Screening." http://www.asge.org/patients/patients.aspx?id=374 (accessed October 14, 2013).

National Cancer Institute. "Colorectal Cancer Screening (PDQ®)." http://www.cancer.gov/cancertopics/pdq/screening/colorectal/Patient (accessed October 14, 2013).

National Digestive Diseases Information Clearinghouse. "Flexible Sigmoidoscopy." National Institute of Diabetes and Digestive and Kidney Diseases. http://digestive.niddk. nih.gov/ddiseases/pubs/sigmoidoscopy (accessed October 14, 2013).

ORGANIZATIONS

American Academy of Family Physicians (AAFP), 11400 Tomahawk Creek Pkwy., Leawood, KS 66211-2680, (913) 906-6000, (800) 274-2237, Fax: (913) 906-6075, http://www.aafp.org.

American Society for Gastrointestinal Endoscopy, 1520 Kensington Rd., Ste. 202, Oak Brook, IL 60523, (630) 573-0600, (866) 353-ASGE (2743), Fax: (630) 573-0691, info@asge.org, http://www.asge.org.

National Digestive Diseases Information Clearinghouse (NDDIC), 2 Information Way, Bethesda, MD 20892-3570, (800) 891-5389, (866) 569–1162, Fax: (703) 738–4929, nddic@info.niddk.nih.gov, http://www.digestive.niddk. nih.gov.

Society of American Gastrointestinal Endoscopic Surgeons (SAGES), 11300 West Olympic Blvd., Ste. 600, Los Angeles, CA 90064, (310) 437-0544, Fax: (310) 437-0585, webmaster@sages.org, http://www. sages.org.

L. Fleming Fallon Jr., MD, DrPH

Simple mastectomy

Definition

Simple **mastectomy** is the surgical removal of one or both breasts. The adjacent lymph nodes and chest muscles are left intact. If a few lymph nodes are removed, the procedure is called an extended simple mastectomy. Breast-sparing techniques may be used to preserve the patient's breast skin and nipple, which is helpful in cosmetic **breast reconstruction**.

Purpose

Removal of a patient's breast is usually recommended when cancer is present in the breast or as a prophylactic when the patient has severe fibrocystic disease and a family history of breast cancer. The choice of a simple mastectomy may be determined by evaluating the size of the breast, the size of the cancerous mass, where the cancer is located, and whether any cancer cells have spread to adjacent lymph nodes or other parts of the body. If the cancer has not been contained within the breast, it calls for a **modified radical mastectomy**, which removes the entire breast and all of the adjacent lymph nodes. Only in extreme circumstances is a radical mastectomy, which also removes part of the chest wall, indicated.

A larger tumor usually is an indication of more advanced disease and will require more extensive surgery such as a simple mastectomy. In addition, if a woman has small breasts, the tumor may occupy more area within the contours of the breast, necessitating a simple mastectomy in order to remove all of the cancer.

Very rapidly growing tumors usually require the removal of all breast tissue. Cancers that have spread to adjacent tissues such as the chest wall or skin make simple mastectomy a good choice. Similarly, multiple sites of cancer within a breast require that the entire breast be removed. In addition, simple mastectomy is also recommended when cancer recurs in a breast that has already undergone a **lumpectomy**, which is a less invasive procedure that just removes the tumor and some surrounding tissue without removing the entire breast.

Sometimes, **surgeons** recommend simple mastectomy for women who are unable to undergo the adjuvant radiation therapy required after a lumpectomy. Radiation treatment is not indicated for pregnant women, those who have had previous therapeutic radiation in the chest area, and patients with collagen vascular diseases such as scleroderma or lupus. In these cases, simple mastectomy is the treatment of choice.

Some women with family histories of breast cancer and who test positive for a cancer-causing gene choose to

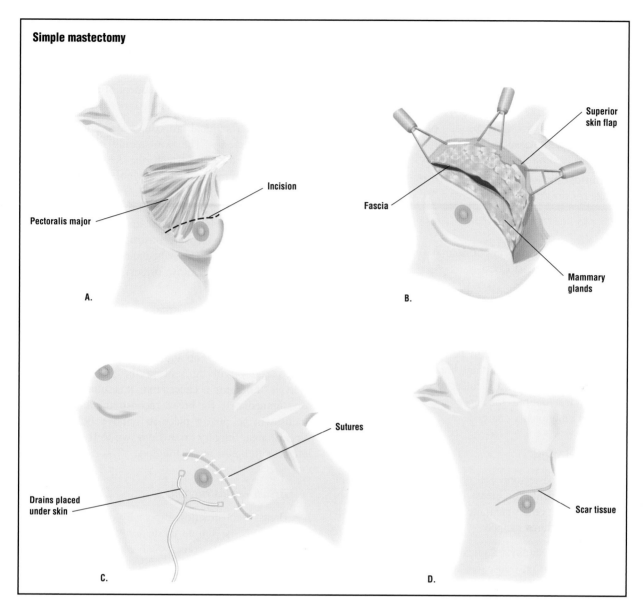

Simple mastectomy

A.

Pectoralis major

Incision

B.

Superior skin flap

Fascia

Mammary glands

C.

Drains placed under skin

Sutures

D.

Scar tissue

In a simple mastectomy, the skin over the tumor is cut open (A). The tumor and tissue surrounding it is removed (B), and the wound is closed (C). *(Illustration by GGS Information Services. Copyright © Cengage Learning®.)*

have one or both of their breasts removed as a preventative for future breast cancer. This procedure is highly controversial. Though prophylactic mastectomy reduces the occurrence of breast cancer by 90% in high-risk patients, it is not a foolproof method. There has been some incidence of cancer occurring after both breasts were removed.

Demographics

According to the American Cancer Society, 232,340 new cases of invasive breast cancer in women were diagnosed in 2013. New cases of breast cancer in men were expected to reach 2,240.

For approximately 80% of women, the first indication of cancer is the discovery of a lump in the breast, found either by themselves in a monthly self-exam, by a partner, or by a mammogram, a special x-ray of the breast that looks for anomalies. Early detection of breast cancer means that smaller tumors are found, which require less intensive surgery and have better treatment outcomes. Simple mastectomy has been the standard treatment of choice for breast cancer for the past 60 years. Newer breast-conserving surgery techniques have gained acceptance since the mid-1980s. For larger hospitals, facilities in urban areas, and health care institutions with a cancer center or high cancer patient volume, these newer techniques are being utilized at a more rapid rate, especially on the East Coast.

In 2003, the National Cancer Institute found that American women were 21% more likely to have a mastectomy than their counterparts in the United Kingdom. Though breast-conserving procedures are available and have proven to be viable options, some physicians and women still think breast removal will also remove all of their risk of cancer recurrence. It is clear that treatment options for cancer are highly individual and often emotionally charged.

Description

Simple mastectomy is one of several types of surgical treatments for breast cancer. Some techniques are rarely used; others are quite common. These common surgical procedures include:

- Radical mastectomy. Radical mastectomy is rarely used, and then only in cases where cancer cells have invaded the chest wall and the tumor is very large. The breast, muscles under the breast, and all of the lymph nodes are removed. This produces a large scar and severe disability to the arm nearest the removed breast.

- Modified radical mastectomy. Modified radical mastectomy was the most common form of mastectomy until the 1980s. The breast is removed along with the lining over the chest muscle and all of the lymph nodes.

- Simple mastectomy. Simple, sometimes called total, mastectomy has been the treatment of choice in the late 1980s and 1990s. Generally, only the breast is removed; though, sometimes, one or two lymph nodes may be removed as well.

- Partial mastectomy. Partial mastectomy is used to remove the tumor, the lining over the chest muscle underneath the tumor, and a good portion of breast tissue, but not the entire breast. This is a good treatment choice for early stage cancers.

- Lumpectomy. Lumpectomy or breast-conserving surgery just removes the tumor and a small amount of tissue surrounding it. Some lymph nodes may be removed as well. This is the most commonly used surgical procedure for the treatment of breast cancer in the early twenty-first century.

Two other surgical procedures are variations on the simple mastectomy. The skin-sparing mastectomy is a surgical procedure in which the surgeon makes an incision, sometimes called a keyhole incision, around the areola. The tumor and all breast tissue are removed, but the incision is smaller and scarring is minimal. About 90% of the skin is preserved and allows a cosmetic surgeon to perform breast reconstruction at the same time as the mastectomy. The subcutaneous mastectomy, or nipple-sparing mastectomy, preserves the skin and the nipple over the breast.

During a simple mastectomy, the surgeon makes a curved incision along one side of the breast and removes the tumor and all of the breast tissue. A few lymph nodes may be removed. The tumor, breast tissue, and any lymph nodes will be sent to the pathology lab for analysis. If the skin is cancer-free, it is sutured in place or used immediately for breast reconstruction. One or two drains will be put in place to remove fluid from the surgical area. Surgery takes from two to five hours; it is longer with breast reconstruction.

Breast reconstruction

Breast reconstruction, especially if it is begun at the same time as the simple mastectomy, can minimize the sense of loss that women feel when having a breast removed. Although there may be other smaller surgeries later to complete the breast reconstruction, there will not be a second major operation nor an additional scar.

If there is not enough skin left after the mastectomy, a balloon-type expander is put in place. In subsequent weeks, the expander is filled with larger amounts of saline (salt water) solution. When it has reached the appropriate size, the expander is removed and a permanent breast implant is installed.

If there is enough skin, an implant is installed immediately. In other instances, skin, fat, and muscle are removed from the patient's back or abdomen and repositioned on the chest wall to form a breast.

None of these reconstructions have nipples at first. Nipples are later reconstructed in a separate surgery. Finally, the areola is tattooed in to make the reconstructed breast look natural.

Breast reconstruction does not prevent a potential recurrence of breast cancer.

Preparation

If a mammogram has not been performed, it is usually ordered to verify the size of the lump the patient has reported. A biopsy of the suspicious lump and/or lymph nodes is usually ordered and sent to the pathology lab before surgery is discussed.

When a simple mastectomy has been determined, preoperative tests such as blood work, a **chest x-ray**, and an electrocardiogram may be ordered. Blood-thinning medications such as **aspirin** should be stopped several days before the surgery date. The patient is also asked to refrain from eating or drinking the night before the operation.

At the hospital, the patient will sign a consent form, verifying that the surgeon has explained what the surgery is and what it is for. The patient will also meet with the anesthesiologist to discuss the patient's medical history and determine the choice of anesthesia.

Aftercare

If the procedure is performed as an **outpatient surgery**, the patient may go home the same day of the surgery. The length of the hospital stay for inpatient mastectomies ranges from one to two days. If breast reconstruction has taken place, the hospital stay may be longer.

The surgical drains will remain in place for five to seven days. Sponge baths will be necessary until the stitches are removed, usually in a week to 10 days. It is important to avoid overhead lifting, strenuous sports, and sexual intercourse for three to six weeks. After the surgical drains are removed, stretching exercises may be begun, though some physical therapists may start a patient on shoulder and arm mobility exercises while in the hospital.

Since breast removal is often emotionally traumatic for women, seeking out a support group is often helpful. Women in these groups offer practical advice about matters such as finding well-fitting bras and swimwear, and emotional support because they have been through the same experience.

For women who chose not to have breast reconstruction, it may be necessary to find the proper fitting breast prosthesis. Some are made of cloth, and others are made of silicone, which are created from a mold from the patient's other breast.

In some case, the patient may be required to undergo additional treatments such as radiation, chemotherapy, or hormone therapy.

Risks

The risks involved with simple mastectomy are the same for any major surgery; however, there may be a need for more extensive surgery once the surgeon examines the tumor, the tissues surrounding it, and the lymph nodes nearby. A biopsy of the lymph nodes is usually performed during surgery and a determination is made whether to remove them. Simple mastectomy usually has limited impact on range of motion of the arm nearest the breast that is removed, but physical therapy may still be necessary to restore complete movement.

There is also the risk of infection around the incision. When the lymph nodes are removed, lymphedema may also occur. This condition is a result of damage to the lymph system. The arm on the side nearest the affected breast may become swollen. It can either resolve itself or worsen.

As in any surgery, the risk of developing a blood clot after a mastectomy is a serious matter. All hospitals use a variety of techniques to prevent blood clots from forming. It is important for the patient to walk daily when at home.

Finally, there is the risk that not all cancer cells were removed. Further treatment may be necessary.

Results

The breast area will fully heal in three to four weeks. If the patient had breast reconstruction, it may take up to six weeks to recover fully. The patient should be able to participate in all of the activities she has engaged in before surgery. If breast reconstruction is done, the patient should realize that the new breast will not have the sensitivity of a normal breast. In addition, dealing with cancer emotionally may take time, especially if additional treatment is necessary.

Morbidity and mortality rates

Deaths due to breast cancer have declined by 1.4% each year between 1989 and 1995, and by 3.2% each year thereafter. The largest decreases have been among younger women, as a result of cancer education campaigns and early screening, which encourage more women to go to their physicians to be checked.

Research performed between 2000 and 2004 demonstrated that the five-year survival rate for cancers confined to the breast is 98%. For cancers that had spread to areas within the chest region, the rate was 83.5%, and it was only 26.7% for cancers occurring in other parts of the body after breast cancer treatment. The best survival rates were for early stage tumors.

Two 20-year longitudinal studies concluded in 2002 indicated that the survival rate for patients with modified

QUESTIONS TO ASK YOUR DOCTOR

- Why is this procedure necessary?
- How big is my tumor?
- Are there other breast-saving or less-invasive procedures for which I might be a candidate?
- What can I expect after surgery?
- Do you work with a cosmetic surgeon?
- Will I have to undergo radiation or chemotherapy after surgery?

radical mastectomy (the removal of the entire breast and all lymph nodes) was no different from that of breast-conserving lumpectomy (the removal of the tumor alone). These studies suggest that the removal of the entire breast may not afford greater protection against future cancer than breast-conserving techniques; however, the majority of cancer recurrences happen within the first five years for both those with mastectomies and those with lumpectomies.

Alternatives

Skin-sparing mastectomy, also called nipple-sparing mastectomy, is becoming a treatment of choice for women undergoing simple mastectomy. In this procedure, the skin of the breast, the areola, and the nipple are peeled back to remove the breast and its inherent tumor. Biopsies of the skin and nipple areas are performed immediately to assure that they do not have cancer cells in them. Then, a cosmetic surgeon performs a breast reconstruction at the same time as the mastectomy. The breast regains its normal contours once prostheses are inserted. Unfortunately, the nipple will lose its sensitivity and, of course, its function, since all underlying tissue has been removed. If cancer is found near the nipple, this procedure cannot be done.

Health care team roles

Simple mastectomy is performed by a general surgeon or a gynecological surgeon. If reconstructive breast surgery is to be done, a cosmetic surgeon performs it. Patients undergo simple mastectomies under **general anesthesia** as an inpatient in a hospital. There is a growing trend, due to reductions in insurance coverage and patient preference, to perform simple mastectomies without reconstructive breast surgery as outpatient procedures.

Resources

BOOKS

Khatri, V. P., and J. A. Asensio. *Operative Surgery Manual.* Philadelphia: Saunders, 2003.

Lentz, Gretchen, et al. *Comprehensive Gynecology.* 5th ed. St. Louis: Mosby/Elsevier, 2012.

Niederhuber, John E., et al. *Abeloff's Clinical Oncology.* 5th ed. Philadelphia: Saunders/Elsevier, 2013.

Townsend, Courtney M., et al. *Sabiston Textbook of Surgery.* 19th ed. Philadelphia: Saunders/Elsevier, 2012.

PERIODICALS

Bugelli, George J., Walid A. Samra, and Karen Stuart-Smith. "Simple Mastectomy and Axillary Lymph Node Biopsy Performed under Paravertebral Block and Light Sedation in a Patient with Severe Cardiorespiratory Comorbidities: Proposed Management of Choice in High-Risk Breast Surgery Patients." *Clinical Breast Cancer* 13, no. 2 (2013): 153–55. http://dx.doi.org/10.1016/j.clbc.2012.12.003 (accessed October 17, 2013).

Johansen, Helge, et al. "Extended Radical Mastectomy versus Simple Mastectomy followed by Radiotherapy in Primary Breast Cancer. A Fifty-Year Follow-Up to the Copenhagen Breast Cancer Randomised Study." *Acta Oncologica* 47, no. 4 (2008): 633–38. http://dx.doi.org/10.1080/02841860801989753 (accessed October 17, 2013).

WEBSITES

American Cancer Society. "What Are the Key Statistics about Breast Cancer?" http://www.cancer.org/cancer/breastcancer/detailedguide/breast-cancer-key-statistics (accessed October 14, 2013).

American Cancer Society. "What Are the Key Statistics about Breast Cancer in Men?" http://www.cancer.org/cancer/breastcancerinmen/detailedguide/breast-cancer-in-men-key-statistics (accessed October 14, 2013).

American Cancer Society. "Surgery for Breast Cancer." http://www.cancer.org/cancer/breastcancer/detailedguide/breast-cancer-treating-surgery (accessed October 14, 2013).

Breastcancer.org. "Skin-Sparing Mastectomy." http://www.breastcancer.org/treatment/surgery/mastectomy/skinsparing (accessed October 17, 2013).

Susan G. Komen for the Cure. "Mastectomy." http://ww5.komen.org/BreastCancer/Mastectomy.html (accessed October 17, 2013).

ORGANIZATIONS

American Cancer Society, 250 Williams St. NW, Atlanta, GA 30303, (800) 227-2345, http://www.cancer.org.

American Society of Plastic Surgeons, 444 E. Algonquin Rd., Arlington Heights, IL 60005, http://www.plasticsurgery.org.

National Cancer Institute, 6116 Executive Blvd., Ste. 300, Bethesda, MD 20892-8322, (800) 4-CANCER (422-6237), http://cancer.gov.

Janie Franz

Single photon emission computed tomography

Definition

Single photon emission **computed tomography** (SPECT) is a type of nuclear medicine scan that uses radioactive materials to generate a high-resolution image of the brain or other parts of the body. SPECT relies on two technologies: computed tomography (CT) and the use of a radioactive material (radionuclide) to label a compound known as a tracer. Tracking the tracer's movement through body tissues and the rate of its radioactive decay allows the doctor to obtain 3-D images of blood flow in the heart, electrical activity in different areas of the brain, or to scan for tumors or bone disease by using a device called a gamma camera contained within the SPECT machine.

Purpose

SPECT is used to diagnose head trauma, epilepsy, dementia, and cerebrovascular disease. Development of a radiotracer called Tc99m (technetium-99) has increased the resolution of brain images generated from SPECT. The images yield very accurate spatial and contrast resolutions. Other radioactive isotopes used in SPECT are iodine-123, xenon-133, thallium-201, and fluorine-18. The resulting sharp images enable the clinician to visualize very small structures within the brain or other parts of the body. The accuracy of SPECT images makes it a very useful clinical and research tool.

Clinically, SPECT is useful for diagnosing the following disease states:

• Cerebrovascular disease or stroke. SPECT is useful to detect ischemia (reduced blood flow), determine causes of stroke, evaluate transient ischemia, determine prognosis, and monitor treatment.

• Such forms of dementia as Alzheimer's disease. SPECT studies can be used effectively to rule out other medical causes of dementia.

• Head trauma. Evidence suggests that SPECT is useful to detect a greater number of lesions following the period after head trauma. It seems that the high resolution and accurate brain images of SPECT can detect lesions in the brain that are not possible to visualize using other techniques such as positron emission tomography (PET) scanning. SPECT images can give clinicians important information concerning prognosis (also sometimes called outcome) and treatment of persons affected with head injury.

• Epilepsy. The radioactive material injected before SPECT imaging concentrates at the seizure locus (the region that contains nerve cells that generate an abnormal impulse). This can help identify the location of seizures and assist clinicians in determining management and treatment outcomes.

• Other brain disorders. SPECT allows clinicians to visualize a specific area of the brain called the corpus striatum, which contains a neurotransmitter (a chemical that communicates nerve impulses from one nerve cell to another) called dopamine. Circuitry in the corpus striatum and interaction with dopamine can help provide valuable information concerning movement disorders, schizophrenia, mood disorders, and hormone diseases (since hormones require control and regulation from the brain in structures called the pituitary gland and hypothalamus).

As a research tool, SPECT imaging seems to be sensitive tool to measure blood flow through the brain (cerebral blood flow) in persons who have psychological disorders such as obsessive-compulsive disorder (higher blood flow) and alcoholism (lower blood flow).

SPECT has also been used in myocardial perfusion imaging (MPI), which is a test done to evaluate patients for coronary artery disease. It is based on the understanding that diseased heart tissue under stress receives less blood than normal heart tissue (myocardium). A special form of technetium-99 known as Tc-sestamibi is injected. The patient's heart is then stressed by either **exercise** or by the administration of a drug, usually dobutamine, adenosine, or dipyridamole. SPECT imaging performed after the stress will reveal the distribution of the Tc-sestamibi within the different regions of the heart muscle. The patient is usually asked to return between one and seven days after the **stress test** for another set of SPECT images taken while he or she is at rest. Doctors then compare the two sets of images. If the images following the stress test are normal, the patient does not have to return for a second SPECT scan.

Other SPECT diagnostic indications and procedures are similar to other imaging studies such as CT, **magnetic resonance imaging** (MRI), and **PET**.

Description

In most cases, the SPECT scan involves injecting the patient with a compound containing the radioactive tracer or administering the tracer through an infusion given intravenously into a vein in the arm. In some cases, the patient may inhale the tracer through the nose. The patient is then asked to lie quietly in a room for 15–30 minutes while the radioactive tracer is absorbed by the body.

In the second phase of the scan, the patient is positioned by the health care team on a table in the room with the SPECT machine. The exact position depends on the part of the patient's body or the organ system that is

KEY TERMS

Gamma camera—A device inside the SPECT machine that forms images of the gamma rays emitted by the radionuclides used in tracers in nuclear medicine.

Gamma rays—Extremely short-wavelength electromagnetic radiation released during the process of radioactive decay.

Myocardium—The medical term for the specialized involuntary muscle tissue found in the walls of the heart.

Nuclear medicine—A branch of medicine that makes use of radioisotopes (also called radionuclides) to evaluate the rate of radioactive decay in diagnosing and treating various diseases.

Radionuclide—An atom with an unstable nucleus that emits gamma rays during the process of its radioactive decay. Radionuclides, also known as radioisotopes, are used to make the tracers used in SPECT. The most common radionuclides used in SPECT are iodine-123, technetium-99m, xenon-133, thallium-201, and fluorine-18.

Tracer—A substance containing a radioisotope, injected into the body and followed in order to obtain information about various metabolic processes in the body.

being investigated. The SPECT machine itself contains a gamma camera, an imaging device that detects gamma rays given off by the radioactive tracer in the patient's body. The SPECT machine rotates around the patient while the gamma camera records a series of two-dimensional images of the patient's body organs. These images are then sent to a computer that produces 3-D images of the organs in question.

Precautions

Women who are pregnant or breast-feeding should not have SPECT scans because the radioactive tracer can be passed to the fetus or the nursing baby. Women of childbearing age may be asked to have a pregnancy test before a SPECT scan.

Preparation

Patients should wear comfortable clothing for a SPECT scan and expect to stay in the hospital for one to three hours. They do not need to fast beforehand or omit the medications they usually take.

Aftercare

Aftercare consists of drinking extra fluids to speed the excretion of the radioactive tracer in the urine. The tracer is usually flushed out in the patient's urine within a few hours after the scan. Any remaining tracer is broken down in the body within the next two days.

Risks

SPECT scans are generally safe and well tolerated by most patients. Some people, however, may experience bruising, bleeding, or pain at the point at which the needle was inserted into their vein. A small number of patients have allergic reactions to the radionuclide.

Results

Typical results of a SPECT scan show which parts of the patient's body or which areas within a specific organ absorbed larger amounts of the radionuclide and which absorbed less of the chemical. The images may be shown in different colors or in various shades of gray.

Resources

BOOKS

Heller, Gary V., April Mann, and Robert C. Hendel, eds. *Nuclear Cardiology: Technical Applications.* New York: McGraw-Hill Medical, 2009.

Levine, Harry III. *Medical Imaging.* Santa Barbara, CA: ABC-CLIO, 2010.

PERIODICALS

Stein, P. D., et al. "SPECT in Acute Pulmonary Embolism." *Journal of Nuclear Medicine* 50 (December 2009): 1999–2007.

Yeo, J. M., et al. "Systematic Review of the Diagnostic Utility of SPECT Imaging in Dementia." *Journal of Neurology, Neurosurgery & Psychiatry* 84, no. 11 (2013): e2. http://dx.doi.org/10.1136/jnnp-2013-306573.88 (accessed October 18, 2013).

WEBSITES

Mayfield Clinic. "SPECT (Single Photon Emission Computed Tomography) Scan." http://www.mayfieldclinic.com/PE-SPECT.htm (accessed October 18, 2013).

Mayo Clinic staff. "SPECT Scan." http://www.mayoclinic.com/health/spect-scan/MY00233 (accessed October 18, 2013).

ORGANIZATIONS

Society of Nuclear Medicine and Molecular Imaging, 1850 Samuel Morse Dr., Reston, VA 20190, (703) 708-9000, http://www.snm.org.

Laith Farid Gulli, MD
Rebecca J. Frey, PhD
Brenda W. Lerner

Sinus x-ray *see* **Skull x-rays**

Skeletal traction *see* **Traction**

Skin biopsy

Definition

A skin biopsy is a procedure in which a small piece of living skin is removed from the body for examination, usually under a microscope. Skin biopsies are usually brief, straightforward procedures performed by a skin specialist (dermatologist) or family physician. It is performed to help the physician make a diagnosis when a skin disorder is suspected. Information from the biopsy also helps the doctor choose the best treatment for the patient.

Purpose

Doctors perform skin biopsies to:

- make a diagnosis
- confirm a diagnosis made from the patient's medical history and a physical examination
- check whether a treatment prescribed for a previously diagnosed condition is working
- check the edges of tissue removed with a tumor to make certain it contains all the diseased tissue

Skin biopsies also can serve a therapeutic purpose. Many skin abnormalities (lesions) can be removed completely during a biopsy procedure.

Description

The first step in a skin biopsy test is obtaining a sample of tissue that best represents the lesion being

---

Skin biopsy

Certain features of skin lesions might be indicative of a need for a skin biopsy. Stay alert for changes in moles over time, especially related to:

Asymmetrical shape
Border
Color
Diameter

SOURCE: Melanoma Research Foundation, "ABCDE's of Melanoma." Available online at: http://www.melanoma.org/learn-more/melanoma-101/abcdes-melanoma.

(Table by PreMediaGlobal. Copyright © 2014 Cengage Learning®.)

---

evaluated. Many biopsy techniques are available. The choice of technique and precise location from which to take the biopsy material are determined by factors such as the type and shape of the lesion. Biopsies can be classified as excisional, when the lesion is completely removed, or as incisional, when a portion of the lesion is removed.

There are four common biopsy techniques:

- In a shave biopsy, the doctor uses a scalpel or razor blade to shave off a thin layer of the lesion parallel to the skin.
- In a punch biopsy, a small cylindrical punch is screwed into the lesion through the full thickness of the skin and a plug of tissue is removed. A stitch or two may be needed to close the wound.
- In a scalpel biopsy, the doctor makes a standard surgical incision or excision to remove tissue. This technique is most often used for large or deep lesions. The wound is closed with stitches.
- In a scissors biopsy, surface (superficial) skin growths or lesions growing from a stem or column of tissue are snipped off with surgical scissors. Such growths are sometimes seen on the eyelids or neck.

After the biopsy tissue is removed, bleeding may be controlled by applying pressure or heat. **Antibiotics** often are applied to the wound to prevent infection. Depending on the type of biopsy performed, stitches may be placed in the wound, or the wound may be bandaged and allowed to heal on its own.

The tissue sample is placed immediately in an appropriate preservative, such as formaldehyde, to prevent drying and structural damage. It is then sent to the laboratory. A variety of laboratory techniques may be used to process the biopsy tissue, including tissue stains and examination with any of several different kinds of microscopes. There are many skin disorders (broadly called dermatosis and dermatitis), so the pathologist studying the sample has had extensive training in their accurate identification. Cases of melanoma, the most malignant kind of skin cancer, have almost tripled in the past 30 years. Because melanoma grows very rapidly in the skin, quick and accurate diagnosis is important.

Precautions

A patient taking **aspirin** or another blood thinner (anticoagulant) may be asked to stop taking it a week or more before the skin biopsy. This adjustment in medication will prevent excessive bleeding during the procedure and allow for normal blood clotting.

Some patients are allergic to lidocaine, the numbing agent most frequently used during a skin biopsy. The doctor can usually substitute another anesthetic agent.

Preparation

The area of the biopsy is cleansed thoroughly with alcohol or a disinfectant containing iodine. Sterile cloths (drapes) may be positioned, and a local anesthetic, usually lidocaine, is injected into the skin near the lesion. Sometimes the anesthetic contains epinephrine, a drug that helps reduce bleeding during the biopsy. Sterile gloves and **surgical instruments** are used in excision procedures to reduce the risk of infection. They are not required for shave or punch biopsies.

Aftercare

If stitches have been placed, they should be kept clean until removed. Sometimes the patient is instructed to put protective ointment on the stitches before or after showering; the doctor should provide specific instructions on how to care for the wound. Stitches are usually removed five to ten days after the biopsy. Wounds that have not been stitched should be cleaned with soap and water daily until they heal. Any adhesive strips should be left in place for two to three weeks. Pain medications usually are not necessary.

Risks

Infection and bleeding rarely occur after skin biopsy. If the skin biopsy may leave a scar, the patient usually is asked to give **informed consent** before the test.

Results

If the biopsy reveals a lesion, it is classified as either benign (noncancerous) or malignant (cancerous). Some benign lesions may require treatment, but all malignant lesions require treatment.

Resources

WEBSITES

A.D.A.M. Medical Encyclopedia. "Skin Lesion Biopsy." MedlinePlus. http://www.nlm.nih.gov/medlineplus/ency/article/003840.htm (accessed August 8, 2013).

UW Health. "Skin Biopsy." University of Wisconsin-Madison. http://www.uwhealth.org/health/topic/medicaltest/skin-biopsy/hw234496.html (accessed August 8, 2013).

ORGANIZATIONS

American Academy of Dermatology, PO Box 4014, Schaumburg, IL 60168-4014, Fax: (847) 240-1859, (866) 503-SKIN (7546), http://www.aad.org.

Collette L. Placek

Skin culture

Definition

A skin culture is a laboratory test used to isolate and identify the microorganism (bacterium, fungus, or virus) causing a skin infection, so the most effective antibiotic or other treatment for the infection can be determined.

Purpose

Skin infections are contagious and, if left untreated, can lead to serious complications. A skin culture helps physicians diagnose and treat skin infections.

Description

Skin infections may involve the top layer of skin (epidermis) only or may involve the deeper dermis, including the sweat glands, oil glands, lymphatics, and hair follicles. Microorganisms can infect healthy skin, but more often they infect skin already damaged by an injury or an abrasion. The lesion produced by the infection is an early indication of which type of microorganism is causing the infection. For example, pustules are associated with impetigo (pyoderma), the most common bacterial skin infection. Pyoderma is most often caused by group A *Streptococcus*. Vesicular skin rashes are commonly caused by herpesviruses as in chickenpox. Scaly rashes are most commonly caused by dermatophytes, fungi that infect the keratinized skin (epidermis).

Types of infections

There are several different causes of skin infections, including:

• Bacterial skin infections are the most common type of infection and can result in ulcers, cellulitis, rashes, boils, abscesses, and other types of lesions. Bacteria are usually introduced through a wound in the skin caused by a bite, decubitus ulcer, burn, trauma, or puncture. Organisms that live in the mouth of dogs and cats can also infect bite wounds.

• Fungal infections include ringworm of the skin, hair, and nails. Candida causes yeast infections. Several other fungi may cause subcutaneous infection.

• Viruses such as rubella (German measles), rubeola (measles), roseola, and herpes varicella zoster (chickenpox) are common causes of viral rashes in children. Herpes simplex 1 and cytomegalovirus may cause more complex infections in immunosuppressed adults. In addition, skin infections can be caused by enteroviruses, poxviruses, and several others.

• Other causes of skin infections include mycobacteria such as *Mycobacterium tuberculosis* and *M. leprae* (the cause of leprosy). Some skin lesions can be caused by parasites when the larva enter the skin.

Collection process

Based on the appearance of the lesion, the physician will order one or more types of skin cultures. Using **aseptic technique**, the physician, nurse, or other health care professional collects the specimen. For open epidermal infections, a sample of the lesion—such as skin cells, pus, or fluid—can be collected using a swab. For crusted or closed lesions, the surface of the vesicle or pustule should be removed with a scalpel blade in order to expose the infected skin before swabbing. Ringworm should be scraped using a

---

KEY TERMS

Antimicrobial—A substance or action that kills or inhibits the growth of microorganisms.

Aseptic technique—Practices performed before, during, and after a clinical procedure to prevent or reduce contamination and postprocedural infection.

Bacteria—Tiny, one-celled forms of life that cause many diseases and infections.

Microorganism—An organism that is too small to be seen with the naked eye.

Pathogen—A disease-causing organism.

Pyoderma—A pus-containing bacterial skin infection.

Sensitivity test—A laboratory test that shows which antibiotics will treat an infection by killing the bacteria.

---

scalpel blade to collect the keratinized skin. Deeper infections should be sampled by aspiration. Swabs for bacterial culture are placed in a sterile container (often containing transport medium such as Stuart or Cary-Blair) before being sent to the laboratory for culture. If anaerobic culture is requested, the specimen is immediately placed in a prereduced oxygen-free transport medium.

Preparation

Before ordering a skin culture, the physician will ask the patient for a complete medical history and perform a **physical examination** to determine the possible causes of the skin infection and whether a skin culture is appropriate. For acute skin infections, immediate treatment is sometimes necessary.

Aftercare

Collection of the specimen may cause slight bleeding at the infection site, which might require attention. Otherwise, no special aftercare is necessary.

Risks

If aseptic technique is not used to collect the specimen, the patient or the health care professionals could develop postprocedure infections. The infection could also be transmitted to other individuals by contaminated hands or objects.

Results

Results for bacterial cultures are usually available in one to three days. Cultures for fungi and viruses may take longer—up to three or more weeks.

Many microorganisms that are found on a person's skin are normally considered to be harmless. When these microorganisms grow on a skin culture, they are reported as "normal flora."

Besides the normal flora, any microorganism that grows on a skin culture is considered to be the cause of the infection if:

• it is the only microorganism or the predominant microorganism

• it grows in large numbers

• it is known to produce infection

Staphylococcus aureus and group A *Streptococcus* cause most bacterial skin infections. *Candida albicans* causes most yeast skin infections, and *Herpes simplex* is the most frequent cause of viral skin infections.

Health care team roles

The patient's physician determines whether a skin culture is needed to diagnose a skin infection and orders the test when appropriate. The physician, a nurse, or another health care professional may collect the specimen and send it to the laboratory. At the lab, a clinical laboratory scientist or medical technologist assumes responsibility for the correct handling, culture, identification, and reporting of the specimen.

Resources

BOOKS

Goldsmith, Lowell A., et al. *Dermatology in General Medicine.* 8th ed. New York: McGraw-Hill, 2012.

Pagana, Kathleen Deska, and Timothy J. Pagana. *Mosby's Diagnostic and Laboratory Test Reference.* 11th ed. St. Louis, MO: Mosby/Elsevier, 2013.

WEBSITES

A.D.A.M. Medical Encyclopedia. "Skin Culture." MedlinePlus. http://www.nlm.nih.gov/medlineplus/ency/article/003762.htm (accessed August 8, 2013).

Healthwise. "Skin and Wound Cultures." University of Michigan Medical System. http://www.uofmhealth.org/health-library/hw5656#hw5659 (accessed August 8, 2013).

ORGANIZATIONS

American Academy of Dermatology, 930 E. Woodfield Rd., Schaumburg, IL 60173, (847) 240-1280, (866) 503-SKIN (7546), http://www.aad.org.

Beverly G. Miller, MT(ASCP)
Nancy J. Nordenson

Skin grafting

Definition

Skin grafting is a surgical procedure in which skin or a skin substitute is placed over a burn or non-healing wound.

Purpose

A skin graft is used to permanently replace damaged or missing skin or to provide a temporary wound covering. This covering is necessary because the skin protects the body from fluid loss, aids in temperature regulation, and helps prevent disease-causing bacteria or viruses from entering the body. Skin that is damaged extensively by burns or non-healing wounds can compromise the health and well-being of the patient.

Demographics

Although anyone can be involved in a fire and need a skin graft, the population groups with a higher risk of fire-related injuries and deaths include:

• children 4 years old and younger

• adults 65 years and older

• African Americans and Native Americans

• low-income Americans

• persons living in rural areas

• persons living in manufactured homes (trailers) or substandard housing

Description

The skin is the largest organ of the human body. It is also known as the integument or integumentary system because it covers the entire outside of the body. The skin consists of two main layers: the outer layer, or epidermis, which lies on and is nourished by the thicker dermis. These two layers are approximately 0.04–0.08 in. (1–2 mm) thick. The epidermis consists of an outer layer of dead cells called keratinocytes, which provide a tough protective coating, and several layers of rapidly dividing cells just beneath the keratinocytes. The dermis contains the blood vessels, nerves, sweat glands, hair follicles, and oil glands. The dermis consists mainly of connective tissue, which is largely made up of a protein called collagen. Collagen gives the skin its flexibility and provides structural support. The fibroblasts that make collagen are the main type of cell in the dermis.

Skin varies in thickness in different parts of the body; it is thickest on the palms and soles of the feet, and thinnest on the eyelids. In general, men have thicker skin than women, and adults have thicker skin than children.

Skin grafting

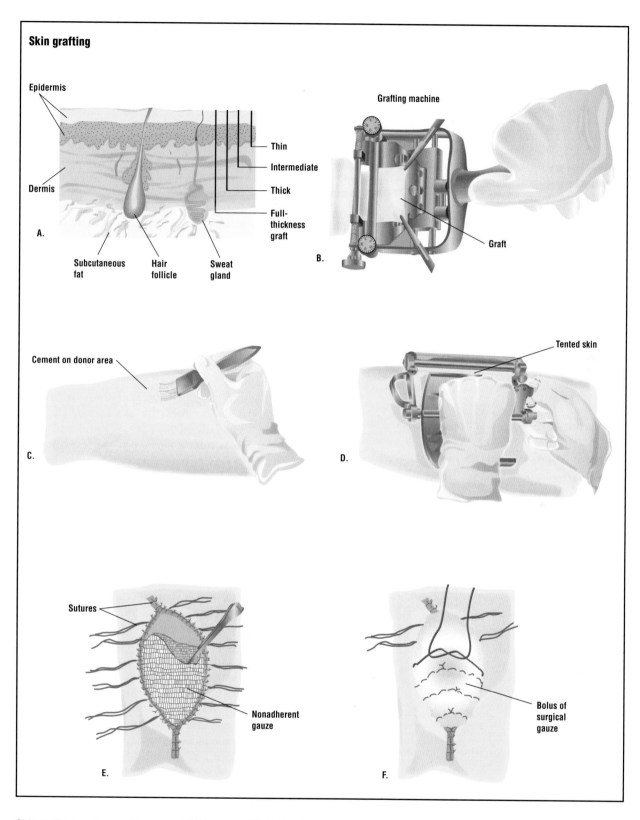

A.
Epidermis
Dermis
Subcutaneous fat
Hair follicle
Sweat gland
Thin
Intermediate
Thick
Full-thickness graft

B.
Grafting machine
Graft

C.
Cement on donor area

D.
Tented skin

E.
Sutures
Nonadherent gauze

F.
Bolus of surgical gauze

Skin grafts may be used in several thicknesses (A). To begin the procedure, a special cement is used on the donor skin area (C). The grafting machine is applied to the area, and a sample is taken (D). After the graft is stitched to the recipient area, it is covered with nonadherent gauze (E) and a layer of fluffy surgical gauze held in place with sutures (F). *(Illustration by GGS Information Services. Copyright © Cengage Learning®.)*

KEY TERMS

Allograft—Tissue that is taken from one person's body and grafted to another person.

Autograft—Tissue that is taken from one part of a person's body and transplanted to a different part of the same person.

Collagen—A protein that provides structural support for the skin. Collagen is the main component of connective tissue.

Contracture—An abnormal persistent shortening of a muscle or the overlying skin at a joint, usually caused by the formation of scar tissue following an injury.

Debridement—The removal of foreign matter and dead or damaged tissue from a traumatic or infected wound until healthy tissue is reached.

Dermatome—A surgical instrument used to cut thin slices of skin for grafts.

Dermis—The underlayer of skin, containing blood vessels, nerves, hair follicles, and oil and sweat glands.

Epidermis—The outer layer of skin, consisting of a layer of dead cells that perform a protective function and a second layer of dividing cells.

Fibroblasts—A type of cell found in connective tissue; produces collagen.

Hematoma—A localized collection of blood in an organ or tissue due to broken blood vessels.

Integument—A covering; in medicine, the skin as a covering for the body. The skin is also called the integumentary system.

Keratinocytes—Dead cells at the outer surface of the epidermis that form a tough protective layer for the skin. The cells underneath divide to replenish the supply.

Xenograft—Tissue that is transplanted from one species to another (e.g., pigs to humans).

After age 50, however, the skin begins to grow thinner again as it loses its elastic fibers and some of its fluid content.

Injuries treated with skin grafts

Skin grafting is sometimes done as part of elective **plastic surgery** procedures, but its most extensive use is in the treatment of burns. For first- or second-degree burns, skin grafting is generally not required, as these burns usually heal with little or no scarring. With third-degree burns, however, the skin is destroyed to its full depth, in addition to damage done to underlying tissues. People who suffer third-degree burns often require skin grafting.

Wounds such as third-degree burns must be covered as quickly as possible to prevent infection or loss of fluid. Wounds that are left to heal on their own can contract, often resulting in serious scarring; if the wound is large enough, the scar can actually prevent movement of limbs. Non-healing wounds, such as diabetic ulcers, venous ulcers, or pressure sores, can be treated with skin grafts to prevent infection and further progression of the wounded area.

Types of skin grafts

The term "graft" by itself commonly refers to either an allograft or an autograft. An autograft is a type of graft that uses skin from another area of the patient's own body if there is enough undamaged skin available, and if the patient is healthy enough to undergo the additional surgery required. An allograft uses skin obtained from another human being. Donor skin from cadavers is frozen, stored, and available for use as allografts. Skin taken from an animal (usually a pig) is called a xenograft because it comes from a nonhuman species. Allografts and xenografts provide only temporary covering because they are rejected by the patient's immune system within 7 to 10 days. They must then be replaced with an autograft.

SPLIT-THICKNESS GRAFTS (STSG). A split-thickness skin graft involves the epidermis and a little of the underlying dermis; the donor site usually heals within several days. The surgeon first marks the outline of the wound on the skin of the donor site, enlarging it by 3%–5% to allow for tissue shrinkage. The surgeon uses a dermatome (a special instrument for cutting thin slices of tissue) to remove a split-thickness graft from the donor site. The wound must not be too deep if a split-thickness graft is going to be successful, since the blood vessels that will nourish the grafted tissue must come from the dermis of the wound itself. The graft is usually taken from an area that is ordinarily hidden by clothes, such as the buttock or inner thigh, and spread on the bare area to be covered. Gentle pressure from a well-padded dressing is then applied, or a few small sutures used to hold the graft in place. A sterile nonadherent dressing is then applied to the raw donor area for approximately three to five days to protect it from infection.

FULL-THICKNESS GRAFTS (FTSG). Full-thickness skin grafts may be necessary for more severe burn injuries. These grafts involve both layers of the skin. Full-thickness autografts are more complicated than partial-thickness grafts, but provide better contour, more natural color, and less contraction at the grafted site. A flap of skin with underlying muscle and blood supply is transplanted to the area to be grafted. This procedure is used when tissue loss is extensive, such as after open fractures of the lower leg, with significant skin loss and underlying infection. The back and the abdomen are common donor sites for full-thickness grafts. The main disadvantage of full-thickness skin grafts is that the wound at the donor site is larger and requires more careful management. Often, a split-thickness graft must be used to cover the donor site.

A composite skin graft is sometimes used, which consists of combinations of skin and fat, skin and cartilage, or dermis and fat. Composite grafts are used in patients whose injuries require three-dimensional reconstruction. For example, a wedge of ear containing skin and cartilage can be used to repair the nose.

A full-thickness graft is removed from the donor site with a scalpel rather than a dermatome. After the surgeon has cut around the edges of the pattern used to determine the size of the graft, he or she lifts the skin with a special hook and trims off any fatty tissue. The graft is then placed on the wound and secured in place with absorbable sutures.

Preparation

The most important part of any skin graft procedure is proper preparation of the wound. Skin grafts will not survive on tissue with a limited blood supply (cartilage or tendons) or tissue that has been damaged by radiation treatment. The patient's wound must be free of any dead tissue, foreign matter, or bacterial contamination. After the patient has been anesthetized, the surgeon prepares the wound by rinsing it with saline solution or a diluted antiseptic (Betadine) and removes any dead tissue by **debridement**. In addition, the surgeon stops the flow of blood into the wound by applying pressure, tying off blood vessels, or administering a medication (epinephrine) that causes the blood vessels to constrict.

Aftercare

Once a skin graft has been put in place, it must be maintained carefully even after it has healed. Patients who have grafts on their legs should remain in bed for seven to ten days with their legs elevated. For several months, the patient should support the graft with an Ace bandage or Jobst stocking. Grafts on other areas of the body should be similarly supported after healing to decrease the amount of contracture.

Grafted skin does not contain sweat or oil glands, and should be lubricated daily for two to three months with mineral oil or another bland oil to prevent drying and cracking.

Aftercare of patients with severe burns typically includes psychological or psychiatric counseling as well as **wound care** and physical rehabilitation, particularly if the patient's face has been disfigured. The severe pain and lengthy period of recovery involved in burn treatment are often accompanied by anxiety and depression. If the patient's burns occurred in combat, a transportation disaster, terrorist attack, or other fire involving large numbers of people, he or she is at high risk of developing post-traumatic stress disorder (PTSD). Anti-anxiety medication may be a helpful adjunct to treatment in these patients. Additionally, because burn patients are at high risk of developing stress ulcers in their gastrointestinal system, with a high rate of bleeding, GI medications that prevent stress ulcers are often given to burn patients.

Risks

The risks of skin grafting include those inherent in any surgical procedure that involves anesthesia. These include reactions to the medications, breathing problems, bleeding, and infection. In addition, the risks of an allograft procedure include transmission of an infectious disease from the donor.

The tissue for grafting and the recipient site must be as sterile as possible to prevent later infection that could result in failure of the graft. Failure of a graft can result from inadequate preparation of the wound, poor blood flow to the injured area, swelling, or infection. The most common reason for graft failure is the formation of a hematoma, or collection of blood in the injured tissues.

Results

A skin graft should provide significant improvement in the quality of the wound site, and may prevent the serious complications associated with burns or non-healing wounds. Normally, new blood vessels begin growing from the donor area into the transplanted skin within 36 hours. Occasionally, skin grafts are unsuccessful or don't heal well. In these cases, repeat grafting is necessary. Even though the skin graft must be protected from trauma or significant stretching for two to three weeks following split-thickness skin grafting, recovery from surgery is usually rapid. A dressing may be necessary for one to two weeks, depending on the location of the graft. Any **exercise** or activity that stretches the graft or puts it at risk for trauma should be avoided for three to four weeks. A one- to two-week hospital stay is most often required in cases of full-thickness grafts, as the recovery period is longer.

Morbidity and mortality rates

According to the American Burn Association, there are more than one million burn injuries in the United States each year that require medical attention. Approximately one-half of these require hospitalization, and roughly 25,000 of those burn patients are admitted to a specialized burn unit. About 4,500 people die from burns each year in the United States.

In the United States, about 500,000 people seek medical treatment for burns every year. About 4,000 people die of their burn injury yearly (including 3,500 due to injuries from residential fires, and 500 due to injuries from fires resulting from a car or airplane crash, and chemical and electrical burns). 40,000 people are admitted to hospitals annually for burn treatment; 25,000 of these are admitted to specialized burn centers.

About 38% of all burn unit admissions are for burns covering more than 10% of the patient's total body surface area. 10% of these admissions are for burns exceeding 30% of the patient's total body surface area. 70% of all burn unit admissions are for male patients, and 30% are for female patients. The source of burns breaks down as follows: 46% from fire or flame, 32% from hot water scalding, 8% from hot object contact, 4% from electrical burns, 3% from chemical burns, and 6% other source of burn. The survival rate for patients admitted to specialized burn centers is about 94.4%.

Treatment for severe burns has improved dramatically in the past 20 years. In the early twenty-first century, patients can survive with burns covering up to about 90% of the body, although they often face permanent physical impairment.

Alternatives

There has been great progress in the development of artificial skin replacement products in the early twenty-first century. Although nothing works as well as the patient's own skin, artificial skin products are important due to the limitation of available skin for allografting in severely burned patients. Unlike allografts and xenografts, artificial skin replacements are not rejected by the patient's body and actually encourage the generation of new tissue. Artificial skin usually consists of a synthetic epidermis and a collagen-based dermis. The artificial dermis consists of fibers arranged in a lattice that acts as a template for the formation of new tissue. Fibroblasts, blood vessels, nerve fibers, and lymph vessels from surrounding healthy tissue grow into the collagen lattice, which eventually dissolves as these cells and structures build a new dermis. The synthetic epidermis, which acts as a temporary barrier during this process, is eventually replaced with a split-thickness autograft or with an

---

epidermis cultured in the laboratory from the patient's own epithelial cells.

Several artificial skin products are available for burns or non-healing wounds, including Integra®, Dermal Regeneration Template® (from Integra Life Sciences Technology), Apligraf® (Novartis), TransCyte® (Advance Tissue Science), and Dermagraft®. Researchers have also obtained promising results growing or cultivating the patient's own skin cells in the laboratory. These cultured skin substitutes reduce the need for autografts and can reduce the complications of burn injuries. Laboratory cultivation of skin cells may improve the prognosis for severely burned patients with third-degree burns over 50% of their body. The recovery of these patients has been hindered by the limited availability of uninjured skin from their own bodies for grafting. Skin substitutes may also reduce treatment costs and the length of hospital stays. In addition, other research has demonstrated the possibility of using stem cells collected from bone marrow or blood for use in growing skin grafts.

Health care team roles

Patients with less severe burns are usually treated in a doctor's office or a hospital emergency room. Patients with any of the following conditions, however, are usually transferred to hospitals with specialized burn units: third-degree burns; partial-thickness burns over 10% of their total body area; electrical or chemical burns; smoke inhalation injuries; or preexisting medical disorders that could complicate management, prolong recovery, or affect mortality. In addition, burned children in hospitals without qualified personnel should be admitted to a hospital with a burn unit. A **surgical team** that specializes in burn treatment and skin grafts will perform the necessary procedures. The team may include neurosurgeons, ophthalmologists, oral **surgeons**, thoracic surgeons, psychiatrists, and trauma specialists as well as plastic surgeons and dermatologists.

Resources

BOOKS

Browner, Bruce D., et al. *Skeletal Trauma: Basic Science, Management, and Reconstruction.* 4th ed. Philadelphia: Saunders/Elsevier, 2009.

Canale, S. T., ed. *Campbell's Operative Orthopaedics.* 12th ed. St. Louis, MO: Mosby, 2012.

Townsend, Courtney M., et al. *Sabiston Textbook of Surgery.* 19th ed. Philadelphia: Saunders/Elsevier, 2012.

PERIODICALS

Farhangkhoee, Hana, Eric Yu Kit Li, and Achilleas Thoma. "Local Anesthetics for Skin Grafting and Local Flaps." *Clinics in Plastic Surgery* 40, no. 4 (2013): 537–49. http://dx.doi.org/10.1016/j.cps.2013.07.004 (accessed October 14, 2013).

WEBSITES

A.D.A.M. Medical Encyclopedia. "Skin Graft." MedlinePlus. http://www.nlm.nih.gov/medlineplus/ency/article/002982.htm (accessed October 14, 2013).

Macmillan Cancer Support. "Skin Grafts for Skin Cancer." http://www.macmillan.org.uk/Cancerinformation/Cancer-types/Skin/Treatingskincancer/Skingrafts.aspx (accessed October 14, 2013).

ORGANIZATIONS

American Burn Association, 311 S. Wacker Dr., Ste. 4150, Chicago, IL 60606, (312) 642-9260, Fax: (312) 642-9130, info@ameriburn.org, http://www.ameriburn.org.

American Society of Plastic Surgeons, 444 E. Algonquin Rd., Arlington Heights, IL 60005, http://www.plasticsurgery.org.

Lisa Christenson, PhD
Crystal H. Kaczkowski, MSc
Rosalyn Carson-DeWitt, MD

Skin smoothing *see* **Dermabrasion**

Skull x-rays

Definition

Skull x-rays are performed to examine the nose, sinuses, and facial bones. These studies may also be referred to as sinus x-rays. X-ray studies produce films, also known as radiographs, by aiming x-rays at soft bones and tissues of the body. X-ray beams are similar to light waves, except their shorter wavelength allows them to penetrate dense substances, producing images and shadows on film.

Purpose

Doctors may order skull x-rays to aid in the diagnosis of a variety of diseases or injuries.

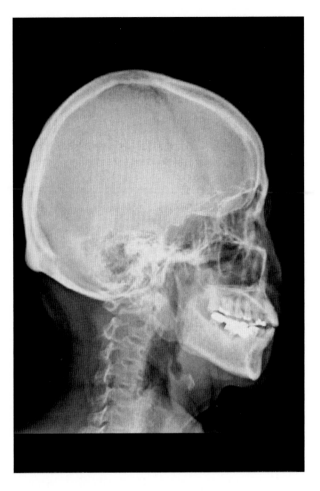

X-ray of the skull. *(momopixs/Shutterstock.com)*

Sinusitis

Sinus x-rays may be ordered to confirm a diagnosis of sinusitis, or sinus infection.

Fractures

A skull x-ray may detect bone fractures resulting from injury or disease. The skull x-ray should clearly show the entire skull, jaw bones, and facial bones.

Tumors

Skull radiographs may indicate tumors in facial bones, tissues, or sinuses. Tumors may be benign (not cancerous) or malignant (cancerous).

Other

Birth defects (referred to as congenital anomalies) may be detected on a skull x-ray by changes in bone structure. Abnormal tissues or glands resulting from various conditions or diseases may also be shown on a skull radiograph.

Description

Skull or sinus x-rays may be performed in a doctor's office that has x-ray equipment and a technologist available. The exam may also be performed in an outpatient radiology facility or a hospital radiology department.

In many instances, particularly for sinus views, the patient will sit upright in a chair, perhaps with the head held stable by a foam vise. A film cassette is located behind the patient. The x-ray tube is in front of the patient and may be moved to allow for different positions and views. A patient may also be asked to move his or her head at various angles and positions.

In some cases, technologists will ask the patient to lie on a table and will place the head and neck at various angles. In routine skull x-rays, as many as five different views may be taken to allow a clear picture of various bones and tissues. The length of the test will vary depending on the number of views taken, but in general, it should last about 10 minutes. The technologist will usually ask a patient to wait while the films are being developed to ensure that they are adequate before going to the radiologist.

Preparation

There is no preparation for the patient prior to arriving at the radiology facility. Patients will be asked to remove jewelry, dentures, or other metal objects that may produce artifacts on the film. The referring doctor or x-ray technologist can answer any questions regarding the procedure. Any woman who is or may be pregnant should tell the technologist.

Aftercare

There is no aftercare required following skull or sinus x-ray procedures.

Risks

There are no common side effects from skull or sinus x-ray. The patient may feel some discomfort in the positioning of the head and neck, but will have no complications. Any x-ray procedure carries minimal radiation risk; children and pregnant women should be protected from radiation exposure to the abdominal or genital areas.

Results

Normal results should indicate sinuses, bones, tissues, and other observed areas are of normal size, shape, and thickness for the patient's age and medical

> ## KEY TERMS
>
> **Radiograph—**The actual picture or film produced by an x-ray study.
>
> **X-ray—**A form of electromagnetic radiation with shorter wavelengths than normal light. X-rays can penetrate most structures.

history. Results, whether normal or abnormal, will be provided to the referring doctor in a written report.

Abnormal results

Abnormal results may include sinusitis, fractures, tumors, or other issues.

SINUSITIS. Air in sinuses will show up on a radiograph as black, but fluid will be cloudy or white (opaque). This helps the radiologist to identify fluid in the sinuses. In chronic sinusitis, the radiologist may also note thickening or destruction of the bony wall of an infected sinus.

FRACTURES. Radiologists may recognize even tiny facial bone fractures as a line of defect.

TUMORS. Tumors may be visible if the bony sinus wall is distorted or destroyed. Abnormal findings may result in follow-up imaging studies.

OTHER. Skull x-rays may also detect disorders that show up as changes in bone structure, such as Paget's disease of the bone or acromegaly (a disorder associated with excess growth hormones from the pituitary gland). Areas of calcification (gathering of calcium deposits) or destruction may indicate a condition such as an infection of bone or bone marrow (osteomyelitis).

Resources

BOOKS

Adam, A., and A. K. Dixon, eds. *Grainger & Allison's Diagnostic Radiology*. 5th ed. Philadelphia: Churchill Livingstone/Elsevier, 2008.

Flint, Paul F., et al. *Cumming's Otolaryngology: Head and Neck Surgery*. 5th ed. rev. Philadelphia: Mosby/Elsevier, 2010.

Mettler, Fred A. Jr. *Essentials of Radiology*. 3rd ed. Philadelphia: Saunders/Elsevier, 2014.

PERIODICALS

Kim, Y. I., J. W. Cheong, and S. H. Yoon. "Clinical Comparison of the Predictive Value of the Simple Skull X-Ray and 3 Dimensional Computed Tomography for Skull Fractures of Children." *Journal of Korean Neurosurgical Society* 52, no. 6 (2012): 528–33.

WEBSITES

A.D.A.M. Medical Encyclopedia. "Skull X-Ray." MedlinePlus. http://www.nlm.nih.gov/medlineplus/ency/article/003802. htm (accessed October 14, 2013).

ORGANIZATIONS

Brain Injury Association of America, 1608 Spring Hill Rd., Ste. 110, Vienna, VA 22182, (703) 761-0750, info@biausa. org, http://www.biausa.org.

Radiological Society of North America (RSNA), 820 Jorie Blvd., Oak Brook, IL 60523-2251, (630) 571-2670, (800) 381-6660, http://www.rsna.org.

Teresa Norris, RN
Lee A. Shratter, MD

Sling procedure

Definition

The sling procedure, or suburethral sling procedure, refers to a particular kind of surgery using ancillary material to aid in closure of the urethral sphincter function of the bladder. It is performed as a treatment of severe urinary incontinence. The sling procedure, also known as the suburethral fascial sling or the pubovaginal sling, has many forms due to advances in the types of material used for the sling. Some popular types of sling material are Teflon® (polytetrafluoroethylene), Gore-Tex®, and rectus fascia (fibrous tissue of the rectum). The surgery can be done through the vagina or the abdomen, and some clinicians perform the procedure using a laparoscope—a small instrument that allows surgery through very small incisions in the belly button and above the pubic hairline. The long-term efficacy and durability of the laparoscopic suburethral sling procedure for management of stress incontinence are undetermined. A new technique, the tension-free vaginal tape sling procedure (TVT), has gained popularity in recent years and early research indicates high success rates and few postoperative complications. This procedure is done under local anesthetic and offers new opportunities for treatment of stress incontinence. However, TVT has not been researched for its long-term effects. Finally, there are many **surgeons** who use the sling procedure for all forms of incontinence.

Purpose

Incontinence is very common and not fully understood. Generally defined as the involuntary loss of urine, incontinence comes in many forms and has many etiologies. Four established types of incontinence, according to the Agency for Healthcare Research and Quality, affect approximately 13 million adults—most of them older women. Actual prevalence may be higher because incontinence is widely under reported and under diagnosed. The four types of incontinence are: stress incontinence, urge incontinence (detrusor overactivity or instability), mixed incontinence, and overflow incontinence. There are also other types of incontinence tied to specific conditions, such as neurogenic bladder in which neurological signals to the bladder are impaired.

Stress incontinence is the most frequently diagnosed form of incontinence and occurs largely with physical activity, laughter and coughing, and sneezing. The inability to hold urine can be due to weakness in the internal and external urinary sphincter or due to a weakened urethra. These two conditions, intrinsic sphincter deficiency (ISD) and urethral hypermobility or genuine stress incontinence (GSI), pertain to the inability of the "gatekeeper" sphincter muscles to stay taut and/or the urethra failing to hold urine under pressure from the abdomen. In women, as the pelvic structures relax due to age, injury, or illness, the uterus prolapses and the urethra becomes hypermobile. This allows the urethra to descend at an angle that permits loss of urine and puts pressure upon the sphincter muscles, both internal and external, allowing the mouth of the bladder to stay open.

Urge incontinence, the other frequent type of incontinence, pertains to overactivity of the sphincter in which the muscle contracts frequently, causing the need to urinate. Stress incontinence is often allied with sphincter overactivity and is often accompanied by urge incontinence.

Severe stress incontinence occurs most frequently in women younger than 60 years old. It is thought to be due to the relaxation of the supporting structures of the pelvis that results from childbirth, obesity, or lack of **exercise**. Some researchers believe that aging, perhaps due to estrogen deficiency, is a major cause of severe urinary incontinence in women, but no link has been found between incontinence and estrogen deficiency. Surgery for stress or mixed incontinence is primarily offered to patients who have failed, are not satisfied with, or are unable to comply with more conservative approaches. It is often performed during other surgeries such as urethra prolapse, cystocele surgery, urethral reconstruction, and **hysterectomy**.

The sling procedure gets its name from the tissue attached under the mid- or proximal urethra and sutured at its ends onto a solid structure like the rectus sheath, pubic bone, or pelvic side walls. The procedure is used in the severest cases of stress incontinence, particularly those that have a concomitant sphincter inadequacy

(ISD). The sling supports the urethra as it receives pressure from the abdomen and helps the internal sphincter muscles to keep the urethral opening closed. The procedure is the most popular because it has the highest success rate of all surgical remedies for severe stress incontinence related to sphincter inadequacies in both men and women.

Demographics

Urinary incontinence (UI) plagues 10%–35% of adults and at least half of the million nursing home residents in the United States. Other studies indicate that between 10% and 30% of women experience incontinence during their lifetimes, compared to about 5% of men. One reason that more women than men have incontinent episodes is the relatively shorter urethras of women. Women have urethras of about 2 in. (5 cm) and men have urethras of 10 in. (25.4 cm). Studies have documented that about 50% of all women have occasional urinary incontinence, and as many as 10% have regular incontinence. Nearly 20% of women over age 75 experience daily urinary incontinence. Incontinence is a major factor in individuals entering long-term care facilities. Women at highest risk are those who have given birth to more than three children and women who were given oxytocin to induce labor. Oxytocin puts more pressure on the pelvic muscles than does ordinary labor. Women who smoke have twice the rate of incontinence, according to one study of 600 women. Those women who do high-impact exercises are at much higher risk for incontinence. According to the medical literature, those at highest risk for urinary leakage are gymnasts, followed by softball, volleyball, and basketball players. Finally, women who have diabetes or are obese have higher rates of incontinence. Women who require sling procedures have often had other surgeries for incontinence, necessitating sling procedure to treat intrinsic sphincter deficiency caused by operative trauma. A rarer cause of stress incontinence in older women is urethral instability. In men, stress incontinence is usually caused by sphincter damage after surgery on the prostate.

Description

Anti-incontinence surgery is used to address the failure of two parts of female urinary continence: loss of support to the bladder neck or central urethra and intrinsic sphincter deficiency (ISD). The surgery does not restore function to the urethra or the ability for closure to the sphincter. It replaces the mechanism for continence with supporting and compressive aids. Stabilizing the supporting elements of the urethra (ligaments, fascia, and muscles) was thought for many years to be the most important factor in curing incontinence. Called anatomic or genuine stress urinary incontinence (SUI), retropubic procedures, like the Burch procedure, sought only to restore the urethra to a fixed position. However, it became clear with the high failure rate of these procedures that ISD was present and unless surgery could confer some added compressive ability to the closure of the bladder, SUI would persist.

The urethral sling procedure is effective in the treatment of the severest types of incontinence (Types II and III) by reestablishing the "hammock effect" of the proximal or central point of the urethra during abdominal straining. The surgery involves the placement of a piece of material under the urethra at its arterial or vesical juncture and anchoring it on either side of the pubic bone or to the abdominal wall or vaginal wall. This technique involves the creation of a sling from a strip of tissue from the patient's own abdominal fascia (fibrous tissue) or from a cadaver. Synthetic slings also are used, but some are prone to break down over time.

The urethral sling procedure is most often performed as open surgery, which involves entering the pelvic area from the abdomen or from the vagina while the patient is under general or regional anesthesia. Broad-spectrum **antibiotics** are offered intravenously. If the patient is fitted with a urethral catheter, ampicillin and gentamicin are administered instead. The patient is placed in stirrups. Surgery takes place as a 6-to-9 cm by 1.5 cm sling is harvested from rectal tissue and sutured under the urethra at each end within the retropubic space (the area that undergirds the urethra). Synthetic tissue or fascia from a donor may also be used.

The goal of the surgery is to create a compression aid to the urethra. This involves an individualized approach to the tension needed on the sling. While the sling procedure is relatively easy to complete, the issue of tension on the sling is hard to determine and involves the use of tests during surgery for determining the compression effect of the sling on the urethra. Some manual tests are performed or a more sophisticated urodynamic test, like cystourethrography, may determine tension. It is important for the surgeon to test tension during surgery because of the high rate of retention of urine (inability to void) after surgery associated with this procedure and the miscalculation of the required tension.

Diagnosis

Candidates for surgical treatment of incontinence must undergo a full clinical, neurological, and radiographic evaluation before there can be direct analysis of the condition to be treated and the desired outcome. Both urethral and bladder functions are evaluated and there is an attempt to determine the conditions associated with stress incontinence. In many women, incontinence may be due to vaginal prolapse. Stress incontinence can be identified by observation of urine during pelvic examination or by a sitting or standing **stress test** where patients are asked to cough or strain and evidence of leakage is obtained. Gynecologists often use a Q-tip test to determine the angle and change in the position of the urethra during straining. Other tests include subtracted cystometry to measure how much the bladder can hold, how much pressure builds up inside the bladder as it stores urine, and how full it is when the patients feels the urge to urinate.

The frequency of stress incontinence as measured by typical symptoms ranges between 33% and 65%. The frequency of stress incontinence is around 12% when measured or defined by cystometric findings. The ability to distinguish SUI as the cause of incontinence, as opposed to ISD, becomes more complicated, but it is a very important factor in the decision to have surgery. A combination of pelvic examination for urethral hypermobility and leak point pressure as measured by coughing or other abdominal straining has been shown to be very effective in distinguishing ISD, and identifying the patient who needs surgery.

Aftercare

IV ketorolac and oral and intravenous pain medication are administered, as are postoperative antibiotics. A general diet is available usually on the evening of surgery. When the patient is able to walk, usually the same day, the urethral catheter is removed. The patient must perform self-catheterization to check urine volume every four hours to protect the urethral wall. If the patient is unwilling to perform catheterization, a tube can be placed suprapubically (in the back of the pubis) for voiding. Catheterization lasts about eight days, with about 98% of patients able to void at three months. Patients are discharged on the second day postoperatively, unless they have had other procedures and need additional recovery time. Patients may not lift heavy objects or engage in strenuous activity for approximately six weeks. Sexual intercourse may be resumed in the fourth week following surgery. Follow-up visits are scheduled for three to four weeks after surgery.

Risks

Although the sling treatment has a very high success rate, it is also associated with a prolonged period of voiding difficulties, intraoperative bladder or urethra injury, infections associated with screw or staple points, rejection of sling material from a donor, or erosion of synthetic sling material. Patients should not be encouraged to undergo a sling procedure unless the risk of long-term voiding difficulty and the need for intermittent self-catheterization are understood. Fascial slings seem to be associated with the fewest complications for sling procedure treatment. Synthetic slings have a greater risk of having to be removed due to erosion and inflammation.

Results

Regardless of the procedure used, a proportion of patients will remain incontinent. Results vary according to the type of sling procedure used, the type of attachment used for the sling, and the type of material used for the sling. Normal results for the sling procedure overall are recurrent stress incontinence of 3%–12% after bladder sling procedures. In general, reported cure rates are lower for second and subsequent surgical procedures. A recent qualitative study published in the *American Journal of Obstetrics and Gynecology* of 57 patients who underwent patient-contributed fascial sling procedures indicates good success with fascial sling procedures. At a median of 42 months after the procedure, the postoperative objective cure rate for stress urinary incontinence was 97%, with 88% of patients indicating that the sling had improved the quality of their lives. Eighty-four percent of patients indicated that the sling relieved their incontinence long term, and 82% of patients stated that they would undergo the surgery again. The study also found that voiding function was a common side effect in 41% of the patients.

QUESTIONS TO ASK YOUR DOCTOR

- Do I have a urethral closure problem as a part of my incontinence?
- How many sling procedures have you performed?
- How soon will I be able to tell if I am going to have urine retention difficulties?
- If this surgery does not work, are there other procedures that will allow me a better quality of life?
- Is patient satisfaction a formal part of your evaluation of the success of the procedure you use?
- What type of material do you use for the sling and why do you choose this material?

Morbidity and mortality rates

The most common complications of sling procedures are voiding problems (10.4%), new detrusor instability (7%–27%), and lower urinary tract damage (3%). Some of the complications depend upon tension issues as well as on the materials used for the sling. There are recent and well designed studies of patient fascia and donor fascia used for slings in five centers with follow-up from 30 to 51 months that report no erosions or vaginal wall complications in any patients. Prolonged retention or voiding issues occurred in 2.3% of patients and de novo or spontaneous urge incontinence developed in 6%. These figures relate only to a large study utilizing patient or donor fascia and one that did not control for other factors like techniques of anchoring. In general, studies of the sling procedure are small and have many variables. There are no long-term studies (over five years) of this most popular procedure.

Alternatives

Alternatives to anti-incontinent sling procedure surgery depend upon the severity of the incontinence and the type. Severe stress incontinence with intrinsic sphincter deficiency can benefit from bulking agents for the urethra to increase compression, as well as external devices like a pessary that is placed in the vagina and holds up the bladder to prevent leakage. Urethral inserts can be placed in the urethra until it is time to use the bathroom. The patient learns to put the insertion in and take it out as needed. There are also urine seals that are small foam pads inserted in garments. Milder forms of incontinence can benefit from an assessment of medication usage, pelvic muscle exercises, bladder retraining, weight loss, and certain devices that stimulate the muscles around the urethra to strengthen them. For mild urethral mobility, procedures for tacking or stabilizing the urethra at the neck called Needle Neck Suspension, as well as procedures to hold the urethra in place with sutures, like the Burch method, are alternative forms of surgery.

Health care team roles

The surgery is performed by a urological surgeon who has trained specifically for this procedure. The surgery takes place in a general hospital.

Resources

BOOKS

Wein, Alan J., et al. *Campbell-Walsh Urology.* 10th ed. Philadelphia: Saunders/Elsevier, 2012.

PERIODICALS

Grigoriadis, C., et al. "Tension-Free Vaginal Tape Obturator versus Ajust Adjustable Single Incision Sling Procedure in Women with Urodynamic Stress Urinary Incontinence." *European Journal of Obstetrics & Gynecology and Reproductive Biology* 170, no. 2 (2013): 563–66. http://dx.doi.org/10.1016/j.ejogrb.2013.07.041 (accessed October 4, 2013).

Kim, Chang Hee, et al. "Modified Distal Urethral Polypropylene Sling (Canal Transobturator Tape) Procedure: Efficacy for Persistent Stress Urinary Incontinence after a Conventional Midurethral Sling Procedure." *International Neurology Journal* 17, no. 1 (2013): 18–23. http://dx.doi.org/10.5213/inj.2013.17.1.18 (accessed October 4, 2013).

WEBSITES

A.D.A.M. Medical Encyclopedia. "Urinary Incontinence—Vaginal Sling Procedures." MedlinePlus. http://www.nlm.nih.gov/medlineplus/ency/article/007376.htm (accessed October 4, 2013).

Mayo Clinic staff. "Urinary Incontinence Surgery: When Other Treatments Aren't Enough." MedlinePlus. http://www.nlm.nih.gov/medlineplus/ency/article/007376.htm (accessed October 4, 2013).

ORGANIZATIONS

Simon Foundation for Continence, PO Box 835, Wilmette, IL 60091, (847) 864-3913, (800) 23-SIMON (237-4666), info@simonfoundation.org, http://simonfoundation.org.

Nancy McKenzie, PhD

Small bowel follow-through (SBFT) *see* Upper gastrointestinal exam

Small bowel resection *see* Bowel resection, small intestine

Small intestine radiography and fluoroscopy *see* Upper gastrointestinal exam

Smoking cessation

Definition

Smoking cessation means quitting smoking or withdrawing from nicotine. Tobacco is highly addictive, and quitting the habit often involves irritability, headache, mood swings, and cravings associated with the sudden cessation or reduction of tobacco use.

Purpose

There are many good reasons to stop smoking, but one of them is that smoking cessation may speed recovery after surgery. Smoking cessation helps a person heal and recover faster, especially in the incision area or if the surgery involved any bones. Research shows that patients who underwent hip and knee replacements or surgery on other bone joints healed better and recovered more quickly if they had quit or cut down their tobacco intake several weeks before the operation. Smoking weakens the bone mineral that keeps the skeleton strong and undermines tissue and vessel health. One study suggested that even quitting tobacco for a few days could improve tissue blood flow and oxygenation, as well as wound healing. Quitting may also reduce wound complications and lower the risk of cardiovascular complications after surgery. If surgery was performed to remove cancerous tumors, quitting will reduce the risk of a second tumor, especially if the cancer was in the lung, head, or neck and has been successfully treated.

Description

The addictive effects of tobacco have been well documented. Tobacco's addictive potential is believed to be comparable to the addictive potentials of alcohol, cocaine, and morphine. Quitting smoking is one of the best things a person can do to increase their life expectancy. On average, male smokers who quit at 35 years old add an estimated seven years on to their life expectancy (from age 69 to 76); women who quit add an additional six years (from age 74 to 80).

Effects of smoking on the body

Nicotine acts as both a stimulant and a depressant on the body. Saliva and bronchial secretions increase along with bowel tone. Newer smokers may experience tremors or even convulsions with high doses of nicotine because of the stimulation of the central nervous system. The respiratory muscles are then depressed following stimulation.

Nicotine causes arousal as well as relaxation from stressful situations. Tobacco use increases the heart rate about 10–20 beats per minute and, because it constricts the blood vessels, increases blood pressure by 5–10 mm Hg; it can also lead to blood clots.

Other side effects of nicotine may include sweating, nausea, and diarrhea, and the hormonal activities of the body are also affected. Nicotine elevates blood glucose levels, increases insulin production, and acts as an appetite suppressant, specifically decreasing the appetite for simple carbohydrates (sweets) and inhibiting the efficiency with which food is metabolized. The fear of weight gain prevents some people from quitting smoking.

Health problems associated with smoking

In general, chronic use of nicotine may cause an acceleration of coronary artery disease, hypertension, reproductive problems, esophageal reflux, peptic ulcer disease, fetal illnesses and death, and delayed wound healing. People who smoke are at greater risk of cancer (especially in the lung, mouth, larynx, esophagus, bladder, kidney, pancreas, and cervix), heart attacks, strokes, and chronic lung disease. Using tobacco during pregnancy increases the risk of miscarriage, premature labor, intrauterine growth retardation (resulting in the birth of an infant small for gestational age), and the infant's risk for sudden infant death syndrome.

Other specific health risks of tobacco use include:

• nicotine addiction
• lung disease
• lung cancer
• emphysema
• chronic bronchitis
• angina
• heart attack
• atherosclerotic and peripheral vascular disease
• aneurysms
• blood clots
• strokes
• oral diseases, including oral cancer

Nonsmokers who are regularly exposed to second-hand smoke may also experience specific health risks, including the development of lung cancer and acute, sudden, and occasionally severe reactions, including eye, nose, throat, and lower respiratory tract symptoms. Children especially are at risk of respiratory infections (e.g., bronchitis and pneumonia), asthma, and decreases in lung function as the lungs mature.

The specific health risks for smokeless tobacco users include many of the diseases of smokers, as well as a 50-

fold greater risk for oral cancer with long-term or regular use.

In people with diabetes who are also taking medication for high blood pressure, smoking may increase the risk of kidney disease and/or kidney failure.

Making a plan to quit

Sometimes surgery is unexpected, but patients planning elective procedures like a joint operation have a good opportunity to stop smoking. Some tips to help with smoking cessation include:

• Set a goal quit date.

• Make a written list of the reasons to quit smoking.

• Consider using an aid to help with quitting, such as a nicotine patch, gum, spray, or inhaler; soft laser therapy; medication; or some other method.

• Limit smoking (initially) to only certain places, preferably outdoors.

• Buy a piggy bank or jar and put the money in it that would normally be spent on cigarettes.

• Do not buy cigarettes by the carton.

• Cut coffee consumption in half.

• Practice putting off lighting up when the urge strikes.

• Go for a walk every day or begin an exercise program.

• Stock up on healthy snacks to help with weight control after quitting.

• Enlist the support of family and friends.

• Clean and put away all ashtrays the day before quitting.

Smokers who are trying to quit should remind themselves that they are doing the right thing and benefiting their health. If a patient has recently quit, he or she should let the attending doctor know. Professional hospital staff can help the patient and offer support. Medical staff may be able to start the patient on nicotine replacement therapy to help control the cravings and increase the chances of quitting permanently.

Methods of quitting

There are many methods to help with quitting smoking:

• Cold turkey, or an abrupt cessation of nicotine, is one way to stop smoking. Quitting cold turkey can provide cost savings because paraphernalia and smoking cessation aids are not required; however, it is very difficult, and not everyone can stop this way.

• Laser therapy is a safe and pain-free form of acupuncture that has been in use since the 1980s. The laser beam is applied to specific energy points on the body, stimulating the production of endorphins. These natural body chemicals produce a calming, relaxing effect. When a person stops smoking, it is the sudden drop in endorphin levels that leads to withdrawal symptoms and physical cravings. Laser treatment not only helps relieve these cravings but helps with stress reduction and lung detoxification. Some studies indicate that laser therapy is the most effective method of smoking cessation.

• Acupuncture—the insertion of small needles or springs into the skin—is another aid in smoking cessation. The needles or springs are sometimes left in the ears and touched lightly by the patient between visits.

• Some smokers find hypnosis particularly useful, especially if the reasons for smoking are associated with psychological issues such as phobias, panic attacks, or weight control.

• Similarly, some people quit smoking through the use of psychotherapy. Cognitive-behavioral therapy (CBT) is considered the most effective form of psychotherapy for smoking cessation. A research team at Yale University reported in the fall of 2007 that CBT was more effective than brief behavioral interventions in helping adolescent smokers stay in a smoking cessation program as well as actually quitting smoking.

• Aversion techniques attempt to make smoking seem unpleasant. This technique reminds a person of the distasteful aspects of smoking, such as the smell, coughing, high cost, and health issues. The most common technique prescribed by psychologists for "thought stopping"—stopping unwanted thoughts—is to wear a rubber band around the wrist. Every time there is an unwanted thought (a craving to smoke), the band is pulled so that it hurts. The thought then becomes associated with pain and gradually neutralized.

• Rapid smoking is a technique in which smoking times are strictly scheduled once a day for the first three days after quitting. Phrases are repeated such as "smoking irritates my throat" or "smoking burns my lips and tongue." This technique causes oversmoking in a way that makes the taste and sensations associated with smoking very unpleasant.

• There are special mouthwashes available that, when used before smoking, give cigarettes a very unpleasant taste. The intention is to create a link in the smoker's mind between cigarettes and a bad taste in the mouth.

• Smoking cessation aids wean a person off nicotine slowly, and the nicotine can be delivered where it does the least bodily harm. Unlike cigarettes, these aids do not introduce other harmful poisons to the body. They can be used for a short period of time; however, nicotine from any source (smoking, nicotine gum, or the nicotine patch) can make some health problems worse. These include heart or circulation problems, irregular heartbeat, chest pain, high blood pressure, overactive thyroid, stomach ulcers, or diabetes.

Smoking cessation aids

The four main brands of the nicotine patch are Nicotrol, Nicoderm, Prostep, and Habitrol. All four transmit low doses of nicotine to the body throughout the day. The patch comes in varying strengths ranging from 7 mg to 21 mg. The patch must be prescribed and used under a physician's care. Package instructions must be followed carefully. Other smoking cessation programs or materials should be used while using the patch.

Nicorette gum allows nicotine to be absorbed through the membrane of the mouth between the cheek and gums. Past smoking habits determine the right strength to choose. The gum should be chewed slowly.

The nicotine nasal spray reduces cravings and withdrawal symptoms, allowing smokers to cut back slowly. The nasal spray acts quickly to stop the cravings, as it is rapidly absorbed through the nasal membranes. One of the drawbacks is a risk of addiction to the spray.

The nicotine inhaler uses a plastic mouthpiece with a nicotine plug, delivering nicotine to the mucous membranes of the mouth. It provides nicotine at about one-third the nicotine level of cigarettes.

Bupropion hydrochloride, sold under the trade name Zyban, is an oral medication used to help smokers quit. It is a treatment for nicotine dependence. Another medication, approved by the U.S. Food and Drug Administration (FDA) in 2006, is varenicline tartrate, sold under the trade name Chantix. Chantix is thought to work by affecting parts of the brain affected by nicotine in two ways: by providing some nicotine effects to ease withdrawal symptoms and by blocking the effects of nicotine from cigarettes if the patient resumes smoking. In November 2007, however, the FDA issued a warning regarding mood changes reported in persons taking Chantix. The drug is still considered safe, but anyone taking it in order to stop smoking should contact their doctor at once if they feel depressed or notice other sudden mood changes.

The nicotine lozenge is another smoking cessation aid recently added to the growing list of tools to combat nicotine withdrawal.

Scientists are researching the possibility of developing medications that inhibit the function of CYP2A6, an enzyme that makes people more susceptible to nicotine addiction. Some people have a genetic variant that decreases the amount of CYP2A6 in the body, which is thought to protect these individuals against nicotine addiction. Thus medications that lower the amount of this enzyme might offer a new approach to smoking cessation.

Withdrawal symptoms

Generally, the longer a person has smoked and the greater the number of cigarettes (and nicotine) consumed, the more likely it is that withdrawal symptoms will occur and the more severe they are likely to be. When a smoker switches from regular to low-nicotine cigarettes or significantly cuts back smoking, a milder form of nicotine withdrawal involving some or all of these symptoms can occur.

Some of the most common withdrawal symptoms include:

• dry mouth
• mood swings
• irritability
• feelings of depression
• excess gas in the digestive tract
• tension
• sleeplessness or sleeping too much
• difficulty in concentration
• intense cravings for a cigarette
• increased appetite and weight gain
• headaches

These side effects are temporary and usually subside in a short time for most people. Symptoms can last from one to three weeks and are strongest during the first week after quitting. Drinking plenty of water during the first week can help detoxify the body and shorten the duration of the withdrawal symptoms. A positive attitude, drive, commitment, and a willingness to get help from health care professionals and support groups will help a smoker kick the habit.

Researchers from the University of California, San Diego strongly suggest that smoking cessation aids should be used in combination with other types of smoking cessation help, such as counseling and/or support programs. These products are not designed to help with the behavioral aspects of smoking, only the cravings associated with them. Counseling and support groups can offer tips on coping with difficult situations that can trigger the urge to smoke.

Morbidity and mortality rates

In a three-year study at the University of Pittsburgh of 202 heart transplant recipients, 71% of the recipients were smokers before surgery. The overall rate of post-transplant smoking was 27%. All but one of the smokers

KEY TERMS

Addiction—Compulsive, overwhelming involvement with a specific activity. The activity may be smoking, gambling, alcohol, or may involve the use of almost any substance, such as a drug.

Appetite suppressant—To decrease the appetite.

Constrict—To squeeze tightly, compress, draw together.

Convulsion—To shake or effect with spasms; to agitate or disturb violently.

Depressant—A drug or other substance that soothes or lessens tension of the muscles or nerves.

Detoxification—To remove a poison or toxin or the effect of such a harmful substance; to free from an intoxicating or addictive substance in the body or from dependence on or addiction to a harmful substance.

Endorphins—Any of a group of proteins with analgesic properties that occur naturally in the brain.

Gestational age—The length of time of growth and development of the young in the mother's womb.

Nicotine—A poisonous, oily alkaloid in tobacco.

Oxygenation—To supply with oxygen.

Psychoactive—Affecting the mind or behavior.

Respiratory infections—Infections that relate to or affect respiration or breathing.

Stimulant—A drug or other substance that increases the rate of activity of a body system.

Tremor—A trembling, quivering, or shaking.

Withdrawal—Stopping of administration or use of a drug; the syndrome of sometimes painful physical and psychological symptoms that follow the discontinuance.

resumed the smoking habit they had before the transplant. The biggest reason for resuming smoking was addiction to nicotine. Smoking is a complex behavior, involving social interactions, visual cues, and other factors. Those who smoked until less than six months before the transplant were much more likely to resume smoking early and to smoke more. One of the major causes of early relapse was the depression and anxiety felt during two months after the transplant. Another strong predictor of relapse was having a caretaker who smoked. The knowledge of these risk factors could help develop strategies for identifying those

in greatest need of early intervention. According to European studies, the five-year survival rate for post-transplant smokers is 37%, compared to 80% for nonsmoking recipients. Smokers can develop inoperable lung cancers within five years after a transplant, resulting in a shorter survival rate. There is an alarming incidence of head and neck cancers in transplant recipients who resume smoking.

Overall, there is a 90% relapse rate in the general population; however, the more times a smoker tries to quit, the greater the chance of success with each new try.

Resources

BOOKS

Perkins, Kenneth A., Cynthia A. Conklin, and Michele D. Levine. *Cognitive-Behavioral Therapy for Smoking Cessation: A Practical Guidebook to the Most Effective Treatments.* New York: Routledge, 2008.

PERIODICALS

Barone, Mauro, Annalisa Cogliandro, and Paolo Persichetti. "Plastic Surgery and Smoking: A Prospective Analysis of Incidence, Compliance, and Complications." *Plastic & Reconstructive Surgery* 132, no. 4 (2013): 686–87e. http://dx.doi.org/10.1097/PRS.0b013e31829fe385 (accessed October 18, 2013).

Cavallo, D. A., et al. "Combining Cognitive Behavioral Therapy with Contingency Management for Smoking Cessation in Adolescent Smokers: A Preliminary Comparison of Two Different CBT Formats." *American Journal on Addictions* 16, no. 6 (November 2007): 468–74.

Lancaster, T., L. Stead, and K. Cahill. "An Update on Therapeutics for Tobacco Dependence." *Expert Opinion on Pharmacotherapy* 9, no. 1 (January 2008): 15–22.

Musallam, K. M., et al. "Smoking and the Risk of Mortality and Vascular and Respiratory Events in Patients Undergoing Major Surgery." *JAMA Surgery* 148, no. 8 (2013): 755–62. http://dx.doi.org/10.1001/jamasurg.2013.2360 (accessed October 18, 2013).

Mwenifumbo, J. C., and R. F. Tyndale. "Genetic Variability in CYP2A6 and the Pharmacokinetics of Nicotine." *Pharmacogenomics* 8, no. 10 (October 2007): 1385–1402.

Taylor, D. H. Jr., et al. "Research and Practice: Benefits of Smoking Cessation for Longevity." *American Journal of Public Health* 92, no. 6 (June 2002): 990–96.

OTHER

Action on Smoking and Health. *Smoking and Surgery.* July 2013. http://www.ash.org.uk/files/documents/ASH_711.pdf (accessed October 18, 2013).

WEBSITES

A.D.A.M. Medical Encyclopedia. "Smoking and Surgery." MedlinePlus. http://www.nlm.nih.gov/medlineplus/ency/patientinstructions/000437.htm (accessed October 18, 2013).

American Academy of Orthopaedic Surgeons. "Surgery and Smoking." OrthoInfo. http://orthoinfo.aaos.org/topic.cfm?topic=A00262 (accessed October 18, 2013).

American Lung Association. "Stop Smoking." http://www.lung.org/stop-smoking (accessed October 18, 2013).

Centers for Disease Control and Prevention. "Quit Smoking." http://www.cdc.gov/tobacco/quit_smoking/index.htm (accessed October 18, 2013).

Centers for Disease Control and Prevention. "Smoking Cessation." http://www.cdc.gov/tobacco/data_statistics/fact_sheets/cessation/quitting/index.htm (accessed October 18, 2013).

MedlinePlus. "Quitting Smoking." U.S. National Library of Medicine, National Institutes of Health. http://www.nlm.nih.gov/medlineplus/quittingsmoking.html (accessed October 18, 2013).

U.S. Department of Health and Human Services and National Institutes of Health. Smokefree.gov. http://smokefree.gov (accessed October 18, 2013).

U.S. Food and Drug Administration. "FDA Drug Safety Communication: Chantix (Varenicline) May Increase the Risk of Certain Cardiovascular Adverse Events in Patients with Cardiovascular Disease." http://www.fda.gov/Drugs/DrugSafety/ucm259161.htm (accessed October 18, 2013).

ORGANIZATIONS

Action on Smoking and Health, 4th St. NW, Washington, DC 20001, (202) 659-4310, info@ash.org, http://ash.org.

American Academy of Orthopaedic Surgeons (AAOS), 6300 N. River Rd., Rosemont, IL 60018-4262, (847) 823-7186, Fax: (847) 823-8125, pemr@aaos.org, http://www.aaos.org.

American Cancer Society, 250 Williams St. NW, Atlanta, GA 30303, (800) 227-2345, http://www.cancer.org.

American Lung Association, 1301 Pennsylvania Ave. NW, Ste. 800, Washington, DC 20004, (202) 785-3355, (800) LUNG-USA (586-4872), http://www.lung.org.

Centers for Disease Control and Prevention, 1600 Clifton Rd., Atlanta, GA 30333, (800) CDC-INFO (232-4636), (888) 232-6348, cdcinfo@cdc.gov, http://www.cdc.gov.

Crystal H. Kaczkowski, MSc
Rebecca Frey, PhD

Snoring surgery

Definition

Snoring is defined as noisy or rough breathing during sleep, caused by vibration of loose tissue in the upper airway. Surgical treatments for snoring include several different techniques for removing tissue from the back of the patient's throat, removing the tonsils and adenoids, removing nasal polyps that block the airway, reshaping the nasal passages or jaw, or preventing the tongue from blocking the airway during sleep. Implanting plastic cylinders in the soft palate to stiffen it so that it prevents vibration can also reduce snoring.

Purpose

The purpose of snoring surgery is to improve or eliminate the medical and social consequences of heavy snoring. Most insurance companies, however, regard surgical treatment of snoring as essentially a cosmetic procedure, which means that patients must cover the expenses themselves. The major exception is surgery to correct a deviated septum or other obstruction in the nose, on the grounds that nasal surgery generally improves the patient's breathing during the day as well as at night.

Demographics

Snoring is a commonplace problem in the general population in North America. About 30% of all Americans snore, and more than half of all middle-aged men snore. Men are more affected than women because of the architecture of their throat, and because of hormonal patterns and how those hormones affect fat distribution and the muscles of the upper airway. About 12% of children over the age of five are reported to snore frequently and loudly. Among adults, 45% snore occasionally, while 25% snore almost every night. The problem usually grows worse as people age; 50% of people over age 65 are habitual snorers.

Problem snoring is worse among males than among females in all age brackets. With regard to racial and ethnic differences, a sleep research study published in 2003 reported that frequent snoring is more common (in the United States) among African American women, Hispanic women, and Hispanic men than in their Caucasian counterparts, even after adjusting for weight and body mass index (BMI). African American, Native American, and Asian American males have the same rates of snoring as Caucasian males. Further research is needed to determine whether these differences are related to variations in the rates and types of health problems in these respective groups.

According to international researchers, heavy snoring appears to be more common in persons of Asian origin than in persons of Middle Eastern, European, or African origin.

Description

Most adults who snore have what is called primary snoring, which means that the loud sounds produced in the upper airway during sleep are *not* interrupted by episodes of breathing cessation. Other terms for primary snoring are simple snoring, benign snoring, rhythmical snoring, continuous snoring, and socially unacceptable snoring (SUS).

Heavy snoring may sometimes indicate a breathing disorder. Obstructive sleep apnea (OSA) is a condition marked by brief stoppages in breathing during sleep resulting from partial blockage of the airway. It is thought to affect about 4% of middle-aged males and 2% of middle-aged females. A person with OSA may stop breathing temporarily as often as 20–30 times per hour. The individual usually snores or makes choking and gasping sounds between these episodes, is not refreshed by nighttime sleep, and may suffer from morning headaches as well as daytime sleepiness. In some cases, people may be misdiagnosed as suffering from clinical depression when the real problem is physical tiredness. In addition, the high levels of carbon dioxide that build up in the blood when a person is not breathing normally may eventually lead to high blood pressure, irregular heartbeat, heart attacks, and stroke. In children, heavy snoring appears to be a major risk factor for attention deficit hyperactivity disorder (ADHD).

Although people with OSA snore, not everyone who snores has OSA. Primary snoring is not associated with severe disorders to the same extent as OSA, but it has been shown to have some negative consequences for health, including such things as chronic daily headaches. A group of Swedish researchers reported that heavy snoring has the same level of negative effects on quality of life among adult males as high blood pressure, chronic obstructive pulmonary disease, heart disease, and similar chronic medical conditions. It may also have social consequences, as people who snore heavily often keep other family members, roommates, or even neighbors from getting a good night's sleep.

Risk factors for snoring

Some people are at higher risk of developing problem snoring than others. Risk factors in addition to gender and age include:

- genetic factors—the size and shape of the uvula, soft palate, tonsils, and other parts of the airway are largely determined by heredity

- family history of heavy snoring

- obesity—being severely overweight increases a person's risk of developing OSA

- lack of exercise—physical activity helps to keep the muscles of the throat firm and strong

- heavy consumption of alcohol and tobacco

- a history of frequent upper respiratory infections or allergies

- trauma to the nose, face, or throat

Types of snoring surgeries

With the exception of uvulopalatopharyngoplasty, all of the surgical treatments for snoring are outpatient or office-based procedures.

UVULOPALATOPHARYNGOPLASTY. Uvulopalatopharyngoplasty, or UPPP, is the oldest and most invasive surgical treatment for snoring. It was first performed in 1982 by Japanese surgeon Dr. Shiro Fujita. UPPP requires **general anesthesia**, one to two nights of inpatient care in a hospital, and a minimum of two weeks of recovery afterward. In a uvulopalatopharyngoplasty, the surgeon resects (removes) the patient's tonsils, part of the soft palate, and the uvula. The procedure works by enlarging the airway and removing some of the soft tissue that vibrates when the patient snores. It is not effective in treating snoring caused by obstructions at the base of the tongue.

UPPP has several drawbacks in addition to its cost and lengthy recovery period. It can result in major complications, including severe bleeding due to removal of the tonsils, as well as airway obstruction. In addition, the results may not be permanent; between 50% and 70% of patients who have been treated with UPPP report that improvements in snoring do not last longer than a year.

LASER-ASSISTED UVULOPALATOPLASTY. Laser-assisted uvulopalatoplasty, or LAUP, is an outpatient surgical treatment for snoring in which a carbon dioxide laser is used to vaporize part of the uvula, a small triangular piece of tissue that hangs from the soft palate above the back of the tongue. The patient is seated upright in a comfortable chair in the doctor's office. The doctor first sprays a local anesthetic—usually lidocaine—over the back of the patient's throat, covering the patient's soft palate, tonsils, and uvula. The second step is the injection of more anesthetic into the muscle tissue in the uvula. After waiting for the anesthetic to take effect, the surgeon uses a carbon dioxide laser to make two vertical incisions in the soft palate on either side of the uvula. A third incision is used to remove the tip of the uvula. The surgeon also usually removes part of the soft palate itself. The total procedure takes about half an hour.

LAUP is typically performed as a series of three to five separate treatments. Additional treatment sessions, if needed, are spaced four to eight weeks apart.

LAUP was developed in the late 1980s by Dr. Yves-Victor Kamami, a French surgeon whose first article on the technique was published in 1990. Kamami claimed a high rate of success for LAUP in treating OSA as well as snoring. The procedure has become controversial because other **surgeons** found it less effective than the first reports indicated, and also because most patients suffer considerable pain for about two weeks after surgery. Although some surgeons report a success rate as high as 85% in treating snoring with LAUP, the effectiveness of the procedure is highly dependent on the surgeon's experience and ability.

SOMNOPLASTY. Somnoplasty, or radiofrequency volumetric tissue reduction (RFVTR), is a newer technique in which the surgeon uses a thin needle connected to a source of radiofrequency signals to shrink the tissues in the soft palate, throat, or tongue. It was approved by the U.S. Food and Drug Administration (FDA) for the treatment of snoring in 1997. The needle is inserted beneath the surface layer of cells and heated to a temperature between 158°F and 176°F (70° and 80°C). The upper layer of cells is unaffected, but the heated tissue is destroyed and gradually reabsorbed by the body over the next four to six weeks. Somnoplasty stiffens the remaining layers of tissue as well as reducing the total volume of tissue. Some patients require a second treatment, but most find that their snoring is significantly improved after only one. The procedure takes about 30 minutes and is performed under **local anesthesia**.

Somnoplasty appears to have a higher success rate (about 85%) than LAUP and is considerably less painful. Most patients report two to three days of mild swelling after somnoplasty, compared to two weeks of considerable discomfort for LAUP.

TONGUE SUSPENSION PROCEDURE. The tongue suspension procedure, originally known as the Repose™ System but now called the AIRvance™ System, is a minimally invasive surgical treatment for snoring that stabilizes the base of the tongue during sleep, preventing it from falling backward and obstructing the airway. This technique was approved by the FDA in 1998. It consists of a titanium screw inserted into the lower jaw on the floor of the mouth and a suture passed through the base of the tongue that is then attached to the screw. The attachment holds the tongue forward during sleep.

The AIRvance™ System is done as an outpatient procedure under total anesthesia. It takes about 30 minutes to complete. The advantages of the tongue suspension procedure include the fact that it is reversible, since no incision is made, and that it can be combined with UPPP, LAUP, or a **tonsillectomy**. Its disadvantages include its relatively long healing time (one to two weeks), and the fact that it appears to be more effective in treating OSA than primary snoring. One team of American and Israeli researchers who conducted a multicenter trial concluded that the tongue suspension procedure requires further evaluation.

INJECTION SNOREPLASTY. Injection snoreplasty was developed by a team of Army physicians at Walter Reed Hospital and introduced to other ear, nose, and throat specialists at a professional conference in 2000. In injection snoreplasty, the surgeon gives the patient a local anesthetic and then injects a hardening agent known as sodium tetradecyl sulfate underneath the skin of the roof of the mouth just in front of the uvula. The chemical, which is also used in sclerotherapy, creates a blister that hardens into scar tissue. The scar tissue pulls the uvula forward, reducing the vibration or flutter that causes snoring.

Preliminary research indicates that injection snoreplasty is safe, has a higher rate of success than LAUP (about 92%), and is also less painful. Most patients need only one treatment, and can manage the discomfort the next day with a mild **aspirin** substitute and throat spray. The primary drawback of injection snoreplasty is that it treats only tissues in the area of the uvula. Snoring caused by tissue vibrations elsewhere in the throat requires another form of treatment. Injection snoreplasty costs about $500 per treatment.

Diagnosis

The most important task in diagnosing a patient's snoring is to distinguish between primary snoring and obstructive sleep apnea. The reason for care in the diagnosis is that surgical treatment without the recommended tests for OSA can complicate later diagnosis of the disorder.

The sounds made when a person snores have a number of different physical causes. Snoring noises may result from one or more of the following:

• An unusually long soft palate and uvula. These structures narrow the airway between the nose and the throat. They act like noisy flutter valves when the person breathes in and out during sleep.

• Too much tissue in the throat. Large tonsils and adenoids can cause snoring, which is one reason why tonsillectomies are sometimes recommended to treat heavy snoring in children.

• Nasal congestion. When a person's nose is stuffy, their attempts to breathe create a partial vacuum in the throat that pulls the softer tissues of the throat together. This suction can also produce a snoring noise. Nasal congestion helps to explain why some people snore only when they have a cold or during pollen season.

• Anatomical deformations of the nose. People who have had their noses or cheekbones fractured or who have a deviated septum are more likely to snore, because their nasal passages develop a twisted or crooked shape and vibrate as air passes through them.

• Sleeping position. People are more likely to snore when they are lying on their backs because the force of gravity draws the tongue and soft tissues in the throat backward and downward, blocking the airway.

• Obesity. Obesity adds to the weight of the tissues in the neck, which can cause partial blockage of the airway during sleep.

• Use of alcohol, sleeping medications, or tranquilizers. These substances relax the throat muscles, which may become soft or limp enough to partially close the airway.

Because snoring may be related to lifestyle factors, upper respiratory infections, seasonal allergies, and sleeping habits as well as the anatomy of the person's airway, a complete medical history is the first step in determining suitable treatments. In some cases, the patient may have been referred by his or her dentist on the basis of findings during a dental procedure. A primary care doctor can take a history and perform a basic examination of the patient's nose and throat. In addition, the primary care doctor may give the patient one or more short questionnaires to evaluate the severity of daytime sleepiness and other problems related to snoring. The test most commonly used is the Epworth Sleepiness Scale (ESS), which was developed by an Australian physician, Dr. Murray Johns, in 1991. The ESS lists eight situations (reading, watching TV, etc.) and asks the patient to rate his or her chances of dozing off in each situation on a four-point scale (0–3, with 3 representing a high chance of falling asleep). A score of 6 or lower indicates that the person is getting enough sleep; a score higher than 9 is a danger sign. The ESS is often used to measure the effectiveness of various treatments for snoring as well as to evaluate patients prior to surgery.

The next stage in the differential diagnosis of snoring problems is a detailed examination of the patient's airway by an otolaryngologist, who is a physician that specializes in diagnosing and treating disorders involving the nose and throat. The American Sleep Apnea Association (ASAA) maintains that no one should consider surgery for snoring until their airway has been examined by a specialist. The otolaryngologist will be able to determine whether the size and shape of the patient's uvula, soft palate, tonsils and adenoids, nasal cartilage, and throat muscles are contributing factors, and to advise the patient on specific procedures. It may be necessary for the patient to undergo more than one type of treatment for snoring, as some surgical procedures correct only one or two structures in the nose or throat.

A complete airway examination includes an external examination of the patient's face and neck, an endoscopic examination of the nasal passages and throat, the use of a laryngeal mirror or magnifying laryngoscope to study the lower portions of the throat, and various imaging studies. The otolaryngologist may use a nasopharyngoscope, which allows for evaluation of obstructions below the palate and the tongue, and may be performed with the patient either awake or asleep. The nasopharyngoscope is a flexible fiberoptic device that is introduced into the airway through the patient's nose. Other imaging studies that may be done include acoustic reflection, **computed tomography** (CT) scans, or **magnetic resonance imaging** (MRI).

In addition to the airway examination, patients considering surgical treatment for snoring must make an appointment for sleep testing in a specialized laboratory. The American Academy of Sleep Medicine recommends this step in order to exclude the possibility that the patient has obstructive sleep apnea. Sleep testing consists of an overnight stay in a special sleep laboratory. Before the patient goes to sleep, he or she will be connected to a polysomnograph, which is an instrument that monitors the patient's breathing, heart rate, temperature, muscle movements, airflow, body position, and other measurements that are needed to evaluate the cause(s) of sleep disorders. A technician records the data in a separate room. Some facilities may use portable polysomnographs that allow patients to connect the device to a computer in their home and transmit the data to the sleep center over an Internet connection.

Preparation

Apart from the extensive diagnostic testing that is recommended, preparation for outpatient snoring surgery is usually limited to taking a mild sedative before the procedure. Preparation for UPPP requires a **physical examination**, EKG, blood tests, and a preoperation interview with the anesthesiologist to evaluate the patient's fitness for general anesthesia.

Aftercare

Aftercare following outpatient snoring surgery consists primarily of medication for throat discomfort, particularly when swallowing. The patient can resume normal work and other activities the same day as the procedure, and speaking is usually not affected.

Risks

Risks associated with the surgical procedure include possible throat swelling, nerve injury, sleepiness, and an allergic reaction to the local anesthetic. Other risks include:

• Severe pain following the procedure that lasts longer than two to three days. This complication occurs more

KEY TERMS

Continuous positive airway pressure (CPAP)—A ventilation device that blows a gentle stream of air into the nose during sleep to keep the airway open.

Deviated septum—An abnormal configuration of the cartilage that divides the two sides of the nose. It can cause breathing problems if left uncorrected.

Injection snoreplasty—A technique for reducing snoring by injecting a chemical that forms scar tissue near the base of the uvula, helping to anchor it and reduce its fluttering or vibrating during sleep.

Obstructive sleep apnea (OSA)—A potentially life-threatening condition characterized by episodes of breathing cessation during sleep alternating with snoring or disordered breathing. The low levels of oxygen in the blood of patients with OSA may eventually cause heart problems or stroke.

Palate—The roof of the mouth.

Polysomnography—A test administered in a sleep laboratory to analyze heart rate, blood circulation, muscle movement, brain waves, and breathing patterns during sleep.

Primary snoring—Simple snoring; snoring that is not interrupted by episodes of breathing cessation.

Somnoplasty—A technique that uses radiofrequency signals to heat a thin needle inserted into the tissues of the soft palate. The heat from the needle shrinks the tissues, thus enlarging the patient's airway. Somnoplasty is also known as radiofrequency volumetric tissue reduction (RFVTR).

Uvula—A triangular piece of tissue that hangs from the roof of the mouth above the back of the tongue. Primary snoring is often associated with fluttering or vibrating of the uvula during sleep.

Uvulopalatopharyngoplasty (UPPP)—An operation to remove the tonsils and other excess tissue at the back of the throat to prevent it from closing the airway during sleep. This procedure may also be performed with a laser.

frequently with LAUP than with somnoplasty or injection snoreplasty.

- Causation or worsening of obstructive sleep apnea. LAUP has been reported to cause OSA in patients who only had primary snoring before the operation.
- Nasal regurgitation. This complication refers to food shooting or leaking through the nose when the patient swallows.
- Dehydration. This complication has been reported with the tongue suspension procedure.
- Permanent change in the quality of the patient's voice.
- Recurrence of primary snoring.

Results

In general, surgical treatment for snoring appears to be most effective in patients whose primary problem is nasal obstruction. The results of snoring surgery depend to a large degree on a good "fit" between the anatomy of a specific patient's airway and the specific procedure performed, as well as on the individual surgeon's skills.

Morbidity and mortality rates

Mortality rates for UPPP are related to complications of OSA rather than to the procedure itself. With regard to the outpatient procedures for snoring, mortality rates are very close to zero because these surgeries are performed under local anesthesia. Complication rates, however, are high with both UPPP and LAUP. According to one European study, as many as 42% of patients have complications following UPPP, with 14% reporting general dissatisfaction with the results of surgery. Specific complication rates for UPPP are: 15% for recurrence of snoring, 13% for nasal regurgitation, 10% for excessive throat secretions, 9% for swallowing problems, and 7% for speech disturbances. Complications for LAUP have been estimated to be: 30%–40% for recurrence of snoring, 30% for causing or worsening of OSA, 5%–10% for persistent nasal regurgitation, and 1% for permanent change in vocal quality.

Alternatives

Oral devices and appliances

Oral appliances are intended to reduce snoring by changing the shape of the oral cavity or preventing the tongue from blocking the airway. There are three basic types of mouthpieces: those that push the lower jaw forward; those that raise the soft palate; and those that restrain the tongue from falling backward during sleep. To work properly, oral appliances should be fitted by an experienced dentist or orthodontist and checked periodically for proper fit. Their major drawback is a low rate of patient compliance; one German study found that only 30% of patients fitted with these devices were still using them after four years. In addition, oral appliances cannot be used by patients with gum disease, **dental implants**, or teeth that are otherwise in poor condition.

Continuous positive airway pressure (CPAP) devices

CPAP devices are masks that fit over the nose during sleep and deliver air into the airway under enough pressure to keep the airway open. If used correctly, CPAP devices can be an effective alternative to surgery. Their main drawback is a relatively low rate of patient compliance; the mask must be worn every night, and some people feel mildly claustrophobic when using it. In addition, patients are often asked to lose weight or stop smoking while using CPAP, which are lifestyle adjustments that some would rather not make.

Lifestyle changes

Patients who snore only occasionally or who are light snorers may be helped by one or more of the following changes without undergoing surgery:

• Losing weight and getting adequate physical exercise.

• Avoiding tranquilizers, sleeping pills, antihistamines, or alcoholic beverages before bedtime.

• Quitting smoking.

• Sleeping on the side rather than the back. One do-it-yourself device that is sometimes recommended to keep the patient turned on his or her side is a tennis ball placed inside a sock and attached to the back of the pajamas or nightgown. This approach seems to work for some patients with simple snoring.

• Tilting the head of the bed upward about 4 in. (10 cm).

Complementary and alternative (CAM) approaches

There are three forms of alternative treatment that have been shown to be helpful in reducing primary snoring in patients with histories of nasal congestion or swollen tissues in the throat. The first is acupuncture. Treatments for snoring usually focus on acupuncture points on the stomach, arms, and legs associated with the production of excess mucus. Insertion of the acupuncture needles at these points is thought to stimulate the body to release the excess moisture or phlegm.

Homeopathy and aromatherapy also appear to benefit some patients whose snoring is related to colds, allergies, or sore throats. Homeopathic remedies for snoring are available as nose drops and throat sprays as well as the traditional pill formulations. Aromatherapy formulas for snoring typically contain marjoram oil, which may be used alone or combined with lavender and other herbs that clear

QUESTIONS TO ASK YOUR DOCTOR

• How often have you performed surgery for primary snoring? Which procedures have you performed most frequently?

• What is your opinion of somnoplasty and injection snoreplasty?

• Am I likely to benefit from lifestyle changes or other less invasive alternatives?

• Should I talk to my dentist about an oral appliance to control snoring?

the nasal passages. Some people find aromatherapy preparations helpful alongside mainstream treatments because their fragrance is pleasant and relaxing.

Health care team roles

Snoring surgery is done by a head and neck surgeon, a plastic surgeon, or an otolaryngologist, who is a doctor with special training in treating disorders of the ear, nose, and throat. UPPP is performed under general anesthesia and requires an overnight hospital stay. LAUP, somnoplasty, the tongue suspension procedure, and injection snoreplasty are performed as **outpatient surgery**, usually in a doctor's office or other outpatient facility.

Prosthetic devices to alter the position of the jaw or restrain the tongue during sleep are prescribed and fitted by general dentists or orthodontists.

Polysomnography as a part of a diagnostic workup is done in a special sleep laboratory by experts who are trained in the use of the equipment and interpretation of the results. Advances in technology, however, may allow patients to be monitored at home with portable polysomnographs and a computer with an Internet connection.

Resources

BOOKS

Friedman, Michael. *Sleep Apnea and Snoring: Surgical and Non-Surgical Therapy*. Philadelphia: Saunders/Elsevier, 2009.

Hörmann, Karl, and Thomas Verse. *Surgery for Sleep Disordered Breathing*. London; New York: Springer, 2010.

Lee, K. J. *Essential Otolaryngology: Head and Neck Surgery*. 10th ed. New York: McGraw-Hill, 2012.

PERIODICALS

Carroll, William, et al. "Snoring Management with Nasal Surgery and Upper Airway Radiofrequency Ablation." *Otorhinolaryngology—Head and Neck Surgery* 146, no. 6 (2012): 1023–27. http://dx.doi.org/10.1177/0194599812436940 (accessed October 9, 2013).

Eckert, Danny Joel, and Magdy K. Younes. "Arousal from Sleep: Implications for Obstructive Sleep Apnea Pathogenesis and Treatment." *Journal of Applied Physiology* (August 29, 2013): e-pub ahead of print. http://dx.doi.org/10.1152/japplphysiol.00649.2013 (accessed October 9, 2013).

WEBSITES

American Association of Oral and Maxillofacial Surgeons. "Snoring and Sleep Apnea." http://www.aaoms.org/conditions-and-treatments/snoring-and-sleep-apnea (accessed October 9, 2013).

American Sleep Apnea Association. "OSA Treatment Options." http://www.sleepapnea.org/treat/treatment-options.html (accessed October 9, 2013).

MedlinePlus. "Snoring." U.S. National Library of Medicine, National Institutes of Health. http://www.nlm.nih.gov/medlineplus/snoring.html (accessed October 9, 2013).

National Heart, Lung, and Blood Institute. "What Is Sleep Apnea?" National Institutes of Health. http://www.nhlbi.nih.gov/health/health-topics/topics/sleepapnea (accessed October 9, 2013).

ORGANIZATIONS

American Academy of Medical Acupuncture, 1970 E. Grand Ave., Ste. 330, El Segundo, CA 90245, (310) 364-0193, jdowden@prodigy.net, http://medicalacupuncture.org.

American Academy of Otolaryngology—Head and Neck Surgery, 1650 Diagonal Rd., Alexandria, VA 22314-2857, (703) 836-4444, http://www.entnet.org.

American Academy of Sleep Medicine, 2510 N. Frontage Rd., Darien, IL 60561, (630) 737-9700, http://www.aasmnet.org.

American Association of Oral and Maxillofacial Surgeons, 9700 W. Bryn Mawr Ave., Rosemont, IL 60018-5701, (847) 678-6200, (800) 822-6637, Fax: (847) 678-6286, http://www.aaoms.org.

American Dental Association, 211 E. Chicago Ave., Chicago, IL 60611, (312) 440-2500, http://www.ada.org.

American Sleep Apnea Association, 6856 Eastern Ave. NW, Ste. 203, Washington, DC 20012, (888) 293-3650, http://www.sleepapnea.org.

National Center on Sleep Disorders Research, 6701 Rockledge Dr., Bethesda, MD 20892, (301) 435-0199, http://www.nhlbi.nih.gov/about/ncsdr/index.htm.

Rebecca Frey, PhD
Tammy Allhoff, CST/CSFA, AAS

Sodium test *see* **Electrolyte tests; Serum sodium level**

Somnoplasty *see* **Snoring surgery**

Sonography *see* **Ultrasound**

SPECT scan *see* **Single photon emission computed tomography**

Sphygmomanometer

Definition

A sphygmomanometer is a device for measuring blood pressure.

Purpose

The sphygmomanometer is designed to monitor blood pressure by measuring the force of the blood in the heart where the pressure is greatest. This occurs during the contraction of the ventricles, when blood is pumped from the heart to the rest of the body (systolic pressure). The minimal force is also measured. This occurs during the period when the heart is relaxed between beats and pressure is lowest (diastolic pressure).

A sphygmomanometer is used to establish a baseline at a healthcare encounter and on admission to a hospital. Checking blood pressure is also performed to monitor the effectiveness of medication and other methods to control hypertension, and as a diagnostic aid to detect various diseases and abnormalities.

Description

A sphygmomanometer consists of a hand bulb pump, a unit that displays the blood pressure reading, and an inflatable cuff that is usually wrapped around a person's upper arm. Care should be taken to ensure that the cuff size is appropriate for the person whose blood pressure is being taken. This improves the accuracy of the reading. Children and adults with arms smaller or larger than average-sized arms require specially sized cuffs. A **stethoscope** is also used in conjunction with the sphygmomanometer to hear the blood pressure sounds. Some devices have the stethoscope already built in.

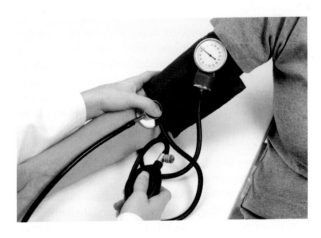

A sphygmomanometer measures blood pressure.
(LeventeGyori/Shutterstock.com)

Aneroid monitor—A monitor that works without fluids (mercury free).

Blood pressure—The tension of the blood in the arteries, measured in millimeters of mercury (mm Hg) by a sphygmomanometer or by an electronic device.

Diastolic—Minimum arterial blood pressure during ventricular relaxation or rest.

Systolic—Maximum arterial blood pressure during ventricular contraction.

A sphygmomanometer may be used or encountered in a variety of settings:

- home
- hospital
- primary care clinic or professional office
- ambulance
- dental office
- pharmacy and other retail establishment

There are three types of equipment in common use for monitoring blood pressure:

- A mercury-based unit has a manually inflatable cuff attached by tubing to the unit that is calibrated in millimeters of mercury. During blood pressure measurement, the unit must be kept upright on a flat surface and the gauge read at eye level. Breakage of the unit may cause dangerous mercury contamination and would require specialist removal for disposal. Due to the hazards of mercury, the use of mercury-based sphygmomanometers has declined sharply since 2000.

- An aneroid unit is mercury free. It consists of a cuff that can be applied with one hand for self-testing, a stethoscope, and a valve that inflates and deflates automatically. The data is displayed on an easy-to-read gauge that will function in any position. The aneroid unit is sensitive and if dropped may require recalibration.

- An automatic unit is also mercury free and is typically battery operated. It has a cuff that can be applied with one hand for self-testing and a valve that automatically inflates and deflates. Units with manual inflation are also available. The reading is displayed digitally and a stethoscope is not required. This is useful for persons who are hearing impaired, for emergency situations when staff is limited, and for automatic input into

instruments for storage or graphic display. A wrist monitor is also available for home testing. Some more expensive models remember and print out recordings. The automatic units tend to be more portable than the mercury devices.

Operation

The flow, resistance, quality, and quantity of blood circulating through the heart and the condition of the arterial walls are all factors that influence blood pressure. If blood flow in the arteries is restricted, the reading will be higher.

Blood pressure should be routinely checked every one to two years. It can be checked at any time, but it is best measured when a person has been resting for at least five minutes so that any exertion prior to the test will not influence the outcome of the reading.

To record blood pressure, the person should be seated with one arm bent slightly, the arm bare or the sleeve loosely rolled up. With an aneroid or automatic unit, the cuff is placed level with the heart and wrapped around the upper arm, one inch above the elbow. Following the manufacturer's guidelines, the cuff is inflated and then deflated while an attendant records the reading.

If the blood pressure is monitored manually, a cuff is placed level with the heart and wrapped firmly but not tightly around the arm one inch (2–3 cm) above the elbow over the brachial artery. Wrinkles in the cuff should be smoothed out. Positioning a stethoscope over the brachial artery in front of the elbow with one hand and listening through the earpieces, the health professional inflates the cuff well above normal levels (to about 200 mm Hg), or until no sound is heard. Alternatively, the cuff should be inflated 10 mm Hg above the last sound heard. The valve in the pump is slowly opened. Air is allowed to escape no faster than 5 mm Hg per second to deflate the pressure in the cuff to the point where a clicking sound is heard over the brachial artery. The reading of the gauge at this point is recorded as the systolic pressure. The sounds continue as the pressure in the cuff is released and the flow of blood through the artery is no longer blocked. At this point, the noises are no longer heard. The reading of the gauge at this point is noted as the diastolic pressure. "Lub-dub" is the sound produced by the normal heart as it beats. Every time this sound is detected, it means that the heart is contracting once. The sounds are created when the heart valves click to close. When one hears "lub," the atrioventricular valves are closing. The "dub" sound is produced by the pulmonic and aortic valves.

With children, the clicking sound does not disappear but changes to a soft muffled sound. Because sounds continue to be heard as the cuff deflates to zero, the reading of the gauge at the point where the sounds change is recorded as the diastolic pressure.

Blood pressure readings are recorded with the systolic pressure first, then the diastolic pressure (e.g., 120 [systolic]/70 [diastolic]).

Maintenance

Devices should be checked and calibrated annually by a qualified technician to ensure accurate readings. This is especially important for automatic sphygmomanometers.

Results

One elevated reading does not mean that hypertension is present. Repeated measurements may be required if hypertension is suspected. The **blood pressure measurement** is recorded and compared with normal ranges for an individual's age and medical condition, and a decision is made on whether any further medical intervention is required.

Resources

BOOKS

Bickley, Lynn S., and Peter G. Szilagyi. *Bates' Guide to Physical Examination & History Taking*. 11th ed. Philadelphia: Wolters Kluwer Health/Lippincott Williams & Wilkins, 2013.

Chan, Paul D., and Peter J. Winkle. *History and Physical Examination*. 10th ed. New York: Current Clinical Strategies, 2002.

Seidel, Henry M. *Mosby's Physical Examination Handbook*. 7th ed. St. Louis, MO: Mosby/Elsevier, 2011.

Swartz, Mark H. *Textbook of Physical Diagnosis: History and Examination*. 6th ed. Philadelphia: Saunders/Elsevier, 2010.

PERIODICALS

Jones, D. W., et al. "Measuring Blood Pressure Accurately: New and Persistent Challenges." *Journal of the American Medical Association* 289, no. 8 (2003): 1027–30.

O'Brien, E. "Demise of the Mercury Sphygmomanometer and the Dawning of a New Era in Blood Pressure Measurement." *Blood Pressure Monitoring* 8, no. 1 (2003): 19–21.

Pickering, T. G. "What Will Replace the Mercury Sphygmomanometer?" *Blood Pressure Monitoring* 8, no. 1 (2003): 23–25.

Stergiou, G. S. "A Perfect Replacement for the Mercury Sphygmomanometer: The Case of the Hybrid Blood Pressure Monitor." *Journal of Human Hypertension* 26 (April 2012): 220–27. http://dx.doi.org/10.1038/jhh.2011.77 (accessed October 23, 2013).

WEBSITES

MedlinePlus. "High Blood Pressure." U.S. National Library of Medicine, National Institutes of Health. http://www.nlm.nih.gov/medlineplus/highbloodpressure.html (accessed May 2, 2013).

National Heart, Lung, and Blood Institute. "How Is Blood Pressure Tested?" National Institutes of Health. http://www.nhlbi.nih.gov/hbp/detect/tested.htm (accessed May 2, 2013).

L. Fleming Fallon Jr., MD, DrPH

Sphygmomanometry *see* **Blood pressure measurement**

Spina bifida surgery *see* **Meningocele repair**

Spinal fluid analysis *see* **Cerebrospinal fluid (CSF) analysis**

Spinal fusion

Definition

Spinal fusion is a procedure that promotes the fusing, or growing together, of two or more vertebrae in the spine.

Purpose

Spinal fusion is performed to:

• straighten a spine deformed by scoliosis, neuromuscular disease, cerebral palsy, or other disorder

• prevent further deformation

• support a spine weakened by infection or tumor

• reduce or prevent pain from pinched or injured nerves

• compensate for injured vertebrae or disks

The goal of spinal fusion is to unite two or more vertebrae to prevent them from moving independently of each other. This may be done to improve posture, increase ability to ventilate the lungs, prevent pain, or treat spinal instability and reduce the risk of nerve damage.

Demographics

According to the American Academy of Orthopaedic Surgeons, approximately a quarter-million spinal fusions are performed each year, half on the upper and half on the lower spine.

Spinal fusion

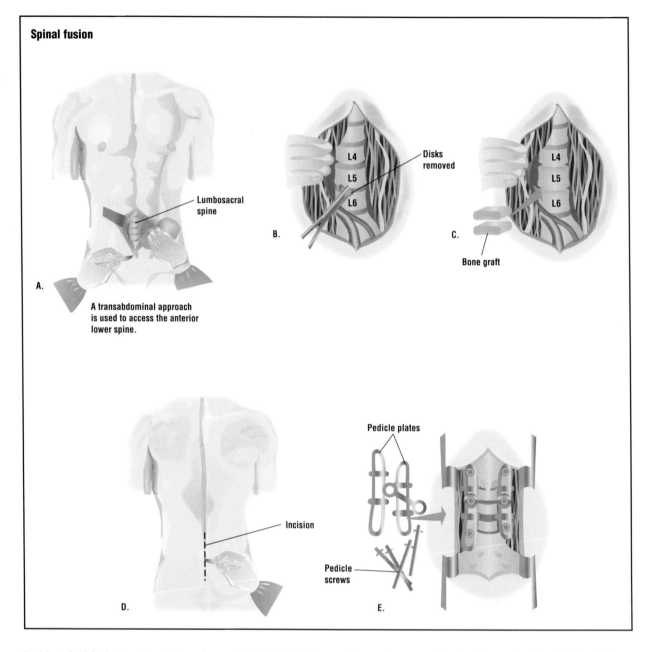

A.

Lumbosacral spine

A transabdominal approach is used to access the anterior lower spine.

B.
L4
L5
L6
Disks removed

C.
L4
L5
L6
Bone graft

D.
Incision

E.
Pedicle plates
Pedicle screws

In this spinal fusion, the surgeon makes an incision in the lower abdomen to access the lumbosacral spine (A). The disks between the vertebrae are removed (B), and bone grafts are inserted into the spaces (C). Another incision is made in the patient's back (D), and the vertebrae are exposed and fixed with pedicle plates and screws (E). *(Illustration by GGS Information Services. Copyright © Cengage Learning®.)*

Description

Spinal anatomy

The spine is a series of individual bones, called vertebrae, separated by cartilaginous disks. The spine is composed of seven cervical (neck) vertebrae, 12 thoracic (chest) vertebrae, five lumbar (lower back) vertebrae, and the fused vertebrae in the sacrum and coccyx that help to form the hip region.

While the shapes of individual vertebrae differ among these regions, each is essentially a short hollow tube containing the bundle of nerves known as the spinal cord. Individual nerves, such as those carrying messages to the arms or legs, enter and exit the spinal cord through gaps between vertebrae.

The spinal disks act as shock absorbers, cushioning the spine, and preventing individual bones from contacting each other. Disks also help to hold the vertebrae together.

Fusion—A union, joining together; e.g., bone fusion.

Herniated disk—A blister-like bulging or protrusion of the contents of the disk out through the fibers that normally hold them in place. Also called ruptured disk, slipped disk, or displaced disk.

Magnetic resonance imaging (MRI)—A test that provides pictures of organs and structures inside the body by using a magnetic field and pulses of radio wave energy to detect tumors, infection, and other types of tissue disease or damage, or conditions affecting blood flow. The area of the body being studied is positioned inside a strong magnetic field.

Vertebra—One of the bones that make up the back bone (spine).

The weight of the upper body is transferred through the spine to the hips and the legs. The spine is held upright through the work of the back muscles, which are attached to the vertebrae.

While the normal spine has no side-to-side curve, it does have a series of front-to-back curves, giving it a gentle "S" shape. The spine curves in at the lumbar region, back out at the thoracic region, and back in at the cervical region.

Surgery for scoliosis, neuromuscular disease, and cerebral palsy

Abnormal side-to-side curvature of the spine is termed scoliosis. An excessive lumbar curve is termed lordosis, and an excessive thoracic curve is kyphosis. "Idiopathic" scoliosis is the most common form of scoliosis; it has no known cause.

Scoliosis and other curves can be caused by neuromuscular disease, including Duchenne muscular dystrophy. Progressive and perhaps uneven weakening of the spinal muscles leads to gradual inability to support the spine in an upright position. The weight of the upper body then begins to collapse the spine, inducing a curve. In addition to pain and disfigurement, severe scoliosis prevents adequate movement of air into and out of the lungs. Scoliosis also occurs in cerebral palsy, due to excess and imbalanced muscle activity pulling on the spine unevenly.

Idiopathic scoliosis, which occurs most often in adolescent girls, is usually managed with a brace that wraps the abdomen and chest, allowing the spine to develop straight. Spinal fusion is indicated in patients whose curves are more severe or are progressing rapidly. The indication for surgery in cerebral palsy is similar to that for idiopathic scoliosis.

Spinal fusion in Duchenne muscular dystrophy is usually indicated earlier than in otherwise healthy adolescents. This is because these patients lose ventilatory function rapidly through adolescence, making the surgery more dangerous as time passes. Surgery should occur before excess ventilatory function is lost.

Surgery for herniated disks, disk degeneration, and pain

As people age, their disks become less supple and more prone to damage. A herniated disk is one that has developed a bulge. The bulge can press against nerves located in the spinal cord or exiting from it, causing pain. Disks can also degenerate, losing mass and thickness, allowing vertebrae to contact each other. This can pinch nerves and cause pain. Disk-related pain is very common in the neck, which is subject to constant twisting forces, and the lower back, which experiences large compressive forces. In these cases, spinal fusion is employed to prevent the nerves from being damaged. The offending disk is removed at the same time. A fractured vertebra may also be treated with fusion to prevent it from causing future problems.

Sometimes, spinal fusion is used to treat back pain even when the anatomical source of the problem cannot be located. This is usually viewed as a last resort for intractable and disabling pain.

The spinal fusion operation

Spinal fusion is performed under **general anesthesia**. During the procedure, the target vertebrae are exposed. Protective tissue layers next to the bone are removed, and small chips of bone are placed next to the vertebrae. These bone chips can either be from the patient's hip or from a bone bank. The chips increase the rate of fusion. Using bone from the patient's hip (an autograft) is more successful than banked bone (an allograft), but it increases the stresses of surgery and loss of blood.

Fusion of the lumbar and thoracic vertebrae is done by approaching from the rear, with the patient lying face down. Cervical fusion is typically performed from the front, with the patient lying on his or her back.

Many spinal fusion patients also receive **spinal instrumentation**. During the fusion operation, a set of rods, wires, or screws will be attached to the spine. This instrumentation allows the spine to be held in place while the bones fuse. The alternative is an external brace applied after the operation.

An experimental treatment, called human recombinant bone morphogenetic protein-2, has shown promise for its ability to accelerate fusion rates without bone chips and instrumentation. This technique is only available through clinical trials at a few medical centers.

Spinal fusion surgery takes approximately four hours. The patient is intubated (tube placed in the trachea), and has an IV line and Foley (urinary) catheter in place. At the end of the operation, a drain is placed in the incision site to help withdraw fluids over the next several days. The fusion process is gradual and may not be completed for months after the operation.

Preparation

A potential candidate for spinal fusion undergoes a long series of medical tests. In patients with scoliosis, x-rays are taken over many months or years to track progress of the curve. Patients with disk herniation or degeneration may receive x-rays, MRI studies, or other tests to determine the location and extent of injury.

Patients in good health may donate several units of their own blood in preparation for surgery. This may be done between six weeks and one week prior to the operation. The patient will probably be advised to take iron supplements to help replace lost iron in the donated blood. Sunburn or sores on the back should be avoided prior to surgery because they increase the risk of infection.

A variety of medical tests will be done shortly before surgery to ensure that the patient is in good health and prepared for the rigors of surgery. Blood and urine tests, x-rays, and possibly photographs documenting the curvature will be done. An electroencephalogram (EEG) may be performed to test nerve function along the spine.

The patient will be admitted to the hospital the evening before surgery. No food is allowed after midnight in order to clear the gastrointestinal tract, which will be immobilized by anesthesia.

Aftercare

The patient will stay in the hospital for four to six days after the operation.

Postoperative pain is managed by intravenous pain medication. Many centers use **patient-controlled analgesia** (PCA) pumps, which allow patients to control the timing of pain medication.

For several days after the operation, the patient is unable to eat or drink because of the lasting effects of the

anesthesia on the bowels. Fluids and nutrition are delivered via the IV line.

The nurse helps the patient sit up several times per day, and assists with other needs as well. Physical therapy begins several days after the operation.

Most activities are restricted for several weeks. Strenuous activities such as bike riding or running are usually resumed after six to eight months. The surgical incision should be protected from sunburn for approximately one year to promote healing of the scar.

Risks

Spinal fusion carries a risk of nerve damage. Rarely, delayed paralysis can occur, probably from loss of oxygen to the spine during surgery. Infection may occur. Bone from the bone bank carries a small risk of infection with transmissible diseases from the bone donor. Anesthesia also poses risks. Unsuccessful fusion (pseudarthrosis) may occur, leaving the patient with the same problem after the operation.

Results

Spinal fusion for scoliosis is usually very successful in partially or completely correcting the deformity. Spinal fusion for pain is less uniformly successful because the cause of the pain cannot always be completely identified.

Morbidity and mortality rates

Unsuccessful fusion may occur in 5%–25% of patients. Neurologic injury occurs in less than 1%–5% of patients. Infection occurs in 1%–8%. Death occurs in less than 1% of patients.

Alternatives

Bracing and "watchful waiting" is the alternative to scoliosis surgery. Disk surgery without fusion is possible for some patients. Strengthening exercises and physical therapy may help some back pain patients avoid back surgery.

Health care team roles

Spinal fusion is performed by an orthopedic surgeon or neurosurgeon in a hospital setting.

Resources

BOOKS

Lane, Michael. *Spinal Fusion: Science and Technique.* New York: Springer, 2012.

PERIODICALS

McClendon, Jamal Jr., et al. "The Impact of Body Mass Index on Hospital Stay and Complications After Spinal Fusion." *Neurosurgery* (October 1, 2013): e-pub ahead of print. http://dx.doi.org/10.1227/NEU.0000000000000195 (accessed October 4, 2013).

Tian, Nai F., et al. "Efficacy of Electrical Stimulation for Spinal Fusion: A Meta-Analysis of Fusion Rate." *The Spine Journal* (August 30, 2013): e-pub ahead of print. http://dx.doi.org/10.1016/j.spinee.2013.06.056 (accessed October 4, 2013).

WEBSITES

MedlinePlus. "Spine Injuries and Disorders." U.S. National Library of Medicine, National Institutes of Health. http://www.nlm.nih.gov/medlineplus/spineinjuriesanddisorders.html (accessed October 4, 2013).

North American Spine Society. "Spinal Fusion." Know YourBack.org. http://www.knowyourback.org/Pages/Treatments/SurgicalOptions/SpinalFusion.aspx (accessed October 4, 2013).

ORGANIZATIONS

National Scoliosis Foundation, 5 Cabot Pl., Stoughton, MA 02072, (800) NSF-MYBACK (673-6922), nsf@scoliosis.org, http://www.scoliosis.org.

North American Spine Society (NASS), 7075 Veterans Blvd., Burr Ridge, IL 60527, (630) 230-3600, (866) 960-6277, Fax: (630) 230-3700, http://www.spine.org.

Richard Robinson

Spinal instrumentation

Definition

Spinal instrumentation is a method of keeping the spine rigid after **spinal fusion** surgery by surgically attaching hooks, rods, and wire to the spine in a way that redistributes the stresses on the bones and keeps them in proper alignment while the bones of the spine fuse.

Purpose

Spinal instrumentation is used to treat instability and deformity of the spine. Instability occurs when the spine no longer maintains its normal shape during movement. Such instability results in nerve damage, spinal deformities, and disabling pain. Scoliosis is a side-to-side spinal curvature. Kyphosis is a front-to-back curvature of the upper spine, while lordosis is an excessive curve of the lower spine. More than one type of curve may be present.

Spinal deformities may be caused by:

- birth defects
- fractures
- Marfan syndrome
- neurofibromatosis
- neuromuscular diseases
- severe injuries
- tumors
- idiopathic scoliosis, or scoliosis of unknown origin (approximately 85% of cases occur in girls between the ages of 12 and 15 experiencing adolescent growth spurts)

Description

Spinal instrumentation provides a stable, rigid column that encourages bones to fuse after spinal fusion surgery. Its purpose is to aid fusion. Without fusion, the metal will eventually fatigue and break, and so instrumentation is not itself a treatment for spine deformity.

Different types of spinal instrumentation are used to treat different spinal problems. Although the details of the insertion of rods, wires, screws, and hooks vary, the purpose of all spinal instrumentation is the same—to correct and stabilize the backbone while the bones of the spine fuse. The various instruments are all made of stainless steel, titanium, or titanium alloy.

The oldest form of spinal instrumentation is the Harrington rod. While it was simple in design, it required a long period of brace wearing after the operation, and did not allow segmental adjustment or correction. The Luque rod was developed to avoid the long postoperative bracing period. This system threads wires into the space within each vertebra. The risk of injury to the nerves and spinal cord is higher than with some other forms of instrumentation. Cotrel-Dubousset instrumentation uses hooks and rods in a cross-linked pattern to realign the spine and redistribute the biomechanical stress. The main advantage of Cotrel-Dubousset instrumentation is that because of the extensive cross-linking, the patient may not have to wear a cast or brace after surgery. The disadvantage is the complexity of the operation and the number of hooks and cross-links that may fail.

Several newer systems use screws that are embedded into the portion of the vertebra called the pedicle. Pedicle screws avoid the need for threading wires, but carry the risk of migrating out of the bone and contacting the spinal cord or the aorta (the major blood vessel exiting the heart). During the late 1990s, pedicle screws were the subject of several high-profile lawsuits. The controversies have since subsided, and pedicle screws remain an indispensable part of the spinal instrumentation. Many operations today are performed with a mix of techniques, such as Luque rods in the lower back and hooks and screws up higher. A physician chooses the proper type of instrumentation based on the type of disorder, the age and health of the patient, and the physician's experience.

The surgeon strips the tissue away from the area to be fused. The surface of the bone is peeled away. A piece of bone is removed from the hip and placed along side the area to be fused. The stripping of the bone helps the bone graft to fuse.

After the fusion site is prepared, the rods, hooks, screws, and wires are inserted. There is much variation in how this is done based on the spinal instrumentation chosen. Once the rods are in place, the incision is closed.

Preparation

Spinal fusion with spinal instrumentation is major surgery. The patient will undergo many tests to determine the nature and exact location of the back problem. These tests are likely to include

- x-rays
- magnetic resonance imaging (MRI)
- computed tomography scans (CT scans)
- myelograms

In addition, the patient will undergo a battery of blood and urine tests, and possibly an electrocardiogram to provide the surgeon and anesthesiologist with information that will allow the operation to be performed safely. In Harrington rod instrumentation, the patient may be placed in **traction** or an upper body cast to stretch contracted muscles before surgery.

Aftercare

After surgery, the patient will be confined to bed. A catheter is inserted so that the patient can urinate without getting up. **Vital signs** are monitored, and the patient's position is changed frequently so that **pressure ulcers** do not develop.

Recovery from spinal instrumentation can be a long, arduous process. Movement is severely limited for a period of time. In certain types of instrumentation, the patient is put in a cast to allow the realigned bones to stay in position until healing takes place. This can be as long as six to eight months. Many patients will need to wear a brace after the cast is removed.

During the recovery period, the patient is taught respiratory exercises to help maintain respiratory function during the time of limited mobility. Physical therapists assist the patient in learning self-care and in performing strengthening and range-of-motion exercises. **Length of hospital stay** depends on the age and health of the patient, as well as the specific problem that was corrected. The patient can expect to remain under a physician's care for many months.

Risks

Spinal instrumentation carries a significant risk of nerve damage and paralysis. The skill of the surgeon can affect the outcome of the operation, so patients should look for a hospital and **surgical team** that has a lot of experience doing spinal procedures.

Since the hooks and rods of spinal instrumentation are anchored in the bones of the back, spinal instrumentation should not be performed on people with serious osteoporosis. To overcome this limitation, techniques are being explored that help anchor instrumentation in fragile bones.

After surgery there is a risk of infection or an inflammatory reaction due to the presence of the foreign material in the body. Serious infection of the membranes covering the spinal cord and brain can occur. In the long term, the instrumentation may move or break, causing nerve damage and requiring a second surgery. Some bone grafts do not heal well, lengthening the time the patient must spend in a cast or brace or necessitating additional surgery. Casting and wearing a brace may take an emotional toll, especially on young people. Patients who have had spinal instrumentation must avoid contact sports, and, for the rest of their lives, eliminate situations that will abnormally put stress on their spines.

Results

Many young people with scoliosis heal with significantly improved alignment of the spine. Results of spinal instrumentation done for other conditions vary widely.

Morbidity and mortality rates

Mortality rate for spinal fusion surgery is less than 1%. Neurologic injury may occur in 1%–5% of cases. Delayed paralysis is possible but rare.

Alternatives

Not all patients require instrumentation with their spinal fusion. For some patients, a rigid external brace can provide the required rigidity to allow the bones to fuse.

Health care team roles

Spinal instrumentation is performed by a neurosurgical and/or orthopedic surgical team with special experience in spinal operations. The surgery is done in a hospital under **general anesthesia**. It is done at the same time as spinal fusion.

Resources

BOOKS

Canale, S. T., ed. *Campbell's Operative Orthopaedics*. 12th ed. St. Louis, MO: Mosby, 2012.

DeLee, Jesse, David Drez, and Mark D. Miller. *DeLee and Drez's Orthopaedic Sports Medicine: Principles and Practice*. 3rd ed. Philadelphia: Saunders/Elsevier, 2010.

PERIODICALS

Gerometta, Antoine, Juan Carlos Rodriguez Olaverri, and Fabian Bitan. "Infections in Spinal Instrumentation." *International Orthopaedics* 36, no. 2 (2012): 457–64. http://dx.doi.org/10.1007%2Fs00264-011-1426-0 (accessed October 18, 2013).

WEBSITES

Piedmont Healthcare. "Spinal Instrumentation." http://www.piedmonthospital.org/medical-care/Spine-Spinal-Instrumentation.aspx (accessed October 18, 2013).

ORGANIZATIONS

National Scoliosis Foundation, 5 Cabot Pl., Stoughton, MA 02072, (800) NSF-MYBACK (673-6922), nsf@scoliosis.org, http://www.scoliosis.org.

North American Spine Society (NASS), 7075 Veterans Blvd., Burr Ridge, IL 60527, (630) 230-3600, (866) 960-6277, Fax: (630) 230-3700, http://www.spine.org.

Tish Davidson, AM
Richard Robinson

Spinal tap *see* **Cerebrospinal fluid (CSF) analysis**

Spirometry

Definition

Spirometry is the measurement of air flow into and out of the lungs.

Purpose

Spirometry measures ventilation, or the movement of air into and out of the lungs. It is the most commonly performed pulmonary function test (PFT) and is often the first test performed when a problem with lung function is suspected. Spirometry may also be suggested by an abnormal x-ray, **arterial blood gas** analysis, or other diagnostic pulmonary test results. The National Lung Health Education Program recommends that regular spirometry tests be performed on persons over 45 years old who have a history of smoking. Spirometry tests are also recommended for persons with a family history of

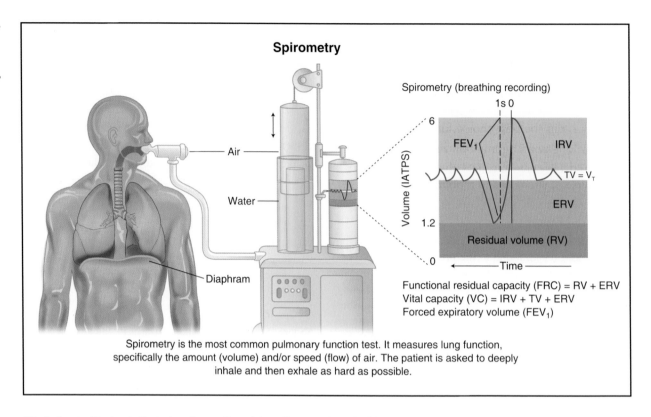

Spirometry

Spirometry (breathing recording)

FEV₁ — FEV_1

IRV

TV = V$_T$

ERV

Residual volume (RV)

Volume (IATPS)

Time

Functional residual capacity (FRC) = RV + ERV
Vital capacity (VC) = IRV + TV + ERV
Forced expiratory volume (FEV₁)

Spirometry is the most common pulmonary function test. It measures lung function, specifically the amount (volume) and/or speed (flow) of air. The patient is asked to deeply inhale and then exhale as hard as possible.

Air

Water

Diaphram

(Illustration by Electronic Illustrators Group. Copyright © Cengage Learning®.)

lung disease, chronic respiratory ailments, and advanced age.

Description

Spirometry is used to assess lung function over time. The patient's nose is pinched off as the patient breathes through a mouthpiece attached to the spirometer. The patient is instructed on how to breathe during the procedure. Three breathing maneuvers are practiced before recording the procedure, and the highest of three trials is used for the evaluation of breathing. This procedure measures air flow by electronic or mechanical displacement principles, and uses a microprocessor and recorder to calculate and plot air flow.

The test produces a recording of the patient's ventilation under conditions involving both normal and maximal effort. The recording, called a spirogram, shows the volume of air moved and the rate at which it travels into and out of the lungs. Spirometry measures several lung capacities. Accurate measurement is dependent upon the patient performing the appropriate maneuver properly. The most common measurements are:

• Vital capacity (VC). This is the amount of air (in liters) moved out of the lungs during normal breathing. The patient is instructed to breathe in and out normally to attain full expiration. Vital capacity is usually about

80% of the total lung capacity. Because of the elastic nature of the lungs and surrounding thorax, a small volume of air will remain in the lungs after full exhalation. This volume is called the residual volume (RV).

• Forced vital capacity (FVC). After breathing out normally to full expiration, the patient is instructed to breathe in with a maximal effort and then exhale as forcefully and rapidly as possible. The FVC is the volume of air that is expelled into the spirometer following a maximum inhalation effort.

• Forced expiratory volume (FEV). At the start of the FVC maneuver, the spirometer measures the volume of air delivered through the mouthpiece at timed intervals of 0.5, 1, 2, and 3 seconds. The sum of these measurements normally constitutes about 97% of the FVC measurement. The most commonly used FEV measurement is FEV-1, which is the volume of air exhaled into the mouthpiece in one second. The FEV-1 should be at least 70% of the FVC.

• Forced expiratory flow 25%–75% (FEF 25–75). This is a calculation of the average flow rate over the center portion of the forced expiratory volume recording. It is determined from the time in seconds at which 25% and 75% of the vital capacity is reached. The volume of air exhaled in liters per second between these two times is the FEF 25–75. This value reflects the status of the medium- and small-sized airways.

- Maximal voluntary ventilation (MVV). This maneuver involves the patient breathing as deeply and as rapidly as possible for 15 seconds. The average air flow (liters per second) indicates the strength and endurance of the respiratory muscles.

Normal values for FVC, FEV, FEF, and MVV are dependent on the patient's age, gender, and height.

Breathing patterns

The spirogram will identify two different types of abnormal ventilation patterns: obstructive and restrictive.

Common causes of an obstructive pattern are cystic fibrosis, asthma, bronchiectasis, bronchitis, and emphysema. These conditions may be collectively referred to by using the acronym CABBE. Chronic bronchitis, emphysema, and asthma result in dyspnea (difficulty breathing) and ventilation deficiency, a condition known as chronic obstructive pulmonary disease (COPD). COPD is the fourth leading cause of death among Americans.

Common causes of a restrictive pattern are pneumonia, heart disease, pregnancy, lung fibrosis, pneumothorax (collapsed lung), and pleural effusion (compression caused by chest fluid).

Obstructive and restrictive patterns can be identified on spirographs using both a "y" and "x" axis. Volume (liters) is plotted on the y-axis versus time (seconds) on the x-axis. A restrictive pattern is characterized by a normal shape showing reduced volumes for all parameters. The reduction in volumes indicates the severity of the disease. An obstructive pattern produces a spirogram with an abnormal shape. Inspiration volume is reduced. The volume of air expelled is normal but the air flow rate is slower, causing an elongated tail to the FVC.

Flow-volume spirogram

A flow-volume loop spirogram is another way of displaying spirometry measurements. This requires the FVC maneuver followed by a forced inspiratory volume (FIV). Flow rate in liters per second is plotted on the y-axis and volume (liters) is plotted on the x-axis. The expiration phase is shown on top and the inspiration phase on the bottom. The flow-volume loop spirogram is helpful in diagnosing upper airway obstruction, and can differentiate some types of restrictive patterns.

Precautions

The patient should inform the physician of any medications he or she is taking, or of any medical

---

KEY TERMS

Bronchodilator—A drug, usually self-administered by inhalation, that dilates the airways.

Forced expiratory volume (FEV)—The volume of air exhaled from the beginning of expiration to a set time (usually 0.5, 1, 2, and 3 seconds).

Forced vital capacity (FVC)—The volume of air that can be exhaled forcibly after a maximal inspiration.

Hemoptysis—Spitting up of blood derived from the lungs or bronchial tubes as a result of pulmonary or bronchial hemorrhage.

Thrombosis—Formation or presence of a thrombus; clotting within a blood vessel that may cause infarction of tissues supplied by the vessel.

Thrombotic—Relating to, caused by, or characterized by thrombosis.

Vital capacity (VC)—The volume of air that can be exhaled following a full inspiration.

---

conditions that are present; these factors may affect the validity of the test. The patient's smoking habits and history should be thoroughly documented. The patient must be able to understand and respond to instructions for the breathing maneuvers. Therefore, the test may not be appropriate for very young, unresponsive, or physically impaired persons.

Spirometry is contraindicated in patients whose condition will be aggravated by forced breathing, including:

- hemoptysis (spitting up blood from the lungs or bronchial tubes)
- pneumothorax (free air or gas in the pleural cavity)
- recent heart attack
- unstable angina
- aneurysm (cranial, thoracic, or abdominal)
- thrombotic condition (such as clotting within a blood vessel)
- recent thoracic or abdominal surgery
- nausea or vomiting

The test should be terminated if the patient shows signs of significant head, chest, or abdominal pain while the procedure is in progress.

Spirometry is dependent upon the patient's full compliance with breathing instructions, especially his or her willingness to extend a maximal effort at forced breathing. Therefore, the patient's emotional state must be considered.

Spirometry is often used to evaluate the efficacy of bronchodilator inhalers such as albuterol. It is important for the patient to refrain from using a bronchodilator prior to the evaluation. Spirometry is performed before and after inhaling the bronchodilator.

Preparation

The patient's age, gender, and race are recorded, and height and weight are measured before the procedure begins. The patient should not have eaten heavily within three hours of the test, and should be instructed to wear clothing that fits loosely over the chest and abdominal area. The respiratory therapist or other testing personnel should explain and demonstrate the breathing maneuvers to the patient. The patient should practice breathing into the mouthpiece until he or she is able to duplicate the maneuvers successfully on two consecutive attempts.

Aftercare

In most cases, special care is not required following spirometry. Occasionally, a patient may become light-headed or dizzy. Such patients should be asked to rest or lie down, and should not be discharged until after the symptoms subside. In rare cases, the patient may experience pneumothorax, intracranial hypertension, chest pain, or uncontrolled coughing. In such cases, additional care directed by a physician may be required.

Results

The results of spirometry tests are compared to predicted values based on the patient's age, gender, and height. For example, a young adult in good health is expected to have the following FEV values:

• FEV-0.5—50%–60% of FVC

• FEV-1—75%–85% of FVC

• FEV-2—95% of FVC

• FEV-3—97% of FVC

In general, a normal result is 80%–100% of the predicted value. Abnormal values are:

• mild lung dysfunction—60%–79%

• moderate lung dysfunction—40%–59%

• severe lung dysfunction—below 40%

For patients using bronchodilator inhalers, a 12% or greater improvement in both FVC and FEV-1, or an increase in FVC by 0.2 liters, is considered a significant improvement for an adult.

QUESTIONS TO ASK YOUR DOCTOR

• What preparation is needed before the test?
• What results are expected?
• When will the results be available?
• What are the risks of the test in this particular case?

Some conditions produce specific signs on the spirogram. Irregular inspirations with rapid frequency are caused by hyperventilation associated with stress. Diffuse fibrosis of the lung causes rapid breathing of reduced volume, which produces a repetitive pattern known as the penmanship sign. Serial reduction in the FVC peaks indicates air trapped inside the lung. A notch and reduced volume in the early segments of the FVC is consistent with airway collapse. A rise at the end of expiration is associated with airway resistance.

Health care team roles

The test can be performed at the bedside, in a physician's office, or in a pulmonary laboratory.

Resources

BOOKS

Bope, E. T. Conn's Current Therapy. Philadelphia: Saunders/Elseier, 2013.

Ferri, Fred, ed. Ferri's Clinical Advisor 2013. Philadelphia: Mosby/Elsevier, 2013.

Goldman, L., and D. Ausiello, eds. Cecil Textbook of Internal Medicine. 24th ed. Philadelphia: Saunders, 2012.

Mason, R. J., et al. Murray & Nadel's Textbook of Respiratory Medicine. 5th ed. Philadelphia: Saunders, 2010.

Rakel, R. Textbook of Family Medicine. 8th ed. Philadelphia: Saunders/Elsevier, 2011.

PERIODICALS

Brunelli, A. "Spirometry: Predicting Risk and Outcome." Liver International 18 (February 1, 2008): 1–8.

Chu, M. W. "Introduction to Pulmonary Function." Otolaryngology Clinics of North America 41 (April 1, 2008): 387–96.

Coates, A. L. "Spirometry in Primary Care." Canadian Respiratory Journal 20, no. 1 (2013): 13–21.

Frith, J. "The Importance of the Assessment of Pulmonary Function in COPD." Medical Clinics of North America 29 (July 1, 2012): 745–52.

WEBSITES

COPD Alliance. "What Is Spirometry?" http://www.copd.org/what-spirometry (accessed July 9, 2013).

ORGANIZATIONS

National Lung Health Education Program, 18000 W. 105th St., Olathe, KS 66061, (913) 895-4631, info@nlhep.org, http://www.nlhep.org.

Robert Harr
Paul Johnson
Mark A. Best

Spleen removal *see* **Splenectomy**

Splenectomy

Definition

A splenectomy is the total or partial surgical removal of the spleen, an organ that is part of the lymphatic system.

Purpose

The human spleen is a dark purple, bean-shaped organ located in the upper left side of the abdomen just behind the bottom of the rib cage. In adults, the spleen is about 4.8 × 2.8 × 1.6 in. (12 × 7 × 4 cm) in size, and weighs about 4–5 oz. (113–141 g). The spleen plays a role in the immune system of the body. It also filters foreign substances from the blood and removes worn-out blood cells. The spleen regulates blood flow to the liver and sometimes stores blood cells—a function known as sequestration. In healthy adults, about 30% of blood platelets are sequestered in the spleen.

Splenectomies are performed for a variety of different reasons and with different degrees of urgency. Most splenectomies are done after a patient has been diagnosed with hypersplenism. Hypersplenism is not a specific disease but a syndrome (group or cluster of symptoms) that may be associated with different disorders. Hypersplenism is characterized by enlargement of the spleen (splenomegaly), defects in the blood cells, and an abnormally high turnover of blood cells. It is almost always associated with such specific disorders as cirrhosis of the liver or certain cancers. The decision to perform a splenectomy depends on the severity and prognosis of the disease that is causing the hypersplenism.

Splenectomy always required

There are two diseases for which a splenectomy is the only treatment—primary cancers of the spleen and a blood disorder called hereditary spherocytosis (HS). In HS, the absence of a specific protein in the red blood cell membrane leads to the formation of relatively fragile cells that are easily damaged when they pass through the spleen. The cell destruction does not occur elsewhere in the body and ends when the spleen is removed. HS can appear at any age, even in newborns, although doctors prefer to put off removing the spleen until the child is five to six years old.

Splenectomy usually required

There are some disorders for which a splenectomy is usually recommended. They include:

- Immune (idiopathic) thrombocytopenic purpura (ITP). ITP is a disease in which platelets are destroyed by antibodies in the body's immune system. A splenectomy is the definitive treatment for this disease and is effective in about 70% of cases of chronic ITP.

- Trauma. The spleen can be ruptured by blunt as well as penetrating injuries to the chest or abdomen. Car accidents are the most common cause of blunt traumatic injury to the spleen.

- Abscesses. Abscesses of the spleen are relatively uncommon but have a high mortality rate.

- Rupture of the splenic artery. This artery sometimes ruptures as a complication of pregnancy.

- Hereditary elliptocytosis. This is a relatively rare disorder. It is similar to HS in that it is characterized by red blood cells with defective membranes that are destroyed by the spleen.

Splenectomy sometimes required

Other disorders may or may not necessitate a splenectomy. These include:

- Hodgkin's disease, a serious form of cancer that causes the lymph nodes to enlarge. A splenectomy is often performed in order to find out how far the disease has progressed.

- Autoimmune hemolytic disorders. These disorders may appear in patients of any age but are most common in adults over 50. The red blood cells are destroyed by antibodies produced by the patient's own body (autoantibodies).

- Myelofibrosis. Myelofibrosis is a disorder in which bone marrow is replaced by fibrous tissue. It produces severe and painful splenomegaly. A splenectomy does not cure myelofibrosis but may be performed to relieve pain caused by the swelling of the spleen.

- Thalassemia. Thalassemia is a hereditary form of anemia that is most common in people of Mediterranean origin. A splenectomy is sometimes performed if the patient's spleen has become painfully enlarged.

Demographics

In the United States, splenomegaly affects as many as 30% of full-term newborns and about 10% of healthy children. Approximately 3% of healthy first-year college

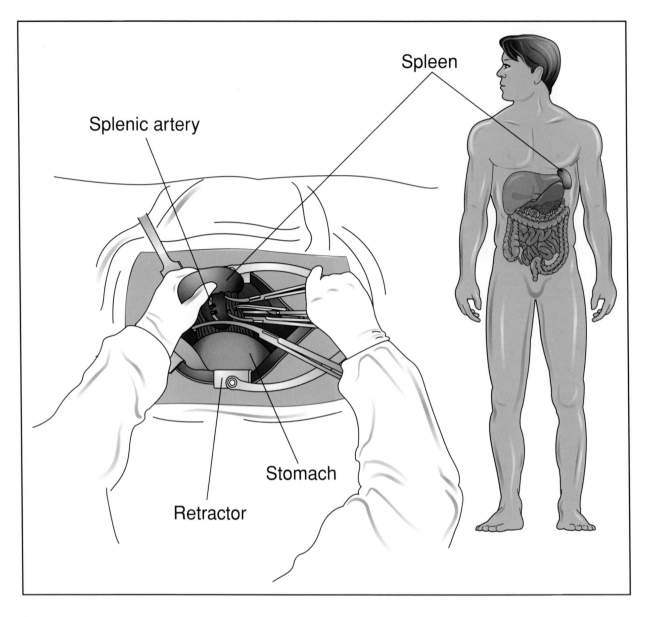

Spleen

Splenic artery

Stomach

Retractor

Splenectomy is the surgical removal of the spleen. This procedure is performed as a last resort in most diseases involving the spleen. *(Illustration by Electronic Illustrators Group. Copyright © Cengage Learning®.)*

students also have spleens that are large enough to be felt when a doctor palpates the abdomen. Some specific causes of splenomegaly are more common in certain racial or ethnic groups. For example, splenomegaly is a common complication of sickle cell disease in patients of African or Mediterranean ancestry. In other parts of the world, splenomegaly is frequently caused by malaria, schistosomiasis, and other infections in areas where these diseases are endemic.

Hereditary spherocytosis (HS) is a disorder that is most common in people of northern European descent but has been found in all races. A family history of HS increases the risk of developing this disorder.

Immune thrombocytopenic purpura (ITP) is much more common in children, with male and female children being equally afflicted. Female predominance begins at puberty and continues in adult patients. Overall, 70% of patients with ITP are female; 72% of women diagnosed with ITP are over 40 years old.

Description

Complete splenectomy

REMOVAL OF ENLARGED SPLEEN. A splenectomy is performed under **general anesthesia**. The most common technique is used to remove greatly enlarged spleens.

KEY TERMS

Computed tomography (CT) scan—An imaging technique that creates a series of pictures of areas inside the body, taken from different angles. The pictures are created by a computer linked to an x-ray machine.

Embolization—A treatment in which foam, silicone, or other substance is injected into a blood vessel in order to close it off.

Endemic—Present in a specific population or geographical area at all times. Some diseases that may affect the spleen are endemic to certain parts of Africa or Asia.

Hereditary spherocytosis—A hereditary disorder that leads to a chronic form of anemia (too few red blood cells) due to an abnormality in the red blood cell membrane.

Idiopathic thrombocytopenia purpura (ITP)—A rare autoimmune disorder characterized by an acute shortage of platelets with resultant bruising and spontaneous bleeding.

Laparoscopy—A procedure in which a laparoscope (a thin, lighted tube) is inserted through an incision in the abdominal wall to evaluate the presence or spread of disease. Tissue samples may be removed for biopsy.

Lymphatic system—The tissues and organs that produce and store cells that fight infection, together with the network of vessels that carry lymph. The organs and tissues in the lymphatic system include the bone marrow, spleen, thymus gland, and lymph nodes.

Palpate—To examine by means of touch.

Platelet—A disk-shaped structure found in blood that binds to fibrinogen at the site of a wound to begin the clotting process.

Sequestration—A process in which the spleen withdraws blood cells from the circulation and stores them.

Spleen—An organ that produces lymphocytes, filters the blood, stores blood cells, and destroys those that are aging. It is located on the left side of the abdomen near the stomach.

Splenomegaly—Enlargement of the spleen.

After the surgeon makes a cut (incision) in the abdomen, the artery to the spleen is tied to prevent blood loss and reduce the size of the spleen. Tying the splenic artery also keeps the spleen from further sequestration of blood cells. The surgeon detaches the ligaments holding the spleen in place and removes the organ. In many cases, tissue samples will be sent to a laboratory for analysis.

REMOVAL OF RUPTURED SPLEEN. When the spleen has been ruptured by trauma, the surgeon approaches the organ from its underside and ties the splenic artery before removing the ruptured organ.

Partial splenectomy

In some cases, the surgeon removes only part of the spleen. This procedure is considered by some to be a useful compromise that reduces pain caused by an enlarged spleen while leaving the patient less vulnerable to infection.

Laparoscopic splenectomy

Laparoscopic splenectomy, or removal of the spleen through several small incisions, has been performed more frequently in recent years. Laparoscopic surgery, which is sometimes called keyhole surgery, is done with smaller surgical instruments inserted through very short incisions, with the assistance of a tiny camera and video monitor. Laparoscopic procedures reduce the **length of hospital stay**, the level of **postoperative pain**, and the risk of infection. They also leave smaller scars. A laparoscopic procedure is contraindicated, however, if the patient's spleen is greatly enlarged. Most **surgeons** will not remove a spleen longer than 20 cm (as measured by a CT scan) by this method.

Diagnosis

The most important part of a medical assessment in disorders of the spleen is the measurement of splenomegaly. The normal spleen cannot be felt when the doctor palpates the patient's abdomen. A spleen that is large enough to be felt indicates splenomegaly. In some cases, the doctor will hear a dull sound when he or she thumps (percusses) the patient's abdomen near the ribs on the left side. Imaging studies that can be used to confirm splenomegaly include **ultrasound** tests, technetium-99m sulfur colloid imaging, and CT scans. The rate of platelet or red blood cell destruction by the spleen can also be measured by tagging blood cells with radioactive chromium or platelets with radioactive indium.

Preparation

Preoperative preparation for a splenectomy procedure usually includes:

• Correction of abnormalities of blood clotting and the number of red blood cells.

• Treatment of any infections.

• Control of immune reactions. Patients are usually given protective vaccinations about a month before surgery. The most common vaccines used are Pneumovax or Pnu-Imune 23 (against pneumococcal infections) and Menomune-A/C/Y/W-135 (against meningococcal infections).

Aftercare

Immediately following surgery, patients are given instructions for **incision care** and medications intended to prevent infection. Blood transfusions may be indicated for some patients to replace defective blood cells. The most important part of aftercare, however, is long-term caution regarding vulnerability to infection. Patients are asked to see their doctor at once if they have a fever or any other sign of infection, and to avoid travel to areas where exposure to malaria or similar diseases is likely. Children with splenectomies may be kept on antibiotic therapy until they are 16 years old. All patients can be given a booster dose of pneumococcal vaccine five to ten years after undergoing a splenectomy.

Risks

The main risk of a splenectomy procedure is overwhelming bacterial infection, or postsplenectomy sepsis. This condition results from the body's decreased ability to clear bacteria from the blood, and lowered levels of a protein in blood plasma that helps to fight viruses (immunoglobulin M). The risk of dying from infection after undergoing a splenectomy is highest in children, especially in the first two years after surgery. The risk of postsplenectomy sepsis can be reduced by vaccinations before the operation. Some doctors also recommend a two-year course of penicillin following splenectomy, or long-term treatment with ampicillin.

Other risks associated with the procedure include inflammation of the pancreas and collapse of the lungs. In some cases, a splenectomy does not address the underlying causes of splenomegaly or other conditions. Excessive bleeding after the operation is an additional possible complication, particularly for patients with ITP. Infection of the incision immediately following surgery may also occur.

Results

Results depend on the reason for the operation. In blood disorders, the splenectomy will remove the cause of the blood cell destruction. Normal results for patients with an enlarged spleen are relief of pain and the complications of splenomegaly. It is not always possible, however, to predict which patients will respond well or to what degree.

Recovery from the operation itself is fairly rapid. Hospitalization is usually less than a week (one to two days for laparoscopic splenectomy), and complete healing usually occurs within four to six weeks. Patients are encouraged to return to such normal activities as showering, driving, climbing stairs, light lifting, and work as soon as they feel comfortable. Some patients may return to work in a few days while others prefer to rest at home a little longer.

Morbidity and mortality rates

The outcome of the procedure varies with the underlying disease or the extent of other injuries. Rates of complete recovery from the surgery itself are excellent, in the absence of other severe injuries or medical problems.

Splenectomy for HS patients is usually delayed in children until the age of five to prevent unnecessary infections; reported outcomes are very good.

Studies of patients with ITP show that 80%–90% of children achieve spontaneous and complete remission in two to eight weeks. A small percentage develop chronic or persistent ITP, but 61% show complete remission by 15 years. No deaths in patients older than 15 have been attributed to ITP.

Alternatives

There are no medical alternatives to removing the spleen.

Splenic embolization is a surgical alternative to splenectomy that is used in some patients who are poor candidates for surgery. Embolization involves plugging or blocking the splenic artery with synthetic substances to shrink the size of the spleen. The substances that are injected during this procedure include polyvinyl alcohol foam, polystyrene, and silicone.

Health care team roles

A splenectomy is performed by a surgeon trained in gastroenterology, the branch of medicine that deals with the diseases of the digestive tract. An anesthesiologist is responsible for administering anesthesia and the operation is performed in a hospital setting.

Resources

BOOKS

Gabrielson, Curt. *Surgical Diseases of the Spleen*. New York: Springer, 2012.
O'Malley, Dennis P. *Atlas of Spleen Pathology*. New York: Springer, 2013.

PERIODICALS

Jankulovski, N., et al. "Laparoscopic versus Open Splenectomy: A Single Center Eleven-Year Experience." *Acta Clinica Croatica* 52, no. 2 (2013): 229–34. http://dx.doi.org/10.1111/hepr.12234 (accessed October 4, 2013).
Nomura, Yoriko, et al. "Influence of Splenectomy in Patients with Liver Cirrhosis and Hypersplenism." *Hepatology Research* (September 3, 2013): e-pub ahead of print. http://dx.doi.org/10.1111/hepr.12234 (accessed October 4, 2013).
Wang, Xin, et al. "Laparoscopic Splenectomy: A Surgeon's Experience of 302 Patients with Analysis of Postoperative Complications." *Surgical Endoscopy* 27, no. 10 (2013): 3564–71. http://dx.doi.org/10.1007/s00464-013-2978-4 (accessed October 4, 2013).

WEBSITES

A.D.A.M. Medical Encyclopedia. "Spleen Removal." Medline Plus. http://www.nlm.nih.gov/medlineplus/ency/article/002944.htm (accessed October 4, 2013).
American Academy of Family Physicians. "Splenectomy." FamilyDoctor.org. http://familydoctor.org/familydoctor/en/drugs-procedures-devices/procedures-devices/splenectomy.html (accessed October 4, 2013).
Platelet Disorder Support Association. "Splenectomy." http://www.pdsa.org/treatments/conventional/splenectomy.html (accessed October 4, 2013).

ORGANIZATIONS

American College of Gastroenterology, 6400 Goldsboro Rd., Ste. 200, Bethesda, MD 20817, (301) 263-9000, info@acg.gi.org, http://gi.org.
American Gastroenterological Association, 4930 Del Ray Ave., Bethesda, MD 20814, (301) 654-2055, Fax: (301) 654-5920, member@gastro.org, http://www.gastro.org.
National Cancer Institute, 6116 Executive Blvd., Ste. 300, Bethesda, MD 20892-8322, (800) 4-CANCER (422-6237), http://cancer.gov.

Teresa Norris, RN
Monique Laberge, PhD

Stapedectomy

Definition

Stapedectomy is a surgical procedure in which the innermost bone (stapes) of the three bones (the stapes, the incus, and the malleus) of the middle ear is removed, and replaced with a small plastic tube surrounding a short length of stainless-steel wire (a prosthesis). The operation was first performed in the United States in 1956.

Purpose

A stapedectomy is performed to improve the movement of sound to the inner ear. It is done to treat progressive hearing loss caused by otosclerosis, a condition in which spongy bone hardens around the base of the stapes. This condition fixes the stapes to the opening of the inner ear, so that the stapes no longer vibrates properly. Otosclerosis can also affect the malleus, the incus, and the bone that surrounds the inner ear. As a result, the transmission of sound to the inner ear is disrupted. Untreated otosclerosis eventually results in total deafness, usually in both ears.

Demographics

Otosclerosis affects about 10% of the U.S. population. It is an autosomal dominant disorder with variable penetrance. These terms mean that a child having one parent with otosclerosis has a 50% chance of inheriting the gene for the disorder, but that not everyone who has the gene will develop otosclerosis. In addition, some researchers think that the onset of the disorder is triggered when a person who has the gene for otosclerosis is infected with the measles virus. This hypothesis is supported by the finding that the incidence of otosclerosis has been steadily declining in countries with widespread measles vaccination.

Otosclerosis develops most frequently in people between the ages of 10 and 30. In most cases, both ears are affected; however, about 10%–15% of patients diagnosed with otosclerosis have loss of hearing in only one ear. The disorder affects women more frequently than men by a ratio of two to one. Pregnancy is a risk factor for onset or worsening of otosclerosis.

With regard to race, Caucasian and Asian Americans are more likely to develop otosclerosis than African Americans.

Description

A stapedectomy does not require any incisions on the outside of the body, as the entire procedure is performed through the ear canal. With the patient under local or **general anesthesia**, the surgeon opens the ear canal and folds the eardrum forward. Using an operating microscope, the surgeon is able to see the structures in detail, and evaluates the bones of hearing (ossicles) to confirm the diagnosis of otosclerosis.

Next, the surgeon separates the stapes from the incus; freed from the stapes, the incus and malleus bones can now move when pressed. A laser or small drill may be used to cut through the tendon and arch of the stapes bone, which is then removed from the middle ear.

The surgeon then opens the window that joins the middle ear to the inner ear and acts as the platform for the stapes bone. The surgeon directs the laser's beam at the window to make a tiny opening, and gently clips the prosthesis to the incus bone. A piece of tissue is taken from a small incision behind the ear lobe and used to help seal the hole in the window and around the prosthesis. The eardrum is then gently replaced and repaired, and held there by absorbable packing ointment or a gelatin sponge. The procedure usually takes about an hour and a half.

Good candidates for the surgery are those who have a fixed stapes from otosclerosis and a conductive hearing loss of at least 20 dB. Patients with a severe hearing loss might still benefit from a stapedectomy, if only to improve their hearing to the point where a hearing aid can be of help. The procedure can improve hearing in more than 90% of cases.

Diagnosis

Diagnosis of otosclerosis is based on a combination of the patient's family history, the patient's symptoms, and the results of hearing tests. Some patients notice only a gradual loss of hearing, but others experience dizziness, tinnitus (a sensation of buzzing, ringing, or hissing in the ears), or balance problems. The hearing tests should be administered by an ear specialist (audiologist or otologist) rather than the patient's family doctor. The examiner will need to determine whether the patient's hearing loss is conductive (caused by a lesion or disorder in the ear canal or middle ear) or sensorineural (caused by a disorder of the inner ear or the eighth cranial nerve).

Two tests that are commonly used to distinguish conductive hearing loss from sensorineural are Rinne's test and Weber's test. In Rinne's test, the examiner holds the stem of a vibrating tuning fork first against the mastoid bone and then outside the ear canal. A person with normal hearing will hear the sound as louder when it is held near the outer ear; a person with conductive hearing loss will hear the tone as louder when the fork is touching the bone.

In Weber's test, the vibrating tuning fork is held on the midline of the forehead and the patient is asked to indicate the ear in which the sound seems louder. A person with conductive hearing loss on one side will hear the sound louder in the affected ear.

A **computed tomography** (CT) scan or x-ray study of the head may also be done to determine whether the patient's hearing loss is conductive or sensorineural.

Preparation

Patients are asked to notify the surgeon if they develop a cold or sore throat within a week of the scheduled surgery. The procedure should be postponed in order to minimize the risk of infection being carried from the upper respiratory tract to the ear.

Some **surgeons** prefer to use general anesthesia when performing a stapedectomy, although an increasing number are using **local anesthesia**. A sedative injection is given to the patient before surgery.

Aftercare

The patient is asked to have a friend or relative drive them home after the procedure. **Antibiotics** are given up to five days after surgery to prevent infection; packing and sutures are removed about a week after surgery.

It is important that the patient not put pressure on the ear for a few days after surgery. Blowing the nose, lifting heavy objects, swimming underwater, descending rapidly in high-rise elevators, or taking an airplane flight should be avoided.

Right after surgery, the ear is usually quite sensitive, so the patient should avoid loud noises until the ear retrains itself to hear sounds properly.

It is extremely important that the patient avoid getting the ear wet until it has completely healed. Water in the ear could cause an infection; most seriously, water could enter the middle ear and cause an infection within the inner ear, which could then lead to a complete hearing loss. When taking a shower, and washing the hair, the patient should plug the ear with a cotton ball or lamb's wool ball soaked in Vaseline. The surgeon should give specific instructions about when and how this can be done.

Usually, the patient may return to work and normal activities about a week after leaving the hospital, although if the patient's job involves heavy lifting, three weeks of home rest is recommend. Three days after surgery, the patient may fly in pressurized aircraft.

Risks

The most serious risk is an increased hearing loss, which occurs in about 1% of patients. Because of this risk, a stapedectomy is usually performed on only one ear at a time.

Less common complications include:

- temporary change in taste (due to nerve damage) or lack of taste
- perforated eardrum
- vertigo that may persist and require surgery
- damage to the chain of three small bones attached to the eardrum
- partial facial nerve paralysis
- ringing in the ears

Severe dizziness or vertigo may be a signal that there has been an incomplete seal between the fluids of the middle and inner ear. If this is the case, the patient needs immediate bed rest, an examination by the ear surgeon, and (rarely) an operation to reopen the eardrum to check the prosthesis.

Results

Most patients are slightly dizzy for the first day or two after surgery, and may have a slight headache. Hearing improves once the swelling subsides, the slight bleeding behind the ear drum dries up, and the packing is absorbed or removed, usually within two weeks. Hearing continues to get better over the next three months.

About 90% of patients will have markedly improved hearing following the procedure, while 8% experience only minor improvement. About half the patients who had tinnitus before surgery will experience significant relief within six weeks after the procedure.

Morbidity and mortality rates

Stapedectomy is a very safe procedure with a relatively low rate of complications. With regard to hearing, about 2% of patients may have additional hearing loss in the operated ear following a stapedectomy; fewer than 1% lose hearing completely in the operated ear. About 9% of patients experience disturbances in their sense of taste. Infection, damage to the eardrum, and facial nerve palsy are rare complications that occur in fewer than 0.1% of patients.

Alternatives

Alternatives to a stapedectomy include:

- Watchful waiting. Some patients with only a mild degree of hearing loss may prefer to postpone surgery.

QUESTIONS TO ASK YOUR DOCTOR

- What is your opinion of medication treatments for otosclerosis?
- Am I a candidate for a stapedotomy without prosthesis?
- What are the chances of my hearing getting worse if I postpone surgery?
- How many stapedectomies have you performed?
- What are the possible complications I could expect following a stapedectomy?

- Medications. Although there is no drug that can cure otosclerosis, some compounds containing fluoride or calcium are reported to be effective in preventing further hearing loss by slowing down abnormal bone growth. The medication most commonly recommended for this purpose is a combination of sodium fluoride and calcium carbonate sold under the trade name Florical. The medication is taken twice a day over a two-year period, after which the patient's hearing is reevaluated. Florical should not be used during pregnancy, however.

- Hearing aids.

- Stapedotomy. A stapedotomy is a surgical procedure similar to a stapedectomy except that the surgeon uses the laser to cut a hole in the stapes in order to insert the prosthesis rather than removing the stapes. In addition, some ear surgeons use the laser to free the stapes bone without inserting a prosthesis. This variation, however, works best in patients with only mild otosclerosis.

Health care team roles

Stapedectomies are usually done by otologists or otolaryngologists, who are surgeons with advanced training in treating ear disorders. A stapedectomy is usually performed as an outpatient procedure in an ambulatory surgery facility or same-day surgery clinic.

Resources

PERIODICALS

Hsu, Griffith S. "Improving Hearing in Stapedectomy with Intraoperative Auditory Brainstem Response." *Otolaryngology—Head and Neck Surgery* 144, no. 1 (2011): 60–63. http://dx.doi.org/10.1177/0194599810390895 (accessed October 4, 2013).

Neilan, Ryan E., et al. "Pediatric Stapedectomy: Does Cause of Fixation Affect Outcomes?" *International Journal of Pediatric Otorhinolaryngology* 77, no. 1 (2013):

1099–102. http://dx.doi.org/10.1016/j.ijporl.2013.04.009 (accessed October 4, 2013).

Stucken, Emily Z., Kevin D. Brown, and Samuel H. Selesnick. "The Use of KTP Laser in Revision Stapedectomy." *Otology & Neurotology* 33, no. 8 (2012): 1297–99. http://dx.doi.org/10.1097/MAO.0b013e3182634e45 (accessed October 4, 2013).

WEBSITES

Ear Surgery Information Center. "Stapedectomy." http://www.earsurgery.org/site/pages/surgery/stapedectomy.php (accessed October 4, 2013).

National Institute on Deafness and Other Communication Disorders. "Otosclerosis." http://www.nidcd.nih.gov/health/hearing/Pages/otosclerosis.aspx (accessed October 4, 2013).

University of Wisconsin-Madison, School of Medicine and Public Health. "Your Care at Home after Stapedectomy." http://www.uwhealth.org/healthfacts/B_EXTRANET_HEALTH_INFORMATION-FlexMember-Show_Public_HFFY_1126664718742.html (accessed October 4, 2013).

ORGANIZATIONS

American Academy of Audiology, 11480 Commerce Park Dr., Ste. 220, Reston, VA 20191, (800) AAA-2336 (222-2336), infoaud@audiology.org, http://www.audiology.org.

American Academy of Otolaryngology—Head and Neck Surgery, 1650 Diagonal Rd., Alexandria, VA 22314-2857, (703) 836-4444, http://www.entnet.org.

Better Hearing Institute, 1444 I St. NW, Ste. 700, Washington, DC 20005, (202) 449-1100, Fax: (202) 216-9646, mail@betterhearing.org, http://betterhearing.org.

National Institute on Deafness and Other Communication Disorders (NIDCD), NIDCD Office of Health Communication and Public Liaison, 31 Center Dr., MSC 2320, Bethesda, MD 20892-2320, (301) 496-7243, (800) 241-1044, (800) 241-1055, nidcdinfo@nidcd.nih.gov, http://www.nidcd.nih.gov.

Carol A. Turkington
Rebecca J. Frey, PhD

Staples *see* **Closures**

STD tests *see* **Sexually transmitted disease cultures**

Stem cell transplantation

Definition

Stem cells are cells that can continuously reproduce themselves and produce other, more specialized cell types of differentiated cells. A stem cell transplant is a procedure that replaces unhealthy stem cells with healthy ones. Stem cells can be harvested from bone marrow, from peripheral blood, and from umbilical cord blood.

Purpose

Physicians use stem cell transplants to treat many diseases that damage or destroy bone marrow, found in the soft fatty tissue inside the bones. Examples of these diseases are leukemia and multiple myeloma. Some patients develop bone marrow disorders because of aggressive cancer treatments or as result of diseases such as aplastic anemia, which causes abnormal blood cell production.

Recent advances in stem cell research have made it a treatment possibility for patients with certain types of lymphomas, genetic disorders, hereditary metabolic disorders, and autoimmune disorders. These stem cells are typically not bone marrow stem cells but other types of stem cells. Researchers are hoping eventually to harvest stem cells to treat diseases such as Parkinson's disease, type 1 diabetes, Alzheimer's disease, liver disease, arthritis, and spinal cord injuries.

Demographics

The number of stem cell transplants performed continues to increase. It is estimated that between 30,000 to 40,000 transplantations are performed on an annual basis worldwide and this number is increasing by up to 20% yearly.

Description

Stem cell transplants sometimes are called hematopoietic stem cell transplants, bone marrow transplants, or cord blood transplants. Nearly 100 years ago, physicians tried to give patients with leukemia and anemia bone marrow by mouth. These treatments were not successful, but led to experiments showing healthy bone marrow transfused into the blood stream could restore damaged bone marrow.

Today, two types of stem cell transplants are performed most often. When a patient's own stem cells are collected (harvested) then returned to the same patient's body, it is called an autologous transplant. Using stem cells from another person, or a donor, is called allogenic transplant. A third type, which is rare, is called a syngeneic transplant, in which the donor is an identical twin. In many cases, donor cells come from a close relative, such as a brother or sister. However, the likelihood that a sibling will match the patient is 25%. Stem cells may need to come from a person not related to the recipient.

To find out if a patient can receive stem cells from a donor, physicians developed human leukocyte antigen

(HLA) testing to match tissue types. The next challenge became finding donors. Throughout the 1980s and 1990s, private individuals, hospitals, foundations, and states worked to set up a nationwide registry of bone marrow donors. The National Marrow Donor Program (NMDP) now has the largest stem cell donor registry in the world. At present, there are more than three million donors registered through the NMDP. However, ethnic minorities represent only a small percentage of the donors to the NMDP, often making it more difficult to provide a donor to a member of an ethnic minority requiring a stem cell transplant.

Stem cell transplants normally take place at specialized centers. Procurement of stem cells from the donor can be accomplished in several ways: from the bone marrow, the peripheral blood, and less commonly, from umbilical cord blood.

Donor cells harvested directly from the bone marrow are taken in an **operating room** while the patient (or the donor) is under regional or **general anesthesia**. Bone marrow normally is harvested from the top of the hip bone. The marrow usually is filtered, treated, and either transplanted immediately or frozen for later use.

Stem cells can also be harvested from a donor's peripheral blood during apheresis once a process called stem cell mobilization has occurred. Hematopoietic stem cells are typically found in low concentrations in the circulating peripheral blood. Stem cells can be mobilized to enter the peripheral blood by administering the hematopoietic growth factor, granulocyte colony-stimulating factor (G-CSF) (filgrastim or lenograstim) to the donor. After about four days, enough stem cells are available in the circulating peripheral blood to be harvested. During a three- to four-hour apheresis collection process, more stem cells can typically be collected than during a bone marrow harvest without the need for general anesthesia and an operating room setting.

Bone marrow transplantation is considered superior to peripheral blood stem cell transplant (PBSCT) for most nonmalignant conditions. Peripheral blood stem cell transplant is considered superior to bone marrow transplant when rapid engraftment of stem cells is needed. PBSCT is also associated with early hospital discharges, decreased relapse rates, and decreased mortality rates. However, PBSCT is associated with increased incidence of graft-versus-host disease (GVHD), a post-transplant complication.

Stem cells are transfused through an intravenous (IV) catheter that physicians insert in the patient's neck or chest. The procedure is usually done in the patient's hospital room. This part of the transplant process is referred to as the "rescue process." The stem cells replace

KEY TERMS

Catheter—A medical device shaped like a tube that physicians can insert into vessels, canals, or passageways to more easily inject or withdraw fluids.

Embryo—A developing human from the time of conception to the end of the eighth week after conception.

Engraftment—The process of transplanted stem cells reproducing new cells.

malignant or defective cells. Transplanted donor cells travel to the bone cavities and begin replacing old bone marrow.

Precautions

The transplant team will weigh many factors when determining if a patient is a candidate for stem cell transplantation, including overall health and function of many vital organ systems. Stem cell transplantation is an aggressive treatment and may not be recommended for some patients, including those with heart, kidney, or lung disorders. If the patient has an aggressive cancer that has spread throughout the body, he or she may not be considered a candidate for a stem cell transplant. It once was thought that stem cell transplants were not safe in patients over age 60, but research shows that some elderly patients can safely receive stem cells from donors.

Many ethical and legal factors are impacting the research and development into stem cell transplantation. Much debate surrounds scientific advances. For example, human embryos, fetal tissues and umbilical cords are sources of stem cells that may be transplanted or used for disease research. Some people have ethical problems with the use of embryos in fertility clinics for stem cell research or transplantation. Some link stem cell transplantation for disease with cloning and want to stop funding for stem cell research over fear of human cloning. A study released in 2005 stated that 63% of Americans back embryonic stem cell research and 70% support federal legislation to promote more research. Meanwhile, scientists continue to develop new and exciting possibilities for transplanting stem cells into the human body that may one day lead to new treatments for previously incurable diseases. Many do so with private funding. However, the most common type of stem cell transplant, with bone marrow, is not controversial.

Preparation

Standard preparation involves eliminating diseased and damaged cells. The exact process depends on the patient and the disease or condition being treated. In many cases when transplantation is done to treat cancer, the patient will receive chemotherapy, often in extremely high doses. Some also receive radiation therapy. Another goal of preparation is to suppress the immune system. This makes it less likely that the patient's body will reject the donated stem cells. This step is called the conditioning regimen and is considered a crucial element in stem cell transplantation. New advances have been made that allow some of the patient's diseased cells to remain and mix with the new cells. Immediately before transplantation, the treating physician and staff will give the patient special instructions and precautions, depending on his or her disease and exact procedure. Many serious side effects are associated with the preparative regimens including nausea, vomiting, hair loss (alopecia), diarrhea, skin rashes, mouth sores, and ulcers, as well as lung, liver, and neurological toxicities. Another serious result of the conditioning regimen is infertility. Sperm banking may be an option for some men. Preservation of female fertility by banking of oocytes (eggs) has not been as successful.

Aftercare

Stem cells take up to three weeks or longer to begin producing new cells or bone marrow, a process called engraftment. Until engraftment is complete, patients may bleed easily and are at high risk for the development of life-threatening infections. To reduce the risk for infection, patients are hospitalized in high-efficiency particulate air (HEPA) filtered rooms that are sealed using positive air pressure. All individuals entering the room should practice strict hand hygiene to minimize the potential for spread of infection. Patients may be required to stay in the hospital for at least one week following transplantation until blood cell counts reach a safe level. Patients who received autologous transplants can often be managed on an outpatient basis. Once home, patients must be closely monitored, must be careful not to risk infection, may be anemic, and may be extremely fatigued. Most patients will receive prophylactic antibiotic and antifungal therapy for 75–100 days after the transplant and will be monitored very closely for the occurrence of graft-versus-host disease and other transplant-related side effects.

Risks

In addition to the risk of a life-threatening infection following a stem cell transplant, patients receiving stem cells from donors risk serious complications from graft-versus-host disease (GVHD). GVHD is caused when the donor's cells react against the patient's (recipient's) tissue. Sometimes, the patient's body simply rejects the new cells. Researchers continue to explore ways to lessen risks of complications following stem cell transplants.

Resources

BOOKS

Rowley, S. D., and H. Benn. "Collection and Processing of Peripheral Blood Stem Cells and Bone Marrow." In *Blood Banking and Transfusion Medicine*, 2nd ed. Edited by C. D. Hillyer, L. E. Silberstein, and P. M. Ness. Philadelphia: Churchill Livingstone/Elsevier, 2007.

PERIODICALS

Copelan, E. A. "Hematopoietic Stem-Cell Transplantation." *New England Journal of Medicine* 354, no. 17 (2006): 1813–26.

Doubek, M., et al. "Autologous Hematopoietic Stem Cell Transplantation in Adult Acute Lymphoblastic Leukemia: Still Not Out of Fashion." *Annnals of Hematology* 88, no. 9 (2009): 881–7.

Lubin, B. H., and W. T. Shearer. "Cord Blood Banking for Potential Future Transplantation." *Pediatrics* 119, no. 1 (2007): 165–70.

WEBSITES

American Cancer Society. "Stem Cell Transplant (Peripheral Blood, Bone Marrow, and Cord Blood Transplants)." http://www.cancer.org/treatment/treatmentsandsideeffects/treatmenttypes/bonemarrowandperipheralbloodstemcelltransplant/bone-marrow-and-peripheral-blood-stem-cell-transplant-toc (accessed October 21, 2013).

Multiple Myeloma Research Foundation. "Treatment Options—Stem Cell Transplantation." http://www.themmrf.org/living-with-multiple-myeloma/patients-starting-treatment/treatment-options/stem-cell-transplantation.html (accessed October 21, 2013).

National Heart, Lung, and Blood Institute. "What Is a Blood and Marrow Stem Cell Transplant?" http://www.nhlbi.nih.gov/health/health-topics/topics/bmsct (accessed October 21, 2013).

National Institutes of Health. "Stem Cell Basics." http://stemcells.nih.gov/info/basics/Pages/Default.aspx (accessed October 21, 2013).

ORGANIZATIONS

International Myeloma Foundation (IMF), 12650 Riverside Dr., Ste. 206, North Hollywood, CA 91607–3421, (800) 452-CURE, http://www.myeloma.org.

National Marrow Donor Program (NMDP), 3001 Broadway St. NE, Ste. 100, Minneapolis, MN 55413–1753, (800) 627-7692, http://www.marrow.org.

Teresa G. Odle
Melinda Granger Oberleitner, RN, DNS, APRN, CNS

Stents, biliary *see* **Biliary stenting**

Stents, coronary *see* **Coronary stenting**

Stents, ureteral *see* **Ureteral stenting**

▌Stereotactic radiosurgery

Definition

Stereotactic radiosurgery uses 3-D computerized imaging to precisely target a narrow x-ray beam and deliver a highly concentrated dose of radiation to an affected area. It does not require an incision, and **general anesthesia** is not often required for adults undergoing treatment.

Purpose

Stereotactic radiosurgery is used to treat brain tumors, arteriovenous malformations and arteriovenous fistulas in the brain, and in some cases, trigeminal neuralgia, benign eye tumors, or other disorders within the brain.

Description

"Radiosurgery" refers to the use of a high-energy beam of radiation. "Stereotactic" refers to the three-

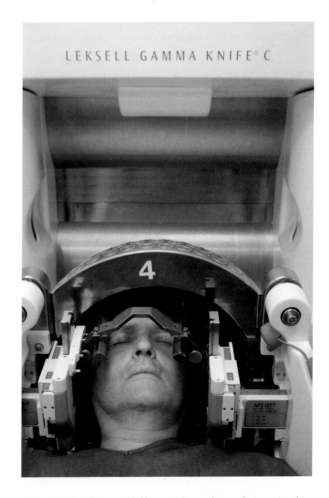

Patient in the Gamma Knife machine, a form of stereotactic radiosurgery that treats small tumors and similar abnormalities. *(UIG via Getty Images)*

dimensional targeting system used to deliver the beam to the precise location desired. Stereotactic radiosurgery delivers concentrated radiation to malformed vessels, causing the abnormal vessels to close off. It is primarily confined to the head and neck, because the patient must be kept completely still during the delivery of the radiation in order to prevent damage to surrounding tissue. The motion of the patient's head and neck are restricted by a stereotactic frame that holds them in place. The stereotactic frame is attached to the patient's head with pins. **Computed tomography** (CT or CAT scan) or **magnetic resonance imaging** (MRI) may then be used to determine the precise location of the tumor within the brain. It is difficult to immobilize other body regions in this way.

The high energy of the radiation beam disrupts the DNA of the targeted cells, killing them. Multiple weak beams are focused on the target area, delivering maximum energy to it while keeping surrounding tissue safe. Since the radiation passes through the skull to its target, there is no need to cut open the skull to perform the surgery. The beam can be focused on any structure in the brain, allowing access to tumors or malformed blood vessels that cannot be reached by open-skull surgery.

Two major forms of stereotactic radiosurgery are used in treating disorders. The Gamma Knife® is a stationary machine that is most useful for small tumors, blood vessels, or similar targets. Because it does not move, it can deliver a small, highly localized, and precise beam of radiation. Gamma Knife treatment is done all at once in a single hospital stay. The second type of radiosurgery uses a movable linear accelerator-based (LINAC) machine that is preferred for larger tumors up to 3.5 centimeters in diameter. This treatment is delivered in several small doses given over several weeks. Radiosurgery that is performed with divided doses is known as fractionated radiosurgery. The total dose of radiation is higher with a linear accelerator-based machine than with Gamma Knife treatment. There are multiple manufacturers that make this type of machine.

Disorders treated by stereotactic radiosurgery include:

- benign brain tumors, including acoustic neuromas and meningiomas
- malignant brain tumors, including gliomas and astrocytomas
- metastatic brain tumors
- trigeminal neuralgia
- Parkinson's disease
- essential tremor
- arteriovenous fistula
- arteriovenous malformations
- pituitary tumors

KEY TERMS

Angiography—A technique for the diagnostic imaging of blood vessels that involves the injection of contrast material.

Arteriovenous fistula—Arteriovenous fistula (AVF) is an abnormal channel or passage between an artery and a vein that results in a disruption of normal blood flow patterns. It can be acquired or congenital.

Arteriovenous malformation—Arteriovenous malformation (AVM) is a web or tangle of abnormal and poorly formed blood vessels including arteries and veins. The blood vessels have a higher rate of bleeding than normal blood vessels.

Fractionated radiosurgery—Radiosurgery in which the radiation is delivered in several smaller doses over a period of time rather than the full amount in a single treatment.

Metastatic—Referring to the spread of cancer from one organ in the body to another not directly connected to it.

Radiosurgery—Surgery that uses ionizing radiation to destroy tissue rather than a surgical incision.

Simulation scan—The process of making a mask for the patient and other images in order to plan the radiation treatment.

Stereotactic—Characterized by precise positioning in space. When applied to radiosurgery, stereotactic refers to a system of three-dimensional coordinates for locating the target site.

Preparation

A patient requiring radiosurgery will undergo neuroimaging studies to determine the precise location of the target area in the brain. These studies may include CT scans, MRI scans, and others. Imaging of the blood vessels (**angiography**) or the brain's ventricles (ventriculography) may be done as well. These require the injection of either a harmless radioactive substance or a contrast dye.

Prior to the procedure, the patient will be fitted with a stereotactic frame or rigid mask to immobilize the head. This part of the treatment may be uncomfortable. The patient may receive a simulation scan to establish the precise relationship of the mask or frame to the head to help plan the treatment.

The patient may be given a sedative and an antinausea agent prior to the simulation scan or treatment.

Aftercare

Stereotactic radiosurgery does not produce some of the side effects commonly associated with radiation treatment, such as reddening of the skin or hair loss. **Bandages** are placed over the pin sites from the stereotactic frame. Some swelling may occur around the insertion sites for the pins. Most patients can return to their usual daily activities following treatment without any special precautions.

Risks

The risks of stereotactic radiosurgery include mild headache, tiredness, nausea and vomiting, and recurrence of the tumor. Minimum bleeding around the pin sites may also occur.

Results

Stereotactic radiosurgery does not cause pain, and because the skull is not opened, there is no long hospital stay or risk of infection. Recovery is very rapid; most patients go home the same day they are treated, although follow-up imaging and retreatment may be necessary in some cases. This form of surgery appears to be quite successful in extending the length of survival in cancer patients. One study found that Gamma Knife radiosurgery controlled tumor growth in 96% of patients with kidney cancer that had spread to the brain, and added an average of 15 months to the patients' survival.

Morbidity and mortality rates

Stereotactic radiosurgery has a low reported rate of serious complications with minimal mortality. One German study reported a 4.8% rate of temporary morbidity in patients under treatment for brain tumors, with no permanent morbidity and no mortality. An American group of researchers found that less than 2% of patients who had eye tumors treated with radiosurgery suffered damage to the optic nerve from the dose of radiation.

Mild side effects following Gamma Knife radiosurgery are not uncommon, however.

Alternatives

With certain types of brain tumors, whole-brain radiation treatment (WBRT) is an option; however, it has a number of severe side effects. Surgical removal of the tumor is another option, but it carries a higher risk of tumor recurrence.

Health care team roles

Stereotactic radiosurgery is performed by a radiosurgeon, who is a neurosurgeon with advanced training

---

> ### QUESTIONS TO ASK YOUR DOCTOR
>
> - What are the alternatives, if any, to radiosurgery for my specific condition?
> - How many radiosurgical procedures have you performed?
> - What is your success rate?
> - What side effects have your patients reported?

in the use of a Gamma Knife or linear accelerator-based machine. The radiosurgeon's dose plan is checked by a physicist before the treatment is administered to the patient. Stereotactic radiosurgery is done in a hospital that has the necessary specialized equipment.

Resources

BOOKS

Benedict, Stanley, Brian D. Kavanagh, and David J. Schlesinger. *Stereotactic Radiosurgery and Radiotherapy.* Boca Raton, FL: CRC Press, 2014.

Lo, Simon S., et al., eds. *Stereotactic Body Radiation Therapy.* Berlin; New York: Springer, 2012.

PERIODICALS

Friedman, W. A. "Expanding Indications for Stereotactic Radiosurgery in the Treatment of Brain Metastases." *Neurosurgery* 60, suppl. 1 (2013): 9–12. http://dx.doi.org/10.1227/01.neu.0000430329.25516.94 (accessed September 8, 2013).

Jung, Edward, et al. "Gamma Knife Radiosurgery in the Management of Brainstem Metastases." *Clinical Neurology and Neurosurgery* (July 18, 2013): e-pub ahead of print. http://dx.doi.org/10.1016/j.clineuro.2013.06.012 (accessed September 8, 2013).

Lippitz, Bodo, et al. "Stereotactic Radiosurgery in the Treatment of Brain Metastases: The Current Evidence." *Cancer Treatment Reviews* (June 28, 2013): e-pub ahead of print. http://dx.doi.org/10.1016/j.ctrv.2013.05.002 (accessed September 8, 2013).

Luther, Neal, et al. "Motor Function after Stereotactic Radiosurgery for Brain Metastases in the Region of the Motor Cortex." *Journal of Neurosurgery* (July 10, 2013): e-pub ahead of print. http://dx.doi.org/10.3171/2013.6.JNS122081 (accessed September 8, 2013).

Pannullo, Susan C., et al. "Stereotactic Radiosurgery: A Meta-Analysis of Current Therapeutic Applications in Neuro-Oncologic Disease." *Journal of Neuro-Oncology* 103, no. 1 (2011): 1–17. http://dx.doi.org/10.1007/s11060-010-0360-0 (accessed September 8, 2013).

Régis, J., et al. "Seeking New Paradigms in Epilepsy: Stereotactic Radiosurgery." *World Neurosurgery* (July 19, 2013): e-pub ahead of print. http://dx.doi.org/10.1016/j.wneu.2013.07.004 (accessed September 8, 2013).

WEBSITES

A.D.A.M. Medical Encyclopedia. "Stereotactic Radiosurgery." MedlinePlus. http://www.nlm.nih.gov/medlineplus/ency/article/007274.htm (accessed July 25, 2013).

A.D.A.M. Medical Encyclopedia. "Stereotactic Radiosurgery—CyberKnife." PubMed Health. http://www.ncbi.nlm.nih.gov/pubmedhealth/PMH0004533 (accessed July 25, 2013).

American Association of Neurological Surgeons. "Stereotactic Radiosurgery." http://www.aans.org/Patient%20Information/Conditions%20and%20Treatments/Stereotactic%20Radiosurgery.aspx (accessed September 5, 2013).

Chabner, Bruce A., and Elizabeth Chabner Thompson. "Modalities of Cancer Therapy." *The Merck Manual for Health Care Professionals* (online). http://www.merckmanuals.com/professional/hematology_and_oncology/principles_of_cancer_therapy/modalities_of_cancer_therapy.html (accessed September 8, 2013).

National Cancer Institute. "Adult Brain Tumors Treatment (PDQ®)." PubMed Health. http://www.ncbi.nlm.nih.gov/pubmedhealth/PMH0032635 (accessed September 8, 2013).

Stanford Medicine Cancer Institute. "Stereotactic Radiotherapy/Radiosurgery." http://cancer.stanford.edu/patient_care/services/radiationTherapy/stereotacticRadiother.html (accessed September 8, 2013).

ORGANIZATIONS

International Radiosurgery Support Association (IRSA), PO Box 5186, Harrisburg, PA 17110, (717) 260-9808, http://www.irsa.org.

National Cancer Institute, 6116 Executive Blvd., Ste. 300, Bethesda, MD 20892-8322, (800) 4-CANCER (422-6237), http://cancer.gov.

Richard Robinson
Tammy Allhoff, CST/CSFA, AAS

Sterilization, female *see* **Tubal ligation**

Sterilization, male *see* **Vasectomy**

Stethoscope

Definition

The stethoscope is an instrument used for auscultation, or listening to sounds produced by the body. It is used primarily to listen to the lungs, heart, and intestinal tract. It is also used to listen to blood flow in peripheral vessels and the heart sounds of developing fetuses in pregnant women.

Purpose

A stethoscope is used to detect and study heart, lung, stomach, and other sounds in humans and animals. Using

---

KEY TERMS

Atrioventricular—Referring to the valves regulating blood flow from the upper chambers of the heart (atria) to the lower chambers (ventricles). There are two such valves, one connecting the right atrium and ventricle and one connecting the left atrium and ventricle.

Auscultation—The act of listening to sounds produced by the body.

Bell—The cup-shaped portion of the head of a stethoscope, useful for detecting low-pitched sounds.

Borborygmi—Sounds created by the passage of food, gas, or fecal material in the stomach or intestines.

Diaphragm—The flat-shaped portion of the head of a stethoscope, useful for detecting high-pitched sounds.

Murmur—The sound made as blood moves through the heart when there is turbulence in the flow of blood through a blood vessel, or if a valve does not completely close.

---

a stethoscope, the listener can hear normal and abnormal respiratory, cardiac, pleural, arterial, venous, uterine, fetal, and intestinal sounds.

Examination with a stethoscope is noninvasive but very useful. It can assist members of the health care team in localizing problems related to the patient's symptoms.

Description

Stethoscopes vary in their design and material. Most are made of Y-shaped rubber tubing. This shape allows sounds to enter the device at one end and travel up the tubes and through to the ear pieces. Many stethoscopes have a two-sided sound-detecting device, or head, that listeners can reverse, depending on whether they need to hear high or low frequencies. Some newer models have only one pressure-sensitive head. The various types of stethoscopes include binaural stethoscopes, which are designed for use with both ears; single stethoscopes, which are designed for use with one ear; differential stethoscopes, which allow listeners to compare sounds at two different body sites; and electronic stethoscopes, which electronically amplify tones. Some stethoscopes are designed specifically for hearing fetal heartbeats or sounds in the esophagus.

Some stethoscopes must be placed directly on the skin, while others can work effectively through clothing. For the stethoscopes with a two-part sound detecting

---

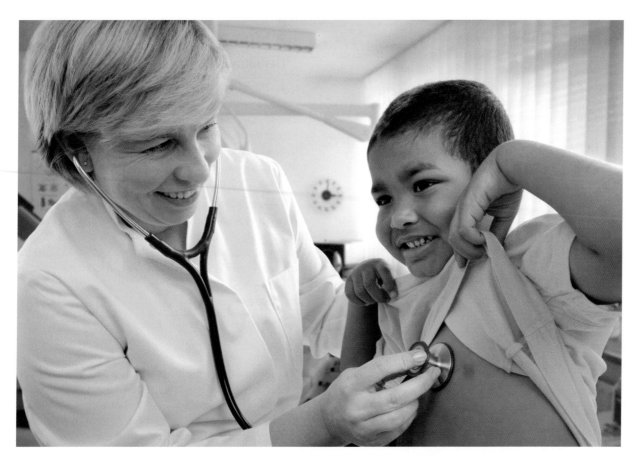

Doctor examining a young child with a stethoscope. *(Alexander Raths/Shutterstock.com)*

device in the bell, listeners press the rim against the skin, using the bowl-shaped side, to hear low-pitched sounds. The other flat side, called the diaphragm, detects high-pitched sounds.

A stethoscope is also used in conjunction with a device to measure blood pressure (**sphygmomanometer**). The stethoscope detects sounds of blood passing though an artery.

Operation

Stethoscope users must learn to assess what they hear. When listening to the heart, the user must listen to the left side of the chest, where the heart is located. Specifically, the heart lies between the fourth and sixth ribs, almost directly below the breast. The stethoscope must be moved around, and the health care provider should listen for different sounds coming from different locations. The diaphragm side of the stethoscope is used to listen to the different areas of the heart. "Lub-dub" is the sound produced by the normal heart as it beats. Every time this sound is detected, it means that the heart is contracting once. The noises are created when the heart valves click to

close. When one hears "lub," the atrioventricular valves are closing. The "dub" sound is produced by the pulmonic and aortic valves. Other heart sounds, such as a quiet "whoosh," are produced by murmurs. These sounds are created when there are irregularities in the path of blood flow through the heart. The sounds reflect turbulence in the flow; if a valve remains closed rather than opening completely, turbulence is created and a murmur is produced. Murmurs are not uncommon; many people have them and are unaffected. They are frequently too faint to be heard and remain undetected.

The lungs and airways require different listening skills from those used to detect heart sounds. The stethoscope must be placed over the chest, and the person being examined must breathe in and out deeply and slowly. Using the bell, the listener should note different sounds in various areas of the chest. Then, the diaphragm should be used in the same way. Crackles or wheezes are abnormal lung sounds. When the lung rubs against the chest wall, it creates friction and a rubbing sound. When there is fluid in the lungs, crackles are heard. A high-pitched whistling sound called a wheeze is often heard when the airways are constricted.

When the stethoscope is placed over the upper left portion of the abdomen, gurgling sounds produced by the stomach and small intestines can usually be heard just below the ribs. The large intestines, in the lower part of the abdomen, can also be heard. The noises they make are called borborygmi and are entirely normal. Borborygmi are produced by the movement of food, gas, or fecal material.

Maintenance

Stethoscopes should be cleaned after each use in order to avoid the spread of infection. This precaution is especially important when they are placed directly onto bare skin.

Health care team roles

Any member of a health care team participating in a **physical examination** uses a stethoscope.

Resources

BOOKS

Bickley, Lynn S., and Peter G. Szilagyi. *Bates' Guide to Physical Examination & History Taking.* 11th ed. Philadelphia: Wolters Kluwer Health/Lippincott Williams & Wilkins, 2013.

Blaufox, M. Donald. *An Ear to the Chest: An Illustrated History of the Evolution of the Stethoscope.* Boca Raton, FL: CRC Press-Parthenon Publishers, 2001.

PERIODICALS

Bhaskar, Anand. "A Simple Electronic Stethoscope for Recording and Playback of Heart Sounds." *Advances in Physiology Education* 36, no. 4 (December 2012): 360–62. http://dx.doi.org/10.1152/advan.00073.2012 (accessed October 23, 2013).

Cheng, Tsung O. "Seeing Is Not Believing, but Hearing Is: The Stethoscope Is Still Useful." *International Journal of Cardiology* 165, no. 1 (April 2013): 1–2. http://dx.doi.org/10.1016/j.ijcard.2012.11.114 (accessed October 23, 2013).

Hanna, Ibrahim R., and Mark E. Silverman. "A History of Cardiac Auscultation and Some of Its Contributors." *American Journal of Cardiology* 90, no. 3 (August 2002): 259–67.

Kamran, Haroon, et al. "Determination of Heart Rate Variability with an Electronic Stethoscope." *Clinical Autonomic Research* 23, no. 1 (February 2013): 41–47. http://dx.doi.org/10.1007/s10286-012-0177-3 (accessed October 23, 2013).

WEBSITES

British Broadcasting Company. *Guessing Tubes.* BBC Radio 4, October 8, 2002. http://www.bbc.co.uk/radio4/science/guessingtubes.shtml (accessed May 2, 2013).

L. Fleming Fallon Jr., MD, DrPH

Stitches *see* **Closures**

Stoma

Definition

A stoma (plural, stomata) is an artificial opening created by surgery between two hollow organs or between an internal hollow organ and the outside environment. The English word *stoma* is simply the Greek word for mouth transliterated into the letters of the Latin alphabet. The surgical procedure that creates a stoma is called an ostomy.

Ostomies are named for the part of the body in which the stoma is created; thus a stoma in the throat is called a tracheostomy; a stoma that connects the colon to the abdominal wall is called a **colostomy**; a stoma created for the urinary tract is called a urostomy; and so on.

Purpose

The purpose of stomata are somewhat different for adults or adolescents and for children. In adults and adolescents, stomata are usually made in order to treat traumatic injuries, cancer of the throat or digestive tract, or disorders of the gastrointestinal tract that cannot be managed with medications, such as Crohn's disease or ulcerative colitis. In addition, most stomata in adults and older teenagers are formed toward the lower end of the digestive tract in the ileum or colon, in order to allow as much of the natural process of digestion as possible to take place before the waste products are eliminated through the stoma. In infants and children, however, stomata may be required at multiple points along the digestive tract because of the variety of congenital as well as acquired disorders that may be present. The most common disorder in infants for which a stoma is created, and the reason for the earliest ostomies in children, is imperforate anus.

Another major difference between the creation of stomata in adults and in children is that most pediatric stomata are temporary; that is, they are created in order to allow burns or traumatic injuries to the anal area or perineum to heal or until the congenital problem can be corrected. In adults, however, while some stomata are reversible or allowed to close when no longer needed (for example, most tracheostomies), most are permanent.

A special type of stoma is used in patients with neurogenic bladder or bowel dysfunction, where the patient passes a clean catheter through the opening to empty the bladder or bowel several times a day.

Description

Surgically created stomata have been used to treat disorders of the urinary or digestive tract since the 1850s, although the specific techniques have changed over the years. Ostomies are no longer unusual or rare procedures; it is estimated that there were about a million people living with stomata in the United States and Canada as of 2013. There are about 70,000 ostomies performed each year in North America.

Stoma creation

TRACHEAL STOMA. A tracheal stoma is an opening made in the front of the neck into the trachea (windpipe) to allow the patient to breathe when the normal passage of air is blocked by traumatic injury to the head or neck; when the patient must be placed on a ventilator for some length of time; or when the larynx (voice box) and nearby lymph nodes must be removed surgically as part of cancer therapy. After cutting through the skin at the lower part of the front of the neck and pulling the muscles aside, the surgeon places a tracheostomy tube into the stoma and secures it with a faceplate, neck strap, and sutures. Unlike abdominal stomata, a tracheal stoma does not protrude from the skin surface. The inside of a tracheal stoma should be moist and glistening, and look like the tissues that line the mouth.

ABDOMINAL STOMA. Abdominal stomata are created during bowel or urinary diversion surgeries, which are performed when cancer or other disorders of the urinary system or digestive tract require urine or stool to be diverted from the urethra or rectum and discharged from the body through a stoma located on the abdomen. An **ileostomy** or colostomy may be performed directly to remove digestive wastes through a stoma. To divert the flow of urine through the digestive tract, the surgeon first performs what is called an anastomosis, joining the ureters (the tubes that convey urine from the kidneys to the bladder) to either the ileum (the final portion of the small intestine) or the colon (large intestine). The next step is the formation of the stoma itself.

To create an abdominal stoma, the surgeon cuts a hole in the abdominal wall at the appropriate location, pulls a section of the ileum or the colon through the hole, turns the end of the bowel section back on itself (similar to a shirt or sweater cuff), and sutures the end of the bowel to the outer wall of the abdomen. This technique explains why an abdominal stoma protrudes from the surface of the skin about an inch. A normal abdominal stoma has no feeling. It is bright red or pink, the normal color of the lining of the intestine. It may be round or oval in shape but should be moist and slightly shiny. The skin around the stoma should be dry.

Basic stoma care

TRACHEAL STOMA. A patient with a tracheal stoma will be instructed to clean the stoma twice a day to prevent infection, and to clean and change the tracheostomy tube. The patient will need to meet with a speech therapist to learn how to use the voice again, particularly if the larynx was removed and the stoma will be permanent. There are several techniques for vocal communication, ranging from learning to use air pressure in the esophagus to form words to having an artificial larynx placed in the throat. The speech therapist will also instruct the patient in learning to strengthen and coordinate the throat muscles so that foods and beverages can be safely taken by mouth.

Other concerns include using a filter in the stoma to prevent dust, pollen, and other particles in the air from reaching the airway, since the air is no longer filtered through the patient's nose. In addition, the patient will also need to use either a heat and moisture exchanger (HME) or a device called a humidivent in the stoma to humidify the air taken in, since it will not be humidified in the normal manner by passing through the moist tissues of the nose and throat before reaching the lungs. In addition, the patient may be taught to use a suction machine to clear mucus and other secretions from the airway, and to use saline solution to cleanse and moisten the stoma.

Last, the patient with a tracheal stoma will need to protect the stoma from water during bathing or outdoor activities on or close to water (fishing, boating, etc.). To cover the stoma when outside the home, patients may wear scarves, jewelry, or turtleneck jerseys. Crocheted bib-like stoma covers are also available through the American Cancer Society. Patients with tracheal stomata should carry medical identification at all times to alert first responders in case of an accident to the fact that they must breathe through the neck.

ABDOMINAL STOMA. Like a tracheal stoma, an abdominal stoma needs to be checked for normal appearance, cleansed carefully, and the surrounding skin dried whenever the patient changes the ostomy pouch. Patients should avoid using soaps with perfumes or oils, and baby wipes that contain oils or moisturizers, as these will interfere with a secure seal for the pouching system. If the skin around the stoma is wet, weepy, or looks inflamed, it may mean that the pouch is not sealed well against the skin. While urine or fecal matter will not irritate the stoma itself, it will cause the surrounding skin to become red and raw. In addition to checking the appearance of the stoma, patients should be instructed never to insert a **thermometer**, suppository, capsule, or any other object inside the stoma.

Selection and proper use of a pouching system is one of the most important aspects of caring for an abdominal stoma. Pouching systems for ileostomies and colostomies come in one- or two-piece versions and in different sizes. In a one-piece pouching system, the pouch that collects the digestive wastes and the skin barrier are attached to the skin around the stoma as a single unit. In a two-piece pouching system, there is a skin barrier that sticks to the skin around the stoma and has a flange for holding the pouch securely against the skin. The skin barrier should be changed every three to five days.

Ostomy pouches may be drainable or closed. They may be opaque or clear. The patient's choice of size will depend on the amount of waste material produced and the level of activity. Small pouches may be more convenient for travel or during **exercise**, although they will require more frequent changes. Some patients wear an ostomy belt to provide extra support for the pouching system or for swimming and other water sports. Urostomy pouching systems are similar to those for ileostomies and colostomies except for the fact that all urostomy pouches are drainable.

Products that may be used to make sure that the pouching system is sealed firmly against the skin include skin barrier pastes and skin sealants. A product that may be used to protect the skin around the stoma from becoming wet or weepy is skin barrier powder. Adhesive remover may be used after removing a skin barrier to make sure that any paste or sticky residue from the skin barrier is gone.

Preparation

Tracheostomy: With the exception of an emergency tracheostomy, which may be performed at the scene of an accident when traumatic injury to the head or neck obstructs the patient's breathing, most tracheostomies are performed in a hospital under **general anesthesia**. The patient will be asked to stop certain medications before the procedure and to avoid food and drink overnight before surgery.

Bowel and urinary diversion ostomies: Prior to surgery, the surgeon (usually assisted by a nurse specialist) will need to mark the location of the stoma to be created very precisely on the patient's abdomen to lower the risk of later complications. The ideal location is on the rectus abdominis muscle, on a flat surface away from scar tissue, bony ridges, and skin creases. The skin around the area should be healthy, and the surgeon will need to allow about 2 inches around the stoma to allow for a pouch appliance to seal properly. The belt line should be avoided whenever possible because stomata located in this area are easily injured. To be sure that the stoma will function properly in any position of the patient's body, the surgeon and the nurse will have the patient sit, stand, lie down, and lean forward before

making the final marking on the abdomen. Further preparation for surgery is similar to that for any other abdominal operation.

Aftercare

Patients usually remain in the hospital for several days after a stoma is created, and then recover at home for three to six weeks before returning to work or school. They should not drive a car for a week after returning home, or as long as they are taking pain medications.

Patient education

Patient education is a critical part of stoma care because of the many specific details related to stoma care, the number of complications that can arise, and the variety of different pouching systems available for abdominal stomata. Patients are instructed in most cases by specialized wound and ostomy nurses, who are experienced in the care of stomata and the use of pouching systems. The patient may also be helped by patient education materials.

Psychosocial adjustment

One of the most difficult adjustments to living with a stoma is coping with its effects on family life, intimate relationships, self-esteem, body image, and employment. Patients' reactions to the stoma may range from shock, denial, and anger to depression to grudging acceptance to gratitude for a life-saving procedure. Common concerns include questions about whom to tell about the stoma and how much to tell them; how to travel safely and pack the necessary supplies; how to deal with fears about odor or leakage from the stoma at work or in public places; how to select clothing or accessories to cover the stoma without injuring it; anxiety about sexual intimacy; anxiety about possible strains on family relationships; and questions about finances and health insurance. Ostomy nurses and support groups that include family members as well as patients can usually help with these concerns.

When to call the doctor

Although problems with skin irritation, skin barriers failing to stick properly, and minor bleeding from the stoma (a few drops) can be handled by consulting the ostomy nurse, some changes in the stoma, the surrounding skin, or the digestive process may indicate a medical emergency. Patients should contact their surgeon *at once* or go to the nearest hospital emergency department if they notice any of the following:

- A deep cut in the stoma.
- A change in color from red or pink to purple or purplish-black; the color change may indicate that the stoma has an inadequate blood supply.
- More than 4 tablespoons of bleeding into the pouch.
- Finding blood in the pouch repeatedly, or finding blood between the edge of the stoma and the skin.
- Continuous nausea and vomiting; this symptom may indicate bowel obstruction.
- Severe breakdown of the skin around the stoma.
- Continuous diarrhea with signs of dehydration.
- Severe abdominal cramps combined with no output from the stoma for four to six hours.

Risks

The creation of a stoma frequently results in various complications. The most common complications of stomata include:

- Improper site selection. A stoma that is poorly sited is more likely to leak, leading to skin irritation and social isolation of the patient. In some cases the patient may require a second operation to relocate the stoma.
- Inadequate blood supply to the stoma. This complication is more likely in obese patients. It can be corrected surgically in a procedure called a stoma revision.
- Retraction. Retraction refers to the sinking inward of the stoma so that it appears to be level with or below the skin surface. While retraction is not a medical emergency, it can make it difficult to get a good seal between the stoma and the pouching system. In severe cases, the stoma will require surgical revision.
- Irritation of the skin around the stoma. This condition may result from leakage, a fungal skin infection, frequent changes of the pouch and skin barrier, allergic reactions to the adhesive backing of the skin barrier, and overly rough removal of the skin barrier during changes of the pouching system. Antifungal medications can be used to treat fungal infections; other causes of skin irritation may require further patient education by the ostomy nurse.
- Infection, abscess, and fistula formation. These complications are more likely in patients with Crohn's disease.
- Parastomal herniation. A parastomal hernia is a condition in which a portion of the intestine pushes through the portion of the abdominal wall that was weakened by the creation of the stoma. It may result in a bowel obstruction, which will cause severe nausea and vomiting on the patient's part. An acute parastomal hernia and bowel obstruction requires emergency surgery, particularly if it occurs shortly after the stoma was created.

KEY TERMS

Anastomosis (plural, anastomoses)—In surgery, the joining together of two hollow organs following removal of a diseased area, or to bypass a diseased section of intestine that cannot be removed.

Congenital—Present at birth.

Fistula—An abnormal passageway or connection between two organs or vessels that are not ordinarily connected.

Ileum—The final section of the small intestine before it joins the large intestine. The ileum in humans is between 6 and 12 feet long.

Ostomy—A surgical procedure in which a new body opening is created. The term usually refers to an opening in the abdomen for the discharge of stool or urine.

Parastomal hernia—A condition in which a portion of the intestine bulges through a weak area in the abdominal wall near a stoma situated in the digestive tract. Parastomal hernias affect almost 30% of all patients with intestinal ostomies.

Perineum—The surface area of the body between the anus and the base of the male or female genitals.

Pouching system—A medical device consisting of a pouch or bag for the collection of digestive wastes or urine that is held against the skin surrounding a stoma by an adhesive skin barrier.

Prolapse—A condition in which an organ falls or slips out of place. In a prolapsed stoma, the bowel protrudes through the opening of the stoma further than was intended at the time of surgery.

Retraction—A condition in which the stoma sinks inward to become level with the skin surface or falls completely below the surface.

Trachea—The medical term for the windpipe.

- Prolapse. A prolapsed stoma is a condition in which the stoma protrudes further than normal from the surrounding skin. A prolapse is not a medical emergency as long as the stoma continues to be red in color and moist in appearance. The patient should, however, notify the surgeon and the ostomy nurse.

Drugs

Patients are usually given medications to relieve pain during the immediate postoperative period, and

antibiotics or antifungal medications if any skin infections develop.

Patients with abdominal stomata should ask their primary care doctor about changes in their regular prescription medications, as drugs that are formulated as capsules or tablets may not be fully absorbed during the shortened process of digestion. Liquid or gel formulations may be needed instead.

Results

Normal results for stoma creation are the maintenance of the stoma's proper size, appearance, and function as an opening for breathing (tracheal stoma) or the discharge of bodily wastes (abdominal stoma), and the absence of infection, prolapse, retraction, or other complications.

Morbidity and mortality rates

Abdominal stomata have a fairly high rate of morbidity, with various studies reporting complication rates ranging between 25% to 67%. This high figure is the result of the number of different complications that can occur with urinary and bowel diversion surgeries.

Alternatives

In some cases of bladder cancer or other bladder disorders, the surgeon can create what is called an orthotopic neobladder from a section of intestine that can hold urine and allow the patient to void through the urethra in the normal fashion. This procedure eliminates the need for a stoma.

An alternative to a standard ileostomy is the creation of an ileoanal reservoir, also called a J-pouch procedure. If the patient's anus is free of disease, the surgeon can remove a diseased large intestine and perform an anastomosis between the lower end of the ileum and the remaining portion of the rectum. The pouchlike structure thus created is called the ileoanal reservoir.

Stool collects in the reservoir and is discharged through the anus rather than through a stoma.

Health care team roles

Stomas are usually created in hospital operating rooms, although tracheostomies are sometimes performed in the field or a hospital emergency department. Tracheal stomata are usually made by otolaryngologists (specialists in head and neck surgery) while abdominal stomata are usually made by gastroenterologists. Anesthesiologists assist with general anesthesia.

Other professionals who assist patients with caring for or learning about stomata include speech therapists for patients who have undergone laryngectomies; ostomy nurses; respiratory therapists; and physical therapists. Patients who are depressed or having other emotional difficulties coping with an ostomy may benefit from individual psychotherapy or a support group.

Resources

BOOKS

Burch, Jennie. *Stoma Care.* Hoboken, NJ: Wiley-Blackwell, 2008.

Fazio, Victor W., James M. Church, and James S. Wu, eds. *Atlas of Intestinal Stomas.* New York: Springer, 2012.

Mullen, Barbara Dorr, and Kerry Anne McGinn. *The Ostomy Book: Living Comfortably with Colostomies, Ileostomies, and Urostomies,* 3rd ed., rev. and updated. Boulder, CO: Bull Publishing, 2008.

PERIODICALS

Brook, I., et al. "Long-term Use of Heat and Moisture Exchangers among Laryngectomees: Medical, Social, and Psychological Patterns." *Annals of Otology, Rhinology, and Laryngology* 122 (June 2013): 358–363.

Coldicutt, P., and B. Hill. "An Overview of Surgical Stoma Construction and Its Effects on the Child and Their Family." *Nursing Children and Young People* 25 (May 2013): 26–35.

Danielsen, A.K., et al. "Learning to Live with a Permanent Intestinal Ostomy: Impact on Everyday Life and Educational Needs." *Journal of Wound, Ostomy, and Continence Nursing* 40 (July–August 2013): 407–412.

Erwin-Toth, P., et al. "Factors Impacting the Quality of Life of People with an Ostomy in North America: Results from the Dialogue Study." *Journal of Wound, Ostomy, and Continence Nursing* 39 (July–August 2012): 417–422.

Martin, S.T., and J.D. Vogel. "Intestinal Stomas: Indications, Management, and Complications." *Advances in Surgery* 46 (2012): 19–49.

Palma, E., et al. "An Observational Study of Family Caregivers' Quality of Life Caring for Patients with a Stoma." *Gastroenterology Nursing* 35 (March-April 2012): 99–104.

Person, B., et al. "The Impact of Preoperative Stoma Site Marking on the Incidence of Complications, Quality of Life, and Patient's Independence." *Diseases of the Colon and Rectum* 55 (July 2012): 783–787.

Watson, A.J., et al. "Complications of Stomas: Their Aetiology and Management." *British Journal of Community Nursing* 18 (March 2013): 111–116.

WEBSITES

American College of Gastroenterology (ACG). "Inflammatory Bowel Disease." http://patients.gi.org/topics/inflammatory-bowel-disease (accessed November 25, 2013).

American College of Surgeons (ACS). *Ostomy Home Care Booklet.* http://www.facs.org/patienteducation/skills/complete-booklet.pdf (accessed August 10, 2013).

Mayo Clinic. "Ostomy: Adapting to Life after Colostomy, Ileostomy or Urostomy." http://www.mayoclinic.com/health/ostomy/SA00072 (accessed August 10, 2013).

Mayo Clinic. "Tracheostomy." (accessed August 10, 2013).

MedlinePlus. "Ileostomy—Care of Your Stoma." http://www.nlm.nih.gov/medlineplus/ency/patientinstructions/000071.htm (accessed August 9, 2013).

Medscape Reference. "Stomas of the Small and Large Intestine." http://emedicine.medscape.com/article/939455-overview (accessed August 9, 2013).

Medscape Reference. "Urinary Diversions and Neobladders." http://emedicine.medscape.com/article/451882-overview (accessed August 11, 2013).

National Institute of Diabetes and Digestive and Kidney Diseases (NIDDK). "Bowel Diversion Surgeries: Ileostomy, Colostomy, Ileoanal Reservoir, and Continent Ileostomy." http://digestive.niddk.nih.gov/ddiseases/pubs/ileostomy/index.aspx (accessed August 10, 2013).

United Ostomy Associations of America (UOAA). "What Is an Ostomy?" http://www.ostomy.org/ostomy_info/whatis.shtml (accessed August 10, 2013).

University of California at Davis Medical Center. "Care of Your Laryngectomy Stoma." http://www.ucdmc.ucdavis.edu/otolaryngology/Health%20Information/CARE_OF_YOUR_LARYNGECTOMY%20STOMA.pdf (accessed August 11, 2013).

Wound, Ostomy and Continence Nurses Society (WOCN). "Teen Chat: You and Your Ostomy." http://c.ymcdn.com/sites/www.wocn.org/resource/collection/A199E33D-CA30-4368-A6EA-911166C669AB/Teen_Chat_You_&_Your_Ostomy_FINAL_%282013%29.pdf (accessed August 10, 2013).

ORGANIZATIONS

American College of Gastroenterology (ACG), 6400 Goldsboro Rd., Ste. 200, Bethesda, MD 20817, (301) 263-9000, info@acg.gi.org, http://gi.org.

American College of Surgeons (ACS), 633 North Saint Clair St., Chicago, IL 60611-3211, (312) 202-5000, Fax: (312) 202-5001, (800) 621-4111, http://www.facs.org/contact/contact.html, http://www.facs.org/index.html.

National Institute of Diabetes and Digestive and Kidney Diseases (NIDDK), Bldg. 31, Room 9A06, 31 Center Drive, MSC 2560, Bethesda, MD 20892-2560, (301) 496-3583, http://www2.niddk.nih.gov/Footer/ContactNIDDK, http://www2.niddk.nih.gov.

United Ostomy Associations of America, Inc. (UOAA), PO Box 512, Northfield, MN 55057-0512, (800) 826-0826, info@ostomy.org, http://www.ostomy.org.

Wound, Ostomy and Continence Nurses Society (WOCN), 15000 Commerce Parkway, Ste. C, Mount Laurel, NJ 08054, Fax: (856) 439-0525, (888) 224-9626, wocn_info@wocn.org, http://www.wocn.org.

Rebecca J. Frey, PhD

Stomach resection *see* **Gastrectomy**

Stomach stapling *see* **Vertical banded gastroplasty**

Stomach tube insertion *see* **Gastrostomy**

Stool culture

Definition

A stool culture is a test to identify bacteria in patients with a suspected infection of the digestive tract. A sample of the patient's feces is placed in a special medium. Any bacteria that grows in the culture are identified using a microscope and biochemical tests. The test may also be referred to as a fecal culture.

Purpose

Stool culture is performed to identify bacteria or other organisms in persons with symptoms of gastrointestinal infection, most commonly diarrhea. Identification of the organism is necessary to determine the proper course of treatment or to trace the cause of an outbreak or epidemic of certain types of diarrhea.

According to the Centers for Disease Control and Prevention (CDC), doctors are most likely to order a stool culture for patients with any of the following characteristics:

• AIDS

• bloody stools

• diarrhea lasting longer than three days

• high fever

• history of recent travel abroad

• severe dehydration

Description

To obtain a specimen for culture, the patient is asked to collect a stool sample into a special sterile container. In some cases, the container may contain a transport solution. Specimens may need to be collected on three consecutive days. It is important to return the specimen to the doctor's office or the laboratory in the time specified by the physician or nurse. Laboratories do not accept stool specimens contaminated with water, urine, or other materials, including toilet paper.

The culture test involves placing a sample of the stool on a special substance, called a medium, that provides nutrients for certain organisms to grow and reproduce. The medium is usually a thick gel-like substance. The culture is done in a test tube or on a flat round culture plate and is incubated at the proper temperature for growth of the bacteria. After a colony of bacteria grows in the medium, the type of bacteria is identified by observing the colony's growth, physical characteristics, and microscopic features. The bacteria may be dyed with special stains that make it easier to identify features specific to particular bacteria.

Although most intestinal infections are caused by bacteria, in some cases a fungal or viral culture may be necessary. The most common bacterial infections of the digestive tract are caused by *Shigella*, *Salmonella*, *Campylobacter*, and *Yersinia*. Patients taking certain **antibiotics** may be susceptible to infection with *Clostridium difficile*. In some cases, as with *Clostridium difficile*, the stool culture is used to detect the toxin (poison or harmful chemical) produced by the bacteria.

Patients with AIDS or other immune system diseases may develop gastrointestinal infections caused by fungi, such as *Candida*, or viral organisms, including cytomegalovirus.

Several intestinal parasites may cause gastrointestinal infection and diarrhea. Parasites are not cultured but are identified microscopically in a stool ova and parasites test, also referred to as a **stool O & P test**.

Preparation

The physician or other healthcare provider will ask the patient for a complete medical history and perform a **physical examination** to determine possible causes of the gastrointestinal problem. Information about the patient's diet, any medications taken, and recent travel may provide clues to the identity of possible infectious organisms.

Stool culture normally does not require any special preparation. Patients do not need to change their diet

---

KEY TERMS

Bismuth—A substance used in medicines to treat diarrhea, nausea, and indigestion.

Enteric—Pertaining to the intestine.

Enterotoxigenic—Refers to an organism that produces toxins in the gastrointestinal tract that cause such things as vomiting, diarrhea, and other symptoms of food poisoning.

Feces—Material excreted by the intestines.

Flora—Refers to normal bacteria found in a healthy person.

Gastrointestinal—Referring to the digestive tract; the stomach and intestines.

Psyllium hydrophilic mucilloid—A plant material contained in some laxatives.

Sterile—Free of microorganisms.

Toxin—A poison; usually refers to protein poisons produced by bacteria, animals, and some plants.

---

before collecting the specimen. Intake of some substances can contaminate the stool specimen and should not be taken the day before collection. These substances include castor oil, bismuth, certain antibiotics, and laxative preparations containing psyllium hydrophilic mucilloid.

Patients may wish to find out ahead of time if their insurance covers stool cultures. This common test is usually covered when ordered by a physician approved by the patient's insurance plan and done at an approved laboratory.

Aftercare

An antibiotic sensitivity test may be done after a specific bacterium is identified. This test shows which antibiotics will be most effective for treating the infection.

Results

The length of time needed to perform a stool culture depends on the laboratory where it is done and the culture methods used. Stool culture usually takes 72 hours or longer to complete. Some organisms may take several weeks to grow in a culture.

Bacteria that are normally found in the intestines include *Pseudomonas* and *Escherichia coli*. These enteric bacteria (bacteria of the gastrointestinal system) are considered normal flora and usually do not cause infection in the digestive tract.

Abnormal results

Bacteria that do not normally inhabit the digestive tract and that are known to cause gastrointestinal infection include *Shigella*, *Salmonella*, *Campylobacter*, and *Yersinia*. *Clostridium difficile* produces a toxin that can cause severe diarrhea. Other bacteria that produce toxins are *Staphylococcus aureus*, *Bacillus cereus*, and enterotoxigenic (producing disease in the digestive system) *Escherichia coli*. Although *Escherichia coli* is a normal bacteria found in the intestines, the enterotoxigenic type of this bacteria can be acquired from consuming contaminated meat, produce, or juice. It produces a toxin that causes severe inflammation and bleeding of the colon.

Alternatives

Newer methods of testing stool samples for specific disease organisms include various forms of polymerase chain reaction (PCR) assays. One type that has been used to test for several different types of intestinal viruses at the same time is the RT-PCR, which stands for reverse transcriptase polymerase chain reaction. This assay measures changes in an organism's messenger ribonucleic acid (RNA). RT-PCR assays have several advantages over standard stool cultures: they require only very small samples of material, they can be performed much more rapidly, and they can be used to test environmental water for virus contamination as well as human stool samples.

Resources

PERIODICALS

Hewison, C. J., C. H. Heath, and P. R. Ingram. "Stool Culture." *Australian Family Physician* 41, no. 10 (2012): 775–79.

WEBSITES

A.D.A.M. Medical Encyclopedia. "Fecal Culture." MedlinePlus. http://www.nlm.nih.gov/medlineplus/ency/article/003758.htm (accessed August 8, 2013).
American Association for Clinical Chemistry. "Stool Culture." Lab Tests Online. http://labtestsonline.org/understanding/analytes/stool-culture (accessed August 8, 2013).
Medical University of South Carolina. "Stool Culture." http://www.muschealth.com/lab/content.aspx?id=150422 (accessed August 8, 2013).

ORGANIZATIONS

Centers for Disease Control and Prevention, 1600 Clifton Rd., Atlanta, GA 30333, (800) CDC-INFO (232-4636), (888) 232-6348, cdcinfo@cdc.gov, http://www.cdc.gov.

Toni Rizzo
Rebecca J. Frey, PhD

▌Stool fat test

Definition

Stool fats, also known as fecal fats or lipids, are fats that are excreted in feces. When secretions from the pancreas and liver are adequate, emulsified dietary fats are almost completely absorbed in the small intestine. When a malabsorption disorder or other condition disrupts this process, excretion of fat in the stool increases.

Purpose

This test evaluates the digestion of fats by determining excessive excretion of lipids in patients exhibiting signs of malabsorption, such as weight loss, abdominal distention, and scaly skin.

Description

Excessive excretion of fecal fat is called steatorrhea, a condition that is suspected when the patient has large, "greasy," and foul-smelling stools. Both digestive and absorptive disorders can cause steatorrhea. Digestive disorders affect the production and release of the enzyme lipase from the pancreas or bile from the liver, which are substances that aid in the digestion of fats. Absorptive disorders disturb the absorptive and enzyme functions of the intestine. Any condition that causes malabsorption or maldigestion is associated with increased fecal fat. As an example, children with cystic fibrosis have mucous plugs that block the pancreatic ducts. The absence or significant decrease of the pancreatic enzymes amylase, lipase, trypsin, and chymotrypsin limits fat protein and carbohydrate digestion, resulting in steatorrhea due to fat malabsorption.

Both qualitative and quantitative tests are used to identify excessive fecal fat. The qualitative test involves staining a specimen of stool with a special dye, then examining it microscopically for evidence of malabsorption, such as undigested muscle fiber and various fats. The quantitative test involves drying and weighing a three-day stool specimen, then using an extraction technique to separate the fats, which are subsequently evaporated and weighed. This measurement of the total output of fecal fat per day is the most reliable test for steatorrhea.

Precautions

Drugs that may increase fecal fat levels include enemas and **laxatives**, especially mineral oil. Drugs that may decrease fecal fat include Metamucil and barium. Other substances that can affect test results include alcohol, potassium chloride, calcium carbonate, neomycin, kanamycin, and other broad-spectrum **antibiotics**.

American Association for Clinical Chemistry. "Fecal Fat." Lab Tests Online. http://labtestsonline.org/understanding/analytes/fecal-fat (accessed August 8, 2013).

Janis O. Flores

KEY TERMS

Enzyme—A protein that changes the rate of a chemical reaction within the body without being depleted in the reaction.

Lipid—Any organic compound that is greasy and insoluble in water but soluble in alcohol. Fats, waxes, and oils are examples of lipids.

Malabsorption—Poor absorption of nutrients.

Preparation

This test requires a 72-hour stool collection. The patient should abstain from alcohol during this time and maintain a high-fat diet (100 grams [g] per day) for three days before the test and during the collection period. The patient should call the laboratory for instructions on how to collect the specimen.

Results

Reference values vary from laboratory to laboratory but are generally found within the range of 5–7 grams per 24-hour period.

It should be noted that children, especially infants, cannot ingest the 100 g/day of fat that is suggested for the test. Therefore, an alternate method determines the difference between ingested fat and fecal fat, expressed as a percentage. The figure, called the fat retention coefficient, is 95% or greater in healthy children and adults. A low value is indicative of steatorrhea.

Abnormal results

Increased fecal fat levels are found in cystic fibrosis; malabsorption secondary to other conditions like Whipple's disease or Crohn's disease; maldigestion secondary to pancreatic or bile duct obstruction; and "short-gut" syndrome secondary to surgical resection, bypass, or congenital anomaly.

Resources

BOOKS

Pagana, Kathleen Deska, and Timothy J. Pagana. *Mosby's Diagnostic and Laboratory Test Reference*. 11th ed. St. Louis, MO: Mosby/Elsevier, 2013.

WEBSITES

A.D.A.M. Medical Encyclopedia. "Fecal Fat." MedlinePlus. http://www.nlm.nih.gov/medlineplus/ency/article/003588.htm (accessed August 8, 2013).

Stool O & P test

Definition

The stool O & P test is the stool ova and parasites test. In this test, a stool sample is examined for the presence of intestinal parasites and their eggs, which are called ova.

Purpose

The ova and parasites test is performed to look for and identify intestinal parasites and their eggs in persons with symptoms of gastrointestinal infection. Patients may have no symptoms, or experience diarrhea, blood in the stools, and other gastrointestinal distress. Identification of a particular parasite indicates the cause of the patient's disease and determines the medication needed to treat it.

Precautions

Stool O & P is performed if an infection of the digestive tract is suspected. The test has no harmful effects.

Description

Examination of the stool for ova and parasites is done to diagnose parasitic infection of the intestines. The test may be done in the doctor's office or a laboratory. The patient collects a stool sample in one or more sterile containers containing special chemical fixatives. The feces should be collected directly into the container. It must not be contaminated with urine, water, or other materials. Three specimens are often needed—collected every other day, or every third day. However, as many as six specimens may be needed to diagnose the amoeba *Entamoeba histolytica*. The specimen does not need to be refrigerated. It should be delivered to the doctor's office or laboratory within 12 hours.

In the laboratory, the stool sample is observed for signs of parasites and their eggs. Some parasites are large enough to be seen without a microscope. For others, microscope slides are prepared with fresh unstained stool, and with stool dyed with special stains. These preparations are observed with a microscope for the presence of parasites or their eggs.

An unstained stool examination for ova and parasites normally only takes a few minutes. If specimen staining and other preparation is done, the test may take longer. When the specimen is sent to a laboratory, the results may take 8 to 24 hours to be reported.

The most common intestinal parasites in North America that cause infections are:

• roundworms: *Ascaris lumbricoides*

• hookworms: *Necator americanus*

• pinworms: *Enterobius follicularis*

• tapeworms: *Diphyllobothrium latum, Taenia saginata,* and *Taenia solium*

• protozoa: *Entamoeba histolytica* (an amoeba), and *Giardia lamblia* (a flagellate)

Numerous other parasites are found in other parts of the world. These may be contracted by travelers to other countries. Patients with acquired immune deficiency syndrome (AIDS) or other immune system disorders are commonly infected with the parasites in the *Microsporidia* family, *Cryptosporidium,* and *Isospora belli.*

Insurance coverage for stool ova and parasites may vary among different insurance plans. This test usually is covered if ordered by a physician approved by the patient's insurance plan, and if it is done at an approved laboratory.

Preparation

The physician, or other healthcare provider, will ask the patient for a complete medical history, and perform a **physical examination** to determine possible causes of the gastrointestinal symptoms. Information about the patient's diet, any medications taken, and recent travel may provide clues to the identity of possible infectious parasites.

Collecting a stool sample for ova and parasite detection normally does not require any special preparation. Patients do not need to change their diet before collecting the specimen. Patients should avoid taking any medications or treatments containing mineral oil, castor oil, or bismuth; magnesium or other antidiarrheal medicines; or **antibiotics** for seven to ten days before collecting the specimen. Sometimes samples taken over multiple days may be required.

Results

Normally, parasites and eggs should not be found in stools. Some parasites are not pathogenic, which means

---

KEY TERMS

Amoeba—A type of protozoa (one-celled animal) that can move or change its shape by extending projections of its cytoplasm.

Bismuth—A substance used in medicines to treat diarrhea, nausea, and indigestion.

Cryptosporidium—A type of parasitic protozoa.

Feces—Material excreted by the intestines.

Flagellate—A microorganism that uses flagella (hair-like projections) to move.

Gastrointestinal—Referring to the digestive tract; the stomach and intestines.

Isospora belli—A type of parasitic protozoa.

Microsporida—A type of parasitic protozoa.

Ova—Eggs.

Parasite—An organism that lives on or inside another living organism (host), causing damage to the host.

Pathogenic—Disease-causing.

Protozoa—One-celled eukaryotic organisms belonging to the kingdom Protista.

Sterile—Free of microorganisms.

---

they do not cause disease. If these are found, no treatment is necessary.

Abnormal results

The presence of any pathogenic parasite indicates an intestinal parasitic infection. Depending on the parasite identified, other tests may need to be performed to determine if the parasite has invaded other parts of the body. Some parasites travel from the intestines to other parts of the body and may already have caused damage to other tissues by the time a diagnosis is made. For example, the roundworm, *A. lumbricoides*, penetrates the intestinal wall and can cause inflammation in the abdomen. It can also migrate to the lungs and cause pneumonia. This kind of injury can occur weeks before the roundworm eggs show up in the stool.

Other types of damage caused by intestinal parasites include anemia due to hemorrhage caused by hookworms, and anemia caused by depletion of vitamin B_{12} through the action of tapeworms.

When a parasite is identified, the patient can be treated with the appropriate medications to eliminate the parasite.

Alternatives

Pinworms may be detected by using a tape test. After waking, the person suspected of having pinworms should place a 1 in. piece of clear cellophane tape over the anus. If eggs are present, they will stick to the tape. The tape should then be placed (sticky-side down) on a glass slide and given to a physician for analysis.

Resources

BOOKS

Daniels, Rick. *Delmar's Manual of Laboratory and Diagnostic Tests: Organized by Type of Test.* 2nd ed. Clifton Park, NY: Delmar/Cengage Learning, 2010.

WEBSITES

A.D.A.M. Medical Encyclopedia. "Pinworm Test." Medline-Plus. http://www.nlm.nih.gov/medlineplus/ency/article/003452.htm (accessed September 2, 2013).

American Association for Clinical Chemistry. "O&P." Lab Tests Online. http://labtestsonline.org/understanding/analytes/op (accessed September 2, 2013).

Centers for Disease Control and Prevention. "Diagnosis of Parasitic Diseases." http://www.cdc.gov/parasites/references_resources/diagnosis.html (accessed September 2, 2013).

Toni Rizzo

Strabismus repair *see* **Eye muscle surgery**

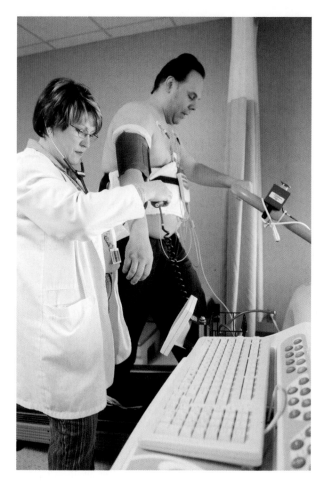

Man undergoing a cardiac stress test. *(BSIP/UIG Via Getty Images)*

pressure, electrocardiogram (ECG), and any symptoms that occur during the test are monitored. The result shows the general physical condition of the patient's circulatory system and, specifically, may show when an abnormal flow of blood is going into or out of the heart. Besides helping to diagnose heart disease, it also provides prognoses after heart attacks.

Stress test

Definition

A stress test is primarily used to identify coronary artery disease. Consequently, it is also sometimes called a cardiac stress test or cardiac diagnostic test. The stress test measures the ability of the heart to react to **exercise** while being monitored in a controlled environment. The test measures the heart at rest and while it is under the stress of exercise. It requires patients to exercise on a treadmill or exercise bicycle while their heart rate, blood

Purpose

The body requires more oxygen during exercise than when it is at rest. To deliver more oxygen during exercise, the heart has to pump more oxygen-rich blood. Because of the increased stress on the heart, exercise can reveal coronary problems that are not apparent when the body is at rest. This is why the stress test, though not perfect, remains the best initial, noninvasive, practical coronary test.

The stress test is particularly useful for detecting ischemia (inadequate supply of blood to the heart muscle) caused by blocked coronary arteries. Less commonly, it is used to determine safe levels of exercise in people with existing coronary artery disease. A stress test may also be given when the following conditions are suspected or present:

- acute chest pain
- acute coronary syndrome (ACS)
- angina
- atypical or non-cardiac chest pain
- cardiac disease (if undergoing emergency non-cardiac surgery)
- coronary artery disease (if disease status changes)
- past coronary revascularization
- newly diagnosed heart failure or cardiomyopathy
- select arrhythmias
- valvular heart disease

Description

A technician affixes electrodes to the patient's chest, using adhesive patches with a special gel that conducts electrical impulses. Typically, electrodes are placed under each collarbone and each bottom rib, and six electrodes are placed across the chest in a rough outline of the heart. Wires from the electrodes are connected to an ECG, which records the electrical activity picked up by the electrodes.

The technician performs resting ECG tests while the patient is lying down, then standing up, and then breathing heavily for half a minute. These baseline tests can later be compared with the ECG tests performed while the patient is exercising. The patient's blood pressure is taken and the blood pressure cuff is left in place so that blood pressure can be measured periodically throughout the test.

The patient begins riding a stationary bicycle or walking on a treadmill. Gradually the intensity of the exercise is increased. For example, if the patient is walking on a treadmill, then the speed of the treadmill increases and the treadmill is tilted upward to simulate an incline. If the patient is on an exercise bicycle, then the resistance or "drag" is gradually increased. The patient continues exercising at increasing intensity until reaching the target heart rate (generally set at a minimum of 85% of the maximal predicted heart rate based on the patient's age) or experiencing severe fatigue, dizziness, or chest pain. During the test, the patient's heart rate, ECG, and blood pressure are monitored.

Sometimes other tests, such as **echocardiography** or thallium scanning, are used in conjunction with the exercise stress test. This is partly because studies suggest that women have a high rate of false negatives (results

showing no problem when one exists) and false positives (results showing a problem when one does not exist) with the stress test. They may benefit from another test, such as exercise echocardiography. People who are unable to exercise may be injected with drugs, such as adenosine, which mimic the effects of exercise on the heart, and then they are given a thallium scan. The thallium scan and echocardiogram are particularly useful when the patient's resting ECG is abnormal. In such cases, interpretation of exercise-induced ECG abnormalities is difficult.

An echocardiogram stress test is performed in a similar fashion to an ECG stress test (the subject rides a bike or walks on a treadmill in both tests). However, in an echocardiogram, sound waves create a moving image of the heart. The image is more detailed than the one produced with an x-ray scan and does not require radiation. The type of echocardiogram that is most often used is a transthoracic echocardiogram (TTE). In the TTE process, a transducer is positioned above or around the heart so that when high-frequency sound waves are emitted, the transducer receives back the sound waves as they bounce off the heart. The waves are transmitted as electrical impulses to the echocardiograph machine, which converts these impulses into two-dimensional or three-dimensional images of the heart. In addition to this, a Doppler echocardiogram records the motion of blood as it passes through the heart.

Radionuclide myocardial perfusion imaging (rMPI) is a nuclear procedure used in medicine that shows the function of the heart muscle. This imaging scan is the most common nuclear medicine procedure used for heart analyses. The scan is performed after a small amount of radioactive material such as thallium (chemical symbol Tl) or technetium (Tc) is injected into a vein of the patient. The radioactive material passes into the patient's heart muscle and images are taken with a special camera to obtain a three-dimensional image. In order to detect coronary heart disease, a stress test is performed along with the scan. The overall test requires two sets of images of the heart and usually two sets of injections. One set of images is obtained immediately after a patient exercises on a treadmill or after stressing the heart with a medication, and the other is taken while the heart is at rest.

The use of rMPI with single-photon emission **computed tomography** (SPECT) or **positron emission tomography** (PET) is well established for the diagnosis of coronary heart disease. SPECT is a nuclear medicine tomographic imaging technique that uses gamma rays to detect the functioning of the heart. In SPECT, a three-dimensional image is produced, one that consists of cross-sectional slices of an organ. PET, also a nuclear medicine tomographic technique, produces three-dimensional images by detecting pairs of gamma rays emitted indirectly by a radionuclide (called a tracer) that gives off tiny positively charged particles (positrons). A camera records the positrons and converts the recording into images on a computer. The tracer is introduced into the body at the beginning of the test. The PET scan is especially useful for determining the flow of blood in and around the heart.

Although exercise stress testing is generally preferred when evaluating the heart, an alternative means of evaluation is sometimes used in patients who cannot properly exercise for the test. The pharmacologic stress test is the evaluation method that does not use exercise as part of its method. It is most often used when patients cannot exercise to an adequate level, which is defined as at least 80% of the workload necessary for their gender and age, or 85% or more of their maximum heart rate for their gender and age.

Preparation

Patients are usually instructed not to eat or smoke for several hours before the test. They should be advised to inform the physician about any medications they are taking, and to wear comfortable sneakers and exercise clothing.

Patients should understand the purpose of the test and the signs and symptoms that indicate the test should be stopped. Physicians, nurses, and ECG technicians can ensure patient safety by encouraging them to immediately communicate discomfort at any time during the stress test.

Aftercare

After the test, the patient should rest until blood pressure and heart rate return to normal. If all goes well, and there are no signs of distress, the patient may return to his or her normal daily activities.

Risks

There is a very slight risk of myocardial infarction (a heart attack) from the exercise, as well as cardiac arrhythmia (irregular heartbeat), angina, or cardiac arrest (about one in 100,000). For this reason, exercise stress tests should be attended by healthcare professionals with immediate access to defibrillators and other emergency equipment.

Patients are cautioned to stop the test should they develop any of the following symptoms:

• unsteady gait
• confusion
• skin that is grayish or cold and clammy
• dizziness or fainting
• a drop in blood pressure

KEY TERMS

Angina—Chest pain from a poor blood supply to the heart muscle due to stenosis (narrowing) of the coronary arteries.

Cardiac arrhythmia—An irregular heart rate (frequency of heartbeats) or rhythm (the pattern of heartbeats).

Defibrillator—A device that delivers an electric shock to the heart muscle through the chest wall in order to restore a normal heart rate.

False negative—Test results showing no problem when one exists.

False positive—Test results showing a problem when one does not exist.

Hypertrophy—The overgrowth of muscle.

Ischemia—Diminished supply of oxygen-rich blood to an organ or area of the body.

• angina (chest pain)
• cardiac arrhythmia (irregular heartbeat)

Results

A normal result of an exercise stress test shows normal electrocardiogram tracings and heart rate, blood pressure within the normal range, and no angina, unusual dizziness, or shortness of breath.

A number of abnormalities may appear on an exercise stress test. Examples of exercise-induced ECG abnormalities are ST segment depression or heart rhythm disturbances. These ECG abnormalities may indicate deprivation of blood to the heart muscle (ischemia) caused by narrowed or blocked coronary arteries. Stress test abnormalities generally require further diagnostic evaluation and therapy.

The Duke Treadmill Score (DTS) is a common prognostic scoring system used for finding a result from a stress test in which a patient has chest pain and is undergoing a treadmill stress test. It predicts coronary heart disease, but is not applicable for patients who already have coronary heart disease. The DTS is a weighted index that incorporates exercise duration, symptoms, and ECG changes based on the following:

• Treadmill Exercise Time (Ex Time): amount of time for treadmill exercise, using the standard Bruce protocol, in minutes, usually from 0 to 15 minutes
• Maximum net ST segment deviation (Max ST): taking into account depression or elevation, in millimeters

QUESTIONS TO ASK YOUR DOCTOR

- What can this stress test tell me about the condition of my heart?
- What type of stress test will I have?
- Will my stress test be an exercise test or will it be one in which I take medication to make my heart pump faster? Why is this type of test being performed on me?
- When will the results of the tests be available?
- Are stress tests different for men than they are for women?
- How accurate is this particular type of stress test?
- What happens if this test shows that my heart is not functioning properly?
- Will I need to perform this stress test on an empty stomach? Is so, when should I stop eating?
- What kind of stress tests are available for me to take?

after 80 milliseconds from the J-Point; usually 0 to 7 millimeters; the ST segment on an electrocardiogram connects the QRS complex and the T wave, and has a duration of 0.080 seconds to 0.120 seconds

- Exercise-induced Treadmill Angina Index (Angina Index): 0 (no angina during exercise), 1 (non-limiting), or 2 (exercise-limiting)

The scoring for DTS consists of the following equation: (treadmill exercise time) minus (five times maximum net ST deviation) minus (four times treadmill angina index); or (Ex Time) − (5 × Max ST) − (4 × Angina Index). A range of scores for the DTS is from −25 to −11 (for highest risk of coronary heart disease), −10 to +4 (moderate risk), and +5 to +15 (lowest risk).

Resources

BOOKS

Adam, Andy, Adrian K. Dixon, Ronald G. Grainger, and David J. Allison. *Grainger & Allison's Diagnostic Radiology: A Textbook of Medical Imaging.* 5th ed. Philadelphia: Churchill Livingstone/Elsevier, 2008.

Bonow, Robert O., et al., eds. *Braunwald's Heart Disease: A Textbook of Cardiovascular Medicine.* 9th ed. Philadelphia: Elsevier Saunders, 2012.

Mettler Jr., Fred A. *Essentials of Radiology.* 3rd ed. Philadelphia: Elsevier/Saunders, 2014.

OTHER

Society of Nuclear Medicine and Molecular Imaging. "Radionuclide Perfusion Imaging of the Heart." http://www.snm.org/docs/PET_PROS/Heart%20Disease%20Fact%20Sheet.pdf (accessed September 18, 2013).

WEBSITES

A.D.A.M. Medical Encyclopedia. "Echocardiogram." MedlinePlus. http://www.nlm.nih.gov/medlineplus/ency/article/003869.htm (accessed September 18, 2013).

A.D.A.M. Medical Encyclopedia. "Nuclear Stress Test." MedlinePlus. http://www.nlm.nih.gov/medlineplus/ency/article/007201.htm (accessed September 18, 2013).

Canadian Society of Echocardiography. "Duke Treadmill Score." http://www.csecho.ca/cardiomath/?eqnHD=stress&eqnDisp=duketsc (accessed September 18, 2013).

Heller, Gary V., Justin B. Lundbye, and Athanasios Kapetanopoulos. "Vasodilator Stress Radionuclide Myocardial Perfusion Imaging: Testing Methodologies and Safety." UpToDate.com. (March 8, 2013). http://www.uptodate.com/contents/vasodilator-stress-radionuclide-myocardial-perfusion-imaging-testing-methodologies-and-safety (accessed September 18, 2013).

Mayo Clinic staff. "Stress Test." MayoClinic.com. http://www.mayoclinic.com/health/stress-test/MY00977 (accessed September 18, 2013).

WebMD. "Heart Disease and Stress Tests." http://www.webmd.com/heart-disease/guide/stress-test (accessed September 18, 2013).

Zunis Foundation. "Duke Treadmill Score: Prediction Of Coronary Heart Disease in a Patient with Chest Pain Undergoing a Treadmill Stress Test." http://www.zunis.org/Duke%20Treadmill%20Score%20-%20CAD%20Predictor.htm (accessed September 18, 2013).

ORGANIZATIONS

American Heart Association, 7272 Greenville Ave., Dallas, TX 75231, (800) AHA-USA-1 (242-8721), http://www.heart.org.

National Heart, Lung, and Blood Institute Information Center, PO Box 30105, Bethesda, MD 20824-0105, (301) 592-8573, Fax: (240) 629-3246, nhlbiinfo@nhlbi.nih.gov, http://www.nhlbi.nih.gov.

Barbara Wexler
Lee A. Shratter, MD
William A. Atkins, BB, BS, MBA

Sulfonamides

Definition

Sulfonamides are a group of anti-infective drugs that prevent the growth of bacteria in the body by interfering with their metabolism. Bacteria are one-celled disease-causing microorganisms that commonly multiply by cell division.

Purpose

Sulfonamides are used to treat many kinds of infections caused by bacteria and certain other microorganisms. Physicians may prescribe these drugs to treat urinary tract infections, ear infections, frequent or long-lasting bronchitis, bacterial meningitis, certain eye infections, *Pneumocystis carinii* pneumonia (PCP), traveler's diarrhea, and a number of other infections. These drugs do not work for colds, flu, and other infections caused by viruses.

Description

Sulfonamides, which are also called sulfa medicines, are available only with a physician's prescription. They are sold in tablet and liquid forms. Some commonly used sulfonamides are sulfisoxazole (Gantrisin) and the combination drug sulfamethoxazole and trimethoprim (Bactrim, Cotrim, Septra).

Although the sulfonamides have been largely replaced by **antibiotics** for treatment of infections, some bacteria have developed resistance to antibiotics but can still be treated with sulfonamides because the bacteria have not been exposed to these drugs in the past.

Silver sulfadiazine, an ointment containing a sulfonamide, is valuable for the treatment of infections associated with severe burns. The combination drug trimethoprim/sulfamethoxazole (TMP-SMZ) remains in use for many infections, including those associated with human immunodeficiency virus (HIV) infection. TMP-SMZ is particularly useful for prevention and treatment of *Pneumocystis carinii* pneumonia, which has been the most dangerous of the infections associated with HIV infection.

Recommended dosage

The recommended dosage depends on the type of sulfonamide, the strength of the medication, and the medical problem for which it is being taken. Patients should check the correct dosage with the physician who prescribed the drug or the pharmacist who filled the prescription.

Patients should always take sulfonamides exactly as directed. To make sure the infection clears up completely, the full course of the medicine must be taken. Patients should not stop taking the drug just because their symptoms begin to improve, because the symptoms may return if the drug is stopped too soon.

Sulfonamides work best when they are at constant levels in the blood. To help keep blood levels constant,

patients should take the medicine in doses spaced evenly throughout the day and night without missing any doses. For best results, sulfa medicines should be taken with a full glass of water, and the patient should drink several more glasses of water every day. This precaution is necessary because sulfa drugs do not dissolve in tissue fluids as easily as some other anti-infective medications. Drinking plenty of water will help prevent some of the medicine's side effects.

Precautions

Symptoms should begin to improve within a few days of beginning to take a sulfa drug. If they do not, or if they get worse, the patient should consult the physician who prescribed the medicine.

Although major side effects are rare, some people have had severe and life-threatening reactions to sulfonamides. These include sudden and severe liver damage; serious blood problems; breakdown of the outer layer of the skin; and a condition called Stevens-Johnson syndrome (erythema multiforme), in which people get blisters around the mouth, eyes, or anus. The patient may be unable to eat and may develop ulcerated areas in the eyes or be unable to open the eyes. It is important to consult a dermatologist and an ophthalmologist as quickly as possible if a patient develops Stevens-Johnson syndrome, to prevent lasting damage to the patient's eyesight. In addition, the syndrome is sometimes fatal.

A physician should be called immediately if any of these signs of a dangerous reaction occur:

- skin rash or reddish or purplish spots on the skin
- such other skin problems as blistering or peeling
- fever
- sore throat
- cough
- shortness of breath
- joint pain
- pale skin
- yellow skin or eyes

Sulfa drugs may also cause dizziness. Anyone who takes sulfonamides should not drive, use machines, or do anything else that might be dangerous until they have found out how these drugs affect them.

Sulfa medications may increase the skin's sensitivity to sunlight. Even brief exposure to sun can cause a severe sunburn or a rash. During treatment with these drugs, patients should avoid exposure to direct sunlight, especially high sun between 10 a.m. and 3 p.m.; wear a hat and tightly woven clothing that covers the arms and legs; use a sunscreen with a skin protection factor (SPF) of at least 15; protect the lips with a lip balm containing sun block; and avoid the use of tanning beds, tanning booths, or sunlamps.

Babies under two months should not be given sulfonamides unless their physician has specifically ordered these drugs.

Surgery

Sulfonamides may cause blood problems that can interfere with healing and lead to additional infections. Patients should try to avoid minor injuries while taking these medicines, and be especially careful not to injure the mouth when brushing or flossing the teeth or using a toothpick. They should not have dental work or surgery done until their blood is back to normal.

Older people may be especially sensitive to the effects of sulfonamides, increasing the chance of such unwanted side effects as severe skin problems and blood disorders. Patients who are taking water pills (**diuretics**) at the same time as sulfonamides may also be more likely to have these problems.

Special conditions

People with certain medical conditions or who are taking other medicines may have problems if they take sulfonamides. Before taking these drugs, the patient must inform the doctor about any other diseases or conditions.

ALLERGIES. Anyone who has had unusual reactions to sulfonamides, diuretics, diabetes medicines, or glaucoma medications in the past should let his or her physician know before taking sulfonamides. The physician should also be told about any allergies to foods, dyes, preservatives, or other substances.

PREGNANCY. Some sulfonamides have been found to cause birth defects in studies of laboratory animals. The drugs' effects on human fetuses have not been studied. Pregnant women are advised not to use sulfa drugs around the time of labor and delivery, because they can cause side effects in the baby. Women who are pregnant or who may become pregnant should check with their physicians about the safety of using sulfonamides during pregnancy.

LACTATION. Sulfonamides pass into breast milk and may cause liver problems, anemia, and other problems in nursing babies whose mothers take the medicine. Because of those problems, women should not breast-feed their babies when they are under treatment with sulfa drugs. Women who are breast-feeding but require treatment with sulfonamides should check with their physicians to find out how long they should stop breast-feeding.

OTHER MEDICAL CONDITIONS. People with any of the following medical problems should make sure their physicians are aware of their conditions before they take sulfonamides:

• anemia or other blood problems
• kidney disease
• liver disease
• asthma or severe allergies
• alcohol abuse
• poor nutrition
• abnormal intestinal absorption
• porphyria
• folic acid deficiency
• deficiency of an enzyme known as glucose-6-phosphate dehydrogenase (G6PD)

Side effects

The most common side effects are mild diarrhea, nausea, vomiting, dizziness, headache, loss of appetite, and tiredness. These problems usually go away as the body adjusts to the drug and do not require medical treatment.

More serious side effects are not common, but may occur. If any of the following side effects occur, the patient should check with a physician immediately:

• itching or skin rash
• reddish or purplish spots on the skin
• such other skin problems as redness, blistering, or peeling
• severe, watery, or bloody diarrhea
• muscle or joint aches
• fever
• sore throat
• cough
• shortness of breath
• unusual tiredness or weakness
• unusual bleeding or bruising
• pale skin
• yellow eyes or skin
• swallowing problems

Other rare side effects may occur. Anyone who has unusual symptoms while taking sulfonamides should get in touch with his or her physician.

Interactions

Sulfonamides may interact with a large number of other medicines. When an interaction occurs, the effects of one or both of the drugs may change or the risk of side effects may be greater. Anyone who takes sulfonamides should give the physician a list of all other medicines that he or she is taking. Among the drugs that may interact with sulfonamides are:

• acetaminophen (Tylenol)

• medicines to treat an overactive thyroid gland

• male hormones (androgens)

• female hormones (estrogens)

• other medicines used to treat infections

• birth control pills

• such medicines for diabetes as glyburide (Micronase)

• warfarin (Coumadin) and other blood-thinning drugs (anticoagulants)

• disulfiram (Antabuse), a drug used to treat alcohol abuse

• amantadine (Symmetrel), used to treat influenza and also Parkinson's disease

• hydrochlorothiazide (HCTZ, HydroDIURIL) and other diuretics

• the anticancer drug methotrexate (Rheumatrex)

• valproic acid (Depakote, Depakene) and other antiseizure medications

Other medications may interact with sulfonamides. Patients should be careful to check with their physician or pharmacist before combining sulfonamides with any other prescription or nonprescription (over-the-counter) medicine, including vitamins and supplements. Some herbs, such as bearberry, parsley, dandelion leaf, and sarsaparilla, have a diuretic effect and should not be used while taking sulfa drugs. Basil, which is commonly used in cooking to flavor salad dressings, stews, and tomato recipes, is reported to affect the absorption of sulfonamides.

Resources

BOOKS

Cohen, Jonathan, William G. Powderly, and Stephen M. Opal. *Infectious Diseases.* 3rd ed. St. Louis: Mosby/Elsevier, 2010.

Mandell, Gerald L., John E. Bennett, and Raphael Dolin. *Principles and Practice of Infectious Diseases.* 7th ed. Philadelphia: Churchill Livingstone, 2010.

WEBSITES

Levison, Matthew E. "Sulfonamides." *The Merck Manual for Health Care Professionals* (online). http://www.merckmanuals.com/home/hormonal_and_metabolic_disorders/acid-base_balance/overview_of_acid-base_balance.html (accessed July 24, 2013).

Micromedex. "Sulfonamide (Oral Route)." http://www.mayoclinic.com/health/drug-information/DR602147 (accessed July 24, 2013).

ORGANIZATIONS

American Society of Health-System Pharmacists, 7272 Wisconsin Ave., Bethesda, MD 20814, (301) 664-8700, (866) 279-0681, custserv@ashp.org, http://www.ashp.org.

U.S. Food and Drug Administration, 10903 New Hampshire Ave., Silver Spring, MD 20993, (888) INFO-FDA (463-6332), http://www.fda.gov.

Nancy Ross-Flanigan
Sam Uretsky, PharmD

Surgeons

Definition

Surgeons are physicians who perform operations to treat injuries, diseases, and malformations. Surgeons have traditionally performed procedures that involve cutting and stitching tissue. However, with the development of new technologies, the distinction between surgery and other medical procedures is not always clearly defined.

Surgical specialties in the United States, 2010	
Specialty	Number of surgeons
Obstetrics and gynecology	34,083
General surgery	24,327
Orthopedic surgery	19,325
Ophthalmology	15,723
Urological surgery	8,606
Otolaryngology	7,964
Plastic surgery	6,180

SOURCE: National Center for Health Statistics, *Health, United States, 2012: With Special Feature on Emergency Care*, Hyattsville, MD: 2013. Available online at: http://www.cdc.gov/nchs/data/hus/hus12.pdf (accessed September 3, 2013).

(Table by PreMediaGlobal. Copyright © 2014 Cengage Learning®.)

Description

More than 53 million surgeries are performed in the United States each year. Surgeons may remove tissues, open blockages, reattach arteries and veins to improve blood flow to parts of the body, graft human or artificial tissues to replace blood vessels or connective tissue, insert metal rods into bones to repair injuries, or transplant organs. Surgeons also perform diagnoses, such as biopsies to remove tissue for examination under a microscope. In emergency situations, surgeons often diagnose and treat patients in a single operation.

Surgeons may be either medical doctors (MDs) or doctors of osteopathic medicine (DOs). Although they use the same surgical procedures, osteopathic surgeons emphasize the musculoskeletal system of the body and may promote preventive care and holistic healing.

Qualities and responsibilities

Surgery is an extremely demanding medical specialty. It requires coping with the unexpected in the **operating room** and making rapid decisions in situations where very short delays can cause serious complications. Surgeons must have good leadership skills and be able to communicate quickly and clearly with all members of the **surgical team**. The chief surgeon may need to direct assistant surgeons, as well as surgical nurses and other operating room personnel. Complex surgeries may require large surgical teams, including multiple surgeons with different specialties. Surgeons also work very closely with anesthesiologists. Studies have found that the leadership behaviors exhibited by surgeons include guidance and support, communication and coordination, and task management. Often, these behaviors are directed at the entire surgical team rather than a specific person.

Demanding behaviors are required much more frequently during highly complex procedures.

Surgery requires very precise physical dexterity and superb attention to detail, since the smallest mistake can have serious consequences. Surgeons must have patience and physical stamina, since operations can last for many hours, and surgeons may spend very long periods standing and bending over a patient.

Although the primary responsibilities of surgeons are in the operating room, they are also involved in many other aspects of patient care. They familiarize themselves with a patient's medical history, current condition, test results, and other treatments. They examine and counsel patients and perform and interpret diagnostic tests. Surgeons typically meet with patients before surgery to explain exactly what will take place, as well as potential risks and complications. Surgeons are required to treat patients with compassion, understanding, and respect.

Surgeons usually study and interpret their patients' imaging results, often in consultation with the radiologist.

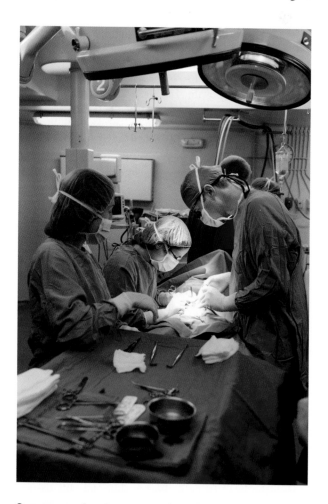

Surgeons performing an operation. *(Franck Boston/ Shutterstock.com)*

Various types of imaging are performed and displayed during surgery. Some surgeons have begun to use three-dimensional (3D) printers to construct plastic models from **computed tomography** (CT) scans. These models can be used in the operating room to reveal details such as the direction of blood vessels or the exact location of a tumor in the liver or kidney. Three-dimensional copies of bones are commonly used to guide **orthopedic surgery**. Oral surgeons are beginning to use 3-D copies of a patient's jaw to plan surgery, and custom templates may even be placed in the patient's mouth during an operation for the precise insertion of implants. The replicas can also help less-experienced surgeons practice with accurate models prior to an actual surgery.

Procedures

Surgeries must always be performed in a sterile environment to reduce the risk of infection. All members of the surgical team wear scrub suits, sterile gowns, booties, caps covering their hair, masks covering their noses and mouths, and sterile gloves. Before donning sterile gowns and gloves, the hands are thoroughly scrubbed with antimicrobial soap or an alcohol-based solution that has persistent and cumulative antimicrobial activity. This removes microorganisms from the fingernails, hands, and forearms; reduces resident microorganisms to the absolute minimum; and slows bacterial growth. The area under the fingernails harbors far more microorganisms than the skin of the hands and forearms. Therefore, fingernails are carefully cleaned with disposable nail cleaners under running water in the scrub sink. Fingernails must never extend beyond the fingertips because the nails could puncture the sterile gloves.

Surgical positioning—safely moving and securing the patient before and during surgery—is very important and is one of the factors that contributes to positive surgical outcomes and the prevention of complications. Once the patient is properly positioned for the surgery on the operating table and before the first incision, the surgeon calls a "time out." This is the signal for the team to confirm the identity of the patient and that the patient is correctly positioned for the surgery. The surgical site is confirmed. The availability of all required instruments and equipment and prophylaxis for preventing infection and blood clots is confirmed. All patient images relevant to the surgery are displayed.

Specialties

Many surgeons practice **general surgery**. General surgeons diagnose, treat, and manage patients with a wide variety of conditions affecting most parts of the body—the head or neck; breast; skin and soft tissues; abdomen; extremities; and gastrointestinal, vascular, and endocrine systems. In addition to establishing or confirming diagnoses, general surgeons provide preoperative, operative, and **postoperative care** and are often responsible for the overall care of trauma and critically ill patients.

After training in general surgery, many surgeons go on to specialize:

- Orthopedic surgeons treat the musculoskeletal system. Some orthopedic surgeons specialize in the foot and ankle, others in the knee and hip, and still other specialize in sports medicine. Hand surgeons are orthopedic surgeons who treat injuries, diseases, and abnormalities of the hand, including microvascular surgery for the reattachment of amputated fingers or hands.

- Neurological surgeons (neurosurgeons) provide both surgical and non-surgical management of disorders of the brain, spinal cord, spinal column, and peripheral nerves, as well as supporting structures and the blood supply. Some neurosurgeons specialize in pediatric neurosurgery.

- Thoracic and cardiovascular surgeons specialize in injuries of the airway and chest, in heart and respiratory diseases, and in coronary artery disease. Vascular surgeons treat the lymphatic system and arteries and veins other than those within the heart and brain.

- Plastic and reconstructive surgeons repair, replace, and reconstruct body coverings and the underlying musculoskeletal system. Subspecialties include hand surgery and plastic surgery of the head and neck. Plastic surgeons may specialize in cosmetic or reconstructive surgery or in pediatric plastic surgery.

- Pediatric surgeons specialize in the treatment of children from birth through adolescence. They may further specialize in prenatal surgery, newborn or neonatal surgery, traumatic injuries, surgical oncology (cancer), or gastrointestinal surgery.

- Critical care surgeons diagnose and treat trauma victims as well as critically ill patients with multi-organ involvement. They often coordinate teams of other doctors and nurses.

- Obstetric and gynecologic surgeons specialize in maternal/fetal medicine for complicated pregnancies, reproductive endocrinology and infertility, gynecological cancers, and female pelvic and reconstructive surgeries.

- Reproductive surgeons treat the reproductive system.

- Endrocrine surgeons treat components of the endocrine system.

- Urology surgeons treat conditions of the adrenal gland and genitourinary system.

- Laparoendoscopic surgeons specialize in laparoscopic surgery.
- Colon and rectal surgeons treat the intestinal tract, colon, rectum, and anus. They may also deal with intestinal diseases that involve the liver or the urinary and female reproductive systems. They may further specialize in abdominal open surgery or in endoscopy or other minimally invasive laparoscopic techniques.
- Gastrointestinal endoscopic surgeons specialize in endoscopic surgery of the digestive tract.
- Ophthalmologic surgeons treat ocular and visual disorders.
- Oral and maxillofacial surgeons specialize in dentistry and care for the health and appearance of the mouth and face.
- Otolaryngologists are head and neck surgeons who operate on the ears, nose, throat, respiratory and upper alimentary systems, and related structures. Subspecialties include neurotology for treating disorders of the ear and temporal bone, plastic surgery of the neck and head, and pediatric otolaryngology.
- Dermatologic surgeons treat skin conditions.

Distractions and errors

The operating room is a high-stress environment. Sharp instruments are a significant hazard for surgeons and staff. Angry outbursts by surgeons are commonplace in TV soap operas and appear frequently throughout the history of surgery. Verbal abuse and even **surgical instruments** have been hurled at nurses and residents. More recently, studies have documented typical operating room distractions and interruptions that can cause surgical trainees to commit errors, particularly later in the day.

"Never events" are surgical mistakes that should never happen—operating on the wrong patient or the wrong site, performing the wrong procedure, or sewing up a patient with an object left inside. A 2013 study found that U.S. surgeons make more than 4,000 such mistakes every year. The study was based on payouts for malpractice claims and the estimate that only 12% of adverse events result in paid claims. Other studies have shown that many patients never file malpractice claims. Furthermore, items left inside a patient are not necessarily discovered unless the patient has a postsurgical complication such as an infection. It is estimated that as many as one in three or four forgotten surgical sponges are never discovered. The time out before initiating surgery was introduced to eliminate errors such as wrong-patient and wrong-site surgeries. New technologies, such as bar codes and scanners, are intended to account for all sponges and other items. Indelible ink can

be used to mark the surgical site before the patient undergoes anesthesia. Such measures appear to be reducing the incidence of surgical errors.

Training and certification

Almost all surgeons have completed at least a four-year undergraduate program, followed by four years of medical school and three to eight years of internships and residencies, depending on the surgical specialty. The first two years of medical school are usually spent in the classroom and laboratory, followed by two years of supervised practical experience in clinics and hospitals, rotating through different specialties. Most medical school graduates carry large amounts of student debt. Surgeons must pass written and practical exams for state licensing, and many also pursue board certification in their particular specialty.

In an effort to reduce preventable errors by sleep-deprived residents, beginning in 2003, residents were

QUESTIONS TO ASK YOUR DOCTOR

- What is your surgical specialty?
- What training have you had in my surgical procedure?
- How many such procedures have you performed?
- What is your success rate with this procedure?
- What exactly will take place during my surgery?

restricted to an 80-hour workweek. Further restrictions on the working hours of surgeons-in-training went into effect in 2011. Studies have found that this resulted in a 26% reduction in surgical experience. Surgical interns reported participating in an average of 66 operations in 2011, compared with 89 in 2007–2010. Surveys of surgical residents show that the majority dislike the restrictions and believe that the quality of their education has declined as a result.

Work settings

Surgeons work in hospitals, clinics, health maintenance organizations (HMOs), group practices, and private offices. Surgeons work very closely with other surgeons, anesthesiologists, and other physicians and staff, including nurses and medical assistants. Complex surgeries may require the combined efforts of surgeons with different specialties. Surgeons often work long and irregular hours, including overnight shifts, and may have to travel frequently among offices, clinics, and hospitals. Increasingly, surgeons share a large number of patients with other doctors, which eases their workloads and permits the coordination of patient care, but reduces individual independence. Surgery is one of the highest paid occupations. In 2010, the mean annual compensation for general surgeons was almost $344,000.

Future outlook

Together, surgeons and other physicians held about 691,000 jobs in the United States in 2010. The number of jobs for physicians and surgeons is expected to increase by 24% between 2010 and 2020. The expansion of the healthcare industry, combined with an aging population, is expected to increase the demand for surgeons. Surgical specialties related to the medical needs of baby boomers, such as heart disease and cancer, are expected to be in particular demand. Despite these demands, the influx of

new medical personnel, along with new technologies and simplified and minimally invasive surgeries, are expected to reduce surgeons' workloads.

Rural and low-income urban areas have difficulty attracting and retaining physicians and surgeons. A 2013 study found that appendicitis more often leads to a ruptured appendix in areas with few general surgeons, because appendectomies are likely to be delayed. Less than three general surgeons per 100,000 population increased the likelihood of a ruptured appendix by 5% compared to areas that had at least five surgeons per 100,000.

Resources

BOOKS

Cooley, Denton A. *100,000 Hearts: A Surgeon's Memoir.* Austin, TX: Dolph Briscoe Center for American History, University of Texas, 2012.

Pickover, Clifford A. *The Medical Book: From Witch Doctors to Robot Surgeons: 250 Milestones in the History of Medicine.* New York: Sterling, 2012.

Ruggieri, Paul. *Confessions of a Surgeon: The Good, the Bad, and the Complicated . . . Life Behind the O.R. Doors.* New York: Berkley, 2012.

Stockinger, Zsolt T. *Fragments from Iraq: Diary of a Navy Trauma Surgeon.* Jefferson, NC: McFarland & Co., 2012.

Youn, Anthony, and Alan Eisenstock. *In Stitches: A Memoir.* New York: Gallery, 2012.

Yount, Lisa. *Alfred Blalock, Helen Taussig, and Vivien Thomas: Mending Children's Hearts.* New York: Chelsea, 2012.

PERIODICALS

Cristancho, Sayra M., et al. "When Surgeons Face Intraoperative Challenges: A Naturalistic Model of Surgical Decision Making." *American Journal of Surgery* 205, no. 2 (February 2013): 156–62.

Gelber, David, and Susan Jensen. "Behind the Mask: The Mystique of Surgery and the Surgeons Who Perform Them." *AORN Journal* 96, no. 3 (September 2012): 347–8.

Jacobs, George, and Rosanne Wille. "Consequences and Potential Problems of Operating Room Outbursts and Temper Tantrums by Surgeons." *Surgical Neurology International* Suppl. 33 (2012): 167–73.

Landro, Laura. "Surgeons Make Thousands of Errors." *Wall Street Journal* (December 20, 2012): A2.

Parker, Sarah Henrickson, et al. "Surgeons' Leadership in the Operating Room: An Observational Study." *American Journal of Surgery* 204, no. 3 (September 2012): 347–54.

WEBSITES

American College of Surgeons. "Looking for a Qualified Surgeon? Here's How." http://www.facs.org/public_info/yourhealth/findadoc.html (accessed September 18, 2013).

Bureau of Labor Statistics. "Occupational Outlook Handbook." http://stats.bls.gov/ooh/Healthcare/Physicians-and-surgeons.htm (accessed September 18, 2013).

Doyle, Kathryn. "Surgeon Shortage Linked to Burst Appendices." MedlinePlus. June 14, 2013. http://www.nlm.nih.gov/medlineplus/news/fullstory_137856.html (accessed September 18, 2013).

Seaman, Andrew M. "Less Practice for Surgeons-in-Training After Restrictions." MedlinePlus. July 10, 2013. http://www.nlm.nih.gov/medlineplus/news/fullstory_138599.html (accessed September 18, 2013).

ORGANIZATIONS

American Academy of Neurological and Orthopaedic Surgeons, 1516 N. Lakeshore Dr., Chicago, IL 60610, (800) 766-3427, Fax: (312) 787-9289, http://www.aanos.org.

American Academy of Orthopaedic Surgeons (AAOS), 6300 N. River Rd., Rosemont, IL 60018-4262, (847) 823-7186, Fax: (847) 823-8125, pemr@aaos.org, http://www.aaos.org.

American Association of Endocrine Surgeons, 5019 W. 147th St., Leawood, KS 66224, (913) 402-7102, Fax: (913) 273-9940, information@endocrinesurgery.org, http://www.endocrinesurgery.org.

American Association of Hip and Knee Surgeons (AAHKS), 6300 N. River Rd., Ste. 615, Rosemont, IL 60018-4237, (847) 698-1200, Fax: (847) 698-0704, helpdesk@aahks.org, http://www.aahks.org.

American Association of Oral and Maxillofacial Surgeons, 9700 W. Bryn Mawr Ave., Rosemont, IL 60018-5701, (847) 678-6200, (800) 822-6637, Fax: (847) 678-6286, http://www.aaoms.org.

American College of Surgeons, 633 N. Saint Clair St., Chicago, IL 60611-3211, (312) 202-5000, (800) 621-4111, Fax: (312) 202-5001, postmaster@facs.org, http://www.facs.org.

American Society of Colon and Rectal Surgeons, 85 W. Algonquin Rd., Ste. 550, Arlington Heights, IL 60005, (847) 290-9184, Fax: (847) 290-9203, ascrs@fascrs.org, http://www.fascrs.org.

American Society of Plastic Surgeons, 444 E. Algonquin Rd., Arlington Heights, IL 60005, http://www.plasticsurgery.org.

American Society of Transplant Surgeons (ASTS), 2461 South Clark St., Ste. 640, Arlington, VA 22202, (703) 414-7870, http://www.asts.org.

The Canadian Society of Plastic Surgeons, 1469 St. Joseph Blvd. E., #4, Montreal, Quebec H2J 1M6, Canada, (514) 843-5415, http://www.plasticsurgery.ca.

Royal College of Surgeons of England, 35/43 Lincoln's Inn Fields, London WC2A 3PE, England, +44 207 405 8074, office@baoms.org.uk, http://www.baoms.org.uk.

The Society of Thoracic Surgeons, 633 N. Saint Clair St., Fl. 23, Chicago, IL 60611, (312) 202-5800, Fax: (312) 202-5801, http://sts.org.

Margaret Alic, PhD

Surgery and the elderly

Definition

Older patients have different physiological needs and risk factors than younger patients, and surgery in the elderly refers to not only surgical procedures but also the specific measures taken before, during, and after surgery to account for the differences in physical and mental functioning between older and younger adults. Geriatric surgery is not considered a distinct surgical specialty, but the phrase is increasingly used to refer to the special requirements associated with surgery in elderly patients.

Although 65 years of age has been used for some time as an arbitrary cutoff point to distinguish seniors from younger adults, doctors recognize that older adults vary widely in their cardiovascular fitness levels, health status, mental alertness, personality traits, and other factors that are now known to affect their readiness for surgery and their ability to recover from it. Chronological age is considered less important than physiological age in determining whether an elderly patient will benefit from a specific surgical procedure. The emphasis is on a careful preoperative assessment of elderly patients that considers all aspects of a patient's well-being, rather than basing the decision on whether or not to operate solely on chronological age.

Purpose

Surgery in the elderly is most often performed to treat a specific disease or condition. The primary goal of geriatric surgery as a field of medicine is to encourage cooperation between specialists in geriatrics and doctors in various surgical specialties to improve surgical outcomes for older adults. There is no surgical procedure unique to elderly humans—older adults receive the same treatments for cancer, cardiovascular disorders, gastrointestinal complaints, musculoskeletal injuries, and disorders of other body systems as younger adults. The field of geriatric surgery seeks to apply knowledge of the aging process in humans across the surgical specialties.

A secondary drive behind geriatric surgery is research. Older adults have traditionally been excluded from clinical trials of various surgical procedures, imaging techniques, anesthetics, and other treatment innovations. As a result, less was known about the effectiveness of newer treatments in the elderly. As of mid-2013, however, there were more than 500 clinical trials of surgical procedures, anesthetics, and postoperative complications in elderly patients registered with the National Institutes of Health (NIH). This new interest in clinical research with elderly subjects should further improve surgeons' understanding of the effects of aging on the human body and mind.

Demographics

The major factor stimulating interest in geriatric surgery is the aging of the U.S. population coupled with a shortage of geriatricians (doctors who specialize in the health care of the elderly). The number of people over 65 in the United States is expected to increase from 35 million in 2013 to 78 million by 2050. The number of seniors over 85 is expected to quadruple in the same time period to 18.2 million, and possibly as high as 30 million. The rapid increase in the population of the elderly is the result of two changes: advances in medical care that enable people to live much longer than previous generations, and the fact that the post–World War II "baby boomers" are now reaching retirement age.

In addition to the increase in the numbers of the elderly, **surgeons** are concerned about the fact that this age group requires a disproportionate number of surgical operations. Although seniors make up only 12% of the U.S. population, they account for 40% of surgical operations—a proportion that will certainly increase when seniors become 20% of the population in North America, projected for 2030. Moreover, technological improvements across a range of procedures—from joint replacements and **spinal fusion** to cataract removal and cardiac catheterization—mean that more elderly patients are candidates for surgery than in the past.

Description

In general, the most important age-related change that affects an older adult's readiness for surgery is decreased functional reserve. This means that while the older adult's baseline functioning may decrease only slightly with age, their body's ability to function at a maximal level under such stress as a major surgical procedure is significantly lower. Elderly people can tolerate major or lengthy operations, but the very largest or most complicated operations will challenge their functional reserve. Other major age-related changes in elderly adults that affect their readiness for surgery include:

- Mental decline. Older adults with cognitive disorders like dementia are at increased risk of postoperative delirium, which in turn is associated with longer hospital stays, functional decline, and increased postoperative mortality. Some studies indicate that dementia by itself increases postoperative mortality by 52%.
- Poor functional status. Functional impairments in the elderly are sometimes referred to as the "geriatric giants"; in addition to intellectual impairment, they include immobility, incontinence, and instability (susceptibility to falling).
- Limited social and housekeeping support at home.

- High severity of the illness to be treated.
- Age itself. One study of abdominal procedures in the elderly reported that the mortality rate for patients aged 80–84 years was 3%, 9% for patients aged 85–89 years, and 25% for patients older than 90.

Preparation

Preparation is the most important stage of surgery in elderly patients because of the potential for complications in this age group as well as the differences in health status among patients. Ideally, older adults considering nonemergency surgery should consult with a geriatrician as well as their surgeon before undergoing surgery. The anesthesiologist may also participate in the consultation. Patients should come prepared with questions for the anesthesiologist as well as the surgeon, and bring a complete list of all prescription medications they take regularly, as well as over-the-counter (OTC) preparations, vitamins, herbal remedies, and supplements.

Preoperative assessment of elderly candidates for surgery

In 2012, the American Geriatrics Society (AGS) and the American College of Surgeons (ACS) compiled a checklist of 13 assessments that should be made in addition to a standard **physical examination** for elderly patients considering surgery:

- Assess the patient's cognitive ability. Cognitive ability includes the patient's capacity to provide informed consent for the procedure, as well as to understand what the surgery involves and why it is recommended. In some cases, family members may be consulted for evidence of recent cognitive decline in the patient. Accurate preoperative assessment of the patient's cognitive ability is important in evaluating the significance of any postoperative cognitive disturbances.
- Screen the patient for depression.
- Identify any risk factors for postoperative delirium. Postoperative delirium is a common complication in elderly patients, ranging from 9% to 52% in some samples, depending on the complexity of the surgery. Risk factors for postoperative delirium include dementia, sleep deprivation, alcohol or substance abuse, depression, anemia, poor nutrition, kidney insufficiency, dehydration, polypharmacy, impaired vision or hearing, and the presence of a urinary catheter.
- Screen the patient for alcohol or substance abuse.
- Perform a preoperative cardiac evaluation.
- Assess risk factors for postoperative pulmonary complications. These include a history of smoking, history of breathing disorders, congestive heart failure,

obstructive sleep apnea, recent unintended weight loss, age above 60 years, and abnormal values on kidney function tests.

- Document the patient's functional status and history of falls (if any).
- Determine the patient's baseline frailty score.
- Assess the patient's nutritional status; consider preoperative treatment if the patient appears to be malnourished.
- Obtain a detailed and complete medication history and make any necessary adjustments before surgery, and also monitor the patient for polypharmacy (the use of five or more prescription drugs on a regular basis). Prescription medications most likely to cause postoperative complications are sleep medications, narcotic pain relievers, antidepressants, and benzodiazepine tranquilizers.
- Evaluate the patient's expectations of and goals for treatment in light of the likely outcome.
- Evaluate the patient's family and social support network.
- Order the appropriate preoperative tests.

Tests

The current ACS/AGS recommendations regarding preoperative tests for elderly surgical patients distinguish between a small group of tests for all such patients and two additional groups of laboratory or functional tests for selected patients.

Preoperative tests recommended for all geriatric surgical patients include:

- hemoglobin test
- kidney function tests—blood urea nitrogen (BUN) and creatinine
- serum albumin

Laboratory tests for selected patients include:

- white blood cell count (WBC), done in case of known or suspected infection or suspected leukopenia from drugs
- platelet count
- coagulation tests, done for known or suspected bleeding disorders or malnutrition, or in patients undergoing cardiac or cancer surgery
- electrolytes, done for patients with kidney insufficiency or congestive heart failure, or for patients taking certain prescription medications (diuretics, digoxin, ACE inhibitors)
- serum glucose, done for patients with obesity or known or suspected diabetes
- urinalysis, done for patients with diabetes or suspected urinary tract infection, or patients undergoing urogenital surgery

Preoperative imaging and function tests for selected patients:

- chest x-ray, done for patients with a history of smoking or lung disease, scheduled for major surgery, or who may require stays in an intensive care unit (ICU)
- electrocardiogram (EKG), done for patients undergoing vascular or intermediate-risk surgery or with a known history of heart disease, previous heart attack, vascular disease, kidney insufficiency, cardiac arrhythmias, prior heart failure, or respiratory disease
- pulmonary function tests (PFT), done for patients undergoing lung resection or with obstructive lung disease or questionable pulmonary function
- noninvasive stress testing, done if a patient has three or more clinical risk factors and poor functional capacity

Aftercare

Aftercare for elderly patients depends on the specific surgical procedure. One of the most important considerations in all patients, however, is pain management. Certain pain relievers, particularly **acetaminophen**, meperidine, and propoxyphene, are avoided in older patients because of the increased risk of toxicity. Other opioid pain relievers also increase the risk of postoperative side effects in elderly patients.

A new trend in many hospitals is the construction of specialized acute-care geriatric units with enhanced patient-centered care. **Postoperative care** in these units focuses on rehabilitation and preserving the patient's ability to return to independent living after discharge rather than being released to a long-term care facility. Patients are encouraged to resume activities of daily living (ADL) as soon as possible.

Very frail elderly patients who undergo major surgery often require prolonged ventilation on an mechanical ventilator in a surgical ICU after the operation.

Alternative

An important part of preoperative as well as postoperative care for some elderly patients is spiritual care. Elderly patients are more likely than their younger counterparts to say that religion plays an important role in their life; for many, their faith community is their most important social support group outside their family. It is appropriate for surgeons and other medical professionals to ask elderly patients about their spiritual needs and to find out whether the hospital or surgical center can provide appropriate pastoral care if the patient's own religious leader cannot visit.

Risks

Elderly patients are at increased risk of postoperative complications, including inadequate nutrition; wound breakdown; and other neurologic, pulmonary, and cardiovascular complications.

- Proper nutrition is important for geriatric patients to assist in wound healing. Elderly patients have frail skin and are prone to pressure ulcers, wound breakdown, and slow healing. Elderly patients sometimes lack the support they need to ensure a balanced diet and may need the help of a nutritionist. Some geriatric patients are advised to drink a diet supplement to get the required number of vitamins to promote wound healing.

- Neurological complications include postoperative delirium and postoperative cognitive dysfunction (POCD). Postoperative delirium is the most common postsurgical complication in the elderly, affecting between 15% and 53% of patients over 65. The patient is confused and disoriented, with some periods of lucidity, for a week to ten days after surgery. The most important risk factors for postoperative delirium are dementia and advanced age. POCD is a condition in which a patient experiences long-term problems with memory, ability to concentrate, and other cognitive functions after surgery. POCD was first observed in patients who had undergone cardiac surgery but may occur after other major operations. The risk of POCD increases in patients over 60 years of age and in those with a history of alcohol or drug abuse. It is thought that the body's inflammatory response to surgery plays a role in the emergence of POCD, but the condition is not yet well understood.

- Pulmonary complications affect about 7% of elderly surgical patients. Patient-related risk factors include advanced age, chronic obstructive pulmonary disease (COPD), congestive heart failure, and poor functional status. With regard to surgery, abdominal, aortic, and thoracic surgery carry the highest risk of pulmonary complications. Other surgery-related risks include emergency surgery, procedure length over three hours, use of general anesthesia, and multiple transfusions during surgery.

- Cardiac complications occur in 12% of older surgical patients. Risk factors include patient age over 65, obesity, emergency surgery, prior cardiac surgery, congestive heart failure, cerebrovascular disease, high blood pressure, procedure length over 3.8 hours, and administration of packed red blood cells during surgery.

Results

The results of surgery in the elderly are influenced by a number of different factors, including the patient's preoperative health status; the patient's previous lifestyle choices (particularly smoking and heavy drinking); the type, location, and complexity of the surgical procedure performed; the surgeon's training and length of experience; the thoroughness of the patient's preoperative assessment; and the number and severity of the patient's comorbid disorders (if any).

Morbidity and mortality rates

Morbidity and mortality following surgery are higher in certain groups of elderly patients, regardless of the specific surgery performed. These include:

- patients who were in nursing homes rather than living independently prior to surgery

- patients with several comorbid chronic health problems, such as diabetes, congestive heart failure, malnutrition, chronic obstructive pulmonary disease, HIV infection, cancer, kidney disorders, or uncontrolled high blood pressure

QUESTIONS TO ASK YOUR DOCTOR

- Have you ever referred patients to a geriatrician prior to surgery?
- Have you ever conducted a detailed preoperative assessment of an elderly patient?
- Have you ever advised a patient to consider alternatives to invasive surgery?
- What is your opinion of specialized geriatric surgical centers or inpatient units?

• patients who are clinically depressed

• patients with dementia

• patients who have no family or social support network

In general, elderly patients have much higher rates of morbidity and mortality following **emergency surgery** than elective procedures—a finding that underscores the importance of preoperative assessment and (when needed) appropriate treatment before the surgery.

Alternatives

Alternatives to surgery in the elderly include the decision not to perform an elective procedure when the stress on the patient's body or a high risk of complications may outweigh any benefits. In some cases, such as gallbladder attacks or appendicitis, the patient may be treated with **antibiotics** or a drain inserted under **local anesthesia** rather than major abdominal surgery. An article published in the *New York Times* in 2012 reported on these alternatives for nursing home residents, who have a much higher risk of postoperative complications than elderly patients living independently.

Another alternative to major surgery in the elderly is the use of less invasive procedures, including minimally invasive spinal surgical techniques as well as laparoscopic procedures for abdominal disorders rather than open abdominal surgery. Several studies have reported that elderly patients have fewer complications following less invasive procedures and recover more quickly than those treated with open surgery.

Health care team roles

Surgery in elderly patients may be performed in outpatient clinics or ambulatory surgical centers as well as in hospitals or specialized geriatric surgery centers. The surgeons, geriatricians, and anesthesiologists who are involved in preoperative assessment and the surgery

itself are assisted by nurses and other medical specialists as needed. The patient's rehabilitation following surgery is carried out by respiratory therapists, physical therapists, and speech therapists. The patient may also need the services of a psychologist, social worker, and nutritionist.

Resources

BOOKS

Kahn, Joseph H., Brendan G. Magauran Jr., and Jonathan S. Olshaker, eds. *Geriatric Emergency Medicine: Principles and Practice*. Cambridge, UK: Cambridge University Press, 2014.

Katlic, Mark R., ed. *Cardiothoracic Surgery in the Elderly*. New York: Springer, 2011.

Rosenthal, Ronnie A., Michael E. Zenilman, and Mark R. Katlic, eds. *Principles and Practice of Geriatric Surgery*, 2nd ed. New York: Springer, 2011.

Spiliotis, John D., and Konstantinos Tepetes, eds. *Cancer Surgery in the Elderly*. New York: Nova Science Publishers, 2011.

Wilmoth, Janet F., and Kenneth F. Ferraro, eds. *Gerontology: Perspectives and Issues*, 4th ed. New York: Springer, 2013.

PERIODICALS

Bartels, K., et al. "Neurocognitive Outcomes after Cardiac Surgery." *Current Opinion in Anaesthesiology* 26 (February 2013): 91–97.

Brown, E. N., and P.L. Purdon. "The Aging Brain and Anesthesia." *Current Opinion in Anesthesiology* 26 (August 2013): 414–19.

Chow, W. B., et al. "Optimal Preoperative Assessment of the Geriatric Surgical Patient: A Best Practices Guideline from the American College of Surgeons National Surgical Quality Improvement Program and the American Geriatrics Society." *Journal of the American College of Surgeons* 215 (October 2012): 453–66.

Jung, S. W. "Indirect Reduction Maneuver and Minimally Invasive Approach for Displaced Proximal Humerus Fractures in Elderly Patients." *Clinics in Orthopedic Surgery* 5 (March 2013): 66–73.

Petre, B.M., et al. "Pain Reporting, Opiate Dosing, and the Adverse Effects of Opiates after Hip or Knee Replacement in Patients 60 Years Old or Older." *Geriatric Orthopaedic Surgery and Rehabilitation* 3 (March 2012): 3–7.

Scarpa, M., et al. "Minimally Invasive Surgery for Colorectal Cancer: Quality of Life and Satisfaction with Care in Elderly Patients." *Surgical Endoscopy* 27 (August 2013): 2911–20.

Shiono, S., et al. "Postoperative Complications in Elderly Patients after Lung Cancer Surgery." *Interactive Cardiovascular and Thoracic Surgery* 16 (June 2013): 819–23.

Sieber, F. E., and S. R. Barnett. "Preventing Postoperative Complications in the Elderly." *Anesthesiology Clinics* 29 (March 2011): 83–97.

Span, Paula. "Avoiding Surgery in the Elderly." *New York Times*, January 25, 2012.

Vacas, S., et al. "The Neuroinflammatory Response of Postoperative Cognitive Decline." *British Medical Bulletin* 106 (2013): 161–78.

WEBSITES

American Geriatrics Society (AGS). "Geriatrics for Specialists: Getting Involved." http://specialists.americangeriatrics.org/involved.php (accessed September 8, 2013).

American Society of Anesthesiologists (ASA). "Seniors and Anesthesia." https://www.asahq.org/sitecore/content/lifeline/anesthesia-topics/seniors-and-anesthesia.aspx (accessed September 8, 2013).

Ersan, Tulay. "Perioperative Management of the Geriatric Patient." Medscape Reference. http://emedicine.medscape.com/article/285433-overview#showall (accessed September 8, 2013).

LifeBridgeHealth. "Dr. Mark Katlic Discusses the Sinai Center for Geriatric Surgery." YouTube video, 3:00. http://www.youtube.com/watch?v=rqijb-ooCto (accessed September 8, 2013).

Merck Manual for Health Care Professionals. "Religion and Spirituality in the Elderly." http://www.merckmanuals.com/professional/geriatrics/social_issues_in_the_elderly/religion_and_spirituality_in_the_elderly.html (accessed September 8, 2013).

ORGANIZATIONS

American Academy of Orthopaedic Surgeons (AAOS), 6300 N River Rd., Rosemont, IL 60018-4262, (847) 823-7186, Fax: (847) 823-8125, orthoinfo@aaos.org, http://www.aaos.org.

American College of Surgeons (ACS), 633 N Saint Clair St., Chicago, IL 60611-3211, (312) 202-5000, Fax: (312) 202-5001, (800) 621-4111, http://www.facs.org/contact/contact.html, http://www.facs.org/index.html.

American Geriatrics Society (AGS), 40 Fulton St., 18th Fl., New York, NY 10038, (212) 308-1414, Fax: (212) 832-8646, info.amger@americangeriatrics.org, http://www.americangeriatrics.org.

American Society of Anesthesiologists (ASA), 520 N Northwest Highway, Park Ridge, IL 60068-2573, (847) 825-5586, Fax: (847) 825-1692, communications@asahq.org, http://www.asahq.org.

National Institute on Aging (NIA), Bldg. 31, Rm. 5C27, 31 Center Dr., MSC 2292, Bethesda, MD 20892, (800) 222-2225, Information Center: niaic@nia.nih.gov, http://www.nia.nih.gov.

Sinai Center for Geriatric Surgery, Sinai Hospital, 2401 W Belvedere Ave., Baltimore, MD 21215, (410) 601-5719, jocolema@lifebridgehealth.org, http://www.lifebridgehealth.org/GeriatricSurgery/GeriatricSurgery1.aspx.

Rebecca J. Frey, PhD

Surgical debridement *see* **Debridement**

Surgical glue *see* **Closures**

Surgical instruments

Definition

Surgical instruments are tools or devices that perform functions such as cutting, dissecting, grasping, holding, retracting, or suturing. Most surgical instruments are made from stainless steel. Other metals, such as titanium, chromium, vanadium, and molybdenum, are also used. The specific usage of the instrument is determined by the design of the instrument.

Purpose

Surgical instruments facilitate a variety of procedures and operations. Specialized surgical sets or trays contain the most common instruments needed for particular surgeries.

In the United States, surgical instruments are used in all hospitals, outpatient facilities, and most professional offices. Users of surgical instruments include **surgeons**, dentists, physicians, and many other health care

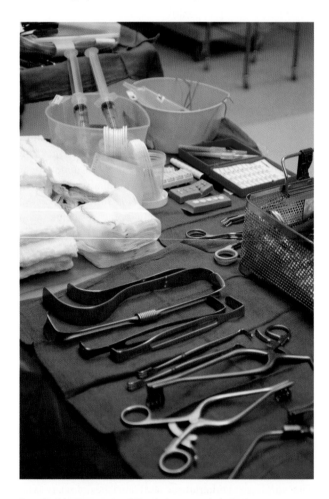

Surgical instruments. *(iStockphoto.com/miralex)*

providers. Millions of new and replacement instruments are sold each year. Many modern surgical instruments have electronic or computerized components.

Description

Basic categories of surgical instruments include specialized implements for the following functions:

- cutting, grinding, and dissecting
- clamping or occluding
- grasping and holding
- probing
- dilating or enlarging
- retracting
- suctioning
- suturing

Scissors are an example of cutting instruments. Dissecting instruments are used to cut or separate tissue. Dissectors may be sharp or blunt. One example of a sharp dissector is a scalpel. Examples of blunt dissectors include the back of a knife handle, curettes, and elevators. Clamps, tenacula, and forceps are grasping and holding instruments. Probing instruments are used to enter natural openings, such as the common bile duct, or fistulas. Dilating instruments expand the size of an opening, such as to the urethra or cervix. Retractors assist in the visualization of the operative field while preventing trauma to other tissues. Suction devices remove blood and other fluids from a surgical or dental operative field. Suturing instruments such as needle holders are used in conjunction with suturing material for occlusion of vessels or approximation of tissue.

Risks

Risks associated with surgical instruments include improper use or technique by an operator, leaving an instrument inside a person after an operation, and transmitting infection or disease due to improper cleaning and sterilization techniques. Improperly cleaned or sterilized instruments may contribute to **postoperative infections** or mortality. Improper use of surgical instruments may contribute to postoperative complications.

Operation

Any tool with a sharp edge (sharps) and all related items should be counted four times: prior to the start of the procedure, before closure of a cavity within a cavity, before wound closure begins, and at skin closure or the end of the procedure. A count should also be performed when adding anything to the sterile set up. In addition, a count should be taken any time surgical personnel are

replaced before, during, or after a procedure. Instruments, sharp tools, and sponges should be counted during all procedures in which there is a possibility of leaving an item inside a patient.

Surgical instruments are maintained and sterilized prior to use and must be kept clean during all procedures. This is accomplished by carefully wiping with a moist sponge. They may also be rinsed in sterile water if they have excessive or dried blood on them. Periodic cleaning during the procedure prevents blood and other tissues from hardening and becoming trapped on the surface of an instrument.

Maintenance

Instruments should always be inspected before, during, and after surgical or dental procedures. Inspection is an ongoing process that must be carried out by all members of a **surgical team**. Surgical scissors, for example, must be sharp and smooth and must cut easily. Their edges must be inspected for chips, nicks, or dents.

Instruments must be promptly rinsed and thoroughly cleaned and sterilized after a procedure. Ultrasonic cleaning and automatic washing often follow the manual cleaning of instruments. Instruments may also be placed into an autoclave after manual cleaning. The manufacturer's instructions must be followed for each type of machine. Staff members responsible for cleaning instruments should wear protective gloves, waterproof aprons, and face shields to protect themselves and maintain instrument sterility.

The staff members responsible for cleaning and disinfecting the instruments should also inspect them. The instruments should be inspected again after cleaning and during packaging. Any instrument that is not in good working order should be sent for repair. Depending on their use, surgical instruments can last for up to ten years, given proper care.

Health care team roles

Patient observation after surgical or dental procedures provides the best indication that correct instrument handling and **aseptic technique** were followed during surgery. After an operation or dental procedure, health care team members should make sure that patients show no evidence of surgical site infection or of retained instruments or sponges.

Training

Instruction in the use and care of surgical instruments may range from the medical training required by physicians and dentists to on-the-job training for orderlies and aides. Surgical instruments are prepared for use according to strict institutional and professional protocols.

Resources

BOOKS

Brunicardi, F. C., D. K. Anderson, D. L. Dunn, J. G. Hunter, and R. E. Pollock. *Schwartz's Manual of Surgery.* 8th ed. New York: McGraw Hill, 2006.

Ellis, Harold, Sir Roy Caine, and Christopher Watson. *General Surgery: Lecture Notes.* 12th ed. Hoboken, NJ: Wiley-Blackwell, 2011.

Lawrence, Peter F., ed. *Essentials of General Surgery.* 5th ed. Philadelphia: Lippincott Williams & Wilkins, 2013.

Townsend, Courtney M., et al. *Sabiston Textbook of Surgery.* 19th ed. Philadelphia: Saunders/Elsevier, 2012.

PERIODICALS

Egorova, N. N., A. Moskowitz, A. Gelijns, A. Weinberg, et al. "Managing the Prevention of Retained Surgical Instruments: What Is the Value of Counting?" *Annals of Surgery* 247, no. 1 (January 2008): 13–18.

Ryu, Jiwon, Jaesoon Choi, and Hee Chan Kim. "Endoscopic Vision-Based Tracking of Multiple Surgical Instruments During Robot-Assisted Surgery." *Artificial Organs* 37, no. 1 (2013): 107–12. http://dx.doi.org/10.1111/j.1525-1594.2012.01543.x (accessed August 12, 2013).

Seavey, Rose. "High-Level Disinfection, Sterilization, and Antisepsis: Current Issues in Reprocessing Medical and Surgical Instruments." *American Journal of Infection Control* 41, suppl. 5 (2013): S111–17. http://dx.doi.org/10.1016/j.ajic.2012.09.030 (accessed August 12, 2013).

WEBSITES

Spartanburg Community College Library. "Basic Surgical Instruments." http://library.sccsc.edu/surgtech/instrument.htm (accessed August 12, 2013).

ORGANIZATIONS

American Board of Surgery, 1617 John F. Kennedy Blvd., Ste. 860, Philadelphia, PA 19103-1847, (215) 568-4000, Fax: (215) 563-5718, http://www.absurgery.org.

American College of Surgeons, 633 N. Saint Clair St., Chicago, IL 60611-3211, (312) 202-5000, (800) 621-4111, Fax: (312) 202-5001, postmaster@facs.org, http://www.facs.org.

Association of periOperative Registered Nurses (AORN), 2170 S. Parker Rd., Ste. 400, Denver, CO 80231-5711, (303) 755-6300, (800) 755-2676, Fax: (800) 847-0045, custsvc@aorn.org, http://www.aorn.org.

Association of Surgical Technologists, 6 West Dry Creek Cir., Ste. 200, Littleton, CO 80120-8031, (303) 694-9130, (800) 637-7433, Fax: (303) 694-9169, http://www.ast.org.

L. Fleming Fallon Jr., MD, DrPH

Surgical mesh

Definition

Surgical mesh is a sterile woven piece of netting that is used in surgical procedures to help repair sites of surgical incision, tissue herniation, or to provide support to internal parts of the body.

Purpose

Surgical mesh is used in many different types of surgical procedures. Hernia repair is one of the most frequently performed general surgeries worldwide, and usually involves the use of surgical mesh. Mesh is also used to assist in surgical correction of urinary incontinence, uterine suspension, vertebral reconstruction, tissue reconstruction, and vaginal prolapse, and for devices implanted to support the heart.

Description

Surgical mesh can be used in many different surgical procedures to provide wound closure or support for internal body parts. Also known as a patch or screen, surgical mesh

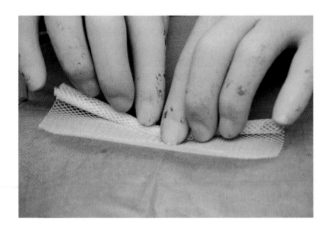

A surgeon prepares surgical mesh for use during surgery.

is implanted in the body for repair or reinforcement. Surgical mesh may be absorbable or nonabsorbable. Some types of repair procedures using surgical mesh may also be called a "Lichtenstein repair," because of a surgeon named Irving Lichtenstein whose influence in the medical field increased the widespread use of surgical mesh. A Lichtenstein repair is a flat piece of surgical mesh used as a patch placed on top of a tissue defect.

Surgical mesh is usually a sterile, woven material made of a type of synthetic plastic. Surgical mesh can be made of various different types of synthetic material, such as Gore-Tex, polypropylene, or knitted polyester. Mesh is very sturdy and strong, yet extremely thin. It is soft and flexible to allow it to easily conform to the movement of the body. Surgical mesh is available in various measurements and can be cut to size for each surgical application. Depending on the type of repair that is needed, a patch of mesh is placed under, over, or within a defect in the body and sewn in place by a few sutures. The mesh acts as a type of scaffold for the body tissue that grows around and into the mesh. It is also used like a sling to support internal body parts and hold them in place.

Once inserted, mesh is eventually incorporated into the surrounding tissue as if it were part of the body. For this reason, mesh is considered a tension-free type of repair, as opposed to sutures. Sutures hold flesh together through the tension they create by pulling tissues together to close a wound. Because sutures create tension in the tissue they repair, too much movement early on in the recovery period after surgery can reopen the repair site and cause internal bleeding. Mesh is different in that it does not rely on tension to hold tissue together; rather, the mesh itself fills the wound and allows tissue to grow into and around it. Patients in whom surgical mesh has been used may resume activity much sooner after the

surgical procedure than is usually seen with tension repair techniques. Surgical mesh may be used in the form of a patch that goes under or over tissues or a plug that goes inside a hole in the tissue. The patient cannot feel the internal mesh and is able to move freely.

Tissue support

Surgical mesh may be used to help physically support body tissues that are weak or damaged. One example of a procedure that may benefit from mesh in this way is uterine suspension. Uterine suspension is necessary when the uterus is tipped out of its normal position and causes medical complications. Uterine suspension is performed to put the uterus back into its normal position. Surgical mesh may be used as a sling to support the uterus and hold it in place. A second example of mesh used for tissue support is as a sling for the urethra in treating some types of urinary incontinence where the urethra has fallen out of its normal position. In surgery done for urinary incontinence, a sling is put in place to lift the urethra back into its normal position and create a type of pressure that helps prevent the incontinence. A mesh sling may be used and attached to the abdominal wall, where the body tissue will grow around and into it to provide strength and support.

Hernia repair

Hernia repair is the most common use for surgical mesh. A hernia is a protrusion of body tissues through a defect in a muscle or other body parts. Mesh may be used to repair the defect that allowed the herniation of body tissue. Hernias used to be commonly repaired using sutures and other types of tension-based tissue closure techniques. However, sutures do not allow for free movement as soon after the surgery. They are associated with a higher postoperative intra-abdominal pressure, consequent breathing problems, and a higher rate of hernia recurrence than mesh. Mesh hernia repair also causes less pain after surgery than suture repair.

Almost all hernia repairs are performed today using tension-free surgical mesh. Polypropylene is one of the most commonly used synthetic meshes in hernia repair, with each type of mesh material having advantages and disadvantages for hernia repair. Some hernia repair techniques using mesh include the Lichtenstien repair, where mesh is placed over the defect in the tissue; the Kugel method, where mesh is placed behind the defect; and the Prolene Hernia System, where two layers of mesh are placed around the defect, one behind and one over the defect. Another method of mesh-based hernia repair is the plug-and-patch method, where mesh is placed like a plug into the tissue defect and then covered over the top with another mesh patch. Hernia repairs using mesh may

Adhesions—Scar tissue.

Intra-abdominal pressure—The pressure present in the abdominal cavity that affects the pressure on the diaphragm and the ability to breathe easily.

Prolapse—A condition where organs fall out of their normal location in the body.

Sutures—Stitches that are used in surgical procedures to bring two pieces of flesh together or close a wound.

Urinary incontinence—Disorder where urination is uncontrolled and involuntary.

Uterine suspension—Procedure that places a sling under the uterus and holds it in place.

Vertebral reconstruction—Procedure for reconstruction and support of the vertebrae of the skeletal system.

be done as same day surgery using only **local anesthesia**. Because surgical mesh is a type of tension-free repair, patients can resume normal physical activity much sooner after the operation.

Risks

While the use of surgical mesh has many advantages over other techniques, it is also associated with the risk of some medical complications. One of the greatest risks of the use of surgical mesh is infection. Mesh infections tend to be resistant to **wound care** techniques and **antibiotics** and are generally removed upon discovery. Removal of infected mesh necessitates a new surgical procedure and the replacement of the mesh with a new repair. Surgical mesh may also cause tissue inflammation, which can be painful. Mesh may cause **adhesions**, or scar tissue, which sometimes cause medical problems in the surrounding area. For example, adhesions in the abdominal cavity may cause obstruction of the bowels, and adhesions in the pelvic region may contribute to infertility in females. All types of hernia repair are associated with the risk of hernia recurrence.

Resources

BOOKS

Kumar, Vinay, et al. *Robbins and Cotran: Pathologic Basis of Disease.* 8th ed. Philadelphia: Saunders/Elsevier, 2010.

PERIODICALS

Corton, Marlene M. "Critical Anatomic Concepts for Safe Surgical Mesh." *Clinical Obstetrics & Gynecology* 56, no.

2 (2013): 247–56. http://dx.doi.org/10.1097/GRF.0b013e31828e629c (accessed August 21, 2013).

Hansen, Nienke Lynn, et al. "First In-Human Magnetic Resonance Visualization of Surgical Mesh Implants for Inguinal Hernia Treatment." *Investigative Radiology* (May 31, 2013): e-pub ahead of print. http://dx.doi.org/10.1097/RLI.0b013e31829806ce (accessed August 21, 2013).

Jonsson Funk, Michele, et al. "Trends in Use of Surgical Mesh for Pelvic Organ Prolapse." *American Journal of Obstetrics & Gynecology* 208, no. 1 (2013): 79.e1–79.e7. http://dx.doi.org/10.1016/j.ajog.2012.11.008 (accessed August 21, 2013).

Menchen, Lindsey C., Alan J. Wein, Ariana L. Smith. "An Appraisal of the Food and Drug Administration Warning on Urogynecologic Surgical Mesh." *Current Urology Reports* 13, no. 3 (2012): 231–39. http://dx.doi.org/10.1007/s11934-012-0244-2 (accessed August 21, 2013).

WEBSITES

U.S. Food and Drug Administration. "FDA Safety Communication: UPDATE on Serious Complications Associated with Transvaginal Placement of Surgical Mesh for Pelvic Organ Prolapse." July 13, 2011. http://www.fda.gov/MedicalDevices/Safety/AlertsandNotices/ucm262435.htm (accessed August 21, 2013).

U.S. Food and Drug Administration. "Hernia Surgical Mesh Implants." http://www.fda.gov/MedicalDevices/ProductsandMedicalProcedures/ImplantsandProsthetics/HerniaSurgicalMesh/default.htm (accessed August 21, 2013).

U.S. Food and Drug Administration. "Surgical Mesh." http://www.fda.gov/MedicalDevices/Safety/AlertsandNotices/ucm142636.htm (accessed August 21, 2013).

ORGANIZATIONS

U.S. Food and Drug Administration, 10903 New Hampshire Ave., Silver Spring, MD 20993, (888) INFO-FDA (463-6332), http://www.fda.gov.

Maria Basile, PhD

Surgical oncology

Definition

Surgical oncology is a specialized area of oncology that engages **surgeons** in the cure and management of cancer.

Purpose

Cancer has become a medical specialty warranting its own surgical area because of advances in the biology, pathophysiology, diagnostics, and staging of malignant tumors. Surgeons have traditionally been involved with the resection and radical surgeries of tumors, leaving the management of the cancer and the patient to other specialists. Advances in the early diagnosis of cancer, the staging of tumors, microscopic analyses of cells, and increased understanding of cancer biology have broadened the range of nonsurgical cancer treatments. These treatments include systematic chemotherapy, hormonal therapy, and radiotherapy as alternatives or adjunctive therapy for patients with cancer. Specialists known as oncologists often work in conjunction with various specialized surgeons for treatment of patients with cancer.

Not all cancer tumors are manageable by surgery, nor does the removal of some tumors or metastases necessarily lead to a cure or longer life. The oncological surgeon looks for the relationship between tumor excision and the risk presented by the primary tumor. He or she is knowledgeable about patient management with more conservative procedures than the traditional excision or resection.

Demographics

According to the American Cancer Society and the National Cancer Institute, about 580,350 people were expected to die of cancer in the year 2013. According to the American Cancer Society, about 1,660,290 new cancer cases were expected to be diagnosed in 2013— 854,790 males and 805,500 females. Cancer is the second most common cause of death in the United States. The specific cases of newly diagnosed cancers estimated for 2013 in males in the United States were:

- prostate (28%)
- lung and bronchus (14%)
- colon and rectum (9%)
- urinary bladder (6%)
- melanoma of the skin (5%)
- kidney and renal pelvis (5%)
- non-Hodgkin's lymphoma (4%)
- oral cavity and pharynx (3%)
- leukemia (3%)
- pancreas (3%)

The newly diagnosed cases of cancers estimated for females in the United States during 2013 were:

- breast (29%)
- lung and bronchus (14%)
- colon and rectum (9%)
- uterine corpus (6%)
- thyroid (6%)
- non-Hodgkin's lymphoma (4%)
- melanoma of the skin (4%)
- kidney and renal pelvis (3%)

- pancreas (3%)
- ovary (3%)

Description

Surgical oncology is guided by principles that govern the routine procedures related to the cancer patient's cure, palliative care, and quality of life. Surgical oncology performs its most efficacious work by local tumor excision, regional lymph node removal, the handling of cancer recurrence (local or widespread), and in rare cases, with surgical resection of metastases from the primary tumor. Each of these areas plays a different role in cancer management.

Excision

Local excision has traditionally been the hallmark of surgical oncology. Excision refers to the removal of the cancer and its effects. Resection of a tumor in the colon can end the effects of obstruction, for instance, or removal of a breast carcinoma can stop the cancer. Resection of a primary tumor also stops the tumor from spreading throughout the body. The cancer's spread into other body systems, however, usually occurs before a local removal, giving resection little bearing upon cells that have already escaped the primary tumor. Advances in oncology through pathophysiology, staging, and biopsy offer a new diagnostic role to the surgeon using excision. These advances provide simple diagnostic information about size, grade, and extent of the tumor, as well as more sophisticated evaluations of the cancer's biochemical and hormonal features.

Regional lymph node removal

Lymph node involvement provides surgical oncologists with major diagnostic information. The sentinel node biopsy is superior to any biological test in terms of prediction of cancer mortality rates. Nodal biopsy offers very precise information about the extent and type of invasive effects of the primary tumor. The removal of nodes, however, may present pain and other morbid conditions for the patient.

Local and regional recurrence

Radical procedures in surgical oncology for local and regional occurrences of a primary tumor provide crucial information on the spread of cancer and prognostic outcomes; however, they do not contribute substantially to the outcome of the cancer. According to most surgical oncology literature, the ability to remove a local recurrence must be balanced by the patient's goals related to aesthetic and pain control concerns.

Historically, more radical procedures have not improved the chances for survival.

Surgery for distant metastases

In general, a cancer tumor that spreads further from its primary site is less likely to be controlled by surgery. According to research, except for a few instances where metastasis is confined, surgical removal of a distant metastasis is not warranted. Since the rapidity of discovering a distant metastasis has little bearing upon cancer survival, the usefulness of surgery is not time dependent. In the case of liver metastasis, for example, a cure is related to the pathophysiology of the original cancer and level of cancer antigen in the liver rather than the size or time of discovery. While surgery of metastatic cancer may not increase life, there may be indications for it such as pain relief, obstruction removal, control of bleeding, and resolution of infection.

Preparation

Surgery removes cancer cells and surrounding tissues. It is often combined with radiation therapy and chemotherapy. It is important for the patient to meet with the surgical oncologist to talk about the procedure and begin preparations for surgery. Oncological surgery may be performed to biopsy a suspicious site for malignant cells or tumor. It is also used for **tumor removal** from organs such as the tongue, throat, lung, stomach, intestines, colon, bladder, ovary, and prostate. Tumors of limbs, ligaments, and tendons may also be treated with surgery. In many cases, the biopsy and surgery to remove the cancer cells or tissues are done at the same time.

The impact of a surgical procedure depends upon the diagnosis and the area of the body that is to be treated by surgery. Many cancer surgeries involve major organs and require open abdominal surgery, which is the most extensive type of surgical procedure. This surgery requires a number of medical tests prior to surgery to assess the overall health of the patient and to make decisions about adjunctive procedures like radiation or chemotherapy. Preparation for cancer surgery requires psychological readiness for a hospital stay, **postoperative pain**, sometimes slow recovery, and anticipation of complications from tumor excision or resection. It also may require consultation with stomal therapists if a section of the urinary tract or bowel is to be removed and replaced with an outside reservoir or conduit, called an ostomy.

Aftercare

After surgery, the type and duration of side effects and the elements of recovery depend on where in the

---

KEY TERMS

Biopsy—The surgical excision of tissue to diagnose the size, type, and extent of a cancerous growth.

Cancer surgery—Surgery in which the goal is to excise a tumor and its surrounding tissue found to be malignant.

Resection—Cutting out and removing tissue to eliminate a cancerous tumor; usually refers to a section of the organ (e.g., colon, intestine, lung, stomach) that must be cut to remove the tumor and its surrounding tissue.

Tumor staging—The method used by oncologists to determine the risk from a cancerous tumor. A number—ranging from 1A–4B—is assigned to predict the level of invasion by a tumor, and offer a prognosis for morbidity and mortality.

---

body the surgery was performed and the patient's general health. Some surgeries may alter basic functions in the urinary or gastrointestinal systems. Recovering full use of function takes time and patience. Surgeries that remove conduits such as the colon, intestines, or urinary tract require appliances for urine and fecal waste and the help of a stomal therapist. Breast or prostate surgeries yield concerns about cosmetic appearance and intimate activities. For most cancer surgeries, basic functions like tasting, eating, drinking, breathing, moving, urinating, defecating, or neurological ability may be changed in the short-term. Resources to attend to deficits in daily activities need to be set up before surgery.

Risks

The type of risks that cancer surgery presents depends almost entirely upon the part of the body being biopsied or excised. Risks of surgery can be great when major organs are involved, such as the gastrointestinal system or the brain. These risks are usually discussed explicitly with the patient when making treatment decisions.

Results

Most cancers are categorized based upon their likelihood of being contained, of spreading, and of recurring. This assessment is referred to as **tumor grading** or tumor staging. The prognosis after surgery depends upon the stage of the disease and the type of cancer cell involved. General results of cancer surgery depend in large part on norms of success based upon the

QUESTIONS TO ASK YOUR DOCTOR

- What are the alternatives to surgery for this cancer?
- What is the likelihood that this surgery will entirely eliminate the cancer?
- What are the risks involved?
- Is this a surgical procedure that is often performed in this hospital or surgical center?
- What type of treatments will be needed following the surgery?
- What are the costs involved?

study of groups of patients with the same diagnosis. The results are often stated in percentages of the chance of cancer recurrence or its spread after surgery. After five disease-free years, patients are usually considered cured. This is because the recurrence rates decline drastically after five years. The benchmark is based upon the percentage of people known to reach the fifth year after surgery with no recurrence or spread of the primary tumor.

Morbidity and mortality rates

Morbidity and mortality of oncological surgery are high if there is organ involvement or extensive excision of major parts of the body. Because there is an ongoing disease process and many patients may be very ill at the time of surgery, the complications of surgery may be quite complex. Each procedure is understood by the surgeon for its likely complications or risks, and these are discussed during the initial surgical consultations.

With any surgery, there are risks associated with the use of general anesthetic and the opening of body cavities. Open surgery has general risks associated with it that are not related to the type of procedure, such as the occurrence of blood clots or cardiac events.

There is an extensive body of literature about the complication and morbidity rates of surgery performed by high-volume treatment centers. Data show that in general, large volumes of surgery affect the quality outcomes of surgery, with smaller hospitals having lower rates of procedural success and higher operative and postoperative complications than larger facilities. It is not known whether the surgeon's experience or the advantages of institutional resources in operative or **postoperative care** contributes to these statistics.

Alternatives

Alternatives to cancer surgery exist for almost every cancer treated in the United States. Research into alternatives has been very successful for some—but not all—cancers. Most organizations dealing with cancer patients suggest alternative treatments. Physicians and surgeons expect to be asked about alternatives to surgery and are usually quite knowledgeable about their use as cancer treatments or as adjuncts to surgery.

Health care team roles

A surgeon who specializes in cancer surgery or oncology performs oncology surgery in a general hospital or cancer research center.

Resources

BOOKS

Casciatio, Dennis A. *Manual of Clinical Oncology*. 7th ed. Philadelphia: Lippincott Williams & Williams/Wolters Kluwer, 2012.

Lee, K. J. *Essential Otolaryngology: Head and Neck Surgery*. 10th ed. New York: McGraw-Hill, 2012.

Lentz, Gretchen, et al. *Comprehensive Gynecology*. 5th ed. St. Louis: Mosby/Elsevier, 2012.

Townsend, Courtney M., et al. *Sabiston Textbook of Surgery*. 19th ed. Philadelphia: Saunders/Elsevier, 2012.

Wein, Alan J., et al. *Campbell-Walsh Urology*. 10th ed. Philadelphia: Saunders/Elsevier, 2012.

PERIODICALS

Begue, Aaron, et al. "Retrospective Study of Multidisciplinary Rounding on a Thoracic Surgical Oncology Unit." *Clinical Journal of Oncology Nursing* 16, no. 6 (2012): E198–202. http://dx.doi.org/10.1188/12.CJON.E198-E202 (accessed July 29, 2013).

Macefield, R. C., K. N. L. Avery, and J. M. Blazeby. "Integration of Clinical and Patient-Reported Outcomes in Surgical Oncology." *British Journal of Surgery* 100, no. 1 (2013): 28–37. http://dx.doi.org/10.1002/bjs.8989 (accessed July 29, 2013).

Menezes, Amber S., et al. "Clinical Research in Surgical Oncology: An Analysis of ClinicalTrials.gov." *Annals of Surgical Oncology* (June 26, 2013): e-pub ahead of print. http://dx.doi.org/10.1245/s10434-013-3054-y (accessed July 29, 2013).

Povoski, Stephen P., and Nathan C. Hall. "Recognizing the Role of Surgical Oncology and Cancer Imaging in the Multidisciplinary Approach to Cancer: An Important Area of Future Scholarly Growth for BMC Cancer." *BMC Cancer* 13, no. 355 (July 23, 2013). http://dx.doi.org/10.1186/1471-2407-13-355 (accessed July 29, 2013).

Shuman, Andrew G., et al. "A New Care Paradigm in Geriatric Head and Neck Surgical Oncology." *Journal of Surgical Oncology* 108, no. 3 (2013): 187–91. http://dx.doi.org/10.1002/jso.23370 (accessed July 29, 2013).

Søreide, Kjetil, and Annbjørg H. Søreide. "Using Patient-Reported Outcome Measures for Improved Decision-Making in Patients with Gastrointestinal Cancer—The Last Clinical Frontier in Surgical Oncology?" *Frontiers in Clinical Oncology* 3, no. 157 (June 2013). http://dx.doi.org/10.3389/fonc.2013.00157 (accessed July 29, 2013).

Veronesi, Umberto, and Vaia Stafyla. "Grand Challenges in Surgical Oncology." *Frontiers in Surgical Oncology* 2, no. 127 (October 2012). http://dx.doi.org/10.3389/fonc.2012.00127 (accessed July 29, 2013).

OTHER

American Cancer Society. *Cancer Facts & Figures 2013.* Atlanta: American Cancer Society, 2013. http://www.cancer.org/Research/CancerFactsStatistics/CancerFactsFigures2013/2013-cancer-facts-and-figures.pdf (accessed July 29, 2013).

American Cancer Society. *Understanding Cancer Surgery.* Atlanta: American Cancer Society, 2011. http://www.cancer.org/Research/CancerFactsStatistics/CancerFactsFigures2013/2013-cancer-facts-and-figures.pdf (accessed July 29, 2013).

WEBSITES

National Cancer Institute. *Cancer Trends Progress Report—2011/2012 Update.* Online. Bethesda, MD: National Institutes of Health, August 2012. http://progressreport.cancer.gov (accessed July 29, 2013).

National Cancer Institute. "SEER (Surveillance Epidemiology and End Results) Stat Fact Sheets: All Sites." http://seer.cancer.gov/statfacts/html/all.html (accessed July 29, 2013).

National Cancer Institute. "What You Need to Know About™ Cancer: Treatment." http://www.cancer.gov/cancertopics/wyntk/cancer/page8 (accessed July 29, 2013).

ORGANIZATIONS

American Cancer Society, 250 Williams St. NW, Atlanta, GA 30303, (800) 227-2345, http://www.cancer.org.

Cancer Research Institute, One Exchange Plz., 55 Broadway, Ste. 1802, New York, NY 10006, (212) 688-7515, (800) 99-CANCER (992-2623), http://cancerresearch.org.

National Breast Cancer Coalition, 1101 17th St. NW, Ste. 1300, Washington, DC 20036, (202) 296-7477, (800) 622-2838, Fax: (202) 265-6854, http://www.breastcancerdeadline2020.org.

National Cancer Institute, 6116 Executive Blvd., Ste. 300, Bethesda, MD 20892-8322, (800) 4-CANCER (422-6237), http://cancer.gov.

Society of Surgical Oncology, 9525 W. Bryn Mawr Ave., Ste. 870, Rosemont, IL 60018, (847) 427-1400, info@surgonc.org, http://surgonc.org.

Nancy McKenzie, PhD
Rosalyn Carson-DeWitt, MD
Tammy Allhoff, CST/CSFA, AAS

Surgical risk

Definition

Surgical risk is the set of potential adverse medical circumstances that may arise from having surgery, or the dangers and harm that may occur. Risk is determined by surgical risk factors, which are any set of circumstances that increase the risk of surgical complications. Surgical complications are any negative medical results that deviate from the normal expected outcomes of surgery or the expected recovery scenario.

Description

By nature, surgery is a risky business. However, those risks have been greatly minimized by modern technology and the high standard of physician **surgical training**. **Surgeons** usually undergo the rigors of nearly a decade of intensive training and education before they perform surgeries on their own. Experience is key to becoming a qualified surgeon and is included even in the early training stages of a surgeon's career. A qualified surgeon is a highly trained and skilled professional who can serve certain patients to improve or even save their lives. It can be overwhelming to read the long list of potential complications that may arise from having surgery. However, it is important to note that most of these complications are anticipated and measures are taken to avoid harm to the patient. Surgery saves many lives each year, and should be viewed in light of the potential benefits as well as the potential risks.

The degree of surgical risk varies between different surgical procedures, as well as with the individual medical aspects associated with each patient. The risk a

---

Surgical risks

Although specific surgeries carry their own risks, some risks are inherent with all types of surgery. Possible risks include:

- Excess bleeding
- Reactions to anesthesia or other drugs
- Problems due to comorbid conditions (e.g., diabetes, obesity)
- Damage to other organs or blood vessels
- Postoperative infection
- Pain
- Deep vein thrombosis (blood clot)

SOURCE: American Cancer Society, "What are the Risks and Side Effects of Surgery?" Available online at: http://www.cancer.org/treatment/treatmentsandsideeffects/treatmenttypes/surgery/surgery-risks-and-side-effects.

(Table by PreMediaGlobal. Copyright © 2014 Cengage Learning®.)

patient takes when having a surgical procedure is a combination of the risks associated with the procedure itself as well as risks associated with specific patient-based factors regarding surgery. Patient-based risk factors are an important part of surgical risk and help determine the likelihood of a surgical complication occurring. The decision to perform any surgical procedure is based on whether or not potential benefits outweigh the sum of the potential risks.

Procedure-based risk

Any patient undergoing surgery is at risk for medical complications that arise from the procedure itself. The specific factors that may potentially cause these complications are called procedure-based risk factors. The surgical procedures associated with the highest level of risk include cardiac surgery, lung surgery, prostate removal, and some major orthopedic surgeries, such as **hip replacement**.

Patient-based risk

Many patient-based factors increase the risk of having complications during or after a surgical procedure. Patient-based factors that generally increase risk include advanced age, obesity, poor physical condition, smoking, a compromised immune system, recent heart attack or unstable heart conditions, and malnourishment. Some specific types of surgical procedures may have their own specific types of patient-based risk factors. Specific complications are also associated with certain patient-based risk factors. For example, obesity increases the risk for wound and pulmonary complications after surgery. **Smoking cessation** for six weeks before surgery decreases the incidence of pulmonary complications.

Excessive bleeding

Excessive bleeding is a risk factor of undergoing surgery. During any surgical procedure, there may be accidental damage to a major blood vessel. If that damage is not effectively repaired, it may result in excessive blood loss. If procedural damage is done to smaller blood vessels as an expected part of the surgery but is not properly controlled, there may be excessive blood loss. Even without surgical damage to blood vessels, if a patient undergoes too much physical activity soon after having a surgical procedure, they may accidentally open some of the internal or external surgical sites and cause bleeding. Excessive bleeding may result in the patient becoming anemic. Anemia, and the resulting fatigue associated with anemia, is a risk of surgical procedures. If a very large amount of blood is lost, it can lead to complications much more serious than anemia. A very large loss of blood risks the patient going into a state of shock.

Disorders of blood clotting predispose a surgical patient to bleeding complications. If the patient's blood has a defective ability to clot, the body cannot properly close small wounds in a normal manner. Instead, even small cuts that are part of the surgical procedure can result in excessive or prolonged bleeding that may be life threatening. If surgery is a necessity in this type of patient, physicians can appropriately manage these conditions prior to the procedure to minimize the risk for bleeding complications.

Seroma formation

A seroma is an internal collection of bodily fluids at a surgical site. Seromas may result from improper wound closure or as a complication of the specific procedure. For example, breast surgery is associated with a high risk of seroma formation, even when performed properly. The presence of a seroma may delay wound healing and also increases the risk of developing an infection. Seromas are more likely to form in obese individuals, or individuals whose body forms an excessive volume of fluids that need to be drained from the surgical site during the recovery period.

Infection

Hospitals may contain types of bacteria, or mutated strains of common bacteria, to which the average person in the United States is not normally exposed. Having surgery and staying in the hospital may increase the risk of being exposed to these types of bacteria. Additionally, the emergence of antibiotic resistant strains of bacteria complicates the risk of infection after surgery. Infections with mutated strains of bacteria that are resistant to available **antibiotics** are especially difficult to prevent, treat, or control.

Risk of infection is associated with any type of surgical procedure. To minimize the chance of a patient contracting a bacterial infection, some surgical procedures involve prophylactic application of antibiotics. Surgical procedures that may involve **antibiotic prophylaxis** include bowel surgery, procedures that include insertion of prosthetic material, surgeries on patients with impaired immune systems, **neurosurgery**, cardiac surgery, and ophthalmic surgery. In addition to antibiotics, proper surgical technique in an appropriately clean **operating room** setting also minimizes risk of infection. Surgeons "scrub in" to surgery, meaning that they follow specific protocols of handwashing and dressing in surgical gowns that minimize risk of infection. The surgical site on the patient's body also needs to be

KEY TERMS

Acquired immunodeficiency syndrome (AIDS)—A disease syndrome in which the patient's immune cells are destroyed by HIV virus, leaving the patient open to opportunistic infections that a healthy immune system could keep at bay.

Anaphylactic—A serious allergic reaction to a foreign protein or other material.

Anemia—A physiological state in which the number of red blood cells or amount of hemoglobin in the blood is abnormally low, leading to a decrease in the capacity of the blood to carry oxygen to the tissues.

Angina—Disease involving decreased oxygen flow to the heart and often constricting chest pain.

Aspiration—The act of inspiring or sucking foreign fluid or vomit into the airways.

Atherosclerosis—Disease involving irregularly deposited fat within the arteries that results in medical complications.

Bell's palsy—One-sided paralysis of the face that may be due to damage to the facial nerve.

Cardiac arrhythmia—An irregular heartbeat.

Cardiac pulmonary bypass—A procedure where heart blood is diverted into an inserted pump in order to maintain appropriate blood flow.

Catheter—A flexible tube inserted into the body to allow passage of fluids in or out.

Central line—A catheter passed through a vein into large blood vessels of the chest or the heart, used in various medical procedures.

Deep venous thrombosis (DVT)—Blood clot that usually forms in the lower extremities after prolonged inactivity.

Delirium—An altered state of consciousness that includes confusion, disorientation, incoherence, agitation, and defective perception (such as hallucinations).

Electrocardiogram (ECG)—A medical tool used to monitor the electrical impulses released by the beating heart. The results are drawn out in graphical fashion to visualize the function of the heart.

Embolus—A plug of blood cell components, bacteria, or foreign body that travels through the bloodstream, lodges, and occludes a blood vessel.

Endotracheal tube—Tube inserted in the throat during general anesthesia to prevent aspiration of gastric contents into the respiratory tract.

Epidural anesthesia—Regional anesthesia produced by injecting the anesthetic agent into an area near the spinal cord.

effectively disinfected before the procedure can be performed. However, even with proper protective measures taken, there is risk of contracting a bacterial infection at surgical sites after having a procedure.

Bacterial infections after surgery may also occur in the urinary tract when a urinary catheter is used, in the respiratory tract if the patient needs to be on a respirator after the procedure, or may be systemic infections that lead to sepsis. Patients with compromised immune systems are at especially high risk of contracting bacterial infections that healthier individuals are usually able to resist. Other patient-based risk factors for post-surgery infection include a pre-existing infection before surgery, low levels of certain non-immune blood components, advanced age, obesity, smoking, diagnosis of diabetes, certain cardiovascular diseases, a physiological state of shock, excessive physical trauma, and requiring a blood **transfusion**. The organism most often associated with infection of surgical sites in the hospital is *Staphylococcus aureus*, which may be resistant to many current antibiotics such as methicillin.

Neurological damage

Surgical procedures may involve risk of neurological damage, or damage to the nervous system. Depending on the type of surgery, nerve damage may be a result of direct injury to the brain, spinal cord, or peripheral nerves. Nerve damage from a surgical procedure may also occur secondary to the administration of spinal, epidural, or regional anesthesia, or from a temporary reduction of oxygen flow to a specific part of the body. Depending on the part of the nervous system that sustains damage, the results may be mild to severe, temporary or permanent. For example, head and neck surgery is associated with risk of injury to numerous delicate nerves, some of which may result in a permanent state of Bell's palsy if damage occurs.

Postoperative delirium

Although most patients experience a temporary state of confusion when they come out of anesthesia, having a surgical procedure may carry the risk of postoperative delirium. Delirium is a severe state of mental confusion,

Epiglottis—A leaf-shaped piece of cartilage lying at the root of the tongue that protects the respiratory tract from aspiration during the swallowing reflex.

Esophageal sphincter—Muscle at the opening to the stomach that keeps the stomach contents from traveling into the esophagus.

Glucose—A form of sugar used by the body for energy.

Hypotension—Low blood pressure.

Hypovolemia—An abnormally low amount of blood in the body.

Intestinal ileus—Mechanical or dynamic obstruction of the bowel causing pain, abdominal distention, vomiting, and often fever.

Laparoscopy—Minimally invasive surgical procedure in which small incisions are made in the abdominal or pelvic cavity and surgical tools are used with a miniature camera for guidance.

Meperidine—A type of narcotic pain killer that may be used after surgical procedures.

Methicillin-resistant *Staphylococcus aureus* (MRSA)—A strain of Staph bacteria that is resistant to methicillin and hence poses a greater health threat because it is difficult to control or kill.

Pancreatitis—Inflammation of the pancreas.

Parathyroid gland—An endocrine gland that modulates calcium in the body.

Platelet—A blood component responsible for normal clotting mechanisms that seal small wounds.

Prophylaxis—The prevention of disease or infection, or of a process that can lead to disease or infection.

Sepsis—A dangerous physiological state of extensive, systemic bacterial infection.

Seroma—A seroma is an internal collection of fluid at a surgical site.

Spinal anesthesia—Regional anesthesia produced by injecting the anesthetic agent into an area directly around the spinal cord.

Thrombus—A blood clot attached to a blood vessel wall.

Trocars—A surgical tool shaped as a hollow cylinder that is sometimes used to make an initial incision into a body cavity and through which other surgical tools are then passed.

White blood cell—A component of the blood involved in the immune response.

---

disorientation, agitation, and general incoherence. Delirium may also include hallucinations. Postoperative delirium is a temporary state of delirium that may be caused by multiple factors relating to the surgical procedure. It may occur if the patient experiences a lack of oxygen, hypotension, or sepsis as a result of the surgical procedure. Patient-based risk factors for postoperative delirium include advanced age, pre-existing dementia, chronic drug or alcohol abuse, certain metabolic disorders, side effects of certain medications such as meperidine, and sleep deprivation. Because individuals of advanced age are at higher risk for postoperative delirium, the mental status of elderly patients is frequently assessed in postoperative recovery. If delirium occurs, the patient's oxygen levels are checked and all non-essential drugs are temporarily discontinued. With proper treatment, postoperative delirium usually goes away within 72 hours.

Anesthesia complications

A patient undergoing **general anesthesia** for a surgical procedure runs the risk of a temporary, minor disturbance in mental function after the procedure. Patients may experience slight confusion, disorientation, and decreased general mental acuity after having anesthesia for a surgical procedure. This mental state may take up to a week to fully dissipate, and may affect the patient's ability to work or operate an automobile. Patient-based factors that increase the likelihood of anesthesia complications include advanced age, obesity, and kidney or liver insufficiencies resulting in poor metabolism of the anesthetic agent.

Cardiac complications

Cardiac complications are another surgical risk factor. Certain types of anesthesia such as halothane may cause a cardiac arrhythmia during the induction of anesthesia. Additionally, there are other factors that may contribute to cardiac complications after surgery. Certain drugs, excessive pain, certain acid-base imbalances, and problems with oxygen delivery during surgery may lead to arrhythmias. Postoperative hypertension may also occur as a result of poor pain management after a surgical procedure. Patient-based risk factors for postoperative hypertension include advanced age, congestive heart failure, and angina.

There is a slight risk of heart attack associated with non-cardiac surgeries, and a greater risk associated with cardiac or vascular surgeries. Risk factors for heart attack associated with surgery are pre-existing congestive heart failure, angina, atherosclerosis, pre-existing anemia, hypotension or anemia as a result of blood loss during surgery, defective oxygen delivery during surgery, and advanced patient age.

Other organ-based complications

Any surgical procedure performed on or around an organ system has some risk of damage to that system. The following are examples of organ-based surgical risk factors. Pancreatitis (inflammation of the pancreas) is a rare complication as a result of surgery. However, within the cases of pancreatitis that do exist, approximately 10% are related to injury during surgical procedures. When a surgical procedure is performed in the physical vicinity of the pancreas, approximately 1%–3% of patients may develop pancreatitis. If the surgical procedure involves maneuvering the actual biliary tract, the incidence of pancreatitis rises. Patient surgical risk factors that predispose to pancreatitis include previous history of pancreatitis, parathyroid surgery that alters blood levels of calcium very quickly and in a short period of time, cardiopulmonary bypass, and renal transplantation.

Surgeries involving the contents of the abdomen have risk for temporarily disrupting the normal movement of the intestines, a condition known as postoperative intestinal ileus. If the intestines are handled too much or are damaged, or certain types of **postoperative pain** medications are overused, the normal propulsive movements of the bowels may cease completely. While this condition is temporary and treatable, the patient cannot eat or drink until normal intestinal movement is restored. Postoperative ileus may cause abdominal distention, pain, constipation, and vomiting; require a prolonged hospital stay; or contribute to a regional bacterial infection.

Vascular complications

Several vascular complications may result from a surgical procedure. If a procedure involves the placement of a central line, air may be introduced into the body cavity outside of the lung, and then collapse the lung. If a catheter is left open, air may enter the blood stream and travel to and affect the proper functioning of the heart.

Deep Venous Thrombosis (DVT) is a condition where a blood clot (thrombus) forms in a blood vessel.

DVT occurs in approximately 40% of postoperative patients. Clots usually form in the lower extremities. To prevent DVT, support hose and compression devices are used during surgical procedures. DVT is dangerous because if a clot becomes an embolus (clot that detaches from the vessel wall and travels through the bloodstream) and goes into the pulmonary system (pulmonary embolus) it can be life threatening. It is one of the most common causes of sudden death in hospitalized patients and is a risk factor if a surgical procedure requires a long period of bed rest during recovery.

Pulmonary emboli may be caused by multiple types of clots in addition to DVT and are a serious surgical risk. Pulmonary emboli may also be caused by fat droplets entering the bloodstream during joint replacement surgery. Patient-based risk factors for a pulmonary embolus during surgery include advanced age, heart disease, obesity, and varicose veins.

Blood transfusions

Patients undergoing some surgical procedures carry the risk of needing a blood transfusion. Blood transfusions may cause a dangerous immune system reaction against the blood type or other blood components of the transfusion. These reactions can make the patient very sick or may even become anaphylactic and life threatening. To prevent the likelihood of an immune reaction, blood is carefully matched to the patient in a way that minimizes risk. Although the blood used for blood transfusions is screened for known viruses, transmission of an unknown virus is a possibility.

Pulmonary complications

Pulmonary complications are a main cause of postoperative illness. Pulmonary complications may be caused by patient-based risk factors or surgical procedure-based risk factors. Many pulmonary complications after surgery involve part of the respiratory system partially collapsing, usually within 48 hours of a surgical procedure. Other potential respiratory or pulmonary complications involve lung infections, difficulty breathing, or aspirating (breathing in) regurgitated gastric secretions while under general anesthesia. While under anesthesia, the parts of the body that normally protect the respiratory system from taking in food or fluids (the epiglottis and esophageal sphincter) are relaxed. Therefore, safeguards have to be set in place for protection. Endotracheal tubes are placed in the throat to minimize the risk of breathing regurgitated stomach contents down into the respiratory tract. If food or fluids from the stomach enter the respiratory tract, it may result in pulmonary complications associated with high mortality rates. In order to avoid these complications, patients are asked to abstain from eating or drinking before surgical procedures requiring general anesthesia, are positioned carefully for surgery, and carefully fitted with an endotracheal tube.

Patient-based risk factors associated with different types of pulmonary complications include advanced age, obesity, pre-existing chronic lung disease, and smoking history. Surgical procedure-based risk factors include procedures requiring a long duration of anesthesia, prolonged **mechanical ventilation**, thoracic or upper abdomen surgery, abdominal distention, inadequate pain control that results in the patient not coughing effectively after the procedure, oversedation due to administration of too much anesthesia, excessive postsurgical pain killer use, or an endotracheal tube that is not positioned correctly.

Tool-based risk

The tools used during surgery pose a risk for damage to organs, nerves, or blood vessels. Scalpels, cauterizers, needles, and clamps may be mishandled and accidentally cut, burn, pierce, or cause blunt trauma to the body. Even minimal access surgeries such as a **laparoscopy** involve tool-based surgical risk. Tool-based risks of laparoscopies include the use of **trocars**, a tool used to make the first incision or entry into the abdominal cavity. If a classic trocar is used in the first "blind jab" into the abdomen before a camera can be inserted, the physician may push too hard on the trocars and damage blood vessels or internal organs. Any surgical tool poses a risk for damage, and is only as safe as the skill of the surgeon wielding it. Proper protocol should be followed at all times in handling and using **surgical instruments** (tools). This includes counts, sterilization, proper usage, and other specific handling protocol.

Risk prevention

Hospitals may perform laboratory tests before admitting a patient for surgery in order to catch patient-based risk factors that predispose for surgical complications and treat them. Pre-surgery tests such as **urinalysis**, chest x-rays, or complete blood counts may identify potential risk factors that could lead to complications. Commonly performed pre-surgery tests include:

- chest x-rays for patients with shortness of breath, chest pain, or a cough

- electrocardiogram (ECG) for patients with chest pain or abnormal heart signs

- urinalysis for patients with urinary problems, side pain, kidney disease, or diabetes

QUESTIONS TO ASK YOUR DOCTOR

- Why do I need a surgical procedure?
- What are alternative options to surgery?
- What are the potential benefits of this procedure?
- What are the potential risks of this procedure?
- What outcomes are anticipated if I do not have the surgical procedure?
- Who would perform the procedure?
- How many times has my surgeon performed this procedure before?
- Are there any patient-based risk factors that could be altered to minimize risk?
- Will any of my medications, over-the-counter medicines, and nutritional or herbal supplements affect my recovery from this procedure?
- How long should recovery be expected to take?
- Will I have to stay in the hospital after the procedure?

- white blood cell count for patients with a suspected infection, or on medications known to affect white blood cell counts

- platelet count for patients with excessive blood loss, alcoholism, or on medications known to affect platelet count

- glucose levels for patients with excessive sweating, tremors, diabetes, cystic fibrosis, an altered mental status, or alcoholism

- potassium levels for patients with congestive heart failure, kidney failure, muscle weakness, diabetes, or on medications known to affect potassium levels

- sodium levels for patients with pulmonary disease, central nervous system disease, congestive heart failure, or some types of liver disease

Resources

BOOKS

McPherson, Richard A., and Matthew R. Pincus, eds. *Henry's Clinical Diagnosis and Management by Laboratory Methods.* 22nd ed. Philadelphia: Saunders/Elsevier, 2011.

Miller, Ronald D., ed. *Miller's Anesthesia.* 7th ed. Philadelphia: Churchill Livingstone/Elsevier, 2010.

Townsend, Courtney M., et al. *Sabiston Textbook of Surgery.* 19th ed. Philadelphia: Saunders/Elsevier, 2012.

PERIODICALS

Chen, Pin-Liang, et al. "Risk of Dementia after Anaesthesia and Surgery." *British Journal of Psychiatry* (July 25, 2013): e-pub ahead of print. http://dx.doi.org/10.1192/bjp. bp.112.119610 (accessed September 4, 2013).

Nakamura, K. M., et al. "Fracture Risk following Bariatric Surgery: A Population-Based Study." *Osteoporosis International* (August 3, 2013): e-pub ahead of print. http://dx. doi.org/10.1007/s00198-013-2463-x (accessed September 4, 2013).

Symons, N. R. A, et al. "Mortality in High-Risk Emergency General Surgical Admissions." *British Journal of Surgery* 100, no. 10 (2013): 1318–25. http://dx.doi.org/10.1002/ bjs.9208 (accessed September 4, 2013).

WEBSITES

American Cancer Society. "What Are the Risks and Side Effects of Surgery?" http://www.cancer.org/treatment/ treatmentsandsideeffects/treatmenttypes/surgery/surgery-risks-and-side-effects (accessed September 4, 2013).

American Society for Aesthetic Plastic Surgery (ASAPS). "Surgical Risks Overview." http://www.surgery.org/ consumers/patient-safety/surgical-risks-overview (accessed September 4, 2013).

Castillo, Michelle. "Surgical Complications and Errors Bring in More Money for Hospitals." CBS News, April 17, 2013. http://www.cbsnews.com/8301-204_162-57580117/surgi-cal-complications-and-errors-bring-in-more-money-for-hospitals (accessed October 23, 2013).

ORGANIZATIONS

American Association for the Surgery of Trauma, 633 N. Saint Clair St., Ste. 2600, Chicago, IL 60611, (800) 789-4006, Fax: (312) 202-5064, aast@aast.org, http://www.aast.org.

American College of Surgeons, 633 N. Saint Clair St., Chicago, IL 60611-3211, (312) 202-5000, (800) 621-4111, Fax: (312) 202-5001, postmaster@facs.org, http://www.facs. org.

American Society for Aesthetic Plastic Surgery (ASAPS), 11262 Monarch St., Garden Grove, CA 92841, (562) 799-2356, (800) 364-2147, Fax: (562) 799-1098, asaps@ surgery.org, http://www.surgery.org.

Maria Basile, PhD
Rosalyn Carson-DeWitt, MD

Surgical site infections *see* **Postoperative infections**

Surgical team

Definition

The surgical team is a group of healthcare providers that assists in providing a continuum of care, beginning with the preoperative phase of care and extending through the intraoperative phase (during the surgery) and postoperative recovery. These three phases of care are referred to collectively as perioperative care.

Purpose

Surgery, whether elective, required, or emergency, is done for a variety of conditions that include:

• cosmetic procedures

• diagnostic and exploratory procedures

• replacement or implantation of artificial or electronic devices

• reposition and enhancement of bone, ligaments, tendons, or organ conduits

• palliative procedures

• reconstructive procedures

• restorative or corrective procedures

• transplantation of organs

• treatment of acute, chronic, and infectious diseases of tissue or organs

The crucial elements of surgery—surgical and operative procedures, invasive and non-invasive procedures, pain control, patient care, patient safety, and blood and wound control—require individual expertise and high levels of concentration, anticipation, and coordination. Through a team effort, patients are carefully treated and monitored throughout the procedure, regardless of the type of operation.

Demographics

According to the Centers for Disease Control and Prevention (CDC) and the National Center for Health Statistics, 51.4 million inpatient surgical procedures were performed in the United States in 2010. Leading surgeries included:

• cardiovascular system surgeries (7.45 million)

• digestive system surgeries (6 million)

• musculoskeletal system surgeries (5.5 million)

• cesarean sections (1.3 million)

• endoscopy of large intestines (1.1 million)

• endoscopy of small intestines (0.5 million)

• eye surgeries (0.8 million)

• injection of agent into spinal canal (0.3 million)

Description

The components of the surgical team depend on the type of surgery, the precise procedures, and the location and type of anesthesia utilized. The team may include

surgeons, anesthesiologists, and nursing and technical staff who are trained in **general surgery** or in a particular surgical specialty. Intense surgeries may require larger teams and more comprehensive recovery care. Even though minimally invasive procedures (e.g., **laparoscopy** or endoscopy) are conducted with small instruments and a video camera probe, they require specialized expertise and high technological knowledge. These procedures utilize smaller teams, create less extensive wounds, and yield quicker healing, but often require more operating time and may result in operative injuries.

Types of surgery

Many surgeries are categorized as general surgery, and are associated primarily with accidents, emergencies, and trauma care. Hospitals have general surgeons that staff their emergency rooms or trauma centers. As surgical technology and knowledge have advanced, other surgical specialties have developed for each function and organ of the body. They involve special surgical techniques and anesthesiology requirements, and sometimes require subspecialists with in-depth knowledge of organ function, operative techniques, complex anesthesiology procedures, and specialized nursing care.

The basic surgical specialties include:

- General surgery. General surgeons manage a broad spectrum of surgical conditions that involve almost any part of the body. They confirm the diagnoses provided by primary care or emergency physicians and radiologists, and perform procedures necessary to correct or alleviate the problem. General surgery may include procedures on the breast, abdominal cavity, abdominal region, neck and extremities, gastrointestinal tract, and biliary system.
- Cardiothoracic surgery. A major surgical specialty with very high demands, the cardiothoracic surgical team oversees the preoperative, operative, and critical care of patients with pathologic conditions within the chest, including the heart and its valves; cancers of the lung, esophagus, and chest wall; and chest vessels.
- Genitourinary surgery. Also referred to as GU or urology, it includes procedures of the urethra, bladder, ureters, kidneys, and male reproductive system.
- Gynecological and obstetrical surgery. Gynecology focuses on treatment and prevention of pathological conditions that affect the female reproductive system, and obstetrics relates to the process of pregnancy and birth.
- Minimally invasive endoscopic and robotic-assisted surgery. This specialty includes procedures performed with an endoscope or robotic-assisted procedures. It encompasses procedures from various specialties.

- Neurosurgery. Neurosurgical teams specialize in surgery of the nervous system, including the brain, spine, and peripheral nervous system, as well as their supporting structures.
- Ophthalmic surgery. Ophthalmic surgeons perform procedures on the external and internal structures of the eye.
- Oral and maxillofacial surgery. This type of surgery involves reconstruction and repair of the facial bones and may include structures of the oral cavity.
- Orthopedic surgery. Orthopedic surgeons perform procedures on the body's connective tissues to treat or correct injuries; congenital anomalies; or diseases of the bones, joints, ligaments, tendons, or muscles.
- Otorhinolaryngology surgery. Also referred to as ear, nose, and throat (ENT) surgery, this specialty includes procedures of the outer, middle, and inner ear, as well as the nose and throat.
- Pediatric surgery. Pediatric surgical teams are specially trained to treat a broad range of conditions affecting infants and children. They work closely with specially trained anesthesiologists and are experts in childhood diseases of the head, neck, chest, and abdomen, with training in birth defects and injuries. Many pediatric surgeons work to increase the use of minimally invasive techniques with children.
- Reconstructive and plastic surgery. Reconstructive surgery is performed on abnormal structures of the body due to injury, birth defects, infection, tumors, or disease. Cosmetic surgery is performed to improve a patient's appearance.
- Transplantation. Transplant surgical teams specialize in specific organ transplant techniques, such as heart and heart-lung transplants, liver transplants, and kidney/pancreas transplants. These highly intricate surgeries require very advanced training and technological support.
- Vascular surgery. Vascular surgery offers diagnosis and treatment of arterial and venous disorders such as aneurysms, lower extremity revascularization, and other circulatory system problems.

Surgical techniques

Open surgeries requiring invasive procedures within the abdominal cavity, brain, or extensive limb areas may require a hospital stay overnight or up to two weeks. Hospitalization allows the clinical staff to monitor patient recovery (and provide medical attention in the case of a complication), while allowing patients to regain organ functions.

Surgery has been revolutionized by new technology. Ambulatory or outpatient surgeries account for an increasing percentage of surgeries in the United States. Imagery with miniature videoscopes that pass into the patient via tiny incisions is an example of how minimally invasive procedures are replacing open surgeries. Minimally invasive surgeries reduce recovery time and increase the speed of healing. Outpatient or ambulatory surgery environments often allow patients to recover and go home the same day. In specialty surgery centers, such as those designed for ophthalmology, surgery is performed as part of a physician's office practice. These centers contain their own operating rooms and recovery areas.

Minimally invasive procedures that involve the use of a videoscope as an exploratory as well as viewing instrument include:

- Arthroscopy allows viewing of the interior of joints, especially the knee joint.
- Cystoscopy is used to examine the urethra and bladder.
- Endoscopy uses an endoscope in gastrointestinal surgeries of the esophagus, stomach, and colon.
- Laparoscopy uses an illuminated tube with a video camera inserted in small incisions in the abdomen.
- Sigmoidoscopy is used for examining the rectum and sigmoid colon.
- Thoracoscopy is used for biopsy of lung tissue.

Types of anesthesia

Surgical procedures and the surgical setting may be associated with different types of anesthesia:

- General anesthesia renders the patient unconscious during surgery. The anesthesia is either inhaled or given intravenously. A breathing tube may be inserted into the windpipe (trachea) to facilitate breathing. This procedure is known as intubation. The patient is carefully monitored and wakes up in the recovery room.
- Regional anesthesia numbs the surgical section of the body. This is usually accomplished via injection through the spinal canal (spinal anesthesia) or through a catheter to the lower part of the back (epidural). Regional anesthetics numb the area of the nerves that provide feeling to the designated part of the body.
- Local anesthesia medicates only the direct operative site, and is administered through injection. The patient remains conscious but may be sedated during the operation.

Surgical team

The basic surgical team consists of experts in operative procedures, pain management, and overall or specific patient care. Team members include the surgeon, surgeon's assistants, anesthesiologist or anesthesia

personnel, **operating room** nurses, and surgical technologists. In teaching hospitals attached to medical schools, the team may be added to by those in training, such as interns, residents, and nursing students.

SURGEON. The surgeon performs the operation, and leads the surgical team. Surgeons have medical degrees, specialized **surgical training** of up to seven years, and, in most cases, have passed national board certification exams. Board certification means that the surgeon has passed written and oral examinations of academic competence. The American Board of Surgery, a professional organization that strives to improve the quality of care for patients, is the certifying board for surgeons. As a peer review organization, the College has advanced standards to certify surgical competence by allowing examined surgeons to become a fellow of the organization. Fellows of the American College of Surgeons (FACS) are the elite members of the profession. An FACS designation after a physician's name and degree denotes attainment of the profession's highest training and expertise. Surgeons' credentials may be explored through the Official American Board of Medical Specialties, available at libraries or online.

ANESTHESIOLOGIST. Anesthesiologists are physicians with at least four years of advanced training in anesthesia. They may attain further specialization in surgical procedures, such as **neurosurgery** or **pediatric surgery**. They are directly or indirectly involved in all three stages of surgery (preoperative, operative, and postoperative) due to their focus on pain management and patient safety.

CERTIFIED REGISTERED NURSE ANESTHETIST (CRNA). The certified nurse anesthetist supports the anesthesiologist and, in an increasing number of hospitals, takes full control of the anesthesia for the operation. Registered nurses must graduate from an approved nursing program and pass a licensing examination. They may be licensed in more than one state. While states determine the training and certification requirements of nurses, the work setting determines their daily responsibilities. Certified registered nurse anesthetists must have advanced education and clinical practice experience in anesthesiology.

OPERATING NURSE. The general nursing staff is a critical feature of the surgical team. The nursing staff performs comprehensive care, assistance, and pain management during each surgical phase. He or she is usually the team member providing the most continuity between the stages of care. The operating nurse is the general assistant to the surgeon during the actual operation phase, and usually has advanced training.

Preparation

The surgical team admits the patient to the hospital or surgery center. Many surgeons and anesthesiologists have privileges at more than one hospital and may admit the patient to a center of the patient's choosing. Surgical preparation is the preoperative phase of surgery, and involves special team activities that include monitoring **vital signs**, and administering medications and tests needed immediately before the procedure. In preparation for surgery, the patient meets with the surgeon, anesthesiologist, and surgical nurse. Each team member discusses his or her role in the surgery, and obtains pertinent information from the patient.

Aftercare

After the surgical procedure has been performed, the patient is brought to a recovery room where post-anesthesia staff take over from the surgical team under the guidance of the surgeon and anesthesiologist. The staff carefully monitors the patient by checking vital signs, the surgical wound and its **dressings**, IV medications, swallowing ability, level of consciousness, and any tubes or drains. Clinical staff also manages the patient's pain and body positioning.

Risks

Because of its risks, surgery should be the option chosen when the benefit includes the removal of life-threatening conditions or improvement in quality of daily life. Radical surgeries for some types of cancer may offer less than a 20% chance of cure, and the operation may pose the same percentage of mortality risk. A failed operation may shorten time with loved ones and friends, or a successful operation may lead to major positive changes in daily life.

Surgery often brings quicker relief from many conditions than other medical treatment. The risks of surgery depend upon a number of factors, including the experience of the surgical team. In a *New England Journal of Medicine* article, researchers found that mortality decreased as patient volume in a surgical setting increased. The study's messages were that patients should choose surgical centers where a large number of the type of surgery they need is performed, and that physicians working in low-volume hospitals should find ways to increase volume and reduce their morbidity and mortality rates.

Mortality rates are lower and the care more extensive in teaching hospitals with a house staff made up of interns and residents in training.

Healthcare facilities keep records of the procedures they perform. By contacting the Joint Commission (formerly the Joint Commission on Accreditation of Healthcare Organizations), a center's success with surgical care, mortality and morbidity rates, and surgical complications can be determined.

The Institute of Medicine estimates that today's anesthesia care is nearly 50 times safer than it was 20 years ago, with one anesthesia-related death per 200,000–300,000 cases. Despite this record of progress, many questions remain about anesthetic safety. Certified registered nurse anesthetists administer over 65% of anesthesia in the United States, and are often the primary anesthetists for rural communities and delivery rooms.

Independent of surgical team expertise and experience, patient status, and the level of technological advancement in surgical procedures, factors such as cardiac events, blood clots, and infection pose surgical risks. These risks accompany all surgeries and, while great progress has been achieved, they remain risks of any invasive surgery and any use of anesthesia.

Alternatives

Alternatives to surgery should be investigated with the referring physician or primary care physician. Many medical conditions benefit from changes in lifestyle, such as losing weight, increasing **exercise**, and undergoing physical rehabilitation. This is especially true for chronic conditions of the gastrointestinal tract, cardiovascular system, urologic system, and bone and joint issues. Other alternatives to surgery include pharmaceutical and medical remedies.

> ## KEY TERMS
>
> **Anesthesiologist**—A physician with advanced training in anesthesia (and sometimes other medical specialties) who administers or oversees the administration of anesthesia to the patient and monitors care after surgery.
>
> **Anesthetist**—A nurse trained in anesthesiology who, working as an assistant to an anesthesiologist, administers the anesthesia in surgery and monitors the patient after surgery.
>
> **Minimally invasive surgery**—Surgical techniques, especially the use of small instruments and tiny video cameras, that allow surgery to take place without a full operative wound.
>
> **Operative nurse**—A nurse specially trained to assist the surgeon and work in all areas of surgery to care for the patient.

Patients should obtain a **second opinion** before undergoing most major surgeries. It is very important that patients understand that a second opinion offers them the ability to obtain a confirming or differing diagnosis as well as new treatment options. A study of New York City employees and retirees who sought second opinions found that 30% of the second opinions differed from the first. Many health plans have mandatory second opinion clauses. Second opinions should involve physicians in other facilities or even other cities. A change in surgeon will mean a change in the surgical team.

Resources

BOOKS

Khatri, V. P., and J. A. Asensio. *Operative Surgery Manual.* 1st ed. Philadelphia: Saunders, 2003.

Miller, Ronald D., ed. *Miller's Anesthesia.* 7th ed. Philadelphia: Churchill Livingstone/Elsevier, 2010.

Townsend, Courtney M., et al. *Sabiston Textbook of Surgery.* 19th ed. Philadelphia: Saunders/Elsevier, 2012.

PERIODICALS

Koenig, Harold G. "Role of the Chaplain on the Medical-Surgical Team." *AORN Journal* 96, no. 3 (2012): 330–32. http://dx.doi.org/10.1016/j.aorn.2012.06.007 (accessed September 19, 2013).

Martinez, Elizabeth A. "Quality, Patient Safety, and the Cardiac Surgical Team." *Anesthesiology Clinics* 31, no. 2 (2013): 249–68. http://dx.doi.org/10.1016/j.anclin.2013.01.004 (accessed September 19, 2013).

Quick, Julie. "The Role of the Surgical Care Practitioner within the Surgical Team." *British Journal of Nursing* 22, no. 13 (2013): 759–64.

Rosqvist, Eerika A., Teuvo J. Antikainen, and Anne K. Mattila. "Training Curriculum and Simulator Training for the Whole Surgical Team: What Do Nurse Assistants Think?" *Simulation in Healthcare: The Journal of the Society for Simulation in Healthcare* 7, no. 3 (2012): 201–2. http://dx.doi.org/10.1097/SIH.0b013e31825d30ba (accessed September 19, 2013).

Schulman, C. I., et al. "Mobile Learning Module Improves Knowledge of Medical Shock for Forward Surgical Team Members." *Military Medicine* 177, no. 11 (2012): 1316–21.

Xu, Rena, et al. "The Teaming Curve: A Longitudinal Study of the Influence of Surgical Team Familiarity on Operative Time." *Annals of Surgery* (February 12, 2013): e-pub ahead of print. http://dx.doi.org/10.1097/SLA.0b013e3182864ffe (accessed September 19, 2013).

WEBSITES

American College of Surgeons. "Surgical Teams Can Reduce Expensive Postoperative Complications by Combining Communications Team Training with an Internationally Recognized Surgical Checklist." Press release, December 5, 2012. http://www.facs.org/news/jacs/teams1212.html (accessed September 19, 2013).

Centers for Disease Control and Prevention, National Center for Health Statistics. "Inpatient Surgery." FastStats. http://www.cdc.gov/nchs/fastats/insurg.htm (accessed September 19, 2013).

ORGANIZATIONS

American Board of Medical Specialties, 222 N. LaSalle St., Ste. 1500, Chicago, IL 60601, (312) 436-2600, http://www.abms.org.

American Board of Surgery, 1617 John F. Kennedy Blvd., Ste. 860, Philadelphia, PA 19103-1847, (215) 568-4000, Fax: (215) 563-5718, http://www.absurgery.org.

American College of Surgeons, 633 N. Saint Clair St., Chicago, IL 60611-3211, (312) 202-5000, (800) 621-4111, Fax: (312) 202-5001, postmaster@facs.org, http://www.facs.org.

American Society of Anesthesiologists (ASA), 520 N. Northwest Hwy., Park Ridge, IL 60068-2573, (847) 825-5586, Fax: (847) 825-1692, communications@asahq.org, http://www.asahq.org.

The Joint Commission, One Renaissance Blvd., Oakbrook Terrace, IL 60181, (630) 792-5800, Fax: (630) 792-5005, http://www.jointcommission.org.

Nancy McKenzie, PhD
Tammy Allhoff, CST/CSFA, AAS

Surgical training

Definition

Surgical training refers to the acquisition of knowledge and skills required for a physician to operate on patients in a safe and successful manner.

Purpose

The purpose of surgical training is to prepare a physician to perform surgery.

Demographics

As of 2013, there were 78,000 fellows in the American College of Surgeons. More males than females tend to enter surgical training; as a result, the great majority of surgeons in the United States are male.

Description

An individual's first formal exposure to surgery occurs during the third year of medical school. Every medical student spends time in a surgical clerkship. During this period, students are exposed to patients with conditions that can be addressed using surgery. Medical

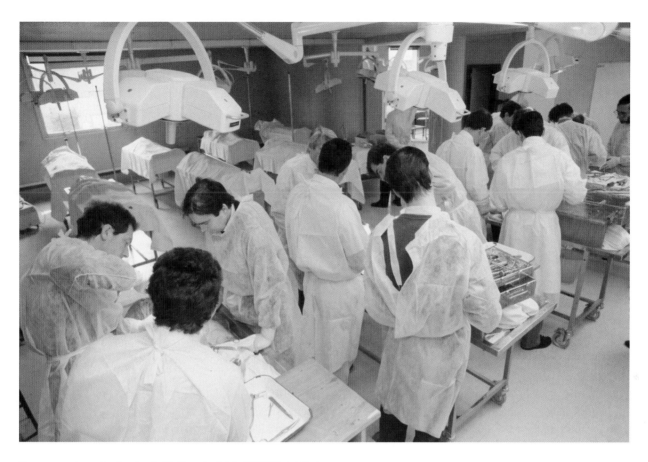

Surgeons at medical school. *(© Boucharlat © BSIP/Phototake)*

students initially accompany surgeons and observe. Gradually, they are allowed to assist with simple activities such as changing **bandages** or wound **dressings** and holding instruments. Under constant direct supervision, they may be allowed to close wounds by placing sutures. During this period, students read about surgery and are taught and quizzed by the surgeons that they are accompanying.

The next phase of surgical training occurs after a physician has graduated from medical school. This phase is called residency training and lasts for five years. The first year of residency training is often referred to as an internship year. During this time, surgical residents receive intensive training in the medical management of patients. Their surgical duties include continued observation of surgical procedures. As their skills improve and their knowledge base grows, they are allowed to perform simple procedures such as establishing a sterile field, making initial incisions, placing drains in wounds, and closing wounds when surgical procedures have been completed.

During the second through fifth years, surgical residents continue to study, acquire additional skills, and manage patients. Throughout these five years of surgical training, residents are constantly observed and evaluated. In the fifth year, trainees spend time as chief residents, which teaches them about leadership. They are responsible for assigning cases (patients) to other surgical residents, instructing other surgical residents, and teaching medical students.

After completing the five years of resident training, trainees must pass an examination. The test involves a written component that covers medical and surgical knowledge and an oral component that covers surgical skills and patient management. Once they pass this examination, they receive Fellowship status in the American College of Surgeons. With this, they are entitled to call themselves surgeons and use the letters FACS after their names. At this point, the surgeons are also considered board certified.

Some surgeons begin regular work in a surgical practice or as employees in a hospital or other similar organization. Other surgeons opt for obtaining additional specialized training and enter fellowships. Fellowship training is focused on a particular aspect of surgery and lasts from one to two years. At the completion of fellowship training, surgeons take another round of examinations. If they successfully complete the written and oral components, they receive an additional board certification as specialists.

Types of surgical fellowship training include:

- cardiac surgery (heart)

- thoracic surgery (lungs)

- plastic surgery (reconstructive and cosmetic surgery)

- orthopedic surgery (bones and joints)

- trauma surgery (especially on the hands or other body parts)

- gynecological surgery (female reproductive system)

- ophthalmic surgery (eyes)

- transplant surgery (especially the kidneys, pancreas, liver, and lungs)

- neurosurgery (brain and nervous system)

Preparation

Prior to entering medical school, individuals interested in becoming surgeons usually complete four years of undergraduate training in a college or university. During their premedical education, future physicians complete a core curriculum that includes a minimum of one year of biology, one year of physics, one year of mathematics (including a semester of calculus), and two years of chemistry (including a year of inorganic chemistry and a year of organic chemistry). Pre-med students often complete a bachelor degree in biology or chemistry, although this is not required. Medical schools seek persons that can think in a logical manner, so students with degrees in any undergraduate major are welcomed as long as they have completed the ten courses of the required core curriculum.

Candidates must take and submit scores from the Medical College Admission Test (MCAT) when applying to medical school.

Risks

Risks associated with surgical training include disappointment for candidates that are unsuccessful in gaining admission to medical school. Risks associated with surgical training from medical school through fellowship training include fatigue and occupational injuries. Occupational injuries associated with surgery include accidental needle sticks, accidental cuts from scalpels or other instruments, and exposure to pathogens acquired from patients. Risks associated with surgical training include fatigue, occupational injuries, and malpractice suits.

KEY TERMS

Fellowship training—Additional specialty training that follows completion of residency training; fellowships are one to two years in length.

Internship—The first year of residency training.

Residency training—A five-year period of additional training that follows completion of medical school.

Surgeon—A physician that has completed surgical residency training, passed all examinations, and is a Fellow of the American College of Surgeons.

Results

The normal result of surgical training is successfully mastering the knowledge presented in medical school and residency, learning the techniques of surgery, and becoming a productive surgeon.

Resources

BOOKS

Lawrence, Peter F., ed. *Essentials of General Surgery*. 5th ed. Philadelphia: Lippincott Williams & Wilkins, 2013.

Townsend, Courtney M., et al. *Sabiston Textbook of Surgery*. 19th ed. Philadelphia: Saunders/Elsevier, 2012.

PERIODICALS

Panting, Allan. "Surgical Training and Assessment: 2013." *ANZ Journal of Surgery* 83, no. 6 (2013): 399–400. http://dx.doi.org/10.1111/ans.12189 (accessed August 12, 2013).

Patel, Anup, et al. "A Multimedia Approach for Surgical Training." *Plastic & Reconstructive Surgery* 132, no. 1 (2013): 188. http://dx.doi.org/10.1097/PRS.0b013e3182910e45 (accessed August 12, 2013).

Tergas, Ana, et al. "A Pilot Study of Surgical Training Using a Virtual Robotic Surgery Simulator." *JSLS (Journal of the Society of Laparoendoscopic Surgeons)* 17, no. 2 (2013): 219–26. http://dx.doi.org/10.4293/108680813X13654754535872 (accessed August 12, 2013).

WEBSITES

American College of Surgeons. "Section III: Surgical Specialties." http://www.facs.org/residencysearch/specialties/specialties.html (accessed August 12, 2013).

U.S. Bureau of Labor Statistics. "How to Become a Physician or Surgeon." U.S. Department of Labor. http://www.bls.gov/ooh/healthcare/physicians-and-surgeons.htm#tab-4 (accessed August 12, 2013).

ORGANIZATIONS

American Academy of Orthopaedic Surgeons (AAOS), 6300 N. River Rd., Rosemont, IL 60018-4262, (847) 823-7186,

Fax: (847) 823-8125, pemr@aaos.org, http://www.aaos.org.

American Association of Neurological Surgeons, 5550 Meadowbrook Dr., Rolling Meadows, IL 60008-3852, (847) 378-0500, (888) 566-AANS (2267), Fax: (847) 378-0600, info@aans.org, http://aans.org.

American Board of Surgery, 1617 John F. Kennedy Blvd., Ste. 860, Philadelphia, PA 19103-1847, (215) 568-4000, Fax: (215) 563-5718, http://www.absurgery.org.

American College of Surgeons, 633 N. Saint Clair St., Chicago, IL 60611-3211, (312) 202-5000, (800) 621-4111, Fax: (312) 202-5001, postmaster@facs.org, http://www.facs.org.

American Society for Aesthetic Plastic Surgery (ASAPS), 11262 Monarch St., Garden Grove, CA 92841, (562) 799-2356, (800) 364-2147, Fax: (562) 799-1098, asaps@surgery.org, http://www.surgery.org.

American Society for Dermatologic Surgery, 5550 Meadowbrook Dr., Ste. 120, Rolling Meadows, IL 60008, (847) 956-0900, Fax: (847) 956-0999, http://www.asds.net.

American Society of Plastic Surgeons, 444 E. Algonquin Rd., Arlington Heights, IL 60005, http://www.plasticsurgery.org.

Association of American Medical Colleges, 2450 N. St. NW, Washington, DC 20037-1126, (202) 828-0400, https://www.aamc.org.

The Society of Thoracic Surgeons, 633 N. Saint Clair St., Fl. 23, Chicago, IL 60611, (312) 202-5800, Fax: (312) 202-5801, http://sts.org.

L. Fleming Fallon Jr, MD, DrPH

Surgical triage

Definition

Triage (from the French verb trier "to sort") is an assessment performed by health care providers to screen for the most critically ill or injured patients out of a group of people. Surgical triage focuses on establishing priority with respect to which surgeries are most critical in a time-sensitive manner. Triage is a necessary process when health care resources are limited and not every patient can be treated at once.

Purpose

Triage is performed to prioritize medical treatment so that the most at-risk patients are treated first, while the number of lives saved is maximized. Triage is especially important in emergency situations when the amount of resources is limited. For example, a patient with a chest wound requiring immediate surgery to maintain life will take priority over a patient who needs surgery for a benign tumor.

Description

Triage is a system of screening, evaluating, and classifying the sick or wounded. It may be done during war, disaster situations, or in the emergency room of a hospital. Regardless of where it is performed, triage for any medical treatment is dependent on the available medical resources. Medical resources include any factors that might limit access to medical treatment, including the availability of medications, **operating room** space, hospital space, **bandages** or other materials, and physicians. Surgical triage takes both the acuity (severity) of the patient's medical condition and the available medical resources into account.

Initial field assessment

In a non-health care setting, the initial assessment of patients may be performed by first responders. To provide a consistent standard of care, first responders may utilize the "ABCDE" assessment, which involves:

• Airway and cervical spine control. The patient's airway needs to be assessed and a functioning airway needs to be maintained. The cervical spine needs to be stabilized to prevent further injury and maintain the airway.

• Breathing and oxygenation. The patient is assessed for thoracic injury such as pneumothorax, flail chest, or hemothorax, which might compromise breathing.

• Circulation and hemorrhage. The degree of blood loss is evaluated, and any hemorrhaging needs to be controlled.

• Dysfunction and disability of the central nervous system. A traumatic brain injury may result in cessation of vital functions.

• Exposure of injuries and environmental control such as thermoregulation. Steps need to be taken to prevent or treat hypothermia.

Emergency surgical triage

There are multiple grading systems or standards for triaging patients in an emergency setting. Each patient is evaluated (including obtaining a brief history when possible) and given a rapid physical exam specifically geared toward assessing **vital signs** and areas of critical injury or illness. The components of the initial triage history include allergies to specific medications; any current medications (in case new medications are indicated); and when the patient last ate, due to the risk of vomiting and breathing in the vomit during **general anesthesia** and the surgical procedure. Establishing an airway and taking basic life support measures are of priority. Other priority items include stopping any arterial bleeding before the patient goes into shock.

Emergency surgery procedures apply the general principles of emergency triage in addition to information about the specific medical condition involved in order to determine which surgeries need to be performed first.

Emergency surgical procedures may be necessary due to trauma (with the patient being critically injured) or a critical phase of a disease state (such as immediately life-threatening heart failure caused by a condition amenable to surgical repair). It is essential that triage be performed rapidly and accurately, because in emergency situations a single minute could make the difference between survival and death. Topics that factor into the order in which patients are triaged includes vital signs, clinical history, mechanism of injury or pre-hospital course of disease, age, comorbid conditions, and whether the airways are open. A patient may be given priority if their vital signs are unstable or if they have a clinical history of cardiac or pulmonary disease, have serious injuries, have closed airways, are very young or very old, have lost consciousness, or are showing signs of neurological injuries.

An initial assessment of the patient involves running a primary survey, during which the patient's airway, breathing, circulation/hemorrhage, and mental capacities are evaluated. If the airway is obstructed, the patient may need to immediately undergo emergency surgery to remove the obstruction. Next, the patient's ability to breathe independently is evaluated. If the patient cannot breathe due to a surgically amenable condition, such as internal bleeding into the chest cavity, they may be triaged into emergency surgery. If the patient has obstructed circulation—such as in cardiac tamponade, where the heart sac is filled with blood and the heart cannot pump properly—emergency surgery may be required. If the patient displays a serious neurological disability due to a head or spinal cord injury, **neurosurgery** may be necessary.

If the patient has not been triaged in the primary survey as having an immediately life-threatening condition, a secondary survey is performed. The secondary survey is a more thorough **physical examination** covering the entire body of the patient. Blood tests may be run to check the basic functioning of the patient's bodily systems. At this point, triage is performed and the patient is prioritized for surgery.

Trauma patients being triaged for surgery may need diagnostic tests, such as a **computed tomography** (CT) scan, to help diagnose what is wrong with them and determine the appropriate surgery. However, if a patient has initially been brought to a smaller hospital without the appropriate surgeon present, this aspect of surgical triage may be temporarily put aside. Diagnostic tools such as CT scans take time and may delay the transfer of the patient to an appropriate trauma facility.

Non-emergency surgical triage

Triage also takes place in non-emergency situations when scheduling operations in the hospital. While non-emergent procedures are generally scheduled on a first-come, first-serve basis, if a patient is identified who medically requires a procedure in a time-sensitive manner, he or she may take precedence over a previously scheduled surgery. For example, if an aggressive tumor that requires surgery is discovered in a patient, a non-emergent procedure may be rescheduled to make room for the patient with the tumor.

Triage systems

Triage systems of classification may have up to five categories into which to place patients. Many U.S. hospitals use three-level systems with the categories of emergency, urgent, and non-urgent. However, studies have shown that five-level systems are the most effective. Five-level systems include the categories of resuscitation (when breathing or pulse is not detected), emergent, urgent, nonurgent, and referred (minimal medical resources are required). One well-known five-level triage system that is employed by emergency departments in the United States is the Emergency Severity Index (ESI). The ESI categorizes patients presenting to the emergency department by both health threat acuity and the resources available. The ESI scale ranges from one to five, with a lower number indicating greater severity. A triage nurse is usually the person who initiates the ESI when a patient presents to the emergency department. The acuity of a patient's medical condition is determined by the stability of the patient's vital signs and the potential for threat to life, limbs, or organs. If the patient meets high acuity level criteria (level 1 or 2), they need immediate treatment, possibly including surgery. If the patient does not meet high acuity level criteria, the triage nurse then proceeds to evaluate the expected resources needed for treatment to help determine a triage level (level 3, 4, or 5). The ESI is a method for emergency departments to triage patients in a validated manner. It is one of the only triage systems that specifically categorizes patients based on the resources available. A general triage system such as the ESI is only one factor in the process of surgical triage, however; patients with high acuity levels and conditions amenable to surgery are then given over to more specific surgical triage done by the appropriate surgical specialty.

Surgical triage after trauma

Triage decisions are based on many factors and may include a trauma score. These scores reflect an assessment of how critical a patient's medical condition is after physical trauma. There are many different trauma-scoring systems that may assist in the process of triage. The Revised Trauma Score (RTS) is one commonly used system to aid triage decisions. The RTS is based on physiological parameters, including blood pressure, respiratory rate, and level of consciousness. Each parameter is worth a certain number of points, with higher points being better. An RTS score lower than 11 requires admission of the patient to a trauma center. Other types of trauma-scoring systems may be geared toward different types of injuries, such as the Injury Severity Score (ISS), Penetrating Abdominal Trauma Index (PATI), Systemic Inflammatory Response Syndrome (SIRS), and ICD-Based Injury Severity Score (ICISS). The Abbreviated Injury Score (AIS) is often used to assist in triage for **trauma surgery**. The AIS is an anatomically based system of grading injuries from one to six, with one being minor injury and six being lethal injury. For trauma conditions that are amenable to surgery, an appropriate trauma-scoring system may greatly influence who is brought to the trauma center and the surgical triage decisions.

Triage coding in disasters

Triage officers in mass casualty situations may utilize the Simple Triage and Rapid Treatment (START) system. The START system is a very simple four-category triage system that categorizes patients as severe, urgent, minor, or beyond medical assistance. In advanced systems, patients triaged in emergency or mass casualty situations are often given a color-coded tag to help identify their status to other health care workers. Triage tag systems vary from country to country. In general, there are four categories, each assigned to a color:

• immediate care required with possible positive outcome anticipated (red)

• urgent care required but may be briefly delayed (yellow)

• care required but may be extensively delayed (green)

• immediate care required but the patient is realistically beyond saving (black)

Red is the color tag used for the group of patients requiring immediate care without which they would not survive. The red triage tag indicates that the patient is in an immediate medical crisis and may be realistically saved given the medical facilities available. Red-tagged triage patients are given top priority over other colored tags. In surgical triage, a red-tagged patient would generally be one requiring immediate surgery to save his or her life. If the medical facilities are substantial

enough, some types of crippling injuries that are not life threatening may be given a red triage tag. For example, amputations may be triaged as red because surgical reattachment of severed or partially severed limbs must take place within minutes of the injury in order for the limbs to be salvaged.

Yellow is the color tag used for patients who require urgent medical care but who are not in immediate danger of losing their life. Yellow triage groups may be able to wait hours for medical treatment, but not days. Yellow is the group known as delayed priority. In surgical triage, yellow-tagged patients may require surgery within a specific time frame in order to maintain life. While yellow-tagged patients may be stable for the moment, triage is a dynamic process, and medical conditions may deteriorate rapidly. A patient in the yellow triage category needs to be monitored while awaiting treatment and re-triaged if necessary.

Green is the color tag used for patients for whom medical care is a minor priority, and who may wait a number of days before treatment without risking life. An example of a green triage condition is a broken bone without compound fracture, which needs to be treated but will not endanger a patient's life. The green category is sometimes referred to as the "walking wounded."

Black is the triage color category that causes the most difficult ethical dilemma. The black triage tag is given to patients who are in immediate danger of losing their lives from injury or disease, but for whom medical treatment is unlikely to be successful. This category of triage is often given lowest priority when medical resources are scarce. The purpose of triage is to maintain the health of the greatest number of people. Resources devoted to black-tagged patients are often considered resources taken away from patients who may have benefited from them. For surgical triage, black-tagged patients are patients for whom surgery is unlikely to salvage. Potential examples of black-tagged surgical triage would be patients with extremely extensive burn injuries or **crush injuries**.

Patients given white tags have such minor injuries that a doctor's care is not required. These patients are dismissed and would not be placed in a surgical triage situation.

Health care team roles

An initial triage officer is a health care professional who performs triage on a patient arriving at the hospital. In the emergency department, the initial triage officer is often a triage nurse, who identifies the critically ill and sends them for further evaluation by a physician. Sometimes the triage officer is a resident, a full medical doctor who is in training for their specialty. For surgical triage, it is often a surgical resident that first determines whether a new patient requires surgery immediately.

Once a patient has undergone a surgical procedure, the triage process continues in the surgical **intensive care unit** (SICU). The SICU is a special hospital unit for patients undergoing surgery to stay in until they are deemed well enough to be transferred to other parts of the hospital or discharged. The surgical specialties of each hospital support the SICU and may include trauma surgery; neurosurgery; cardiothoracic surgery; **transplant surgery**; **orthopedic surgery**; **ear, nose, and throat surgery**; **plastic surgery**; **vascular surgery**; **general surgery**; and obstetrics and gynecological surgery. While the SICU is run by numerous types of health care providers, some systems utilize a surgical intensivist to triage which patients need to stay in the SICU and which may leave. A surgical intensivist is an MD who is both a general surgeon and has special training in intensive care practices.

In addition to the triage needs of each individual patient, the surgical intensivist must also manage a balance between the supply and demand of factors such as operating room time, **post-anesthesia care unit** availability, and bed space. It is a challenge for the surgical intensivist to properly assess which patients require SICU admission and which ones can be either denied admission or discharged safely for home. Patients who are inappropriately judged ready for discharge have been associated with a higher level of mortality, so triage on this level has a critical impact on healthcare. The surgical intensivist's triage decisions may be supported by the **surgeons** on the patient's primary surgical care team.

Ethical considerations

Triage systems have been developed to ensure that the greatest number of people requiring medical care survive disease or injury. Unfortunately, medical resources are often limited, and there are not enough to give each and every patient ideal medical care. For black-tagged triage patients who are unlikely to survive despite medical care, this dilemma is especially poignant. Physicians are generally trained to see any patient under their care as one to whom the physician demonstrates fidelity by acting in the best interests of the patient over the interests of others. However, in emergency triage situations, it is necessary for triage officers to assign priority based on established guidelines. Although physicians may greatly desire to treat any patient that requires help, in emergency situations they may need to put certain patients aside so as to save the lives of others. Since a physician's time is considered a limited medical resource, especially in emergency or mass casualty situations, a patient may even be coded with a black

KEY TERMS

ABCDE—A survey standard that is followed by first responders to do an initial assessment of patients in a non-health care setting.

Cardiac tamponade—A condition in which the sac around the heart is filled with blood and keeps the heart from functioning properly.

Cardiothoracic surgery—Surgery involving the chest body cavity known as the thoracic cavity.

Comorbid conditions—Diseases or disorders that exist simultaneously in one patient.

Computed tomography (CT scan)—A computer uses x-rays across many different directions on a given cross section of the body, and combines all the cross sections to create one image. CT scans can be used to visualize bodily organs including the brain, blood vessels, bones, and the spinal cord. Contrast dye is sometimes administered to the patient to help visualize structures.

Flail chest—Occurs when a section of the thoracic wall such as the rib cage separates from the rest of the chest wall.

Hemorrhage—Excessive blood loss through blood vessel walls.

Hemothorax—A condition in which blood accumulates in the pleural cavity, commonly as a result of traumatic injury.

Neurological—Pertaining to the nervous system: peripheral nervous system, brain, and spinal cord.

Physiological—Pertaining to the normal vital life functions of a living organism.

Pneumothorax—An accumulation of gas or air in the pleural cavity.

Pulmonary disease—Any disease involving the lungs.

Trauma surgery—Surgery performed as a result of injury.

Vital signs—The physiological aspects of body function basic to life: temperature, pulse, breathing rate, and blood pressure.

tag if the amount of time necessary to save them is very long. With limited time to save as many as possible, a 24-hour procedure for one person may mean losing five others that could have been treated in the same time period. Triage is essentially designed to do the greatest good for the greatest number of patients in any given situation. However, accomplishing this goal often puts physicians in difficult ethical situations and an emotionally painful decision-making process.

Resources

PERIODICALS

Iserson, K. V., and J. C. Moskop. "Triage in Medicine, Part I: Concept, History, and Types." *Annals of Emergency Medicine* 49, no. 3 (2007): 275–81.

Iserson, K. V., and J. C. Moskop. "Triage in Medicine, Part II: Underlying Values and Principles." *Annals of Emergency Medicine* 49, no. 3 (2007): 282–87.

Marsden, J., J. Windle, and K. Mackway-Jones. "Emergency Triage." *Emergency Nurse* 21, no. 4 (2013): 11.

Rigal, Sylvain, and François Pons. "Triage of Mass Casualties in War Conditions: Realities and Lessons Learned." *International Orthopaedics* 37, no. 8 (2013): 1433–38. http://dx.doi.org/10.1007/s00264-013-1961-y (accessed August 13, 2013).

Smith, Anita. "Using a Theory to Understand Triage Decision Making." *International Emergency Nursing* 21, no. 2 (2013): 113–17. http://dx.doi.org/10.1016/j.ienj.2012.03.003 (accessed August 13, 2013).

Sprung, Charles L., et al. "Triage of Intensive Care Patients: Identifying Agreement and Controversy." *Intensive Care Medicine* (August 8, 2013): 113–17. http://dx.doi.org/10.1007/s00134-013-3033-6 (accessed August 13, 2013).

Wolfson, Nikolaj. "Orthopaedic Triage during Natural Disasters and Mass Casualties: Do Scoring Systems Matter?" *International Orthopaedics* 37, no. 8 (2013): 1439–41. http://dx.doi.org/10.1007/s00264-013-1997-z (accessed August 13, 2013).

OTHER

Gilboy, Nicki, et al. *Emergency Severity Index: A Triage Tool for Emergency Department Care.* 2012 ed. AHRQ publication no. 12-0041. Rockville, MD: Agency for Healthcare Research and Quality, November 2011. http://www.ahrq.gov/professionals/systems/hospital/esi/esihandbk.pdf (accessed August 13, 2013).

WEBSITES

Centers for Disease Control and Prevention. "Guidelines for the Field Triage of Injured Patients." http://www.cdc.gov/FieldTriage (accessed August 13, 2013).

Dries, David J. "Initial Evaluation of the Trauma Patient." Medscape Reference. http://emedicine.medscape.com/article/434707-overview (accessed August 13, 2013).

ESI Triage Research Team. "Areas of ESI Algorithm." http://www.esitriage.org/algorithm.asp (accessed August 13, 2013).

Pohlman, Timothy H. "Trauma Scoring Systems." Medscape Reference. http://emedicine.medscape.com/article/434076-overview (accessed August 13, 2013).

Maria Basile, PhD

Sutures *see* **Closures**

Sweat test *see* **Electrolyte tests**

Sympathectomy

Definition

Sympathectomy is a surgical procedure that destroys nerves in the sympathetic nervous system. The procedure is performed to increase blood flow and decrease long-term pain in certain diseases that cause narrowed blood vessels. It can also be used to decrease excessive sweating. This surgical procedure cuts or destroys the sympathetic ganglia, which are collections of nerve cell bodies in clusters along the thoracic or lumbar spinal cord.

Purpose

The autonomic nervous system controls involuntary body functions such as breathing, sweating, and blood pressure. It is subdivided into two components, the sympathetic and the parasympathetic nervous systems.

The sympathetic nervous system speeds the heart rate, narrows (constricts) blood vessels, and raises blood pressure. Blood pressure is controlled by means of nerve cells that run through sheaths around the arteries. The sympathetic nervous system can be described as the "fight or flight" system because it allows humans to respond to danger by fighting off an attacker or running away. When danger threatens, the sympathetic nervous system increases heart and respiratory rates and blood flow to muscles, and decreases blood flow to other areas such as skin, digestive tract, and limb veins. The net effect is an increase in blood pressure.

Sympathectomy is performed to relieve intermittent constricting of blood vessels (ischemia) when the fingers, toes, ears, or nose are exposed to cold (Raynaud's phenomenon). In Raynaud's phenomenon, the affected extremities turn white, then blue, and red as the blood supply is cut off. The color changes are accompanied by numbness, tingling, burning, and pain. Normal color and feeling are restored when heat is applied. The condition sometimes occurs without direct cause but is more often caused by an underlying medical condition, such as rheumatoid arthritis. Sympathectomy is usually less effective when Raynaud's syndrome is caused by an underlying medical condition. Narrowed blood vessels in the legs that cause painful cramping (claudication) are also treated with sympathectomy.

Sympathectomy may be helpful in treating reflex sympathetic dystrophy (RSD), a condition that sometimes develops after injury. In RSD, the affected limb is painful (causalgia) and swollen. The color, temperature, and texture of the skin changes. These symptoms are related to prolonged and excessive sympathetic nervous system activity.

Sympathectomy is also effective in treating excessive sweating (hyperhidrosis) of the palms, armpits, or face.

Demographics

Experts estimate that 10,000–20,000 sympathectomy procedures are performed each year in the United States.

Description

Sympathectomy for hyperhidrosis is accomplished by making a small incision under the armpit and introducing air into the chest cavity. The surgeon inserts a fiberoptic tube (endoscope) that projects an image of the operation on a video screen. The ganglia are cut with fine scissors attached to the endoscope. Laser beams may also be used to destroy the ganglia.

If only one arm or leg is affected, it may be treated with a percutaneous radiofrequency technique. In this technique, the surgeon locates the ganglia by a combination of x-ray and electrical stimulation. The ganglia are destroyed by applying radio waves through electrodes on the skin.

Diagnosis

A reversible block of the affected nerve cell (ganglion) determines if sympathectomy is needed. This procedure interrupts nerve impulses by injecting the ganglion with a steroid and anesthetic. If the block has a positive effect on pain and blood flow in the affected area, the sympathectomy will probably be helpful. The surgical procedure should be performed only if conservative treatment has not been effective. Conservative treatment includes avoiding exposure to stress and cold, and the use of physical therapy and medications.

Sympathectomy is most likely to be effective in relieving reflex sympathetic dystrophy if it is performed soon after the injury occurs. The increased benefit of early surgery must be balanced against the time needed to promote spontaneous recovery and responses to more conservative treatments.

Preparation

Patients should discuss expected results and possible risks with their **surgeons**. They should inform their surgeons of all medications they are taking, and provide a complete medical history. Candidates for surgery should have good general health. To improve general health, a surgical candidate may be asked to lose weight, give up smoking or alcohol, and get the proper amount of sleep and **exercise**. Immediately before the surgery, patients will not be permitted to eat or drink, and the surgical site will be cleaned and scrubbed.

KEY TERMS

Causalgia—A severe burning sensation sometimes accompanied by redness and inflammation of the skin. Causalgia is caused by injury to a nerve outside the spinal cord.

Claudication—Cramping or pain in a leg caused by poor blood circulation, frequently caused by hardening of the arteries (atherosclerosis). Intermittent claudication occurs only at certain times, usually after exercise, and is relieved by rest.

Fiberoptics—In medicine, fiberoptics uses glass or plastic fibers to transmit light through a specially designed tube inserted into organs or body cavities where it transmits a magnified image of the internal body structures.

Hyperhidrosis—Excessive sweating. Hyperhidrosis can be caused by heat, overactive thyroid glands, strong emotion, menopause, or infection.

Parasympathetic nervous system—The division of the autonomic (involuntary) nervous system that slows heart rate, increases digestive and glandular activity, and relaxes the sphincter muscles that close off body organs.

Percutaneous—Performed through the skin. It is derived from two Latin words, *per* (through) and *cutis* (skin).

Pneumothorax—A collection of air or gas in the chest cavity that causes a lung to collapse. Pneumothorax may be caused by an open chest wound that admits air.

Aftercare

The surgeon informs the patient about specific aftercare needed for the technique used. Doppler ultrasonography, a test using sound waves to measure blood flow, can help to determine whether sympathectomy has had a positive result.

The operative site must be kept clean until the incision closes.

Risks

Side effects of sympathectomy may include decreased blood pressure while standing, which may cause fainting. After sympathectomy in men, semen is sometimes ejaculated into the bladder, possibly impairing fertility. After a sympathectomy is performed by inserting an endoscope in the chest cavity, some persons may experience chest pain with deep breathing. This procedure may be performed under **local anesthesia** in an outpatient surgical facility.

Resources

BOOKS

Bland, K. I., et al. *General Surgery: Principles and International Practice*. London: Springer, 2009.

Brunicardi, F. Charles, et al. *Schwartz's Principles of Surgery*. 10th ed. New York: McGraw-Hill, 2014.

Henry, Michael M., and Jeremy N. Thompson. *Clinical Surgery*. Edinburgh: Saunders/Elsevier, 2012.

Townsend, Courtney M., et al. *Sabiston Textbook of Surgery*. 19th ed. Philadelphia: Saunders/Elsevier, 2012.

PERIODICALS

Aoki, Hiroshi, et al. "Extent of Sympathectomy Affects Postoperative Compensatory Sweating and Satisfaction in Patients with Palmar Hyperhidrosis." *Journal of Anesthesia* (August 8, 2013): e-pub ahead of print. http://dx.doi.org/10.1007/s00540-013-1692-7 (accessed October 4, 2013).

Ng, Calvin S. H., et al. "Evolving Techniques of Endoscopic Thoracic Sympathectomy: Smaller Incisions or Less?" *The Surgeon* 11, no. 5 (2013): 290–91. http://dx.doi.org/10.1016/j.surge.2013.06.006 (accessed October 4, 2013).

Rajendram, R., and A. Hayward. "Ultrasound-Guided Digital Sympathectomy Using Botulinum Toxin." *Anaesthesia* 68, no. 10 (2013): 1077. http://dx.doi.org/10.1111/anae.12416 (accessed October 4, 2013).

WEBSITES

A.D.A.M. Medical Encyclopedia. "Endoscopic Thoracic Sympathectomy." MedlinePlus. http://www.nlm.nih.gov/medlineplus/ency/article/007291.htm (accessed October 4, 2013).

The Society of Thoracic Surgeons. "Hyperhidrosis." http://www.sts.org/patient-information/other-types-surgery/hyperhidrosis (accessed October 4, 2013).

Stanford School of Medicine, Department of Thoracic Surgery. "Thoracoscopic (VATS) Sympathectomy for Hyperhidrosis." http://thoracicsurgery.stanford.edu/patient_care/hyperhidrosis.html (accessed October 4, 2013).

ORGANIZATIONS

American Academy of Neurology, 201 Chicago Ave., Minneapolis, MN 55415, (612) 928-6000, (800) 879-1960, Fax: (612) 454-2746, memberservices@aan.com, http://www.aan.com.

American Board of Surgery, 1617 John F. Kennedy Blvd., Ste. 860, Philadelphia, PA 19103-1847, (215) 568-4000, Fax: (215) 563-5718, http://www.absurgery.org.

American College of Surgeons, 633 N. Saint Clair St., Chicago, IL 60611-3211, (312) 202-5000, (800) 621-4111, Fax: (312) 202-5001, postmaster@facs.org, http://www.facs.org.

The Society of Thoracic Surgeons, 633 N. Saint Clair St., Fl. 23, Chicago, IL 60611, (312) 202-5800, Fax: (312) 202-5801, http://sts.org.

L. Fleming Fallon Jr., MD, DrPH

---

problem usually disappears within two weeks. They may also experience pneumothorax (air in the chest cavity).

Results

Studies show that sympathectomy relieves hyperhidrosis in more than 90% of cases and causalgia in up to 75% of cases. The less invasive procedures cause very little scarring. Most persons stay in the hospital for less than one day and return to work within a week.

Morbidity and mortality rates

In 30% of cases, surgery for hyperhidrosis may cause increased sweating on the chest. In 2% of cases, the surgery may cause increased sweating in other areas, including increased facial sweating while eating. Less frequent complications include Horner's syndrome, a condition of the nervous system that causes the pupil of the eye to close, the eyelid to droop, and sweating to decrease on one side of the face. Other rare complications are nasal blockage and pain to the nerves supplying the skin between the ribs. Mortality is extremely rare, and usually attributable to low blood pressure.

Alternatives

Nonsurgical treatments include physical therapy, medications, and avoidance of stress and cold. These measures reduce or remove the likelihood of triggering a problem mediated by the sympathetic nervous system.

Health care team roles

A sympathectomy is usually performed by a general surgeon, neurosurgeon, or surgeon with specialty training in head and neck surgery.

Sympathectomy was traditionally performed on an inpatient under **general anesthesia**. An incision was made on the mid-back, exposing the ganglia to be cut. Recent techniques are less invasive. As a result, the

Sympathomimetic drugs *see* **Adrenergic drugs**

Syndactyly surgery *see* **Webbed finger or toe repair**

Syringe and needle

Definition

Syringes and needles are sterile devices used to inject solutions into or withdraw secretions from the body. A syringe is a calibrated glass or plastic cylinder with a plunger at one end and an opening that attaches to a needle at the other. The needle is a hollow metal tube with a pointed tip.

Purpose

A syringe and needle assembly is used to administer drugs when a small amount of fluid is to be injected; when a person cannot take the drug by mouth; or when the drug would be destroyed by digestive secretions. A syringe and needle may also be used to withdraw various types of body fluids, most commonly tissue fluid from swollen joints or blood from veins.

Description

The modern hypodermic needle was invented in 1853 by Alexander Wood, a Scottish physician, and independently in the same year by Charles Pravaz, a French surgeon. Today, there are many different types and sizes of syringes used for a variety of purposes. Syringe sizes may vary from 0.25 mL to 450 mL, and can be made from glass or assorted plastics. Latex-free syringes eliminate the exposure of health care professionals and patients to allergens to which they may be sensitive. The most common type of syringe is the piston syringe. Pen, cartridge, and dispensing syringes are also extensively used.

One common type of syringe consists of a hollow barrel with a piston at one end and a nozzle at the other end that connects to a needle. Other syringes have a needle already attached. These devices are often used for subcutaneous injections of insulin and are single-use (i.e., disposable). Syringes have markings etched or printed on their sides, showing the graduations (in milliliters) for accurate dispensing of drugs or removal of body fluids. Cartridge syringes are intended for multiple uses, and are often sold in kits containing a pre-filled drug cartridge with a needle inserted into the piston syringe. Syringes may also have anti-needlestick features, as well as positive stops that prevent accidental pullouts.

There are three types of nozzles:

- Luer-lock, which locks the needle onto the nozzle of the syringe.
- Slip tip, which secures the needle by compressing the slightly tapered hub onto the syringe nozzle.
- Eccentric, which secures with a connection that is almost flush with the side of the syringe.

A hypodermic needle is a hollow metal tube, usually made of stainless steel and sharpened at one end. It has a female connection at one end that fits into the male connection of a syringe or intravascular administration set. The size of the diameter of the

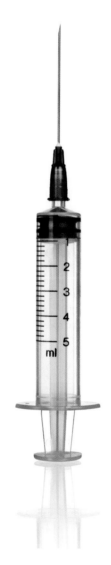

Syringe and needle. *(urfin/Shutterstock.com)*

KEY TERMS

Aseptic—Free from infection or diseased material; sterile.

Bevel—The slanted opening on one side of the tip of a needle.

Hypodermic—Applied or administered beneath the skin. The modern hypodermic needle was invented to deliver medications below the skin surface.

Piston—The plunger that slides up and down inside the barrel of a syringe.

Sharps—A general term for needles, lancets, scalpel blades, and other medical devices with points or sharp edges requiring special disposal precautions.

Sterile—Free from living microorganisms.

Subcutaneous—Beneath the skin.

Vacutainer—A tube with a rubber top from which air has been removed.

Z-track injection—A special technique for injecting a drug into muscle tissue so that the drug does not leak (track) into the layers of tissue just beneath the skin.

needle ranges from the largest gauge (13) to the smallest (27). The length of the needle ranges from 3.5 in. (8 cm) for the 13-gauge to 0.25 in. (0.6 cm) for the 27-gauge. The needle consists of a hub with a female connection at one end that attaches to the syringe. The bevel, which is a slanted opening on one side of the needle tip, is located at the other end.

Needles are almost always disposable. Reusable needle assemblies are available for home use.

Operation

Syringes and needles are used for injecting or withdrawing fluids from a person. The most common procedure for removing fluids is venipuncture or drawing blood from a vein. In this procedure, the syringe and a needle of the proper size are used with a vacutainer. A vacutainer is a tube with a rubber top from which air has been removed. Fluids enter the container without pressure applied by the person withdrawing the blood. A vacutainer is used to collect blood as it is drawn. The syringe and needle can be left in place while the health care provider changes the vacutainer,

allowing for multiple samples to be drawn during a single procedure.

Fluids can be injected by intradermal injection, subcutaneous injection, intramuscular injection, or Z-track injection. For all types of injections, the size of syringe should be chosen based on the amount of fluid being delivered; the gauge and length of needle should be chosen based on the size of the patient and type of medication. A needle with a larger gauge may be chosen for drawing up the medication into the syringe, and a smaller-gauge needle used to replace the larger one for administering the injection. Proper procedures for infection control should be strictly followed for all injections.

Maintenance

Syringes and needles are normally sterile products and should be stored in appropriate containers. Care should be taken prior to using them. The care provider should ensure that the needles have not been blunted and that the packaging is not torn, as poor handling or storage exposes the contents to air and allows contamination by microorganisms.

Safety

All health care personnel must be offered vaccines against such bloodborne infections as hepatitis B and C.

Used syringes and needles should be discarded quickly in appropriate containers. If a needlestick injury occurs, it must be reported immediately and proper treatment administered to the injured person.

Training

Health care instructors should ensure that staff members are skilled in up-to-date methods of **aseptic technique** as well as the correct handling and use of syringes and needles. All persons administering injections should be aware of current methods of infection prevention.

Teaching the correct use of syringes and needles, as well as their disposal, is important to protect medical staff and people receiving injections from needlestick injuries and contamination from bloodborne infections. Some of the more serious infections are human immunodeficiency virus (HIV), hepatitis B (HBV), and hepatitis C (HCV).

Needles are defined as "sharps" for purposes of public health regulation, and must be broken or otherwise "rendered unrecognizable" before being placed in a puncture-proof container labeled with the universal biohazard symbol. This precaution is intended to prevent drug addicts from reusing the needles as well as to protect the hospital environment from contamination by medical waste.

Resources

BOOKS

Nettina, Sandra M. *Lippincott Manual of Nursing Practice.* 10th ed. Philadelphia: Wolters Kluwer Health/Lippincott Williams & Wilkins, 2013.

Perry, Anne G., and Patricia A. Potter. *Clinical Nursing Skills & Techniques.* 7th ed. St. Louis, MO: Mosby/Elsevier, 2010.

PERIODICALS

Eisler, Peter. "Dirty Medical Needles Put Tens of Thousands at Risk in USA." *USA Today*, March 6, 2013. http://oneandonlycampaign.org/safe_injection_practices (accessed October 4, 2013).

WEBSITES

Centers for Disease Control and Prevention. "Injection Safety." http://www.cdc.gov/injectionsafety (accessed October 4, 2013).

Centers for Disease Control and Prevention and Safe Injection Practices Coalition. "Safe Injection Practices." One & Only Campaign. http://oneandonlycampaign.org/safe_injection_practices (accessed October 4, 2013).

U.S. Food and Drug Administration. "Needles and Other Sharps (Safe Disposal Outside of Health Care Settings)." http://www.fda.gov/MedicalDevices/ProductsandMedical Procedures/HomeHealthandConsumer/ConsumerProducts/ Sharps/default.htm (accessed October 4, 2013).

ORGANIZATIONS

American Academy of Family Physicians (AAFP), 11400 Tomahawk Creek Pkwy., Leawood, KS 66211-2680, (913) 906-6000, (800) 274-2237, Fax: (913) 906-6075, http://www.aafp.org.

American Nurses Association, 8515 Georgia Ave., Ste. 400, Silver Spring, MD 20910-3492, (800) 274-4ANA (4262), http://nursingworld.org.

Centers for Disease Control and Prevention, 1600 Clifton Rd., Atlanta, GA 30333, (800) CDC-INFO (232-4636), (888) 232-6348, cdcinfo@cdc.gov, http://www.cdc.gov.

L. Fleming Fallon Jr., MD, DrPH

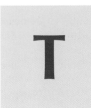

Talking to the health care provider

Definition

Talking to the health care provider refers to the exchange of information between a patient and his or her healthcare provider. It includes communicating private or potentially sensitive information and requires a climate of trust. Without trust and accurate information, treatment and healing are difficult.

Purpose

The purpose of talking to a health care provider is to exchange information and obtain relief from pain and suffering. It requires an atmosphere of openness and mutual confidence.

Description

Talking to a health care provider should be easy, but for many people, this is not the case. Patients may avoid asking their healthcare providers questions or revealing symptoms because they feel nervous, scared, or even guilty. This hesitation may also be fueled by a sense of hurry and urgency on behalf of the healthcare professional; patients may feel uncomfortable when they sense that they are being rushed. Additional barriers may include not being a native English speaker or depending on a family member or caregiver to represent needs (such as for a small child or elderly patient).

Establishing trust

Trust requires time to develop, but it is also a two-way interaction. People seeking the advice of a health care provider may reveal only a portion of their symptoms at first. While it is the health care provider's task to elicit relevant information, the patient who is answering the questions must be open and willing to share.

In some situations, health care providers often assume that patients do not give completely honest answers—for example, women typically understate their body weight, while men overstate their strength. Smokers rarely admit to the true number of cigarettes that they smoke per day, and drinkers underestimate the amount of alcohol that they consume.

Preparation

Important elements of any healthcare provider-patient conversation are honesty and openness. Inaccurate or incomplete information may lead the health care provider to make an incorrect diagnosis or treatment decision. While some patients feel concerned that their healthcare provider may not approve of all the choices they have made to treat their conditions or optimize their health, it is crucial to good medical care that patients are made to feel comfortable in revealing all of the OTC medications, herbal preparations, and any other complementary and alternatives modalities they utilize to treat heath issues or to maintain their physical or mental health.

Bringing records from visits to other healthcare providers is very useful to a health care provider. The number of people who have known their health care providers for long periods of time is declining. Providing a new health care provider with a personal medical history saves time and usually improves diagnostic accuracy. For example, old photographs are especially invaluable when evaluating skin problems.

Results

Preventive care should be part of the interaction between health care provider and patient. A frank exchange of information is one form of prevention. The passage of time, repeated positive interactions, and good outcomes from the information provided by the patient help to establish mutual trust, which then enhances the therapeutic interaction. The result may be better health for the patient.

Resources

BOOKS

Berger, Zackary. *Talking to Your Doctor: A Patient's Guide to Communication in the Exam Room and Beyond.* Lanham, MD: Rowman & Littlefield, 2013.

PERIODICALS

Beach, Mary Catherine, et al. "A Multicenter Study of Physician Mindfulness and Health Care Quality." *Annals of Family Medicine* 11, no. 5 (2013): 421–28. http://dx. doi.org/10.1370/afm.1507 (accessed September 19, 2013).

Farberg, Aaron S., et al. "Dear Doctor: A Tool to Facilitate Patient-Centered Communication." *Journal of Hospital Medicine* (August 28, 2013): e-pub ahead of print. http://dx.doi.org/10.1002/jhm.2073 (accessed September 19, 2013).

Karkowsky, Chavi Eve, and Cynthia Chazotte. "Simulation: Improving Communication with Patients." *Seminars in Perinatology* 37, no. 3 (2013): 157–60. http://dx.doi.org/10.1053/j.semperi.2013.02.006 (accessed September 19, 2013).

OTHER

National Institute on Aging. *Talking With Your Doctor: A Guide for Older People.* NIH Publication no. 05-3452. Bethesda, MD: National Institutes of Health/U.S. Department of Health and Human Services, August 2010. http://www.nia.nih.gov/sites/default/files/talking_with_your_doctor.pdf (accessed September 19, 2013).

WEBSITES

Agency for Healthcare Research and Quality. "Quick Tips—When Talking with Your Doctor." http://www.ahrq.gov/patients-consumers/diagnosis-treatment/diagnosis/doctalk/index.html (accessed September 19, 2013).

American Academy of Family Physicians. "Tips for Talking to Your Doctor." http://familydoctor.org/familydoctor/en/healthcare-management/working-with-your-doctor/tips-for-talking-to-your-doctor.html (accessed September 19, 2013).

American Heart Association. "Heart-to-Heart: Talking to Your Doctor." http://www.heart.org/HEARTORG/Conditions/More/ConsumerHealthCare/Heart-to-heart-Talking-to-Your-Doctor_UCM_323844_Article.jsp (accessed September 19, 2013).

Consumer Reports. "How to Talk to Your Doctor." http://www.consumerreports.org/cro/2013/06/how-to-talk-to-your-doctor/index.htm (accessed September 19, 2013).

MedlinePlus. "Talking with Your Doctor." U.S. National Library of Medicine, National Institutes of Health. http://www.nlm.nih.gov/medlineplus/talkingwithyourdoctor.html (accessed September 19, 2013).

National Institute on Aging and the U.S. National Library of Medicine. "Talking with Your Doctor." NIHSeniorHealth.gov. http://nihseniorhealth.gov/talkingwithyourdoctor/planningyourdoctorvisit/01.html (accessed September 19, 2013).

National Institutes of Health. "Talking to Your Doctor." http://nih.gov/clearcommunication/talktoyourdoctor.htm (accessed September 19, 2013).

Nemours Foundation. "Talking to Your Doctor." TeensHealth.org. teenshealth.org/teen/your_body/medical_care/talk_doctor.html (accessed September 19, 2013).

ORGANIZATIONS

American Academy of Family Physicians (AAFP), 11400 Tomahawk Creek Pkwy., Leawood, KS 66211-2680, (913) 906-6000, (800) 274-2237, Fax: (913) 906-6075, http://www.aafp.org.

American Academy of Pediatrics, 141 Northwest Point Blvd., Elk Grove Village, IL 60007-1098, (847) 434-4000, (800) 433-9016, Fax: (847) 434-8000, http://www.aap.org.

American College of Physicians (ACP), 190 N. Independence Mall West, Philadelphia, PA 19106-1572, (215) 351-2400, (800) 523-1546, http://www.acponline.org.

American College of Surgeons, 633 N. Saint Clair St., Chicago, IL 60611-3211, (312) 202-5000, (800) 621-4111, Fax: (312) 202-5001, postmaster@facs.org, http://www.facs.org.

L. Fleming Fallon, Jr., MD, DrPH
Rosalyn Carson-DeWitt, MD

Tarsorrhaphy

Definition

Tarsorrhaphy is a rare procedure in which the eyelids are partially sewn together to narrow the opening.

Purpose

The eye needs the lid for protection. It also needs tears and periodic blinking to cleanse it and keep it moist. There are many conditions that impair these functions and threaten the eye, specifically the cornea, with drying. Sewing the eyelids partially together helps protect the eye until the underlying condition can be corrected.

Some of the conditions that can improve with tarsorrhaphy include:

• Paralysis or weakness of the eyelids that may prevent the eyelids from closing adequately. Bell's palsy is a nerve condition that weakens the muscles of the face, including the eyelids. It is usually temporary. Myasthenia gravis also weakens facial muscles, but it is usually

KEY TERMS

Cornea—The clear part of the front of the eye through which vision occurs.

Enophthalmos—A condition in which the eye falls back into the socket and inhibits proper eyelid function.

Exophthalmos—A condition in which the eyes bulge out of their sockets and inhibit proper eyelid function.

Palpebral fissure—Eyelid opening.

Sjögren's syndrome—A connective tissue disease that hinders the production of tears and other body fluids.

QUESTIONS TO ASK YOUR DOCTOR

• How long will the eyes be closed with sutures?
• Will it be painful?
• Will the condition be remedied after the procedure?

treatable. A stroke can also weaken eyelids so that they do not close.

• Exophthalmos (eyes bulging out of their sockets) occurs with Graves' disease of the thyroid, and with tumors behind the eyes. If the eyes bulge out too far, the lids cannot close over them.

• Enophthalmos is a condition in which the eye falls back into the socket, making the eyelid ineffective.

• Several eye and corneal diseases cause swelling of the cornea, and require temporary added protection until the condition resolves.

• Sjögren's syndrome reduces tear flow to the point where it can endanger the cornea.

• Dendritic ulcers of the cornea caused by viruses may need to be covered with the eyelid while they heal.

Demographics

People of all ages can suffer from paralysis or corneal diseases that may benefit from tarsorrhaphy. For that reason, physicians can perform tarsorrhaphy on patients of any age. However, it is viewed as a last alternative for many patients, and is not indicated until after other treatments (e.g., patching and eye ointments) have been attempted.

Description

Tarsorrhaphy is an outpatient procedure done under local anesthetic. Stitches are carefully placed at the corners of the eyelid opening (palpebral fissure) to narrow the opening. This provides the eye with improved lubrication and less air exposure. Eyeball motion can help bathe the cornea in tears when it rolls up under the lid.

Preparation

The use of eye drops and contact lenses to moisten and protect the eyes must be considered before tarsorrhaphy is performed. Special preparation is not necessary.

Aftercare

Patients should avoid rubbing the eye and refrain from wearing make-up until given permission from the physician. Driving should be restricted until approval from the ophthalmologist.

Pathways in the home should be cleared of obstacles, and patients should be aware of peripheral vision loss. They will need to compensate by turning their head fully when looking at an object.

An analgesic may be used to ease pain, but severe pain is not normal, and the physician must be alerted. Sutures will be removed in two weeks.

Eye drops or ointment may still be needed to preserve the cornea or treat accompanying disease.

Risks

Tarsorrhaphy carries few risks, but complications may include minor eyelid swelling and superficial infection.

Results

A successful tarsorrhaphy procedure protects the eye and helps it retain moisture.

Morbidity and mortality rates

This is a safe procedure. Only superficial infections have been reported.

Alternatives

Eye drops and contact lenses are widely used to treat conditions that once warranted tarsorrhaphy. The procedure is now considered a last option for treatment.

Health care team roles

Ophthalmologists perform the procedure on an outpatient basis in a hospital, or sometimes in their offices.

Resources

BOOKS

Cassel, Gary H., Michael D. Billig, and Harry G. Randall. *The Eye Book: A Complete Guide to Eye Disorders and Health*. Baltimore, MD: Johns Hopkins University Press, 1998.

Daly, Stephen, ed. *Everything You Need to Know About Medical Treatments*. Springhouse, PA: Springhouse, 1996.

Hersh, Peter, and Bruce Zagelbaum. *Ophthalmic Surgical Procedures*. 2nd ed. New York: Thieme, 2009.

PERIODICALS

Weyns, Marlies, Carina Koppen, and Marie-José Tassignon. "Scleral Contact Lenses as an Alternative to Tarsorrhaphy for the Long-Term Management of Combined Exposure and Neurotrophic Keratopathy." *Cornea* 32, no. 3 (2013): 359–61. http://dx.doi.org/10.1097/ICO.0b013e31825 fed01 (accessed October 4, 2013).

WEBSITES

Palo Alto Medical Foundation. "Lower Eyelid Suspension Surgery." http://www.pamf.org/cosmeticsurgery/procedures/eyelid_suspension.html (accessed October 4, 2013).

ORGANIZATIONS

National Eye Institute, NEI Information Office, 31 Center Dr., MSC 2510, Bethesda, MD 20892-2510, (301) 496-5248, 2020@nei.nih.gov, http://www.nei.nih.gov.

J. Ricker Polsdorfer, MD
Mary Bekker

Tattoo removal

Definition

Although tattoos are considered to be permanent, it is possible to safely remove unwanted tattoos using one of several techniques.

Purpose

A growing number of people, especially the young, are getting tattoos. It is estimated that almost a quarter of all U.S. college students have at least one tattoo.

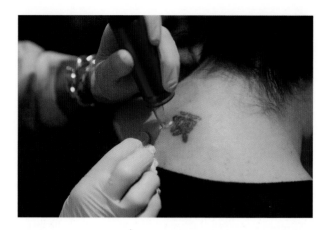

Woman during a tattoo removal session. *(Boston Globe/Getty Images)*

However, one study found that approximately half of all people with permanent tattoos eventually attempt to have them removed.

There are many reasons—personal, cultural, and physical—why people decide to have a tattoo removed. As people age, their self-image may change such that their tattoos no longer reflect who they feel they are. As fashions change, a particular tattoo may no longer be in style. Tattoos commemorating a particular person or relationship may become inappropriate if the relationship ends—divorce is one of the most common reasons for tattoo removal. Sometimes people must have tattoos removed for a new job. Tattoos may fade or blur. Finally, some people experience allergic reactions to the ink in their tattoos or other physical complications from a tattoo.

Description

Tattoo removal may be accomplished with laser treatments, **dermabrasion**, or surgery. Tattoo removal costs anywhere between several hundred to several thousand dollars—often far more than the cost of the original tattoo. Because tattoo removal is considered an aesthetic or cosmetic procedure, it is usually not covered by medical insurance. The cost of tattoo removal depends on a number of factors, including the age of the tattoo, the number of laser treatments required to remove it, the type of anesthesia used for surgical removal, and whether skin grafts are required.

Other factors also affect the cost, safety, and effectiveness of tattoo removal. These factors should be carefully considered before getting a permanent tattoo:

• the type of tattoo

• the size of the tattoo

- its location on the body
- the colors and types of tattoo pigments used

Laser removal

Laser removal—also called **laser surgery**, laser therapy, laser vaporization, or laser rejuvenation—has become the most common method of tattoo removal. It is considered safer and more effective than other methods, with less risk of infection. The U.S. Food and Drug Administration (FDA) has approved several types of lasers for tattoo removal. The most common type is a handheld Q-switched laser (QSL), which delivers short pulses of very high intensity light to the outer layers of the skin. These pulses of energy quickly superheat the tattoo ink, shattering it into smaller fragments. The laser wavelength is then switched to destroy different colors until the entire tattoo has been removed. This is a slow process. Multiple treatments are usually required in order to break down the pigments into particles that are small enough to be recognized as foreign bodies by the cells of the immune system. Eventually, the particles are removed from the body by the lymphatic system. Each treatment lasts only a few minutes, but the entire process usually takes several months. There is a new tattoo ink on the market, however, that is designed to be removable with only one or two laser treatments. Lasers usually remove tattoos without leaving a scar because the laser beam is precisely aimed to avoid damaging the skin surrounding the tattoo.

Some tattoo colors respond better than others to laser treatment. Dark blue, some lighter blues, red, and green inks tend to respond best. The wavelength of laser light is precisely tuned to each different pigment color, either by using different lasers or different settings on the same laser:

- Black tattoos on light-colored skin are the easiest to remove. Black ink responds to most wavelengths, but 1064 nanometers (nm) is most often used.
- Green ink responds best to 755 nm, although 694 nm or 650 nm can also be effective.
- Blue ink responds to 585 nm.
- Red ink responds to 532 nm.

A new type of laser, called a picosecond alexandrite laser, received FDA approval for marketing at the end of 2012. A small study suggested that it could remove tattoos with four or fewer treatments—far fewer than are generally needed with a Q-switched laser.

Dermabrasion

Dermabrasion, also known as surgical skin planing, is the traditional method for tattoo removal and may be less expensive than other methods. It is a skin-resurfacing procedure that uses a high-speed rotary instrument with an abrasive wheel or brush to sand down the surface and middle layers of the tattooed skin. This allows the tattoo ink to leach out of the body.

Surgical removal

In the past, surgical excision was the only way to remove a tattoo. Surgical tattoo removal involves physically removing the tattooed skin with a scalpel and then stitching the edges of the skin back together. It is the most invasive method of tattoo removal. However, it is the easiest and most effective method for removing some small tattoos, since it can be performed with high precision. Large tattoos are generally not good candidates for surgical removal.

Preparation

A dermatologist should be consulted before proceeding with tattoo removal. The dermatologist will explain the removal options and suggest which method is likely to be most effective. For example, some tattoo inks do not respond well to laser treatment. The doctor will probably review the patient's medical history and perform a physical exam, as well as explain the potential risks and likely outcome of the chosen removal procedure.

Prior to laser removal, it is extremely important to avoid tanning the area that will be treated. It is also important to avoid sun exposure for several weeks before surgical tattoo removal. Precautions include:

- using a high sun protection factor (SPF) sunblock every day and reapplying frequently when in the sun
- staying in the shade
- avoiding outdoor activities between 10 a.m. and 3 p.m.
- covering the skin with long sleeves and a hat
- wearing a bandage over the tattoo when out in the sun

Blood-thinning medications that contain **aspirin** or **nonsteroidal anti-inflammatory drugs** (NSAIDs) such as ibuprofen (Advil) should be avoided before any type of tattoo removal, since these can cause bruising or bleeding after the treatment. Medications that can cause the skin to darken (hyperpigmentation) should also be avoided.

Laser removal is often more painful than the original tattooing. The pain has been compared to being snapped repeatedly with a rubber band. A nonaspirin pain reliever such as **acetaminophen** (Tylenol) may be taken prior to the procedure. Many patients use an anesthetic cream one to two hours prior to treatment. The skin may or may not be numbed by injection with a local anesthetic. The skin is cleaned immediately before treatment.

Prior to dermabrasion, patients may be given medication to help them relax, and the tattooed area is sprayed to freeze or numb the skin. Prior to surgical tattoo removal, the treatment area is numbed by injection of a local anesthetic.

Aftercare

Following a laser treatment, the skin may be temporarily swollen and white. Blistering or bleeding is possible. The area may redden and form a scab. The wound must be cleaned gently, without scrubbing or rubbing, and kept protected from the sun. An antibacterial ointment can promote healing.

Following dermabrasion, the treated area may be sore and raw for up to ten days. An antibacterial ointment may be needed, and the area may need to be covered with a special bandage. Recovery time is usually two to three weeks. The treated area will be temporarily pink or red, with the color fading in 8 to 12 weeks. Patients must avoid the sun and regularly use sunscreen when outside for three to six months after dermabrasion, because exposure to sunlight can cause excessive scarring.

Following surgical tattoo removal, the skin may feel sunburned or tight. Pain medications or **antibiotics** may be prescribed. An ice pack and a dressing may be applied. The area must be kept clean with repeated application of antibacterial ointment, as directed by the doctor. It is usually possible to bathe or shower the day after surgery, but the treated area should not be scrubbed. A bandage or patch should be applied or, if left uncovered, sunscreen with an SPF factor of 30 or higher should be used when outside to avoid excessive scarring. The doctor also may prescribe a moisturizing cream or lotion.

Risks

Tattoo removal should never be attempted by people with certain types of autoimmune disorders, pigmentation problems, active acne or warts, uncontrolled or unstable diabetes, active rosacea, or undiagnosed lesions.

Surgery is the only method guaranteed to completely remove a tattoo, and it will leave a scar. Some scarring, infection, and skin discoloration—including temporary or permanent hyperpigmentation or lightening (hypopigmentation) of the tattooed skin—are risks with any method of tattoo removal.

Laser tattoo removal usually requires multiple treatments every few weeks, which can add up to several

KEY TERMS

Dermabrasion—Surgical sanding to remove tattoos from the skin.

Hyperpigmentation—Excessive pigmentation or color on part of the skin.

Hypopigmentation—Decreased pigmentation or color on a portion of the skin.

Immune system—The specialized cells and substances that help remove foreign particles, including ink particles, from the body.

Laser—A device that emits electromagnetic radiation at specific wavelengths, usually in the ultraviolet, visible, or infrared regions of the spectrum.

Lymphatic system—The part of the circulatory system responsible for immune responses, consisting of lymphatic fluid and vessels, lymph nodes, lymphocytes, and the thymus, spleen, bone marrow, tonsils, and adenoids.

Q-switched laser (QSL)—The type of laser generally used for tattoo removal.

thousand dollars, and it may not be successful. Dermabrasion also may not completely remove the tattoo. In addition to the above risks, dermabrasion may cause redness, swelling, and bleeding. Scarring may occur if the dermabrasion penetrates too deeply into the skin. Infections are rare but possible with dermabrasion. In addition to the above risks, surgery may fail to completely remove all of the tattoo pigment, and a raised or thickened scar may develop three to six months after tattoo removal.

Home remedies

Do-it-yourself tattoo removal creams and other home treatments are dangerous and unlikely to be effective. These products are acid-based and are not approved by the FDA. They can cause serious skin irritation and other reactions. Attempting to remove tattoos at home by other methods can lead to infection, serious complications, or even death.

Results

The results of tattoo removal vary greatly, and completely removing a tattoo can be very difficult. Multiple laser treatments or dermabrasion may only succeed in lightening the tattoo. Complete removal depends on many factors, including the age and size of

QUESTIONS TO ASK YOUR DOCTOR

- What tattoo removal method do you recommend?
- How much will my tattoo removal cost?
- If I have Q-switched laser removal, how many treatments will be required and what will be the interval between treatments?
- How likely is it that my tattoo will be completely removed?
- What are the potential risks, side effects, or complications of tattoo removal?

the tattoo and the types and colors of the inks. Sometimes more recent tattoos are more difficult to remove than older tattoos. However, sometimes older tattoos are more difficult to remove because the ink has penetrated deeper into the skin over time. Fluorescent colors are the most difficult to remove, and darker colors may be more difficult than lighter colors. Professional tattoos done with some of the newer inks and pastels may be difficult to entirely remove. Professional tattoos tend to have more uniform penetration of the deeper skin layers, which facilitates surgical removal of the inked skin to the same depth; however, many laser treatments may be required for removal of deeply penetrating pigment. Amateur tattoos fade more easily because they have generally been applied with less ink. However, if the ink has been applied unevenly, the tattoo may be more difficult to remove completely. Although surgical removal is usually effective, it leaves a scar and may be appropriate only for small tattoos. In contrast, dermabrasion usually results in new skin that is smoother and rejuvenated in appearance.

A recent study of laser tattoo removal found that success was more likely with nonsmokers and with tattoos smaller than 12 in. (30 cm) in size. Smoking reduced the likelihood of successful tattoo removal with ten laser treatment sessions by 70%, possibly because smoking interferes with wound healing. Tattoos on the feet or legs were less likely to be effectively removed than tattoos elsewhere on the body. Black and red pigments were the easiest to remove. Colors such as blue or yellow were less likely to be effectively removed. Tattoos that were all black had a removal rate of 58%. Black and red tattoos had a 51% success rate after ten treatments, since black and red absorb the laser wavelengths better than other colors. Colors such as green, yellow, or blue lowered the effective removal rate

by up to 80%. Intervals of eight weeks or less between laser treatments were not as effective as longer intervals between treatments.

Alternatives

An alternative to tattoo removal may be a second tattoo that covers the undesired tattoo.

Health care team roles

Although some tattoo shops remove tattoos, it is much safer to have them removed by a medical doctor trained in tattoo removal procedures. All tattoo removal methods are generally performed by dermatologic **surgeons** as an outpatient procedure in the surgeon's office or in an outpatient surgical clinic.

Resources

BOOKS

Adatto, M. A., S. Halachmi, and M. Lapidoth. "Laser Tattoo Removal." In *Basics in Dermatological Laser Applications*, edited by Inja Bogdan Allemann and David J. Goldberg. New York: Karger, 2011.

Kirby, William, Francisco Kartono, and Rebecca Small. "Tattoo Removal with Lasers." In *Dermatologic and Cosmetic Procedures in Office Practice*, edited by Richard Usatine. Philadelphia: Elsevier/Saunders, 2012.

Spalding, Frank. *Erasing the Ink: Getting Rid of Your Tattoo*. New York: Rosen, 2012.

PERIODICALS

Adatto, M. A., et al. "Tattoo Removal." *Current Problems in Dermatology* 42 (2011): 97.

Bencini, Pier Luca, et al. "Removal of Tattoos by Q-Switched Laser: Variables Influencing Outcome and Sequelae in a Large Cohort of Treated Patients." *Archives of Dermatology* 148, no. 12 (December 2012): 1364.

Bowers, Jan. "Rebellion and Remorse: More Americans Getting—and Getting Rid of—Tattoos." *Dermatology World*, April 2, 2012. http://www.aad.org/dw/monthly/2012/april/rebellion-and-remorse (accessed September 2, 2013).

Dooren, Jennifer Corbett. "Color, Size, and Smoking Affect Tattoo Removal." *Wall Street Journal*, September 18, 2012. http://online.wsj.com/article/SB10000872396390443995604578002543545271044.html (accessed September 20, 2013).

WEBSITES

American Society for Dermatologic Surgery. "Unwanted Tattoos."http://www.asds.net/TattooRemovalInformation.aspx (accessed September 2, 2013).

Mayo Clinic staff. "Tattoo Removal." MayoClinic.com. http://www.mayoclinic.com/health/tattoo-removal/MY01066 (accessed September 2, 2013).

Mozes, Alan. "Studies Show Limits, Promise of Laser Removal of Tattoos." *HealthDay.* September 17, 2012. http://health.usnews.com/health-news/news/articles/2012/09/17/studies-show-limits-promise-of-laser-removal-of-tattoos (accessed September 2, 2013).

Nemours Foundation. "Tattoos." TeensHealth.org. http://teenshealth.org/teen/your_body/skin_stuff/safe_tattooing.html (accessed September 2, 2013).

ORGANIZATIONS

American Academy of Dermatology, PO Box 4014, Schaumburg, IL 60168, (866) 503-SKIN (7546), http://www.aad.org.

American Society for Dermatologic Surgery, 5550 Meadowbrook Drive, Ste. 1220, Rolling Meadows, IL 60008, (847) 956-0900, Fax: (847) 956-0999, http://www.asds.net.

U.S. Food and Drug Administration, 10903 New Hampshire Avenue, Silver Spring, MD 20993-0002, (888) INFO-FDA (463-6332), http://www.fda.gov.

Margaret Alic, PhD

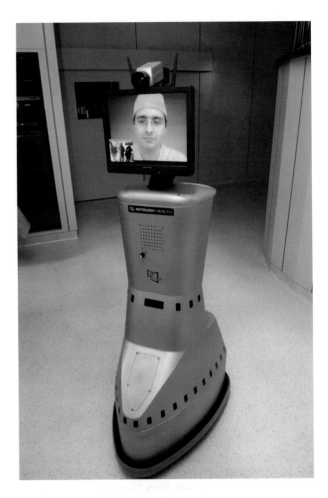

A surgeon consults on a procedure in a different hospital by way of a robotic video system. *(Pool DEMANGE/MARCHI/ Getty Images)*

Telesurgery

Definition

Telesurgery, also called remote surgery, is surgery directed from a site removed from the patient. The word telesurgery is derived from the Greek words *tele*, meaning "far off," and *cheirourgia*, meaning "working by hand." Surgical tasks are directly performed by a robotic system controlled by a surgeon at the remote site.

Description

In the early 2000s, several projects investigating the practicality of telesurgery were successful in performing complete surgical procedures on human patients from remote locations.

Technological basis of telesurgery

Telesurgery became a possibility with the advent of laparoscopic surgery in the late 1980s. **Laparoscopy** (also called minimally invasive surgery) is a surgical procedure in which a laparoscope (a thin, lighted tube) and other instruments are inserted into the body through small incisions. The internal operating field may then be visualized on a video monitor connected to the scope. In certain cases, the technique may be used in place of more invasive surgical procedures that require more extensive incisions and longer recovery times.

Computer-assisted surgery premiered in the mid-1990s; it was the next step toward the goal of remote surgery. The ZEUS Surgical System, developed in 1995 by Computer Motion, Inc., was approved by the U.S. Food and Drug Administration (FDA) in 2002 for use in general and laparoscopic surgeries with the patient and surgeon in the same room. ZEUS comprises three table-mounted robotic arms—one holding the AESOP endoscope positioner, which provides a view of the internal operating field, and the others holding **surgical instruments**. The robotic arms are controlled by the surgeon, who sits at a console several meters away. Visualization of the operating field is controlled by voice activation, while the robotic arms are controlled by movements of the surgeon's hands and wrists.

Computer-assisted surgery, which is generally called telerobotic surgery, has a number of advantages over traditional laparoscopic surgery. The computer interface provides a method for filtering out the normal hand tremors of the surgeon. Two- and three-dimensional visualization of the operating field is possible. The surgeon can perform a maneuver on the console, review it to be sure of its safety and efficacy, then instruct the remote device to perform the task. The surgeon is also seated in an ergonomic position with arms supported by armrests for the duration of the operation. One limitation on telerobotic surgery is the cost of the robots, which can run to more than $1 million.

Operation Lindbergh

The major constraint of telesurgery is time delay, which could lead to disastrous results. In the case of computer-assisted surgery, the computer console and remote surgical device are directly connected by several feet (meters) of cable; there is, therefore, virtually no delay in the transmission of data from the console to the surgical device and back to the console. The surgeon views his or her movements on the computer interface as they are happening. If the surgical system were removed to a more distant site, however, it would introduce a time delay. Visualization of the operating field could be milliseconds or even seconds behind the real-time manipulations of the surgeon. Studies showed that a delay of more than 150–200 milliseconds would be dangerous; satellite transmission, for example, would introduce a delay of more than 600 milliseconds.

In order to make telesurgery a reality, expert **surgeons** needed to work with the telecommunication industry to develop secure, reliable, high-speed transmission of data over large distances with imperceptible delays. In January 2000, such a project, labeled Operation Lindbergh, began under the direction of Dr. Jacques Marescaux, director of the European Institute of Telesurgery; Moji Ghodoussi, project manager at Computer Motions, Inc.; and communication experts from France Télécom. Testing began on a prototype remote system (a modified version of the ZEUS Surgical System called ZEUS TS) in September 2000, with data being relayed between Paris and Strasbourg, France—a distance of approximately 625 miles (mi.) (1,000 kilometers [km]). Once an acceptable length of time delay was established, trials began in July 2001 between New York City and Strasbourg.

On September 7, 2001, Operation Lindbergh culminated in the first complete remote surgery on a human patient (a 68-year-old female), performed over a distance of 4,300 mi. (7,000 km). The patient and surgical system were located in an **operating room** in Strasbourg, while the surgeon and remote console were situated in a high-rise building in downtown New York. A team of surgeons remained at the patient's side to step in if need arose. The procedure performed was a laparoscopic **cholecystectomy** (gallbladder removal),

considered the standard of care in minimally invasive surgery. The established time delay during the surgery was 135 ms—remarkable considering that the data traveled a distance of more than 8,600 mi. (14,000 km) from the surgeon's console to the surgical system and back to the console. The patient left the hospital within 48 hours—a typical stay following laparoscopic cholecystectomy—and had a successful recovery.

Limitations that still need to be overcome in order to make telesurgery more widely available include the establishment of international compatibility of equipment and training to overcome linguistic difficulties. Another concern is the need for a backup human surgeon at the remote location in case the robot malfunctions or there is an interruption in telecommunications.

Applications

Operation Lindbergh has paved the way for wide-ranging applications of telesurgery technology. On February 28, 2003, the first hospital-to-hospital telerobotic-assisted surgery took place in Ontario, Canada, over a distance of 250 mi. (400 km). Two surgeons worked together to perform a Nissen fundoplication (surgery to treat chronic acid reflux), with one situated at the patient's side and the other controlling a robotic surgical system from a remote hospital site. Such a scenario may eventually allow surgeons in rural areas to receive expert assistance during minimally invasive procedures. Since the first telesurgery in Canada, Dr. Mehran Anvari, the founder of the Centre for Minimal Access Surgery (CMAS) in Ontario, has performed a number of remote surgeries between St. Joseph's Hospital in Hamilton, Ontario, and a community hospital in North Bay, about 250 miles from Hamilton. Dr. Anvari uses a virtual private network (VPN) over a nondedicated fiber-optic connection that shares bandwidth with regular telecommunications data.

Other applications of telesurgery include:

• Training new surgeons. CMAS has developed a program in advanced minimal access surgery for Canadian surgeons, which combines lectures, laboratory sessions, and live surgery.

• Assisting and training surgeons in developing countries.

• Treating injured soldiers on or near the battlefield.

• The expanded use of telerobotic surgery. Telerobotic surgery offers the advantages of allowing surgery to be performed during an epidemic (such as the SARS outbreak of 2002–2003) without having to bring patients from remote and uninfected communities into cities affected by the epidemic.

• Performing surgical procedures in space or underwater. CMAS joined forces in 2006 with the National

QUESTIONS TO ASK YOUR DOCTOR

- Will a surgeon be with me in person in the operating room in case something goes wrong?
- How much experience do you have with telesurgery?
- How many of these remote robotic operations has the surgeon controlling the robot done?
- How long will I have to stay in the hospital?
- Will my insurance cover remote surgery?

Aeronautics and Space Administration (NASA), the U.S. Army Telemedicine and Advanced Technology Research Center (TATRC), and the National Space Biomedical Research Institute (NSBRI) to work on NASA's Extreme Environment Mission Operation 9, or NEEMO 9. Dr. Anvari at CMAS tested remote surgery with a next-generation surgical robot and a patient simulator in the Aquarius Undersea Habitat, an underwater laboratory operated by the National Undersea Research Center at the University of North Carolina at Wilmington (UNCW) for the National Oceanic and Atmospheric Administration (NOAA). The laboratory is located on the ocean floor off Key Largo in the Florida Keys, 70 feet beneath the surface. The mission lasted 18 days. A two-second time delay was built into the telecommunications system to simulate the time delay that would be present in a manned lunar exploration mission.

- Collaboration and mentoring during surgery by surgeons around the globe. Telementoring has been used in Canada since 2004 with financial assistance from a government partnership program. Telementoring involves an experienced surgeon in an advanced treatment facility in a major city using a two-way telecommunications link to guide the remote surgeon during an operation.

Resources

BOOKS

Liverneaux, Philippe A., et al., eds. *Telemicrosurgery: Robot Assisted Microsurgery*. New York: Springer, 2013.

PERIODICALS

Gambadauro, Pietro, and Rafael Torrejón. "The 'Tele' Factor in Surgery Today and Tomorrow: Implications for Surgical Training and Education." *Surgery Today* 43, no. 2 (Feb. 2013): 115–22. http://dx.doi.org/10.1007/s00595-012-0267-9 (accessed October 23, 2013).

Saliba, Vanessa, et al. "Telemedicine Across Borders: A Systematic Review of Factors that Hinder or Support Implementation." *International Journal of Medical Informatics* 81, no. 2 (Dec. 2012): 793–809. http://dx.doi.org/10.1016/j.ijmedinf.2012.08.003 (accessed September 5, 2013).

Santomauro, M., et al. "Telementoring in Robotic Surgery." *Current Opinion in Urology* 23, no. 2 (2013): 141–45. http://dx.doi.org/10.1097/MOU.0b013e32835d4cc2 (accessed September 5, 2013).

Stark, Michael, Emilio Ruiz Morales, and Stefano Gidaro. "Telesurgery is Promising but Still Need Proof through Prospective Comparative Studies." *Journal of Gynecological Oncology* 23, no. 2 (April 2012): 134–35. http://dx.doi.org/10.3802/jgo.2012.23.2.134 (accessed September 5, 2013).

WEBSITES

Hemsworth, Wade. "Medicine's Future." theSpec.com, March 18, 2011. http://www.thespec.com/news-story/2197125-medicine-s-future (accessed September 5, 2013).

Kay, Sharon. "Light Speed: Remote Surgery." PBS Innovation. http://www.pbs.org/wnet/innovation/episode7_essay1.html (accessed September 5, 2013).

Malik, Tariq. "NASA's NEEMO 9: Remote Surgery and Mock Moonwalks on the Sea Floor." SPACE.com, April 19, 2006. http://www.space.com/businesstechnology/060419_neemo9_techwed.html (accessed September 5, 2013).

Scoble, Robert. "Robots Help with Remote Surgery, Part 1 (Part of SRI International Tour)." March 5, 2011. YouTube video, 14:30. http://www.youtube.com/watch?v=bioGAH1KnME (accessed September 5, 2013).

ORGANIZATIONS

Centre for Minimal Access Surgery (CMAS), 50 Charlton Ave. E., HamiltonOntarioCanada L8N 4A6, (905) 522-1155, ext. 35144, Fax: (905) 521-6924, info@cmas.ca, http://www.cmas.ca.

European Institute of TeleSurgery (EITS), Hôpitaux Universitaires 1, place de l'Hôpital, Strasbourg Cedex, France 67091, +33 (0)3 88 11 90 00, info@eits.fr, http://www.eits.fr.

Stephanie Dionne Sherk
Rebecca Frey, PhD
Tish Davidson, AM

Temperature measurement

Definition

Temperature measurement is the quantification of a person's body temperature, which is an important indicator of a person's physiological state. Temperature measurement is done to assess whether body temperature is within a narrow, safe range. An abnormally high temperature is a fever, a sign that the body is mounting an immune response.

Purpose

Temperature measurement is done to monitor a person's body temperature. Body temperature, heart rate, breathing rate, and blood pressure are all considered **vital signs**. If body temperature is abnormal, it is an important indicator of the physiological state of the body. A fever is the body mounting an immune defense against a foreign invader to help fight infection or disease. A fever can be a critical sign that the body is fighting a battle, such as a postsurgical bacterial infection or cancer. It can also be used to assess whether a treatment is working, such as an antibiotic. The extent of a fever does not necessarily correlate with the severity of the illness. However, temperature measurement is still an important tool used in the hospital to monitor a patient's health.

Measuring and monitoring body temperature can be done at specific time points in the process of diagnosing and treating illness. Physicians sometimes use repeated temperature measurements to follow patterns in body temperature, such as how frequently a fever occurs and how long it lasts. These measurements may provide diagnostic insights into body processes during illness. Temperature measurement is especially important for the management of critically ill patients, where trends in body temperature are significant. Careful temperature measurement is also essential in the health management of elderly people. Because the elderly may have difficulty mounting a high fever as an immune response against infection, a low-grade fever is often the only early sign that something is wrong. Elderly people are also more prone to hypothermia than younger individuals.

Description

When humans become too warm, blood vessels in the skin increase in diameter (dilate). The purpose is to carry the excess heat to the surface of the skin. In turn, this causes the body to begin to perspire. As the perspiration evaporates, it helps to cool the body. When the body becomes too cold, the blood vessels decrease in diameter (contract) so that blood flow to the skin is reduced in an attempt to conserve body heat. This often causes people to start shivering. This involves rapid, involuntary contractions of muscles. Shivering helps to generate additional heat through muscle activity. Under normal conditions, these activities maintain human body temperature within a narrow, healthy range.

Normal body temperature varies from person to person. Gender, age, recent physical activity, having a meal, and the menstrual cycle all affect body temperature within the normal range. Body temperature measurement also varies based on which part of the body it is taken from. The average normal body temperature is 98.6 degrees Fahrenheit (F) or 37 degrees Celsius (C) when taken orally. However, body temperature may vary slightly more than one degree higher or lower and still be in the normal range. Normal body temperature can range from 97°F to 100°F (36.1°C to 37.8°C). A temperature higher than normal is considered a fever (hyperthermia). A temperature lower than 96°F is considered a state of hypothermia.

Temperature varies with the age of a person. Younger people tend to have higher body temperatures. Temperature also varies by the time of day it is taken. Body temperature is usually lowest in the morning and highest in the evening. Temperature can also be elevated by **exercise**, stress or strong emotions, eating food, heavy clothing, certain medications, or high room temperature. All of these factors need to be taken into account when temperature is measured because they affect the interpretation of temperature-measurement results.

In the hospital, routine temperature measurement takes place twice a day. The first measurement is usually done in the morning between 7 and 10 am. The second measurement takes place in the afternoon around 2 pm. If a patient is suspected to have an illness causing fever or is critically ill, temperature measurement may be performed up to four times an hour to closely monitor the situation. Interpretation of temperature measurement is influenced by when the measurement is taken. In the early morning, normal adult body temperature may be as low as 96.4°F (35.8°C). In the evening, normal temperature may be as high as 99.1°F (37.3°C).

Locations for body temperature measurement

ORAL. Temperature is often measured orally by placing a **thermometer** in the heat pocket under the tongue in the back of the mouth. The mouth is closed and the patient breathes through their nose for several minutes until the temperature is measured. Oral temperatures that are 1 to 1.5°F above a patient's normal body temperature are considered a fever.

RECTAL. The most accurate method of assessing body temperature is rectally using a glass or electronic digital thermometer. A lubricated electronic probe is inserted about 1 to 1.5 inches into the anal canal. Normal rectal temperature is usually 0.5 to 1.0°F higher than oral temperature. A rectal body temperature above 100.5°F is considered a fever in adults. In infants and children, a normal rectal temperature may approach 101°F. Rectal temperature measurement is a convenient alternative for patients who are unable to hold an oral thermometer in a closed mouth due to illness or being unconscious. It is also used for infants or very young children who cannot safely hold a thermometer in their mouth.

ARMPIT. Another temperature measurement method sometimes employed by pediatricians is placing a thermometer in the armpit. While less invasive than rectal temperature measurement, this location is the least accurate and takes the longest time to measure. Normal temperature in the armpit tends to be 0.5 to 1.0°F lower than oral temperature.

EAR. Thermometers made for the ear can be used to assess the body's core temperature, which approximates the temperature of the internal organs. Ear thermometers may measure the temperature of the eardrum or the ear canal. Normal ear temperature tends to be about 1.4°F higher than oral temperature.

Types of thermometers

MERCURY THERMOMETERS. Traditionally temperature was measured orally with a graded glass thermometer containing mercury. The level to which the mercury would rise on the graded scale was an indication of temperature. According to the Environmental Protection Agency (EPA), mercury is a toxic substance that is poisonous to both humans and the environment. The dangers associated with mercury if the thermometer breaks in a patient's body and the cost of disposing of mercury led to the development of modern mercury-free thermometers that do not pose such health risks.

ELECTRONIC DIGITAL THERMOMETERS. Digital thermometers with an electronic probe are far more accurate at measuring body temperature than the old mercury thermometers. They are usually a lightweight plastic and shaped like a broad pencil, with the electronic temperature probe at the tip. A digital temperature display window at the other end measures temperature down to a tenth of a decimal point. Electronic thermometers are designed for use in the mouth, rectum, or armpit. Rectal thermometers may have a colored probe to help distinguish them from silver-tipped oral thermometers. They are accurate and easy to use in the hospital. In addition to antiseptic, disposable protective guards are often used to cover the probe to help prevent the spread of infection between patients.

INFRARED EAR THERMOMETERS. Digital ear thermometers use infrared energy to measure body temperature instead of an electronic probe. They are made in different shapes. One design has a small cone-shaped end that is placed within the ear. An infrared beam is then aimed at the eardrum. Ear thermometers only take seconds to measure body temperature, whereas other types of thermometers require minutes for accurate temperature measurement.

DISPOSABLE THERMOMETERS. Hospitals often use disposable thermometers to decrease risk of transmitting infection from patient to patient. Disposable thermometers are thin pieces of plastic with a colored grid of dots representing temperature on one end. The color change displayed in the grid is how temperature measurement is visualized. Disposable thermometers are accurate and safe since they contain no glass or mercury. One thermometer can be reused on the same patient until it is no longer needed. Disposable thermometers are designed for use in the mouth, armpit, or rectum. A disposable thermometer in patch form has been designed for use on infants whose temperature needs to be monitored for long periods of time.

Preparation

Preparation for taking a body temperature consists of ensuring that the thermometer is clean and disinfected.

Aftercare

Aftercare consists of ensuring that the thermometer is clean and disinfected. Electronic thermometers must be turned off to conserve their batteries.

Risks

Taking a body temperature involves little risk. Inserting a thermometer into the rectum can occasionally be painful. Breaking a thermometer that contains mercury causes exposure to a toxic substance (mercury).

Results

An abnormally high body temperature means that the patient has a fever. Fever is not an illness itself but rather a defense mechanism of the body to fight disease or infection. Higher body temperatures are less hospitable for most bacteria and viruses, and also allow the body's immune system to mobilize against disease more readily. However, if the body temperature is raised too high for a prolonged period of time, then fever may pose a threat to the body. In infants and children, a very high fever may occur even in response to minor infections.

Potential causes of abnormally high body temperature include:

• infection by bacteria, viruses, or parasites

• medications

KEY TERMS

Autoimmune disorders—Disorder in which the immune system mounts a response against some aspect of its own body.

Hyperthyroidism—Disease of the thyroid gland involving overproduction of thyroid hormones. Hyperthyroidism affects body temperature.

Hypothermia—State of abnormally low body temperature that can be fatal if left untreated.

Hypothyroidism—Disease of the thyroid gland involving underproduction of thyroid hormones. Hypothyroidism affects body temperature.

Immune response—Any response of the immune system against something identified by the immune system as being foreign.

Infrared—A type of energy wave given off as heat.

Physiological state—The status of the normal vital life functions of a living organism.

Vital signs—The physiological aspects of body function basic to life. They are temperature, pulse, breathing rate, and blood pressure.

- response to surgical procedures without having an infection
- drugs used during surgery
- metabolic disorders such as hyperthyroidism
- heat stroke
- extreme dehydration
- cancer
- inflammatory conditions and autoimmune disorders
- physical trauma
- certain blood disorders

Potential causes of abnormally low body temperature include:

- hypothermia from cold exposure
- medications
- metabolic disorders such as hypothyroidism
- excessive alcohol intake
- starvation

Resources

BOOKS

Bickley, Lynn S. *Bates' Guide to Physical Examination and History Taking.* 10th ed. Philadelphia: Wolters Kluwer Health/Lippincott Williams & Wilkins, 2009.

Goldman, Lee, and Andrew I. Schafer. *Goldman's Cecil Medicine.* 24th ed. Philadelphia: Saunders/Elsevier, 2012.

Longo, Dan, et al. *Harrison's Principles of Internal Medicine.* 18th ed. New York: McGraw-Hill, 2012.

WEBSITES

A.D.A.M. Medical Encyclopedia. "Temperature Measurement." MedlinePlus. http://www.nlm.nih.gov/medlineplus/ency/article/003400.htm (accessed October 17, 2013).

Maria Basile, PhD

Temporal lobectomy *see* **Lobectomy, cerebral**

Tendon repair

Definition

Tendon repair refers to the surgical repair of damaged or torn tendons, which are cord-like structures made of strong fibrous connective tissue that connect muscles to bones. The shoulder, elbow, knee, and ankle are the joints most commonly affected by tendon injuries.

Purpose

The goal of tendon repair is to restore the normal function of joints or their surrounding tissues following a tendon laceration.

Demographics

Tendon injuries are widespread in the general adult population. They are more common among people whose occupations or recreational athletic activities require repetitive motion of the shoulder, knee, elbow, or ankle joints. Injuries to the tendons in the shoulder often occur among baseball players, window washers, violinists, dancers, carpenters, and some assembly line workers. Rowers are at increased risk for injuries to the forearm tendons. The repetitive stresses of classical ballet, running, and jogging may damage the Achilles tendon at the back of the heel. So-called tennis elbow, which occurs in many construction workers, highway crews, maintenance workers, and baggage handlers as well as professional golfers and tennis players, is thought to affect 5% of American adults over the age of 30.

Women in all age brackets are at greater risk than men for injuries to the tendons in the elbow and knee joints. It is thought that injuries in these areas are related to the slightly greater looseness of women's joints compared to those in men.

Tendon repair

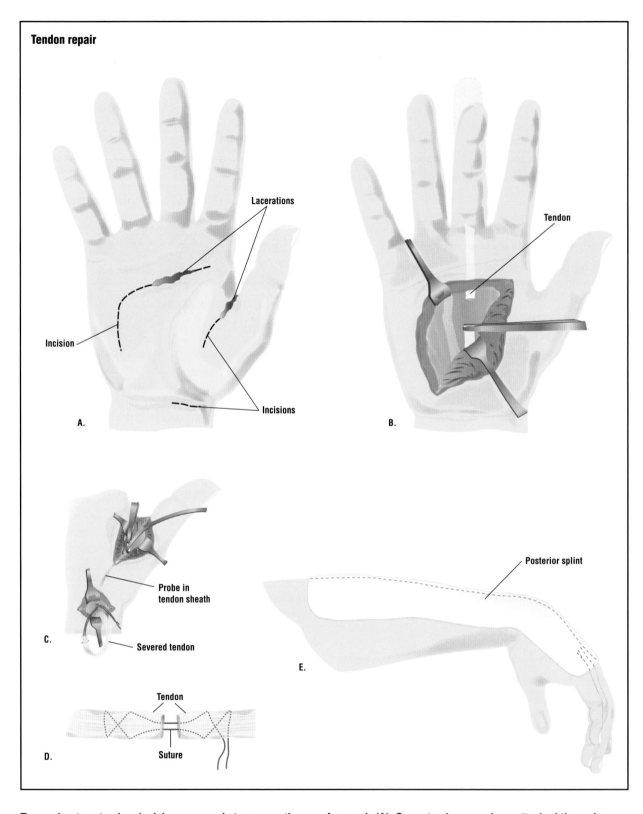

To repair a torn tendon, incisions are made to expose the area for repair (A). Some tendons can be reattached through one incision (B), while others require two to access the severed point and the remaining tendon (C). The tendon is stitched back together (D), and a special splint that minimizes stretching the tendons may be worn after surgery (E). *(Illustration by GGS Information Services. Copyright © Cengage Learning®.)*

Anesthesia—Loss of normal sensation or feeling induced by anesthetic drugs.

Collagen—Any of a group of about 14 proteins found outside cells. Collagens are a major component of connective tissue, providing its characteristic strength and flexibility.

Contracture—A condition of high resistance to the passive stretching of a muscle, resulting from the formation of fibrous tissue in a joint or from a disorder of the muscle tissue itself.

Fibroblast—A type of cell found in connective tissue involved in collagen production as well as tendon formation and healing.

Laceration—A physical injury that results in a jagged tearing or mangling of the skin.

Meniscus (plural, menisci)—One of two crescent-shaped pieces of cartilage attached to the upper surface of the tibia. The menisci act as shock absorbers within the knee joint.

Prolotherapy—A technique for stimulating collagen growth in injured tissues by the injection of glycerin or dextrose.

Tendon—A fibrous cord of strong connective tissue that connects muscle to bone.

Description

Local, regional or **general anesthesia** is administered to the patient depending on the extent and location of tendon damage. With a general anesthetic, the patient is asleep during surgery. With a regional anesthetic, a specific region of nerves is anesthetized; with a local anesthetic, the patient remains alert during the surgery, and only the incision location is anesthetized.

After the overlying skin has been cleansed with an antiseptic solution and covered with a sterile drape, the surgeon makes an incision over the injured tendon. When the tendon has been located and identified, the surgeon sutures the damaged or torn ends of the tendon together. If the tendon has been severely injured, a tendon graft may be required. This is a procedure in which a piece of tendon is taken from the foot or other part of the body and used to repair the damaged tendon. If required, tendons are reattached to the surrounding connective tissue. The surgeon inspects the area for injuries to nerves and blood vessels, and closes the incision.

Diagnosis

Diagnosis of a tendon injury is usually made when the patient consults a doctor about pain in the injured area. The doctor will usually order radiographs and other imaging studies of the affected joint as well as taking a history and performing an external **physical examination** in the office. In some cases, fluid will be aspirated (withdrawn through a needle) from the joint to check for signs of infection, bleeding, or arthritis.

Preparation

In the hours prior to surgery, the patient is asked not to eat or drink anything, even water. A few days before the operation, patients are also instructed to stop taking such over-the-counter (OTC) pain medications as **aspirin** or ibuprofen. If the patient has a splint or cast, it is removed before surgery.

To prepare for surgery, the patient typically reports to a preoperative nursing unit. Next, the patient is taken to a preoperative holding area, where an anesthesiologist administers an intravenous sedative. The patient is then taken to the **operating room**.

Aftercare

Healing may take as long as six weeks, during which the injured part may be immobilized in a splint or cast. Patients are asked not to use the injured tendon until the physician gives permission. The physician will decide how long to rest the tendon. It should not be used for lifting heavy objects or walking. Patients are also asked to avoid driving until the physician gives the go-ahead. To reduce swelling and pain, they should keep the injured limb lifted above the level of the heart as much as possible for the first few days after surgery.

Splints or **bandages** should be left in place until the next checkup. Patients are advised to keep bandages clean and dry. If patients have a cast, they are asked not to get it wet. Fiberglass casts that get wet may be dried with a hair dryer. Patients are also instructed not to push or lean on the cast to avoid breaking it. If patients have a splint that is held in place with an Ace bandage, they are instructed to ensure that the bandage is not too tight. They are also asked to ensure that splints remain in exactly the same place. Medications prescribed by the doctor should be taken exactly as directed. Patients who have been given **antibiotics** should take the complete course even if they feel well; this precaution is needed to minimize the risk of drug resistance developing in the disease organism. If patients are taking medicine that makes them feel drowsy, they are advised against driving or using heavy equipment.

Aftercare may also include physical therapy for the affected joint. There are a variety of exercises, wraps, splints, braces, bandages, ice packs, massages, and other treatments that physical therapists may recommend or use in helping a patient recover from tendon surgery.

Risks

Tendon repair surgery includes the risks associated with any procedure requiring anesthesia, such as reactions to medications and breathing difficulties. Risks associated with any surgery are also present, such as bleeding and infection. Additional risks specific to tendon repair include formation of scar tissue that may prevent smooth movements (adequate tendon gliding), nerve damage, and partial loss of function in the involved joint.

Results

Tendon injuries represent a difficult and frustrating problem. Conservative treatment has little if any chance of restoring optimal range of motion in the injured area. Even after surgical repair, a full range of motion is usually not achieved. Permanent loss of motion, joint contractures, and weakness and stiffness may be unavoidable. Scar tissue tends to form between the moving surfaces within joints, resulting in **adhesions** that hamper motion. The surgical repair may also split apart or loosen. Revision surgery may be required to remove scar tissue, insert tendon grafts, or perform other reconstructive procedures. Thus, successful tendon repair depends on many factors. Recovery of the full range of motion is less likely if there is a nerve injury or a broken bone next to the tendon injury; if a long period of time has elapsed between the injury and surgery; if the patient's tissues tend to form thick scars; and if the damage was caused by a crush injury. The location of the injury is also an important factor in determining how well a patient will recover after surgery.

Morbidity and mortality rates

Mortality rates for tendon repairs are very low, partly because some of these procedures can be performed with local or regional anesthesia, and partly because most patients with tendon injuries are young or middle-aged adults in good general health. Morbidity varies according to the specific tendon involved; ruptures of the Achilles tendon or shoulder tendons are more difficult to repair than injuries to smaller tendons elsewhere in the body. In addition, some postoperative complications result from patient noncompliance; in one study, two out of 50 patients in the study sample had new injuries within three weeks after surgery because they did not follow the

QUESTIONS TO ASK YOUR DOCTOR

- What happens on the day of surgery?
- What type of anesthesia will be used?
- How long will it take to recover from the surgery?
- Can I expect normal flexibility in the affected area?
- What are the risks associated with tendon repair surgery?
- How many tendon repair procedures do you perform in a year?
- Will there be a scar?

surgeon's recommendations. In general, tendon repairs performed in the United States are reported as having an infection rate of about 1.9%, with other complications ranging between 5.8% and 9.5%.

Alternatives

There are no alternatives to surgery for tendon repair; however, research is providing encouraging findings. Although there is no presently approved drug that targets this notoriously slow and often incomplete healing process, a cellular substance recently discovered at the Lawrence Berkeley National Laboratory may lead to a new drug that would improve the speed and durability of healing for injuries to tendons and ligaments. The substance, called Cell Density Signal-1, or CDS-1, by its discoverer, cell biologist Richard Schwarz, acts as part of a chemical switch that turns on procollagen production. Procollagen is a protein manufactured in large amounts by embryonic tendon cells. It is transformed outside the cell into collagen, the basic component of such connective tissues as tendons, ligaments or bones. Amgen Inc. is planning to use genetic engineering to bring CDS-1 into mass production.

Prolotherapy represents a less invasive alternative to surgery. It is a form of treatment that stimulates the repair of injured or damaged structures. It involves the injection of dextrose or natural glycerin at the exact site of an injury to stimulate the immune system to repair the area. Thus, prolotherapy causes an inflammatory reaction at the exact site of injuries to such structures as ligaments, tendons, menisci, muscles, growth plates, joint capsules, and cartilage to stimulate these structures to heal. Specifically, prolotherapy causes fibroblasts to multiply rapidly. Fibroblasts are the cells that actually make up ligaments and tendons. The rapid production of new fibroblasts means that strong, fresh collagen tissue is formed, which is what is needed to repair injuries to ligaments or tendons.

Health care team roles

Tendon repairs are usually performed in an outpatient setting. Hospital stays, if any, are short—no longer than a day. Tendon repairs are performed by orthopedic **surgeons**. Orthopedics is the medical specialty that focuses on the diagnosis, care and treatment of patients with disorders of the bones, joints, muscles, ligaments, tendons, nerves and skin.

Resources

BOOKS

Browner, Bruce D., et al. *Skeletal Trauma: Basic Science, Management, and Reconstruction.* 4th ed. Philadelphia: Saunders/Elsevier, 2009.

Canale, S. T., ed. *Campbell's Operative Orthopaedics.* 12th ed. St. Louis, MO: Mosby, 2012.

DeLee, Jesse, David Drez, and Mark D. Miller. *DeLee and Drez's Orthopaedic Sports Medicine: Principles and Practice.* 3rd ed. Philadelphia: Saunders/Elsevier, 2010.

PERIODICALS

Ozsoy, Mehmet Hakan, et al. "Minimally Invasive Achilles Tendon Repair: A Modification of the Achillon Technique." *Foot & Ankle International* (September 17, 2013): 1712–17. http://dx.doi.org/10.1177/1071100713505754 (accessed October 17, 2013).

Starr, H. M., et al. "Flexor Tendon Repair Rehabilitation Protocols: A Systematic Review." *Journal of Hand Surgery* 38, no. 9 (2013): 1712–17. http://dx.doi.org/10.1016/j.jhsa.2013.06.025 (accessed October 17, 2013).

OTHER

Massachusetts General Hospital. *Achilles Tendon Rupture.* http://www.massgeneral.org/ortho/services/sports/rehab/Achilles%20repair%20rehabilitation%20protocol.pdf (accessed October 17, 2013).

WEBSITES

American Academy of Orthopaedic Surgeons. "Flexor Tendon Injuries." OrthoInfo. http://orthoinfo.aaos.org/topic.cfm?topic=a00015 (accessed October 17, 2013).

Aurora Health Care. "Tendon Repair." http://www.aurora-healthcare.org/yourhealth/healthgate/getcontent.asp?URLhealthgate=%2214869.html%22 (accessed October 17, 2013).

NHS (UK National Health Service). "Tendon Repair, Hand." http://www.nhs.uk/conditions/tendonhand/Pages/Introduction.aspx (accessed October 17, 2013).

ORGANIZATIONS

American Academy of Orthopaedic Surgeons (AAOS), 6300 N. River Rd., Rosemont, IL 60018-4262, (847) 823-7186,

Fax: (847) 823-8125, pemr@aaos.org, http://www.aaos.org.

American Physical Therapy Association, 1111 N. Fairfax St., Alexandria, VA 22314-1488, (703) 684-APTA (2782), TTY: (703) 683-6748, (800) 999-APTA (2782), http://www.apta.org.

Monique Laberge, PhD

Tenotomy

Definition

Tenotomy is the cutting of a tendon. This and related procedures are also called tendon release, tendon lengthening, and heel-cord release (for tenotomy of the Achilles tendon).

Purpose

Tenotomy is performed in order to lengthen a muscle that has developed improperly, or become shortened and is resistant to stretch. It is performed most often in infants with clubfoot, a common developmental deformity in which the foot is turned inward, with shortening of one or more of the muscles controlling the foot and possibly some bone deformity as well. It is also performed in older patients who develop contractures or subluxations from neuromuscular disease, the upper motor neuron syndrome, or other disorders.

A muscle can become shortened and resistant to stretch when it remains in a shortened position for many months. When this occurs, the tendon that attaches muscle to bone can shorten, and the muscle itself can develop fibrous tissue within it, preventing it from stretching to its full range of motion. This combination of changes is called contracture.

Contracture commonly occurs in upper motor neuron syndrome, following spinal cord injury, traumatic brain injury, stroke, multiple sclerosis, or cerebral palsy. Damage to the nerves controlling muscles lead to an imbalance of opposing muscle forces across a joint, which may allow one muscle to pull harder than another. For instance, excess pull from the biceps, unless opposed by the triceps, can bend the elbow joint. If the shortened bicep remains in this position, it will develop contracture, becoming resistant to stretching. Tenotomy is performed to lengthen the tendon, allowing the muscle to return to its normal length and allowing the joint to straighten.

When one muscle pulls much more strongly than its opposing muscle, it may cause the joint to become partially dislocated, which is called subluxation. Tenotomy is also performed to prevent or correct subluxation, especially of the hip joint in cerebral palsy.

Chronic pain or bone deformity may prevent a person from moving a joint through its full range of motion, leading to contracture.

Contracture also occurs in a variety of neuromuscular diseases, including muscular dystrophies and polio. Degeneration of one muscle can allow the opposing muscle to pull too hard across the joint, shortening the muscle.

Description

During a tenotomy, the tendon is cut entirely or partway through, allowing the muscle to be stretched. Tenotomy may be performed through the skin (percutaneous tenotomy) or by surgically exposing the tendon (open tenotomy). The details of the operation differ for each tendon.

During a percutaneous lengthening of the Achilles tendon, a thin blade is inserted through the skin to partially sever the tendon in two or more places. This procedure is called a Z-plasty, and is very rapid, requiring only a few minutes. It may be performed under **local anesthesia**.

More severe contracture may be treated with an open procedure. In this case, the tendon may be cut lengthwise, and the two pieces joined lengthwise to form a single longer tendon. This procedure takes approximately half an hour. This type of tenotomy is usually performed under **general anesthesia**.

If multiple joints are to be treated (for example, ankle, knee, and hip), these are often performed at the same time.

Diagnosis

Patients requiring tenotomy are those with contracture or developmental deformity leading to muscle shortening that has not responded sufficiently to treatment with casts, splints, stretching exercises, or medication. Tests performed before surgery include determining the range of motion of the joint involved, and possibly x-rays to determine if there is a bone deformity impeding movement or subluxation.

Preparation

Patients undergoing general anesthesia will probably be instructed not to eat anything for up to 12 hours before the procedure.

Aftercare

After tenotomy, the patient may receive pain medication. This may range from over-the-counter (OTC) **aspirin** to intravenous morphine, depending on the severity of the pain. Ice packs may also be applied. The patient will usually spend the night in the hospital, especially children with swallowing or seizure disorders, who need to be monitored closely after anesthesia.

Casts are applied to the limb receiving the surgery. Before the cast is applied, the contracted muscle is stretched to its normal or near-normal extension. The cast then holds it in that position while the tendon regrows at its extended length. Braces or splints may also be applied.

After the casts come off (typically two to three weeks), intensive physical therapy is prescribed to strengthen the muscle and keep it stretched out.

Risks

Tenotomy carries a small risk of excess bleeding and infection. Tenotomy performed under general anesthesia carries additional risks associated with the anesthesia itself.

Results

Tenotomy allows the muscle to stretch out, proving more complete range of motion to the affected joint. This promotes better posture and movement and may improve the ability to walk, stand, reach, or perform other activities, depending on the location of the procedure. Pain may be reduced as well. Clubfoot is usually completely fixed by proper treatment. Contracture and subluxation may be only partially remedied, depending on the degree of muscle shortening and fibrotic changes within the muscle before the procedure.

Morbidity and mortality rates

Properly performed, tenotomy does not carry the risk of mortality. It may cause temporary pain and bleeding, but these are usually easily managed.

Alternatives

Tenotomy is usually recommended only after other treatments have failed, or when the rate and severity of contracture or subluxation progression indicates no other, more conservative treatment is likely to be effective. Aggressive stretching programs can sometimes prevent or delay development of contracture.

Health care team roles

Tenotomy is performed by an orthopedic surgeon in a hospital.

Resources

BOOKS

Browner, Bruce D., et al. *Skeletal Trauma: Basic Science, Management, and Reconstruction.* 4th ed. Philadelphia: Saunders/Elsevier, 2009.

Canale, S. T., ed. *Campbell's Operative Orthopaedics.* 12th ed. St. Louis, MO: Mosby, 2012.

DeLee, Jesse, David Drez, and Mark D. Miller. *DeLee and Drez's Orthopaedic Sports Medicine: Principles and Practice.* 3rd ed. Philadelphia: Saunders/Elsevier, 2010.

PERIODICALS

Niki, H., et al. "Effect of Achilles Tenotomy on Congenital Clubfoot-Associated Calf-Muscle Atrophy: An Ultrasonographic Study." *Journal of Orthopaedic Science* 18, no. 4 (2013): 552–56. http://dx.doi.org/10.1007/s00776-013-0398-x (accessed October 17, 2013).

Slenker, N. R., et al. "Biceps Tenotomy Versus Tenodesis: Clinical Outcomes." *Arthroscopy: The Journal of Arthroscopic and Related Surgery* 28, no. 4 (2012): 576–82. http://dx.doi.org/10.1016/j.arthro.2011.10.017 (accessed October 17, 2013).

WEBSITES

Global Clubfoot Initiative. "Achilles Tenotomy (Percutaneous Heel Cord Tenotomy)." http://globalclubfoot.org/ponseti/achilles-tenotomy (accessed October 17, 2013).

Richard Robinson

Testicular cancer surgery *see* **Orchiectomy**

Testicular torsion repair *see* **Orchiopexy**

Tetracyclines

Definition

Tetracyclines are broad-spectrum **antibiotics** that kill bacteria, which are one-celled disease-causing microorganisms. Many bacteria developed resistance to the older classes of tetracyclines, but a new group known as glycylcyclines was introduced in 2005 to treat infections that are resistant to other antibiotics, including the older tetracyclines. The name tetracycline comes from the four (*tetra* in Greek) hydrocarbon rings found in the chemical structure of these antibiotics.

Purpose

Tetracyclines are called broad-spectrum antibiotics because they can be used to treat a wide variety of infections. Physicians may prescribe these drugs to treat eye infections, pneumonia, gonorrhea, syphilis, chlamydia, bubonic plague, anthrax, brucellosis, malaria, Rocky Mountain spotted fever, urinary tract infections, travelers' diarrhea, Lyme disease, and other infections caused by bacteria. These drugs are also used to treat acne and rosacea (a chronic inflammatory skin condition marked by flushing and redness). Tigecycline is used to treat skin and soft-tissue infections, as well as infections inside the abdomen. Tetracyclines do not treat colds, flu, and other infections caused by viruses.

Surgery

Tetracyclines have been used for treatment of gum infections in dental surgery. In **orthopedic surgery**, they have been used as markers to identify living bone. They may also be mixed with bone cement for prevention of infection in bone surgery. In nasal surgery, tetracycline ointments have been used to help prevent postsurgical infections.

Description

Tetracyclines are available only with a physician's prescription. They are sold in capsule, tablet, liquid, and injectable forms. Some commonly used medicines in this group are tetracycline (Achromycin V, Sumycin), demeclocycline (Declomycin), minocycline (Minocin), oxytetracycline (Terramycin), and doxycycline (Doryx, Vibramycin, Vivox). Tigecycline (Tygacil) is not available in oral form and must be given as a slow intravenous infusion over a period of 30–60 minutes.

Origins

Tetracyclines are classified as antibiotics, which are chemical substances produced by a microorganism that are able to kill other microorganisms without being toxic to the person, animal, or plant being treated. They were first discovered in the 1940s when a scientist at Lederle Laboratories isolated chlortetracycline from a bacterium in the soil known as *Streptomyces aureofaciens*; the drug was given the trade name Aureomycin. Oxytetracycline (Terramycin) was then derived from the bacterium *Streptomyces rimosus*. After the chemical structure of oxytetracycline was worked out, researchers were able to make synthetic tetracyclines in the laboratory. One of these semi-synthetic drugs, minocycline, was used to develop tigecycline (Tygacil), the first glycylcycline to receive regulatory approval for use in the United States. Tigecycline was the first new tetracycline to be approved since the early 1980s.

Recommended dosage

The recommended dosage depends on the specific tetracycline, its strength, and the disease agent and severity of infection for which it is being taken. Patients should check with the physician who prescribed the drug or the pharmacist who filled the prescription for the correct dosage.

To make sure an infection clears up completely, patients should take the full course of antibiotic medication. It is important to not stop taking the drug just because symptoms begin to improve.

Tetracyclines are most effective at constant levels in the blood. To keep blood levels constant, the medicine should be taken in doses spaced evenly throughout the day and night. It is important not to miss any doses.

These medicines work best when taken on an empty stomach with a full glass of water. The water will help prevent irritation of the stomach and esophagus (the tube-like structure that runs from the throat to the stomach). If the medicine still causes stomach upset, the patient may take it with food. Tetracyclines should never be taken with milk or milk products, however, as these foods may prevent the drugs from working properly. Patients should not drink or eat milk or dairy products within one to two hours of taking tetracyclines (except doxycycline and minocycline).

Precautions

There are specific warnings that apply to tetracycline preparations taken by mouth to treat infections; they do not apply to topical ointments or tetracyclines mixed with bone cement. Also, these warnings apply primarily to tetracycline itself. Some members of the tetracycline family, particularly doxycycline and minocycline, have different adverse effects and precautions. Patients should consult their physician or pharmacist about these specific drugs.

Taking outdated tetracyclines can cause serious side effects, particularly damage to the kidneys. Patients should not take these medicines when:

• the color, appearance, or taste has changed

• the drug has been stored in a warm or damp area

• the expiration date on the label has passed

Expired medication should be thrown out. Patients should check with their physician or pharmacist if they have any doubts about the effectiveness of their drugs.

Patients should not take antacids, calcium supplements, such salicylates as Magan or Trilisate, magnesium-containing **laxatives**, or sodium bicarbonate (baking soda) within one to two hours of taking tetracyclines. Patients should also not take any medicines that contain iron (including multivitamin and mineral supplements) within two to three hours of taking tetracyclines.

Some people feel dizzy when taking these drugs. Tetracyclines may also cause blurred vision or interfere with color vision. Because of these possible side effects, anyone who takes these drugs should not drive, use machines, or do anything else that might be dangerous until they have found out how the drugs affect them.

Birth control pills may not work properly while tetracyclines are being taken. To prevent pregnancy, women should use alternative methods of birth control while taking tetracyclines.

Tetracyclines may increase the skin's sensitivity to sunlight. Even brief exposure to sun can cause severe sunburn or a rash. During treatment with these drugs, patients should avoid exposure to direct sunlight, especially high sun between 10 a.m. and 3 p.m.; wear a hat and tightly woven clothing that covers the arms and legs; use a sunscreen with a skin protection factor (SPF) of at least 15; protect the lips with a lip balm containing sun block; and avoid the use of tanning beds, tanning booths, or sunlamps. Sensitivity to sunlight and sunlamps may continue for two weeks to several months after stopping the medicine, so patients must continue to be careful about sun exposure.

Tetracyclines may permanently discolor the teeth of people who took the medicine in childhood. The drugs may also slow down the growth of children's bones. Tetracyclines should not be given to infants or children under eight years of age unless directed by the child's physician.

Special conditions

People with certain medical conditions or who are taking other medicines may have problems if they take tetracyclines. Before taking these drugs, the patient must inform the doctor about any of these conditions.

FOOD OR MEDICATION ALLERGIES. Anyone who has had unusual reactions to tetracyclines in the past should inform his or her physician before taking the drugs again. The physician should also be told about any allergies to foods, dyes, preservatives, or other substances.

(2013). http://dx.doi.org/10.1186/1756-0500-6-194 (accessed October 23, 2013).

WEBSITES

Health Care Without Harm. "Mercury: Laws and Resolutions." http://www.hcwh.org/us_canada/issues/toxins/mercury/laws.php (accessed May 21, 2013).

U.S. Environmental Protection Agency. "Phase-Out of Mercury Thermometers Used in Industrial and Laboratory Settings." http://www.epa.gov/hg/thermometer.htm (accessed May 21, 2013).

World Health Organization and Health Care Without Harm. Mercury-Free Health Care (homepage). http://www.mercuryfreehealthcare.org (accessed May 21, 2013).

ORGANIZATIONS

Health Care Without Harm, 12355 Sunrise Valley Dr., Ste. 680, Reston, VA 20191, (703) 860-9790, Fax: (703) 860-9795, http://noharm.org.

U.S. Environmental Protection Agency, Ariel Rios Bldg., 1200 Pennsylvania Ave., NW, Washington, DC 20460, (202) 272-0167 (202) 272-0165, http://www.epa.gov.

L. Fleming Fallon, Jr., MD, DrPH

Thoracentesis

Definition

Also known as pleural fluid analysis, thoracentesis is a procedure that removes fluid or air from the chest through a needle or tube.

Purpose

Thoracentesis is performed to remove excess fluid from the pleural cavity. It may also be performed as a diagnostic measure; in these cases, only small amounts of material need to be withdrawn.

Thoracentesis was traditionally used to remove blood from the chest cavity. This is rare now that the placement of a thoracostomy tube has proven to be a more effective and safer method.

Description

The lungs are lined on the outside with two thin layers of tissue called pleura. The space between these two layers is called the pleural space or pleural cavity. Normally, there is only a small amount of lubricating fluid in this space. Excess liquid and/or air can accumulate as a result of many conditions. The excess liquid is known as a pleural effusion; excess air is referred to as pneumothorax. Most pleural effusions are complications from metastatic malignancy (movement of cancer cells from one part of the body to another). The effusions are detected and controlled by thoracentesis.

Symptoms of a pleural effusion include breathing difficulty, chest pain, fever, weight loss, cough, and edema. The removal of air is often an emergency procedure to prevent suffocation from pressure on the lungs. Negative air pressure within the chest cavity allows normal respiration, but the accumulation of air or fluid within the pleural space can disrupt breathing and the movement of air within the chest cavity. Fluid removal is performed to reduce the pressure in the pleural space and to analyze the liquid.

Thoracentesis often provides immediate abatement of symptoms. However, fluid can begin to reaccumulate. A majority of patients will ultimately require additional therapy beyond thoracentesis.

Pleural effusion

There are two types of liquid in the pleural space, one having more protein in it than the other. More watery liquids are called transudates; thicker fluids are called exudates. On the basis of this difference, the cause of the effusion can more easily be determined.

TRANSUDATES. Transudate is a thin, watery fluid that oozes into the chest either because back pressure from circulation squeezes it out or because the blood has lost some of its osmotic pressure. Many conditions may cause transudate to accumulate, including:

• Heart failure creates back pressure in the veins as blood must wait to be pumped through the heart.

• A pulmonary embolism is a blood clot in the lung. It will create back pressure in the blood flow and also damage a part of the lung so that it leaks fluid.

• Cirrhosis is a type of liver disease that affects the liver's ability to make enough protein for the blood and also restricts the flow of blood through it.

• Nephrosis is a collection of kidney disorders that change the osmotic pressure of blood and allow liquid to seep into body cavities.

• Myxedema is a disease caused by too little thyroid hormone.

EXUDATES. Exudate is a thicker, more viscous fluid that usually accumulates due to greater damage to tissues, allowing blood proteins as well as water to seep out. Causes of exudate accumulation include:

• Pneumonia, caused by viruses and by bacteria, damages lung tissue and can open the way for exudates to enter the pleural space.

- Tuberculosis can infect the pleura as well as the lungs and cause them to leak liquid.
- Cancers of many types settle in the lungs or the pleura and leak liquids from their surface.
- Depending upon its size and the amount of damage it has done, a pulmonary embolism can produce an exudate.
- An esophagus perforated by cancer, trauma, or other conditions can spill liquids and even food into the chest. The irritation creates exudate in the pleural space.
- Pancreatic disease can cause massive fluid build-up in the abdomen, which can then find its way into the chest.
- Pericarditis is an inflammation of the sac that contains the heart. It can ooze fluid from both sides—into the heart's space and into the chest.
- Radiation to treat cancer or from accidents with radioactive materials can damage the pleura and lead to exudates.
- A wide variety of autoimmune diseases can attack the pleura, including rheumatoid arthritis and systemic lupus erythematosus (SLE).
- Many other rare conditions can also lead to exudates.

BLOOD. Blood in the chest (hemothorax) is infrequently seen outside of two conditions:

- Major trauma can sever blood vessels in the chest, causing them to bleed into the pleural space.
- Cancers can ooze blood as well as fluid, although they do not usually bleed massively.

CHYLE. Occasionally, the liquid that comes out of the chest is neither transparent nor bloody, but milky. This is due to a tear of the large lymphatic channel—the thoracic duct carrying lymph fluid from the intestines to the heart. It is milky because it is transporting fats absorbed in the process of digestion. The major causes of chylothorax are:

- injury from major trauma, such as an automobile accident
- cancers eroding into the thoracic duct

Pneumothorax

Air in the pleural space is called pneumothorax. Air can enter the pleural space either directly through a hole between the ribs or from a hole in the lungs. Holes in the lungs may be spontaneous, due to a traumatic injury, or the result of disease.

Performing thoracentesis

The usual place to tap the chest is below the armpit (axilla). Under sterile conditions and **local anesthesia**, a needle, a through-the-needle-catheter, or

an over-the-needle catheter may be used to perform the procedure. Overall, the catheter techniques may be safer. Fluid or air is withdrawn, and any fluid is sent to the laboratory for analysis. If the air or fluid continues to accumulate, a tube is left in place and attached to a one-way system so that it can drain without sucking air into the chest.

Precautions

Care must be taken not to puncture the lung when inserting the needle. Thoracentesis should never be performed by inserting the needle through an area with an infection. An alternative site needs to be found in these cases. Patients who are on **anticoagulant drugs** should be carefully considered for the procedure, as they are at increased risk of bleeding.

Preparation

The location of the fluid is pinpointed through x-ray or **ultrasound**. Ultrasound is a more accurate method when the effusion is small. A sedative may be administered in some cases but is generally not recommended. Oxygen should be given to the patient.

Aftercare

As long as the tube is in the chest, the patient must lie still. After it is removed, x-rays will determine if the effusion or air is reaccumulating—though some researchers and clinicians believe chest x-rays do not need to be performed after routine thoracentesis.

Risks

Reaccumulation of fluid or air is a possible complication, as are hypovolemic shock (shock caused by a lack of circulating blood) and infection. Patients are at increased risk for poor outcomes if they have a recent history of anticoagulant use, very small effusions, significant amounts of fluid, poor health leading into this condition, positive airway pressure, or **adhesions** in the pleural space. A pneumothorax can sometimes be caused by the thoracentesis procedure. The use of ultrasound to guide the procedure can reduce the risk of pneumothorax.

Thoracentesis can also result in hemothorax, or bleeding within the thorax. In addition, such internal structures as the diaphragm, spleen, or liver can be damaged by needle insertion. Repeat thoracentesis can increase the risk of developing hypoproteinemia (a decrease in the amount of protein in the blood).

Resources

BOOKS

Goldman, Lee, and Andrew I. Schafer. *Goldman's Cecil Medicine.* 24th ed. Philadelphia: Saunders/Elsevier, 2012.
Niederhuber, John E. *Abeloff's Clinical Oncology.* 5th ed. Philadelphia: Saunders/Elsevier, 2014.

PERIODICALS

Berg, Dale, et al. "The Development of a Validated Checklist for Thoracentesis: Preliminary Results." *American Journal of Medical Quality* 28, no. 3 (2013): 220–26. http://dx.doi.org/10.1177/1062860612459881 (accessed August 12, 2013).
Patel, Pankaj A., Frank R. Ernst, and Candace L. Gunnarsson. "Ultrasonography Guidance Reduces Complications and Costs Associated with Thoracentesis Procedures." *Journal of Clinical Ultrasound* 40, no. 3 (2012): 135–41. http://dx.doi.org/10.1002/jcu.20884 (accessed August 12, 2013).

WEBSITES

A.D.A.M. Medical Encyclopedia. "Thoracentesis." Medline-Plus. http://www.nlm.nih.gov/medlineplus/ency/article/003420.htm (accessed August 12, 2013).
Cleveland Clinic. "Thoracentesis." https://www.clevelandclinic.org/thoracic/Chest/dia_Thoracentesis.htm (accessed August 12, 2013).

Lechtzin, Noah. "Thoracentesis." *The Merck Manual for Health Care Professionals* (online). http://www.merckmanuals.com/professional/pulmonary_disorders/diagnostic_pulmonary_procedures/thoracentesis.html (accessed August 12, 2013).
National Heart, Lung, and Blood Institute. "What Is Thoracentesis?" National Institutes of Health. http://www.nhlbi.nih.gov/health/health-topics/topics/thor (accessed August 12, 2013).

ORGANIZATIONS

National Heart, Lung, and Blood Institute Information Center, PO Box 30105, Bethesda, MD 20824-0105, (301) 592-8573, Fax: (240) 629-3246, nhlbiinfo@nhlbi.nih.gov, http://www.nhlbi.nih.gov.

Mark A. Mitchell, MD

Thoracic surgery

Definition

Thoracic surgery is any surgery performed in the chest (thorax).

Purpose

The purpose of thoracic surgery is to treat diseased or injured organs in the thorax, including the esophagus (muscular tube that passes food to the stomach), trachea (windpipe that branches to form the right bronchus and the left bronchus), pleura (membranes that cover and protect the lung), mediastinum (area separating the left and right lungs), chest wall, diaphragm, heart, and lungs.

General thoracic surgery is a field that specializes in diseases of the lungs and esophagus. The field also encompasses accidents and injuries to the chest, esophageal disorders (esophageal cancer or esophagitis), lung cancer, **lung transplantation**, and surgery for emphysema.

Description

The most common diseases requiring thoracic surgery include lung cancer, chest trauma, esophageal cancer, emphysema, and lung transplantation.

Lung cancer

Lung cancer is one of the most significant public health problems in the world. Approximately 228,190 new cases of lung and bronchial cancer will be diagnosed in 2013. It is the second most common type of cancer, and the leading cause of cancer deaths among both men and women, killing about 160,340 people annually. The overall five-year survival rate for all types of lung cancer is about 16.3%, as compared to 65.2% for colon cancer, 90% for breast cancer, and 99.9% for prostate cancer.

Lung cancer develops primarily by exposure to toxic chemicals. Cigarette smoking is the most important risk factor responsible for the disease. Other environmental factors that may predispose a person to lung cancer include industrial substances such as arsenic, nickel, chromium, asbestos, radon, organic chemicals, air pollution, and radiation.

Most cases of lung cancer develop in the right lung because it contains the majority (55%) of lung tissue. Additionally, lung cancer occurs more frequently in the upper lobes of the lung than in the lower lobes. The tumor receives blood from the bronchial artery (a major artery in the pulmonary system).

Adenocarcinoma of the lung is the most frequent type of lung cancer, accounting for 45% of all cases. This type of cancer can spread (metastasize) earlier than another type of lung cancer called squamous cell carcinoma (which occurs in approximately 30% of lung cancer patients). Approximately 66% of squamous cell carcinoma cases are centrally located. They expand against the bronchus, causing compression. Small-cell carcinoma accounts for 20% of all lung cancers; the majority (80%) are centrally located. Small-cell carcinoma is a highly aggressive lung cancer, with early metastasis to distant sites such as the brain and bone marrow (the central portion of certain bones, which produce formed elements that are part of blood).

Most lung tumors are not treated with thoracic surgery since patients seek medical care later in the disease process. Chemotherapy increases the rate of survival in patients with limited (not advanced) disease. Surgery may be useful for staging or diagnosis. Pulmonary resection (removal of the tumor and neighboring lymph nodes) can be curative if the tumor is less than or equal to 1.8 in. (3 cm), and presents as a solitary nodule. Lung tumors spread to other areas through neighboring lymphatic channels. Even if thoracic surgery is performed, postoperative chemotherapy may also be indicated to provide comprehensive treatment (i.e., to kill any tumor cells that may have spread via the lymphatic system).

Genetic engineering has provided insights related to the growth of tumors. A genetic mutation called a k-ras mutation frequently occurs, and is implicated in 90% of genetic mutations for adenocarcinoma of the lung. Mutations in the cancer cells make them resistant to chemotherapy, necessitating the use of multiple chemotherapeutic agents.

Chest trauma

Chest trauma is a medical/surgical emergency. Initially, the chest should be examined after an airway is maintained. The mortality (death) rate for trauma patients with respiratory distress is approximately 50%. This figure rises to 75% if symptoms include both respiratory distress and shock. Patients with respiratory distress require **endotracheal intubation** (passing a plastic tube from the mouth to the windpipe) and mechanically assisted ventilator support. Invasive thoracic procedures are necessary in emergency situations.

Trauma requiring urgent thoracic surgery may include any of the following problems: a large clotted hemothorax, massive air leak, esophageal injury, valvular cardiac (heart) injury, proven damage to blood vessels in the heart, or chest wall defect.

Esophageal cancer

The number of new cases of esophageal cancer is slowly rising, with about 17,990 people diagnosed annually. While the cause of esophageal cancer is not precisely known, the greatly increased rate of esophageal cancer seems to be tied to the epidemic of obesity in the United States. Obesity results in acid reflux into the esophagus, chronic esophageal irritation, and progression to abnormal cell types that result in esophageal cancer, specifically of adenocarcinoma of the esophagus. Smoking and alcohol seem to also result in chronic esophageal irritation, leading to an association with squamous cell carcinoma of the esophagus.

Difficulty swallowing (dysphagia) is the cardinal symptom of esophageal cancer. Radiography, endoscopy, computerized axial tomography (CT scan), and ultrasonography are part of a comprehensive diagnostic evaluation. The standard operation for patients with resectable esophageal carcinoma includes removal of the tumor from the esophagus, a portion of the stomach, and the lymph nodes (within the cancerous region).

Emphysema

Lung volume reduction surgery (LVRS) is the term used to describe surgery for patients with emphysema. LVRS is intended to help persons whose disabling dyspnea (difficulty breathing) is related to emphysema and does not respond to medical management. Breathlessness is a result of the structural and functional pulmonary and thoracic abnormalities associated with emphysema. Surgery will assist the patient, but the primary pathogenic process that caused the emphysema is permanent because lung tissues lose the capability of elastic recoil during normal breathing (inspiration and expiration).

Patients are usually transferred out of the **intensive care unit** (ICU) within one day of surgery. Physical therapy and rehabilitation (coughing and breathing exercises) begin soon after surgery, and the patient is discharged when deemed clinically stable.

Lung transplantation

There are various types of lung transplantations: unilateral (one lung, the most common type); bilateral (both lungs); heart-lung; and living donor lobe transplantation.

The survival rate for persons receiving a single lung transplant is more than 80% at one year, almost 70% at three years, and more than 55% at five years. Double-lung transplants have similar success rates: 82% at one year, 64% at three years, and 48% at five years. A successful outcome is highly dependent on the patient's general medical condition. Those who have symptomatic osteoporosis (severe disease of the musculoskeletal system) or are users of **corticosteroids** may not have favorable outcomes.

The death rate occurs due to infections (pulmonary infections) or chronic rejection (bronchiolitis obliterans) if the donor lung was not a perfect genetic match. Patients are given postoperative **antibiotics** to prevent bacterial infections during the early period following surgery.

Bacterial pneumonia is usually severe. A bacterial genus known as *Pseudomonas* accounts for 75% of post-transplant pneumonia cases. Patients can also acquire viral and fungal infections, and an infection caused by a cell parasite known as *Pneumocystis carinii*. Infections are treated with specific medications intended to destroy the invading microorganism. Viral infections require treatment of symptoms.

Acute (quick onset) rejection is common within the first weeks after lung transplantation. Acute rejection is treated with steroids (bolus given intravenously), and is effective in 80% of cases. Chronic rejection is the most common problem, and typically begins with symptoms of fatigue and a vague feeling of illness. Treatment is difficult, and the results are unrewarding. There are several immunosuppressive protocols currently utilized for cases of chronic rejection. The goal of immunosuppressive therapy is to prevent the host's immune reaction from destroying the genetically foreign organ.

Preparation

The surgeon may use two common incisional approaches: sternotomy (incision through and down the breastbone) or via the side of the chest (**thoracotomy**).

An operative procedure known as video-assisted thoracoscopic surgery (VATS) is minimally invasive. During VATS, a lung is collapsed and the thoracoscope and **surgical instruments** are inserted into the thorax through any of three or four small incisions in the chest wall.

Another approach involves the use of a mediastinoscope or bronchoscope to visualize the internal anatomical structures during thoracic surgery or diagnostic procedures.

Preoperative evaluation for most patients (except emergency cases) must include cardiac tests, blood chemistry analysis, and **physical examination**. Like most operative procedures, the patient should not eat or drink food 10–12 hours prior to surgery. Patients who undergo thoracic surgery with the video-assisted approach tend to have shorter inpatient hospital stays.

Aftercare

Patients typically experience severe pain after surgery, and are given appropriate pain medications. In uncomplicated cases, chest and urine (Foley catheter) tubes are usually removed within 24–48 hours. A highly trained and comprehensive team of respiratory therapists and nurses is vital for **postoperative care** that results in improved lung function via deep breathing and coughing exercises.

Risks

Precautions for thoracic surgery include coagulation blood disorders (disorders that prevent normal blood clotting) and previous thoracic surgery. Risks include hemorrhage, myocardial infarction (heart attack), stroke, nerve injury, embolism (blood clot or air bubble that obstructs an artery), and infection. Total lung collapse can occur from fluid or air accumulation, as a result of chest tubes that are routinely placed after surgery for drainage.

Health care team roles

Thoracic surgery is performed in a hospital by a specialist in **general surgery** who has received advanced training in thoracic surgery.

Resources

BOOKS

Goldman, Lee, and Andrew I. Schafer. *Goldman's Cecil Medicine.* 24th ed. Philadelphia: Saunders/Elsevier, 2012.

Mason, Robert J., et al. *Murray & Nadel's Textbook of Respiratory Medicine.* 5th ed. Philadelphia: Saunders/ Elsevier, 2010.

McKenna, Robert J. Jr., Ali Mahtabifard, and Scott J. Swanson. *Atlas of Minimally Invasive Thoracic Surgery (VATS).* Philadelphia: Saunders/Elsevier, 2011.

Townsend, Courtney M., et al. *Sabiston Textbook of Surgery.* 19th ed. Philadelphia: Saunders/Elsevier, 2012.

PERIODICALS

Nelems, Bill. "Palliative Care Principles for Thoracic Surgery." *Thoracic Surgery Clinics* 23, no. 3 (2013): 443–46. http://dx.doi.org/10.1016/j.thorsurg.2013.04.006 (accessed September 19, 2013).

Rupp, Michael, Helen Miley, and Kathleen Russell-Babin. "Incentive Spirometry in Postoperative Abdominal/ Thoracic Surgery Patients." *AACN Advanced Critical Care* 24, no. 3 (2013): 255–63. http://dx.doi.org/10.1097/ NCI.0b013e31828c8878 (accessed September 19, 2013).

Zhang, Guangjian, et al. "Video-Assisted Thoracic Surgery Right Upper Lobectomy and Lymph Node Dissection." *Journal of Thoracic Disease* 5, suppl. 3 (2013): S328–30. http://dx.doi.org/10.3978/j.issn.2072-1439.2013.08.58 (accessed September 19, 2013).

WEBSITES

Harvard Medical School. "Video-Assisted Thoracic Surgery." http://www.health.harvard.edu/diagnostic-tests/video-assisted-thoracic-surgery.htm (accessed September 19, 2013).

The Society of Thoracic Surgeons. "What Is a Thoracic Surgeon?" http://www.sts.org/patient-information/what-thoracic-surgeon (accessed September 19, 2013).

ORGANIZATIONS

American Association for Thoracic Surgery, 500 Cummings Ctr., Ste. 4550, Beverly, MA 01915, (978) 927-8330, http://aats.org.

American Thoracic Society, 25 Broadway, New York, NY 10004, (212) 315-8600, Fax: (212) 315-6498, atsinfo@thoracic.org, http://www.thoracic.org.

The Society of Thoracic Surgeons, 633 N. Saint Clair St., Fl. 23, Chicago, IL 60611, (312) 202-5800, Fax: (312) 202-5801, http://sts.org.

Laith Farid Gulli, MD, MS
Abraham F. Ettaher, MD
Nicole Mallory, MS, PA-C

Thoracoscopy

Definition

Thoracoscopy is the insertion of an endoscope, a narrow-diameter tube with a viewing mirror or camera attachment, through a very small incision (cut) in the chest wall.

Purpose

Thoracoscopy makes it possible for a physician to examine the lungs or other structures in the chest cavity, without making a large incision. It is an alternative to **thoracotomy** (opening the chest cavity with a large incision). Many surgical procedures, especially taking tissue samples (biopsies), can also be accomplished with thoracoscopy. The procedure is done to:

- assess lung cancer
- take a biopsy for study
- determine the cause of fluid in the chest cavity
- introduce medications or other treatments directly into the lungs
- treat accumulated fluid, pus (empyema), or blood in the space around the lungs
- treat recurrent or persistent pneumothorax
- perform a pulmonary resection
- evacuate a blood clot following trauma or injury

For many patients, thoracoscopy replaces thoracotomy. It avoids many of the complications of open chest surgery and reduces pain, hospital stay, and recovery time.

Precautions

Because one lung is partially deflated during thoracoscopy, the procedure cannot be done on patients whose lung function is so poor that they do not receive enough oxygen with only one lung. Patients who have had previous surgery that involved the chest cavity, or who have blood clotting problems, are not good candidates for this procedure.

Thoracoscopy gives physicians a good but limited view of the organs, such as lungs, in the chest cavity. Endoscope technology is being refined every day, as is what physicians can accomplish by inserting scopes and instruments through several small incisions instead of making one large cut.

Description

Thoracoscopy is most commonly performed in a hospital, and **general anesthesia** is used. Some of the procedures are moving toward outpatient services and **local anesthesia**. More specific names are sometimes applied to the procedure, depending on what the target site of the effort is. For example, if a physician intends to examine the lungs, the procedure is often called pleuroscopy. The procedure takes two to four hours.

The surgeon makes two or three small incisions in the chest wall, often between the ribs. By making the incisions between the ribs, the surgeon minimizes damage to muscle and nerves and the ribs themselves. A tube is inserted in the trachea and connected to a ventilator, which is a mechanical device that assists the patient with inhaling and exhaling.

The most common reason for a thoracoscopy is to examine a lung that has a tumor or a metastatic growth of cancer. The lung to be examined is deflated to create a space between the chest wall and the lung. The patient breathes with the other lung with the assistance of the ventilator.

A specialized endoscope, or narrow-diameter tube, with a video camera or mirrored attachment, is inserted through the chest wall. Instruments for taking necessary tissue samples are inserted through other small incisions. After tissue samples are taken, the lung is reinflated. All incisions except one are closed. The remaining open incision is used to insert a drainage tube. The tissue samples are sent to a laboratory for evaluation.

Preparation

Prior to thoracoscopy, the patient will have several routine tests, such as blood, urine and **chest x-ray**. Older patients must have an electrocardiogram (a trace record of the heart activity) because the anesthesia and the lung deflation put a big load on the heart muscle. The patient should not eat or drink from midnight the night before the thoracoscopy. The anesthesia used can cause vomiting, and, because anesthesia also causes the loss of the gag reflex, a person who vomits is in danger of moving food into the lungs, which can cause serious complications and death.

Aftercare

After the procedure, a chest tube will remain in one of the incisions for several days to drain fluid and release residual air from the chest cavity. Hospital stays range from two to five days. Medications for pain are given as needed. After returning home, patients should do only light lifting for several weeks.

Risks

The main risks of thoracoscopy are those associated with the administration of general anesthesia. Prolonged air leak is also a risk following thoracoscopy. Sometimes excessive bleeding, or hemorrhage, occurs, necessitating a thoracotomy to stop it. Another risk comes when the drainage tube is removed, and the patient is vulnerable to lung collapse (pneumothorax).

Resources

PERIODICALS

Dhooria, S., et al. "A Randomized Trial Comparing the Diagnostic Yield of Rigid and Semirigid Thoracoscopy in Undiagnosed Pleural Effusions." *Respiratory Care* (October 8, 2013): e-pub ahead of print. http://dx.doi.org/10.4187/respcare.02738 (accessed October 18, 2013).

WEBSITES

University of Southern California Keck School of Medicine. "A Patient's Guide to Lung Surgery." http://www.cts.usc.edu/lpg-thoracoscopy.html (accessed October 18, 2013).

ORGANIZATIONS

The Society of Thoracic Surgeons, 633 N. Saint Clair St., Fl. 23, Chicago, IL 60611, (312) 202-5800, Fax: (312) 202-5801, http://sts.org.

Tish Davidson, AM

Thoracotomy

Definition

Thoracotomy is the process of making of an incision (cut) into the chest wall.

Thoracotomy

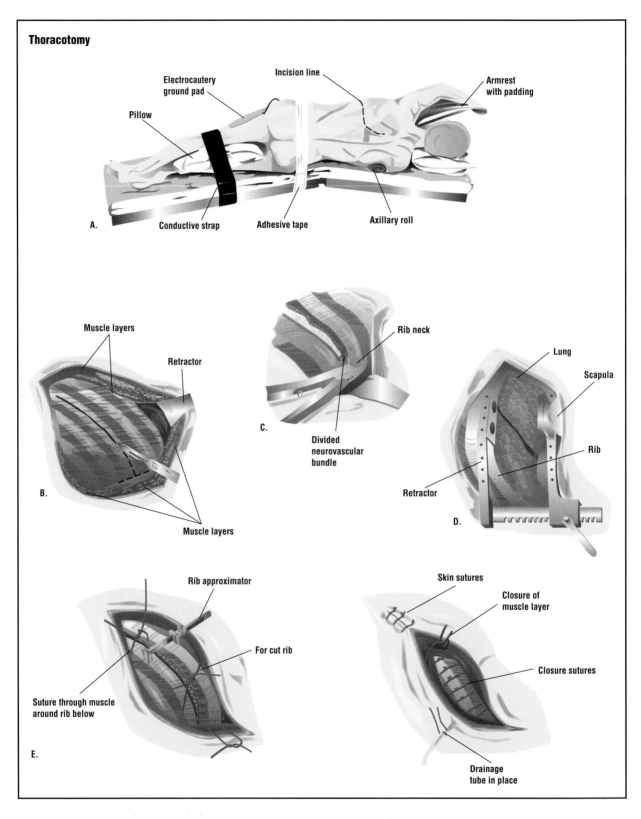

A. — Pillow / Electrocautery ground pad / Incision line / Armrest with padding / Conductive strap / Adhesive tape / Axillary roll

B. — Muscle layers / Retractor / Muscle layers

C. — Rib neck / Divided neurovascular bundle

D. — Lung / Scapula / Rib / Retractor

E. — Rib approximator / For cut rib / Suture through muscle around rib below / Skin sutures / Closure of muscle layer / Closure sutures / Drainage tube in place

For a thoracotomy, the patient lies on his or her side with one arm raised (A). An incision is cut into the skin of the rib cage (B). Muscle layers are cut, and a rib may be removed to gain access to the cavity. (C). Retractors hold the ribs apart, exposing the lung (D). After any repairs are made, the cut rib is replaced and held in place with special materials (E). Layers of muscle and skin are stitched. *(Illustration by GGS Information Services. Copyright © Cengage Learning®.)*

Purpose

A physician gains access to the chest cavity (called the thorax) by cutting through the chest wall. Reasons for the entry are varied. Thoracotomy allows for study of the condition of the lungs; removal of a lung or part of a lung; removal of a rib; and examination, treatment, or removal of any organs in the chest cavity. Thoracotomy also provides access to the heart, esophagus, diaphragm, and the portion of the aorta that passes through the chest cavity.

Lung cancer is the most common cancer requiring a thoracotomy. Tumors and metastatic growths can be removed through the incision (a procedure called resection). A biopsy, or tissue sample, can also be taken through the incision, and examined under a microscope for evidence of abnormal cells.

A resuscitative or emergency thoracotomy may be performed to resuscitate a patient who is near death as a result of a chest injury. An emergency thoracotomy provides access to the chest cavity to control injury-related bleeding from the heart, cardiac compressions to restore a normal heart rhythm, or to relieve pressure on the heart caused by cardiac tamponade (accumulation of fluid in the space between the heart's muscle and outer lining).

Demographics

Thoracotomy may be performed to diagnose or treat a variety of conditions; therefore, no data exist as to the overall incidence of the procedure. Lung cancer, a common reason for thoracotomy, is diagnosed in approximately over 196,000 people each year and affects more men than women (108,355 diagnoses in men compared to 87,897 in women).

Description

The thoracotomy incision may be made on the side, under the arm (axillary thoracotomy); on the front, through the breastbone (median sternotomy); slanting from the back to the side (posterolateral thoracotomy); or under the breast (anterolateral thoracotomy). The exact location of the cut depends on the reason for the surgery. In some cases, the physician is able to make the incision between ribs (called an intercostal approach) to minimize cuts through bone, nerves, and muscle. The incision may range from just under 5–10 in. (12.7–25 cm).

During the surgery, a tube is passed through the trachea. It usually has a branch to each lung. One lung is deflated for examination and surgery, while the other one is inflated with the assistance of a mechanical device (a ventilator).

A number of different procedures may be commenced at this point. A lobectomy removes an entire lobe or section of a lung (the right lung has three lobes and the left lung has two). It may be done to remove cancer that is contained by a lobe. A **segmentectomy**, or wedge resection, removes a wedge-shaped piece of lung smaller than a lobe. Alternatively, the entire lung may be removed during a **pneumonectomy**.

In the case of an emergency thoracotomy, the procedure performed depends on the type and extent of injury. The heart may be exposed so that direct cardiac compressions can be performed; the physician may use one hand or both hands to manually pump blood through the heart. Internal paddles of a defibrillating machine may be applied directly to the heart to restore normal cardiac rhythms. Injuries to the heart causing excessive bleeding (hemorrhaging) may be closed with staples or stitches.

Once the procedure that required the incision is completed, the chest wall is closed. The layers of skin, muscle, and other tissues are closed with stitches or staples. If the breastbone was cut (as in the case of a median sternotomy), it is stitched back together with wire.

Preparation

Patients are told not to eat after midnight the night before surgery. They must tell their physicians about all known allergies so that the safest anesthetics can be selected. Older patients must be evaluated for heart ailments before surgery because of the additional strain on the heart.

Aftercare

Opening the chest cavity means cutting through skin, muscle, nerves, and sometimes bone. It is a major procedure that often involves a hospital stay of five to seven days. The skin around the drainage tube to the thoracic cavity must be kept clean, and the tube must be kept unblocked.

The pressure differences that are set up in the thoracic cavity by the movement of the diaphragm (the large muscle at the base of the thorax) make it possible for the lungs to expand and contract. If the pressure in the chest cavity changes abruptly, the lungs can collapse. Any fluid that collects in the cavity puts a patient at risk for infection and reduced lung function, or even collapse (called a pneumothorax). Thus, any entry to the chest usually requires that a chest tube remain in place for several days after the incision is closed.

The first two days after surgery may be spent in the **intensive care unit** (ICU) of the hospital. A variety of tubes, catheters, and monitors may be required after surgery.

Risks

The rich supply of blood vessels to the lungs makes hemorrhage a risk; a blood **transfusion** may become necessary during surgery. **General anesthesia** carries risks such as nausea, vomiting, headache, blood pressure issues, or allergic reaction. After a thoracotomy, there may be drainage from the incision. There is also the risk of infection; the patient must learn how to keep the incision clean and dry as it heals.

After the chest tube is removed, the patient is vulnerable to pneumothorax. Physicians strive to reduce the risk of collapse by timing the removal of the tube. Doing so at the end of inspiration (breathing in) or the end of expiration (breathing out) poses less risk. Deep breathing exercises and coughing should be emphasized as an important way that patients can improve healing and prevent pneumonia.

Results

The results following thoracotomy depend on the reasons why it was performed. If a biopsy was taken during the surgery, a normal result would indicate that no cancerous cells are present in the tissue sample. The procedure may indicate that further treatment is necessary; for example, if cancer was detected, chemotherapy, radiation therapy, or more surgery may be recommended.

QUESTIONS TO ASK YOUR DOCTOR

- Why is thoracotomy being recommended?
- What diagnostic tests will be performed to determine if thoracotomy is necessary?
- What type of incision will be used and where will it be located?
- What type of procedure will be performed?
- How long is the recovery time and what is expected during this period?
- If a biopsy is the only reason for the procedure, is a thoracoscopy or a guided needle biopsy an option (instead of thoracotomy)?

Morbidity and mortality rates

One study following lung cancer patients undergoing thoracotomy found that 10%–15% of patients experienced heartbeat irregularities, readmittance to the ICU, or partial or full lung collapse; 5%–10% experienced pneumonia or extended use of the ventilator (greater than 48 hours); and up to 5% experienced wound infection, accumulation of pus in the chest cavity, or blood clots in the lung. The mortality rate in the study was 5.8%, with patients dying as a result of the cancer itself or of postoperative complications.

Alternatives

Video-assisted **thoracic surgery** (VATS) is a less invasive alternative to thoracotomy. Also called **thoracoscopy**, VATS involves the insertion of a thoracoscope (a thin, lighted tube) into a small incision through the chest wall. The surgeon can visualize the structures inside the chest cavity on a video screen. Instruments such as a stapler or grasper may be inserted through other small incisions. Although initially used as a diagnostic tool (to visualize the lungs or to remove a sample of lung tissue for further examination), VATS is being increasingly used to remove some lung tumors, and is usually appropriate for those under 2.4 in. (6 cm). In some practices, as many as 8% of all lobectomies are now performed using VATS technique.

An alternative to emergency thoracotomy is a tube thoracostomy, a tube placed through chest wall to drain excess fluid. Over 80% of patients with a penetrating chest wound can be successfully managed with a thoracostomy.

Health care team roles

Thoracotomy may be performed by a thoracic surgeon, a medical doctor who has completed **surgical training** in the areas of **general surgery** and surgery of the chest area, or an emergency room physician (in the case of emergency thoracotomy). The procedure is generally performed in a hospital **operating room**, although emergency thoracotomies may be performed in an emergency department or trauma center.

Resources

BOOKS

Khatri, V. P., and J. A. Asensio. *Operative Surgery Manual.* Philadelphia: Saunders, 2003.

Mason, Robert J., et al. *Murray & Nadel's Textbook of Respiratory Medicine.* 5th ed. Philadelphia: Saunders/Elsevier, 2010.

Townsend, Courtney M., et al. *Sabiston Textbook of Surgery.* 19th ed. Philadelphia: Saunders/Elsevier, 2012.

PERIODICALS

Matsutani, Noriyuki, and Masafumi Kawamura. "Successful Management of Postoperative Pain with Pregabalin after Thoracotomy." *Surgery Today* (September 27, 2013): e-pub ahead of print. http://dx.doi.org/10.1007/s00595-013-0743-x (accessed October 17, 2013).

Yao, S., et al. "Incidence and Risk Factors for Acute Lung Injury after Open Thoracotomy for Thoracic Diseases." *Journal of Thoracic Disease* 5, no. 4 (2013): 455–60. http://dx.doi.org/10.3978/j.issn.2072-1439.2013.08.20 (accessed October 17, 2013).

OTHER

American College of Surgeons. *Thoracotomy in the Emergency Department.* http://www.facs.org/trauma/publications/thoracotomy.pdf (accessed October 17, 2013).

University of Michigan Health System, Department of Thoracic Surgery. *Preparing for Your Thoracotomy.* http://www.med.umich.edu/1libr/surgery/thoracicsurgery/Thoracotomy.pdf (accessed October 17, 2013).

WEBSITES

American Cancer Society. "Lung Cancer." http://www.cancer.org/cancer/lungcancer/index (accessed October 17, 2013).

Brohi, Karim. "Emergency Department Thoracotomy." Trauma.org. http://www.trauma.org/archive/thoracic/EDTintro.html (accessed October 17, 2013).

ORGANIZATIONS

American Cancer Society, 250 Williams St. NW, Atlanta, GA 30303, (800) 227-2345, http://www.cancer.org.

National Cancer Institute, 6116 Executive Blvd., Ste. 300, Bethesda, MD 20892-8322, (800) 4-CANCER (422-6237), http://cancer.gov.

The Society of Thoracic Surgeons, 633 N. Saint Clair St., Fl. 23, Chicago, IL 60611, (312) 202-5800, Fax: (312) 202-5801, http://sts.org.

Diane M. Calabrese
Stephanie Dionne Sherk

Thrombectomy

Definition

Thrombectomy is the surgical dissolution and/or extraction of a blood clot in a vein or artery.

Purpose

Thrombectomy is one method of treating a blood clot. Clotting is a normal process that prevents excessive blood loss from a wound. Once the injury is healed, the clot normally dissolves. Sometimes, however, clots form in uninjured blood vessels or fail to dissolve properly. Blood clots in arteries are usually caused by atherosclerosis—the narrowing and hardening of the arteries due to a buildup of plaque. Blood pressure in an artery can cause plaque to rupture, and the body reacts by forming a clot. A clot inside an artery can block the flow of blood and oxygen to a tissue, damaging or killing it. A clot that blocks blood flow to the heart or brain can cause a heart attack or ischemic stroke. If a clot blocks blood flow in a vein, blood is unable to flow back toward the heart, causing swelling and pain in the part of the body behind the clot. Deep vein thrombosis (DVT) is usually a clot in a major vein of the lower leg, although it can also occur in another large vein, such as in the thigh, pelvis, or arm. If the clot dislodges and travels through the veins to the lungs, it can cause a pulmonary embolism (PE). More than 250,000 Americans are hospitalized for DVT each year, and about 100,000 people die within the first hour of a PE, making it the third most common cause of cardiovascular-related mortality, following heart attack and stroke.

In the United States, thrombectomies are most often performed in life-threatening emergencies, when a clot in a blood vessel in the brain is causing an ischemic stroke or when a clot has a high risk of dislodging and causing a heart attack, stroke, or PE. Thrombectomy is frequently used to restore flow in a threatened limb or to treat a clot that is resistant to break up (thrombolysis) with clot-busting drugs called thrombolytics. Thrombectomy may also be used:

• for DVT higher up in the leg in active, healthy individuals who have been having severe symptoms for less than seven days and have no serious associated conditions

• for a rare complication of DVT called phlegmasia cerulea dolens (PCD) that has not responded to other therapies or that is threatening a limb with gangrene

• in patients who cannot tolerate thrombolytics; for example, because they are at high risk for hemorrhage (excessive bleeding)

• for patients who have not responded to anticoagulants that prevent clots from forming or enlarging

• to avoid lengthy, expensive infusions with thrombolytics in an intensive care unit

• to reduce the dosage and infusion time of thrombolytics

• for clots in pregnant women

• to treat vascular insufficiency, in which improper blood valve function causes the blood to flow backward through one-way valves, pooling in the legs, ankles, or feet and increasing the likelihood of a blood clot

• to remove dangerous clots before angioplasty (opening up of a narrowed blood vessel), thereby increasing the safety and effectiveness of angioplasty

The first thrombectomy for PCD was performed in 1939. In the United States, thrombectomies have been largely superceded by other procedures, especially catheter-directed thrombolysis, in which clot-busting thrombolytics are delivered directly to the clot.

Description

Thrombectomy is performed in conjunction with **angiography** or venography to map the blood vessels and locate the clot. A contrast dye injected into an artery or vein allows the blood vessels and the procedure to be visualized on an x-ray screen. For venography, the dye is injected through a short tube called a catheter sheath inserted through a small incision in the femoral vein in the groin or the popliteal vein below the knee. Minimally invasive percutaneous mechanical thrombectomy is the most common surgery for breaking up and removing blood clots. Surgical thrombectomy is much less common. Thrombectomies generally take two to three hours and may be performed under local or **general anesthesia**.

Percutaneous mechanical thrombectomy

For percutaneous thrombectomy, a soft guide wire is inserted through the catheter sheath and threaded through the blood vessel past the clot. A catheter with a thrombectomy device at its tip is then passed over the wire to the clot as shown on the x-rays.

There are several types of thrombectomy devices:

• Thromboaspiration is the simplest type of mechanical thrombectomy. A device reminiscent of a miniature vacuum cleaner suctions or aspirates the clot out through the sheath. It may be threaded into the pulmonary artery for treating PE.

• Recirculation devices destroy a clot by continuous mixing to create a vortex. Recirculation devices have been approved by the U.S. Food and Drug Administration (FDA) for treating DVT and for clots in coronary and peripheral arteries.

• Ultrasonic thrombectomy liquefies the clot with an ultrasound device at the tip of the catheter.

• Fragmentation devices have tiny surgical instruments that cut, chop, or brush the clot into small pieces that can be sucked out of the blood vessel.

• Angiojet thrombectomy pumps a saline solution through high-pressure or low-pressure jets directly into the clot. This creates a strong vacuum that breaks up the clot. The pieces are then pumped out through the catheter. The jetting takes just a few minutes, and the entire procedure takes about one hour.

• Balloon maceration isolates the clotted segment between two balloons, and a rotating filament disrupts the clot while injecting a thrombolytic.

Percutaneous mechanical thrombectomy is most often used with catheter-directed thrombolysis, in which the thrombectomy device also injects a precise dose of a thrombolytic directly into the clot. The powerful natural thrombolytic tissue plasminogen activator (tPa) softens the clot for destruction by the device and dissolves the clot fragments.

Percutaneous thrombectomy is also often performed in conjunction with **angioplasty**, in which a balloon catheter is used to open up narrowed blood vessels, and/or stenting, in which tiny plastic, metal, or fabric tubes are placed in the vessel to hold it open. An inferior vena cava (IVC) filter may be implanted to prevent additional clots from reaching the heart or lungs. A temporary pacemaker may be inserted in the left groin by a cardiologist to keep the heart beating regularly during the procedure.

Surgical thrombectomy

With a surgical thrombectomy, the clot is located by angiography/venography, a larger incision is made over the vessel with the clot, and the clot is removed with a catheter. For an iliofemoral thrombosis—a clot in a deep vein in the groin—the leg is enclosed in a sterile stockinette. Vessels around the clot are clamped, the vessel is partially opened, and the clot is partially extracted with forceps. A thrombectomy catheter with a balloon at its tip is inserted and removes the remainder of the clot, and the vessel is flushed out with an anticoagulant irrigation solution. The vessel, tissue layers, and skin are stitched closed.

Thrombectomy for subclavian thrombosis—a clot in the artery under the collarbone—is performed under general anesthesia. An incision is made along the clavicle, the subclavian artery is opened, and the clot is removed. A catheter is not required.

Preparation

Imaging techniques—ultrasound, CT or MRI scans, or angiography/venography—are used to diagnose and locate blood clots, which may or may not have symptoms. A blood test for "D-dimer," which is a sign of active recent clotting, may be performed to diagnose DVT.

As with any surgery, patients should not eat or drink after midnight on the day of the thrombectomy. An intravenous (IV) line into the arm administers fluids, sedatives, and heparin to prevent the blood from clotting during the procedure. The groin is cleaned with an antiseptic, and the site or sites of catheter insertion are shaved. The insertion site is numbed with a local anesthetic, and a tiny incision is made in the appropriate vein. Contrast dye is injected for angiography/venography.

Aftercare

Following percutaneous thrombectomy, the catheter is removed, and pressure is applied to stop bleeding. After some procedures, the patient must remain flat or hold a treated arm or leg straight for several hours. Following a procedure on a leg, compression **bandages** or stockings are applied to reduce swelling, and the patient may be asked to walk for 15 minutes and rest for 45 minutes for up to six hours. IV heparin is usually administered during recovery. The patient may be given fluids, **antibiotics**, and/or painkillers.

Patients are closely monitored for heart rate, blood pressure, medication rate, signs of bleeding, and complications at the insertion site. Monitoring is especially vigilant if thrombolytic infusions are continued after the procedure. Blood tests and imaging scans may be repeated. If **vital signs** are normal, the patient may be discharged. Patients should not lift more than about 10 lb. (4.5 kg) for several days. They should drink plenty of water to flush out the contrast dye. Patients may shower after 24 hours but should not bathe for several days. The physician should be notified immediately if there are any signs of excessive bleeding. Patients usually take the blood-thinner warfarin (Coumadin) to prevent future clots. If an IVC filter was implanted, it may eventually be removed.

Risks

In addition to the very small risk that accompanies anesthesia, mechanical thrombectomy carries a risk of damaging, puncturing, or tearing the lining of blood vessels or the valves. However, blood vessel damage is unlikely because the procedure is monitored with x-rays. There is also a risk of fragmenting the clot, which could result in PE or a heart attack if a fragment travels to the lungs or heart. As blood clots break down, chemicals are released that may temporarily affect kidney function or, rarely, the heart. There is also a very rare risk of an allergic reaction to the contrast dye. Surgical thrombectomy carries an increased risk of bleeding and infection.

Venous thrombectomy is controversial because it is sometimes associated with repeated clotting. Post-thrombotic syndrome (PTS), which includes leg swelling and discoloration and ulcers around the ankles, PCD, excessive bleeding, and stroke are other potential complications of thrombectomy. There is a risk of occlusion or blocking of more distal arteries in an affected extremity or swelling after blood flow is restored. Patients older than 65, with a tendency to bleed, or with high blood pressure, congestive heart failure, or poor kidney function are at increased risk of complications. Thus, thrombectomy carries additional risk and expense compared to other treatments for clots.

Drugs

A 2013 study found that patients who were administered the anticlotting medication tirofiban with mechanical thrombectomy for acute ischemic stroke were at higher risk for fatal intracerebral hemorrhage and poor outcomes.

Results

Prompt thrombectomy—before prolonged obstruction of blood flow and tissue death—usually has a good outcome. When combined with thrombolysis, anticoagulants, placement of an IVC filter, and/or angioplasty/stenting, venous thrombectomy has a success rate of 70%–100%. A study of balloon maceration reported a 97% success rate with a single treatment, and no bleeding complications in more than 700 patients. Initial and 24-hour success rates of 74%–100% have been reported with various other thrombectomy devices, although complete clot removal varied from 23% to 100%. Thrombolytic infusion in combination with thrombectomy appears to improve outcomes and reduces the thrombolytic treatment, which lowers the risk of bleeding. Thrombectomy and catheter-driven thrombolysis both appear to reduce the incidence and severity of PTS compared with anticoagulant treatment alone.

Thrombectomy

KEY TERMS

Angiography—X-ray visualization of arteries after the injection of a radiopaque contrast dye.

Angioplasty—Opening up of a narrowed blood vessel; often performed in conjunction with thrombectomy and/or stenting.

Anticoagulant—Blood-thinner; a medication such as heparin or warfarin that prevents coagulation or clotting of the blood.

Atherosclerosis—Thickening and hardening of the inner layer of arteries due to the accumulation of plaque.

Catheter-driven thrombolysis—A procedure performed in conjunction with or in place of thrombectomy that delivers a thrombolytic directly into a blood clot.

Deep-vein thrombosis (DVT)—A clot in a deep vein, as in the leg or pelvis.

Inferior vena cava (IVC) filter—A device implanted in the IVC—the largest vein in the body—to prevent clots or clot fragments from reaching the heart or lungs during or after thrombectomy.

Ischemic stroke—A stroke caused by the obstruction of blood supply to the brain, as from a clot.

Phlegmasia cerulea dolens (PCD)—A rare, very severe complication of a blood clot that is treated by thrombectomy.

Plaque—Deposits of fatty and other substances that accumulate in the lining of artery walls.

Post-thrombotic syndrome (PTS)—Leg swelling, discoloration, and ulcers resulting from deep-vein thrombosis.

Pulmonary embolism (PE)—A blood clot that travels to the pulmonary artery, usually from a vein in the leg or pelvis.

Stenting—The insertion of a plastic mesh or metal tube into an artery to hold it open.

Thrombolysis—The dissolving of a blood clot.

Thrombolytic—Clot-buster; a medication that dissolves blood clots.

Thrombosis—The formation of a blood clot within a blood vessel.

Tissue plasminogen activator (PA)—A genetically engineered form of a natural human thrombolytic.

Venography—X-ray visualization of veins after the injection of a radiopaque contrast dye.

However, if the vessel wall is distorted, as from plaque or an aneurysm, re-occlusion is more likely and may require a bypass graft. The outcome of thrombectomy for mesenteric venous thrombosis—a blood clot in a major vein draining the intestine—depends on the cause of the thrombosis and whether intestinal tissue has died.

One analysis found that aspiration thrombectomy before angioplasty/stenting reduced major cardiac events in heart attack patients, but did not affect the ultimate amount of damaged tissue. Although aspiration thrombectomy improved restoration of blood flow to the heart and reduced mortality, mechanical thrombectomy devices appeared to increase the risk of death. Thus, thrombectomy under these conditions remains controversial.

Mechanical thrombectomy for acute ischemic stroke is also controversial. A study of nearly 4,000 acute ischemic stroke patients who underwent thrombectomy reported that 75% either died in the hospital or were discharged to long-term-care facilities. Although trials suggested that thrombectomy improved outcomes, and FDA approval of the devices led to their widespread use, other studies have not supported the routine use of thrombectomy for stroke or found no difference between IV tPA alone and tPA followed by thrombectomy. The American College of Chest Physicians issued an evidence-based guideline against the use of mechanical thrombectomy for acute ischemic stroke.

Alternatives

There are multiple alternatives to thrombectomy. The most common alternative is to leave the clot in place and administer either heparin injections or oral warfarin, which prevents the clot from increasing in size and other clots from forming. Systemic thrombolysis delivers a thrombolytic through a vein to break up clots throughout the body. Catheter-driven thrombolysis delivers the clot-buster directly to the clot over a period of hours or days. These methods are used much more often than thrombectomy. For DVT, physicians usually recommend anticoagulants, beginning with heparin injections followed by several months of oral warfarin, the wearing of graduated compression stockings, and elevating the legs.

Health care team roles

Thrombectomies are usually performed by cardiovascular **surgeons**. They are also performed by

- Why do you recommend a thrombectomy rather than another treatment for my blood clot?
- Will you perform any other procedures during the thrombectomy?
- What exactly will occur during the thrombectomy?
- Will I be treated with any drugs before and/or after the thrombectomy?
- What are the alternatives to a thrombectomy?

interventional radiologists. Several other physicians may be involved, including a cardiologist and sometimes a hematologist. A lung specialist may monitor blood oxygen levels when the procedure is performed for PE. Thrombectomies are performed in a hospital **operating room**, interventional radiology suite, or catheterization laboratory.

Resources

BOOKS

Gan, Huili. *Pulmonary Embolism and Pulmonary Thromboendarterectomy.* New York: Nova Science, 2011.
Jansen, Olav, and Hartmut Brückmann, eds. *Interventional Stroke Therapy.* New York: Thieme, 2013.
Kern, Morton J. *The Interventional Cardiac Catheterization Handbook.* Philadelphia: Elsevier/Saunders, 2013.
Malgor, Rafael, Antonios Gasparis, and Nicos Labropoulos. "Endovenous Thrombectomy and Thrombolysis." In *Atlas of Endovascular Surgery*, edited by Jose I. Almeida. Philadelphia: Elsevier/Saunders, 2012.

PERIODICALS

Chimowitz, Marc I. "Endovascular Treatment for Acute Ischemic Stroke—Still Unproven." *New England Journal of Medicine* 368, no. 10 (March 7, 2013): 952–5.
Ferrell, Andrew, and Gavin Britz. "Developments on the Horizon in the Treatment of Neurovascular Problems." *Surgical Neurology International* 4, suppl. 2 (2013): 31–7.
Gorelick, Philip B. "Assessment of Stent Retrievers in Acute Ischaemic Stroke." *Lancet* 380, no. 9849 (October 6, 2012): 1208–10.

WEBSITES

A.D.A.M. Medical Encyclopedia. "Mesenteric Venous Thrombosis." MedlinePlus. http://www.nlm.nih.gov/medlineplus/ency/article/001157.htm (accessed September 18, 2013).
American Society of Hematology. "Blood Clots." http://www.hematology.org/Patients/Blood-Disorders/Blood-Clots/5233.aspx (accessed September 18, 2013).
Boggs, Will. "Aspiration Thrombectomy May Improve Angioplasty After Acute MI." Medscape Today News. May 13, 2013. http://www.medscape.com/viewarticle/804021 (accessed September 18, 2013).
Great Ormond Street Hospital for Children. "Thrombolysis and Thrombectomy." http://www.gosh.nhs.uk/medical-conditions/procedures-and-treatments/thrombolysis-and-thrombectomy (accessed September 18, 2013).
Leighton Heart & Vascular Center. Memorial Hospital of South Bend. "Angiojet Thrombectomy." http://www.qualityoflife.org/memorialcms/index.cfm/heart/procedures/catheterization-lab/angiojet-thrombectomy (accessed September 18, 2013).
New Mexico Heart Institute. "Venous Thrombectomy." http://www.nmhi.com/ourservices/viewprocedure.cfm?pid=46D3D17D-E0CB-91F4-21843CE1D35A7C6A (accessed September 18, 2013).
Schreiber, Donald. "Percutaneous Transcatheter Treatment of Deep Venous Thrombosis." Medscape Reference. March 20, 2011. http://emedicine.medscape.com/article/1921338-overview#a1 (accessed September 18, 2013).
Vascular Disease Foundation. "DVT Treatment." http://vasculardisease.org/deep-vein-thrombosis-venous-disease/dvt-treatment (accessed September 18, 2013).
Vascular Disease Foundation. "John Bunch's Profile." http://vasculardisease.org/media/patient-profiles/john-bunchs-profile (accessed September 18, 2013).
Vascular Disease Foundation. "Venous Thromboembolism (VTE): What You Need to Know About Risk Factors, Symptoms, and Treatment." http://vasculardisease.org/flyers/focus-on-blood-clots-flyer.pdf (accessed September 18, 2013).

ORGANIZATIONS

American Society of Hematology, 2021 L St. NW, Ste. 900, Washington, DC 20036, (202) 776-0544, Fax: (202) 776-0545, http://www.hematology.org.
U.S. Food and Drug Administration, 10903 New Hampshire Avenue, Silver Spring, MD 20993-0002, (888) INFO-FDA (463-6332), http://www.fda.gov.
Vascular Disease Foundation, 550 M Ritchie Highway, PMB-281, Severna Park, MD 21146, (443) 261-5564, robert.greenberg@vdf.org, http://vasculardisease.org.

Margaret Alic, PhD

Thrombocyte count *see* **Complete blood count**

Thrombolytic therapy

Definition

Thrombolytic therapy is the use of drugs that dissolve blood clots. The name "thrombolytic" comes from two Greek words that mean "clot" and "loosening."

Purpose

Blood clots are a risk after surgery. When a blood clot forms in a blood vessel, it may cut off or severely reduce blood flow to parts of the body that are served by that blood vessel. This event can cause serious damage to those parts of the body. If the clot forms in an artery that supplies blood to the heart, for example, it can cause a heart attack. A clot that cuts off blood to the brain can cause a stroke. Thrombolytic therapy is used to dissolve blood clots that could cause serious and possibly life-threatening damage if they are not removed.

In heart attacks, thrombolytic therapy is an alternative to stenting, a procedure in which a spring-like device is inserted into a blocked blood vessel. Stenting is the preferred treatment, since it both removes the clot and opens the blood vessel, which may have internal cholesterol deposits. Thrombolytic therapy only removes the clot, but it can be administered in hospitals with fewer resources than are required for insertion of a stent.

Thrombolytic therapy is also used to dissolve blood clots that form in catheters or tubes put into patients' bodies for medical treatments, such as dialysis or chemotherapy.

Description

Thrombolytic therapy uses drugs called thrombolytic agents, such as alteplase (Activase), anistreplase (Eminase), streptokinase (Streptase, Kabikinase), urokinase (Abbokinase), and tissue plasminogen activator (TPA) to dissolve clots. These drugs are given as injections and are given only under physician supervision.

Recommended dosage

The physician supervising the thrombolytic therapy decides on the proper dose for each patient. He or she will take into account the type of drug, the purpose for which it is being used, and in some cases, the patient's weight.

Precautions

For thrombolytic therapy to be effective in treating stroke or heart attack, prompt medical attention is very important. The drugs must be given within a few hours of the beginning of a stroke or heart attack. This type of treatment is not right, however, for every patient who has a heart attack or a stroke. Only a qualified medical professional can decide whether a thrombolytic agent should be used. To increase the chance of survival and reduce the risk of serious permanent damage, anyone who has signs of a heart attack or stroke should get immediate medical help.

Thrombolytic therapy may cause bleeding in other parts of the body. This side effect is usually not serious, but severe bleeding does occur in some patients, especially older people. Some people have had minor hemorrhagic strokes in which there has been a small amount of bleeding into the brain. These hemorrhagic strokes have been blocked by clots that would be broken up by use of a thrombolytic agent, so that removal of the harmful clot would cause equally dangerous bleeding. To lower the risk of serious bleeding, people who are given thrombolytic medications should move around as little as possible and not try to get up on their own unless told to do so by their health care professional. Following all the instructions of the health care providers in charge is very important.

Thrombolytic therapy may be more likely to cause serious bleeding in people who have certain medical conditions or have recently had certain procedures. Before taking a thrombolytic agent, patients with any of these problems or conditions should make sure their prescribing physician is aware:

- blood disease or current or past bleeding problems in any part of the body
- heart or blood vessel disease
- stroke (recent or in the past)
- high blood pressure
- brain tumor or other brain disease
- stomach ulcer or colitis
- severe liver disease
- active tuberculosis
- recent falls, injuries, or blows to the body or head
- recent injections into a blood vessel
- recent surgery, including dental surgery
- tubes recently placed in the body for any reason
- recent delivery of a baby

In addition, anyone who has had a recent streptococcal (strep) infection should tell the physician. Some thrombolytic agents may not work properly in people who have just had a strep infection, so the physician may want to use a different drug.

People who take certain medicines may be at greater risk for severe bleeding when they are given a thrombolytic agent.

Women who are pregnant should tell the physician in charge before being given a thrombolytic agent. There is a slight chance that women undergoing thrombolytic therapy during the first five months of pregnancy will miscarry. Streptokinase and urokinase, however, have both been used without problems in pregnant women.

After being treated with thrombolytic therapy, women who are breast-feeding should check with their physicians before starting to breast-feed again.

Side effects

Anyone who develops a fever or who notices bleeding or oozing from their gums, from cuts, or from the site where the thrombolytic agent was injected should immediately tell their health care provider.

People who are given thrombolytic therapy should also be alert to the signs of bleeding inside the body and should check with a physician immediately if any of the following symptoms occur:

• blood in the urine
• blood in the stool or black, tarry stools
• constipation
• coughing up blood
• vomiting blood or material that looks like coffee grounds
• nosebleeds
• unexpected or unusually heavy vaginal bleeding
• dizziness
• sudden, severe, or constant headaches
• pain or swelling in the abdomen or stomach
• back pain or backache
• severe or constant muscle pain or stiffness
• stiff, swollen, or painful joints

Other side effects of thrombolytic agents are possible. Anyone who has unusual symptoms during or after thrombolytic therapy should tell their health care professional.

Interactions

People who take certain medicines may be at greater risk for severe bleeding when they receive a thrombolytic agent. Anyone who is given a thrombolytic agent should tell the physician in charge about all other prescription or nonprescription (over-the-counter) medicines he or she is taking, including vitamins and supplements. Medicines that may increase the chance of bleeding include:

• aspirin and other medicines for pain and inflammation
• blood thinners (anticoagulants)
• antiseizure medicines, including divalproex (Depakote) and valproic acid (Depakene)
• cephalosporins, including cefamandole (Mandol), cefoperazone (Cefobid), and cefotetan (Cefotan)

In addition, anyone who has been treated with anistreplase or streptokinase within the past year should tell the physician. These drugs may not work properly if they are given again, so the physician may want to use a different thrombolytic agent.

Patients who are taking thrombolytic medications should not take vitamin E supplements or certain herbal preparations without consulting their doctor. High doses of vitamin E can increase the risk of hemorrhagic stroke. Ginger, borage, angelica, dong quai, feverfew, and other herbs can intensify the anticlotting effect of thrombolytic medications and increase the risk of bleeding.

Resources

BOOKS

Karch, Amy M. *2014 Lippincott's Nursing Drug Guide.* Ambler, PA: Lippincott Williams & Wilkins, 2014.

Townsend, Courtney M., et al. *Sabiston Textbook of Surgery.* 19th ed. Philadelphia: Saunders/Elsevier, 2012.

Wecker, Lynn, et al. *Brody's Human Pharmacology: Molecular to Clinical.* 5th ed. Philadelphia: Mosby/Elsevier, 2010.

WEBSITES

A.D.A.M. Medical Encyclopedia. "CO2 blood test." University of Maryland Medical Center. http://www.nlm.nih.gov/medlineplus/ency/article/003469.htm (accessed August 12, 2013).

Society for Vascular Surgery. "Thrombolytic Therapy." VascularWeb. http://www.vascularweb.org/vascular health/Pages/thrombolytic-therapy.aspx (accessed August 12, 2013).

ORGANIZATIONS

American Society of Health-System Pharmacists, 7272 Wisconsin Ave., Bethesda, MD 20814, (301) 664-8700, (866) 279-0681, custserv@ashp.org, http://www.ashp.org.

U.S. Food and Drug Administration, 10903 New Hampshire Ave., Silver Spring, MD 20993, (888) INFO-FDA (463-6332), http://www.fda.gov.

Nancy Ross-Flanigan
Sam Uretsky, PharmD

Thyroid function tests

Definition

Thyroid function tests are blood tests used to evaluate how effectively the thyroid gland is working. These tests include the thyroid-stimulating hormone test (TSH), the thyroxine test (T_4), the triiodothyronine test (T_3), the thyroxine-binding globulin test (TBG), the triiodothyronine resin uptake test (T_3RU), and the long-acting thyroid stimulator test (LATS).

Purpose

Thyroid function tests are used to:

- help diagnose an underactive thyroid (hypothyroidism) and an overactive thyroid (hyperthyroidism)
- evaluate thyroid gland activity
- monitor response to thyroid therapy

Description

Most doctors consider the sensitive thyroid-stimulating hormone (TSH) test to be the most accurate measure of thyroid activity. It is used to diagnose primary hypothyroidism, as well as to monitor the effects of exogenous thyroid replacement or suppression therapy. Because this test is so sensitive, abnormalities in thyroid function can be determined before a patient complains of symptoms.

TSH "tells" the thyroid gland to secrete the hormones thyroxine (T_4) and triiodothyronine (T_3). Before TSH tests were used, standard blood tests measured levels of T_4 and T_3 to determine if the thyroid gland was working properly. The triiodothyronine (T_3) test measures the amount of this hormone in the blood.

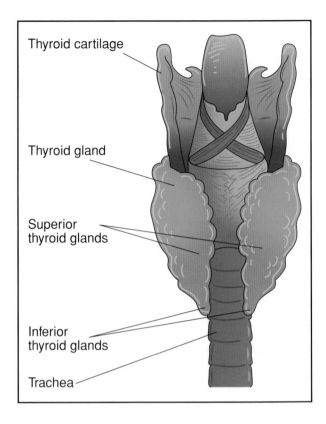

Parathyroidectomy refers to the surgical removal of one or more of the parathyroid glands due to hyperparathyroidism (an abnormal over-functioning of the parathyroid glands). It is usually done after other nonsurgical methods have failed to control or correct the condition. *(Illustration by Electronic Illustrators Group. Copyright © Cengage Learning®.)*

T_3 is normally present in very small amounts but has a significant impact on metabolism and is the active component of thyroid hormones.

The thyroxine-binding globulin (TBG) test measures blood levels of this substance, which is manufactured in the liver. TBG binds to T_3 and T_4, prevents the kidneys from flushing the hormones from the blood, and releases them when and where they are needed to regulate body functions.

The triiodothyronine resin uptake (T_3RU) test measures blood T_4 levels. Laboratory analysis of this test takes several days, and it is used less often than tests whose results are available more quickly.

The long-acting thyroid stimulator (LATS) test shows whether blood contains long-acting thyroid stimulator. Not normally present in blood, LATS causes the thyroid to produce and secrete abnormally high amounts of hormones. The LATS test is useful in diagnosing Graves' disease.

It takes only minutes for a nurse or medical technician to collect the blood needed for these blood tests. A needle is inserted into a vein, usually in the forearm, and a small amount of blood is collected and sent to a laboratory for testing. The patient will usually feel minor discomfort from the "stick" of the needle.

Precautions

Thyroid treatment must be stopped one month before blood is drawn for a thyroxine (T_4) test.

Steroids, propranolol (Inderal), cholestyramine (Questran), and other medications that may influence thyroid activity are usually stopped before a triiodothyronine (T_3) test.

Estrogens, anabolic steroids, phenytoin (Dilantin), and thyroid medications may be discontinued prior to a thyroxine-binding globulin (TBG) test. The laboratory analyzing the blood sample must be told if the patient cannot stop taking any of these medications. Some patients will be told to take these medications as usual so that the doctor can determine how they affect thyroxine-binding globulin.

Patients are asked not to take estrogens, androgens, phenytoin, salicylates (e.g., **aspirin**), and thyroid medications before having a triiodothyronine resin uptake (T_3RU) test.

Prior to taking a long-acting thyroid stimulant (LATS) test, the patient will probably be told to stop taking all drugs that could affect test results.

Preparation

There is no need to make any changes in diet or activities. The patient may be asked to stop taking certain medications until after the test is performed.

Aftercare

Warm compresses can be used to relieve swelling or discomfort at the site of the puncture. With a doctor's approval, the patient may start taking medications stopped before the test.

Results

Not all laboratories measure or record thyroid hormone levels the same way. Each laboratory will provide a range of values for each test.

Normal

TSH. Normal TSH levels for adults are 0.5–5.0 mU/L.

T_4. Normal T_4 levels for adults are 4.5–12.6 ug/dL, according to the National Institute of Diabetes and Digestive and Kidney Diseases (NIDDK). Results may vary slightly based on the laboratory methods used. Levels are typically higher at birth and then gradually decrease to the normal range.

Normal T_4 levels do not necessarily indicate normal thyroid function. T_4 levels can register within normal ranges in a patient who:

- is pregnant
- has recently had contrast x-rays
- has nephrosis (kidney disease) or cirrhosis (liver disease)

T_3. Normal T_3 levels are:

- 90–170 ng/dL at birth
- 115–190 ng/dL at 6 to 12 years
- 110–230 ng/dL in adulthood

TBG. Normal TBG levels are:

- 1.5–3.4 mg/dL or 15–34 mg/L in adults
- 2.9–5.4 mg/dL or 29–54 mg/L in children

T_3RU. Between 25% and 35% of T_3 should bind to or be absorbed by the resin added to the blood sample. The test indirectly measures the amount of thyroid binding globulin (TBG) and thyroid-binding prealbumin (TBPA) in the blood.

LATS

Long-acting thyroid stimulator is found in the blood of only 5% of healthy people.

Abnormal results

T_4. Elevated T_4 levels can be caused by:

- acute thyroiditis
- birth control pills
- clofibrate (Altromed-S), a medication used to lower cholesterol and triglyceride levels
- contrast x-rays using iodine
- estrogen therapy
- heparin, a medication used to prevent blood clots
- heroin
- hyperthyroidism
- pregnancy
- thyrotoxicosis
- toxic thyroid adenoma

Cirrhosis and severe non-thyroid disease can raise T_4 levels slightly.

Reduced T_4 levels can be caused by:

- anabolic steroids
- androgens

- antithyroid drugs
- cretinism
- hypothyroidism
- kidney failure
- lithium (Lithane, Lithonate)
- myxedema
- phenytoin
- propranolol

T₃. Although T_3 levels usually rise and fall when T_4 levels do, T_3 toxicosis causes T_3 levels to rise while T_4 levels remain normal. T_3 toxicosis is a complication of:

- Graves' disease
- toxic adenoma
- toxic nodular goiter

T_3 levels normally rise when a woman is pregnant or using birth-control pills. Elevated T_3 levels can also occur in patients who use estrogen, methadone, or who have:

- certain genetic disorders that do not involve thyroid malfunction
- hyperthyroidism
- thyroiditis
- T_3 thyrotoxicosis
- toxic adenoma

Low T_3 levels may be a symptom of:

- acute or chronic illness
- hypothyroidism
- kidney or liver disease
- starvation

Decreased T_3 levels can also be caused by using:

- anabolic steroids
- androgens
- phenytoin
- propranolol
- reserpine (Serpasil)
- salicylates in high doses

TBG. TBG levels, normally high during pregnancy, are also high in newborns. Elevated TBG levels can also be symptoms of:

- acute hepatitis, a disease characterized by inflammation of the liver
- acute intermittent porphyria, an inherited disease affecting the liver and bone marrow
- hypothyroidism
- inherited thyroid hormone abnormality

KEY TERMS

Cretinism—Severe hypothyroidism that is present at birth and characterized by severe intellectual disability.

Graves' disease—The most common form of hyperthyroidism, characterized by bulging eyes, rapid heart rate, and other symptoms.

Hyperthyroidism—Overactive thyroid gland; symptoms include irritability/nervousness, muscle weakness, tremors, irregular menstrual periods, weight loss, sleep problems, thyroid enlargement, heat sensitivity, and vision/eye problems. The most common type of this disorder is called Graves' disease.

Hypothyroidism—Underactive thyroid gland; symptoms include fatigue, difficulty swallowing, mood swings, hoarse voice, sensitivity to cold, forgetfulness, and dry/coarse skin and hair.

Myxedema—Hypothyroidism, characterized by thick, puffy features, an enlarged tongue, and lack of emotion.

Nodular goiter—An enlargement of the thyroid (goiter) caused when groups of cells collect to form nodules.

Thyroid gland—A butterfly-shaped gland in front and to the sides of the upper part of the windpipe; influences body processes like growth, development, reproduction, and metabolism.

Thyroiditis—Inflammation of the thyroid gland.

Thyrotoxicosis—A condition resulting from high levels of thyroid hormones in the blood.

Toxic thyroid adenoma—Self-contained concentrations of thyroid tissue that may produce excessive amounts of thyroid hormone.

TBG levels can also become high by using:

- anabolic steroids
- birth control pills
- anti-thyroid agents
- clofibrate
- estrogen therapy
- phenytoin
- salicylates in high doses
- thiazides (diuretics)
- thyroid medications
- warfarin (Coumadin)

(2013): 282–86. http://dx.doi.org/10.7861/clinmedicine. 13-3-282 (accessed September 2, 2013).

QUESTIONS TO ASK YOUR DOCTOR

- What type of thyroid disorder do I have?
- What treatments do you recommend?
- Will I have to take medication for the rest of my life?
- What are the side effects of treatment?

TBG levels can be raised or lowered by inherited liver disease whose cause is unknown.

Low TBG levels can be a symptom of:

- acromegaly, a disorder characterized by increased growth in bone and soft tissue

- acute hepatitis or other acute illness

- hyperthyroidism

- kidney disease

- malnutrition

- marked hypoproteinemia, characterized by abnormally low levels of protein in the blood

- uncompensated acidosis, a condition in which blood and tissues are unusually acidic

T₃RU. A high degree of resin uptake and high thyroxine levels indicate hyperthyroidism. A low degree of resin uptake, coupled with low thyroxine levels, is a symptom of hypothyroidism.

Thyroxine and triiodothyronine resin uptake that are not both high or low may be a symptom of a thyroxine-binding abnormality.

LATS

Long-acting thyroid stimulator, not usually found in blood, is present in the blood of 80% of patients with Graves' disease. It is a symptom of this disease whether or not symptoms of hyperthyroidism are detected.

Resources

BOOKS

Brent, Gregory A. *Thyroid Function Testing.* New York: Springer, 2010.

Harvard Health Publications. *Thyroid Disease: Understanding Hypothyroidism and Hyperthyroidism.* Boston: Harvard, 2010.

PERIODICALS

Levy, M. J., O. Koulouri, and M. Gurnell. "How to Interpret Thyroid Function Tests." *Clinical Medicine* 13, no. 3

OTHER

American Thyroid Association. *Thyroid Function Tests.* http://www.thyroid.org/wp-content/uploads/patients/brochures/FunctionTests_brochure.pdf (accessed September 2, 2013).

Rugge, Bruin, et al. *Screening and Treatment of Subclinical Hypothyroidism or Hyperthyroidism.* Comparative Effectiveness Reviews 24. Rockville, MD: Agency for Healthcare Research and Quality, October 2011. http://www.ncbi.nlm.nih.gov/pubmedhealth/n/cer24/pdf (accessed September 2, 2013).

WEBSITES

A.D.A.M. Medical Encyclopedia. "Hypothyroidism." PubMed Health. http://www.ncbi.nlm.nih.gov/pubmedhealth/PMH0001393 (accessed September 2, 2013).

Institute for Quality and Efficiency in Health Care. "Fact Sheet: Understanding Thyroid Gland Tests." PubMed Health. http://www.ncbi.nlm.nih.gov/pubmedhealth/PMH0010400 (accessed September 2, 2013).

Mayo Clinic staff. "Hyperthyroidism (Overactive Thyroid)." MayoClinic.com. http://www.mayoclinic.com/health/hyperthyroidism/DS00344 (accessed September 2, 2013).

MedlinePlus. "Thyroid Diseases." U.S. National Library of Medicine, National Institutes of Health. http://www.nlm.nih.gov/medlineplus/thyroiddiseases.html (accessed September 2, 2013).

National Endocrine and Metabolic Diseases Information Service. "Graves' Disease." National Institute of Diabetes and Digestive and Kidney Diseases (NIDDK). http://endocrine.niddk.nih.gov/pubs/graves/index.aspx (accessed September 2, 2013).

National Endocrine and Metabolic Diseases Information Service. "Thyroid Function Tests." National Institute of Diabetes and Digestive and Kidney Diseases (NIDDK). http://www.endocrine.niddk.nih.gov/pubs/thyroidtests/index.aspx (accessed September 2, 2013).

ORGANIZATIONS

American Thyroid Association, 6066 Leesburg Pike, Ste. 550, Falls Church, VA 22041, (703) 998-8890, thyroid@thyroid.org, http://www.thyroid.org.

National Endocrine and Metabolic Diseases Information Service, 6 Information Way, Bethesda, MD 20892-3569, (888) 828-0904, Fax: (703) 738-4929, endoandmeta@info.niddk.nih.gov, http://www.endocrine.niddk.nih.gov.

Maureen Haggerty

Thyroid gland removal *see* **Thyroidectomy**

Thyroidectomy

Definition

Thyroidectomy is a surgical procedure in which all or part of the thyroid gland is removed. The thyroid gland is located in the forward (anterior) part of the neck just under the skin and in front of the Adam's apple. The thyroid is one of the body's endocrine glands, which means that it secretes its products inside the body, into the blood or lymph. The thyroid produces several hormones that have two primary functions: they increase the synthesis of proteins in most of the body's tissues, and they raise the level of the body's oxygen consumption.

Purpose

All or part of the thyroid gland may be removed to correct a variety of abnormalities. If a person has a goiter, which is an enlargement of the thyroid gland that causes swelling in the front of the neck, the swollen gland may cause difficulties with swallowing or breathing. Hyperthyroidism (overactivity of the thyroid gland) produces

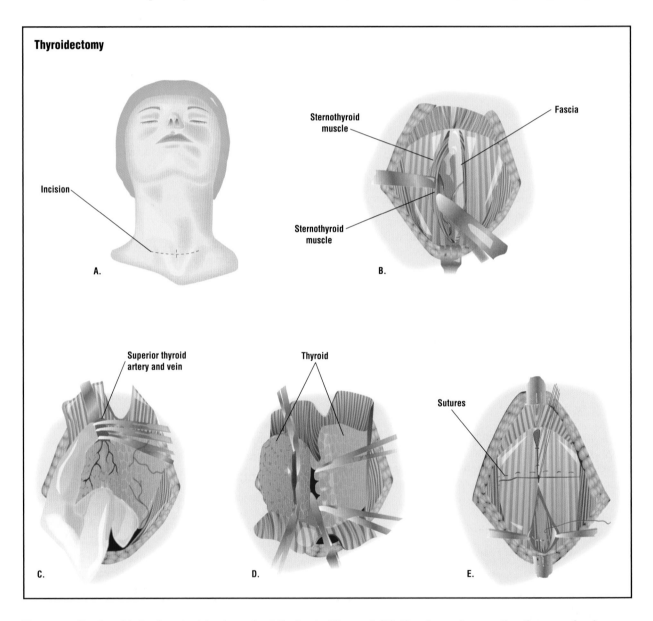

Thyroidectomy

Incision

Sternothyroid muscle

Sternothyroid muscle

Fascia

A.

B.

Superior thyroid artery and vein

Thyroid

Sutures

C.

D.

E.

To remove the thyroid gland, an incision is made at the front of the neck **(A)**. Muscles and connecting tissue, or fascia, are divided **(B)**. The veins and arteries above and below the thyroid are severed **(C)**, and the gland is removed in two parts **(D)**. The tissues and muscles are repaired before the skin incision is closed **(E)**. *(Illustration by GGS Information Services. Copyright © Cengage Learning®.)*

hypermetabolism, a condition in which the body uses abnormal amounts of oxygen, nutrients, and other materials. A thyroidectomy may be performed if the hypermetabolism cannot be adequately controlled by medication, or if the condition occurs in a child or pregnant woman. Both cancerous and noncancerous tumors (frequently called nodules) may develop in the thyroid gland. These growths must be removed, in addition to some or all of the gland itself.

Demographics

According to the American Thyroid Association, about 20 million people in the United States have a type of thyroid disorder, with up to 60% being undiagnosed. Many people with abnormal levels of thyroid hormone do not have any disease symptoms. Females are somewhat more likely than males to require a thyroidectomy.

Description

A thyroidectomy begins with **general anesthesia** administered by an anesthesiologist. The anesthesiologist injects drugs into the patient's veins and then places an airway tube in the windpipe to ventilate (provide air for) the person during the operation. After the patient has been anesthetized, the surgeon makes an incision in the front of the neck at the level where a tight-fitting necklace would rest. The surgeon locates and takes care not to injure the parathyroid glands and the recurrent laryngeal nerves, while freeing the thyroid gland from these surrounding structures. The next step is clamping off the blood supply to the portion of the thyroid gland that is to be removed. Next, the surgeon removes all or part of the gland. If cancer has been diagnosed, all or most of the gland is removed. If other diseases or nodules are present, the surgeon may remove only part of the gland. The total amount of glandular tissue removed depends on the condition being treated. The surgeon may place a drain, which is a soft plastic tube that allows tissue fluids to flow out of an area, before closing the incision. The incision is closed with either sutures (stitches) or metal clips. A dressing is placed over the incision and the drain, if one has been placed.

People generally stay in the hospital one to four days after a thyroidectomy.

Diagnosis

Thyroid disorders do not always develop rapidly; in some cases, the patient's symptoms may be subtle or difficult to distinguish from the symptoms of other disorders. Patients suffering from hypothyroidism are sometimes misdiagnosed as having a psychiatric

KEY TERMS

Endocrine—A type of organ or gland that secretes hormones or other products inside the body, into the bloodstream or the lymphatic system. The thyroid is an endocrine gland.

Endocrinologist—A physician who specializes in treating persons with diseases of the thyroid, parathyroid, adrenal glands, and the pancreas.

Goiter—An enlargement of the thyroid gland due to insufficient iodine in the diet.

Hyperthyroidism—Abnormal overactivity of the thyroid gland. People with hyperthyroidism are hypermetabolic, lose weight, exhibit nervousness, have muscular weakness and fatigue, sweat heavily, and have increased urination and bowel movements. This condition is also called thyrotoxicosis.

Hypothyroidism—Abnormal underfunctioning of the thyroid gland. People with hypothyroidism have a lowered body metabolism, gain weight, and are sluggish.

Parathyroid glands—Two pairs of smaller glands that lie close to the lower surface of the thyroid gland. They secrete parathyroid hormone, which regulates the body's use of calcium and phosphorus.

Recurrent laryngeal nerve—A nerve that lies very near the parathyroid glands and serves the larynx or voice box.

Thyroid storm—An unusual complication of thyroid function that is sometimes triggered by the stress of thyroid surgery. It is a medical emergency.

depression. Before a thyroidectomy is performed, a variety of tests and studies are usually required to determine the nature of the thyroid disease. Laboratory analysis of blood determines the levels of active thyroid hormones circulating in the body. The most common test is a blood test that measures the level of thyroid-stimulating hormone (TSH) in the bloodstream. Sonograms and **computed tomography** scans (CT scans) help to determine the size of the thyroid gland and location of abnormalities. A nuclear medicine scan may be used to assess thyroid function or to evaluate the condition of a thyroid nodule, but it is not considered a routine test. A needle biopsy of an abnormality or aspiration (removal by suction) of fluid from the thyroid gland may also be performed to help determine the diagnosis.

Preparation

If the diagnosis is hyperthyroidism, a person may be asked to take antithyroid medication or iodides before the operation. Continued treatment with antithyroid drugs may be the treatment of choice. Otherwise, no other special procedure must be followed prior to the operation.

Aftercare

A thyroidectomy incision requires little to no care after the dressing is removed. The area may be bathed gently with a mild soap. The sutures or the metal clips are removed three to seven days after the operation.

Risks

There are definite risks associated with the procedure. The thyroid gland should be removed only if there is a pressing reason or medical condition that requires it.

As with all operations, people who are obese, smoke, or have poor nutrition are at greater risk for developing complications related to the general anesthetic itself.

Hoarseness or voice loss may develop if the recurrent laryngeal nerve is injured or destroyed during the operation. Nerve damage is more apt to occur in people who have large goiters or cancerous tumors.

Hypoparathyroidism (underfunctioning of the parathyroid glands) can occur if the parathyroid glands are injured or removed at the time of the thyroidectomy. Hypoparathyroidism is characterized by a drop in blood calcium levels resulting in muscle cramps and twitching.

Hypothyroidism (underfunctioning of the thyroid gland) can occur if all or nearly all of the thyroid gland is removed. Complete removal, however, may be intentional when the patient is diagnosed with cancer. If a person's thyroid levels remain low, thyroid replacement medications may be required for the rest of his or her life.

A hematoma is a collection of blood in an organ or tissue, caused by a break in the wall of a blood vessel. The neck and the area surrounding the thyroid gland have a rich supply of blood vessels. Bleeding in the area of the operation may occur and be difficult to control or stop. If a hematoma occurs in this part of the body, it may be life-threatening. As the hematoma enlarges, it may obstruct the airway and cause a person to stop breathing. If a hematoma does develop in the neck, the surgeon may need to perform drainage to clear the airway.

Wound infections can occur. If they do, the incision is drained, and there are usually no serious consequences.

QUESTIONS TO ASK YOUR DOCTOR

- Which parts of the thyroid will be removed?
- What will my neck look like after surgery?
- Is the surgeon a board certified otolaryngologist?
- How many radical neck procedures has the surgeon performed?
- What is the surgeon's complication rate?
- Will I need any medications after surgery?

Results

Most patients are discharged from the hospital one to four days after a thyroidectomy. Most resume their normal activities two weeks after the operation. People who have cancer may require subsequent treatment by an oncologist or endocrinologist.

Morbidity and mortality rates

The mortality of thyroidectomy is essentially zero. Hypothyroidism is thought to occur in 12%–50% of persons in the first year after a thyroidectomy. Late-onset hypothyroidism develops among an additional 1%–3% of persons each year. Although hypothyroidism may recur many years after a partial thyroidectomy, 43% of recurrences occur within five years.

Mortality from thyroid storm, an uncommon complication of thyroidectomy, is in the range of 20%–30%. Thyroid storm is characterized by fever, weakness and wasting of the muscles, enlargement of the liver, restlessness, mood swings, change in mental status, and in some cases, coma. Thyroid storm is a medical emergency requiring immediate treatment. After a partial thyroidectomy, thyroid function returns to normal in 90%–98% of persons.

Alternatives

Injections of radioactive iodine were used to destroy thyroid tissue in the past. This alternative is rarely performed.

Health care team roles

Thyroidectomies are usually performed by **surgeons** with specialized training in otolaryngology, head and neck surgery. Occasionally, a general surgeon will perform a thyroidectomy. The procedure is performed in a hospital under general anesthesia.

Resources

BOOKS

Bland, K. I., et al. *General Surgery: Principles and International Practice*. London: Springer, 2009.

Brunicardi, F. Charles, et al. *Schwartz's Principles of Surgery*. 10th ed. New York: McGraw-Hill, 2014.

Ruggieri, Paul, and Scott Isaacs. *A Simple Guide to Thyroid Disorders: From Diagnosis to Treatment*. Omaha, NE: Addicus Books, 2010.

Townsend, Courtney M., et al. *Sabiston Textbook of Surgery*. 19th ed. Philadelphia: Saunders/Elsevier, 2012.

PERIODICALS

Rogers, H. "Do Low Grade Thyroid Cancers Really Require Thyroidectomy?" *BMJ* 347 (September 25, 2013): f5734. http://dx.doi.org/10.1136/bmj.f5734 (accessed October 4, 2013).

Romero Arenas, Minerva A. "The Role of Thyroidectomy in Metastatic Disease to the Thyroid Gland." *Annals of Surgical Oncology* (October 1, 2013): e-pub ahead of print. http://dx.doi.org/10.1245/s10434-013-3282-1 (accessed October 4, 2013).

Shinall, Myrick C. "Total Thyroidectomy for Graves' Disease: Compliance with American Thyroid Association Guidelines May Not Always Be Necessary." *Surgery* (September 27, 2013): e-pub ahead of print. http://dx.doi.org/10.1016/j.surg.2013.04.064 (accessed October 4, 2013).

WEBSITES

A.D.A.M. Medical Encyclopedia. "Thyroid Gland Removal." MedlinePlus. http://www.nlm.nih.gov/medlineplus/ency/article/002933.htm (accessed October 4, 2013).

American Thyroid Association. "General Information/Press Room." http://www.thyroid.org/media-main/about-hypothyroidism (accessed October 4, 2013).

Mayo Foundation for Medical Education and Research. "Robotic Thyroidectomy." http://www.mayoclinic.org/medicalprofs/robotic-thyroidectomy-new.html (accessed October 4, 2013).

Zanocco, Kyle, and Cord Sturgeon. "Thyroidectomy for Graves'—Surgical Option." Graves' Disease and Thyroid Foundation. http://www.gdatf.org/about/about-graves-disease/patient-education/thyroidectomy-for-graves-surgical-option (accessed October 4, 2013).

ORGANIZATIONS

American Academy of Otolaryngology—Head and Neck Surgery, 1650 Diagonal Rd., Alexandria, VA 22314-2857, (703) 836-4444, http://www.entnet.org.

American College of Surgeons, 633 N. Saint Clair St., Chicago, IL 60611-3211, (312) 202-5000, (800) 621-4111, Fax: (312) 202-5001, postmaster@facs.org, http://www.facs.org.

American Osteopathic Colleges of Otolaryngology—Head and Neck Surgery, 4764 Fishburg Rd., Ste. F, Huber Heights, OH 45424, (800) 455-9404, info@aocoohns.org, http://www.aocoohns.org.

American Thyroid Association, 6066 Leesburg Pike, Ste. 550, Falls Church, VA 22041, (703) 998-8890, thyroid@thyroid.org, http://www.thyroid.org.

L. Fleming Fallon Jr., MD, DrPH

Tissue plasminogen activator *see* **Thrombolytic therapy**

Tissue typing *see* **Human leukocyte antigen (HLA) test**

Tongue removal *see* **Glossectomy**

Tonometry

Definition

Tonometry is a procedure that is done by a qualified eye care professional to measure the pressure of the fluid inside the eye, known as intraocular pressure or IOP. The English word comes from two Greek words that mean "tension" and "measure." Ocular tonometry requires a special instrument called a tonometer, which measures the IOP in millimeters of mercury (mm Hg).

Purpose

Tonometry is used as part of a complete eye examination or to screen patients at risk for glaucoma. Glaucoma is an eye disorder caused by fluid pressure on the optic nerve that can lead to permanent damage of the optic nerve and eventual blindness.

Intraocular pressure is a measurement of the production of aqueous humor within the eye compared with its rate of outflow. The aqueous humor is a watery gelatinous fluid secreted by the ciliary epithelium; it flows into the anterior chamber—the space between the iris of the eye and the cornea. The aqueous humor serves to protect the eye against dust, pollen, and other contaminants; to nourish tissues in the eye that are not well supplied with blood vessels; and to keep the globe of the eye inflated. The aqueous humor flows out of the anterior chamber through the trabecular meshwork, an area of spongy tissue located around the base of the cornea. Intraocular pressure is determined by the rate of production of aqueous humor divided by the rate of outflow through the trabecular meshwork. A high IOP can be caused by overproduction of aqueous humor, by inadequate outflow, or both.

Tonometry may also be used to monitor the effectiveness of medications used to treat high IOP, or to evaluate patients presenting in the emergency department with closed-angle glaucoma—a form of the disorder that can appear suddenly and cause severe pain along with visual disturbances.

Tonometry is only one portion of a comprehensive eye examination for glaucoma. It is insufficient by itself because some people can develop glaucoma with normal IOP, while others have a high IOP without any apparent damage to the optic nerve or visual disturbances; this condition is known as ocular hypertension. Still others have eyes with such anatomical features as an irregularly shaped or unusually thin cornea, which may yield misleading results with tonometry.

Other tests that are done to detect glaucoma include a slit lamp examination of the back of the eye following dilation of the eye with special mydriatic eye drops; this test allows the doctor to examine the retina and the optic nerve for indications of damage. The doctor may also perform pachymetry, which is a test that involves the use of an ultrasonic device to measure the thickness of the cornea; or gonioscopy, which involves the use of a special prism or lens together with the slit lamp to measure the angle between the iris of the eye and the cornea. Gonioscopy allows the doctor to determine whether the angle between the iris and the cornea is wide enough to permit adequate drainage of the aqueous humor.

Description

There are several different types of tonometers; some involve direct contact with the cornea of the eye while others do not.

Applanation tonometers

Applanation tonometers require direct contact between the instrument and the cornea of the eye. Applanation is a term that refers to the flattening of the cornea, and applanation tonometers work by temporarily flattening the surface of the cornea with a special sterilized probe. To use an applanation tonometer, the ophthalmologist or optometrist applies anesthetic eye drops to the patient's eyes, followed by the application of a fluorescein dye. The patient sits upright in front of a special microscope called a slit lamp with his or her chin resting on a chin rest and the forehead against a head band. The doctor looks through the eyepiece of the slit lamp to measure how much pressure is required to flatten the cornea. This type of tonometer is considered the most accurate and is the standard by which other types of tonometers are measured.

The two most common types of applanation tonometers are the Goldmann, first introduced in 1950,

and the Perkins. The Perkins tonometer is portable and is used with children, patients who cannot sit upright, or patients who are heavily anesthetized and must lie flat.

Electronic indentation tonometers

Electronic indentation tonometers, like applanation tonometers, require direct contact with the patient's cornea. They are also known as dynamic contour tonometers. Electronic tonometers resemble a pen somewhat in appearance, with rounded tips covered by a sterile film that is replaced after each use; common brand names are Tono-Pen and AccuPen. They can be used by primary practice physicians or paraoptometric technicians as well as by ophthalmologists or optometrists.

The practitioner administers anesthetic eye drops to the patient before using the tonometer. The patient is instructed to look straight ahead or upward while the physician or technician touches the electronic tonometer to the tear film on the surface of the cornea to obtain IOP readings. The device will click each time a reading is obtained and beep when enough readings have been recorded to obtain an average score. The score is displayed in a small panel on the side of the instrument.

Electronic indentation tonometers are also widely used by veterinarians to test for glaucoma in dogs and cats, as both species are predisposed to this eye disorder. Veterinary electronic tonometers take less than eight seconds to provide a readout.

Schiotz indentation tonometers

The Schiotz tonometer is an older form of indentation tonometer; it is also called an impression tonometer. Like applanation and electronic indentation tonometers, a Schiotz tonometer requires the administration of anesthetic eye drops to the patient prior to use. Named for the Norwegian physician who invented it in 1881, the Schiotz tonometer has a free-floating barrel with a footplate that is wider than the radius of the human cornea when resting on it. A hole in the center of the footplate allows a weighted plunger to move downward through the hole until it touches the cornea. As the plunger indents the cornea, it moves a mechanical pointer over a scale at the top of the tonometer. The physician converts the scale reading into millimeters of mercury by using a graph or conversion chart.

The patient is required to lie flat on an examining table when a Schiotz tonometer is used. The doctor will instruct the patient to avoid blinking or squeezing the eyes shut while the tonometer is resting on the cornea. This form of tonometry requires only a few seconds.

Rebound tonometers

Rebound tonometers are small handheld instruments that use an induction coil to magnetize a sterile plastic-tipped probe and release it against the patient's cornea. The probe bounces (rebounds) against the cornea and returns back into the device. As it returns, it creates an induction current that allows the tonometer to calculate the IOP. The most common brand name of this type of tonometer is Icare. Rebound tonometers can be used by technicians or primary care physicians without specialized training in ophthalmology or optometry. Although rebound tonometers do involve direct contact with the cornea, they do not require the use of anesthetic eye drops for the patient's comfort. The sterile plastic probe is discarded after use.

Air puff tonometers

Also known as pneumotonometers or noncontact tonometers (NCTs), air puff tonometers do not require the use of anesthetic eye drops. The patient sits in front of the instrument and rests his or her chin on a padded support. The tonometer releases a jet or puff of air toward the patient's eye, and records the change in the light reflected from the cornea as it is slightly flattened by the stream of air. The instrument then calculates the IOP on the basis of the time required to flatten a predetermined area of the cornea. Patients usually experience the puff of air as a slight cooling of the eye surface. Air puff tonometers are particularly useful in screening children and patients who have had **LASIK** surgery, which involves reshaping the patient's cornea and consequently affects the accuracy of IOP scores obtained with contact tonometers.

Preparation

Risk factors for glaucoma

Patients should be prepared to tell the doctor about any risk factors they may have for glaucoma. These risk factors include:

- Age over 60 for the general population
- Age over 40 for African Americans
- Family history of glaucoma
- Personal history of eye injury or eye surgery
- Anatomical characteristics of the eye that increase the difficulty of the outflow of aqueous humor
- Congenital disorders of the eye, including Sturge-Weber syndrome
- Personal history of eye cataracts
- Diabetes mellitus

- Use of steroid medications, nasal sprays, eye patches, or injections
- Personal history of eye infections, including herpes zoster (shingles), herpes simplex, or toxoplasmosis
- Extreme nearsightedness
- An unusually thin cornea

Contraindications

Conditions that preclude tonometry or that may yield unhelpful results include:

- an active eye infection
- recent injury to the eye
- a history of LASIK or other laser refractive surgery on the eye
- an irregularly shaped cornea
- extreme nearsightedness
- history of major eye surgery

Other preparations

To improve the accuracy of the results, patients should prepare for tonometry as follows:

- Do not smoke marijuana for 24 hours before the test, and do not drink alcoholic beverages for 12 hours before the test.
- Do not drink more than 2 cups of water for 4 hours before the test.
- Wear clothing and jewelry that is loose around the neck, as tight collars or a close-fitting necklace can increase the pressure on the veins in the neck and increase the IOP.
- Remove contact lenses before the test.

Aftercare

Patients who have been given anesthetic eye drops prior to contact tonometry should avoid rubbing their eyes for about half an hour after the procedure or until the anesthetic has worn off. Contact lenses should not be replaced until two hours after the examination.

Patients who have been given drops to dilate the pupil of the eye as the second part of a slit lamp examination will need someone to drive them home afterward, and will need to wear sunglasses for a few hours if they go outside or into a brightly lit room.

Risks

The use of a contact tonometer carries a small risk of scratching the patient's cornea. There may be some discomfort with a corneal scratch, but it should go away in a day or so. There is also a small risk of infection or an

Anterior chamber—The fluid-filled space at the front of the eye between the iris and the inner surface of the cornea.

Applanation tonometry—A type of tonometry that involves flattening a portion of the patient's cornea to obtain a reading of intraocular pressure. The two most widely used applanation tonometers are the Goldmann tonometer and the Perkins tonometer.

Aqueous humor—A watery gelatinous fluid that is secreted by the ciliary epithelium and flows into the anterior chamber (the space between the lens of the eye and the cornea). The aqueous humor flows out of the anterior chamber through the trabecular meshwork, an area of spongy tissue located around the base of the cornea. Intraocular pressure is determined by the rate of production of aqueous humor divided by the rate of outflow through the trabecular meshwork.

Cornea—The clear front portion of the eye that covers the pupil and the colored iris.

Gonioscopy—A technique for measuring the adequacy of the outflow of aqueous humor through the trabecular meshwork. It involves the use of a special lens or prism that allows the doctor to view the angle between the iris and the cornea of the eye through a slit lamp.

Laser-assisted in situ keratomileusis (LASIK) surgery—A type of refractive eye surgery that uses an excimer laser to reshape the cornea of the eye in order to correct nearsightedness, farsightedness, or astigmatism.

Miotics—A class of drugs given to constrict the size of the pupil. They are used to treat glaucoma because they cause the muscles around the iris to constrict, which in turn allows aqueous humor to

flow out through the trabecular meshwork more rapidly, thus lowering IOP.

Mydriatics—A class of drugs that are administered to dilate the pupil of the eye before a slit lamp examination.

Ocular hypertension—A condition in which a person has an IOP above 21 mm Hg without damage to the optic nerve or visual field loss.

Ophthalmologist—A physician who specializes in treating diseases and disorders of the eye. Ophthalmologists are qualified to practice eye surgery as well as prescribe medicines for eye disorders. They hold the degree of either doctor of medicine (MD) or doctor of osteopathic medicine (DO).

Optometrist—A health care professional who is trained to prescribe and fit corrective lenses to improve vision, and to diagnose and treat various eye diseases. Optometrists in the United States and Canada hold the degree of doctor of optometry (OD).

Pachymetry—A test performed to measure the thickness of the cornea. It may be done as part of glaucoma screening or prior to LASIK surgery.

Sclera—The opaque fibrous protective outer layer of the eye, also known as the white of the eye.

Slit lamp—An instrument that combines a binocular microscope with a high-powered light source that can be focused to shine a thin sheet (slit) of light into the eye.

Tear film—The coating of fluid on the surface of the cornea that serves to lubricate the eye and remove bacteria from the cornea. The tear film consists of three layers: a mucous layer, a liquid layer, and an oily or lipid layer. It is also called the precorneal film.

allergic reaction to the anesthetic eye drops used with contact tonometry.

There is no risk of a corneal scratch or infection with air puff tonometry, but as noted, noncontact tonometry is considered less reliable than the contact methods.

Tonometry should *not* cause severe pain or visual disturbances. Patients should tell the doctor at once during the test if they experience significant pain. They should also call the doctor if the discomfort of a scratch on the cornea lasts for 48 hours or if they experience vision problems.

Drugs

The local anesthetics most often used with applanation or other contact forms of tonometry are proxymetacaine (also called proparacaine) and tetracaine (also called amethocaine). Drugs given to dilate the pupil of the eye are called mydriatics; the most common drug in this class that is used for glaucoma examinations is tropicamide (Mydriacyl).

Drugs given to reduce IOP work either by reducing the production of aqueous humor or by improving its drainage. Drugs that reduce the production of aqueous humor include beta blockers, carbonic anhydrase inhibitors, and adrenergic agonists. Drugs that increase the outflow of aqueous humor include miotics and prostaglandins. Most of these preparations are used as eye drops, although the carbonic anhydrase inhibitors are also available as oral medications. Eye drop formulations to lower IOP are preferred to oral forms because the side effects of the oral medications can be severe.

Results

Normal IOP usually falls between 10 and 21 mm Hg, with 15–16 mm Hg being an average score. IOP fluctuates between 3 and 6 mm Hg in normal eyes during the day, however, and is usually higher just before arising. Women tend to have a slightly higher IOP than men, and IOP increases in both sexes as people age.

An IOP reading above 21 mm Hg is considered high. Some people have an IOP consistently above 21 mm Hg, however, without apparent damage to the optic nerve or any vision problems; as noted, this condition is known as ocular hypertension. Between 5 and 10 million adults in the United States have ocular hypertension. A reading of 27 mm Hg or higher indicates that the patient is at serious risk of glaucoma unless he or she takes medications to lower the IOP. The different types of medications that may be prescribed were outlined in the previous section.

Alternatives

One alternative to corneal tonometry is known as transpalpebral tonometry because it involves measuring IOP through the eyelid with the patient's eyes closed. A handheld device known as the Diaton tonometer measures the response of a falling rod as it strikes the sclera of the eye through the eyelid. While notably less accurate than applanation tonometry, this method may be useful in evaluating patients who are fearful of contact tonometers, or patients who have unusually thin corneas—which usually result in inaccurate IOP measurements with applanation tonometers.

An older method, which is unreliable unless performed by a highly skilled and experienced optometrist or ophthalmologist, is digital tonometry, also known as palpation. The doctor gently presses his or her index finger against the cornea through the eyelid of the patient's closed eye. This method is not recommended except in emergencies.

A newer form of noncontact tonometry that is under development is tonometry utilizing optical coherence tomography or OCT. OCT is a technique that resembles **ultrasound** in providing high-resolution images of subsurface tissues and structures except that it uses light

rather than sound waves. However, OCT tonometry is considered experimental.

Another innovation is a contact lens sensor that would allow for 24-hour monitoring of IOP in patients at high risk for glaucoma. Known as the Sensimed Triggerfish, the device is a single-use soft silicone contact lens containing a sensor that transmits changes in IOP to a portable recorder worn by the patient. At the end of the 24-hour recording period, the contact lens is removed and the data uploaded from the recorder to the physician's computer. The Triggerfish is made in Switzerland and was not available for use in the United States as of 2013.

Health care team roles

Tonometry is most often done in the office of an ophthalmologist or optometrist as it requires only **local anesthesia** or no anesthesia at all. It may also be done in the emergency department of a hospital for patients who present with acute angle-closure glaucoma. The procedure may be performed by a certified paraoptometric technician (CPOT) under the supervision of an optometrist as well as by an optometrist, ophthalmologist, or emergency room physician. CPOTs are trained to perform certain clinical procedures in optometry, including tonometry, as well as to take patient histories and perform vision screening tests.

Resources

BOOKS

DuBois, Lindy. *Clinical Skills for the Ophthalmic Examination: Basic Procedures*, 2nd ed. Thorofare, NJ: SLACK, 2006.

Eperjesi, Frank, Hannah Bartlett, and Mark Dunne. *Ophthalmic Clinical Procedures: A Multimedia Guide.* New York: Elsevier/Butterworth Heinemann, 2007.

QUESTIONS TO ASK YOUR DOCTOR

- How often should I have a complete eye examination?
- I don't have any risk factors for glaucoma. Is air puff tonometry sufficiently accurate in my case?
- What are the advantages of contact tonometers?
- What is your opinion of new devices for 24-hour monitoring of IOP?
- Have you ever used a rebound tonometer to evaluate a patient's IOP?

Tonometry

PERIODICALS

Anton, A., et al. "Comparative Measurement of Intraocular Pressure by Icare Tonometry and Airpuff Tonometry in Healthy Subjects and Patients Wearing Therapeutic Soft Contact Lenses." *Graefe's Archive for Clinical and Experimental Ophthalmology* 251 (July 2013): 1791–1795.

Cook, J. A., et al. "Systematic Review of the Agreement of Tonometers with Goldmann Applanation Tonometry." *Ophthalmology* 119 (August 2012): 1552–1557.

Doherty, M. D., et al. "Diaton Tonometry: An Assessment of Validity and Preference against Goldmann Tonometry." *Clinical and Experimental Ophthalmology* 40 (May-June 2012): e171–e175.

Mansouri, K., and R. N. Weinreb. "Meeting an Unmet Need in Glaucoma: Continuous 24-h Monitoring of Intraocular Pressure." *Expert Review of Medical Devices* 9 (May 2012): 225–231.

Nessim, M., et al. "The Relationship Between Measurement Method and Corneal Structure on Apparent Intraocular Pressure in Glaucoma and Ocular Hypertension." *Contact Lens and Anterior Eye* 36 (April 2013): 57–61.

Schweier, C., et al. "Repeatability of Intraocular Pressure Measurements with Icare Pro Rebound, Tono-Pen AVIA and Goldmann Tonometers in Sitting and Reclining Positions." *BMC Ophthalmology* 13 (September 5, 2013): 44.

Stamper, R. L. "A History of Intraocular Pressure and Its Measurement." *Optometry and Vision Science* 88 (January 2011): e16–E28.

WEBSITES

American Academy of Ophthalmology (AAO). "Glaucoma Diagnosis." http://www.geteyesmart.org/eyesmart/diseases/glaucoma-diagnosis.cfm (accessed October 1, 2013).

American Optometric Association (AOA). "Comprehensive Eye and Vision Examination." http://www.aoa.org/patients-and-public/caring-for-your-vision/comprehensive-eye-and-vision-examination (accessed October 1, 2013).

Emergency Eye Examination Module, Part 4. "Using a Tonometer." http://www.youtube.com/watch?v=sBosdQ6o1oY (accessed October 2, 2013).

MedicineNet. "Tonometry." http://www.medicinenet.com/tonometry/article.htm (accessed October 1, 2013).

Medscape Reference. "Glaucoma, Suspect, Adult." http://emedicine.medscape.com/article/1205421-overview (accessed October 1, 2013).

National Eye Institute (NEI). "National Eye Institute Statement on Detection of Glaucoma and Adult Vision Screening." http://www.nei.nih.gov/nehep/programs/glaucoma/detection.asp (accessed October 1, 2013).

National Library of Medicine (NLM). "How to Measure Intraocular Pressure: Applanation Tonometry." http://www.ncbi.nlm.nih.gov/pmc/articles/PMC2206330 (accessed October 1, 2013).

San Antonio Eye Center. "The Icare Rebound Tonometer." http://www.youtube.com/watch?v=WXNsTK8t_o8 (accessed October 2, 2013).

WebMD. "Tonometry." http://www.webmd.com/eye-health/tonometry (accessed October 1, 2013).

ORGANIZATIONS

American Academy of Ophthalmology (AAO), PO Box 7424, San Francisco, CA 94120-7424, (415) 561-8500, Fax: (415) 561-8533, http://www.aao.org.

American Optometric Association (AOA), 243 N. Lindbergh Blvd., Floor 1, St. Louis, MO 63141-7881, (800) 365-2219, http://www.aoa.org/about-the-aoa/contact-aoa, http://www.aoa.org.

National Eye Institute (NEI), NEI Information Office, 31 Center Drive, MSC 2510, Bethesda, MD 20892-2510, (301) 496-5248, 2020@nei.nih.gov, http://www.nei.nih.gov.

Rebecca J. Frey, PhD

Tonsil removal *see* **Tonsillectomy**

Tonsillectomy

Definition

Tonsillectomy is a surgical procedure to remove the tonsils. The tonsils are part of the lymphatic system, which is responsible for fighting infection.

Purpose

Tonsils are removed when a person, most often a child, has any of the following conditions:

- obstruction

- sleep apnea (a condition in which an individual snores loudly and stops breathing temporarily at intervals during sleep)

- inability to swallow properly because of enlarged tonsils

- a breathy voice or other speech abnormality due to enlarged tonsils

- recurrent or persistent abscesses or throat infections

Physicians are not in complete agreement on the number of sore throats that necessitate a tonsillectomy. Most would agree that four cases of strep throat in any one year; six or more episodes of tonsillitis in one year; or five or more episodes of tonsillitis per year for two years indicate that the tonsils should be removed.

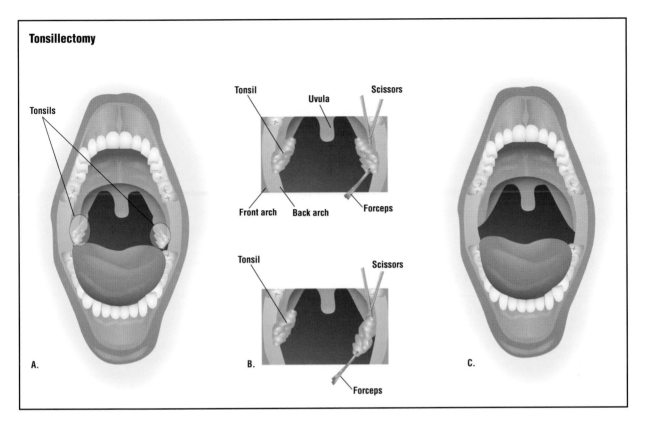

Tonsillectomy

In a tonsillectomy, the tonsils are removed through the mouth (A). The surgeon uses scissors to cut the tonsils and a forceps to pull them away (B). *(Illustration by GGS Information Services. Copyright © Cengage Learning®.)*

Demographics

A tonsillectomy is one of the most common surgical procedures among children. It is uncommon among adults. More than 400,000 tonsillectomies are performed each year in the United States. Approximately 70% of surgical candidates are under age 18.

Description

A tonsillectomy is usually performed under **general anesthesia**, although adults may occasionally receive a local anesthetic. The surgeon depresses the tongue in order to see the throat, and removes the tonsils with an instrument resembling a scoop or scissors.

Alternate methods for removing tonsils are being investigated, including lasers and other electronic devices.

Preparation

Tonsillectomy procedures are not performed as frequently today as they once were. One reason for a more conservative approach is the risk involved when a person is put under general anesthesia.

In some cases, a tonsillectomy may need to be modified or postponed. Bleeding disorders must be adequately controlled prior to surgery, and any cases of acute tonsillitis should be successfully treated prior to surgery. Treatment may postpone the surgery three to four weeks.

Aftercare

Persons are turned on their side after the operation to prevent the possibility of blood being drawn into the lungs (aspirated). **Vital signs** are monitored. Patients can drink water and other non-irritating liquids when they are fully awake.

Adults are usually warned to expect a very sore throat and some bleeding after the operation. They are given **antibiotics** to prevent infection, and some receive pain-relieving medications. For at least the first 24 hours, individuals are instructed to drink fluids and eat soft, pureed foods.

People are usually sent home the day of surgery. They are given instructions to call their surgeon if there is bleeding or earache, or fever that lasts longer than three days. They are told to expect a white scab to form in the throat between five and ten days after surgery.

KEY TERMS

Abscess—A localized area of tissue destruction and pus formation.

Sleep apnea—A condition marked by loud snoring during sleep and periodic episodes of suspended breathing.

Tonsils—Oval masses of lymphoid tissue on each side of the throat.

QUESTIONS TO ASK YOUR DOCTOR

- What will be the resulting functional status of the body after the operation?
- Is the surgeon board certified in head and neck surgery?
- How many tonsillectomy procedures has the surgeon performed?
- What is the surgeon's complication rate?
- Has the surgeon operated on children?

Risks

There is a chance that children with previously normal speech will develop a nasal-sounding voice. In addition, children younger than five years may be emotionally upset by the hospital experience. There are risks associated with any surgical procedure, including postoperative infection and bleeding.

Results

Normal results include the correction of the condition for which the surgery was performed.

Morbidity and mortality rates

Morbidity other than minor postsurgical infection is uncommon. About one in every 15,000 tonsillectomies ends in death, either from the anesthesia or bleeding five to seven days after the operation.

Alternatives

There are no alternatives to surgical removal of the tonsils. Drug therapy may be used for recurrent infections involving the tonsils.

Health care team roles

A tonsillectomy is performed in an outpatient facility associated with a hospital by a general surgeon or otolaryngologist (physician who specializes in treating disorders of the ear, nose, and throat).

Resources

BOOKS

Bland, K. I., et al. *General Surgery: Principles and International Practice*. London: Springer, 2009.

Brunicardi, F. Charles, et al. *Schwartz's Principles of Surgery*. 10th ed. New York: McGraw-Hill, 2014.

Goldman, Lee, and Andrew I. Schafer. *Goldman's Cecil Medicine*. 24th ed. Philadelphia: Saunders/Elsevier, 2012.

Longo, Dan, et al. *Harrison's Principles of Internal Medicine*. 18th ed. New York: McGraw-Hill, 2012.

Townsend, Courtney M., et al. *Sabiston Textbook of Surgery*. 19th ed. Philadelphia: Saunders/Elsevier, 2012.

PERIODICALS

Fedorowicz, Z., et al. "Oral Rinses, Mouthwashes and Sprays for Improving Recovery following Tonsillectomy." *Cochrane Database of Systematic Reviews* 9, art. no. CD007806 (September 10, 2013). http://dx.doi.org/10.1002/14651858.CD007806.pub4 (accessed October 4, 2013).

Gysin, C. "Indications of Pediatric Tonsillectomy." *ORL* 75, no. 3 (2013): 193–202. http://dx.doi.org/10.1159/000342329 (accessed October 4, 2013).

Larrosa, Francisco, et al. "The Cost Associated with Interstitial Thermotherapy for Tonsil Reduction vs. Standard Tonsillectomy." *European Archives of Oto-Rhino-Laryngology* (September 22, 2013): e-pub ahead of print. http://dx.doi.org/10.1007/s00405-013-2705-8 (accessed October 4, 2013).

WEBSITES

A.D.A.M. Medical Encyclopedia. "Tonsillectomy." MedlinePlus. http://www.nlm.nih.gov/medlineplus/ency/article/003013.htm (accessed October 4, 2013).

American Academy of Otolaryngology—Head and Neck Surgery. "Fact Sheet: Tonsillectomy Procedures." http://www.entnet.org/healthinformation/tonsillectomyprocedures.cfm (accessed October 4, 2013).

HealthDay. "After Tonsillectomy, Over-the-Counter Painkillers Suffice, Study Says." U.S. News & World Report, October 3, 2013. http://health.usnews.com/health-news/news/articles/2013/10/03/after-tonsillectomy-over-the-counter-painkillers-suffice-study-says (accessed October 4, 2013).

Nemours Foundation. "Tonsils and Tonsillitis." KidsHealth.org. http://kidshealth.org/parent/medical/ears/tonsil.html (accessed October 4, 2013).

ORGANIZATIONS

American Academy of Otolaryngology—Head and Neck Surgery, 1650 Diagonal Rd., Alexandria, VA 22314-2857, (703) 836-4444, http://www.entnet.org.

American Cancer Society, 250 Williams St. NW, Atlanta, GA 30303, (800) 227-2345, http://www.cancer.org.

American College of Surgeons, 633 N. Saint Clair St., Chicago, IL 60611-3211, (312) 202-5000, (800) 621-4111, Fax: (312) 202-5001, postmaster@facs.org, http://www.facs.org.

American Osteopathic Colleges of Otolaryngology—Head and Neck Surgery, 4764 Fishburg Rd., Ste. F, Huber Heights, OH 45424, (800) 455-9404, info@aocoohns.org, http://www.aocoohns.org.

L. Fleming Fallon Jr., MD, DrPH

Tooth extraction

Definition

Tooth extraction is the removal of a tooth from its socket in the bone.

Purpose

Extraction is performed for positional, structural, or economic reasons. Teeth are often removed because they are impacted. Teeth become impacted when they are prevented from growing into their normal position in the mouth by gum tissue, bone, or other teeth. Impaction is a common reason for the extraction of wisdom teeth. Extraction is the only known method that will prevent further problems with impaction.

Teeth may also be extracted to make more room in the mouth prior to straightening the remaining teeth (orthodontic treatment), or because they are so badly positioned that straightening is impossible. Extraction may be used to remove teeth that are so badly decayed or broken that they cannot be restored. In addition, some patients choose extraction as a less expensive alternative to filling or placing a crown on a severely decayed tooth.

Demographics

Exact statistics concerning tooth extraction are not available. Experts estimate that over 20 million teeth are extracted each year in the United States. Many of these are performed in conjunction with orthodontic procedures. Some extractions are due to tooth decay.

Description

Tooth extraction can be performed with **local anesthesia** if the tooth is exposed and appears to be easily removable in one piece. The dentist or oral surgeon uses an instrument called an elevator to luxate, or loosen, the tooth; widen the space in the underlying bone; and break the tiny elastic fibers that attach the tooth to the bone. Once the tooth is dislocated from the bone, it can be lifted and removed with forceps.

If the extraction is likely to be difficult, a general dentist may refer the patient to an oral surgeon. Oral **surgeons** are specialists who are trained to administer nitrous oxide (laughing gas), an intravenous sedative, or a general anesthetic to relieve pain. Extracting an impacted tooth or a tooth with curved roots typically requires cutting through gum tissue to expose the tooth. It may also require removing portions of bone to free the tooth. Some teeth must be cut and removed in sections. The extraction site may or may not require one or more stitches (sutures) to close the incision.

Precautions

In some situations, tooth extractions may be temporarily postponed:

- Infection that has progressed from the tooth into the bone complicates administering anesthesia. Infections must be treated with antibiotics before extraction.
- Patients taking blood thinners, such as warfarin (Coumadin) and aspirin, should stop using these medications for three days prior to extraction.
- People who have had certain medical procedures—heart valve replacement, open heart surgery, prosthetic joint replacement, or placement of a medical shunt—in the past six months may be given antibiotics to reduce the risk of bacterial infection spreading from the mouth to other parts of the body.

Preparation

Before extracting a tooth, the dentist will take the patient's medical history, noting allergies and other prescription medications that the patient is taking. A dental history is also recorded. Particular attention is given to previous extractions and reactions to anesthetics. The dentist may then prescribe **antibiotics** or recommend stopping certain medications prior to the extraction. The tooth is x-rayed to determine its full shape and position, especially if it is impacted.

Patients scheduled for deep anesthesia should wear loose clothing with sleeves that are easily rolled up to allow the dentist to place an intravenous line. They should not eat or drink anything for at least six hours before the procedure. Arrangements should be made for a friend or relative to drive them home after the surgery.

Tooth extraction

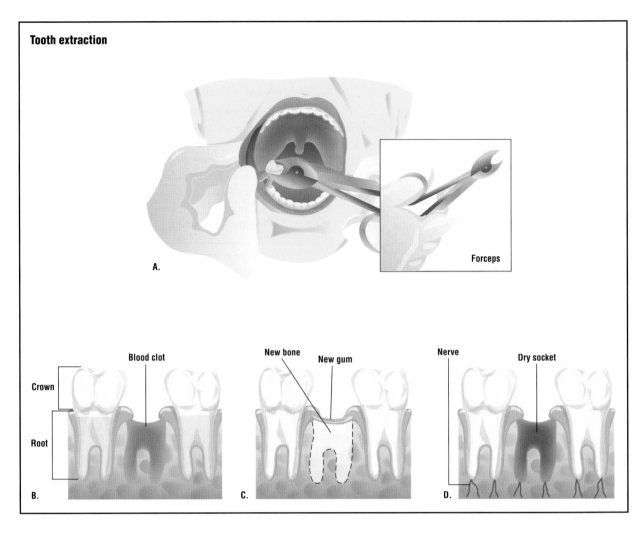

A dental surgeon uses special forceps to extract a tooth (A). In its place, a blood clot forms (B), which becomes new bone with gum tissue over the top (C). If the blood clot does not form or falls out, a dry socket occurs (D). No new bone forms, and the nerves are exposed, causing pain. *(Illustration by GGS Information Services. Copyright © Cengage Learning®.)*

Aftercare

An important aspect of aftercare is encouraging a clot to form at the extraction site. The patient should put pressure on the area by biting gently on a roll or wad of gauze for several hours after surgery. Once the clot is formed, it should not be disturbed. The patient should not rinse, spit, drink with a straw, or smoke for at least 24 hours after the extraction and preferably longer. He or she should also avoid vigorous **exercise** for the first three to five days after the extraction.

For the first two days after the procedure, the patient should drink liquids without using a straw and eat soft foods. Any chewing must be done on the side away from the extraction site. Hard or sticky foods should be avoided. The mouth may be gently cleaned with a toothbrush, but the extraction area should not be scrubbed.

Wrapped ice packs can be applied to reduce facial swelling. Swelling is a normal part of the healing process; it is most noticeable in the first 48–72 hours after surgery. As the swelling subsides, the patient's jaw muscles may feel stiff. Moist heat and gentle exercise will restore normal jaw movement. The dentist or oral surgeon may prescribe medications to relieve **postoperative pain**.

Risks

Potential complications of tooth extraction include postoperative infection, temporary numbness from nerve irritation, jaw fracture, and jaw joint pain. An additional complication is called dry socket. When a blood clot does not properly form in the empty tooth socket, the bone beneath the socket is exposed to air and contamination by

KEY TERMS

Dry socket—A painful condition following tooth extraction in which a blood clot does not properly fill the empty socket. Dry socket leaves the underlying bone exposed to air and food particles.

Extraction site—The empty tooth socket following removal of a tooth.

Impacted tooth—A tooth that is growing against another tooth, bone, or soft tissue.

Luxate—To loosen or dislocate a tooth from its socket.

Nitrous oxide—A colorless, sweet-smelling gas used by dentists for mild anesthesia. It is sometimes called laughing gas because it makes some people feel giddy or silly.

Oral surgeon—A dentist who specializes in surgical procedures of the mouth, including extractions.

Orthodontic treatment—The process of realigning and straightening teeth to correct their appearance and function.

QUESTIONS TO ASK YOUR DOCTOR

- Why are you suggesting a tooth extraction?
- What will my mouth look like after surgery?
- Is the oral surgeon board certified in maxillofacial surgery?
- How many teeth extractions has the oral surgeon performed?
- What is the oral surgeon's complication rate?
- Will I need medication after surgery?

food particles; as a result, the extraction site heals more slowly than is normal or desirable.

Results

The wound usually closes in about two weeks after a tooth extraction, but it takes three to six months for the bone and soft tissue to be restructured. Such complications as infection or dry socket may prolong the healing process.

Morbidity and mortality rates

Mortality from tooth extraction is very rare. Complications include a brief period of pain and swelling; post-extraction infections; and migration of adjacent teeth into the empty space created by an extraction. Most people experience some pain and swelling after having a tooth extracted. With the exception of removing wisdom teeth, migration into the empty space is common. Braces or orthodontic appliances usually control this problem.

Alternatives

Alternatives to tooth extraction depend on the reason for the extraction. Postponing or canceling an extraction to correct tooth crowding will cause malocclusion and an undesirable appearance. Not removing an impacted wisdom tooth may cause eventual misalignment,

although it may have no impact. Not removing a decayed or abscessed tooth may lead to septicemia and other complications.

Health care team roles

Teeth are most often extracted by maxillofacial or oral surgeons. Occasionally, a general dentist will extract a tooth. Teeth are most commonly removed in an outpatient facility adjacent to a hospital under **general anesthesia**.

Resources

BOOKS

Harris, Norman O., Franklin García-Godoy, and Christine Nielsen Nathe. *Primary Preventative Dentistry*. 8th ed. Boston: Pearson, 2014.

Hupp, James R., Edward Ellis, and Myron R Tucker. *Contemporary Oral and Maxillofacial Surgery*. 6th ed. St. Louis, MO: Elsevier/Mosby, 2014.

Scully, Crispian. *Oral and Maxillofacial Medicine: The Basis of Diagnosis and Treatment*. New York: Churchill Livingstone/Elsevier, 2013.

Tronstad, Leif. *Clinical Endodontics*. 3rd ed. New York: Thieme, 2009.

PERIODICALS

Adeyemo, Wasiu L., et al. "Oral Health-Related Quality of Life following Non-Surgical (Routine) Tooth Extraction: A Pilot Study." *Contemporary Clinical Dentistry* 3, no. 4 (2012): 427–32. http://dx.doi.org/10.4103/0976-237X.107433 (accessed October 4, 2013).

Saund, D., and T. Dietrich. "Minimally-Invasive Tooth Extraction: Doorknobs and Strings Revisited!" *Dental Update* 40, no. 4 (2013): 325–26, 328–30. http://dx.doi.org/10.4103/0976-237X.107433 (accessed October 4, 2013).

WEBSITES

Academy of General Dentistry. "How to Prevent Dry Socket." http://www.knowyourteeth.com/infobites/abc/article/?abc=%20&iid=340&aid=4154 (accessed October 4, 2013).

American Association of Endodontists. "Treatment Options for the Diseased Tooth." http://www.aae.org/patients/treatments-and-procedures/implants/treatment-options-for-the-diseased-tooth.aspx (accessed October 4, 2013).

American Dental Association. "Extractions." MouthHealthy.org. http://www.mouthhealthy.org/en/az-topics/e/extractions (accessed October 4, 2013).

ORGANIZATIONS

American Association of Endodontists, 211 E. Chicago Ave., Ste. 1100, Chicago, IL 60611-2691, (312) 266-7255, (800) 872-3636, info@aae.org, http://aae.org.

American Association of Oral and Maxillofacial Surgeons, 9700 W. Bryn Mawr Ave., Rosemont, IL 60018-5701, (847) 678-6200, (800) 822-6637, Fax: (847) 678-6286, http://www.aaoms.org.

American Dental Association, 211 E. Chicago Ave., Chicago, IL 60611, (312) 440-2500, http://www.ada.org.

British Association of Oral and Maxillofacial Surgeons, Royal College of Surgeons of England, 35/43 Lincoln's Inn Fields, London WC2A 3PE, England, +44 207 405 8074, office@baoms.org.uk, http://www.baoms.org.uk.

L. Fleming Fallon Jr., MD, DrPH

Tooth replantation

Definition

Tooth replantation is the reinsertion and splinting of a tooth that has been avulsed (knocked or torn out) of its socket.

Purpose

Teeth are replanted to prevent permanent loss of the tooth, and to restore the landscape of the mouth so that the patient can eat and speak normally.

Demographics

According to the National Center for Health Statistics, about five million teeth are accidentally avulsed in the United States each year. Most teeth that are replanted are lost through trauma, usually falls and other types of accidents. The most common traumata resulting in tooth avulsion are sports accidents that result in falls or blows to the head. The mandatory use of mouth guards, which are plastic devices that protect the upper teeth, has prevented approximately 200,000 oral injuries each year in football alone. The American Dental Association recommends the use of mouth guards for any sport that involves speed, contact, or the potential for falls. These categories include not only contact sports

like football, wrestling, and boxing, but also gymnastics, baseball, hockey, bicycling, skateboarding, and skiing. Without a mouth guard, a person is 60 times more likely to experience dental trauma if he or she participates in these sports.

Other common causes of trauma to the mouth resulting in avulsed teeth include motor vehicle accidents, criminal assaults, and fist fights. Domestic violence is the most common cause of avulsed teeth in women over the age of 21.

Description

In most cases, only permanent teeth are replanted. Primary teeth (baby teeth) do not usually have long enough roots for successful replantation. The only exception may be the canine teeth, which have longer roots and therefore a better chance of staying in place. In some cases, however, the dentist may choose to replant a child's primary tooth because there is risk to the permanent tooth that has not yet emerged.

To replant a tooth, the dentist or oral surgeon will first administer a local anesthetic to numb the patient's gums. He or she will then reinsert the avulsed tooth in its socket and anchor it within the mouth by installing a splint made of wire and composite resin. Some dentists remove the root canal nerve of the tooth and replace it with a plastic material before reinserting the tooth. The splint holds the tooth in place for two to six weeks. At that time, the splint can be removed and the tooth examined for stability.

Preparation

When a tooth is dislodged, it is critical to recover the tooth, preserve it under proper conditions, and get the patient to a dentist immediately. The tooth should be handled carefully; it should be picked up or touched by its crown (the top part of the tooth), not by its root. The tooth should be rinsed and kept moist, but not cleaned or brushed. The use of toothpaste, soap, mouthwash, or other chemicals can remove the fibroblasts clinging to the root of the tooth. Fibroblasts are connective tissue cells that act as a glue between teeth and the underlying bone.

The avulsed tooth can be placed in milk or a special Save-a-Tooth® kit, which is a tooth-preserving cup that contains a medium for preserving the fibroblasts around the tooth. The tooth and the patient should go to the dentist within 30 minutes of the accident since fibroblasts begin to die within that time. Rapid treatment improves the chances for successful replantation. In some cases, artificial fibroblasts can be substituted for the patient's own connective tissue cells.

If the tooth is a primary tooth, it should be rinsed and kept moist. The dentist should be consulted to determine whether the tooth should be replanted by examining the gums and the emergent tooth. The dentist will take a set of x-rays to determine how soon the permanent tooth is likely to emerge. Sometimes an artificial spacer is placed where the primary tooth was lost until the permanent tooth comes in.

Any injury to the gum is treated before the tooth is replanted. The dentist may give the patient an antibiotic medication to reduce the risk of infection. Cold compresses can reduce swelling. Stitches may be necessary if the gum is lacerated. The dentist may also take x-rays of the mouth to see if there are other injuries to the jawbone or nearby teeth.

Aftercare

The patient may take **aspirin** or **acetaminophen** for pain. **Antibiotics** may also be given for infection. The patient should avoid rinsing the mouth, spitting, or smoking for the first 24 hours after surgery. He or she should limit food to a soft diet for the next few days.

Beginning 24 hours after surgery, the patient should rinse the mouth gently with a solution of salt and lukewarm water every one to two hours. The salt helps to reduce swelling in the tissues around the tooth.

QUESTIONS TO ASK YOUR DOCTOR

- How should I take care of the replanted tooth?
- How long will it take to assess the results of treatment?
- What can be done if the tooth cannot be replanted?
- Where can I be fitted for a mouth guard?

Any kind of traumatic injury always carries the risk of infection. Patients with heart disease or disorders of the immune system should be monitored following tooth replantation. Dentists recommend consulting a physician within 48 hours of the dental surgery to determine the risk of tetanus, particularly if the patient has not received a tetanus booster within the past five years.

Adults with replanted teeth should have periodic checkups. According to the American Association of Endodontists, it takes about two to three years after replantation before the dentist can fully evaluate the outcome of treatment.

Risks

In addition to infection, tooth replantation carries the risks of excessive bleeding and rejection of the tooth. Rejection is a rare complication. An additional risk is that the root of the tooth may become fused to the underlying bone.

Results

Most permanent tooth replantations are successful when the patient acts quickly (within two hours). If the tooth is rejected, the dentist may attach the tooth to the bone with tissue glue. The rate of complications varies according to the circumstances of the injury, the patient's age, and his or her general health. A history of smoking increases the risk of rejection of the tooth, as well as infection.

Alternatives

There are no effective medical alternatives to **oral surgery** for replanting an avulsed tooth. Over-the-counter **analgesics** (pain relievers), prescription antibiotics, and some herbal preparations may be useful in relieving pain, reducing swelling, or preventing infection.

Herbal preparations that have been found useful as mouthwashes following oral surgery include calendula (*Calendula officinalis*) and clove (*Eugenia caryophyllata*).

Health care team roles

Tooth replantations are performed by general dentists, endodontists, and oral **surgeons**, usually as office or outpatient procedures. In some cases, the patient may be treated in the emergency room of a hospital.

Resources

BOOKS

Marx, John A., et al. *Rosen's Emergency Medicine: Concepts and Clinical Practice.* 7th ed. Philadelphia: Mosby, 2010.

Roberts, James R., and Jerris R. Hedges. *Clinical Procedures in Emergency Medicine.* 5th ed. Philadelphia: Saunders/Elsevier, 2010.

PERIODICALS

Kabashima, H., et al. "The Usefulness of Three-Dimensional Imaging for Prognostication in Cases of Intentional Tooth Replantation." *Journal of Oral Science* 54, no. 4 (2012): 355–58.

WEBSITES

International Association of Dental Traumatology. "Avulsion—First Aid for Avulsed Teeth." The Dental Trauma Guide. http://www.dentaltraumaguide.org/permanent_avulsion_treatment.aspx (accessed October 17, 2013).

ORGANIZATIONS

American Academy of Pediatric Dentistry, 211 E. Chicago Ave., Ste. 1700, Chicago, IL 60611-2637, (312) 337-2169, http://www.aapd.org.

American Association of Endodontists, 211 E. Chicago Ave., Ste. 1100, Chicago, IL 60611-2691, (312) 266-7255, (800) 872-3636, info@aae.org, http://aae.org.

American Association of Oral and Maxillofacial Surgeons, 9700 W. Bryn Mawr Ave., Rosemont, IL 60018-5701, (847) 678-6200, (800) 822-6637, Fax: (847) 678-6286, http://www.aaoms.org.

American Dental Association, 211 E. Chicago Ave., Chicago, IL 60611, (312) 440-2500, http://www.ada.org.

Janie Franz

Topical antibiotics *see* **Antibiotics, topical**

Total hip replacement *see* **Hip replacement**

Total knee replacement *see* **Knee replacement**

Total parenteral nutrition

Definition

Total parenteral nutrition (TPN) is a way of supplying all the nutritional needs of the body by bypassing the digestive system and administering a nutrient solution directly into a vein. Other terms used synonymously with TPN include parenteral nutrition and hyperalimentation.

Purpose

TPN is used when individuals cannot or should not get their nutrition through eating, such as when the intestines are obstructed, the small intestine is not absorbing nutrients properly, or a gastrointestinal fistula (abnormal connection) is present. It is also used when the bowels need to rest and should not have any food passing through them. Bowel rest may be necessary in Crohn's disease, pancreatitis, ulcerative colitis, and prolonged bouts of diarrhea in young children. TPN is also used for individuals with severe burns, multiple fractures, and in malnourished individuals to prepare them for major surgery, chemotherapy, or radiation treatment. Individuals with AIDS, widespread infection (sepsis), or other medical conditions may also benefit from the administration of TPN.

Description

TPN is normally given through a large central vein. A catheter is inserted into the vein in the chest area under **local anesthesia** and sterile conditions. Placement may be done in an **operating room** to decrease the chance of infection. Several different types of catheters are used based on the reason TPN is needed and the expected length of treatment. Catheters are made of silicone or similar materials. Once the catheter is in place, a **chest x-ray** is done to make sure the placement is correct.

TPN is normally administered in a hospital, but under certain conditions and with proper patient and caregiver education, it may also be used at home for long-term therapy. TPN solution is mixed daily under sterile conditions. Maintaining sterility is essential for preventing infection. For this reason, the outside tubing leading from the bag of solution to the catheter is changed daily, and special **dressings** covering the catheter are changed daily as well.

The contents of the TPN solution are determined based on the patient's age, weight, height, and medical condition. All solutions contain sugar (dextrose) for energy and protein (amino acids). Fats (lipids) may also

KEY TERMS

Catheter—A hollow tube that is inserted into veins or other passages in the body to insert or remove fluid.

Electrolyte—An ion such as potassium, sodium, or chloride dissolved in fluid that helps to regulate metabolic activities of cells.

Fistula—An abnormal passage that connects one organ to another or that connects the organ to the outside of the body.

be added to the solution. Electrolytes such as potassium, sodium, calcium, magnesium, chloride, and phosphate are also included, as these are essential to the normal functioning of the body. Trace elements such as zinc, copper, manganese, and chromium are also needed. Vitamins can be included in the TPN solution, and insulin, a hormone that helps the body use sugar, may need to be added. Adults need approximately two liters of TPN solution daily, although this amount varies with age, size, and health of the individual. Special solutions have been developed for individuals with reduced liver and kidney function. The solution is infused slowly at first to prevent fluid imbalances, then the rate is gradually increased. The infusion process takes several hours.

Successful TPN requires frequent, often daily, monitoring of the individual's weight, glucose (blood sugar) level, blood count, blood gases, fluid balance, urine output, waste products in the blood (plasma urea), and electrolytes. Liver and **kidney function tests** may also be performed. Contents of the solution are individualized based on the results of these tests.

Precautions

Individuals need to tell their doctor if they have any allergies; what medications they are taking, including over-the-counter drugs and dietary supplements; if they have diabetes or have ever had liver, kidney, heart, lung, or hormonal disorder; and if they are pregnant. All these factors can affect the type and amount of TPN required.

Preparation

Preparation to insert the catheter involves creating a sterile environment. Other special preparations are not normally necessary.

QUESTIONS TO ASK YOUR DOCTOR

- How long will I need TPN?
- What are the possible signs of complications?

Aftercare

During the time the catheter is in place, patients and caregivers must stay alert to any signs of infection such as redness, swelling, fever, drainage, or pain.

Risks

TPN requires close monitoring. Two types of complications can develop. Infection, air in the lung cavity (pneumothorax), and blood clot formation (thrombosis) all can develop as a result of inserting the catheter into a vein. Metabolic and fluid imbalances can occur if the contents of the nutritional fluid are not properly balanced and monitored. The most common metabolic imbalance is hypoglycemia (low blood sugar), caused by abruptly discontinuing a solution high in sugar. Minor risks associated with TPN include mouth sores, poor night vision, and skin changes.

Most of the time, TPN is administered through an infusion pump so that delivery of the fluids can be precisely monitored and calculated.

Results

The goal of TPN is to provide all required nutrients in the correct quantity to allow the body to function normally.

Resources

PERIODICALS

Thibault, R., and C. Pitchard. "Parenteral Nutrition in Critical Illness: Can It Safely Improve Outcomes?" *Critical Care Clinics* 26, no. 3 (2010): 467–80.

Winkler, M. F., et al. "An Exploration of Quality of Life and the Experience of Living with Home Parenteral Nutrition." *Journal of Parenteral and Enteral Nutrition* 34, no. 4 (2010): 387–94.

WEBSITES

AHFS Consumer Medication Information. "Total Parenteral Nutrition." American Society of Health-System Pharmacists. Available from: http://www.nlm.nih.gov/medlineplus/druginfo/meds/a601166.html (accessed October 18, 2013).

American Society for Parenteral and Enteral Nutrition. "What is Parenteral Nutrition?" http://www.nutritioncare.org/wcontent.aspx?id=270 (accessed October 18, 2013).

ORGANIZATIONS
American Society for Parenteral and Enteral Nutrition, 8630 Fenton St., Ste. 412, Silver Spring, MD 20910, (301) 587-6315, (800) 727-4567, aspen@nutr.org, https://www. nutritioncare.org.

Tish Davidson, AM
Melinda Granger Oberleitner, RN, DNS, APRN, CNS

Total shoulder replacement *see* **Shoulder joint replacement**

Total wrist replacement *see* **Wrist replacement**

Toxicology screen

Definition

A toxicology screen, also known as a tox screen or drug test, is a test or set of tests done on body fluids, tissues, or organs to determine the type and amount(s) of prescription drugs, alcohol, drugs of abuse, heavy metals, or other toxic substances in the body. The examiner may test for one substance at a time or up to 30 different drugs at once.

Screening for the type of substance(s) involved is known as qualitative testing; examination of the amount(s) involved is called quantitative testing. Qualitative testing is the most common form of analysis in toxicology screening; quantitative testing is performed most often as a follow-up procedure to confirm the results of qualitative testing.

Purpose

The drugs most commonly tested during toxicology screens include:

- ethanol (beverage alcohol)
- barbiturates, methaqualone, and other sleep medications
- benzodiazepines and other tranquilizers
- antidepressants
- date rape drugs
- cocaine
- THC (the active compound in marijuana)
- narcotics (opium and opioid painkillers, including heroin, propoxyphene, morphine, oxycodone, and hydrocodone)
- phencyclidine (PCP or angel dust)
- antipsychotic drugs
- acetaminophen and other non-narcotic pain relievers
- amphetamines
- steroids

There are many different reasons for tox screens:

- Toxicology screens are frequently performed in the emergency department of a hospital to evaluate patients with symptoms of drug or alcohol intoxication or overdose; to distinguish between substance abuse or intoxication and psychiatric or medical conditions such as psychosis, dementia, or delirium; and to determine the appropriate course of treatment.
- Toxicology screens are often used to screen job applicants prior to employment for abuse of alcohol or illegal drugs, or for random testing of current employees. Workplace drug testing is particularly common in industries and occupations in which the safety of other workers or the general public may be affected by drug abuse, such as transportation, construction, mining, demolition, health care, and retail.
- Tox screens are performed in sports medicine to test student and professional athletes for the use of performance-enhancing drugs (doping), including anabolic steroids, human growth hormone, erythropoietin, and androstenedione. The screens are done not only to guarantee the fairness of athletic competition, but also to protect participants against the long-term side effects of these drugs, which include infertility, delayed growth (in adolescents), liver disorders, high blood pressure, psychiatric disorders, and heart problems.
- Drug testing is sometimes performed to monitor a patient's compliance with prescribed medications, particularly barbiturates, amphetamines, and opiates and other drugs given for pain management. Tox screens may also be done as part of addiction treatment. In some cases, a drug screen may be done to find out whether a patient's body is absorbing and processing prescription medications properly.
- Newborn infants whose mothers are known or suspected to have abused alcohol or illicit drugs during pregnancy can be tested shortly after birth for the presence of these substances or their metabolites (breakdown products). In addition to blood or urine samples, the infant's meconium (the first stool produced after delivery) can be tested for drugs of abuse. Meconium testing is presently considered the most accurate method of screening for maternal drug abuse during pregnancy.
- Drivers suspected of operating a motor vehicle under the influence of alcohol, marijuana, or other drugs may be asked to take a breathalyzer test or provide a blood sample at the police station or a medical facility.

• Women who have been sexually assaulted may be given a urine test at the hospital to assess the presence of drugs like flunitrazepam (Rohypnol), ketamine, or gamma-hydroxybutyric acid (GHB), often referred to as date rape drugs.

• Toxicology screening is used during the process of drug development to study the ways that drugs are metabolized in the body, their interactions with other drugs, their side effects, their potential for dependence or addiction, and the difference between a therapeutic dose and a toxic or lethal one.

• Toxicology screening may used on people affected by the venom from an animal bite or sting; this type of screen falls within the field of veterinary toxicology.

• Toxicology screens may also be run postmortem if drugs or other substances are suspected in the cause of death. This type of screening is known as forensic toxicology.

Description

A toxicology screen has two steps: sample collection and laboratory analysis. Clinical toxicology screens are performed on one or more samples of body fluids or tissues, including blood, urine, saliva, stomach contents, hair, and sweat.

Sample collection

BLOOD. Blood samples are usually obtained by venipuncture, typically from a vein in the forearm near the elbow. The blood is drawn by a trained professional through a needle into a vacuum tube and sent to a laboratory for analysis.

URINE. The person being tested is asked to go into a bathroom to provide what is called a clean catch urine sample; that is, a sample collected from the middle of the urinary stream. The person is instructed to wash his or her hands, clean the external genitalia with an antiseptic towelette, and begin to urinate into the toilet for a few seconds. The person should then collect about three ounces of midstream urine in the container provided by the test center, cover the container with its lid, and return it to the nurse or lab technician. Urine samples must be refrigerated if they cannot be tested within an hour of collection.

ORAL FLUID (SALIVA). There are two methods for collecting oral fluid for testing. In the first, the examiner swabs the inside of the patient's cheek with an absorbent material. In the second method, the person being tested is asked to spit into a collection tube.

STOMACH CONTENTS. Stomach contents in living patients are usually tested only in hospital emergency departments, when the person being examined for drug use or overdose has recently swallowed a toxic or potentially lethal dose of one or more drugs. The contents of the stomach are obtained by gastric lavage (stomach pumping), which involves passing a tube through the mouth or nose into the stomach, administering small quantities of warm water or saline solution, and withdrawing the contents of the stomach.

HAIR. Hair can be tested for most drugs of abuse, including alcohol, amphetamines, narcotics, cocaine, PCP, marijuana, and methamphetamines. The advantage of hair testing is that human hair retains evidence of drug use for as long as a year—much longer than body fluids. The hair can be taken from any part of the body, including the head, arms, legs, underarms, face, and pubic area. Head hair taken for sampling is cut close to the scalp; between 80 and 120 strands are needed for a toxicology screen.

SWEAT. Sweat is tested for drug use by applying a patch of absorbent material to a person's skin, leaving it in place for up to 14 days, and removing the patch for laboratory testing. The advantage of sweat testing is that it can be used when urine testing is not practical, and it is relatively resistant to tampering. The drawback of sweat testing is that it is more expensive than other screening methods and can be used for only a limited number of drugs.

Laboratory testing

Laboratory testing of body fluid or tissue samples is usually performed in two stages. The first is the screening test and uses immunoassay to detect the presence of alcohol or other drugs. If the sample tests positive for any substances, the laboratory performs a second test to confirm the results of the immunoassay. This confirmation test is most often either gas chromatography or mass spectrometry. Samples that test positive during the confirmation test may be stored in the laboratory for a period of months or even years in case of lawsuits or disputed results. Confirmation tests are particularly important in forensic toxicology because they can detect much smaller quantities of drugs in test samples than the immunoassay method.

Preparation

When possible, a patient should prepare for a toxicology screen by making a list of all prescription drugs, nonprescription medications, alcoholic beverages, illicit drugs (if any), herbal remedies, vitamins, and dietary supplements taken within the last four days. This information is important to proper interpretation of the test results. Friends or family members accompanying a person affected by drugs or alcohol to a hospital emergency department should also be prepared to describe the drugs taken and the approximate quantities, if possible.

The patient should also prepare for the test by discussing any concerns with the doctor, such as the need for the test, any risks involved, the types of samples that will be taken, and the significance of the test results.

Workplace drug testing, athletic testing, and sobriety testing typically require the persons being tested to sign a consent form stating that they understand the risks of the testing and agree to have it done. Consent forms for teenage athletes usually require parents' signatures as well as the athlete's.

Persons scheduled for workplace or athletic drug testing should *not* drink large quantities of water before the test in the belief that the water will dilute the urine and prevent detection of drug use. Heavy water consumption will not only not affect the test results, but can also pose a danger to health.

Aftercare

Aftercare following venipuncture consists of applying pressure, a gauze pad, and adhesive tape to the puncture site. The phlebotomist or other health care professional will instruct the patient to hold the arm straight and upward for a few seconds, continue to apply pressure, and keep the bandage on the site for a few hours after the test.

No aftercare is needed for the other types of tests.

Risks

Risks associated with venipuncture include pain when the needle is inserted in the vein, a feeling of lightheadedness or dizziness, and swelling or a bruise (hematoma) at the site of the venipuncture. More serious risks include excessive bleeding and infection. Risks associated with gastric lavage include nosebleed, mechanical damage to the stomach, electrolyte imbalances, and laryngospasm. Serious complications, however, are rare. There are no known risks associated with urine, hair, oral fluid, or sweat testing.

Persons arrested on suspicion of driving under the influence (DUI) risk more severe legal penalties for refusing a drug test than for taking the test and failing it.

Results

The results of toxicology screens can be affected by a range of factors, including:

• the person's age, sex, race or ethnicity, or overall health condition

• regular use of prescription, over-the-counter, and herbal medications or preparations

• smoking

• the length of time elapsed between drug or alcohol use and collection of the test samples

• improper collection or storage of the test samples prior to analysis

• the specific method(s) of analysis used by the laboratory that receives the test samples

• recent use of cough or cold medicines (which may produce a false positive for narcotics)

• the consumption of certain food items, such as poppy seeds or certain spices

• the presence of blood in the urine

• a scanty urine sample

Normal results include no unexpected drugs or substances in the samples and normal (therapeutic) levels of known prescription and nonprescription medications.

Abnormal results include the presence of alcohol or illicit drugs in the samples or abnormally low or high levels of prescription and nonprescription drugs in the blood, urine, or saliva. Values that are too low may indicate that the patient is not taking prescribed medications as directed or that his or her body is not metabolizing the medications normally. Values that are too high may indicate that the patient is overdosing on the medication.

In some cases, the toxicology test may fail to detect drugs taken by the patient; this is known as a false negative result. In other cases, the test may indicate the presence of a drug that the patient did not use; this is called a false positive result. Because of the possible legal and financial consequences of false positives, any test results that suggest the presence of alcohol or drug abuse should always be confirmed by a different test method.

Abnormal results may also occur if evidence suggests that the patient attempted to tamper with the sample. Suspicious urine results, for example, include urine with an abnormal temperature, gravity, or pH level, among other factors.

Morbidity and mortality rates

There are occasional case reports of uncontrolled bleeding or nerve damage during venipuncture; one Danish study reported a rate of 443 complications per 100,000 blood withdrawals. No complications have been reported with urine, saliva, hair, or sweat tests.

False negative—A test result that fails to detect a drug that the patient has used.

False positive—A test result that suggests that the patient has taken a drug that has not, in fact, been used.

Forensic—Pertaining to matters of interest to civil or criminal law.

Gas chromatography—A method for separating the various chemicals in a test sample by vaporizing a portion of a sample, mixing it with a carrier gas (usually nitrogen), and passing the mixture through a long column of adsorbent material. The different chemicals in the sample will pass through the column at different rates of speed and can then be identified.

Immunoassay—A biochemical test that measures the presence of a substance in a body fluid sample through the use of an immunoglobulin or an antibody.

Mass spectrometry—A method of analyzing a test sample by converting a portion of the sample into charged ions and measuring the electric current produced when the charged ions strike a detector. Mass spectrometry can be used to measure the quantity as well as the identity of a substance in the test sample.

Metabolite—In medicine, any substance produced during digestion or the breakdown of a drug in the body.

Pathologist—A physician with specialized training in the diagnosis of disease based on the anatomical, microscopic, chemical, or immunologic examination of tissues, organs, or entire bodies.

Phlebotomist—A person specially trained to withdraw blood from a vein for testing, research, or transfusion.

Postmortem—After death.

Screen—In medicine, any test or technique used to detect patients with a high likelihood of having a specific disease, or to detect one or more substances in body fluids or tissues.

Toxicology—The branch of science that deals with the study of drugs, poisons, and other chemicals, and their effects on human and animal bodies.

Venipuncture—The withdrawal of blood from a patient's vein for purposes of testing or research. The most common procedure used in adults involves the withdrawal of blood from the medial cubital vein near the elbow using a hypodermic needle and a vacuum tube.

Alternatives

There are no useful alternatives to toxicology screens.

Health care team roles

A toxicology screen may involve a number of different health professionals, depending on the location of the test, its purpose, the patient's condition, and the legal implications of the test, if any:

- Nurses may administer or supervise the collection of urine, hair, sweat, or oral fluid samples; they are also qualified to perform venipuncture to collect a blood sample.

- A phlebotomist is a healthcare worker with specialized training in venipuncture (the collection of blood from a vein for purposes of testing or research). Phlebotomists may work in hospitals, outpatient clinics, or diagnostic testing facilities.

- Emergency physicians have specialized training in the assessment, diagnosis, and treatment of patients brought to a hospital emergency department, including those with suspected drug or alcohol intoxication or overdose.

- A medical toxicologist is a physician with advanced training in diagnosing and treating adverse drug reactions, poisoning, and occupational exposure to toxins, as well as drug abuse and overdoses. Medical toxicologists may work in occupational medicine and pediatrics as well as in hospital emergency departments.

- Medical review officers are licensed physicians who are in charge of reviewing the laboratory results for employer drug testing programs. They determine if there are any legitimate medical explanations for positive or abnormal tests and maintain the confidentiality of the information.

- Medical technologists and clinical chemists are professionals with specialized training in testing samples of human body fluids and tissues. Clinical chemists hold a doctoral degree in chemistry and are certified by either the American Board of Clinical Chemistry or the American Board of Forensic Toxicology.

Resources

BOOKS

Corbett, Jane Vincent, and Angela Denise Banks. *Laboratory Tests and Diagnostic Procedures with Nursing Diagnoses.* 8th ed. Upper Saddle River, NJ: Pearson, 2013.

Frone, Michael R. *Alcohol and Illicit Drug Use in the Workforce and Workplace.* Washington, DC: American Psychological Association, 2013.

Gupta, Ramesh C., ed. *Veterinary Toxicology: Basic and Clinical Principles.* 2nd ed. Boston: Elsevier, 2012.

Luch, Andreas, ed. *Molecular, Clinical and Environmental Toxicology.* New York: Springer, 2012.

Magnani, Barbarajean, Michael G. Bissell, and Tai C. Kwong, eds. *Clinical Toxicology Testing: A Guide for Laboratory Professionals.* Northfield, IL: College of American Pathologists, 2011.

PERIODICALS

Cotten, S. W. "Drug Testing in the Neonate." *Clinics in Laboratory Medicine* 32 (September 2012): 449–66.

Frederick, D. L. "Toxicology Testing in Alternative Specimen Matrices." *Clinics in Laboratory Medicine* 32 (September 2012): 467–92.

Gambelunghe, C., et al. "Sweat Testing to Monitor Drug Exposure." *Annals of Clinical and Laboratory Science* 43 (2013): 22–30.

Jürschik, S., et al. "Rapid and Facile Detection of Four Date Rape Drugs in Different Beverages Utilizing Proton Transfer Reaction Mass Spectrometry (PTR-MS)." *Journal of Mass Spectrometry* 47 (September 2012): 1092–97.

Kronstrand, R., et al. "A Screening Method for 30 Drugs in Hair Using Ultrahigh-Performance Liquid Chromatography Time-of-Flight Mass Spectrometry." *Therapeutic Drug Monitoring* 35 (June 2013): 288–95.

Lee, H., et al. "Rapid Screening and Determination of Designer Drugs in Saliva by a Nib-assisted Paper Spray-Mass Spectrometry and Separation Technique." *Journal of Separation Science* 35 (October 2012): 2822–25.

Milone, M. C. "Laboratory Testing for Prescription Opioids." *Journal of Medical Toxicology* 8 (December 2012): 408–16.

Roman, M., et al. "Liquid Chromatography/Time-of-flight Mass Spectrometry Analysis of Postmortem Blood Samples for Targeted Toxicological Screening." *Analytical and Bioanalytical Chemistry* 405 (May 2013): 4107–25.

Rosano, T. G., et al. "Postmortem Drug Screening by Non-targeted and Targeted Ultra-performance Liquid Chromatography-Mass Spectrometry Technology." *Journal of Analytical Toxicology* 35 (September 2011): 411–23.

Schamasch, P., and O. Rabin. "Challenges and Perspectives in Anti-Doping Testing." *Bioanalysis* 4 (July 2012): 1691–1701.

WEBSITES

A.D.A.M. Medical Encyclopedia. "Toxicology Screen." PubMed Health. http://www.ncbi.nlm.nih.gov/pubmedhealth/PMH0004045 (accessed September 2, 2013).

College of American Pathologists (CAP). "Toxicology Information." http://www.cap.org/apps/cap.portal?_nfpb=true&cntvwrPtlt_actionOverride=%2Fportlets%2FcontentViewer%2Fshow&_windowLabel=cntvwrPtlt&cntvwrPtlt{actionForm.contentReference}=fact_sheets%2Ftoxicology_info.html (accessed September 23, 2013).

Healthwise. "Toxicology Tests." WebMD. http://www.webmd.com/a-to-z-guides/toxicology-tests (accessed September 2, 2013).

Mayo Clinic staff. "Performance-Enhancing Drugs: Know the Risks." MayoClinic.com. http://www.mayoclinic.com/health/performance-enhancing-drugs/HQ01105 (accessed September 2, 2013).

Office on Women's Health. "Date Rape Drugs Fact Sheet." U.S. Department of Health and Human Services. http://www.womenshealth.gov/publications/our-publications/fact-sheet/date-rape-drugs.cfm (accessed September 2, 2013).

Quest Diagnostics. "Prescription Drug Monitoring: Available Tests." https://www.questdiagnostics.com/home/physicians/testing-services/by-test-name/prescription-drug-monitoring/available-tests.html (accessed September 2, 2013).

ORGANIZATIONS

American Academy of Clinical Toxicology (AACT), 6728 Old McLean Village Dr., McLean, VA 22101, (703) 556-9222, Fax: (703) 556-8729, admin@clintox.org, http://www.clintox.org.

American College of Medical Toxicology (ACMT), 10645 N. Tatum Blvd., Ste. 200-111, Phoenix, AZ 85028, (623) 533-6340, Fax: (623) 533-6520, info@acmt.net, http://www.acmt.net.

College of American Pathologists, 325 Waukegan Rd., Northfield, IL 60093-2750, (847) 832-7000, (800) 323-4040, Fax: (847) 832-8000, http://www.cap.org.

Society of Toxicology, 1821 Michael Faraday Dr., Ste. 300, Reston, VA 20190, (703) 438-3115, sothq@toxicology. org, http://www.toxicology.org.

U.S. Food and Drug Administration (FDA), National Center for Toxicological Research (NCTR), 3900 NCTR Rd., Jefferson, AR 72079, (870) 543-7000, NCTRinformation @fda.hhs.gov, http://www.fda.gov/AboutFDA/Centers Offices/OC/OfficeofScientificandMedicalPrograms/ NCTR/default.htm.

Rebecca J. Frey, PhD

T-PA *see* **Thrombolytic therapy**

Trabeculectomy

Definition

Trabeculectomy is a surgical procedure that removes part of the trabecular meshwork in the eye to relieve pressure caused by glaucoma.

Purpose

Glaucoma is a disease that injures the optic nerve, causing progressive vision loss. Glaucoma is a major cause of blindness in the United States. If caught early, glaucoma-related blindness is easily prevented. However, because it does not produce symptoms until late in its cycle, periodic tests for the disease are necessary.

Glaucoma is usually associated with an increase in the pressure inside the eye, called intraocular pressure (IOP). This increase occurs in front of the iris in a fluid called the aqueous humor. Aqueous humor exits through tiny channels between the iris and the cornea, in an area called the trabecular meshwork. When this area is blocked, pressure from the build up of aqueous humor either increases rapidly with pain and redness, or builds slowly with no symptoms until there is a significant loss of vision. Trabeculectomy is the last treatment employed for either type of glaucoma. It is used only after medications and laser trabeculoplasty have failed to alleviate IOP.

Demographics

Glaucoma can develop at any age, but people over 45 are at higher risk. African Americans are more likely to develop glaucoma, especially primary open-angle glaucoma. Other factors, such as a family history of glaucoma, greatly increase the risk of contracting the disease. Diabetes and previous eye injury also increase chances of developing glaucoma.

Description

The procedure is performed in an **operating room**, usually under local anesthetic. However, some ophthalmologists give patients only a topical anesthetic. A trabeculectomy involves removing a tiny piece of the eyeball, where the cornea connects to the sclera, to create a flap that allows fluid to escape the anterior chamber without deflating the eye. After the procedure, fluid can flow out onto the eye's surface, where it is absorbed by the conjunctiva, the transparent membrane that lines the sclera and the eyelids.

Sometimes, an additional piece is taken from the iris so that anterior chamber fluid can also flow backward into the vitreous. This procedure is called an **iridectomy**.

Preparation

The procedure is fully explained and any alternative methods to control intraocular pressure are discussed. Antiglaucoma drugs are prescribed before surgery. Added pressure on the eye caused from coughing or sneezing should be avoided.

Several eye drops are applied immediately before surgery. The eye is sterilized, and the patient draped. A speculum is inserted to keep the eyelids apart during surgery.

Aftercare

Eye drops, and perhaps patching, will be needed until the eye is healed. Driving should be restricted until the ophthalmologist grants permission. The patient may experience blurred vision. Severe eye pain, light sensitivity, and vision loss should be reported to the physician.

Antibiotic and anti-inflammatory eye drops must be used for at least six weeks after surgery. Additional medicines may be prescribed to reduce scarring.

Risks

Infection and bleeding are risks of any surgery. Scarring can cause the drainage to stop. One-third of trabeculectomy patients will develop cataracts.

Results

Trabeculectomy will delay the progression of glaucoma. In many cases, people still require medication to lower IOP.

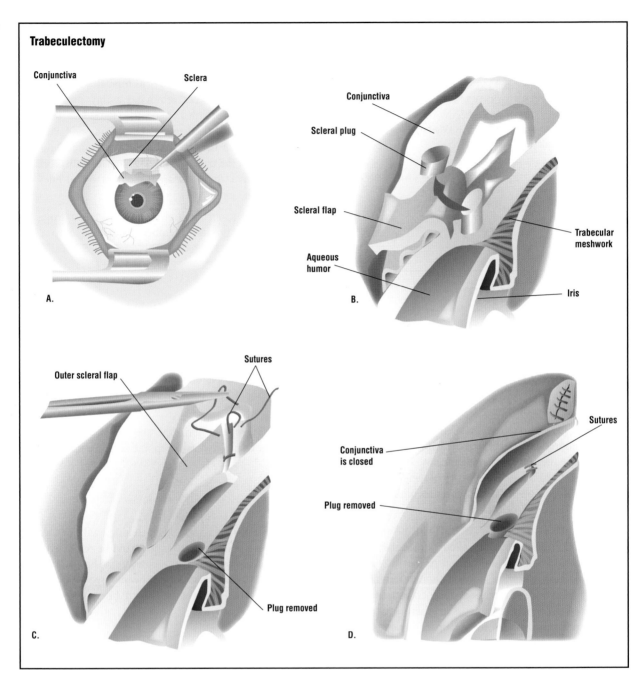

Trabeculectomy

A.
Conjunctiva
Sclera

B.
Conjunctiva
Scleral plug
Scleral flap
Aqueous humor
Trabecular meshwork
Iris

C.
Outer scleral flap
Sutures
Plug removed

D.
Sutures
Conjunctiva is closed
Plug removed

During a trabeculectomy, the patient's eye is held open with a speculum (A). The outer layer (conjunctiva) and the white of the eye (sclera) are cut open (A). A superficial scleral flap is created, and a plug of sclera and the underlying trabecular network are removed (B). This allows the fluid in the eye to circulate, relieving pressure. The scleral flap is closed and sutured (C), and the conjunctiva is closed (D). *(Illustration by GGS Information Services. Copyright © Cengage Learning®.)*

Morbidity and mortality rates

Trabeculectomy is considered a safe procedure. Infection is a complication that could lead to more serious medical problems; however, it is controllable with eye drops.

Alternatives

Physicians will first try to lower IOP with glaucoma medications. Several types of eye drops are effective for this use. Sometimes a patient must instill more than one eye drop, several times a day. Compliance is very

KEY TERMS

Cornea—Transparent film that covers the iris and pupil.

Iris—Colored part of the eye, which is suspended in aqueous humor and perforated by the pupil.

Sclera—White, outer coating of the eyeball.

Trabeculoplasty—Laser surgery that creates perforations in the trabecular meshwork, to drain built-up aqueous humor and relieve pressure.

QUESTIONS TO ASK YOUR DOCTOR

- Will IOP-lowering medication be needed after the surgery?
- How long will it take to determine if the surgery was a success?
- Can cataracts be treated in conjunction with glaucoma surgery?
- When will vision return to normal?

important when using these eye drops; missed dosages will raise IOPs.

Lasers are now used to treat both closed-angle and open-angle glaucoma. Peripheral iridectomy is used for people with acute angle-closure glaucoma attacks and chronic closed-angle glaucoma. The procedure creates a hole to improve the flow of aqueous humor.

Laser trabeculoplasty uses an argon laser to create tiny burns on the trabecular meshwork, which lowers IOP. The effects, however, are not permanent, and the patient must be retreated.

Transscleral cyclophotocoagulation treats the ciliary body with a laser to decrease production of aqueous humor, which reduces IOP.

A tube shunt might be implanted to create a drainage pathway in patients who are not candidates for trabeculectomy.

Health care team roles

Ophthalmologists and optometrists may detect and treat glaucoma; however, only ophthalmologists can perform surgery. Ophthalmologists who are glaucoma

subspecialists may have an additional two years of fellowship training.

The **outpatient surgery** is performed in a hospital or surgery suite designed for ophthalmic surgery.

Resources

BOOKS

Cassel, Gary H., Michael D. Billig, and Harry G. Randall. *The Eye Book: A Complete Guide to Eye Disorders and Health*. Baltimore, MD: Johns Hopkins University Press, 1998.

Giaconi, JoAnn A., et al. *Pearls of Glaucoma Management*. Berlin: Springer, 2010.

PERIODICALS

Kirwan, James F., et al. "Trabeculectomy in the 21st Century: A Multicenter Analysis." *Ophthalmology* (September 24, 2013): e-pub ahead of print. http://dx.doi.org/10.1016/j.ophtha.2013.07.049 (accessed October 4, 2013).

Landers, John, et al. "A Twenty-Year Follow-up Study of Trabeculectomy: Risk Factors and Outcomes." *Ophthalmology* 119, no. 4 (2012): 694–702. http://dx.doi.org/10.1016/j.ophtha.2011.09.043 (accessed October 4, 2013).

Murdoch, Ian. "Post-Operative Management of Trabeculectomy in the First Three Months." *Community Eye Health Journal* 25, nos. 79–80 (2012): 73–75.

WEBSITES

Chen, Teresa C. "Glaucoma Filtration Surgery (Trabeculectomy)." *Digital Journal of Ophthalmology*. http://www.djo.harvard.edu/site.php?url=/patients/pi/420 (accessed October 4, 2013).

EyeCare America. "Glaucoma Filtration Surgery." American Academy of Ophthalmology. http://eyecareamerica.org/eyecare/treatment/glaucoma-filtration (accessed October 4, 2013).

University of Wisconsin-Madison, School of Medicine and Public Health. "Glaucoma Surgery—Trabeculectomy." http://www.uwhealth.org/healthfacts/B_EXTRANET_HEALTH_INFORMATION-FlexMember-Show_Public_HFFY_1105110068675.html (accessed October 4, 2013).

ORGANIZATIONS

American Academy of Ophthalmology, 655 Beach St., San Francisco, CA 94109, (415) 561-8500, Fax: (415) 561-8533, http://www.aao.org.

The Glaucoma Foundation, 80 Maiden Ln., Ste. 700, New York, NY 10038, (212) 285-0080, info@glaucoma foundation.org, http://www.glaucomafoundation.org.

J. Ricker Polsdorfer, MD
Mary Bekker

Tracheoesophageal fistula repair *see* **Esophageal atresia repair**

Tracheostomy *see* **Tracheotomy**

Tracheotomy

Definition

A tracheotomy is a surgical procedure that opens up the windpipe (trachea). It is performed in emergency situations, in the **operating room**, or at bedside of critically ill patients. The term tracheostomy is sometimes used interchangeably with tracheotomy. Strictly speaking, however, tracheostomy usually refers to the opening itself while a tracheotomy is the actual operation.

Purpose

A tracheotomy is performed if enough air is not getting to the lungs, or if the person cannot breathe without help or is having problems with mucus and other secretions getting into the windpipe because of difficulty swallowing. There are many reasons why air cannot get to the lungs. The windpipe may be blocked by a swelling; a severe injury to the neck, nose, or mouth; a large foreign object; paralysis of the throat muscles; or a tumor. The patient may be in a coma, or need a ventilator to pump air into the lungs for a long period of time.

Description

There are two different procedures that are called tracheotomies. The first is done only in emergency situations and can be performed quite rapidly. The emergency room physician or surgeon makes a cut in a thin part of the voice box (larynx) called the cricothyroid

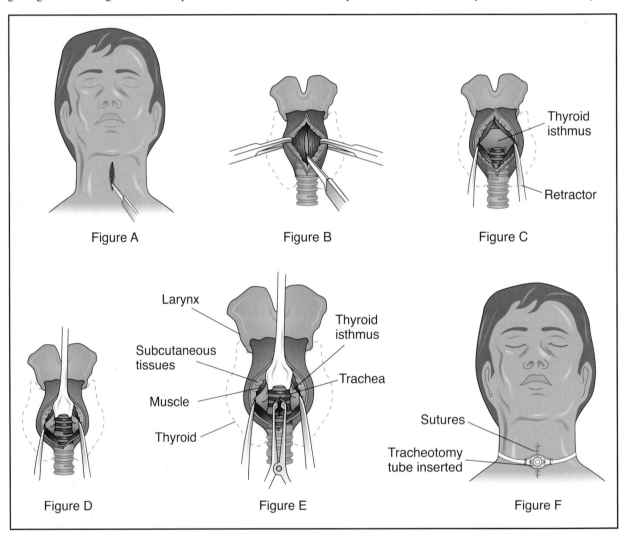

Tracheotomy is a surgical procedure in which an opening is made in the windpipe or trachea. A vertical incision is made through the skin (A), and another incision is made through the subcutaneous tissues and muscles of the neck (B). The neck muscles are separated using retractors (C). The thyroid isthmus is either cut or retracted (D). The surgeon identifies the rings of cartilage that make up the trachea and cuts into the walls (E). A metal or plastic tube is inserted into the opening, and sutures are used to hold the tube in place (F). *(Illustration by Electronic Illustrators Group. Copyright © Cengage Learning®.)*

membrane. A tube is inserted and connected to an oxygen bag. This emergency procedure is sometimes called a **cricothyroidotomy**.

The second type of tracheotomy takes more time and is usually done in an operating room. The surgeon first makes a cut (incision) in the skin of the neck that lies over the trachea. This incision is in the lower part of the neck between the Adam's apple and top of the breastbone. The neck muscles are separated and the thyroid gland, which overlies the trachea, is usually cut down the middle. The surgeon identifies the rings of cartilage that make up the trachea and cuts into the tough walls. A metal or plastic tube, called a tracheotomy tube, is inserted through the opening. This tube acts like a windpipe and allows the person to breathe. Oxygen or a mechanical ventilator may be hooked up to the tube to bring oxygen to the lungs. A dressing is placed around the opening. Tape or stitches (sutures) are used to hold the tube in place.

After a nonemergency tracheotomy, the patient usually stays in the hospital for three to five days, unless there is a complicating condition. It takes about two weeks to recover fully from the surgery.

Preparation

In the emergency tracheotomy, there is no time to explain the procedure or the need for it to the patient. The patient is placed on his or her back with face upward (supine), with a rolled-up towel between the shoulders. This positioning of the patient makes it easier for the doctor to feel and see the structures in the throat. A local anesthetic is injected across the cricothyroid membrane.

In a nonemergency tracheotomy, there is time for the doctor to discuss the surgery with the patient, to explain what will happen and why it is needed. The patient is then put under **general anesthesia**. The neck area and chest are then disinfected and surgical drapes are placed over the area, setting up a sterile surgical field.

Aftercare

Postoperative care

A **chest x-ray** is often taken, especially in children, to check whether the tube has become displaced or if complications have occurred. The doctor may prescribe **antibiotics** to reduce the risk of infection. If the patient can breathe without a ventilator, the room is humidified; otherwise, if the tracheotomy tube is to remain in place, the air entering the tube from a ventilator is humidified. During the hospital stay, the patient and his or her family members will learn how to care for the tracheotomy tube, including suctioning and clearing it. Secretions are

removed by passing a smaller tube (catheter) into the tracheotomy tube.

It takes most patients several days to adjust to breathing through the tracheotomy tube. At first, it will be hard even to make sounds. If the tube allows some air to escape and pass over the vocal cords, then the patient may be able to speak by holding a finger over the tube. Special tracheotomy tubes are also available that facilitate speech.

The tube will be removed if the tracheotomy is temporary. Then the wound will heal quickly and only a small scar may remain. If the tracheotomy is permanent, the hole stays open and, if it is no longer needed, it will be surgically closed.

Home care

After the patient is discharged, he or she will need help at home to manage the tracheotomy tube. Warm compresses can be used to relieve pain at the incision site. The patient is advised to keep the area dry. It is recommended that the patient wear a loose scarf over the opening when going outside. He or she should also avoid contact with water, food particles, and powdery substances that could enter the opening and cause serious breathing problems. The doctor may prescribe pain medication and antibiotics to minimize the risk of infections. If the tube is to be kept in place permanently, the patient can be referred to a speech therapist in order to learn to speak with the tube in place. The tracheotomy tube may be replaced four to ten days after surgery.

Patients are encouraged to go about most of their normal activities once they leave the hospital. Vigorous activity is restricted for about six weeks. If the tracheotomy is permanent, further surgery may be needed to widen the opening, which narrows with time.

Risks

Immediate risks

There are several short-term risks associated with tracheotomies. Severe bleeding is one possible complication. The voice box or esophagus may be damaged during surgery. Air may become trapped in the surrounding tissues or the lung may collapse. The tracheotomy tube can be blocked by blood clots, mucus, or the pressure of the airway walls. Blockages can be prevented by suctioning, humidifying the air, and selecting the appropriate tracheotomy tube. Serious infections are rare.

Long-term risks

Over time, other complications may develop following a tracheotomy. The windpipe itself may become damaged for a number of reasons, including pressure from the tube, infectious bacteria that form scar tissue, or friction from a tube that moves too much. Sometimes the opening does not close on its own after the tube is removed. This risk is higher in tracheotomies with tubes remaining in place for 16 weeks or longer. In these cases, the wound is surgically closed. Increased secretions may occur in patients with tracheostomies, which require more frequent suctioning.

High-risk groups

The risks associated with tracheotomies are higher in the following groups of patients:

• children, especially newborns and infants

• smokers

• alcoholics

• obese adults

• persons over 60

• persons with chronic diseases or respiratory infections

• persons taking muscle relaxants, sleeping medications, tranquilizers, or cortisone

Results

Normal results include uncomplicated healing of the incision and successful maintenance of long-term tube placement.

QUESTIONS TO ASK YOUR DOCTOR

● How do I take care of my tracheostomy?

● How many of your patients use noninvasive ventilation?

● Am I a candidate for noninvasive ventilation?

Morbidity and mortality rates

The overall risk of death from a tracheotomy is less than 5%.

Alternatives

For most patients, there is no alternative to emergency tracheotomy. Some patients with pre-existing neuromuscular disease (such as ALS or muscular dystrophy) can be successfully managed with emergency noninvasive ventilation via a face mask, rather than with tracheotomy. Patients who receive nonemergency tracheotomy in preparation for **mechanical ventilation** may often be managed instead with noninvasive ventilation, with proper planning and education on the part of the patient, caregiver, and medical staff.

Health care team roles

Tracheotomy is performed by a surgeon in a hospital. In an emergency, a tracheotomy may be performed on the scene by another medical professional.

Resources

BOOKS

Esquinas, Antonio Matias. *Noninvasive Mechanical Ventilation: Theory, Equipment, and Clinical Applications.* Berlin; London: Springer, 2010.

Seidman, Peggy A., Elizabeth Sinz, and David Goldenberg. *Tracheotomy Management: A Multidisciplinary Approach.* Cambridge: Cambridge University Press, 2011.

PERIODICALS

Byrd, J. Kenneth, et al. "Predictors of Clinical Outcome after Tracheotomy in Critically Ill Obese Patients." *The Laryngoscope* (August 8, 2013): e-pub ahead of print. http://dx.doi.org/10.1002/lary.24347 (accessed October 4, 2013).

Lawrason, Amy, and Katherine Kavanagh. "Pediatric Tracheotomy: Are the Indications Changing?" *International Journal of Pediatric Otorhinolaryngology* 77, no. 6 (2013): 922–25. http://dx.doi.org/10.1016/j.ijporl.2013.03.007 (accessed October 4, 2013).

"No Benefit from Early Tracheotomy in Mechanically Ventilated ICU Patients?" *BMJ* 346 (June 4, 2013): f3582. http://dx.doi.org/10.1136/bmj.f3582 (accessed October 4, 2013).

Shan, L., R. Zhang, and L. D. Li. "Effect of Timing of Tracheotomy on Clinical Outcomes: An Update Meta-analysis Including 11 Trials." *Chinese Medical Sciences Journal* 28, no. 3 (2013): 159–66. http://dx.doi.org/10.1136/bmj.f3582 (accessed October 4, 2013).

WEBSITES

American Speech-Language-Hearing Association. "Frequently Asked Questions (FAQ) About Tracheotomy and Swallowing." http://www.asha.org/slp/clinical/frequently-asked-questions-on-tracheotomy-and-swallowing (accessed October 4, 2013).

Eastern Virginia Medical School, Department of Otolaryngology. "Tracheotomy Tubes." http://www.evmsent.org/tracheotomy.asp (accessed October 4, 2013).

ORGANIZATIONS

American College of Surgeons, 633 N. Saint Clair St., Chicago, IL 60611-3211, (312) 202-5000, (800) 621-4111, Fax: (312) 202-5001, postmaster@facs.org, http://www.facs.org.

Jeanine Barone, Physiologist
Richard Robinson

Traction

Definition

Traction is force applied by weights or other devices to treat bone or muscle disorders or injuries.

Purpose

Traction treats fractures, dislocations, or muscle spasms in an effort to correct deformities and promote healing.

Description

Traction is referred to as a pulling force to treat muscle or skeletal disorders. There are two major types of traction: skin and skeletal traction, within which there are a number of treatments.

Skin traction

Skin traction includes weight traction, which uses lighter weights or counterweights to apply force to fractures or dislocated joints. Weight traction may be employed short term (e.g., at the scene of an accident) or on a temporary basis (e.g., when weights are connected to a pulley located above the patient's bed). The weights, typically weighing five to seven pounds, attach to the skin using tape, straps, or boots. They bring together the fractured bone or dislocated joint so that it may heal correctly.

In obstetrics, weights pull along the pelvic axis of a pregnant woman to facilitate delivery. In elastic traction, an elastic device exerts force on an injured limb.

Skin traction also refers to specialized practices, such as Dunlop's traction, used on children when a fractured arm must maintain a flexed position to avoid circulatory and neurological problems. Buck's skin traction stabilizes the knee, and reduces muscle spasm for knee injuries not involving fractures. In addition, splints, surgical collars, and corsets also may be used.

Skeletal traction

Skeletal traction requires an invasive procedure in which pins, screws, or wires are surgically installed for use in longer term traction requiring heavier weights. This is the case when the force exerted is more than skin traction can bear, or when skin traction is not appropriate for the body part needing treatment. Weights used in skeletal traction generally range from 25–40 lb. (11–18 kg). It is important to place the pins correctly because they may stay in place for several months, and are the hardware to which weights and pulleys are attached. The pins must be clean to avoid infection. Damage may result if the alignment and weights are not carefully calibrated.

Other forms of skeletal traction are tibia pin traction, for fractures of the pelvis, hip, or femur; and overhead arm traction, used in certain upper arm fractures. Cervical traction is used when the neck vertebrae are fractured.

Proper care is important for patients in traction. Prolonged immobility should be avoided because it may cause **pressure ulcers** and possible respiratory, urinary, or circulatory problems. Mobile patients may use a

Traction

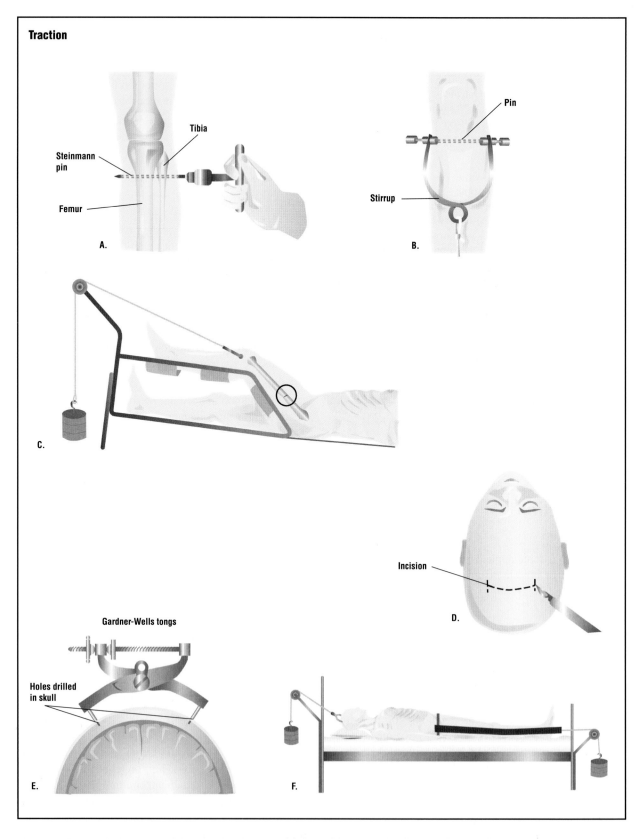

For tibial traction, a pin is surgically placed in the lower leg (A). The pin is attached to a stirrup (B) and weighted (C). In cervical traction, an incision is made into the head (D). Holes are drilled into the skull, and a halo or tongs are applied (E). Weights are added to pull the spine into place (F). *(Illustration by GGS Information Services. Copyright © Cengage Learning®.)*

trapeze bar, giving them the option of controlling their movements. An **exercise** program instituted by caregivers will maintain the patient's muscle and joint mobility. Traction equipment should be checked regularly to ensure proper position and exertion of force. With skeletal traction, it is important to check for inflammation of the bone, a sign of foreign matter introduction (potential source of infection at the screw or pin site).

Preparation

Both skin and skeletal traction require x-rays prior to application. If skeletal traction is required, standard preoperative surgical tests are conducted, such as blood and urine studies. X-rays may be repeated over the course of treatment to ensure that alignment remains correct, and that healing is proceeding.

Research and general acceptance

There have been few scientific studies on the effects of traction. Criteria (such as randomized controlled trials and monitored compliance) do exist, but an outcome study incorporating all of them has not yet been done. Some randomized controlled trials emphasize that traction does not significantly influence long-term outcomes of neck pain or lower back pain.

Resources

BOOKS

"Cervical Spine Traction." In *Noble: Textbook of Primary Care Medicine*. 3rd ed. St. Louis, MO: Mosby, 2001.

PERIODICALS

De Clerck, Hugo J., et al. "Orthopedic Traction of the Maxilla With Miniplates: A New Perspective for Treatment of Midface Deficiency." *Cochrane Database of Systematic Reviews* 67, no. 10 (2009): 2123–29. http://dx.doi.org/10.1016/j.joms.2009.03.007 (accessed October 4, 2013).

Wegner, Inge, et al. "Traction for Low-Back Pain with or without Sciatica." *Cochrane Database of Systematic Reviews* 8, art. no. CD003010 (August 19, 2013). http://dx.doi.org/10.1002/14651858.CD003010.pub5 (accessed October 4, 2013).

WEBSITES

AO Foundation. "Temporary Skeletal Traction." https://www2.aofoundation.org/wps/portal/surgery/?showPage=redfix&bone=Femur&segment=Distal&classification=33-C1&treatment=&method=Provisional+treatment&implantstype=Temporary+skeletal+traction&redfix_url= (accessed October 4, 2013).

NHS (UK National Health Service). "Traction." http://www.nhs.uk/conditions/Traction/Pages/Introduction.aspx (accessed October 4, 2013).

ORGANIZATIONS

American Academy of Orthopaedic Surgeons (AAOS), 6300 N. River Rd., Rosemont, IL 60018-4262, (847) 823-7186, Fax: (847) 823-8125, pemr@aaos.org, http://www.aaos.org.

Orthopaedic Trauma Association, 6300 N. River Rd., Ste. 727, Rosemont, IL 60018-4226, (847) 698-1631, OTA@aaos.org, http://www.ota.org.

Nancy McKenzie, PhD

Tranquilizers *see* **Antianxiety drugs**

Transfusion

Definition

Transfusion is the process of transferring blood or blood components from a donor to a recipient.

Purpose

Transfusions are given to restore lost blood, to improve clotting time, and to improve the ability of the blood to deliver oxygen to the body's tissues. About 40,000 pints of donated blood are transfused each day in the United States.

In the United States, blood collection is strictly regulated by the U.S. Food and Drug Administration (FDA), which has rules for the collection, processing, storage, and transportation of blood and blood products. In addition, the American Red Cross, the American Association of Blood Banks (AABB), and most states have specific rules for the collection and processing of blood. The main purpose of regulation is to ensure the quality of transfused blood and to prevent the transmission of infectious diseases through donated blood. Before blood and blood products are used, they are extensively tested for such infectious agents as hepatitis and human immunodeficiency virus (HIV).

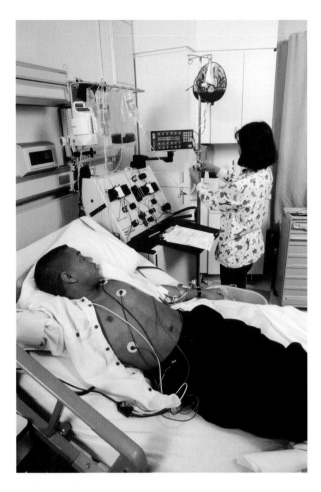

A male patient with sickle-cell anemia receives a blood transfusion. *(Spencer Grant/Photo Researchers, Inc)*

Demographics

In order to donate blood, an individual must be at least 17 years old, weigh at least 110 lb. (50 kg), and be in generally good health. The average blood donor is a white, married, college-educated male between the ages of 30 and 50, although the Red Cross states that 50% of their blood donors are male and 50% are female. Twenty-five percent of people receiving blood transfusions are over the age of 65, although the elderly constitute only 13% of the population. Fewer than 5% of Americans donate blood each year.

Description

Either whole blood or its components can be used for transfusion. Most blood collected from donors is broken down (fractionated) into components that are used to treat specific problems or diseases. Treating patients with fractionated blood is the most efficient way to use the blood supply.

Whole blood

Whole blood is used exactly as received from the donor. Blood components are parts of whole blood, such as red blood cells (RBCs), white blood cells (WBCs), plasma, platelets, clotting factors, and immunoglobulins. Whole blood is used only when needed or when fractionated components are not available, because too much whole blood can raise the recipient's blood pressure. Use of blood components is a more efficient way to use the blood supply, because blood that has been fractionated can be used to treat more than one person.

Whole blood is generally used when a person has lost a large amount of blood. Such blood loss can be caused by injury or surgical procedures. Whole blood is given to help restore the blood volume, which is essential for maintaining blood pressure. It is also given to ensure that the body's tissues are receiving enough oxygen. Whole blood is occasionally given when a required blood fraction is unavailable in isolated form.

Red blood cells

Red blood cells (RBCs) carry oxygen throughout the body. They pick up oxygen as they pass through the lungs, and give up oxygen to the other tissues of the body as they are pumped through the arteries and veins. When patients do not have enough RBCs to properly oxygenate their tissues, they can be given a transfusion with RBCs obtained from donors. This type of transfusion will increase the amount of oxygen carried to the tissues of the body. RBCs are recovered from whole blood after donation. They are then typed, removed from the watery blood plasma to minimize their volume (packed), and stored. RBCs are given to people with anemia (including thalassemia), whose bone marrow does not make enough RBCs, or who have other conditions that decrease the number of RBCs in the blood. Occasionally, red blood cells from rare blood types are frozen. Once frozen, RBCs can survive for as long as ten years. Packed RBCs are given in the same manner as whole blood.

White blood cells

White blood cells (WBCs) are another infection-fighting blood component. On rare occasions, white blood cells are given by transfusion to treat life-threatening infections. Such transfusions are given when the WBC count is very low or when the patient's WBCs are not functioning normally. Most of the time, however, **antibiotics** are used in these cases.

Plasma

Plasma is the clear yellowish liquid portion of blood. It contains many useful proteins, especially clotting factors and immunoglobulins. After plasma or plasma factors are processed, they are usually frozen. Some plasma fractions are freeze-dried. These fractions include clotting factors I through XIII. Some people have an inherited disorder in which the body produces too little of the clotting factors VIII (hemophilia A) or IX (hemophilia B). Transfusions of these clotting factors help to stop bleeding in people with hemophilia. Frozen plasma must be thawed before it is used; freeze-dried plasma must be mixed with liquid (reconstituted). In both cases, these blood fractions are usually small in volume and can be injected with a **syringe and needle**.

Platelets

Platelets are small disk-shaped structures in the blood that are essential for clotting. People who do not have enough platelets (a condition called thrombocytopenia) have bleeding problems. People who have lymphoma or leukemia and people who are receiving cancer therapy do not make enough platelets. Platelets have a very short shelf life; they must be used within five days of **blood donation**. After a unit of blood has been donated and processed, the platelets in it are packed into bags. A platelet transfusion is given in the same manner as whole blood.

Immunoglobulins

Immunoglobulins are the infection-fighting fractions in blood plasma. They are also known as gamma globulin, antibodies, and immune sera. Immunoglobulins are given to people who have difficulty fighting infections, especially people whose immune systems have been depressed by such diseases as AIDS. Immunoglobulins are also used to prevent tetanus after a cut has been contaminated, to treat animal bites when rabies is suspected, or to treat severe childhood diseases. Generally, the volume of immunoglobulins used is small, and it can be injected.

Transfusion process

Blood is collected from the donor by inserting a large needle into a vein in the arm, usually one of the larger veins near the inside of the elbow. A tourniquet is placed on the upper arm to increase the pressure in the arm veins, which makes the veins swell and become more accessible. Once the nurse or technician has identified a suitable vein, she or he sterilizes the area where the needle will be inserted by scrubbing the skin with a soap solution or an antiseptic that contains iodine. Sometimes both solutions are used. The donor lies on a bed or cot during the procedure, which usually takes between 10 and 20 minutes. Generally, an 18-gauge needle is used. This size of needle fits easily into the veins and yet is large enough to allow blood to flow easily. Human blood will sometimes clot in a smaller needle and stop flowing. The donor's blood is collected in a sterile plastic bag that holds one pint (450 mL). The bags contain an anticoagulant to prevent clotting and preservatives to keep the blood cells alive. A sample of the donator's blood is collected at the time of donation and tested for infectious diseases. The blood is not used until the test results confirm that it is safe. Properly handled and refrigerated, whole blood can last for 42 days.

The recipient of a transfusion is prepared in much the same way as the blood donor. The site for the needle insertion is carefully washed with a soap-based solution followed by an antiseptic containing iodine. The skin is then dried and the transfusion needle inserted into the vein. During the early stages of a transfusion, the recipient is monitored closely to detect any adverse reactions. If no signs of adverse reaction are evident, the patient is monitored occasionally for the duration of the transfusion period. Upon completion of the transfusion, a compress is placed over the needle insertion site to prevent extensive bleeding.

Blood typing

All donated blood is typed, which means that it is analyzed to determine which of several major and minor blood types (also called blood groups) it belongs to. Blood types are genetically determined. The major types are classified by the ABO system. This system groups blood with reference to two substances in the red blood cells called antigen A and antigen B. The four ABO blood types are A, B, AB, and O. Type A blood has the A antigen, type B has the B antigen, type AB has both, and type O has neither. These four types of blood are further classified by the Rh factor. The Rh, or Rhesus factor, is also an antigen in the red blood cells. A person who has the Rh factor is Rh positive; a person who does not have the factor is Rh negative. If a person has red blood cells with both the B and the Rh antigens, that person is said to have a B positive (B+) blood type. Blood types determine which kinds of donated blood a patient can receive. Generally, patients are limited to receiving only blood of the exact same ABO and Rh type as their own. For example, a person with B+ blood can receive blood or blood cells only from another person with B+ blood. An exception is blood type O. Individuals with type O blood are called universal donors, because people of all blood types can accept their blood.

Blood can also be typed with reference to several other minor antigens, such as Kell, Kidd, Duffy, and Lewis. These minor antigens can become important when a patient has received many transfusions. These patients tend to build up an immune response to the minor blood groups that do not match their own. They may have an adverse reaction upon receiving a transfusion with a mismatched minor blood group. A third group of antigens that may cause a reaction are residues from the donor's plasma attached to the RBCs. To eliminate this problem, the RBCs are rinsed to remove plasma residues. These rinsed cells are called washed RBCs.

Other transfusion procedures

Autologous transfusion is a procedure in which patients donate blood for their own use. Patients who are to undergo surgical procedures requiring a blood transfusion may choose to donate several units of blood ahead of time. The blood is stored at the hospital for the patient's exclusive use. Autologous donation assures that the blood type is an exact match. It also assures that no infection will be transmitted through the blood transfusion. Autologous donation accounts for 5% of blood use in the United States each year.

Directed donors are family or friends of the patient who needs a transfusion. Some people think that family and friends provide a safer source of blood than the general blood supply. Studies do not show that directed donor blood is any safer. Blood that is not used for the identified patient becomes part of the general blood supply.

Apheresis is a special procedure in which only certain specific components of a donor's blood are collected. The remaining blood fractions are returned to the donor. A special blood-processing instrument is used in apheresis. It fractionates the blood, saves the desired component, and pumps all the other components back into the donor. Because donors give only part of their blood, they can donate more frequently. For example, people can give almost ten times as many platelets by apheresis as they could give by donating whole blood. The donation process takes about one to two hours.

Preparation

The first step in blood donation is the taking of the donor's medical history. Blood donors are questioned about their general health, their lifestyle, and any medical conditions that might disqualify them. These conditions include hepatitis, AIDS, cancer, heart disease, asthma, malaria, bleeding disorders, and high blood pressure. Screening prevents people from donating who might transmit diseases or whose medical condition would place them at risk if they donated blood. Some geographical areas or communities have a high rate of hepatitis or AIDS. Blood collection in most of these areas has been discontinued indefinitely.

The blood pressure, temperature, and pulse of donors are taken to ensure that they are physically able to donate blood. One pint (450 mL) of blood is usually withdrawn, although it is possible to donate smaller amounts. The average adult male has 10–12 pints of blood in his body; the average adult female has 8–9 pints in hers. Within hours after donating, most people's bodies have replaced the fluid lost with the donated blood, which brings their blood volume back to normal. Replacement of the blood cells and platelets, however, can take several weeks. Pregnant women and people with low blood pressure or anemia should not donate blood or should limit the amount of blood they give. Generally, people are allowed to donate blood only once every two months. This restriction ensures the health of the donor and discourages people from selling their blood. The former practice of paying donors for blood has essentially stopped. Donors who sell blood tend to be at high risk for the transmission of blood-borne diseases.

Aftercare

Recipients of blood transfusion are monitored during and after the transfusion for signs of an adverse reaction. Blood donors are generally given fluids and light refreshments to prevent such possible side effects as dizziness and nausea. They are also asked to remain in the donation area for 15–20 minutes after giving blood to make sure that they are not likely to faint when they leave.

Risks

Risks for donors

For donors, the process of giving blood is very safe. Only sterile equipment is used and there is no chance of catching an infection from the equipment. There is a slight chance of infection at the puncture site if the skin is not properly cleaned before the collection needle is inserted. Some donors feel lightheaded when they sit up or stand for the first time after donating. Occasionally, a donor may faint. Donors are encouraged to drink plenty of liquids to replace the fluid lost with the donated blood. It is important to maintain the fluid volume of the blood so that the blood pressure will remain stable. Strenuous **exercise** should be avoided for the rest of the day. It is normal to feel some soreness or to find a small bluish bruise at the site of the needle insertion. Most donors have very slight symptoms or no symptoms at all after giving blood.

Risks for recipients

A number of precautions must be taken for transfusion recipients. Donated blood must be matched with the recipient's blood type, as incompatible blood types can cause a serious adverse reaction (transfusion reaction). Blood is introduced slowly by gravity flow directly into the veins (intravenous infusion) so that medical personnel can observe the patient for signs of adverse reactions. People who have received many transfusions may develop an immune response to some factors in foreign blood cells. This immune reaction must be evaluated before the patient is given new blood. Some transfusion reaction can be avoided or controlled through premedication with medications like steroids and/or antihistamines.

Transfusion reactions include:

- Allergic reactions, in which some allergen in the donated blood reacts with antibodies in the recipient's blood. This can lead to itching, hives, or severe reactions involving respiratory distress.

- Acute hemolytic transfusion reaction is a severe and immediate reaction due to mismatch of donor and recipient blood type, in which the donated blood cells are rapidly destroyed by the recipient's immune system, leading to more severe symptoms such as fever, pain, and kidney failure.

- Delayed hemolytic transfusion reaction occurs some hours or days (up to almost a month) after a transfusion. Like an acute hemolytic reaction, the recipient's body produces antibodies that attack and destroy the donated red cells. Symptoms of this delayed response, however, tend to be more mild than those of the acute reaction or may even go unnoticed, and they can only be diagnosed during blood testing. This variant is called delayed serologic transfusion reaction.

- Febrile non-hemolytic transfusion reaction is the most frequently encountered transfusion reaction. No hemolysis (red blood cell breakdown) takes place, but the patient experiences symptoms of fever and chills.

- Hypotensive transfusion reaction occurs when the blood recipient's blood pressure drops suddenly and severely. Blood pressure rebounds once the transfusion is stopped.

- Post-transfusion purpura usually strikes about 5–12 days after transfusion, when the recipient of platelets begins to produce antibodies against the donor platelets. This results in destruction of both the donor AND the recipient platelets, leading to a potentially fatal low platelet count.

Adverse reactions to mismatched blood (transfusion reaction) is a major risk of blood transfusion. Transfusion reaction occurs when antibodies in the recipient's blood react to foreign blood cells introduced by the transfusion. The antibodies bind to the foreign cells and destroy them. This destruction is called a hemolytic reaction. In addition, a transfusion reaction may also cause a hypersensitivity of the immune system that may in turn result in tissue damage within the patient's body. The patient may also have an allergic reaction to mismatched blood.

The first symptoms of transfusion reaction are a feeling of general discomfort and anxiety. Breathing difficulties, flushing, and a sense of pressure in the chest or back pain may also be present. Evidence of a hemolytic reaction can be seen in the urine, which will be colored from the hemoglobin leaking from the destroyed red blood cells. Severe hemolytic reactions are occasionally fatal. Reactions to mismatches of minor factors are milder. These symptoms include itchiness, dizziness, fever, headache, rash, and swelling. Sometimes the patient will experience breathing difficulties and muscle spasms. Most adverse reactions from mismatched blood are not life-threatening.

Infectious diseases can also be transmitted through donated blood and constitute another major risk of blood transfusion. The infectious diseases most often acquired from blood transfusion in the United States are hepatitis and HIV.

Patients who are given too much blood can develop high blood pressure, a concern for people who have heart disease. Very rarely, an air embolism is created when air is introduced into a patient's veins through the tubing used for intravenous infusion. The danger of embolism is greatest when infusion is begun or ended. Care must be taken to ensure that all air is bled out of the tubing before infusion begins, and that the infusion is stopped before air can enter the patient's blood system.

Results

Most individuals will feel only a slight sting from the needle used during the blood donation process, and will not experience any side effects after the procedure is over. Plasma is regenerated by the body within 24 hours, and red blood cells within a few weeks. Patients who receive a blood transfusion will usually experience mild or no side effects.

Morbidity and mortality rates

The risk of acquiring an infectious disease from a blood transfusion is very low. The risk of HIV transmission is one in 2,135,000 units of blood; hepatitis B virus (HBV), one in 205,000 units; and hepatitis C virus (HCV), one in 1,935,000 units. Bacterial contamination (a cause of infection) is identified in one in 500,000 for red blood cell units and one in 15,400 for apheresis platelet units. In about one in 600,000 to 800,000 transfusions a "fatal misidentification error"

ABO blood groups—A system in which human blood is classified according to the A and B antigens found in red blood cells. Type A blood has the A antigen, type B has the B antigen, AB has both, and O has neither.

Antibody—A simple protein produced by the body to destroy bacteria, viruses, or other foreign bodies. The production of each antibody is triggered by a specific antigen.

Antigen—A substance that stimulates the immune system to manufacture antibodies (immunoglobulins). The function of antibodies is to fight off such intruder cells as bacteria or viruses. Antigens stimulate the blood to fight other blood cells that have the wrong antigens. If a person with blood type A is given a transfusion with blood type B, the A antigens will fight the foreign blood cells as though they were an infectious agent.

Apheresis—A procedure in which whole blood is withdrawn from a donor, a specific blood component is separated and collected, and the remainder is reinfused into the patient.

Autologous blood—The patient's own blood, drawn and set aside before surgery for use during surgery in case a transfusion is needed.

Fractionation—The process of separating the various components of whole blood.

Hemoglobin—The red pigment in red blood cells that transports oxygen.

Hemolysis—The destruction of red blood cells through disruption of the cell membrane, resulting in the release of hemoglobin. A hemolytic transfusion reaction is one that results in the destruction of red blood cells.

Immunoglobulin—An antibody.

Infusion—Introduction of a substance directly into a vein or tissue by gravity flow.

Injection—Forcing a fluid into the body by means of a needle and syringe.

Plasma—The liquid portion of blood, as distinguished from blood cells. Plasma constitutes about 55% of blood volume.

Platelets—Disk-shaped structures found in blood that play an active role in blood clotting. Platelets are also known as thrombocytes.

Rh (Rhesus) factor—An antigen present in the red blood cells of 85% of humans. A person with Rh factor is Rh positive (Rh+); a person without it is Rh negative (Rh-). The Rh factor was first identified in the blood of a rhesus monkey.

Serum (plural, sera)—The clear fluid that separates from blood when the blood is allowed to clot completely. Blood serum can also be defined as blood plasma from which fibrinogen has been removed.

occurs, and in about one in 12,000 to 19,000 cases a non-fatal error occurs.

Alternatives

There are several alternatives to blood transfusion. These include:

- Volume expanders. Certain fluids (saline, Ringer's lactate solution, dextran, etc.) may be used to increase the patient's blood volume without adding additional blood cells.

- Blood substitutes. Much research is currently being done into compounds that can replace some or all of the functions of blood components. One such compound, called HBOC-201 or Hemopure, is hemoglobin derived from bovine (cow) blood. Hemopure shows promise as a substitute for red blood cell transfusion.

- Bloodless surgery. It may be possible to avoid excessive blood loss through careful planning prior to surgery. Specialized instruments can minimize the amount of blood lost during a procedure. It is also possible to collect some of the blood lost during surgery and reinfuse it into the patient at the end of the operation.

Health care team roles

Blood may be donated at hospital donor centers, Red Cross chapter houses, or other locations where special blood drives have been organized (churches, places of business, schools, colleges, etc.). The procedure of blood donation is generally performed by a nurse or phlebotomist (a person who has been trained to draw blood). Blood transfusions are generally administered in a hospital or emergency center with a blood bank.

QUESTIONS TO ASK YOUR DOCTOR

- Why is a transfusion recommended for my condition?
- Do I have the option of donating my own blood for future use?
- Will I need a transfusion of whole blood or blood components?
- What alternatives to blood transfusion are available to me?

Resources

BOOKS

Hoffman, Ronald, et al. *Hematology: Basic Principles and Practice.* 6th ed. Philadelphia: Saunders/Elsevier, 2013.

PERIODICALS

Carson, Jeffrey L., et al. "Red Blood Cell Transfusion: A Clinical Practice Guideline from the AABB*." *Annals of Internal Medicine* 157, no. 1 (2012): 49–58. http://dx.doi.org/10.7326/0003-4819-157-1-201206190-00429 (accessed October 18, 2013).

WEBSITES

A.D.A.M. Medical Encyclopedia. "Transfusion Reaction—Hemolytic." MedlinePlus. http://www.nlm.nih.gov/medlineplus/ency/article/001303.htm (accessed October 18, 2013).

Centers for Disease Control and Prevention. "Blood Safety." http://www.cdc.gov/bloodsafety/basics.html (accessed October 18, 2013).

MedlinePlus. "Blood Transfusion and Donation." U.S. National Library of Medicine, National Institutes of Health. http://www.nlm.nih.gov/medlineplus/bloodtransfusionanddonation.html (accessed October 18, 2013).

National Heart, Lung, and Blood Institute. "What Is a Blood Transfusion?" http://www.nhlbi.nih.gov/health/health-topics/topics/bt (accessed October 18, 2013).

ORGANIZATIONS

AABB (American Association of Blood Banks), 8101 Glenbrook Rd., Bethesda, MD 20814-2749, (301) 907-6977, Fax: (301) 907-6895, aabb@aabb.org, http://www.aabb.org.

American Red Cross, 2025 E St., Washington, DC 20006, (800) RED CROSS (733-2767), http://www.redcross.org.

America's Blood Centers, 725 15th St. NW, Ste. 700, Washington, DC 20005, (202) 393-5725, Fax: (202) 393-1282, abc@americasblood.org, http://www.americasblood.org.

National Heart, Lung, and Blood Institute Information Center, PO Box 30105, Bethesda, MD 20824-0105, (301) 592-8573, Fax: (240) 629-3246, nhlbiinfo@nhlbi.nih.gov, http://www.nhlbi.nih.gov.

John T. Lohr, PhD
Stephanie Dionne Sherk

Transplant surgery

Definition

Transplant surgery is the surgical removal of organs, tissue, or blood products from a donor in order to surgically place or infuse them into a recipient. There are four categories of transplantation, classified by tissue origin: autograft (donor and recipient are the same person); isograft or syngeneic graft (donor and recipient are genetically identical, as in identical twins); allograft or homograft (donor and recipient are genetically unrelated but belong to the same species—i.e., both are human beings) and xenograft or heterograft (donor and recipient belong to different species—e.g., chimpanzee or rabbit tissues have been used in humans on an experimental basis).

Purpose

Transplant surgery is a treatment option for diseases or conditions that have not improved with other medical treatments and have led to organ failure or injury. Transplant surgery is generally reserved for people with end-stage disease who have no other options.

National transplant waiting list by organ type (as of July 10, 2013)

Organ needed	Persons waiting
Kidney	96,708
Liver	15,733
Heart	3,536
Kidney/Pancreas	2,069
Lung	1,644
Pancreas	1,194
Intestine	270
Heart/Lung	45

SOURCE: U.S. Department of Health and Human Services, Organ Procurement and Transplantation Network. Available online at: http://optn.transplant.hrsa.gov/data/default.asp (accessed July 10, 2013).

(Table by PreMediaGlobal. Copyright © 2014 Cengage Learning®.)

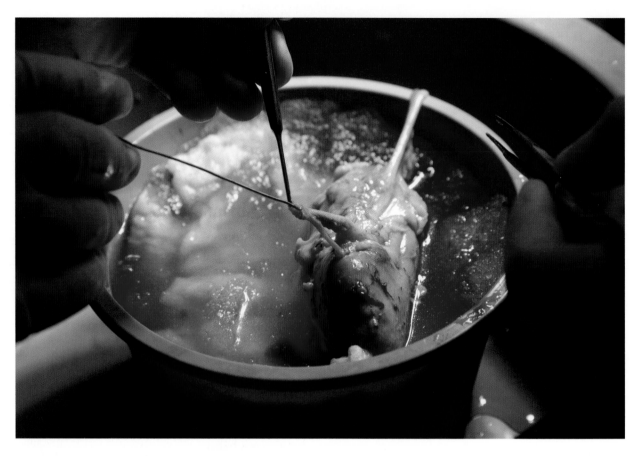

A surgeon dilates the renal artery in a donor kidney during kidney transplantation. *(© B. Slaven/Custom Medical Stock Photo—All rights reserved.)*

The decision to perform transplant surgery is based on the patient's age, general physical condition, specific diagnosis, and stage of the disease. Transplant surgery is not recommended for patients who have liver, lung, or kidney problems; poor leg circulation; cancer; or chronic infections.

Demographics

The typical cut-off age for a transplant recipient used to range between 40 and 55 years; however, a person's general health is usually a more important factor. Currently, many organs can be transplanted into an individual up to the age of 65, as long as their health (aside from the problem requiring transplantation) is good. In some cases, transplants are done in even older individuals.

On average, 79 people receive transplants every day from either a living or deceased donor. In 2012, 28,051 transplants were performed in the United States; unfortunately, the organ shortage is so extreme that 18 people die daily awaiting a suitable organ.

The national waiting list for most transplanted organs continues to grow every year, even though the number of recipients waiting for a heart transplant has leveled off in recent years, and the waiting list for heart-lung transplants has decreased over the past few years. As of September 2013, there were about 119,679 eligible recipients waiting for an organ transplant in the United States.

Description

Organ donors

Organ donors are classified as living donors or cadaveric (non-living) donors. All donors are carefully screened to make sure there is a suitable blood type match and to prevent any transmissible diseases or other complications.

LIVING DONORS. Living donors may be family members or biologically unrelated to the recipient. From 1992 to 2001, the number of biologically unrelated living donors increased tenfold. Living donors must be physically fit, in good general health, and have no existing disorders such as diabetes, high blood pressure, cancer, kidney disease, or heart disease. Of all the organs transplanted in 2011, about 21% came from living donors. Organs that can be donated from living donors include:

• Single kidneys. In 2012, 34% of all kidney transplants came from living donors. There is little risk in living with one kidney because the remaining kidney compensates for and performs the work of both.

• Liver. Living donors can donate segments of the liver because the organ can regenerate and regain full function. The number of living donor liver transplants has doubled since 1999.

• Lung. Living donors can donate lobes of the lung although lung tissue does not regenerate.

• Pancreas. Living donors can donate a portion of the pancreas even though the gland does not regenerate.

Organs donated from living donors eliminate the need to place the recipient on the national waiting list. Transplant surgery can be scheduled at a mutually acceptable time rather than performed under emergency conditions. In addition, the recipient can begin taking immunosuppressant medications two days before the transplant surgery to prevent the risk of rejection. Living donor transplants are often more successful than cadaveric donor transplants because there is a better tissue match between the donor and recipient. The living donor's medical expenses are usually covered by the organ recipient's insurance company, but the amount of coverage may vary.

CADAVERIC OR DECEASED DONORS. Organs from cadaveric donors come from people who have recently died and have willed their organs before death by signing an organ donor card, or are brain-dead. The donor's family must give permission for organ donation at the time of death or diagnosis of brain death. Cadaveric donors may be young adults with traumatic head injuries, or older adults suffering from a stroke. The majority of deceased donors are older than the general population.

Transplant procedures

ORGAN HARVESTING. Harvesting refers to the process of removing cells or tissues from the donor and preserving them until they are transplanted. If the donor is deceased, the organ or tissues are harvested in a sterile **operating room**. They are packed carefully for transportation and delivered to the recipient via ambulance, helicopter, or airplane. Organs from deceased donors should be transplanted within a few hours of harvesting. After the recipient is notified that an organ has become available, he or she should not eat or drink anything.

When the organ is harvested from a living donor, the recipient's transplant surgery follows immediately after the donor's surgery. The recipient and the donor should not eat or drink anything after midnight the evening before the scheduled operation.

PREOPERATIVE PROCEDURES. After arriving at the hospital, the recipient will have a complete physical and such other tests as a **chest x-ray**, blood tests, and an electrocardiogram (EKG) to evaluate his or her fitness for surgery. If the recipient has an infection or major medical problem, or if the donor organ is found to be unacceptable, the operation will be canceled.

The recipient will be prepared for surgery by having the incision site shaved and cleansed. An intravenous tube (IV) will be placed in the arm to deliver medications and fluids, and a sedative will be given to help the patient relax.

TRANSPLANT SURGERY. After the patient has been brought to the operating room, the anesthesiologist will administer a general anesthetic. A central venous catheter may be placed in a vein in the patient's arm or groin. A breathing tube will be placed in the patient's throat. The breathing tube is attached to a mechanical ventilator that expands the lungs during surgery.

Patient's receiving heart and/or lung transplants will then be connected to a heart-lung bypass machine, also called a cardiopulmonary bypass pump, which takes over for the heart and lungs during the surgery. The heart-lung machine removes carbon dioxide from the blood and replaces it with oxygen. A tube is inserted into the patient's aorta to carry the oxygenated blood from the bypass machine back to the heart for circulation to the body. A nasogastric tube is placed to drain stomach secretions, and a urinary catheter is inserted to drain urine during the surgery.

The surgeon carefully removes the diseased organ and replaces it with the donor organ. The blood vessels of the donated organ are connected to the patient's blood vessels, allowing blood to flow through the new organ.

Preparation

Pre-transplant evaluation

Several tests are performed before the transplant surgery to make sure that the patient is eligible to receive the organ and to identify and treat any problems ahead of time. The more common pre-transplant tests include:

• tissue typing

• blood tests

• chest x-ray

• pulmonary function tests

- computed tomography (CT) scan
- heart function tests (electrocardiogram, echocardiogram, and cardiac catheterization)
- sigmoidoscopy
- bone densitometry test

The pre-transplant evaluation usually includes a dietary and social work assessment. In addition, the patient must undergo a complete dental examination to reduce the risk of infection from bacteria in the mouth.

Insurance considerations

Organ transplantation is an expensive procedure. Insurance companies and health maintenance organizations (HMOs) may not cover all costs. Many insurance companies require precertification letters of medical necessity. As soon as transplantation is discussed as a treatment option, the patient should contact his or her insurance provider as soon as possible to determine what costs will be covered. There are, however, organizations that can assist with raising funds to cover the cost of transplantation, such as the National Foundation for Transplants and the National Transplant Assistance Fund and Catastrophic Injury Program.

Patient education and lifestyle changes

Before undergoing transplant surgery, the transplant team will ensure that the patient understands the potential benefits and risks of the procedure. In addition, a team of health care providers will review the patient's social history and psychological test results to ensure that he or she is able to comply with the regimen that is needed after transplant surgery. An organ transplant requires major lifestyle changes, including dietary adjustments, complex drug treatments, and frequent examinations. The patient must be committed to making these changes in order to become a candidate for transplant. Most transplant centers have extensive patient education programs.

Smoking cessation is an important consideration for patients who use tobacco. Many transplant programs require the patient to be a nonsmoker for a certain amount of time (usually six months) before he or she is eligible to participate in the pre-transplant screening evaluation. The patient must also be committed to avoid tobacco products after the transplant.

Informed consent

Patients are legally required to sign an **informed consent** form prior to transplant surgery. Informed consent signifies that the patient is a knowledgeable participant in making healthcare decisions. The doctor will discuss all of the following with the patient before he or she signs the form: the nature of the surgery; reasonable alternatives to the surgery; and the risks, benefits, and uncertainties of each option. Informed consent also requires the doctor to make sure that the patient understands the information that has been given.

Finding a donor

After the patient has completed the pre-transplant evaluation and has been approved for transplant surgery, the next step is locating a donor. Organs from cadaveric donors are located through a computerized national waiting list maintained by the United Network for Organ Sharing (UNOS) to assure equal access to and fair distribution of organs. When a deceased organ donor is identified, a transplant coordinator from an organ procurement organization enters the donor's data in the UNOS computer. The computer then generates a list of potential recipients. This list is called a match run. Factors affecting a potential organ recipient's ranking on the match run list include: tissue match, blood type, size of the organ, length of time on the waiting list, immune status, and the geographical distance between the recipient and donor. For some transplants, such as heart, liver, and intestinal segments, the degree of medical urgency is also taken into consideration.

The organ is offered to the transplant team of the first person on the ranked waiting list. The recipient must be healthy enough to undergo surgery, available, and willing to receive the organ transplant immediately. The matching process involves cross matching, performing an antibody screen, and a host of other tests.

Donor searching can be a long and stressful process. A supportive network of friends and family is important to help the patient cope during this time. The healthcare provider or social worker can also put the patient in touch with support groups for transplant patients.

Contact and travel arrangements

The patient must be ready to go to the hospital as soon as possible after being notified that an organ is available. A suitcase should be kept packed at all times. Transportation arrangements should be made ahead of time. If the recipient lives more than a 90-minute drive from the transplant center, the transplant coordinator will help make transportation arrangements for the recipient and one friend or family member.

Because harvested organs cannot be preserved for more than a few hours, the transplant team must be able to contact the patient at all times. Some transplant programs offer a pager rental service, to be used only for receiving the call from the transplant center. The patient should clear travel plans with the transplant coordinator before taking any trips.

Blood donation and conservation

Some transplant centers allow patients to donate their own blood before surgery, which is known as autologous donation. Autologous blood is the safest blood for **transfusion**, since there is no risk of disease transmission. Preoperative donation is an option for patients receiving an organ from a living donor, since the surgery can be scheduled in advance. In autologous donation, the patient donates blood once a week for one to three weeks before surgery. The blood is separated and the blood components needed are reinfused during the operation.

In addition to preoperative donation, there are several techniques for minimizing the patient's blood loss during surgery:

• Intraoperative blood collection. The blood lost during surgery is processed, and the red blood cells are reinfused during or immediately after surgery.

• Immediate preoperative hemodilution. The patient donates blood immediately before surgery to decrease the loss of red blood cells during the operation. The patient is then given fluids to restore the volume of the blood.

• Postoperative blood collection. The blood lost from the incision following surgery is collected and reinfused after the surgical site has been closed.

Aftercare

Inpatient recovery

A transplant recipient can expect to spend three to four weeks in the hospital after surgery. Immediately following the operation, the patient is transferred to an **intensive care unit** (ICU) for close monitoring of his or her **vital signs**. When the patient's condition is stable, he or she is transferred to a hospital room, usually in a specialized transplant unit. The IV in the patient's arm, the urinary catheter, and a dressing over the incision remain in place for several days. A chest tube may be placed to drain excess fluids. Special stockings may be placed on the patient's legs to prevent blood clots in the deep veins of the legs. A breathing aid called an incentive spirometer is used to help keep the patient's lungs clear and active after surgery.

Medications to relieve pain will be given every three to four hours, or through a device known as a PCA (**patient-controlled analgesia**). The PCA is a small pump that delivers a dose of medication into the IV when the patient pushes a button. The transplant recipient will

also be given immunosuppressive medications to prevent the risk of organ rejection. These medications are typically taken by the recipient for the rest of his or her life.

A 2–4 week waiting period is necessary before the transplant team can evaluate the success of the procedure. Visitors are limited during this time to minimize the risk of infection. The patient will be given intravenous antibiotic, antiviral, and antifungal medications, as well as blood and platelet transfusions to help fight off infection and prevent excessive bleeding. Blood tests are performed daily to monitor the patient's kidney and liver function, as well as his or her nutritional status. Other tests are performed as needed.

Outpatient recovery

After leaving the hospital, the transplant recipient will be monitored through home or outpatient visits for as long as a year. Medication adjustments are often necessary, but barring complications, the recipient can return to normal activities about 6–8 months after the transplant.

Proper outpatient care includes:

• taking medications exactly as prescribed

• attending all scheduled follow-up visits

• contacting the transplant team at the first signs of infection or organ rejection

• having blood drawn regularly

• following dietary and exercise recommendations

• avoiding rough contact sports and heavy lifting

• taking precautions against infection

• avoiding pregnancy for at least a year

Risks

Short-term risks following an organ transplant include pneumonia and other infectious diseases; excessive bleeding; and liver disorders caused by blocked blood vessels. In addition, the new organ may be rejected, which means that the patient's immune system is attacking the new organ. Characteristic signs of rejection include fever, rash, diarrhea, liver problems, and a compromised immune system. Transplant recipients are given immunosuppressive medications to minimize the risk of rejection. In most cases, the patient will take these medications for the rest of his or her life.

Long-term risks include an elevated risk of cancer, particularly skin cancer. Transplant patients carry twice the risk of developing cancer over their lifetime as compared to the general population.

KEY TERMS

Antibody—A substance produced by the immune system in response to specific antigens, thereby helping the body fight infection and foreign substances. An antibody screen involves mixing the white blood cells of the donor with the serum of the recipient to determine if antibodies in the recipient react with the antigens of the donor.

Autologous blood—The patient's own blood, drawn and set aside for use during surgery in case a transfusion is needed.

Bone densitometry test—A test that quickly and accurately measures the density of bone.

Brain death—Irreversible cessation of brain function. Patients with brain death have no potential capacity for survival or for recovery of any brain function.

Cadaveric donor—An organ donor who has recently died of causes not affecting the organ intended for transplant.

Compatible donor—A person whose tissue and blood type are the same as the recipient's.

Confirmatory typing—Repeat tissue typing to confirm the compatibility of the donor and patient before transplant.

Donor—A person who supplies organ(s), tissue, or blood to another person for transplantation.

Harvesting—The process of removing tissues or organs from a donor and preserving them for transplantation.

Hemodilution—A technique in which the fluid content of the blood is increased without increasing the number of red blood cells.

Human leukocyte antigen (HLA)—A group of protein molecules located on bone marrow cells that can provoke an immune response. A donor's and a recipient's HLA types should match as closely as possible to prevent the recipient's immune system from attacking the donor's marrow as a foreign material that does not belong in the body.

Immunosuppression—The use of medications to suppress the immune system to prevent organ rejection.

Organ procurement—The process of donor screening, and the evaluation, removal, preservation, and distribution of organs for transplantation.

Pulmonary function test—A test that measures the capacity and function of the lungs as well as the blood's ability to carry oxygen. During the test, the patient breathes into a device called a spirometer.

Rejection—An immune response that occurs when a transplanted organ is viewed as a foreign substance by the body. If left untreated, rejection can lead to organ failure and even death.

There is a very small risk of infection from a transplanted organ, even though donors in the United States and Canada are carefully screened. In 2007, the Centers for Disease Control and Prevention (CDC) reported a case in which four organ recipients in the Chicago area developed hepatitis C and HIV infection from a high-risk donor. The diseases did not show up on screening tests because the donor contracted them about three weeks before his death, when there were not enough antibodies in his blood to be detected by present tests.

Results

In a successful organ transplant, the patient returns to a more normal lifestyle with increased strength and stamina.

Morbidity and mortality rates

Mortality figures for transplant surgery include recipients who die before a match with a suitable donor can be found. About 18 patients die every day in the United States waiting for a transplant.

In 2011, the Scientific Registry of Transplant Recipients reported the first-year survival rates for transplant surgery as follows:

- 97.8% of pancreas transplant recipients
- 95.6% of deceased donor kidney transplant recipients
- 98.5% of living donor kidney transplant recipients
- 89.3% of intestine transplant patients
- 88.4% of deceased donor liver transplant patients
- 91% of living donor liver transplant patients
- 88.3% of heart transplant patients
- 83.3% of lung transplant patients
- 80.6% of heart-lung transplant patients

Five-year survival rates are:

- 88.7% of pancreas transplant recipients
- 81.9% of deceased donor kidney transplant recipients

- 91% of living donor kidney transplant recipients
- 89.3% of intestine transplant patients
- 73.8% of deceased donor liver transplant patients
- 79% of living donor liver transplant patients
- 88.3% of heart transplant patients
- 54.4% of lung transplant patients
- 44.9% of heart-lung transplant patients

As of 2013, about 461,776 people in the United States were living with a transplanted organ, with almost 120,000 awaiting a life-saving transplant operation.

Alternatives

Clinical trials

Available alternatives to transplant surgery depend upon the individual patient's diagnosis and severity of illness. Some patients may be eligible to participate in clinical trials, which are research programs that evaluate a new medical treatment, drug, or device.

Complementary and alternative (CAM) therapies

Complementary therapies can be used along with standard treatments to help alleviate the patient's pain; strengthen muscles; and decrease depression, anxiety, and stress. Before trying a complementary treatment, however, patients should check with their doctors to make sure that it will not interfere with standard therapy or cause harm. Alternative approaches that have helped transplant recipients maintain a positive mental attitude both before and after surgery include meditation, biofeedback, and various relaxation techniques. Massage therapy, music therapy, aromatherapy, and hydrotherapy are other types of treatment that can offer patients some pleasant sensory experiences as well as relieve pain. Acupuncture has been shown in a number of NIH-sponsored studies to be effective in relieving nausea and headache, as well as chronic muscle and joint pain. Some insurance carriers cover the cost of acupuncture treatments.

Health care team roles

A transplant surgeon, along with a multidisciplinary team of transplant specialists, should perform the transplant surgery. Transplant **surgeons** are usually board-certified by the American Board of Surgery, as well as certified by the medical specialty board or boards related to the type of organ transplant performed. Members of transplant teams include infectious disease specialists, pharmacologists, psychiatrists, advanced care registered nurses, and transplant coordinators in addition to the surgeons and anesthesiologists.

> ## QUESTIONS TO ASK YOUR DOCTOR
>
> - Who performs the transplant surgery? How many other transplant surgeries has this surgeon performed?
> - Where will my organ come from?
> - What is the typical waiting period before a donor is found?
> - Will my insurance provider cover the expenses of my transplant?
> - What types of precautions must I follow before and after my transplant?
> - What are the signs of infection and rejection, and what types of symptoms should I report to my doctor?
> - When will I find out if the transplant was successful?

Organ transplants are performed in special transplant centers, which should be members of the United Network for Organ Sharing (UNOS) as well as of state-level accreditation organizations.

Resources

BOOKS

Hamilton, David. *A History of Organ Transplantation: Ancient Legends to Modern Practice*. Pittsburgh, PA: University of Pittsburgh Press, 2012.

Townsend, Courtney M., et al. *Sabiston Textbook of Surgery*. 19th ed. Philadelphia: Saunders/Elsevier, 2012.

Trzepacz, Paula T., and Andrea F. DiMartini, et al. *The Transplant Patient: Biological, Psychiatric and Ethical Issues in Organ Transplantation*. New York: Cambridge University Press, 2011.

PERIODICALS

Giacomoni, A., et al. "Initial Experience with Robot-Assisted Nephrectomy for Living-Donor Kidney Transplantation: Feasibility and Technical Notes." *Transplantation Proceedings* 45, no. 7 (2013): 2627–31. http://dx.doi.org/10.1016/j.transproceed.2013.07.038 (accessed September 20, 2013).

Lai, J. C., et al. "Reducing Infection Transmission in Solid Organ Transplantation Through Donor Nucleic Acid Testing: A Cost-Effectiveness Analysis." *American Journal of Transplantation* (August 22, 2013): e-pub ahead of print. http://dx.doi.org/10.1111/ajt.12429 (accessed September 20, 2013).

Panocchia, N., et al. "Ethical Evaluation of Risks Related to Living Donor Transplantation Programs." *Transplantation Proceedings* 45, no. 7 (2013): 2601–3. http://dx.doi.org/10.1016/j.transproceed.2013.07.026 (accessed September 20, 2013).

Samstein, B., et al. "Totally Laparoscopic Full Left Hepatectomy for Living Donor Liver Transplantation in Adolescents and Adults." *American Journal of Transplantation* 13, no. 9 (2013): 2462–66. http://dx.doi.org/10.1111/ajt.12360 (accessed September 20, 2013).

Varotti, G., et al. "Impact of Model for End-Stage Liver Disease Score on Transfusion Rates in Liver Transplantation." *Transplantation Proceedings* 45, no. 7 (2013): 2684–88. http://dx.doi.org/10.1016/j.transproceed.2013.07.006 (accessed September 20, 2013).

WEBSITES

Division of Transplantation, U.S. Department of Health and Human Services. Organdonor.gov. http://www.organdonor.gov (accessed September 20, 2013).

The Gift of a Lifetime: Organ & Tissue Transplantation in America. http://www.organtransplants.org (accessed September 20, 2013).

MedlinePlus. "Organ Transplantation." U.S. National Library of Medicine, National Institutes of Health. http://www.nlm.nih.gov/medlineplus/organtransplantation.html (accessed September 20, 2013).

Organ Procurement and Transplantation Network, U.S. Department of Health and Human Services. http://optn.transplant.hrsa.gov (accessed September 20, 2013).

World Health Organization. "Human Organ Transplantation." http://www.who.int/transplantation/organ/en (accessed September 20, 2013).

ORGANIZATIONS

American Society of Transplant Surgeons (ASTS), 2461 South Clark St., Ste. 640, Arlington, VA 22202, (703) 414-7870, http://www.asts.org.

Children's Organ Transplant Association (COTA), 2501 West COTA Dr., Bloomington, IN 47403, (800) 366-2682, cota@cota.org, http://www.cota.org.

Donate Life America, 701 E. Byrd St., 16th Fl., Richmond, VA 23219, (804) 377-3580, donatelifeamerica@donatelife.net, http://donatelife.net.

HelpHOPELive, Two Radnor Corporate Ctr., 100 Matsonford Rd., Ste. 100, Radnor, PA 19087, (610) 727-0612, (800) 642-8399, http://www.helphopelive.org.

Musculoskeletal Transplant Foundation, 125 May St., Edison, NJ 08837, (732) 661-0202, (800) 946-9008, http://www.mtf.org.

National Foundation for Transplants, 5350 Poplar Ave., Ste. 430, Memphis, TN 38119, (901) 684-1697, (800) 489-3863, info@transplants.org, http://www.transplants.org.

Transplant Foundation, 701 SW 27th Ave., Ste. 705, Miami, FL 33135, (305) 817-5645, (866) 900-3172, http://transplantfoundation.org.

Transplant Recipients International Organization (TRIO), 2100 M St. NW, #170-353, Washington, DC 20037-1233, (202) 293-0980, (800) TRIO-386 (874-6386), info@trioweb.org, http://www.trioweb.org.

TransWeb.org, University of Michigan Transplant Center, 3868 Taubman Ctr., 1500 E. Medical Center Dr., SPC 5391, Ann Arbor, MI 48109-5391, (734) 232-1113, transweb@umich.edu, http://www.transweb.org.

United Network for Organ Sharing (UNOS), 700 N. 4th St., Richmond, VA 23219, (804) 782-4800, http://www.unos.org.

Angela M. Costello
Rebecca Frey, PhD
Rosalyn Carson-DeWitt, MD

Transposition of the great arteries *see* **Heart surgery for congenital defects**

Transurethral bladder resection

Definition

Transurethral bladder resection is a surgical procedure used to view the inside of the bladder, remove tissue samples, and/or remove tumors. Instruments are passed through a cystoscope (a slender tube with a lens and a light) that has been inserted through the urethra into the bladder.

Purpose

Transurethral resection is the initial form of treatment for bladder cancers. The procedure is performed to remove and examine bladder tissue and/or a tumor. It may also serve to remove lesions, and it may be the only treatment necessary for noninvasive tumors. This procedure plays both a diagnostic and therapeutic role in the treatment of bladder cancers.

Demographics

According to the American Cancer Society (ACS), there were 72,570 new cases of bladder cancer in the United States in 2013, with approximately 15,210 deaths from the disease.

Industrialized countries such as the United States, Canada, France, Denmark, Italy, and Spain have the highest incidence rates for bladder cancer. Rates are lower in England, Scotland, and Eastern Europe. The lowest rates occur in Asia and South America.

Smoking is a major risk factor for bladder cancer; it increases a person's cancer risk by two to five times and

KEY TERMS

Biopsy—The removal and microscopic examination of a small sample of body tissue to see whether cancer cells are present.

Bladder irrigation—To flush or rinse the bladder with a stream of liquid (as in removing a foreign body or medicating).

Bladder tumor marker studies—A test to detect specific substances released by bladder cancer cells into the urine using chemicals or immunology (using antibodies).

Bladder washing—A procedure in which bladder washing samples are taken by placing a salt solution into the bladder through a catheter (tube) and then removing the solution for microscopic testing.

Chemotherapy—The treatment of cancer with anti-cancer drugs.

Cystoscopy—A procedure in which a slender tube with a lens and a light is placed into the bladder to view the inside of the bladder and remove tissue samples.

Immunotherapy—A method of treating allergies in which small doses of substances that a person is allergic to are injected under the skin.

Interstitial radiation therapy—The process of placing radioactive sources directly into the tumor. These radioactive sources can be temporary (removed after the proper dose is reached) or permanent.

Intravenous pyelogram—An x-ray of the urinary system taken after injecting a contrast solution that enables the doctor to see images of the kidneys, ureters, and bladder.

Metastatic—A change of position, state, or form; as a transfer of a disease-producing agency from the site of disease to another part of the body; a secondary growth of a cancerous tumor.

Noninvasive tumors—Tumors that have not penetrated the muscle wall and/or spread to other parts of the body.

Radiation therapy—The use of high-dose x-rays to destroy cancer cells.

Retrograde pyelography—A test in which dye is injected through a catheter placed with a cystoscope into the ureter to make the lining of the bladder, ureters, and kidneys easier to see on x-rays.

Ureters—Two thin tubes that carry urine downward from the kidneys to the bladder.

Urethra—The small tube-like structure that allows urine to empty from the bladder.

Urine culture—A test which tests urine samples in the lab to see if bacteria are present.

Urine cytology—The examination of the urine under a microscope to look for cancerous or precancerous cells.

accounts for approximately 50% of bladder cancers found in men and 30% found in women. If cigarette smokers quit, their risk declines in two to four years. Exposure to a variety of industrial chemicals also increases the risk of developing this disease. Occupational exposures may account for approximately 25% of all urinary bladder cancers.

Men have a 1-in-30 chance of developing bladder cancer; women have a 1-in-90 chance of developing bladder cancer. The incidence of bladder cancer in the Caucasian population is almost twice that of the African American population. For other ethnic and racial groups in the United States, the incidence of bladder cancer falls between that of Caucasians and African Americans.

There is a greater incidence of bladder cancer with advancing age. Of newly diagnosed cases in both men and women, approximately 80% occur in people aged 60 years and older.

Description

Cancer begins in the lining layer of the bladder and grows into the bladder wall. Transitional cells line the inside of the bladder. Cancer can begin in these lining cells.

During transurethral bladder resection, a cystoscope is inserted through the urethra into the bladder. A clear solution is infused to maintain visibility and the tumor or tissue to be examined is cut away using an electric current. A biopsy is taken of the tumor and muscle fibers in order to evaluate the depth of tissue involvement, while avoiding perforation of the bladder wall. Every attempt is made to remove all visible tumor tissue, along with a small border of healthy tissue. The resected tissue is examined under the microscope for diagnostic purposes. An indwelling catheter may be inserted to ensure adequate drainage of the bladder postoperatively. At this time, interstitial radiation therapy may be initiated, if necessary.

Diagnosis

If there is reason to suspect a patient may have bladder cancer, the physician will use one or more methods to determine if the disease is actually present. The doctor first takes a complete medical history to check for risk factors and symptoms, and does a **physical examination**. An examination of the rectum and vagina (in women) may also be performed to determine the size of a bladder tumor and to see if and how far it has spread. If bladder cancer is suspected, the following tests may be performed, including:

• biopsy
• cystoscopy
• urine cytology
• bladder washing
• urine culture
• intravenous pyelogram
• retrograde pyelography
• bladder tumor marker studies

Most of the time, the cancer begins as a superficial tumor in the bladder. Blood in the urine is the usual warning sign. Based on how they look under the microscope, bladder cancers are graded using Roman numerals 0 through IV. In general, the lower the number, the less the cancer has spread. A higher number indicates greater severity of cancer.

Because it is not unusual for people with one bladder tumor to develop additional cancers in other areas of the bladder or elsewhere in the urinary system, the doctor may biopsy several different areas of the bladder lining. If the cancer is suspected to have spread to other organs in the body, further tests will be performed.

Because different types of bladder cancer respond differently to treatment, the treatment for one patient could be different from that of another person with bladder cancer. Doctors determine how deeply the cancer has spread into the layers of the bladder in order to decide on the best treatment.

Aftercare

As with any surgical procedure, blood pressure and pulse will be monitored. Urine is expected to be blood-tinged in the early postoperative period. Continuous bladder irrigation (rinsing) may be used for approximately 24 hours after surgery. Most operative sites should be completely healed in three months. The patient is followed closely for possible recurrence with visual examination, using a special viewing device (cystoscope) at regular intervals. Because bladder cancer has a high rate of recurrence, frequent screenings are recommended.

Normally, screenings would be needed every three to six months for the first three years, and every year after that, or as the physician considers necessary. **Cystoscopy** can catch a recurrence before it progresses to invasive cancer, which is difficult to treat.

Risks

All surgery carries some risk due to heart and lung problems or the anesthesia itself, but these risks are generally extremely small. The risk of death from **general anesthesia** for all types of surgery, for example, is only about one in 1,600. Bleeding and infection are other risks of any surgical procedure. If bleeding becomes a complication, bladder irrigation may be required postoperatively, during which time the patient's activity is limited to bed rest. Perforation of the bladder is another risk, in which case the urinary catheter is left in place for four to five days postoperatively. The patient is started on antibiotic therapy preventively. If the bladder is lacerated, accompanied by spillage of urine into the abdomen, an abdominal incision may be required.

Results

The results of transurethral bladder resection will depend on many factors, including the type of treatment used, the stage of the patient's cancer before surgery, complications during and after surgery, the age and overall health of the patient, as well as the recurrence of the disease at a later date. The chances for survival are improved if the cancer is found and treated early.

Morbidity and mortality rates

After a diagnosis of bladder cancer, up to 95% of patients with superficial tumors survive for at least five years. Patients whose cancer has grown into the lining of the bladder but not into the muscle itself, and is not in any lymph nodes or distant sites, have a five-year survival rate as high as 85%. The five-year survival rate may be as high as 55% for patients whose tumors have invaded the bladder muscle, but not spread through the muscle into the surrounding fatty tissue. When the cancer has grown totally through the bladder muscle into the surrounding fatty tissue, and perhaps into nearby tissues such as the prostate, uterus, or vagina, the five-year survival rate is about 38%. For patients whose cancer has spread through the bladder wall to the pelvis or abdominal wall or has spread distantly to lymph nodes or other organs (such as the bones, liver, or lungs), the five-year survival rate is 16%.

The five-year survival rate refers to the percentage of patients who live at least five years after their cancer is found, although many people live much longer. Five-year relative survival rates do not take into account patients who die of other diseases. Every person's situation is unique and the statistics cannot predict exactly what will happen in every case; these numbers provide an overall picture.

Mortality rates are two to three times higher for men than women. Although the incidence of bladder cancer in the Caucasian population exceeds that of the African American population, African American women die from the disease at a greater rate. This is due to a larger proportion of these cancers being diagnosed and treated at an earlier stage in the Caucasian population. The mortality rates for Hispanic and Asian men and women are only about one-half those for Caucasians and African Americans. Over the past 30 years, the age-adjusted mortality rate has decreased in both races and genders. This may be due to earlier diagnosis, better therapy, or both.

Alternatives

Surgery, radiation therapy, immunotherapy, and chemotherapy are the main types of treatment for cancer of the bladder. One type of treatment or a combination of these treatments may be recommended, based on the stage of the cancer.

After the cancer is found and staged, the cancer care team discusses the treatment options with the patient. In choosing a treatment plan, the most significant factors to consider are the type and stage of the cancer. Other factors to consider include the patient's overall physical health, age, likely side effects of the treatment, and the personal preferences of the patient.

In considering treatment options, a **second opinion** may provide more information and help the patient feel more confident about the treatment plan chosen.

Alternative methods are defined as unproved or disproved methods, rather than evidence-based or proven methods to prevent, diagnose, and treat cancer. For some cancer patients, conventional treatment is difficult to tolerate and they may decide to seek a less unpleasant alternative. Others are seeking ways to alleviate the side effects of conventional treatment without having to take more drugs. Some do not trust traditional medicine, and feel that with alternative medicine approaches, they are more in control of making decisions about what is happening to their bodies.

A cancer patient should talk to the doctor or nurse before changing the treatment or adding any alternative methods. Some methods can be safely used along with standard medical treatment. Others may interfere with standard treatment or cause serious side effects.

The American Cancer Society (ACS) encourages people with cancer to consider using methods that have been proven effective or those that are currently under

---

QUESTIONS TO ASK YOUR DOCTOR

- What benefits can I expect from this operation?
- What are the risks of this operation?
- What are the normal results of this operation?
- What happens if this operation does not go as planned?
- Are there any alternatives to this surgery?
- What is the expected recovery time?

---

study. They encourage people to discuss all treatments they may be considering with their physician and other health care providers. The ACS acknowledges that more research is needed regarding the safety and effectiveness of many alternative methods. Unnecessary delays and interruptions in standard therapies could be detrimental to the success of cancer treatment.

At the same time, the ACS acknowledges that certain complementary methods such as aromatherapy, biofeedback, massage therapy, meditation, tai chi, or yoga may be very helpful when used in conjunction with conventional treatment.

Health care team roles

Transurethral bladder resections are usually performed in a hospital by a urologist, a medical doctor who specializes in the diagnosis and treatment of diseases of the urinary systems in men and women and also treats structural problems, tumors, and stones in the urinary system. Urologists can prescribe medications and perform surgery. If a transurethral bladder resection is required by a female patient, and there are complicating factors, an urogynecologist may perform the surgery. Urogynecologists treat urinary problems involving the female reproductive system.

Resources

BOOKS

Miller, Ronald D., et al. *Miller's Anesthesia.* 7th ed. Philadelphia: Churchill Livingstone/Elsevier, 2010.

Raghavan, Derek, and Michael Bailey. *Bladder Cancer.* Abingdon, UK: Health Press, 2006.

Wein, Alan J., et al. *Campbell-Walsh Urology.* 10th ed. Philadelphia: Saunders/Elsevier, 2012.

WEBSITES

American Cancer Society. "Surgery for Bladder Cancer." http://www.cancer.org/cancer/bladdercancer/detailedguide/bladder-cancer-treating-surgery (accessed October 17, 2013).

American Cancer Society. "What Are the Key Statistics about Bladder Cancer?" http://www.cancer.org/cancer/bladdercancer/detailedguide/bladder-cancer-key-statistics (accessed October 14, 2013).

National Cancer Institute. "Bladder Cancer." http://www.cancer.gov/cancertopics/types/bladder (accessed October 14, 2013).

University of Cincinnati Cancer Institute. "Treating Bladder Cancer: TUR (Transurethral Resection)." http://cancer.uc.edu/CancerInfo/TypesOfCancer/BladderCancer/TransurethralResection.aspx (accessed October 14, 2013).

ORGANIZATIONS

American Cancer Society, 250 Williams St. NW, Atlanta, GA 30303, (800) 227-2345, http://www.cancer.org.

National Cancer Institute, 6116 Executive Blvd., Ste. 300, Bethesda, MD 20892-8322, (800) 4-CANCER (422-6237), http://cancer.gov.

National Comprehensive Cancer Network (NCCN), 275 Commerce Dr., Ste. 300, Fort Washington, PA 19034, (215) 690-0300, Fax: (215) 690-0280, http://www.nccn.org.

Kathleen D. Wright, RN
Crystal H. Kaczkowski, MSc
Rosalyn Carson-DeWitt, MD

Transurethral resection of the prostate

Definition

Transurethral resection of the prostate (TURP) is a surgical procedure in which portions of the prostate gland are removed through the urethra.

Purpose

The prostate is a gland that is part of the male reproductive system. It consists of three lobes and surrounds the neck of the bladder and urethra (a tube that channels urine from the bladder to the outside through the tip of the penis). The prostate weighs approximately 1 oz. (28 g) and is walnut-shaped. It is partly muscular and partly glandular, with ducts opening into the urethra. It secretes an antigen called prostate-specific antigen (PSA), and a slightly alkaline fluid that forms part of the seminal fluid (semen) that carries sperm.

The prostate gland undergoes several changes as a man ages. The pea-size gland at birth grows only slightly during puberty and reaches its normal adult shape and size when a male is in his early 20s. The prostate gland remains stable until the mid-40s. At that time, in most men, the number of cells begins to multiply and the gland starts to enlarge.

Enlargement of the prostate causes a common disorder called benign (i.e., noncancerous) prostatic hyperplasia (BPH) or benign prostatic enlargement (BPE). BPH occurs due to hormonal changes in the prostate, and is characterized by the enlargement or overgrowth of the gland because of an increase in the number of its constituent cells. BPH can raise PSA levels two to three times higher than normal. Men with increased PSA levels have a higher chance of developing prostate cancer.

BPH usually affects the innermost part of the prostate first, and enlargement frequently results in a gradual squeezing of the urethra at the point where it runs through the prostate. The squeezing sometimes causes urinary symptoms (referred to as lower urinary tract symptoms, LUTS), which often include:

- straining when urinating
- hesitation before urine flow starts
- dribbling at the end of urination or leakage afterward
- weak or intermittent urinary stream
- painful urination
- inability to completely empty the bladder

Other symptoms (called storage symptoms) sometime appear, and may include:

- urgent need to urinate
- bladder pain when urinating
- increased frequency of urination, especially at night
- bladder irritation during urination

The cause of BPH is not fully understood. It is thought to be caused by a hormone that the prostate gland synthesizes from testosterone called dihydrotestosterone (DHT).

Until the mid 1980s, transurethral resection of the prostate was the treatment of choice for BPH, and the most common surgery performed by urologists. By the mid-2000s, TURP surgery was being performed less frequently because of less invasive alternatives such as microwave therapy and prostatic **laser surgery**. Transurethral refers to the procedure being performed through the urethra. Resection means surgical removal.

Demographics

Before age 40, a small amount of prostatic hyperplasia is present in 80% of males, and about 10% of males under age 40 have fully developed BPH.

Transurethral resection of the prostate

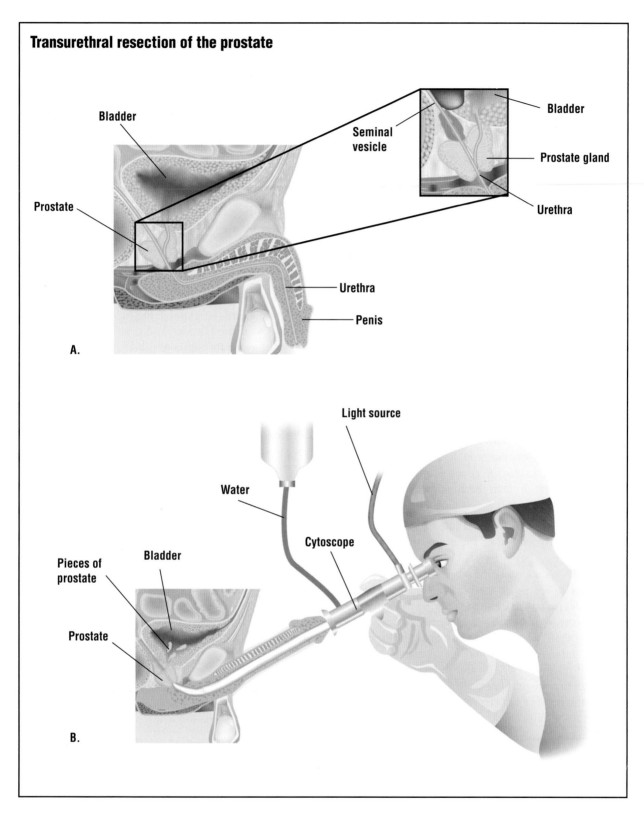

Bladder

Seminal
vesicle

Bladder

Prostate gland

Prostate

Urethra

Urethra

Penis

A.

Light source

Water

Cytoscope

Pieces of
prostate

Bladder

Prostate

B.

An enlarged prostate can cause urinary problems due to its location around the male urethra (A). In TURP, the physician uses a cystoscope to gain access to the prostate through the urethra (B). The prostate material that has been restricting urine flow is cut off in pieces, which are washed into the bladder with water from the scope (B). *(Illustration by GGS Information Services. Copyright © Cengage Learning®.)*

Approximately 8%–31% of males experience moderate to severe LUTS in their fifties. By age 80, about 80% of men have LUTS. A risk factor is the presence of normally functioning testicles; research indicates that castration can minimize prostatic enlargement. It appears that the glandular tissues that multiply abnormally use male hormones produced in the testicles differently than the normal tissues do.

Approximately ten million American men and 30 million men worldwide have symptoms of BPH. It is more prevalent in the United States and Europe, and less common among Asians. BPH is more common in men who are married rather than single, and there is a strong inherited component to the disorder. A man's chance for developing BPH is greater if three of more family members have the condition. The average age of men having TURP surgery is 69.

Description

TURP is a type of surgery that does not involve an external incision. The surgeon reaches the prostate by inserting an instrument through the urethra. In addition to TURP, two other types of transurethral surgery are commonly performed: transurethral incision of the prostate (TUIP), and transurethral laser incision of the prostate (TULIP). The TUIP procedure widens the urethra by making small cuts in the bladder neck (where the urethra and bladder meet) and in the prostate gland itself. In TULIP, a laser beam directed through the urethra melts the tissue.

The actual TURP procedure is simple. It is performed under general or **local anesthesia**. After an intravenous line (IV) is inserted, the surgeon examines the patient with a cystoscope, an instrument that allows him or her to see inside the bladder. The surgeon then inserts a device up the urethra via the penis opening, and removes the excess capsule material that has been restricting the flow of urine. The density of the normal prostate differs from that of the restricting capsule, making it relatively easy for the surgeon to tell exactly how much to remove. After excising the capsule material, the surgeon inserts a catheter into the bladder through the urethra for the subsequent withdrawal of urine.

Diagnosis

Common BPH symptoms include:

• increase in urination frequency

• the need to urinate during the night

• difficulty starting urine flow

• a slow, interrupted flow and dribbling after urinating

• sudden, strong urges to pass urine

KEY TERMS

Benign prostatic hyperplasia (BPH)—Also called benign prostatic enlargement (BPE). Noncancerous enlargement of the prostate gland as a result of an increase in the number of its constituent cells.

Benign tumor—An abnormal growth that is not cancerous (malignant), and does not spread to other areas of the body.

Cryoprostatectomy—Freezing of the prostate through the use of liquid nitrogen probes guided by transrectal ultrasound of the prostate.

Digital rectal exam (DRE)—Procedure in which the physician inserts a gloved finger into the rectum to examine the rectum and the prostate gland for signs of cancer.

Prostate gland—A gland in the male that surrounds the neck of the bladder and urethra. The prostate contributes to the seminal fluid.

Prostatitis—Inflammation of the prostate gland that may be accompanied by discomfort, pain, frequent urination, infrequent urination, and fever.

Protozoan—A single-celled, usually microscopic organism that is eukaryotic and, therefore, different from bacteria (prokaryotic).

Transurethral surgery—Surgery in which no external incision is needed. For prostate transurethral surgery, the surgeon reaches the prostate by inserting an instrument through the urethra.

Urethra—The tube that channels urine from the bladder to the outside. In the female, it measures 1–1.5 in. (25–38 mm); in the male, 9.8 in. (25 cm).

• a sensation that the bladder is not completely empty

• pain or burning during urination

In evaluating the prostate gland for BPH, the physician usually performs a complete **physical examination** as well as the following procedures:

• Digital rectal examination (DRE). Recommended annually for men over age 50, the DRE is an examination performed by a physician who feels the prostate through the wall of the rectum. Hard or lumpy areas may indicate the presence of cancer.

• Prostate-specific antigen (PSA) test. Also recommended annually for men over the age of 50, the PSA test measures the levels of prostate-specific antigen secreted by the prostate. It is normal to observe small quantities of PSA in the blood. PSA levels vary with age, and tend to increase gradually in men over age 60. They also tend to rise as a result of infection (prostatitis), BPH, or cancer.

If the results of the DRE and PSA tests suggest a significant prostate disorder, the examining physician usually refers the patient to a urologist, a medical doctor who specializes in diseases of the urinary tract and male reproductive system. The urologist performs additional tests, including blood and urine studies, to establish a diagnosis.

Patients should select an experienced TURP surgeon to perform the procedure.

Aftercare

When the patient awakens in the recovery room after the procedure, he will already have a catheter in his penis and will be receiving pain medication via the IV line inserted prior to surgery. The initial recovery period lasts approximately one week, and includes some pain and discomfort from the urinary catheter. Spastic convulsions of the bladder and prostate are expected as they respond to the surgical changes.

The following medications or ones similar in function may be prescribed after TURP:

• B&O suppository (belladonna and opium). This medication has the dual purpose of providing pain relief and reducing the ureter and bladder spasms that follow TURP surgery. It is a strong medication that must be used only as prescribed.

• Bulk-forming laxative. Because of the surgical trauma and large quantities of liquids that patients are required to drink, they may need some form of laxative to promote normal bowel movements.

• Detrol. This pain reliever is not as strong as B&O. There may be wide variations in its effectiveness and the patient's response. It also controls involuntary bladder contractions.

• Macrobid. This antibiotic helps prevent urinary tract infections.

• Pyridium. This medication offers symptomatic relief from pain, burning, urgency, frequency, and other urinary tract discomfort.

When discharged from the hospital, patients are advised to avoid weight lifting or strenuous **exercise**. They should check their temperature and report any fever to the physician, and drink plenty of liquids.

Risks

Serious complications have become less common for prostate surgery patients because of advances in operative methods. Nerve-sparing surgical procedures help prevent permanent injury to the nerves that control erection, as well as injury to the opening of the bladder. However, there are risks associated with prostate surgery. The first is the possible development of incontinence (the inability to control urination), which may result in urine leakage or dribbling, especially immediately after surgery. Normal control usually returns within several weeks, but 3% of patients still experience incontinence three months after surgery. There is also a risk of impotence. For a month or so after surgery, most men are not able to become erect. Eventually, approximately 90% of men who were able to have an erection before surgery will be able to have an erection sufficient for sexual intercourse.

Other risks associated with TURP include blood loss requiring **transfusion**, and postoperative urinary tract infections.

TUR syndrome effects about 2% of TURP patients. Symptoms may include temporary blindness due to irrigation fluid entering the bloodstream. On very rare occasions, this can lead to seizures, coma, and even death. The syndrome may also include toxic shock due to bacteria entering the bloodstream, as well as internal hemorrhage.

Results

TURP patients usually notice urine flow improvement as soon as the catheter is removed. Other improvements depend on the condition of the patient's prostate before TURP, his age, and overall health status. Patients are told to expect the persistence of some pre-surgery symptoms. In fact, some new symptoms may appear following TURP, such as occasional blood and tissue in the urine, bladder spasms, pain when urinating, and difficulty judging when to urinate. TURP represents a major adaptation for the body, and healing requires some time. Full recovery may take up to one year. Patients are almost always satisfied with their TURP outcome, and the adaptation to new symptoms is offset by the disappearance of previous problems. For example, most patients no longer have to take daily prostate medication and quickly learn to gradually increase the time between urinating while enjoying uninterrupted and more restful sleep at night.

Normal postoperative symptoms, some of which are often temporary, include:

• urination at night and reduced flow

• mild burning and stinging sensation while urinating

• reduced semen at ejaculation

• bladder control problems

- mild bladder spasm
- fatigue
- urination linked to bowel movements

To eliminate these symptoms, patients are advised to exercise, retrain their bladders, take all medications that were prescribed, and get plenty of rest to facilitate the post-surgery healing process.

Morbidity and mortality rates

TURP improves symptoms in about 90% of BPH patients. Overall, 90-day TURP mortality rates are less than 1.5%. The most common cause of death is an overwhelming systemic infection (sepsis). Following surgery, inadequate relief of BPH symptoms occurs in 20%–25% of patients, and 15%–20% require another operation within ten years. Urinary incontinence affects about 3%, and about 10% of TURP patients become impotent.

Alternatives

Conventional surgical alternatives for BPH patients include:

- Interstitial laser coagulation. In this procedure, a laser beam inserted in the urethra via a catheter heats and destroys the extra prostate capsule tissue.
- Transurethral needle ablation (TUNA). It uses radio waves to heat and destroy the enlarged prostate through needles positioned in the gland. It is generally less effective than TURP for reducing symptoms and increasing urine flow.
- Transurethral electrovaporization. This procedure is a modified version of TURP, and uses a device that produces electronic waves to vaporize the enlarged prostate.
- Photoselective vaporization of the prostate (PVP). This procedure uses a strong laser beam to vaporize the tissue in a 20–50 minute outpatient operation.
- Transurethral incision of the prostate (TUIP). In this procedure, a small incision is made in the bladder, followed by a few cuts into the sphincter muscle to release some of the tension.
- Transurethral microwave thermotherapy (TUMT). TUMT uses microwave heat energy to shrink the enlarged prostate through a probe inserted into the penis to the level of the prostate. This outpatient procedure takes about one hour. The patient can go home the same day, and is able to resume normal activities within a day or two. TUMT does not lead to immediate improvement, and it usually takes up to four weeks for urinary problems to completely resolve.

QUESTIONS TO ASK YOUR DOCTOR

- What are the alternative treatments for benign prostatic hyperplasia?
- What are the risks involved with TURP?
- How long will it take to recover from the surgery?
- How painful is the TURP surgery?
- When and how often will the catheter require flushing?
- How long will it take to feel improvement?
- What are the postoperative problems?
- How will the surgery affect the ability to achieve erection?
- How many TURP procedures does the surgeon perform in a year?
- Will the surgery have to be repeated?

- Water-induced thermotherapy (WIT). WIT is administered via a closed-loop catheter system, through which heated water is maintained at a constant temperature. WIT is usually performed using only a local anesthetic gel to anesthetize the penis, and is very well tolerated. The procedure is FDA approved.
- Balloon dilation. In this procedure, a balloon is inserted in the urethra up to where the restriction occurs. At that point, the balloon expands to push out the prostate tissue and widen the urinary path. Improvements with this technique may only last a few years.

Some BPH patients have experienced improved prostate health from the following:

- Zinc supplements. This mineral plays an important role in prostate health because it decreases prolactin secretion and protects against heavy metals such as cadmium. Both prolactin and cadmium have been associated with BPH.
- Saw palmetto. Saw palmetto has long been used by Native Americans to treat urinary tract disturbances without causing impotence. It shows no significant side effects. A number of recent European clinical studies have also shown that fat soluble extracts of the berry help increase urinary flow and relieve other urinary problems resulting from BPH.
- Garlic. Garlic is believed to contribute to overall body and prostate health.
- Pumpkin seed oil. This oil contains high levels of zinc and has been shown to help most prostate disorders.

Eating raw pumpkin seeds each day has long been a folk remedy for urinary problems, but German health authorities have recently recognized pumpkin seeds as a legitimate BPH treatment.

• Pygeum bark. The bark of the *Pygeum africanus* tree has been used in Europe since early times in the treatment of urinary problems. In France, 81% of BPH prescriptions are for Pygeum bark extract.

Health care team roles

Transurethral resection of the prostate is performed in hospitals by experienced urologic **surgeons** who specialize in prostate disorders and in performing the TURP procedure.

Resources

BOOKS

Blute, Michael, ed. *Mayo Clinic on Prostate Health*. 2nd ed. Rochester, MN: Mayo Clinic, 2003.

Katz, Aaron E. *The Definitive Guide to Prostate Cancer: Everything You Need to Know about Conventional and Integrative Therapies*. New York: Rodale, 2011.

Scardino, Peter T., and Judith Kelman. *Dr. Peter Scardino's Prostate Book: The Complete Guide to Overcoming Prostate Cancer, Prostatitis, and BPH*. 2nd ed. New York: Avery, 2010.

PERIODICALS

Lattouf, J. B. "Antibiotic Use Prior to Transurethral Resection of the Prostate: Are We Doing What We Think We Are Doing?" *Canadian Urological Association Journal* 7, nos. 7–8 (2013): E543.

Omar, M. I. "Systematic Review and Meta-Analysis of the Clinical Effectiveness of Bipolar Compared to Monopolar Transurethral Resection of the Prostate." *BJU International* (June 13, 2013): e-pub ahead of print. http://dx.doi.org/10.1111/bju.12281 (accessed October 17, 2013).

WEBSITES

A.D.A.M. Medical Encyclopedia. "Transurethral Resection of the Prostate." MedlinePlus. http://www.nlm.nih.gov/medlineplus/ency/article/002996.htm (accessed October 17, 2013).

Johns Hopkins Medicine. "Transurethral Resection of the Prostate (TURP)." http://www.hopkinsmedicine.org/healthlibrary/test_procedures/urology/transurethral_resection_of_the_prostate_turp_92,P09349 (accessed October 17, 2013).

Mayo Clinic staff. "Transurethral Resection of the Prostate (TURP)." MayoClinic.com. http://www.mayoclinic.com/health/turp/MY00633 (accessed October 17, 2013).

ORGANIZATIONS

American Prostate Society, 10 E. Lee St., Ste. 1504, Baltimore, MD 21202, (410) 837-3735, Fax: (410) 837-8510, info@americanprostatesociety.com, http://americanprostatesociety.com.

Urology Care Foundation, 1000 Corporate Blvd., Linthicum, MD 21090, (410) 689-3700, (800) 828-7866, Fax: (410) 689-3998, info@urologycarefoundation.org, http://auafoundation.org.

Monique Laberge, PhD
Tish Davidson, AM

▌Trauma surgery

Definition

Trauma surgery is the invasive treatment of serious or life-threatening physical injuries, usually in an emergency situation. In the United States, trauma surgery as a specialty now often encompasses emergency **general surgery** and critical care surgery and is referred to as acute care surgery (ACS).

Purpose

The purpose of trauma surgery is to save lives and minimize long-term effects from injuries resulting from accidents, manmade and natural disasters, and combat. Trauma surgery is required for severe penetrating or blunt injuries, typically caused by automobile accidents, explosions, gunshot or knife wounds, falls, beatings, or burns. Patients transported to trauma centers generally have multiple injuries involving several organ systems. Thus, trauma surgery may involve several different body parts including internal organs, the brain, and/or the

Common causes of trauma, 2012	
Motor-vehicle related	312,983
Falls	309,543
Lacerations	35,193
Firearms	33,649
Burns (including open flames and hot objects/substances)	17,272
Bicycle accidents	14,342
Machine related	7,833
Natural/environmental (including animal bites and stings)	7,558
Overexertion	2,595
Other	32,331

SOURCE: American College of Surgeons, *National Trauma Data Bank 2012 Annual Report*, 2012. Available online at: http://www.facs.org/trauma/ntdb/pdf/ntdb-annual-report-2012.pdf (accessed September 3, 2013).

(Table by PreMediaGlobal. Copyright © 2014 Cengage Learning®.)

extremities. In large-scale emergencies or disasters, trauma surgery may mobilize all available **surgeons** and hospitals in the region.

Demographics

Worldwide, traumatic injury is the leading cause of death in people up to age 45, accounting for almost six million deaths and 100 million hospitalizations annually. Approximately 1.2 million people die in traffic accidents yearly, 90% of them in low-income and middle-income countries. By 2030, road accidents are expected to be the fifth leading cause of death worldwide and the third leading cause of disability. In the United States, there are more than 150,000 deaths from injury every year, including almost 40,000 suicides and homicides, and more than three million nonfatal accidents.

In the United States, traumatic brain injury (TBI) affects one million people annually. It is the number one cause of death from trauma, accounting for one-third of all trauma deaths. Every year, 230,000 people are hospitalized for TBI, and 80,000–90,000 suffer long-term disabilities. More than five million people in the United States are living with disabilities due to TBI.

Description

Trauma surgery includes a wide variety of general, thoracic, orthopedic, and vascular surgeries, as well as **neurosurgery** and all aspects of critical and intensive care medicine. Whether to perform surgery for head trauma is often one of the first decisions a trauma surgeon must make. Evidence of hemorrhage, penetration by a foreign object, or depressed skull fractures are among the indications for trauma surgery. **Craniotomy** is the opening of the skull to reduce pressure on the brain and remove blood clots. Craniectomy is the removal of part of the skull to allow the brain to swell. Craniectomy may be performed in conjunction with blood clot removal. The bone is usually replaced several months later.

In addition to TBI, hemorrhagic shock from excessive bleeding and severe musculoskeletal injury are major aspects of acute trauma. Hemorrhagic shock is the cause of most preventable trauma-related deaths. However, most trauma surgery is now concerned with musculoskeletal injury, which is the cause of much trauma-related disability. The prevalence of musculo-skeletal trauma surgery is due, in part, to advanced treatments for traumatic neck, chest, and abdominal injuries that do not involve surgery. This reduction in the need for trauma surgery not related to the musculoskeletal system has led many U.S. trauma surgeons to devote at least a portion of their practice to general **emergency surgery**.

Other common trauma surgeries include:

- tracheotomy—an incision in the throat over the trachea for the insertion of a breathing tube to replace a temporary breathing tube through the mouth; often performed at the patient's bedside
- suction to remove secretions from the mouth and lungs and suction lines implanted during surgery to remove fluid from the body
- thoracotomy to open the chest
- gastrostomy to open up the stomach for placement of a temporary feeding tube; often performed at the patient's bedside
- jejunostomy—creating an opening for a feeding tube in the small intestine
- laparotomy—opening of the abdomen for examination and treatment of organs, arteries, or other blood vessels

For abdominal injuries, trauma surgeons may use a prescribed order of procedures known as "damage control":

- recognition of hemorrhagic shock
- abbreviated initial abdominal surgery (laparotomy) for control of bleeding and contamination
- subsequent re-examination of the abdominal organs, including relief of symptoms, restoration of the continuity of the gastrointestinal tract, and temporary or permanent closing of the abdominal wall
- final reconstruction of the gastrointestinal tract, if necessary

Mass trauma—the Boston Marathon bombings

Automobile accidents and incidents such as gunshot wounds generally involve only one or a few trauma victims requiring surgery. Natural disasters, airplane crashes, terrorist attacks, and combat can generate large numbers of victims, requiring all of the community's trauma resources. The terrorist bombs that exploded near the finish line of the Boston Marathon on April 15, 2013, killing three and injuring 264 people, required the mobilization of all of the city's trauma facilities and surgeons. Many lives were saved because of the large number of first responders and medical personnel already on location to treat overheated and injured runners; their ability to apply tourniquets to the injured at the scene prevented countless deaths from fatal bleeding. The immediate decision to utilize all 27 nearby hospitals avoided overwhelming individual trauma centers. The hospitals responded by clearing out their emergency departments, sending patients home or to beds elsewhere in the buildings. The hospitals also cleared out their ICUs. Surgeons and other operating and emergency department personnel throughout the city were called in with text messages, since cell phone service was curtailed to prevent the detonation of any additional bombs.

The response to the mass casualties of the Boston Marathon bombings has been described as exemplary. Trauma surgeons reported that the assessment of patients—some arriving two to an ambulance—was calm and efficient. Some victims were sent directly to trauma surgery for stabilization and to halt bleeding; others went directly to ICUs. Using a tactic adopted by military trauma surgeons in Iraq, patients' **vital signs** and injuries were written on their chests in felt markers—far away from leg injuries—to guard against charts being lost between the emergency department and the **operating room**.

The Boston injuries were similar to those seen in battlefield casualties, with limbs blown off, extensive blood loss, and burns. There were also many head and chest wounds. Because the bombs exploded on the ground and were filled with ball bearings, shrapnel, and nails, most of the victims had leg injuries that included shredded tissue, shattered bones, and debris buried deep in tissues. Although most Boston trauma surgeons had treated shattered limbs, few had ever treated so many at once; nor had most of the surgeons treated bomb blast victims. Surgeons were forced to make instant decisions about whether to amputate or attempt to save a limb. In some cases, limbs had to be amputated to stop the bleeding; in other cases, there was too little left to save. Experienced trauma surgeons can usually recognize from artery or nerve damage which legs cannot be saved. Although a leg may be saved temporarily, this might only delay an **amputation** that eventually takes place after multiple failed surgeries and much pain and suffering. Combat casualties have indicated that about 20% of severe traumatic leg injuries require amputation. Nevertheless, the surgeons tried desperately to save the legs of children. They also worked hard to preserve knees, because a prosthesis is much more effective with an intact knee joint. The mobility provided by prostheses improves the chances of long-term survival, since mobility reduces stress on the heart and lungs. Since the Boston trauma rooms had multiple surgeons, there were often two surgeons to concur on each decision. In addition to amputating or repairing shattered legs, the Boston trauma surgeons removed as many as 40 nails, ball bearings, and metal and glass fragments from patient's legs. Victims with large blast wounds required **plastic surgery**.

Preparation

Hospitals, trauma surgeons, emergency personnel, and first responders practice disaster preparedness, often under the direction of the U.S. Centers for Disease Control and Prevention (CDC). Disaster drills for different

scenarios are conducted on local, regional, and national levels. Coordination among trauma facilities and physicians is one of the top priorities of disaster preparedness.

Aftercare

Recovery from trauma surgery and subsequent rehabilitation is often a long and difficult process. About 25% of the Boston Marathon victims whose legs were saved faced multiple future surgeries and the continued risk of infection. Many of the Boston victims required additional surgeries on subsequent days following the attack.

Level 1 trauma centers generally have psychiatric services available for trauma surgery patients, and a 2013 study documented a significant need for such services. Among 25 patients examined at a surgical follow-up clinic, 13 met the criteria for post-traumatic stress disorder (PTSD), 11 met the criteria for moderate-to-severe depression, and five appeared to have alcohol-related problems. On an assessment tool for violence, 15 characterized themselves as victims of violence and 12 as perpetrators of violence.

Results

Recent decades have seen significant improvements in trauma systems, resuscitation, assessment of trauma victims, and emergency care. There has also been significant progress in understanding the physiological processes and underlying molecular changes that occur within minutes or seconds of a traumatic injury, and the ways in which these processes are affected by resuscitation and surgery and are closely associated with patient outcomes. One of the results of improved trauma care has been a significant reduction in trauma surgeries. Nevertheless, the U.S. Institute of Medicine has identified a crisis in the distribution of and access to emergency care that may affect the efficiency and effectiveness of trauma care. For example, although traumas can occur anywhere, most trauma surgeons in the United States are located at larger medical centers. Furthermore, fewer new doctors are choosing to specialize in trauma surgery. The decision to redefine trauma surgery in the United States as acute care surgery came about, in part, because competence in trauma surgery has been declining. This appears to be due to the neglect of trauma surgery by medical school curricula and improvements in traffic and occupational safety that have reduced the need for trauma surgery.

Health care team roles

Trauma surgery requires complex decision-making, usually with very little time and incomplete information. Trauma surgeons are responsible for the initial resuscitation and stabilization of patients. The process of prioritizing diagnostic and surgical procedures begins immediately upon arrival in the emergency department. Patients are initially evaluated according to set protocols called triage for diagnosing and addressing life-threatening conditions first. Triage for prioritizing injuries and conditions is the responsibility of a trauma surgeon. After any life-threatening conditions have been either ruled out or treated, other injuries and conditions are addressed. Diagnostic and treatment procedures initiated in the emergency department are continued in the operating room and **intensive care unit** (ICU) and upon transfer to the appropriate hospital floor. The design of the overall treatment plan is the responsibility of the trauma surgeon.

Trauma surgeons typically operate on injuries to the neck, chest, abdomen, and extremities. In the United States and the United Kingdom, trauma orthopedic surgeons treat skeletal injuries, and maxillofacial surgeons may treat facial injuries. In much of Europe, trauma surgeons treat most musculoskeletal injuries, whereas neurosurgeons treat injuries to the central nervous system. Other specific types of trauma surgery may be performed

QUESTIONS TO ASK YOUR DOCTOR

- Do I need surgery?
- How soon will I have surgery?
- Who will perform the surgery?
- What will happen in the surgery?
- What is my prognosis?

by cardiothoracic surgeons, plastic surgeons, vascular surgeons, and interventional radiologists.

The attending trauma surgeon is in charge of the entire trauma team, which includes critical care nurses, support staff, and resident physicians. Trauma surgeons have usually completed a residency in general surgery and often have additional fellowship training in trauma or critical care surgery. The roles of trauma surgeons differ from those of other surgeons, in part, because of the greater emphasis on intensive care. Trauma surgeons perform many more bedside surgeries, such as tracheostomies and gastrostomies. Approximately 20% of trauma surgeries are performed at the patient's bedside. In contrast, general surgeons perform virtually no bedside surgeries.

Resources

BOOKS

Britt, L. D., and Andrew B. Peitzman. *Acute Care Surgery.* Philadelphia: Wolters Kluwer Health/Lippincott Williams & Wilkins, 2012.

Gadsden, Jeff. *Regional Anesthesia in Trauma: A Case-Based Approach.* Cambridge, UK: Cambridge University, 2012.

Giannoudis, Peter V., and Hans-Christoph Pape. *Practical Procedures in Orthopaedic Trauma Surgery.* Cambridge, UK: Cambridge University, 2014.

Mattox, Kenneth L., Ernest Eugene Moore, and David V. Feliciano. *Trauma.* 7th ed. New York: McGraw-Hill Medical, 2013.

Moore, Laura J., Krista L. Turner, and S. Rob Todd. *Common Problems in Acute Care Surgery.* New York: Springer, 2013.

Peitzman, Andrew B. *The Trauma Manual: Trauma and Acute Care Surgery.* 4th ed. Philadelphia: Wolters Kluwer Health/Lippincott Williams & Wilkins, 2013.

PERIODICALS

Conrad, Erich J., et al. "Assessment of Psychiatric Symptoms at a Level I Trauma Center Surgery Follow-up Clinic: A Preliminary Report." *American Surgeon* 79, no. 5 (May 2013): 492–4.

Kolata, Gina, Jeré Longman, and Mary Pilon. "Saving Lives, if Not Legs, With No Time to Fret." *New York Times* (April 17, 2013): A1.

Montgomery, David, Mary Beth Sheridan, and Lenny Bernstein. "Shrapnel Shredded Victims' Legs, Feet." *Washington Post* (April 17, 2013): A8.

OTHER

University of Arizona Medical Center. *A Guide for Family and Friends of Trauma Patients.* December 2012. http://surgery.arizona.edu/sites/surgery.arizona.edu/files/docs/Trauma%20Patient%20Guide.pdf (accessed October 23, 2013).

WEBSITES

Kaplan, Lewis J. "Critical Care Considerations in Trauma." Medscape Reference. http://emedicine.medscape.com/article/434445-overview (accessed September 23, 2013).

Trauma Survivors Network at Vanderbilt. "Common Trauma Surgery Procedures." http://www.vanderbilthealth.com/traumasurvivors/24840 (accessed September 23, 2013).

ORGANIZATIONS

American Association for the Surgery of Trauma, 633 North Saint Clair St., Ste. 2600, Chicago, IL 60611, (800) 789-4006, aast@aast.org, http://www.aast.org.

American Trauma Society, 201 Park Washington Court, Falls Church, VA 22046, (703) 538-3544, Fax: (703) 241-5603, (800) 556-7890, info@amtrauma.org, http://www.amtrauma.org.

International Association for Trauma Surgery and Intensive Care, Secretariat IATSIC c/o ISS/SIC, Seltisbergerstrasse 16, Lupsingen, Switzerland CH-4419, 41 61 815 96 66, Fax: 41 61 811 47 75, iatsic@iss-sic.ch, http://www.iatsic.org.

U.S. Centers for Disease Control and Prevention, 1600 Clifton Rd., Atlanta, GA 30333, (800) CDC-INFO (232-4636), cdcinfo@cdc.gov, http://www.cdc.gov.

Margaret Alic, PhD

Traumatic amputation *see* **Amputation**

Treadmill stress test *see* **Stress test**

Treatment refusal

Definition

Treatment refusal is the guaranteed right of mentally competent adults to decline medical, psychological, or psychiatric treatment and to express their end-of-life treatment preferences with an advance healthcare directive and appointment of a healthcare proxy decision-maker should they be unable to make their own healthcare decisions. Under some circumstances, medical personnel may also refuse treatment to a patient.

Purpose

There are many reasons why people refuse medical treatments for themselves or their children:

- Religious or cultural beliefs may preclude certain types of treatment; for example, some religions have prohibitions against blood transfusions.

- People may disagree with the treatment recommended by their healthcare provider, decide to pursue an alternative treatment, or be unwilling to undergo a treatment that is considered experimental.

- People may be misinformed, as when parents refuse to have their children immunized because they mistakenly believe that routine childhood vaccines are harmful.

- Patients may be unwilling to risk the side effects of a treatment, particularly if the treatment will diminish their quality of life or will not significantly extend their life. Many people have advance directives for refusing treatments that would keep them alive when there is little hope for recovery, including do not resuscitate (DNR) orders. Many people may prefer to die peacefully and painlessly rather than undergo certain treatments.

- Patients with mental disorders such as schizophrenia may refuse treatments because of the side effects of psychiatric drugs or because the drugs exacerbate other medical problems.

- People may refuse treatment because of financial concerns.

There are also various reasons why medical personnel may refuse treatment requested by patients or their families, although these often pose difficult ethical dilemmas. For example, a physician may believe that there would be no benefit or the strong likelihood of additional harm from a treatment requested by a patient. Physicians may decide against placing patients in an **intensive care unit** (ICU), where they would receive aggressive and focused medical intervention, on the basis that they are "too sick to benefit" from intensive care. Some treatment requests may conflict with the religious or moral beliefs of a healthcare provider. These might include requests for contraception, abortion, sterilization, reproductive technologies, gender-reversing treatments or surgeries, or physician-assisted suicide. Some physicians may refuse treatment to patients who are obese or who continue to smoke, arguing that such patients must first make lifestyle changes.

Description

Treatment refusal by patients

The fundamental right of a competent adult to refuse any and all medical treatments, including life-sustaining treatments, is central to medical ethics and supported in law, provided that the patient understands the significance and possible consequences of treatment refusal. In part, this current consensus emerged as a reaction to the paternalistic form of medicine that was often practiced in the past, in which the physician made unilateral treatment decisions. It is now generally recognized that patients are better positioned to understand how treatments may affect their lives than are doctors who may not know their patients well.

According to medical ethics and the law, parents also have the right to refuse treatment for their children. However, authorities sometimes overrule parental rights for the common good. For example, newborns are usually required to be tested for certain medical conditions even without parental consent. Routine immunizations are usually required for children entering school, although parents are often able to opt out of this requirement for religious or other reasons. In some cases, courts may void parental rights to save a child's life; for example, if parents refuse permission for a lifesaving blood **transfusion**. In other cases, courts have allowed older adolescents, referred to as "maturing minors," to refuse treatments that their parents and physicians want for them. For example, courts have sometimes ruled that adolescents with cancer can refuse further chemotherapy that might prolong their lives, if they appear to have the knowledge and experience to make an informed decision.

INFORMED CONSENT. **Informed consent** is designed to ensure that a patient has enough information to decide whether to accept or refuse a treatment. It means that the healthcare providers have explained the treatment and patients have understood:

• their medical condition and the reasons for the treatment

• the treatment procedure

• the risks of the treatment and the likelihood that side effects or complications might occur

• the likelihood that the treatment will be effective

• other treatment options and their risks and benefits

• unknown risks or possible delayed side effects of the treatment

• whether the treatment is needed immediately

Some treatments require written informed consent, meaning that the patient or guardian has read a description of the treatment and signed a form agreeing to it. Written informed consent is required for:

• most surgeries

• advanced or complex procedures such as endoscopy or a needle biopsy

• radiation or chemotherapy for treating cancer

• most vaccines

• some blood tests, such as HIV testing in some states

When patients are unable to make an informed decision—for example, if they are comatose or have advanced Alzheimer's disease—the healthcare provider will attempt to obtain informed consent from a family member or other decision-maker. If a treatment is refused, healthcare providers may tell patients or their proxies that they believe they are not making the best choice, but they should not try to force treatment on patients. Informed consent is not required in emergencies in which any delay in treatment would be dangerous for the patient.

LIFE-SUSTAINING TREATMENTS. Major advances in life-sustaining medical technologies have made treatment refusal a very important issue. Circulatory, respiratory, and other treatments can stave off death, but are not necessarily in a patient's best interest. While life-support or life-prolonging treatments improve conditions for many patients, complications such as kidney failure or serious brain damage may mean that a patient will continue to deteriorate with no hope of recovery despite life-sustaining treatment. Such patients may refuse life-sustaining treatments while continuing to receive palliative care, including pain management and supportive care. Patients also have the right to refuse life-sustaining artificial nutrition and hydration when they can no longer take food and fluids by mouth. However, if there is uncertainty about a patient's preferences, as in the absence of an advance directive, treatment usually continues. If a patient's end-of-life choices are known, doctors must honor those preferences or transfer the patient's care to another doctor. Patients also have the right to suspend life-sustaining treatments at any time. Refusing artificial nutrition and hydration or other life-sustaining treatments at the end of life is not considered an act of suicide.

Patients who cannot make their own decisions do not lose the right to refuse life-sustaining treatment; rather, there is a hierarchy of surrogate decision-makers who must be consulted in the following order:

• the legal guardian

• the spouse

• an adult son or daughter

• a parent

- an adult sibling
- an adult grandchild
- a close friend
- the executor of the patient's estate

Treatment refusal by physicians

A voluntary relationship between physicians and patients is central to medical ethics in the United States—physicians should be free to choose who they treat and patients should be free to choose who treats them. However, this is not always the case. Hospitals cannot allow physicians to refuse to treat admitted patients, and emergency rooms are required to treat all patients in need of immediate care.

If possible, physicians are usually required to consult with patients as to whether they want to be resuscitated after respiratory or cardiac failure and to follow the end-of-life decisions of patients or their surrogate decision-makers. However, there are cases in which physicians believe that requested resuscitation would be inappropriate. They may believe that resuscitation will fail or leave the patient with an extremely poor quality of life.

Physicians routinely make other treatment refusal decisions. An oncologist may refuse to provide further chemotherapy or a surgeon may refuse to perform heart surgery if the risks of complications or death outweigh the chance of any benefit from the treatment. In such cases, patients have the option of consulting another doctor. However, in cases where ICU clinicians want to remove life support from an elderly, comatose patient with a fatal disease, over the objections of the family, the patient has no opportunity to decide or to choose another physician. Such a patient is considered vulnerable and is granted additional protections under medical ethics and the law.

Preparation

If at all possible, treatment refusal decisions should be made by advance directive. Emergency personnel are obligated to stabilize patients for transfer to a hospital, at which point **advance directives** take effect.

Living wills and healthcare proxies

Living wills—also called directives to physicians, healthcare declarations, or medical directives—are written descriptions of end-of-life decisions for medical treatment in the event that people are unable to communicate their decisions directly. They define for families and physicians the medical treatments that are to be implemented and those that are to be refused. Across the United States, there are varying rules as to how living wills are to be applied, and people can write their own living wills or add further instructions to a state-supplied document.

Healthcare proxies—also called **power of attorney** for health care or appointment of a healthcare agent—identify who will make all treatment decisions in the event that patients are unable to speak for themselves. The designation applies to both temporary and permanent incapacitation from illness or injury. Healthcare proxies are often combined with living wills.

KEY TERMS

Against medical advice (AMA)—Treatment refusal by leaving a hospital or other medical facility without being discharged.

Anorexia—A serious eating disorder that can lead to severe weight loss, malnutrition, and death.

Cardiac arrest—Abrupt cessation of the heartbeat.

Cardiopulmonary resuscitation (CPR)—An emergency procedure for restoring breathing and circulation.

Do not resuscitate (DNR)—Instructions to all medical personnel, including emergency medical technicians, that a patient is not to be resuscitated in case of cardiac or respiratory arrest.

Healthcare proxy—Power of attorney for health care through the appointment of a healthcare agent; a document that names a particular person to make medical decisions in the event that patients are incapable of expressing their own preferences.

Informed consent—Patient consent to undergo a medical treatment after being informed of the details of the procedure and the potential risks and benefits.

Intensive care unit (ICU)—A medical facility with specialized care and monitoring for severely ill patients.

Intubation—The insertion of a tube to supply oxygen to the lungs and heart.

Living will—A document that states end-of-life decisions concerning medical treatment.

Palliative care—Care that focuses on relieving pain and suffering at the end of life.

Respiratory arrest—Cessation of breathing due to failure of the lungs to contract.

Resuscitation—Revival after apparent death.

DNR orders

Resuscitation after cardiac or respiratory arrest is one of the most common end-of-life treatment decisions. The success of **cardiopulmonary resuscitation** (CPR) is heavily dependent on how quickly it is initiated and the patient's underlying medical conditions. CPR can disrupt the natural dying process of a person who is already fatally ill. A non-hospital or pre-hospital **DNR order** applies to the stoppage of the heart or breathing, and it is the only advance directive that emergency medical technicians are allowed to follow. CPR will not be performed on anyone with a valid DNR order signed by a physician. Individuals, family members, or appointed healthcare agents can request a DNR order, but it must have a physician's signature. A DNR is not a refusal for any treatment other than resuscitation. A non-hospital DNR is usually an official form, but it may be issued as a bracelet, necklace, or wallet card. It applies only to emergency medical providers; it does not prevent a bystander from attempting resuscitation.

Sometimes patients obtain do-not-intubate orders as well as DNRs. Intubation may prevent cardiac or respiratory arrest when a patient is having difficulty breathing or getting enough oxygen to the heart.

Psychiatric advance directives

Psychiatric advance directives have recently emerged to address the rights and desires of psychiatric patients. Although all 50 states have laws authorizing healthcare directives, some of these specifically exclude decisions involving certain types of psychiatric treatment. In states that authorize psychiatric advance directives, people with mental disorders can indicate their acceptance or refusal of some or all forms of psychiatric treatment prior to periods of mental incapacitation. These directives can also allow for treatment intervention before a condition deteriorates into an emergency situation. Psychiatric advance directives may help avoid court proceedings over involuntary psychiatric treatment. They may also be used to refuse life-sustaining treatment for conditions caused by some psychiatric disorders, such as end-stage anorexia.

Psychiatric advance directives must be drafted when patients are legally competent and can only be used when patients are not competent to make their own decisions; however, determining competence and incompetence can sometimes be difficult. Furthermore, a patient could theoretically revoke an advance directive when incompetent. For example, a directive that specified preferred medications and identified a proxy for treatment decisions could be revoked while the patient was mentally incompetent, and the patient could then refuse all treatment. A

patient could also potentially use a psychiatric advance directive to refuse all treatment under any circumstances. Although U.S. courts have not ruled conclusively on how these directives are to be used, it is likely that directives refusing all treatment could be overridden if patients posed a danger to themselves or others.

Risks

Treatment refusals on the part of either patients or physicians carry obvious risks. Patients may not fully understand the consequences of refusing a treatment. Physicians may make misjudgments when refusing treatments to patients.

Alternatives

Some patients refuse treatment by simply leaving the hospital against medical advice (AMA). They may be forced to sign a statement that they are leaving AMA, or they may simply walk out of the hospital. Leaving AMA could result in a patient's health insurance carrier refusing to cover the hospital stay.

Health care team roles

Patients should talk with the members of their health care team about all of the risks and benefits before deciding to refuse treatment. Hospital ethics committees often provides consultation for patients considering treatment refusal, as well as mediation services for families experiencing disagreements over treatment choices.

Resources

BOOKS

Weller, Penelope. *New Law and Ethics in Mental Health Advance Directives: The Convention on the Rights of Persons with Disabilities and the Right to Choose.* New York: Routledge, 2013.

PERIODICALS

Campbell, Amy T., and Mark P. Aulisio. "The Stigma of 'Mental' Illness: End Stage Anorexia and Treatment Refusal." *International Journal of Eating Disorders* 45, no. 5 (July 2012): 627.

Cordella, Marisa. "Negotiating Religious Beliefs in a Medical Setting." *Journal of Religion and Health* 51, no. 3 (September 2012): 837–53.

Courtwright, Andrew. "Who is 'Too Sick to Benefit.'" *Hastings Center Report* 42, no. 4 (July/August 2012): 41–7.

Goldman, Larry S. "The Role of the Consulting Psychiatrist in Assessment of Patient Decision-Making Capacity." *Psychiatric Annals* 43, no. 2 (February 2013): 72–7.

Horn, Ruth. "Euthanasia and End-of-Life Practices in France and Germany: A Comparative Study." *Medicine, Health Care, and Philosophy* 16, no. 2 (2013): 197–209.

Mirkes, Renée, and Edward A. Morse. "Conscience and Competing Liberty Claims." *Ethics & Medicine* 29, no. 1 (Spring 2013): 23–39.

Omer, Saad B., Walter A. Orenstein, and Jeffrey P. Koplan. "Go Big and Go Fast—Vaccine Refusal and Disease Eradication." *New England Journal of Medicine* 368, no. 15 (April 11, 2013): 1374–6.

Schaefer, Gabrielle R., et al. "Financial Responsibility of Hospitalized Patients Who Left Against Medical Advice: Medical Urban Legend?" *Journal of General Internal Medicine* 27, no. 7 (July 2012): 825–30.

White, Douglas B., and Mark Wisclair. "Limits on Clinicians' Discretion to Unilaterally Refuse Treatment." *American Journal of Critical Care* 21, no. 5 (2012): 361–64.

WEBSITES

A.D.A.M. Medical Encyclopedia. "Informed Consent—Adults." MedlinePlus. http://www.nlm.nih.gov/medlineplus/ency/patientinstructions/000445.htm (accessed September 23, 2013).

Honberg, Ronald S. "Advance Directives." National Alliance on Mental Illness. http://www.nami.org/PrinterTemplate.cfm?Template=/ContentManagement/HTMLDisplay.cfm&ContentID=31398 (accessed September 23, 2013).

New York Methodist Hospital. "Ethics Committee." http://www.nym.org/About-Us/Ethics-Committee.aspx (accessed September 23, 2013).

University of Illinois at Chicago College of Medicine, Ethics in Clerkships. "Duty to Treat." http://www.uic.edu/depts/mcam/ethics/duty.htm (accessed September 23, 2013).

University of Illinois at Chicago College of Medicine, Ethics in Clerkships. "Withdrawal or Limitation of Treatment." http://www.uic.edu/depts/mcam/ethics/withdrawal.htm (accessed September 23, 2013).

ORGANIZATIONS

Agency for Healthcare Research and Quality, 540 Gaither Rd., Ste. 2000, Rockville, MD 20850, (301) 427-1104, http://www.ahrq.gov.

National Alliance on Mental Illness, 3803 North Fairfax Drive, Ste. 100, Arlington, VA 22203, (703) 524-7600, Fax: (703) 524-9094, (800) 950-NAMI (6264), http://www.nami.org.

National Hospice and Palliative Care Organization, 1731 King St., Ste. 100, Alexandria, VA 22314, (703) 837-1500, Fax: (703) 837-1233, (800) 646-6460, nhpco_info@nhpco.org, http://www.nhpco.org.

Margaret Alic, PhD

Tremor reduction surgery *see* **Deep brain stimulation; Pallidotomy**

Triage *see* **Surgical triage**

Triglyceride test *see* **Cholesterol and triglyceride tests**

Trisegmentectomy *see* **Hepatectomy**

Trocars

Definition

A trocar is a surgical instrument. It is a hollow cylinder into which fits another piece called an obturator, which has a pointed or blunt end. It is used to insert various surgical implements into a blood vessel or body cavity. Trocars were originally three-sided pointed instruments, but they are now made in multiple designs with varying degrees of sharpness. Sometimes only the obturator portion is referred to as the trocar and the entire apparatus is referred to as trocar and cannula.

Purpose

Trocars may be used to insert **surgical instruments** during **laparoscopy**, a procedure that allows for examination of the peritoneal cavity with minimal cutting

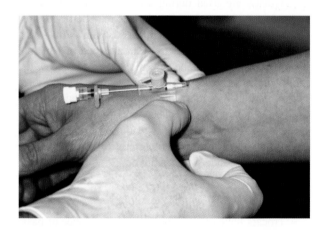

Trocars are used to insert medical equipment into the body—in this case, a thin tube known as a cannula that allows the passage of fluid. *(Science PR/Getty Images)*

of the body wall. Laparoscopic procedures in which trocars are used include **hysterectomy**, endometriosis ablation, and salpingectomy. Trocars can be used to help insert an intravenous cannula (flexible tube) into a blood vessel to allow for the administration of fluids or medication. Trocars may also be used on human cadavers during embalming to assist in draining bodily fluids (a process known as aspiration).

Description

The first trocar used in any laparoscopic procedure is called the primary trocar. The primary trocar is inserted into the peritoneal cavity, and the obturator portion is withdrawn. The insertion of the primary trocar into the peritoneal cavity requires enough force to penetrate the body wall with the obturator, but without damaging the underlying organs. Appropriate training and skill is required to properly insert the primary trocar with guided force, known as a "controlled jab." The cannula remains in the insertion site and is used as an access port through which to put other instruments in place. Through the cannula, the laparoscope (camera) or other surgical tool may be inserted into the body cavity. Once the laparoscope is inserted, the surgeon can view the internal structures of the body. However, when the primary trocar is inserted, it is usually done without being able to view the structures lying just underneath it—sometimes referred to as a "blind jab." Potential for damage to internal organs is decreased by inflating the abdominal cavity with carbon dioxide gas before trocar insertion, to hold the body wall away from the organs. Multiple trocars may be used for each procedure. Laparoscopies commonly require two to five trocars for completion.

Embalming

Trocars are used during the embalming of human cadavers to insert tubes for drainage of bodily fluids. Once the blood has been replaced with embalming chemicals, the trocar is inserted and attached to a suction hose for aspiration. The insertion is made near the umbilicus in order to aspirate the main body cavities. Once the fluid is drained, the trocar is detached from the aspirating hose and attached to a bottle of cavity-embalming fluid. The trocar is then used to fill the body cavities with the fluid. The trocar puncture is sealed with a plastic plug called a trocar button.

Trocar designs

Trocars have evolved from a small number of basic designs to many, with more than 100 different brand names. Trocars may be pointed with a cutting blade at the tip, blunt and bladeless, fitted with a protective shield, or

contain a tiny camera for guided, optical entry into the body.

CUTTING. Cutting trocars have sharp tips designed to create incisions in the body wall and facilitate the insertion of cannulas into the peritoneal cavity. Sharp trocar ends may be conical or three-sided and pyramidal. Multiple types of cutting trocars exist, most of which require blind entry into the peritoneal cavity. Cutting trocars require the least amount of force to insert into the body cavity. However, they cause the greatest amount of post-insertion site pain, scarring, and sometimes hernia formation. Cutting trocars pose the greatest risk for damage to a major blood vessel or puncture of internal organs such as the intestines. Cutting trocars are associated with the greatest number of life-threatening injuries, especially in patients for whom trocar insertion is difficult to perform.

Cutting trocars are positioned onto the ends of some types of drain tubing for ease of insertion following surgical procedures. After insertion, the trocar is cut off so the drain can be attached to a reservoir. Cutting trocars are also sometimes used in conjunction with a purse-string suture in organs such as the gallbladder or stomach for decompression. The trocar is first inserted into the organ and then connected to a suction apparatus.

SHIELDED CUTTING. Shielded cutting trocars have a retractable, protective shield that covers the pointed tip before and after insertion into the peritoneal cavity. The shield was added to trocar designs in 1984 in an attempt to protect the abdominal and pelvic blood vessels and organs from accidental puncture with the trocar tip. For this reason, shielded tips were originally called "safety trocars." However, whether or not the shielded tip is actually effective is controversial. Serious injuries as well as deaths have been associated with shielded trocars. According to trocar safety reviews done by the U.S. Food and Drug Administration (FDA), shielded trocars may have a somewhat improved safety profile if used properly. However, a concern is a mistaken sense of security on the part of the surgeon, leading to inadvertent injury despite the shield. The shield itself has been shown to damage blood vessels, and shielded trocars can still cause life-threatening injury.

BLADELESS. Trocars have also been designed in varying degrees of bluntness to help prevent accidental damage to blood vessels or internal organs. A Hasson trocar is very blunt and pushes through the layers of the abdominal wall instead of cutting them. The tissue fibers are merely separated instead of sliced and can reposition naturally after the trocar is removed. Compared with cutting trocars, the blunt trocars require more force to insert into the peritoneal cavity. However, they create smaller trocar insertion tissue defects that take less time to heal, decrease the incidence of hernia formation, cause less scarring, and cause less pain. Bladeless trocars were designed in an attempt to minimize trocar-related injury or puncture of internal structures.

A Hasson trocar is inserted using the Hasson "cut-down" or "open" technique. Hasson trocars are so blunt-ended that they can only be inserted into the peritoneal cavity after the surgeon makes a small 2 to 3 cm incision through which to push the trocar. Since the surgeon can see the area through which the trocar is penetrating, the procedure does not require blind insertion. The Hasson trocar can then be used along with retractors to introduce other tools such as a laparoscope into the body cavity. The Hasson technique offers the advantage over traditional cutting trocars of being an open technique (as opposed to blind) and so may further minimize risk to blood vessels and internal organs. Whether or not the Hasson technique has succeeded as such is a matter of controversy, with studies especially differing on whether there is any real advantage regarding organ injury. Some types of blunt trocars expand radially upon entry of the abdominal cavity to lift the abdominal wall up and away from the internal structures. Whether this design of trocar confers greater safety margins and reduces risk of injury is also under debate.

OPTICAL. In 1994, a new type of trocar was developed that had a tiny viewing "window" positioned at its tip for a laparoscope. This design eliminates the need for a blind initial puncture by enabling the surgeon to observe the primary trocar insertion through the laparoscope. The surgeon can actually view each tissue layer being penetrated by the trocar device, as well as the underlying abdominal cavity and internal structures. While this design is an improvement over blind insertion trocars, injuries are still reported with optical trocars.

Risks

Trocar use is associated with the risk of life-threatening injury. The most common types of trocar injury are blood vessel damage leading to hemorrhage and bowel injury leading to peritoneal infection. Injuries most commonly occur during the initial insertion of the primary trocar, often a blind insertion. The risk is that the force being applied to penetrate the abdominal wall may accidentally propel the trocar into a blood vessel or puncture an internal organ. Blood vessel hemorrhage or life-threatening bacterial infections may result. Each patient and circumstance requires a different amount of force to be applied for trocar insertion. It requires skill and experience on the part of the surgeon to insert the trocar with sufficient force to penetrate the abdominal cavity, while still maintaining enough control to stop the

movement of the trocar once inserted. The safety margin between the force required for trocar insertion and trocar injury is very slim, especially for children and lean adults. Blunt trocars require more force for insertion than cutting trocars. Despite the blunt edges of these trocars, the extra force required for penetration contributes to the risk of propelling the trocar into and injuring the bowels. Additionally, the larger a trocar is, the greater the risk of injury to the patient. For each patient, **surgeons** use the smallest trocar possible.

Patients who have had prior abdominal surgery have a higher risk of trocar injury. After abdominal surgery, the internal organs and other structures of the abdominal cavity sometimes develop scar tissue that causes adherence to the abdominal wall. If internal structures are attached to the site of trocar entry, even filling the abdomen with carbon dioxide gas is not sufficient to keep them out of the path of injury upon primary trocar insertion. For this reason, blind insertion trocars should not be used on patients with a history of abdominal surgery. If lower abdominal surgery is included in patient history, there is a location that may be safely used for trocar insertion known as Palmer's point. Palmer's point is located in the upper left quadrant of the abdomen and usually does not contain internal structures. Other people at higher risk for injury with blind trocar insertion include children and patients with small and lean body types, alterations in abdomen skin due to multiple pregnancies, or atrophied abdominal musculature. All trocars need to be disposed of properly after the procedure, following established safety precautions.

Potential signs and symptoms of internal hemorrhage into the abdominal cavity include:

- anemia, fatigue, and pallor
- low-grade fever
- increased heart rate
- low blood pressure
- shoulder pain
- dizziness
- faintness
- nausea
- lack of appetite

Potential signs and symptoms of untreated bowel injury include:

- tender abdomen
- pain
- fever and chills
- loss of appetite
- nausea and vomiting
- increased breathing rate

- increased heart rate
- low blood pressure
- decreased urine production
- inability to pass gas or feces

Morbidity and mortality rates

The morbidity and mortality of trocar-related injuries increases when not caught early on. A delay in recognition or treatment of trocar injuries can be fatal for the patient. Injuries occur most frequently with insertion of the primary trocar, which may be the step in laparoscopic procedures associated with the greatest risk.

Trocar use requires extensive training, experience, manual skill, muscular strength, control, and knowledge of the associated risks for each type of patient. Morbidity and mortality are due to a combination of the surgeon's skill level, the type of trocar, and patient-based risk factors. Whether on the part of the patient or the doctor, the failure to recognize the symptoms of injury in a timely manner contribute much to the morbidity and mortality risks of trocar usage.

Alternatives

Some alternatives to procedures with blind trocar insertion include:

- laparotomy
- Hasson open technique
- radially expanding and optical-access trocars
- use of Palmer's point for trocar insertion (for patients with a history of prior abdominal surgery)

Resources

PERIODICALS

Kuru, Timur H., et al. "Improving Accuracy in Image-Guided Prostate Biopsy by Using Trocar-Sharpened Needles." *Urologia Internationalis* (July 2, 2013): e-pub ahead of print. http://dx.doi.org/10.1159/000350653 (accessed August 13, 2013).

Rajab, Taufiek Konrad. "Modified Trocar with Laser Diode for Instrument Guidance." *Surgical Innovation* (June 21, 2013): e-pub ahead of print. http://dx.doi.org/10.1177/1553350613492022 (accessed August 13, 2013).

WEBSITES

Fuller, Janie, et al. "Laparoscopic Trocar Injuries: A Report from a U.S. Food and Drug Administration (FDA) Center for Devices and Radiological Health (CDRH) Systematic Technology Assessment of Medical Products (STAMP) Committee." Silver Spring, MD: FDA, 2003. http://www.fda.gov/MedicalDevices/Safety/AlertsandNotices/ucm197339.htm (accessed August 13, 2013).

ORGANIZATIONS

U.S. Food and Drug Administration, 10903 New Hampshire Ave., Silver Spring, MD 20993, (888) INFO-FDA (463-6332), http://www.fda.gov.

Maria Basile, PhD
Tammy Allhoff, CST/CSFA, AAS

Troponins test *see* **Cardiac marker tests**

Tubal ligation

Definition

Tubal ligation is a permanent voluntary form of birth control (contraception) in which a woman's fallopian

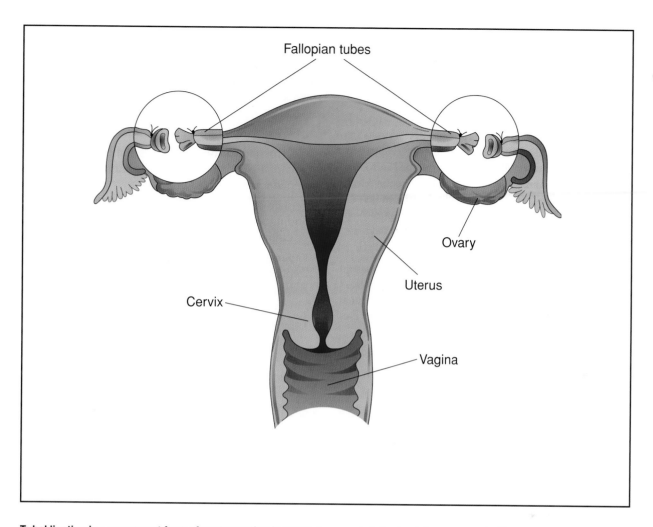

Fallopian tubes

Ovary

Uterus

Cervix

Vagina

Tubal ligation is a permanent form of contraception in which a woman's fallopian tubes are surgically cut, cauterized, tied, or blocked to prevent pregnancy. This procedure blocks the pathway the sperm take to fertilize an egg. *(Illustration by Electronic Illustrators Group. Copyright © Cengage Learning®.)*

tubes are surgically cut, tied, or blocked off to prevent pregnancy. It is important that women understand that tubal ligation prevents only pregnancy, not sexual transmitted infections (STI). Barrier methods are still needed to prevent STIs.

Purpose

Tubal ligation is performed in women who want to prevent future pregnancies. It is frequently chosen by women who do not want more children, but who are still sexually active and potentially fertile and want to be free of the limitations of other types of birth control. Women who should not become pregnant for health concerns or other reasons may also choose this birth control method.

Demographics

Tubal ligation is one of the leading methods of contraception. This form of contraception is chosen by about 650,000–700,000 annually in the United States. The typical tubal ligation patient is over age 30, is married, and has already had two or three children.

Description

Tubal ligation refers to female sterilization, the surgery that ends a woman's ability to conceive. The operation is performed on the patient's fallopian tubes. These tubes, which are about 4 in. (10 cm) long and 0.2 in. (0.5 cm) in diameter, are found on the upper outer sides of the uterus. They open into the uterus through small channels. It is within the fallopian tube that fertilization, the joining of the egg and the sperm, takes place. During tubal ligation, the tubes are cut or blocked in order to close off the sperm's access to the egg.

Normally, tubal ligation takes about 20–30 minutes, and is performed under **general anesthesia**, spinal anesthesia, or **local anesthesia** with sedation. The surgery can be performed on either hospitalized patients within 24 hours after childbirth or on outpatients. The woman can usually leave the hospital the same day.

The most common surgical approaches to tubal ligation include **laparoscopy** and mini-laparotomy. In a laparoscopic tubal ligation, a long, thin telescope-like surgical instrument called a laparoscope is inserted into the pelvis through a small cut about 0.5 in. (1 cm) long near the navel. Carbon dioxide gas is pumped in to help move the abdominal wall to give the surgeon easier access to the tubes. Often, the **surgical instruments** are inserted through a second incision near the pubic hair line. An instrument may be placed through the vagina to hold the uterus in place.

In a mini-laparotomy, a 1.2–1.6 in. (3–4 cm) incision is made just above the pubic bone or under the navel. A larger incision, or laparotomy, is rarely used today. Tubal ligation can also be performed at the time of a **cesarean section**.

Surgical tubal ligation itself is performed in several ways, including:

• Electrocoagulation. A heated needle connected to an electrical device is used to cauterize or burn the tubes. Electrocoagulation is the most common method of tubal ligation.

• Falope ring. In this technique, an applicator is inserted through an incision above the bladder and a plastic ring is placed around a loop of the tube.

• Hulka clip. The surgeon places a plastic clip across a tube held in place by a steel spring.

• Silicone rubber bands. A band placed over a tube forms a mechanical block to sperm.

Tubal ligation costs between $1,500 and $6,000 when performed by a private physician, but is less expensive when performed at a family planning clinic. Most insurance plans cover treatment costs.

Precautions

Tubal ligation should be postponed if the woman is unsure about her decision. While the procedure is sometimes reversible, it should be considered permanent and irreversible. As many as 10% of sterilized women regret having had the surgery, and about 1% seek treatment to restore their fertility.

Preparation

Preparation for tubal ligation includes patient education and counseling. Before surgery, it is important that the woman understands the permanent nature of tubal ligation as well as the risks of anesthesia and

KEY TERMS

Contraception—The prevention of the union of the male's sperm with the female's egg.

Ectopic pregnancy—The implantation of a fertilized egg in a fallopian tube instead of the uterus.

Electrocoagulation—The coagulation or destruction of tissue through the application of a high-frequency electrical current.

Female sterilization—The process of permanently ending a woman's ability to conceive by tying off or cutting apart the fallopian tubes.

Laparoscopy—Abdominal surgery performed through a laparoscope, which is a thin telescopic instrument inserted through an incision near the navel.

Laparotomy—A procedure in which the surgeon opens the abdominal cavity to inspect the patient's internal organs.

Vasectomy—Surgical sterilization of the male, done by removing a portion of the tube that carries sperm to the urethra.

surgery. Her medical history is reviewed, and a **physical examination** and laboratory testing are performed. The patient is not allowed to eat or drink for several hours before surgery.

Aftercare

After surgery, the patient is monitored for several hours before she is allowed to go home. She is instructed on care of the surgical wound, and what signs to watch for, such as fever, nausea, vomiting, faintness, or pain. These signs could indicate that complications have occurred.

Risks

While major complications are uncommon after tubal ligation, there are risks with any surgical procedure. Possible side effects include infection and bleeding. After laparoscopy, the patient may experience pain in the shoulder area from the carbon dioxide used during surgery, but the technique is associated with less pain than mini-laparotomy, as well as a faster recovery period. Mini-laparotomy results in a higher incidence of pain, bleeding, bladder injury, and infection compared with laparoscopy. Patients normally feel better after three to four days of rest, and are able to resume sexual activity at that time.

The possibility for treatment failure is very low—about 5 women per 1,000 will become pregnant during the first year after sterilization. The failure rate increases over time, so that ten years after the procedure, the failure rate is 18 women per 1,000. Failure can happen if the cut ends of the tubes grow back together; if the tube was not completely cut or blocked off; if a plastic clip or rubber band has loosened or come off; or if the woman was already pregnant at the time of surgery.

Results

After having her tubes tied, a woman does not need to use any form of birth control to avoid pregnancy. Tubal ligation is almost 100% effective for the prevention of conception.

Morbidity and mortality rates

About 1%–4% of patients experience complications following tubal ligation. There is a low risk (less than 1%, or 7 per 1,000 procedures) of a later ectopic pregnancy. Ectopic pregnancy is a condition in which the fertilized egg implants in a place other than the uterus, usually in one of the fallopian tubes. Ectopic pregnancies are more likely to happen in younger women, and in women whose tubes were closed off by electrocoagulation.

Rarely, death may occur as a complication of general anesthesia if a major blood vessel is cut. The mortality rate of tubal ligation is about 4 in 100,000 sterilizations.

Post-ligation regret is a very real issue for some women. Women under the age of 20 have rates as high as 20%, while those over 30 have 6% regret rates. Because of these issues, it is crucial that women receive adequate and sensitive counseling prior to undergoing tubal ligation.

Alternatives

There are numerous options available to women who wish to prevent pregnancy. Oral contraceptives are the second most common form of contraception—the first being female sterilization—and have a success rate of 95%–99.5%. Other methods of preventing pregnancy include **vasectomy** (99.9% effective) for the male partner; the male condom (86%–97% effective); the diaphragm or cervical cap (80%–94% effective); the female condom (80%–95% effective); and abstinence.

Fallopian tube implants

Another nonsurgical but permanent method of contraception is fallopian tube implants, which involves inserting metal springs into the fallopian tubes to block the passage of an egg. Over the course of about three months, this implant stimulates an inflammatory and fibrotic response that results in blockage of the tubes, preventing sperm from reaching and fertilizing the eggs. The procedure is done on an outpatient basis and does not usually take more than 30–60 minutes. During the procedure, the woman is placed in the same position as during a yearly pelvic exam. On occasion a physician may insert laminaria into the cervix several hours prior to the procedure to gradually open the cervix. Laminaria are small sticks of dehydrated seaweed that slowly absorb moisture and gradually expand to open the cervix. If laminaria is not used prior to the procedure, then during the procedure, instruments are used to gradually open the cervix. A catheter is placed through the cervical opening and into the fallopian tube, where the small metal spring is placed. This is repeated for the other fallopian tube. After the procedure, an x-ray is performed to make sure that both implants are properly placed, and a follow-up visit should be scheduled for three months after insertion. Fallopian tube implant placement requires the use of other contraceptive methods for at least three months. A diagnostic test is then performed to verify that the tubes are completely blocked, and that adjunct contraceptive methods are no longer necessary.

Health care team roles

Tubal ligation is generally performed by an obstetrician/gynecologist, a medical doctor who has completed specialized training in the areas of women's general health, pregnancy, labor and childbirth, **prenatal testing**, and genetics. The procedure is performed in a hospital or family planning clinic, and usually as an outpatient procedure.

QUESTIONS TO ASK YOUR DOCTOR

- How many tubal ligations do you perform each year?
- What method of ligation will you use?
- What form of anesthesia will be used?
- How long will the procedure take?
- What side effects or complications might I expect?
- What is your failure rate?

Resources

BOOKS

Lentz, Gretchen, et al. *Comprehensive Gynecology.* 5th ed. St. Louis: Mosby/Elsevier, 2012.

WEBSITES

Centers for Disease Control and Prevention. "Female Sterilization: Risk of Ectopic Pregnancy After Tubal Sterilization Fact Sheet." http://www.cdc.gov/reproductivehealth/UnintendedPregnancy/EctopicPreg_factsheet.htm (accessed October 21, 2013).

MedlinePlus. "Tubal Ligation." U.S. National Library of Medicine, National Institutes of Health. http://www.nlm.nih.gov/medlineplus/tuballigation.html (accessed October 21, 2013).

ORGANIZATIONS

American Congress of Obstetricians and Gynecologists, 409 12th St. SW, Washington, DC 20024-2188, (202) 638-5577, (800) 673-8444, resources@acog.org, http://www.acog.org.

International Planned Parenthood Federation, 4 Newhams Row, London, SE1 3UZ, United Kingdom, +44 20 7939 8200, info@ippf.org, http://ippf.org.

Planned Parenthood Federation of America, 434 W. 33rd St., New York, NY 10001, (212) 541-7800, (800) 230-PLAN (7526), Fax: (212) 245-1845, http://www.plannedparenthood.org.

Mercedes McLaughlin
Stephanie Dionne Sherk
Rosalyn Carson-DeWitt, MD

Tube enterostomy

Definition

Tube enterostomy, or tube feeding, is a form of enteral or intestinal site feeding that employs a **stoma** or semi-permanent surgically placed tube to the small intestines.

Purpose

Many patients are unable to take in food by mouth, esophagus, or stomach. A number of conditions can render a person unable to take in nutrition through the normal pathways. Neurological conditions or injuries, injuries to the mouth or throat, obstructions of the stomach, cancer or ulcerative conditions of the gastrointestinal tract, and certain surgical procedures can make it impossible for a person to receive oral nutrition. Tube feeding is indicated for patients unable to ingest adequate nutrition by mouth, but who may have a cleared passage

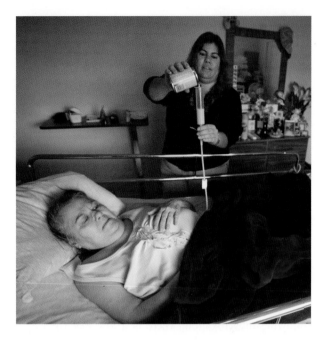

A woman feeds her mother through the use of tube enterostomy. *(MCT via Getty Images)*

in the esophagus and stomach, and even partial functioning of the gastrointestinal tract. Enteral nutrition procedures that utilize the gastrointestinal tract are preferred over intravenous feeding or parenteral nutrition because they maintain the function of the intestines, provide for immunity to infection, and avoid complications related to intravenous feeding.

Tube enterostomy, a feeding tube placed directly into the intestines or jejunum, is one such enteral procedure. It is used if the need for enteral feeding lasts longer than six weeks, or if it improves the outcomes of drastic surgeries such as removal or resection of the intestines. Recently, it has become an important technique for use in surgery in which a gastrectomy—resection of the intestinal link to the esophagus—occurs. The procedure makes healing easier, and seeks to retain the patient's nutritional status and quality of life after **reconstructive surgery**. Some individuals have a tube enterostomy surgically constructed, and successfully utilize it for a long period of time.

There are a variety of enteral nutritional products, liquid feedings with the nutritional quality of solid food. Patients with normal gastrointestinal function can benefit from these products. Other patients must have nutritional counseling, monitoring, and precise nutritional diets developed by a health care professional.

Demographics

Tube enterostomy provides temporary enteral nutrition to patients with injuries as well as inflammatory,

KEY TERMS

Enteral nutritional support—Nutrition utilizing an intact gastrointestinal tract, but bypassing another organ such as the stomach or esophagus.

Parenteral nutritional support—Intravenous nutrition that bypasses the intestines and its contribution to digestion.

Stoma—A portal fashioned from the side of the abdomen that allows for ingestion into or drainage out of the intestines or urinary tract.

Tube feeding—Feeding or nutrition through a tube placed into the body through the esophagus, nose, stomach, intestines, or via a surgically constructed artificial orifice called a stoma.

obstructive, and other intestinal, esophageal, and abdominal conditions. Other uses include patients with pediatric abnormalities, and those who have had surgery for cancerous tumors of the gastroesophageal junction (many of these cases are associated with Barrett's epithelium). Intestinal cancers in the United States have declined since the 1950s. However, this endemic form of gastric cancer is one of the most common causes of death from malignant disease, with an estimated 798,000 annual cases worldwide; 21,900 in the United States. As gastric cancer has declined, esophageal cancers have increased, requiring surgeries that resect and reconstruct the passage between the esophagus and intestine.

Description

Tube enterostomy refers to placement via a number of surgical approaches:

• laparoscopy

• esophagostomy (open surgery via the esophagus)

• stomach (gastrostomy or PEG)

• upper intestines or jejunum (jejunostomy)

The appropriate method depends on the clinical prognosis, anticipated duration of feeding, risk of aspirating or inhaling gastric contents, and patient preference. Whether through a standard operation or with laparoscopic surgical techniques, the surgeon fashions a stoma or opening into the esophagus, stomach, or intestines, and inserts a tube from the outside through which nutrition will be introduced. These tubes are made of silicone or polyurethane, and contain weighted tips and insertion features that facilitate placement. The surgery is fairly simple to perform, and most patients have good outcomes with stoma placement.

Preparation

A number of conditions necessitate tube enterostomy for nutritional support. Many are chronic and require a complete medical evaluation including history, **physical examination**, and extensive imaging tests. Some conditions are critical or acute, and may emerge from injuries or serious inflammatory conditions in which the patient is not systematically prepared for the surgery. In many cases, the patient undergoing this type of surgery has been ill for a period of time. Sometimes the patient is a small child or adult who accidentally swallowed a caustic substance. Some are elderly patients who have obstructive carcinoma of the esophagus or stomach.

Optimal preparation includes an evaluation of the patient's nutritional status, and his or her potential requirements for blood transfusions and **antibiotics**. Patients who do not have gastrointestinal inflammatory or obstructive conditions are usually required to undergo **bowel preparation** that flushes the intestines of all material. The bowel preparation reduces the chances of infection.

The patient's acceptance of tube feeding as a substitute for eating is of paramount importance. Health care providers must be sensitive to these problems, and offer early assistance and feedback in the self-care that the tube enterostomy requires.

In preparation for surgery, patients learn that the tube enterostomy will be an artificial orifice placed outside the abdomen through which they will deliver their nutritional support. Patients are taught how to care for the stoma, cleaning and making sure it functions optimally. In addition, patients are prepared for the loss of the function of eating and its place in their lives. They must be made aware that their physical body will be altered, and that this may have social implications and affect their intimate activities.

Aftercare

Tube enterostomy requires monitoring the patient for infection or bleeding, and educating him or her on the proper use of the enterostomy. According to the type of surgery—minimally invasive or open surgery—it may take several days for the patient to resume normal functioning. Fluid intake and urinary output must be monitored to prevent dehydration.

Risks

Tube enterostomies are not considered high risk surgeries. Insertions have been completed in over 90% of attempts. Possible complications include diarrhea, skin irritation due to leakage around the stoma, and difficulties with tube placement.

QUESTIONS TO ASK YOUR DOCTOR

- How long will the tube enterostomy remain in place?
- How much assistance will be given in adjusting to the stoma and the special diet?
- If the condition does not improve, what other surgical alternatives are available?
- How long can a person live safely and comfortably with a tube enterostomy?

Tube enterostomy is becoming more frequent due to great advances in minimally invasive techniques and new materials used for stoma construction. However, one recent radiograph study of 289 patients who had jejunostomy found that 14% of patients suffered one or more complications, 19% had problems related to the location or function of the tube, and 9% developed thickened small-bowel folds.

Results

Recovery without complications is the norm for this surgery. The greatest challenge is educating the patient on proper stoma usage and types of nutritional support that must be used.

Morbidity and mortality rates

Some feeding or tube stomas have the likelihood of complications. A review of 1,000 patients indicated that PEG tube placement has mortality in 0.5%, with major complications (stomal leakage, peritonitis [infection in the abdomen], traumatized tissue of the abdominal wall, and gastric [stomach] hemorrhage) in 1% of cases. Wound infection, leaks, tube movement or migration, and fever occurred in 8% of patients. In a review of seven published studies, researchers found that a single intravenous dose of a broad-spectrum antibiotic was very effective in reducing infections with the stoma. Open surgery always carries with it a small percentage of cardiac complications, blood clots, and infections. Many gastric stoma patients have complicated diseases that increase the likelihood of surgical complications.

Alternatives

Oral routes are always the preferred method of providing nutritional intake. Intravenous fluid intake can be used as an eating substitute, but only for a short period of time. It is the preferred alternative when adequate protein and calories cannot be provided by oral or other enteral routes, or when the gastrointestinal system is not functioning.

Health care team roles

Gastrointestinal **surgeons** and surgical oncologists perform this surgery in general hospital settings.

Resources

BOOKS

Feldman, M., et al. *Sleisenger & Fordtran's Gastrointestinal and Liver Disease*. 9th ed. Philadelphia: Saunders/Elsevier, 2010.

Townsend, Courtney M., et al. *Sabiston Textbook of Surgery*. 19th ed. Philadelphia: Saunders/Elsevier, 2012.

PERIODICALS

Best, C. "Maintaining Hydration in Enteral Tube Feeding." *Nursing Times* 109, no. 26 (2013): 16–17.

Orrevall, Ylva, et al. "A National Observational Study of the Prevalence and Use of Enteral Tube Feeding, Parenteral Nutrition and Intravenous Glucose in Cancer Patients Enrolled in Specialized Palliative Care." *Nutrients* 5, no. 1 (2013): 267–82. http://dx.doi.org/10.3390/nu5010267 (accessed October 4, 2013).

Rajab, T. K., and J. Watkins. "Anatomic Site of Tube Feeding Influences Glycemic Control—An Evidence-Based Hypothesis." *Surgery* 153, no. 5 (2013): 608–10. http://dx.doi.org/10.1016/j.surg.2012.08.069 (accessed October 4, 2013).

OTHER

California Dietetic Association. *The Selection and Care of Enteral Feeding Tubes*. http://www.dietitian.org/d_cvd/docs/kc_enteral_feeding.pdf (accessed October 4, 2013).

WEBSITES

ALS Association. "Information About Feeding Tubes." http://www.alsa.org/als-care/resources/publications-videos/factsheets/feeding-tubes.html (accessed October 4, 2013).

ORGANIZATIONS

American Society for Parenteral and Enteral Nutrition, 8630 Fenton St., Ste. 412, Silver Spring, MD 20910, (301) 587-6315, (800) 727-4567, aspen@nutr.org, https://www.nutritioncare.org.

United Ostomy Associations of America, Inc. (UOAA), PO Box 512, Northfield, MN 55057-0512, (800) 826-0826, info@ostomy.org, http://www.ostomy.org.

Nancy McKenzie, PhD

Tube feeding *see* **Tube enterostomy**

Tuberculosis test *see* **Mantoux test**

Tube-shunt surgery

Definition

Tube-shunt surgery, or Seton glaucoma surgery, is a surgical method to treat glaucoma. Glaucoma is a potentially blinding disease affecting 2%–3% of the United States population. The major known cause of glaucoma is a relative increase in intraocular pressure, or IOP. The purpose of glaucoma treatment, whether medical or surgical, is to lower the IOP.

Aqueous fluid is made continuously, and circulates throughout the eye before draining though channels in the eye's anterior chamber. When too much fluid is made, or it is not drained sufficiently, the IOP rises. This fluid build-up can lead to glaucoma. Normal intraocular pressure is under 21 mm/Hg. Glaucoma develops at IOPs higher than 21 mm/Hg. However, approximately 20% of glaucoma patients never have pressures higher than 21 mm/Hg.

Seton tube implants are also called glaucoma drainage tubes or implants. The Seton implant is comprised of two parts:

- A portion of tubing is implanted along the inside of the front of the eye. The distal (furthest from the center) end of the tubing protrudes through the anterior (front) or less commonly, the posterior (rear), chamber of the eye.
- An attached reservoir, called a plate, is placed under the conjunctiva of the eye at its equator, or midpoint.

Purpose

The function of the implant is to lower the intraocular pressure by filtering excess aqueous fluid out of the eye. During the first few weeks after surgery, a bleb of fibrous tissue and collagen forms around the plate of the implant. The formation of a filtration bleb is essential for filtering the excessive aqueous fluid. The thickness of the bleb, as well as the size or number of plates, determines the rate at which aqueous flows out of the anterior chamber of the eye. The excess aqueous fluid is shunted through the tubing of the implant, and passes through the space that develops between the bleb and the plate. By diffusion, the fluid flows into the capillaries where it exits the eye and enters general circulation. The IOP is lowered as a result of this decrease in fluid.

There are various types of implants used in glaucoma surgery. They fall into two categories: the non-valved (free-flow implants) and valved (resisted-flow implants). One of the first free-flow implants was the Molteno implant, which consists of one or two polypropylene reservoirs connected to a silicone tube.

The non-valved Baerveldt implant is larger than the Molteno, and is available in three sizes.

The restrictive implants, which include the Krupin and Ahmed implant, have valves that automatically close if the intraocular pressure is too low. This is important because in the first few weeks after surgery (before the bleb forms), the aqueous fluid can flow unimpeded through the implant. As a result, hypotony (low level of fluid in the eye) can develop.

Newer implants such as the Express shunt and the Gore-Tex tube shunt are in early stages of use.

Demographics

Seton tube implants are employed to treat all forms of glaucoma, but are primarily used in patients with elevated IOP despite aggressive medical treatment. They are also used when other types of surgery, such as conventional filtration, or **trabeculectomy**, have not been successful, or would not be recommended. A trabeculectomy should not be performed on patients with neovascular glaucoma, as well as those who have ocular complications caused by previous glaucoma surgeries.

Implants are often placed in the eyes of patients with uveitic glaucoma (fluctuating IOP). The surgeon implants a tube with a ligature, and manipulates the ligature to control pressure. Seton tubes are also used in young patients with aniridia, who often develop glaucoma. These tubes should not be used for patients who have silicon oil implants for the treatment of retinal detachment.

Description

A Seton implant is usually inserted under **local anesthesia**, but may be done under **general anesthesia** for an anxious patient or child. Since implantation may be painful for some children, drugs may be given intravenously during surgery.

After anesthesia is administered, the eye is draped and retractors are placed on the eye to hold it in place. An incision is made on the conjunctiva, a thin membrane layer that lies above the sclera (white of the eye). The implant plate is placed under the conjunctiva and sutured to the sclera, carefully avoiding damage to the recti muscles in the area. Incisions may be made in two quadrants of the eye if a double plate implant is inserted.

If the tubing is implanted into the anterior chamber, that portion of the eye is drained of excess fluid. If the tube is placed in the posterior chamber of the eye, all or part of the vitreous is removed. A needle puncture is made at the limbus where the cornea and the sclera meet, and the tubing is passed through this hole into one of the chambers of the eye. This opening is sealed with a donor scleral patch, which may be autologous (from the patient's own tissue). If a free-flow implant is used, the tubing is ligated with either a disposable suture, or the ligature is positioned such that it can be removed with a minor incision after a few weeks. As an alternative, the

non-valved implant may be inserted in two stages. The plate is first implanted, and the tube is attached during a second surgery after the bleb has formed.

Preparation

Prior to surgery, the patient's eye is examined with a slit-lamp biomicroscope. It is important that the conjunctiva in which the plate is placed is not scarred; that the cornea is clear; and that there are no attachments of the iris to the lens behind it or to the cornea in front of it. An **ultrasound** of pediatric patients is done to assess the size of the eye because not all implants are small enough to fit into a child's eye.

Antibiotic drops may be given for up to three days prior to surgery. The patient will continue most glaucoma medication until the day of surgery.

Informed consent must be given for the procedure. This includes consent for surgery and a list of risks for the Seton tube implant. It is important for the patient to understand that any vision loss acquired prior to surgery cannot be corrected.

Aftercare

For several weeks postoperatively, the patient is given **topical antibiotics** and steroids. In addition, oral steroids may be given to patients who had ocular inflammation prior to surgery. Some **surgeons** use atropine to maintain the eye in a temporary dilated state. Glaucoma medication may be continued for a few months due to possible IOP fluctuation during the early postoperative period. Follow-up visits are scheduled for one day after the surgery, weekly during the first month, twice a month during the second month, and again at three months. Patients can resume normal daily activities within a few days. The sutures may cause a foreign body sensation, which decreases as the stitches dissolve. This does not usually require treatment.

Aftercare in the surgeon's office involves monitoring for the signs of hypotony and lowered IOP. The treatment for postoperative hypotony is to tighten the tube of a non-valved implant. As the bleb forms, adjustments are made in the tubing ligature to increase flow through the ligature. If the pressure continues to rise, the tube may be blocked, and excess fluid may have to be tapped. Tube blockage may occasionally occur. Hypotony may also be caused by leakage from the conjunctival wound site.

Risks

This surgery has intraoperative and postoperative risks. During the procedure, an extraocular muscle can be severed. This is particularly true if the implant is placed in the inferior nasal section of the eye. Strabismus and double vision may follow. Also, the cornea may become scarred, hemorrhaging can occur within the eye, and the iris and lens can be damaged by the protruding tube.

Early postoperative complications include hyphema (blood clots in the anterior chamber of the eye), hypotony, tube obstruction, suture rupture with wound leakage, movement of the implanted plate, corneal edema, and detachment of the retina. Because of the position of the implant plate, retinal detachments are difficult to treat successfully if a Seton implant is present. Double vision during the early postoperative period may be due to swelling in the area, and often will resolve as the orbital edema decreases.

In the late postsurgical period, strabismus as well as orbital cellulitis, a condition that can spread to the central nervous system, can develop. Other long-term risks of glaucoma implant surgery include cataract formation, proptosis (bulging of the eye), and phthisis bulbi (a dangerous situation in which the eye is devoid of all fluid).

Surgical intervention is required for choroidal detachments, strabismus, and if tubing blocks or comes in contact with other structures of the eye, particularly the cornea. If the tube is blocked by blood clots, tissue plasminogen activator may dissolve them. A laser can cut strands of vitreous or iris that may clog the tubing. If bleb enlargement impinges on a muscle, causing strabismus, the implant may be removed and replaced with a smaller type. If the tubing continually rubs on the back or endothelium of the cornea, decomposition of the cornea is possible and a corneal transplant may be required if vision is comprised. In this case, the tubing will have to be relocated to the posterior chamber, and a vitrectomy performed.

Loss of vision is possible with this and all glaucoma surgery. For Seton tube implants, hypotony is the primary cause of vision loss. Other causes include retinal detachment, vitreous bleeding, and macular edema.

Results

Usually the IOP is lower within two weeks of Seton tube placement. At two months, the pressure is stabilized at 16–18 mm/Hg. Glaucoma medication must still be taken. The IOP in 85% of patients with a non-valved implant is lower than 21 mm/Hg without additional medication intervention. Only 50% of patients with a Krupin valve implant have an IOP lower than 21 mm/Hg without added medical treatment.

Morbidity and mortality rates

For 70%–90% of patients, the implant is functional one year after surgery. After three years, 60% remain functional. The failure rate for Seton implants is 4%–8% per year, and differ for valved and non-valved implants. For the non-valved implants, the success rate is 90% at one year, but drops to 60% at two years. At least 66% of valved Seton tube implants are effective at one year, but this drops to 34% at six years. Choroidal detachment is a complication in one-third of these patients.

Strabismus is more common with the Krupin valve as opposed to the Ahmed valve, possibly because it is larger.

For high-risk glaucoma patients, the success rate for Seton tube surgery is approximately 50%. The rate of failure increases 10% with each year. High-risk patients include those who are aphakic (have no intraocular lens), have neovascular glaucoma (which develops from uncontrolled diabetes and hypertension), have congenital glaucoma, or who have had other unsuccessful glaucoma surgeries. Although the success rate for neovascular glaucoma is 56% at 18 months, eventually 31% of neovascular glaucoma patients will lose all vision except for light perception.

Alternatives

Trabeculectomy is another surgical filtration technique used to treat glaucoma. Trabeculectomy surgery is performed by making a flap in the sclera of the eye, which serves as an alternative drainage site for aqueous fluid. Patients who receive this treatment are not as high risk as those undergoing an implant procedure. Overall, they have a lower IOP, but may have more advanced glaucoma. If vascularization of the iris is present, as in neovascular glaucoma, a trabeculectomy is not performed. For patients who do not have neovascular glaucoma, the failure rate for trabeculotomy is similar to that of drainage tube implants.

Cyclodestruction is another alternative to Seton tube implants. Freezing temperatures or lasers are used to destroy the ciliary body, the part of the eye where the aqueous fluid is produced. When compared to the YAG laser cyclophotocoagulation, tube shunts are twice as successful.

Health care team roles

Tube implants are performed by ophthalmologists as outpatient procedures in a hospital **operating room**. The implantation of a Seton tube takes about two hours. An ophthalmologist is a physician with advanced training in the treatment of eye disease. If general anesthesia or extra

QUESTIONS TO ASK YOUR DOCTOR

- Which implant will be used?
- Is a tube implant the best surgical approach for this case?
- How many of these procedures has the surgeon performed?
- When will it be determined if the surgery has been successful?
- What are the risks for this surgery?
- Will glaucoma eye drops still be required after surgery?

pain medication is administered, an anesthesiologist may be present during surgery.

Resources

BOOKS

Healey, Paul R., and Ravi Thomas. *Fast Facts: Glaucoma.* Oxford: Health Press, 2010.

Rhee, Douglas J. *Color Atlas and Synopsis of Clinical Ophthalmology.* Philadelphia: Lippincott Williams & Wilkins, 2012.

Spaeth, George L., et al. *Ophthalmic Surgery: Principles and Practice.* Edinburgh: Saunders/Elsevier, 2012.

PERIODICALS

Gross, Ronald L. "Glaucoma Filtration Surgery: Trabeculectomy or Tube Shunt?" *American Journal of Ophthalmology* 153, no. 5 (2012): 787–88. http://dx.doi.org/10.1016/j.ajo.2011.11.036 (accessed October 4, 2013).

WEBSITES

Glaucoma Research Foundation. "Glaucoma Implant Surgery." http://www.glaucoma.org/treatment/glaucoma-implants.php (accessed October 4, 2013).

Massachusetts Eye and Ear. "Glaucoma Tube Shunt Procedures." http://www.masseyeandear.org/specialties/ophthalmology/glaucoma/treatment/tube-shunt-procedures (accessed October 4, 2013).

ORGANIZATIONS

Glaucoma Research Foundation, 251 Post St., Ste. 600, San Francisco, CA 94108, (415) 986-3162, grf@glaucoma.org, http://glaucoma.org.

Martha Reilly, OD

Tummy tuck *see* **Abdominoplasty**

Tumor grading

Definition

Tumor grading is an estimate of a tumor's malignancy and aggressiveness based on how the tumor cells appear under a microscope and the number of malignant characteristics they possess. It is a way to predict how quickly a tumor is likely to grow and spread in the body, and is used when planning a specific treatment plan for a cancer patient. Different tumor grading systems are used depending on the type of cancer being described.

Purpose

Tumor grading, together with the stage of the tumor, assists doctors in planning treatment strategies. Grading is a part of describing most cancers, and it is extremely important in helping to determine the course of treatment for specific cancers such as soft tissue sarcomas, brain tumors, lymphomas, and breast and prostate cancer. Generally, higher grade and higher stage tumors require more intensive therapy than lower grade and lower stage tumors. Tumor grade and stage also help doctors estimate the prognosis for the patient. Patients with lower grade and stage tumors usually have a more positive prognosis than patients with higher grade and stage tumors. Patients should thoroughly discuss the grade and stage of their tumor with their physician and ask about necessary treatments and prognosis.

Description

Before a tumor can be assigned a grade, a sample of tissue must be removed for microscopic evaluation. Tissue samples can be obtained through one of various types of biopsy or through exfoliative **cytology** (e.g., Pap smear). A pathologist analyzes various characteristics of the tissue, such as the size and shape of the nucleus, the

Gleason tumor scoring system	
Gleason X	Cannot be determined
Gleason 2–6	Well differentiated
Gleason 7	Moderately differentiated
Gleason 8–10	Poorly differentiated or undifferentiated

SOURCE: National Cancer Institute, "Tumor Grade," National Institutes of Health. Available online at: http://www.cancer.gov/cancertopics/factsheet/Detection/tumor-grade.

(Table by PreMediaGlobal. Copyright © 2014 Cengage Learning®.)

ratio of the volume of the nucleus to the volume of the cytoplasm, the relative number of dividing cells (the mitotic index), the organization of the tissue, the boundary of the tumor, and how well-differentiated the cells appear—how close to normal the cells seem in maturity and function.

Benign tumors have normal-looking cells. That is, they have small and regular-shaped nuclei, small nuclear volume relative to the rest of the cellular volume, a relatively low number of dividing cells, and normal and well-differentiated tissue that has a well-defined tumor boundary. However, malignant tumors generally have all or several of the following characteristics: large and pleomorphic (irregular-shaped) nuclei, large nuclear volume compared to the rest of the cellular volume, a high number of dividing cells, and disorganized and anaplastic (poorly differentiated) tissue that has a poorly defined tumor boundary.

Depending on the number of malignant characteristics present, the American Joint Commission on Cancer recommends that tumors be given a grade using G0 through G4:

• G0: A benign lesion or tumor.

• G1: Well-differentiated (Low-grade and less aggressive).

• G2: Moderately well-differentiated (Intermediate-grade and moderately aggressive).

• G3: Poorly differentiated (High-grade and moderately aggressive).

• G4: Undifferentiated (High-grade and aggressive).

Alternatively, Roman numerals I through IV, respectively, may be used. Low-grade tumors are assigned lower Roman numerals (e.g., grade I), indicating that the tumor is less aggressive. High-grade tumors are assigned higher Roman numerals (e.g., grade IV), indicating that the tumor is very aggressive, growing and spreading quickly. This description is stated as:

• I: Well-differentiated (Low-grade and less aggressive).

• II: Moderately well-differentiated (Intermediate-grade and moderately aggressive).

• III: Poorly differentiated (High-grade and moderately aggressive).

• IV: Undifferentiated (High-grade and aggressive).

Some cancers have their own specific grading convention. For example, the Gleason system is a unique grading system that was developed to describe adenocarcinoma of the prostate. Pathologists analyze prostate tissue and give a Gleason score ranging from 2 to 10, subject to the number of malignant characteristics observed. Well-differentiated, less aggressive prostate

tumors with only a few malignant characteristics are given lower Gleason numbers, while poorly differentiated, more aggressive prostate tumors that possess many malignant characteristics are assigned higher Gleason numbers.

Breast cancer tumors

Breast cancers are graded using a system called the Nottingham system. It is also called the Bloom-Richardson grading system, a modification of the Bloom-Richardson-Elston grading system (sometimes known as the modified Bloom-Richardson-Elston system) that originated in 1957. The Nottingham system also goes by such names as the Modified Bloom-Richardson, Scarff-Bloom-Richardson, SBR Grading, and BR Grading. Breast tumors, specifically the cells and tissue structure of the breast, are assessed to determine the state of the cancer. A pathologist examines a sample of breast tissue under a microscope, and the tumors are analyzed (and scored) based on the following three features:

• degree of tubule (gland) formation—the amount of tubule structure that is present

• nuclear grade (pleomorphism)—cell size and appearance, and uniformity of individual cells

• mitotic rate—amount of activity of cell division

Each feature is assigned a score from 1 to 3 based on the following:

• 1: slow cell growth rate

• 2: intermediate cell growth rate

• 3: fast cell growth rate

Cells and tissue structure that look normal are assigned lower scores, while abnormal-looking cells and structure are given higher scores. The scoring, based on the above three features, ranges from 3 (least serious) to 9 (most serious) on the Nottingham system. The total feature score is graded as follows:

- total points 3 to 5: grade 1 tumor—well-differentiated, appears normal, growing slowly, not aggressive

- total points 6 to 7: grade 2 tumor—moderately differentiated, appears semi-normal, growing moderately fast

- total points 8 to 9: grade 3 tumor—poorly differentiated, appears abnormal, growing quickly, aggressive

As an example, the pathologist might give 1 point to degree of tubule formation, 2 points for nuclear grade, and 1 point for mitotic rate, for a total of 4 points. In this case, the tumor is classified as a grade 1 tumor. The higher-grade tumors are treated more aggressively, because they spread faster and are associated with a lower survival rate. Lower-grade tumors have a much higher survival rate for women, so they are treated in a less aggressive manner.

Results

Once a grading system has been used to determine the severity of the tumor, doctors will use that tumor grade, along with other relevant information, to develop a treatment plan for the patient. The grading system also helps to determine a prognosis for the patient, including how aggressive the treatment needs to be, the likely chance for recovery, the likelihood that the cancer will reoccur, and other important concerns. Once a tumor's grade has been determined, it is important that patients discuss these results with their doctor so an effective course of action can be taken.

Resources

BOOKS

Damjanov, Ivan, and Fang Fan, eds. *Cancer Grading Manual.* Berlin: Springer, 2013.

Epstein, Jonathan I. *The Gleason Grading System: A Complete Guide for Pathologists and Clinicians.* Philadelphia: Wolters Kluwer Health/Lippincott Williams & Wilkins, 2013.

Weinberg, Robert A. *The Biology of Cancer.* New York: Garland Science, 2014.

WEBSITES

American Brain Tumor Association. "Grading and Staging." http://www.abta.org/understanding-brain-tumors/diagnosis/grading-and-staging.html (accessed September 27, 2013).

California Cancer Registry. "Bloom-Richardson Grade for Breast Cancer." http://www.ccrcal.org/DSQC_Pubs/V1_2013_Online_Manual/Part_V_Tumor_Data/V_3_5_8_Bloom_Richardson_Grade_for_Breast_Cancer.htm (accessed September 25, 2013).

Johns Hopkins Medicine, Johns Hopkins University. "Overview of Histologic Grade: Nottingham Histologic Score (Elston Grade)." http://pathology.jhu.edu/breast/grade.php (accessed September 25, 2013).

National Cancer Institute. "Tumor Grade." http://www.cancer.gov/cancertopics/factsheet/detection/tumor-grade (accessed September 25, 2013).

Susan G. Komen Foundation. "Tumor Grade." http://ww5.komen.org/BreastCancer/TumorGrade.html (accessed September 27, 2013).

ORGANIZATIONS

American Cancer Society, 250 Williams St. NW, Atlanta, GA 30303, (800) 227-2345, http://www.cancer.org.

Cancer Research Institute, One Exchange Plz., 55 Broadway, Ste. 1802, New York, NY 10006, (212) 688-7515, (800) 99-CANCER (992-2623), http://cancerresearch.org.

National Cancer Institute, 6116 Executive Blvd., Ste. 300, Bethesda, MD 20892-8322, (800) 4-CANCER (422-6237), http://cancer.gov.

Sally C. McFarlane-Parrott
William A. Atkins, BB, BS, MBA

Tumor marker tests

Definition

Tumor markers are a group of proteins, hormones, enzymes, receptors, and other cellular products that are overexpressed (produced in higher than normal amounts) by malignant cells. Tumor markers are usually normal cellular constituents that are present at normal or very low levels in the blood of healthy persons. If the substance in question is produced by the tumor, its levels will be increased either in the blood or in the tissue of origin.

Purpose

The majority of tumor markers are used to detect the possible presence of a tumor, to diagnose a malignant condition (usually only in conjunction with other diagnostic tests), and to monitor patients for response to treatment or for a recurrence of tumors following treatment. In addition, some markers are associated with a more aggressive course and higher relapse rate and have value in staging and prognosis of the cancer. Most tumor markers are not useful for screening because levels found in early malignancy overlap the range of levels found in healthy persons. The levels of most tumor markers are elevated in conditions other than malignancy, and are therefore not useful in establishing a diagnosis.

Description

Physicians use changes in tumor marker levels to follow the course of a patient's disease, to measure the effect of treatment, and to check for recurrence of certain cancers. Tumor markers have been identified in several types of cancer, including malignant melanoma; multiple myeloma; and bone, breast, colon, gastric, liver, lung, ovarian, pancreatic, prostate, renal, and uterine cancers. Serial measurements of a tumor marker are often an effective means to monitor the course of therapy. Some tumor markers can provide physicians with information used in staging cancers, and some help predict the response to treatment. A decrease in the levels of the tumor marker during treatment indicates that the therapy is having a positive effect on the cancer, while an increase indicates that the cancer is growing and not responding to the therapy.

Types of tumor markers

There are five basic types of tumor markers.

ENZYMES. Many enzymes that occur in certain tissues are found in blood plasma at higher levels when the cancer involves that tissue. Enzymes are usually measured by determining the rate at which they convert a substrate to an end product, while most tumor markers of other types are measured by a test called an immunoassay. Some examples of enzymes whose levels rise in cases of malignant diseases are acid phosphatase, alkaline phosphatase, amylase, creatine kinase, gamma glutamyl transferase, lactate dehydrogenase, and terminal deoxynucleotidyl transferase.

TISSUE RECEPTORS. Tissue receptors, which are proteins associated with the cell membrane, are another type of tumor marker. These substances bind to hormones and growth factors, and therefore affect the rate of tumor growth. Some tissue receptors must be measured in tissue samples removed for a biopsy, while others are secreted into the extracellular fluid (fluid outside the cells) and may be measured in the blood. Some important receptor tumor markers are estrogen receptor, progesterone receptor, interleukin-2 receptor, and epidermal growth factor receptor.

ANTIGENS. Oncofetal antigens are proteins made by genes that are very active during fetal development but function at a very low level after birth. The genes become activated when a malignant tumor arises and produce large amounts of protein. Antigens comprise the largest class of tumor marker and include the tumor-associated glycoprotein antigens. Important tumor markers in this class are alpha-fetoprotein (AFP), carcinoembryonic antigen (CEA), prostate specific antigen (PSA), cathepsin-D, HER-2/neu, CA-125, CA-19-9, CA-15-3, nuclear matrix protein, and bladder tumor-associated antigen.

ONCOGENES. Some tumor markers are the product of oncogenes, which are genes that are active in fetal development and trigger the growth of tumors when they are activated in mature cells. Some important oncogenes are BRAC-1, myc, p53, RB (retinoblastoma) gene, and Ph[1] (Philadelphia chromosome).

HORMONES. The fifth type of tumor marker consists of hormones. This group includes hormones that are normally secreted by the tissue in which the malignancy arises as well as those produced by tissues that do not normally make the hormone (ectopic production). Some hormones associated with malignancy are adrenal corticotropic hormone (ACTH), calcitonin, catecholamines, gastrin, human chorionic gonadotropin (hCG), and prolactin.

Tumor markers in clinical use

Currently, there are over 60 analytes that are used as tumor markers. All of the enzymes and hormones mentioned have been approved as tumor markers by the U.S. Food and Drug Administration (FDA), but most of the others are not; they have been designated for investigation purposes only. The following list describes the most commonly used tumor markers approved by the FDA for screening, diagnosis, or monitoring of cancer.

- Alpha-fetoprotein (AFP): AFP is a glycoprotein produced by the developing fetus, but blood levels of alpha-fetoprotein decline after birth. Healthy adults who are not pregnant rarely have detectable levels of AFP in their blood. The maternal serum AFP test (AFP triple screen or AFP Tetra screen) is primarily used to screen for spina bifida and other open fetal abnormalities, such as an abdominal wall defect. Very rarely a very high level of alpha-fetoprotein may be associated with congenital Finnish nephrosis. Lower than average levels of AFP in maternal serum may increase the risk for fetal Down syndrome or other chromosome abnormalities. In adult males and nonpregnant females, an AFP above 300 ng/L is often associated with cancer, although levels in this range may be seen in nonmalignant liver diseases. Levels above 1,000 ng/L are almost always associated with cancer. AFP has been approved by the FDA for the diagnosis and monitoring of patients with non-seminoma testicular cancer. It is elevated in almost all yolk sac tumors and 80% of malignant liver tumors. An elevated AFP level in the maternal circulation during pregnancy warrants further discussion and possible further testing, but usually is not an indication of fetal anomaly, as it can be elevated in normal pregnancies. An elevated level may indicate problems other than fetal anomalies, such as placental problems that may lead to premature delivery or low birth weight.

• CA-125: Measurement of this tumor marker is FDA-approved for the diagnosis and monitoring of women with ovarian cancer. Approximately 75% of persons with ovarian cancer shed CA-125 into the blood and have elevated serum levels. This figure includes approximately 50% of persons with stage I disease and 90% with stage II or higher. Elevated levels of CA-125 are also found in approximately 20% of persons with pancreatic cancer. Other cancers detected by this marker include malignancies of the liver, colon, breast, lung, and digestive tract. Test results, however, are affected by pregnancy and menstruation. Benign diseases detected by the test include endometriosis, ovarian cysts, fibroids, inflammatory bowel disease, cirrhosis, peritonitis, and pancreatitis. CA-125 levels correlate with tumor mass; consequently, this test is used to determine whether recurrence of the cancer has occurred following chemotherapy. Some patients, however, have a recurrence of their cancer without a corresponding increase in the level of CA-125.

• Carcinoembryonic antigen (CEA): CEA is a glycoprotein that is part of the normal cell membrane. It is shed into blood serum and reaches very high levels in colorectal cancer. Over 50% of persons with breast, colon, lung, gastric, ovarian, pancreatic, and uterine cancer have elevated levels of CEA. CEA levels in plasma are monitored in patients with tumors that secrete this antigen to determine if second-look surgery should be performed. CEA levels may also be elevated in inflammatory bowel disease (IBD), pancreatitis, and liver disease. Heavy smokers and about 5% of healthy persons have elevated plasma levels of CEA.

• Prostate specific antigen (PSA): PSA is a small glycoprotein with protease activity that is specific for prostate tissue. The antigen is present in low levels in all adult males, which means that an elevated level may require additional testing to confirm that cancer is the cause. High levels are seen in prostate cancer, benign prostatic hypertrophy, and inflammation of the prostate. PSA is approved as a screening test for prostatic carcinoma. PSA has been found to be elevated in more than 60% of persons with Stage A and more than 70% with Stage B cancer of the prostate. It has replaced the use of prostatic acid phosphatase for prostate cancer screening because it is far more sensitive. Most PSA is bound to antitrypsin in plasma but some PSA circulates unbound to protein (free PSA). Persons with a borderline total PSA (4–10 ng/L) but who have a low free PSA are more likely to have malignant prostate disease.

• Estrogen receptor (ER): ER is a protein found in the nucleus of breast and uterine tissues. The level of ER in the tissue is used to determine whether a person with breast cancer is likely to respond to estrogen therapy with tamoxifen, which binds to the receptors blocking the action of estrogen. Women who are ER-negative have a greater risk of recurrence than women who are ER-positive. Tissue levels are measured using one of two methods. The tissue can be homogenized into a cytosol, and an immunoassay used to measure the concentration of ER receptor protein. Alternatively, the tissue is frozen and thin-sectioned. An immunoperoxidase stain is used to detect and measure the estrogen receptors in the tissue.

• Progesterone receptor (PR): PR consists of two proteins, like the estrogen receptor, which are located in the nuclei of both breast and uterine tissues. PR has the same prognostic value as ER, and is measured by similar methods. Tissue that does not express the PR receptors is less likely to bind estrogen analogs used to treat the tumor. Persons who test negative for both ER and PR have less than a 5% chance of responding to endocrine therapy. Those who test positive for both markers have greater than a 60% chance of tumor shrinkage when treated with hormone therapy.

• Human chorionic gonadotropin (hCG): hCG is a glycoprotein produced by cells of the trophoblast and developing placenta. Very high levels are produced by trophoblastic tumors and choriocarcinoma, which is an aggressive tumor that arises from cells that help to attach the fetus to the uterine wall. About 60% of testicular cancers secrete hCG. hCG is also produced less frequently by a number of other tumors. Some malignancies cause an increase in alpha and/or beta hCG subunits in the absence of significant increases in intact hCG. For this reason, separate tests have been developed for alpha and beta hCG, and most laboratories use these assays as tumor marker tests. Most EIA tests for pregnancy are specific for hCG, but detect the whole molecule and are called intact hCG assays.

• Nuclear matrix protein (NMP22) and bladder tumor-associated analytes (BTA): NMP22 is a structural nuclear protein that is released into the urine when bladder carcinoma cells die. Approximately 70% of bladder carcinomas are positive for NMP22. BTA is comprised of type IV collagen, fibronectin, laminin, and proteoglycan, which are components of the basement membrane that are released into the urine when bladder tumor cells attach to the basement membrane of the bladder wall. These products can be detected in urine using a mixture of antibodies to the four components. BTA is elevated in about 30% of persons with low-grade bladder tumors and over 60% of persons with high-grade tumors.

Precautions

Tumor markers are sometimes elevated in nonmalignant conditions. Not every tumor will cause a rise in the level of its associated marker, especially in the early stages of some cancers. When a marker is used for cancer screening or diagnosis, the physician must confirm a positive test result by using imaging studies, tissue biopsies, and other procedures. False positive results may occur in laboratory tests when the patient has cross-reacting antibodies that interfere with the test.

Preparation

Determination of the circulating level of tumor markers requires a blood test performed by a laboratory scientist. A nurse or phlebotomist usually draws the patient's blood; he or she ties a tourniquet above the patient's elbow, locates a vein near the inner elbow, cleanses the skin overlying the vein with an antiseptic solution, and inserts a sterile needle into that vein. The blood is drawn through the needle into an attached vacuum tube. Collection of a blood sample takes only a few minutes.

Tissue samples are collected by a physician at the time of surgical or needle biopsy. A urine sample is collected by the patient, using the midstream void technique.

Aftercare

Aftercare following a blood test consists of routine care of the area around the puncture site. Pressure is applied for a few seconds and the wound is covered with a bandage. If a bruise or swelling develops around the

---

KEY TERMS

Analyte—A material or chemical substance subjected to analysis.

Antitrypsin—A substance that inhibits the action of trypsin.

Biopsy—The removal of living tissue from the body, done in order to establish a diagnosis.

Glycoprotein—Any of a group of complex proteins that consist of a carbohydrate combined with a simple protein. Some tumor markers are glycoproteins.

Immunoassay—A laboratory method for detecting the presence of a substance by using an antibody that reacts with it.

Multiple myeloma—An uncommon disease that occurs more often in men than in women and is associated with anemia, hemorrhage, recurrent infections, and weakness. Ordinarily it is regarded as a malignant neoplasm that originates in bone marrow and involves mainly the skeleton.

Oncogene—A gene that is capable under certain conditions of triggering the conversion of normal cells into cancer cells.

Oncologist—A physician who specializes in the development, diagnosis, treatment, and prevention of tumors.

Overexpression—Production in abnormally high amounts.

Serum (plural, sera)—The clear, pale yellow liquid part of blood that separates from a clot when the blood coagulates.

Staging—The classification of cancerous tumors according to the extent of the tumor.

Substrate—A substance acted upon by an enzyme.

---

puncture site, the area is treated with a moist warm compress.

Risks

The risks associated with drawing blood include dizziness, bruising, swelling, or excessive bleeding from the puncture site. As previously mentioned, the results of blood tests should be interpreted with caution. A single test result may not yield clinically useful information. Several laboratory reports over a period of months may be needed to evaluate treatment and identify recurrence. Positive results must be interpreted cautiously because some tumor markers are increased in nonmalignant diseases and in a small number of apparently healthy persons. In addition, false negative results may occur because the tumor does not produce the marker, and because levels seen in healthy persons may overlap those seen in the early stages of cancer. A false positive result occurs when the value is elevated even though cancer is not present. A false negative result occurs when the value is normal but cancer is present.

Results

Reference ranges for tumor markers will vary from one laboratory to another because different antibodies and calibrators are used by various test systems. The values below are representative of normal values or cutoffs for commonly measured tumor markers.

- Alpha-fetoprotein (AFP): Less than 15 ng/L in men and nonpregnant women. Levels greater than 1,000 ng/L indicate malignant disease (except in pregnancy).
- CA125: Less than 35 U/mL.
- Carcinoembryonic antigen (CEA): Less than 3 μg/L for nonsmokers and less than 5 μg/L for smokers.
- Estrogen receptor: Less than 6 fmol/mg protein is negative; greater than 10 fmol/mg protein is positive.
- Human chorionic gonadotropin (hCG): Less than 20 IU/L for males and nonpregnant females. Greater than 100,00 IU/L indicates trophoblastic tumor.
- Progesterone receptor: Less than 6 fmol/mg protein is negative. Greater than 10 fmol/mg protein is positive.
- Prostate specific antigen (PSA): Less than 4 ng/L.

Resources

BOOKS

Goldman, Lee, and Andrew I. Schafer. *Goldman's Cecil Medicine*. 24th ed. Philadelphia: Saunders/Elsevier, 2012.

McPherson, Richard A., and Matthew R. Pincus, eds. *Henry's Clinical Diagnosis and Management by Laboratory Methods*. 22nd ed. Philadelphia: Saunders/Elsevier, 2011.

Niederhuber, John E., et al. *Abeloff's Clinical Oncology*. 5th ed. Philadelphia: Saunders/Elsevier, 2013.

PERIODICALS

Chan, K. C. Allen. "Scanning for Cancer Genomic Changes in Plasma: Toward an Era of Personalized Blood-Based Tumor Markers." *Clinical Chemistry* (July 10, 2013): e-pub ahead of print. http://dx.doi.org/10.1373/clinchem.2013.207381 (accessed September 20, 2013).

Duffy, M. J., et al. "Tumor Markers in Colorectal Cancer, Gastric Cancer and Gastrointestinal Stromal Cancers: European Group on Tumor Markers 2014 Guidelines Update." *International Journal of Cancer* (August 27, 2013): e-pub ahead of print. http://dx.doi.org/10.1002/ijc.28384 (accessed September 20, 2013).

Wang, W. J., et al. "Clinical Observations on the Association between Diagnosis of Lung Cancer and Serum Tumor Markers in Combination." *Asian Pacific Journal of Cancer Prevention* 14, no. 7 (2013): 4369–71.

WEBSITES

American Association for Clinical Chemistry. "AFP Tumor Markers." Lab Tests Online. http://labtestsonline.org/understanding/analytes/afp-tumor (accessed September 20, 2013).

American Cancer Society. "Tumor Markers." http://www.cancer.org/treatment/understandingyourdiagnosis/examsandtestdescriptions/tumormarkers (accessed September 20, 2013).

National Cancer Institute. "Tumor Markers." http://www.cancer.gov/cancertopics/factsheet/Detection/tumor-markers (accessed September 20, 2013).

ORGANIZATIONS

American Association for Clinical Chemistry, 1850 K St. NW, Ste. 625, Washington, DC 20006, (800) 892-1400, Fax: (202) 887-5093, custserv@aacc.org, http://www.aacc.org.

American Cancer Society, 250 Williams St. NW, Atlanta, GA 30303, (800) 227-2345, http://www.cancer.org.

American Society of Clinical Oncology (ASCO), 318 Mill Rd., Ste. 800, Alexandria, VA 22314, (571) 483-1300, (888) 282-2552, http://www.asco.org.

National Cancer Institute, 6116 Executive Blvd., Ste. 300, Bethesda, MD 20892-8322, (800) 4-CANCER (422-6237), http://cancer.gov.

U.S. Food and Drug Administration, 10903 New Hampshire Ave., Silver Spring, MD 20993, (888) INFO-FDA (463-6332), http://www.fda.gov.

Victoria E. DeMoranville
Mark A. Best
Renee Laux, MS

Tumor removal

Definition

A tumor is an abnormal growth in the body that is caused by the uncontrolled division of cells. Benign tumors do not have the potential to spread to other parts of the body (a process called metastasis) and are curable by surgical removal. Malignant or cancerous tumors, however, may metastasize to other parts of the body and will ultimately result in death if not successfully treated by surgery and/or other methods.

Purpose

Surgical removal is one of four main ways that tumors are treated; the other treatment options include chemotherapy, radiation therapy, and biological therapy. There are a number of factors used to determine which methods will best treat a tumor. Because benign tumors do not have the potential to metastasize, they are often treated successfully with surgical removal alone. Malignant tumors, however, are most often treated with a combination of surgery and chemotherapy and/or radiation therapy (in about 55% of cases). In some instances, non-curative surgery may make other treatments more effective. Debulking a cancer—making it smaller by surgical removal of a large part of it—is thought to make radiation and chemotherapy more effective.

Surgery is often used to accurately assess the nature and extent of a cancer. Most cancers cannot be adequately identified without examining a sample of the abnormal tissue under a microscope. Such tissue samples are procured during a surgical procedure. Surgery may also be used to determine exactly how far a tumor has spread and to establish its margins.

There are a few standard methods of comparing one cancer to another for the purposes of determining appropriate treatments and estimating outcomes. These methods are referred to as staging. The most commonly used method is the TNM system:

• **T** stands for tumor, and reflects the size of the tumor.

• **N** represents the spread of the cancer to lymph nodes, largely determined by those nodes removed at surgery that contain cancer cells. Since cancers spread mostly through the lymphatic system, this is a useful measure of a cancer's ability to disperse.

• **M** refers to metastasis, and indicates if metastases are present and how far they are from the original cancer.

Staging is particularly important with such lymphomas as Hodgkin's disease, which may appear in many places in the lymphatic system. Surgery is a useful tool for staging such cancers and can increase the chance of a successful cure, since radiation treatment is often curative if all the cancerous sites are located and irradiated.

Demographics

The American Cancer Society estimates that approximately 1,660,290 cases of cancer will be diagnosed in the United States in 2013. Seventy-eight percent of cancers are diagnosed in men and women over the age of 55, although cancer may affect individuals of any age. Men develop cancer more often than women; one in two men will be diagnosed with cancer during his lifetime, compared to one in three women. Additionally, men are

KEY TERMS

Aspiration—A technique for obtaining a piece of tissue for biopsy by using suction applied through a needle attached to a syringe.

Biopsy—The removal of living tissue from the body, done in order to establish a diagnosis.

Debulking—Surgical removal of a major portion of a tumor so that there is less of the cancer left for later treatment by chemotherapy or radiation.

Mammogram—A set of x-rays taken of the front and side of the breast; used to diagnose various abnormalities of the breast.

Metastasis (plural, metastases)—A growth of cancer cells at a site in the body distant from the primary tumor.

Oncologist—A physician who specializes in the diagnosis and treatment of tumors.

Palliative—Offering relief of symptoms, but not a cure.

Pap test—The common term for the Papanicolaou test, a simple smear method of examining stained cells to detect cancer of the cervix.

Staging—The classification of cancerous tumors according to the extent of the tumor.

more likely to die of cancer. Cancer affects individuals of all races and ethnicities, although incidence may differ among these groups by cancer type.

Description

Surgery may be used to remove tumors for diagnostic or therapeutic purposes.

Diagnostic tumor removal

A biopsy is a medical procedure that obtains a small piece of tissue for diagnostic testing. The sample is examined under a microscope by a doctor who specializes in the effects of disease on body tissues (a pathologist) to detect any abnormalities. A definitive diagnosis of cancer cannot be made unless a sample of the abnormal tissue is examined histologically (under a microscope).

There are four main biopsy techniques used to diagnose cancer:

• In an aspiration biopsy, a needle is inserted into the tumor and a sample is withdrawn. This procedure may be performed under local anesthesia or with no anesthesia at all.

• For a needle biopsy, a special cutting needle is inserted into the core of the tumor and a core sample is cut out. Local anesthesia is most often administered.

• With an incisional biopsy, a portion of a large tumor is removed, usually under local anesthesia in an outpatient setting.

• In an excisional biopsy, an entire cancerous lesion is removed along with surrounding normal tissue (called a clear margin). Local or general anesthesia may be used.

Therapeutic tumor removal

Once surgical removal has been decided, a surgical oncologist will remove the entire tumor, taking with it a large section of the surrounding normal tissue. The healthy tissue is removed to minimize the risk that abnormal tissue is left behind. Tumors may be removed by cutting with steel instruments, by the use of a laser beam, by radiofrequency ablation (the use of radio-frequency energy to destroy tissue), by cryoablation (the use of extreme cold to freeze and thus destroy the tumor), or by injecting alcohol into the tumor.

When surgical removal of a tumor is unacceptable as a sole treatment, a portion of the tumor is removed to debulk the mass; this process is called cytoreduction. Cytoreductive surgery aids radiation and chemotherapy treatments by increasing the sensitivity of the tumor and decreasing the number of necessary treatment cycles.

Certain types of skin tumors can be removed by a technique called Mohs micrographic surgery, developed in the late 1930s by Dr. Frederick E. Mohs. The Mohs method involves four steps: surgical removal of the tumor, making a slide of the removed tissue and examining it for cancer cells (called mapping the tissue), interpreting the microscope slides and removing more tissue if necessary until no more cancer cells are found, and performing **reconstructive surgery** to cover the wound.

A newer technique for removing some tumors of the spinal cord involves the use of a suction tip rather than a scalpel. The newer technique appears to have a wider margin of safety when working around the delicate structures of the central nervous system.

In some instances, the purpose of tumor removal is not to cure the cancer, but to relieve the symptoms of a patient who cannot be cured. This approach is called palliative surgery. For example, a patient with advanced cancer may have a tumor causing significant pain or bleeding; in such a case, the tumor may be removed to ease the patient's pain or other symptoms even though a cure is not possible.

Seeding

The surgical removal of malignant tumors demands special considerations. There is a danger of spreading cancerous cells during the process of removing abnormal tissue (called seeding). Presuming that cancer cells can implant elsewhere in the body, the surgeon must minimize the dissemination of cells throughout the operating field or into the bloodstream.

Special techniques called block resection and no-touch are used. Block resection involves taking the entire specimen out as a single piece. The no-touch technique involves removing a specimen by handling only the normal tissue surrounding it; the cancer itself is never touched. These approaches prevent the spread of cancer cells into the general circulation. The surgeon takes great care to clamp off the blood supply first, preventing cells from leaving by that route later in the surgery.

Diagnosis

A tumor may first be palpated (felt) by the patient or by a healthcare professional during a **physical examination**. A tumor may be visible on the skin or protrude outward from the body. Still other tumors are not evident until their presence begins to cause such symptoms as weight loss, fatigue, or pain. In some instances, tumors are located during routine tests (e.g., a yearly mammogram or Pap smear).

Aftercare

Retesting and periodical examinations are necessary to ensure that a tumor has not returned or metastasized after total removal.

Risks

Each tumor removal surgery carries certain risks that are inherent to the procedure. There is always a risk of misdiagnosing a cancer if an inadequate sample was procured during biopsy, or if the tumor was not properly located. There is a chance of infection of the surgical site, excessive bleeding, or injury to adjacent tissues. The possibility of metastasis and seeding are risks that have to be considered in consultation with an oncologist.

Results

The results of a tumor removal procedure depend on the type of tumor and the purpose of the treatment. Most benign tumors can be removed successfully with no risk of the abnormal cells spreading to other parts of the body

QUESTIONS TO ASK YOUR DOCTOR

- What type of tumor do I have and where is it located?
- What procedure will be used to remove the tumor?
- Is there evidence that the tumor has metastasized?
- What diagnostic tests will be performed prior to tumor removal?
- What method of anesthesia/pain relief will be used during the procedure?
- Will the tumor recur?
- When will I be able to return to normal activities?

and little risk of the tumor returning. Malignant tumors are considered successfully removed if the entire tumor can be removed, if a clear margin of healthy tissue is removed with the tumor, and if there is no evidence of metastasis. The normal results of palliative tumor removal are a reduction in the patient's symptoms with no impact on length of survival.

Morbidity and mortality rates

The recurrence rates of benign and malignant tumors after removal depend on the type of tumor and its location. The rate of complications associated with tumor removal surgery differs by procedure, but is generally very low.

Despite low rates of complication for the actual tumor removal procedures, cancer itself remains the second most frequent cause of death among Americans, responsible for about 25% of all deaths. In 2013, about 580,350 people in the United States were expected to die of cancer—about 1,600 deaths daily.

Alternatives

If a benign tumor shows no indication of harming nearby tissues and is not causing the patient any symptoms, surgery may not be required to remove it. Chemotherapy, radiation therapy, and biological therapy are treatments that may be used alone or in conjunction with surgery.

Health care team roles

Tumors are usually removed by a general surgeon or surgical oncologist. The procedure is frequently done in a hospital setting, but specialized outpatient facilities may sometimes be used.

Resources

BOOKS

Niederhuber, John E., et al. *Abeloff's Clinical Oncology.* 5th ed. Philadelphia: Saunders/Elsevier, 2013.

PERIODICALS

Arata, Jumpei, et al. "Neurosurgical Robotic System for Brain Tumor Removal." *International Journal of Computer-Assisted Radiology and Surgery* 6, no. 3 (2011): 375–85. http://dx.doi.org/10.1007/s11548-010-0514-8 (accessed September 19, 2013).

WEBSITES

MedlinePlus. "Benign Tumors." U.S. National Library of Medicine, National Institutes of Health. http://www.nlm. nih.gov/medlineplus/benigntumors.html (accessed September 19, 2013).

MedlinePlus. "Cancer." U.S. National Library of Medicine, National Institutes of Health. http://www.nlm.nih.gov/ medlineplus/cancer.html (accessed September 19, 2013).

ORGANIZATIONS

American Cancer Society, 250 Williams St. NW, Atlanta, GA 30303, (800) 227-2345, http://www.cancer.org.

National Cancer Institute, 6116 Executive Blvd., Ste. 300, Bethesda, MD 20892-8322, (800) 4-CANCER (422-6237), http://cancer.gov.

Society of Surgical Oncology, 9525 W. Bryn Mawr Ave., Ste. 870, Rosemont, IL 60018, (847) 427-1400, info@surgonc.org, http://surgonc.org.

J. Ricker Polsdorfer, MD
Stephanie Dionne Sherk
Rebecca Frey, PhD

Tumor staging

Definition

Tumor staging is the process of defining at what point in the natural history of the malignant disease the patient is when the diagnosis is made. The organ and cell type in which the malignancy has developed defines the type of malignancy. For example, adenocarcinoma of the lung defines that the cancer originated in the mucus-secreting cells lining the airways of the lung. Staging is different than defining the type of cancer; it is the process of defining the degree of advancement of the specific type of malignancy in the patient at the time of presentation (the time when the diagnosis is made).

Example of TNM staging (pancreatic cancer)

Stage 0	Cancer has been identified in the top layer of cells but has not reached deeper tissues.
Stage IA	The cancer is no larger than 2 cm and has not spread beyond the pancreas.
Stage IB	The cancer has grown larger than 2 cm but has not spread.
Stage IIA	The cancer has spread beyond the pancreas but has not reached large blood vessels or lymph nodes.
Stage IIB	The cancer has spread to nearby lymph nodes but not to large blood vessels, nerves, or other parts of the body.
Stage III	The cancer has spread to large blood vessels or nerves but has not reached other parts of the body.
Stage IV	The cancer has spread to other parts of the body.

SOURCE: American Cancer Society, "How is Pancreatic Cancer Staged?" Available online at: http://www.cancer.org/cancer/pancreaticcancer/detailedguide/pancreatic-cancer-staging.

(Table by PreMediaGlobal. Copyright © 2014 Cengage Learning®.)

Because there are many different types of malignancy arising from many different organs in the body, the specifics of staging systems vary.

Purpose

Staging fulfills an organizational role that is central to the treatment of cancer. After the tumor is staged, the treatment team knows to what degree the cancer has evolved in its natural history. This knowledge will provide the information necessary to formulate a plan of treatment and will allow an estimate of the success of that treatment (prognosis). Finally, by establishing uniform criteria for staging, people with the same type of malignancy presenting at the same stage can be treated equivalently. If a new treatment is tested that improves the long-term prognosis then that treatment will become the new standard of care. Thus, staging is vital to the processes of research and scientific reporting.

Prognosis

The first question that most patients want answered when they find they have cancer is "What am I going to do?" They want to know the ultimate outcome—their prognosis. Because of the existing research on the natural history, or progression of the disease, this information is available on a statistical basis. Staging, then, helps define the patient's prognosis. Intuitively, one would think that those presenting with an earlier stage have a better prognosis. For the most part, that is correct.

Scientific reporting and research

When a patient develops a life-threatening disease such as cancer, the physicians and other members of the treatment team intervene in an effort to improve the prognosis. Treatment regimens are defined as good or bad based on how they influence the prognosis of the disease. Staging allows medical professionals to interpret whether or not their efforts are favorably influencing the natural history of the disease. Once a patient's cancer stage has been established, a baseline exists against which to measure the efficacy of the cancer treatment that follows for that patient.

Staging plays a similar "baseline" role when considering a large group of cancer patients. In order to gauge accurately the effectiveness of any cancer treatment, researchers must know if the patients' conditions really are comparable. If they are, comparisons between treatments are fair. If the patients' conditions vary at the outset of a study, then comparing the outcomes of different treatments is not useful.

Staging provides that useful, objective standard so that researchers can accurately compare specific treatments in certain stages of particular cancers. Staging allows uniformity in treatment protocol and reporting of the data related to outcome. As new treatment protocols are developed, they can be tested on patients with the same type and stage of cancer and the two groups compared. If there is improvement with a new treatment protocol, that treatment regimen will be adopted as standard. Physicians can use these established best practices to determine treatments for their patients.

Criteria for staging

As it became apparent to medical professionals that staging of malignancies was necessary for accurate assessment of treatment regimens and defining the treatment recommendations themselves, criteria for staging needed to be developed. Initially this was done for individual tumors separately. Because of the need for uniformity, a universal set of criteria was desired. The TNM system of staging has been adopted for the most part for this reason. It has been developed and updated by The American Joint Committee on Cancer (AJCC). Some of the types of malignancy do not fit well into the TNM criteria and others have older systems that are still in use because they are effective and are deeply established in scientific literature.

TNM system

This system of staging is the general format used for staging cancer of all types and is updated and maintained by the AJCC. The "T" stands for tumor size. The "N" stands for spread to lymph nodes (nodal metastasis). The "M" stands for metastasis (spread of the cancer to sites in the body other than the organ of origin). When the diagnosis of cancer is made, a **physical examination**, along with laboratory testing and imaging studies, will be performed to define the TNM status of the patient. The TNM status will define the stage.

The tumor size, "T," will be assessed by physical examination or various imaging modalities depending on the accessibility of the tumor. The "T" value is generally defined as 1 through 4 on the basis of size and whether or not the tumor is invading structures that surround it. In cancer so early that it is felt to be incapable of spreading, it is assigned a "T" value of 0. The "T" value is, in essence, a description of the tumor in its local place of origin. As time passes and the staging system is continually updated, the "T" value is being subdivided in certain types of cancer. The subdivisions are indicated by letters "a" through "d" and also have a graduated value system. For example: T1 breast cancer is a tumor sized 2 cm or less in greatest dimension. T1a is less than 0.5 cm, T1b is 0.5 to 1.0 cm, and T1c is 1.0 to 2.0 cm.

In many cancers, there seems to be a progression from the place of primary origin, then to the regional lymph nodes, and then throughout the body. Lymph nodes can be thought of as filters that drain tissue fluid coming from a particular organ. If that organ has developed a cancer and some of the cells flow away with the tissue fluid to the lymph node filter that is draining that organ, the cancer may begin to grow there also. Assessment of lymph node involvement thus becomes the next step in staging and defines the "N" value. Since the word metastasis means that the cancer has spread from its point of origin to somewhere else in the body and the lymph nodes are in the region, the "N" value defines presence of regional metastasis. The assessment is performed by physical examination and imaging studies of the region involved. "N" is assigned a value of 0 for no nodes involved, or depending on the anatomic nature of the region, values 1 through 3.

"M" stands for distant metastasis. As mentioned previously, metastasis is the spread of the primary tumor to elsewhere in the body. When that spread or metastasis is outside the region of the primary tumor, the patient has distant metastasis. The "M" value is assessed by physical exam, laboratory studies, and imaging studies. Different cancers have different typical patterns of metastasis. Common areas of metastatic involvement are lung, liver, bone, and brain. The "M" value is assigned either 0 or 1. Another term used to describe the patient who has distant metastasis is having systemic disease. In the TNM system, virtually all patients with an "M" value of 1 have stage IV disease. The "M" value may also have a subscript defining the organ of metastatic involvement.

After the values for TNM have been determined as accurately as possible, the values are grouped together and a stage value is assigned. The stage value is usually I through IV (written in Roman numerals). Each stage may be subdivided if it is useful for treatment recommendations and reporting. In general, stage I implies the tumor is confined to its source of origin and stage IV implies distant metastasis or systemic disease. Because of different anatomical, prognostic, and treatment considerations, the intermediate stages are defined by different tumor sizes, the presence or absence of local invasion of the tumor into surrounding structures, or the number and/or presence of involved lymph nodes. Treatment recommendations and expected outcome are both defined to a large extent by stage. The specific criteria for each stage are contained in the *AJCC Cancer Staging Manual*.

Special staging systems

In the development of staging systems it has been recognized that some malignancies do not fit well into the scheme of the TNM system or that the system in place reflects the same information as the TNM system. Thus, there are a few special staging systems in use for specific organs of involvement. The goal is the same for these schema as for TNM—to define the point in the natural history of the cancer at presentation, to allow establishment of prognosis and treatment recommendations, and to facilitate scientific research and reporting.

OVARIAN CANCER. Ovarian cancer is staged using FIGO, which stands for the International Federation of Gynecology and Obstetrics. This organization developed staging criteria for the various gynecologic malignancies and ovarian cancer. In the FIGO system, ovarian cancer is staged I through IV similar to the TNM scheme, and then each stage is subdivided into A, B, or C, depending on defined criteria. TNM may also be used, but FIGO is more common.

LYMPHOMA. Anatomically, the lymph system and its nodes are found throughout the body. Malignancies involving the lymph system (lymphomas), do not fit the typical TNM scheme well. The Ann Arbor staging criteria are instead utilized to classify this group of malignancies. The goals of the Ann Arbor lymphoma staging system are to define the degree of advancement of the disease so that treatment recommendations can be made, prognosis can be estimated, and consistent reporting and research can be facilitated.

The Ann Arbor system classifies lymphoma into four stages based on anatomic lymph nodal group involvement. Disease confined to one nodal group or location defines stage I. Disease limited to one side of the diaphragm (the muscle separating the chest from the abdomen) defines stage II. Stage III patients have disease on both sides of the diaphragm and stage IV patients once again have disseminated disease. Consideration of involvement of the liver, spleen, and bone marrow are also considered in this system. Finally, the stage is subdivided into categories of A and B depending on the presence of symptoms of itching, weight loss, fever, and night sweats. Those having symptoms receive the designation "B" and have a worse prognosis.

LEUKEMIA. Leukemia is a type of malignancy that begins in the cells of the marrow that produce the cellular components of blood, the progenitor cells. These malignancies are truly systemic from their outset and do not fit any form of the TNM system. Still, there is a need to categorize the presenting features of the patients with these diseases to help make treatment recommendations, estimate prognosis, and to facilitate scientific research and reporting. The type of method used depends on the type of leukemia:

- Acute lymphocytic leukemia (ALL) is classified based upon the lymphocyte of origin (B-cell or T-cell).
- Acute myeloid leukemia is classified using the French-American-British (FAB) classification system. The World Health Organization (WHO) has developed a new system that takes more factors into consideration, but FAB is still common.
- Chronic lymphocytic leukemia is staged using the Rai system in the United States and the Binet system in Europe.
- Chronic myeloid leukemia is described as being in various phases rather than stages. Classification is based on a variety of factors, including disease progression, patient age, and white blood cell count.

LUNG CANCER, SMALL CELL. Unlike other types of lung cancer, the staging of small cell lung cancer is relatively simple. This is because approximately 70% of patients already have metastatic disease when they are diagnosed, and small differences in the amount of tumor found in the lungs do not change the prognosis. Small cell lung cancer is usually divided into three stages:

- Limited stage: The cancer is found only in one lung and in lymph nodes close to the lung.
- Extensive stage: The cancer has spread beyond the lungs to other parts of the body.
- Recurrent stage: The cancer has returned following treatment.

Defining the stage

The process of defining a stage is quite simple. First, the diagnosis is established by study of the patient and by tissue biopsy. Once the cell type and organ of origin are established, the staging criteria are reviewed. The patient will undergo a series of diagnostic tests to define the various parameters of the staging criteria. The results of these tests define the extent of the disease and establish the stage. The known typical natural history of the disease dictates the types of testing done. The tests differ for each type of malignancy.

KEY TERMS

Adenocarcinoma—Malignant cancers that originate in the tissues of glands or that form glandular structures.

Biopsy—A diagnostic procedure in which a small sample of tissue is obtained and examined to determine the type and stage of a disease.

Cancer—A disease caused by uncontrolled growth of the body's cells.

Lymph nodes—Small masses of tissue that are located throughout the body and contain clusters of cells called lymphocytes. They filter out and destroy bacteria, foreign particles, and cancerous cells from the blood.

Malignant—Cancerous.

Metastasis—The spread of cancer cells from one part of the body to another.

Pathologic—Characterized by disease or the structural and functional changes due to disease.

TNM—A system used for cancer staging. "T" stands for tumor, "N" stands for spread to lymph nodes, and "M" stands for metastasis.

Tumor—An abnormal proliferation of cells that can spread to other sites.

Special concerns

Clinical vs. pathological stage

The stage of the patient's disease may be categorized into clinical or pathological. As mentioned, the known natural history of the disease and the staging criteria are utilized to define the stage of the patient at the time of presentation. The investigations performed often involve an initial degree of uncertainty when they are based on clinical grounds alone. For example, the physical exam or the imaging of a particular group of lymph nodes may show that they are enlarged, but the enlargement may not accurately define whether they are truly involved with cancer. This issue may only be resolved by removing some or all of the suspect enlarged nodes, sometimes by biopsy before treatment or sometimes by the removal of the questionable nodes at the time of definitive treatment.

The evaluation under the microscope of the clinically enlarged nodes will define whether they are really involved with cancer or merely enlarged. When staging criteria are based on clinical assessment alone, it is referred to as the clinical stage. Once the results of the microscopic evaluation are known, the true stage or pathologic stage may be assigned.

Stage is uniform and accurate

One of the main goals of staging is to facilitate communication so that like patients are compared to like patients. It is imperative that the adopted staging criteria are rigidly adhered to or inaccurate comparisons may be made and the results of research to develop better treatment regimens will be difficult to interpret.

Tumor grade

When the tissue obtained for diagnosis is evaluated under the microscope for cell type, another index called grade is often defined. As the pathologist analyzes the malignant cells, attention will be given to how close to a normal cell the malignant cells appear to be. If they are very similar, the malignant cells are not felt to be too aggressive and a low grade value is assigned. The more atypical the malignant cells appear to be, the more aggressive the tumor is and a higher grade value is assigned. Grade is usually assigned a value of I through IV, though more levels can be assigned depending on the particular cancer.

The estimate of grade is just that—an estimation. It is subjective in nature and cannot be determined quantitatively. Though useful in predicting prognosis, the correlation is not exact. Rather, grade is included as only one of the factors influencing prognosis. Grade may be included as part of the actual staging criteria; however, it usually is not part of the scheme.

Tumor boards

A tumor board is a body of specialists in the treatment of cancer that convenes to discuss the aspects of patients presenting with cancer. The AJCC encourages the development of tumor boards throughout the nation to facilitate the use of staging and reporting of cancer statistics from region to region throughout the country. In addition to allowing the collection of vital cancer statistics, local tumor boards create a forum where the clinical aspects of a patient's cancer may be discussed to provide recommendations or to play a role in education.

Resources

BOOKS

Casciato, Dennis A., ed. *Manual of Clinical Oncology.* 7th ed. Philadelphia: Lippincott Williams & Wilkins, 2012.

Compton, Caryolyn C., et al., eds. *AJCC Cancer Staging Atlas: A Companion to the Seventh Editions of the AJCC Cancer Staging Manual and Handbook.* 2nd ed. New York: Springer, 2012.

DeVita, Vincent T. Jr., et al., eds. *DeVita, Hellman, and Rosenberg's Cancer: Principles and Practice of Oncology.* 9th ed. Philadelphia: Lippincott Williams & Wilkins, 2011.

Edge, Stephen B., et al., eds. *AJCC Cancer Staging Handbook.* 7th ed. New York: Springer, 2010.

PERIODICALS

Al-Hawary, Mahmoud M., et al. "Staging of Pancreatic Cancer: Role of Imaging." *Seminars in Roentgenology* 48, no. 3 (2013): 245–52. http://dx.doi.org/10.1053/j.ro.2013.03.005 (accessed September 25, 2013).

"Current FIGO Staging for Cancer of the Vagina, Fallopian Tube, Ovary, and Gestational Trophoblastic Neoplasia." *International Journal of Gynaecology and Obstetrics* 105, no. 1 (2009): 3–4.

Ghafoori, M., et al. "Value of MRI in Local Staging of Bladder Cancer." *Urology Journal* 10, no. 2 (2013): 866–72.

Heitz, F., P. Harter, A. du Bois. "Staging Laparoscopy for the Management of Early-Stage Ovarian Cancer: A Meta-analysis." *American Journal of Obstetrics & Gynecology* (June 2013): e-pub ahead of print. http://dx.doi.org/10.1016/j.ajog.2013.06.035 (accessed September 25, 2013).

Nordholm-Carstensen, Andreas, et al. "Indeterminate Pulmonary Nodules at Colorectal Cancer Staging: A Systematic Review of Predictive Parameters for Malignancy." *Annals of Surgical Oncology* (June 2013): e-pub ahead of print. http://dx.doi.org/10.1245/s10434-013-3062-y (accessed September 25, 2013).

Peng, Chun-Wei, et al. "Evaluation of the Staging Systems for Gastric Cancer." *Journal of Surgical Oncology* (June 28, 2013): e-pub ahead of print. http://dx.doi.org/10.1002/jso.23360 (accessed September 25, 2013).

WEBSITES

American Cancer Society. "How is Acute Lymphocytic Leukemia Classified?" http://www.cancer.org/cancer/leukemia-acutelymphocyticallinadults/detailedguide/leukemia-acute-lymphocytic-classified (accessed September 25, 2013).

American Cancer Society. "How is Acute Myeloid Leukemia Classified?" http://www.cancer.org/cancer/leukemia-acutemyeloidaml/detailedguide/leukemia-acute-myeloid-myelogenous-classified (accessed September 25, 2013).

American Cancer Society. "How is Chronic Lymphocytic Leukemia Staged?" http://www.cancer.org/cancer/leukemia-chroniclymphocyticcll/detailedguide/leukemia-chronic-lymphocytic-staging (accessed September 25, 2013).

American Cancer Society. "How is Chronic Myeloid Leukemia Staged?" http://www.cancer.org/cancer/leukemia-chronicmyeloidcml/detailedguide/leukemia-chronic-myeloid-myelogenous-staging (accessed September 25, 2013).

American Cancer Society. "How is Colorectal Cancer Staged?" http://www.cancer.org/cancer/colonandrectumcancer/detailedguide/colorectal-cancer-staged (accessed September 25, 2013).

American Cancer Society. "Staging." http://www.cancer.org/treatment/understandingyourdiagnosis/staging (accessed September 25, 2013).

American Joint Committee on Cancer. "What Is Cancer Staging?" http://www.cancerstaging.org/mission/whatis.html (accessed September 25, 2013).

American Lung Association. "Staging." http://www.lung.org/lung-disease/lung-cancer/learning-more-about-lung-cancer/diagnosing-lung-cancer/staging.html (accessed September 25, 2013).

BreastCancer.org "Stages of Breast Cancer." http://www.breastcancer.org/symptoms/diagnosis/staging (accessed September 25, 2013).

National Cancer Institute. "Cancer Staging." http://www.cancer.gov/cancertopics/factsheet/detection/staging (accessed September 25, 2013).

Target Ovarian Cancer. "International Federation of Obstetricians and Gynaecologists (FIGO) Staging System for Ovarian Cancer." http://www.targetovariancancer.org.uk/page.asp?section=131 (accessed September 25, 2013).

ORGANIZATIONS

American Cancer Society, 250 Williams St. NW, Atlanta, GA 30303, (800) 227-2345, http://www.cancer.org.

American Joint Committee on Cancer (AJCC), 633 N. St. Clair St., Chicago, IL 60611-3211, (312) 202-5205, ajcc@facs.org, http://www.cancerstaging.org.

Cancer Research Institute, One Exchange Plz., 55 Broadway, Ste. 1802, New York, NY 10006, (212) 688-7515, (800) 99-CANCER (992-2623), http://cancerresearch.org.

International Federation of Gynecology and Obstetrics (FIGO), FIGO House, Ste. 3, Waterloo Ct., 10 Theed St., London, SE1 8ST, United Kingdom, +44 20 7928 1166, http://www.figo.org.

National Cancer Institute, 6116 Executive Blvd., Ste. 300, Bethesda, MD 20892-8322, (800) 4-CANCER (422-6237), http://cancer.gov.

Richard A. McCartney, MD

TURP *see* **Transurethral resection of the prostate**

Tylenol *see* **Acetaminophen**

Tympanoplasty

Definition

Tympanoplasty, also called eardrum repair, refers to surgery performed to reconstruct a perforated tympanic membrane (eardrum) or the small bones of the middle ear. Eardrum perforation may result from chronic infection or, less commonly, from trauma to the eardrum.

Purpose

The tympanic membrane of the ear is a three-layer structure. The outer and inner layers consist of epithelium cells. Perforations occur as a result of defects in the middle layer, which contains elastic collagen fibers. Small perforations usually heal spontaneously. However, if the defect is relatively large, or if there is a poor blood supply or an infection during the healing process, spontaneous repair may be hindered. Eardrums may also be perforated as a result of trauma, such as an object in the ear, a slap on the ear, or an explosion.

The purpose of tympanoplasty is to repair the perforated eardrum, and sometimes the middle ear bones (ossicles) that consist of the incus, malleus, and stapes. Tympanic membrane grafting may be required. If needed, grafts are usually taken from a vein or fascia (muscle sheath) tissue on the lobe of the ear. Synthetic materials may be used if patients have had previous surgeries and have limited graft availability.

Demographics

In the United States, ear disorders leading to hearing loss affect all ages. Over 60% of the population with hearing loss is under the age of 65, although nearly 25% of those above age 65 have a hearing loss that is considered significant. Causes include: birth defect (4.4%), ear infection (12.2%), ear injury (4.9%), damage due to excessive noise levels (33.7%), advanced age (28%), and other problems (16.8%).

Description

There are five basic types of tympanoplasty procedures:

• Type I tympanoplasty is called myringoplasty and involves the restoration of the perforated eardrum by grafting.

Tympanoplasty

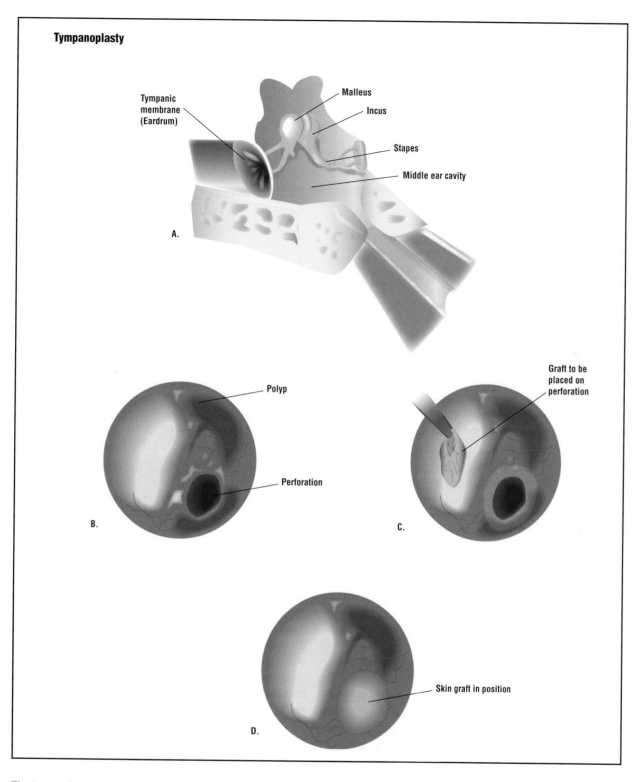

Tympanic membrane (Eardrum)

Malleus

Incus

Stapes

Middle ear cavity

A.

Polyp

Perforation

B.

Graft to be placed on perforation

C.

Skin graft in position

D.

The tympanic membrane, or eardrum, may need surgical repair when punctured (A). During a type I tympanoplasty, a perforation in the eardrum is visualized (B). A tissue graft is placed over the perforation (C) and held in place by the existing eardrum (D). *(Illustration by GGS Information Services. Copyright © Cengage Learning®.)*

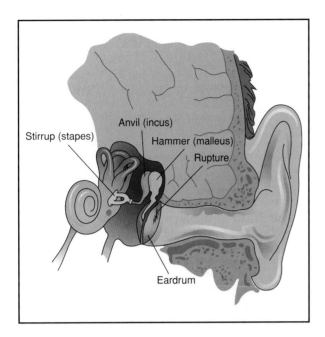

Perforated eardrum. *(Illustration by Electronic Illustrators Group. Copyright © Cengage Learning®.)*

KEY TERMS

Audiogram—A test of hearing at a range of sound frequencies.

Epithelium—The covering of internal and external surfaces of the body, including the lining of vessels and other small cavities. It consists of cells joined by small amounts of cementing substances.

Fistula test—Compression or rarefaction of the air in the external auditory canal.

Mastoid process—The nipple-like projection of part of the temporal bone (the large irregular bone situated in the base and side of the skull).

Mastoidectomy—Hollowing out the mastoid process by curetting, gouging, drilling, or otherwise removing the bony partitions forming the mastoid cells.

Myringoplasty—Surgical restoration of a perforated tympanic membrane by grafting.

Ossicles—Small bones of the middle ear, called stapes, malleus, and incus.

Ossiculoplasty—Surgical insertion of an implant to replace one or more of the ear ossicles. Also called ossicular replacement.

Otoscopy—Examination of the ear with an otoscope, an instrument designed to evaluate the condition of the ear.

Tinnitus—Noises or ringing in the ear.

- Type II tympanoplasty is used for tympanic membrane perforations with erosion of the malleus. It involves grafting onto the incus or the remains of the malleus.

- Type III tympanoplasty is indicated for destruction of two ossicles, with the stapes still intact and mobile. It involves placing a graft onto the stapes, and providing protection for the assembly.

- Type IV tympanoplasty is used for ossicular destruction, which includes all or part of the stapes arch. It involves placing a graft onto or around a mobile stapes footplate.

- Type V tympanoplasty is used when the footplate of the stapes is fixed.

Depending on its type, tympanoplasty can be performed under local or **general anesthesia**. In small perforations of the eardrum, Type I tympanoplasty can be easily performed under **local anesthesia** with intravenous sedation. An incision is made into the ear canal and the remaining eardrum is elevated away from the bony ear canal and lifted forward. The surgeon uses an operating microscope to enlarge the view of the ear structures. If the perforation is very large or the hole is far forward and away from the view of the surgeon, it may be necessary to perform an incision behind the ear. This elevates the entire outer ear forward, providing access to the perforation. Once the hole is fully exposed, the perforated remnant is rotated forward, and the bones of hearing are inspected. If scar tissue is present, it is removed either with micro hooks or laser.

Tissue is then taken either from the back of the ear, the tragus (small cartilaginous lobe of skin in front of the ear), or from a vein. The tissues are thinned and dried. An absorbable gelatin sponge is placed under the eardrum to support the graft. The graft is then inserted underneath the remaining eardrum remnant, which is folded back onto the perforation to provide closure. Very thin sheeting is usually placed against the top of the graft to prevent it from sliding out of the ear when the patient sneezes.

If it was opened from behind, the ear is then stitched together. Usually, the stitches are buried in the skin and do not have to be removed later. A sterile patch is placed on the outside of the ear canal and the patient returns to the recovery room.

Diagnosis

The examining physician performs a complete physical with diagnostic testing of the ear, which includes an audiogram and history of the hearing loss, as well as any vertigo or facial weakness. A microscopic exam is also performed. Otoscopy is used to assess the mobility of the tympanic membrane and the malleus. A fistula test can be performed if there is a history of dizziness or a marginal perforation of the eardrum.

Preparation

Preparation for surgery depends upon the type of tympanoplasty. For all procedures, however, blood and urine studies and hearing tests are conducted prior to surgery.

Aftercare

Generally, the patient can return home within two to three hours. **Antibiotics** are given, along with a mild pain reliever. After ten days, the packing is removed and the ear is evaluated to see if the graft was successful. Water is kept away from the ear, and nose blowing is discouraged. If there are allergies or a cold, antibiotics and a decongestant are usually prescribed. Most patients can return to work after five or six days, or two to three weeks if they perform heavy physical labor. After three weeks, all packing is completely removed under the operating microscope. It is then determined whether or not the graft has been completely successful.

Postoperative care is also designed to keep the patient comfortable. Infection is generally prevented by soaking the ear canal with antibiotics. To heal, the graft must be kept free from infection, and must not experience shearing forces or excessive tension. Activities that change the tympanic pressure are forbidden, such as sneezing with the mouth shut, using a straw to drink, or heavy nose blowing. A complete hearing test is performed four to six weeks after the operation.

Risks

Possible complications include failure of the graft to heal, causing recurrent eardrum perforation; narrowing (stenosis) of the ear canal; scarring or **adhesions** in the middle ear; perilymph fistula and hearing loss; erosion or extrusion of the prosthesis; dislocation of the prosthesis; and facial nerve injury. Other problems such as recurrence of cholesteatoma may or may not result from the surgery.

Tinnitus (noises in the ear), particularly echo-type noises, may be present as a result of the perforation itself. Usually, with improvement in hearing and closure of the eardrum, the tinnitus resolves. In some cases, however, it may worsen after the operation. It is rare for the tinnitus to be permanent after surgery.

QUESTIONS TO ASK YOUR DOCTOR

- Are there any other options aside from tympanoplasty?
- How will the surgery impact hearing?
- How long will it take to recover from the surgery?
- What are the possible complications?
- How many tympanoplasty surgeries does the surgeon perform each year?
- How successful is tympanoplasty in restoring normal hearing?

Results

Tympanoplasty is successful in over 90% of cases. In most cases, the operation relieves pain and infection symptoms completely. Hearing loss is minor.

Morbidity and mortality rates

There can be imbalance and dizziness immediately after this procedure. Dizziness, however, is uncommon in tympanoplasties that only involve the eardrum. Besides failure of the graft, there may be further hearing loss due to unexplained factors during the healing process. This occurs in less than 5% of patients. A total hearing loss from tympanoplasty surgery is rare, occurring in less than 1% of operations. Mild postoperative dizziness and imbalance can persist for about a week after surgery. If the ear becomes infected after surgery, the risk of dizziness increases. Generally, imbalance and dizziness completely disappears after a week or two.

Alternatives

Myringoplasty is another operative procedure used in the reconstruction of a perforation of the tympanic membrane. It is performed when the middle ear space, its mucosa, and the ossicular chain are free of active infection. Unlike tympanoplasty, there is no direct inspection of the middle ear during this procedure.

Health care team roles

Tympanoplasty is usually performed on an outpatient basis by an otolaryngologist, a physician specialized in the diagnosis and treatment of disorders and diseases of the ears, nose, and throat. For most adults, Type I tympanoplasty is performed in the office of the otolaryngologist with topical anesthesia at the tympanic membrane site, and subcutaneous local anesthesia injection at the graft donor site. An overnight stay is recommended if the tympanoplasty involves ossicular replacement.

Resources

BOOKS

Fisch, U., John May, and Thomas Linder. *Tympanoplasty, Mastoidectomy, and Stapes Surgery.* 2nd ed. New York: Thieme, 2008.

Tos, Mirko. *Cartilage Tympanoplasty.* New York: Thieme, 2009.

PERIODICALS

Leong, A. C., and D. A. Bowdler. "A Simple Method to Prevent the Obstruction of Post-Tympanoplasty Ventilation Tubes." *The Journal of Laryngology & Otology* 127, no. 9 (2013): 922–23. http://dx.doi.org/10.1017/S002221511300159X (accessed October 4, 2013).

Tarabichi, M., et al. "Endoscopic Management of Chronic Otitis Media and Tympanoplasty." *Otolaryngologic Clinics of North America* 46, no. 2 (2013): 155–63. http://dx.doi.org/10.1016/j.otc.2012.12.002 (accessed October 4, 2013).

WEBSITES

A.D.A.M. Medical Encyclopedia. "Eardrum Repair." MedlinePlus. http://www.nlm.nih.gov/medlineplus/ency/article/003014.htm (accessed October 4, 2013).

University of Wisconsin-Madison. "Tympanoplasty." MedlinePlus. http://www.uwhealth.org/healthfacts/B_EXTRANET_HEALTH_INFORMATION-FlexMember-Show_Public_HFFY_1117547740636.html (accessed October 4, 2013).

ORGANIZATIONS

American Academy of Otolaryngology—Head and Neck Surgery, 1650 Diagonal Rd., Alexandria, VA 22314-2857, (703) 836-4444, http://www.entnet.org.

American Hearing Research Foundation, 8 S. Michigan Avenue, Ste. 814, Chicago, IL 60603, (312) 726-9670, http://american-hearing.org.

Monique Laberge, PhD

Type and screen

Definition

Blood typing is a laboratory test that identifies blood group antigens (substances that stimulate an immune response) belonging to the ABO blood group system. The test classifies blood into the four major groups designated A, B, AB, and O. Antibody screening is a test

Blood type compatibility

Donor blood type	Recipient blood type			
	A	B	AB	O
A	X		X	
B		X	X	
AB			X	
O	X	X	X	X

SOURCE: American Red Cross, "Blood Types." Available online at: http://www.redcrossblood.org/learn-about-blood/blood-types.

(Chart by PreMediaGlobal. Copyright © 2014 Cengage Learning®.)

to detect atypical antibodies in the serum that may have been formed as a result of **transfusion** or pregnancy. An antibody is a protein produced by lymphocytes (nongranular white blood cells) that binds to an antigen, facilitating its removal by phagocytosis (or engulfing by macrophages) or lysis (cell rupture or decomposition). The type and screen (T&S) is performed on persons who may need a transfusion of blood products. These tests are followed by the compatibility test (crossmatch). This test ensures that no antibodies are detected in the recipient's serum that will react with the donor's red blood cells.

Purpose

Blood typing and screening are most commonly performed to ensure that people who need transfusions will receive blood that matches (is compatible with) their own, and that clinically significant antibodies are identified if present. People must receive blood of the same blood type; otherwise, the recipient's immune system will recognize the antigen in the donor blood as foreign. Antibodies will attack the donor blood, damaging and bursting the donor red blood cells. This can result in high serum levels of hemoglobin spilling from the burst red blood cells (called hemoglobinemia), disseminated intravascular coagulation or DIC (a condition in which clotting factors are used up very rapidly, resulting in the potential for severe, uncontrollable bleeding), kidney failure, and eventually complete cardiovascular collapse (a combination of heart attack, shock, and lack of blood flow to all major organs and tissues).

Prenatal care

Parents who are expecting a baby have their blood typed to diagnose and prevent hemolytic disease of the newborn (HDN), a type of anemia also known as erythroblastosis fetalis. Babies who have a blood type different from their mother's are at risk for developing this disease.

Determination of paternity

Children inherit factors or genes from each parent that determine their blood type. This fact makes blood typing useful in paternity testing. The blood types of the child, mother, and alleged father are compared to determine paternity.

Forensic investigations

Legal investigations may require typing of blood or other body fluids such as semen or saliva to identify criminal suspects. In some cases, typing is used to identify the victims of crime or major disasters.

Description

Blood typing and screening tests are performed in a blood bank laboratory by technologists trained in blood bank and transfusion services. The tests are performed on blood after it has been separated into cells and serum (the yellow liquid left after the blood cells are removed). Costs for both tests are covered by insurance when the tests are determined to be medically necessary.

Blood bank laboratories are usually located in blood center facilities, such as those operated by the American Red Cross, that collect, process, and supply blood that is donated. Blood bank laboratories are also found in most hospitals and other facilities that prepare blood for transfusion. These laboratories are regulated by the United States Food and Drug Administration (FDA) and are inspected and accredited by a professional association such as the American Association of Blood Banks (AABB).

Blood typing and screening tests are based on the reaction between antigens and antibodies. An antigen can be anything that triggers the body's immune response. The body produces a special protein called an antibody, which combines with the antigen to neutralize it. A person's body normally does not produce antibodies against its own antigens.

The antigens found on the surface of red blood cells are important because they determine a person's blood type. When red blood cells having a certain blood type antigen are mixed with serum containing antibodies that react against that antigen, the antibodies combine with and stick to the antigen. In a test tube, this reaction is visible as clumping or aggregating.

Although there are over 600 known red blood cell antigens organized into 22 blood group systems, routine blood typing is usually concerned with only two systems:

the ABO and Rh blood group systems. Antibody screening helps to identify antibodies against several other groups of red blood cell antigens.

Blood typing

THE ABO BLOOD GROUP SYSTEM. In 1901, Karl Landsteiner, an Austrian pathologist, randomly combined the serum and red blood cells of his colleagues. From the reactions he observed in test tubes, he developed the ABO blood group system, which earned him the 1930 Nobel Prize in Medicine. A person's ABO blood type—A, B, AB, or O—is based on the presence or absence of the A and B antigens on the red blood cells. The A blood type has only the A antigen and the B blood type has only the B antigen. The AB blood type has both A and B antigens, and the O blood type has neither the A nor the B antigen.

By the age of six months, a person will have developed antibodies against the antigens that his or her red blood cells lack. That is, a person with A blood type will have anti-B antibodies, and a person with B blood type will have anti-A antibodies. A person with AB blood type will have neither antibody, but a person with O blood type will have both anti-A and anti-B antibodies. Although the distribution of each of the four ABO blood types varies among racial groups, O is the most common and AB is the least common in all groups.

FORWARD AND REVERSE TYPING. ABO typing is the first test done on blood when it is tested for transfusion. A person must receive ABO-matched blood because ABO incompatibilities are the major cause of fatal transfusion reactions. To guard against these incompatibilities, typing is done in two steps. In the first step, called forward typing, the patient's blood is mixed with serum that contains antibodies against type A blood, then with serum that contains antibodies against type B blood. A determination of the blood type is based on whether or not the blood clots in the presence of these sera.

In reverse typing, the patient's blood serum is mixed with blood that is known to be either type A or type B. Again, the presence of clotting is used to determine the type.

An ABO incompatibility between a pregnant woman and her baby is a common cause of HDN but seldom requires treatment. This is because the majority of ABO antibodies are immunoglobulin M (IgM), which are too large to cross the placenta. It is the immunoglobulin G (IgG) component that may cause HDN, and this is most often present in the plasma of group O mothers.

Paternity testing compares the ABO blood types of the child, mother, and alleged father. The alleged father cannot be the biological father if the child's blood type requires a gene that neither he nor the mother have. For example, a child with blood type B whose mother has blood type O requires a father with either AB or B blood type; a man with blood type O cannot be the biological father.

In some people, ABO antigens can be detected in body fluids other than blood, such as saliva, sweat, or semen. People whose body fluids contain detectable amounts of antigens are known as secretors. ABO typing of these fluids provides clues in legal investigations.

THE RH BLOOD GROUP SYSTEM. The Rh, or Rhesus, system was first detected in 1940 by Landsteiner and Wiener when they injected blood from rhesus monkeys into guinea pigs and rabbits. More than 50 antigens have since been discovered that belong to this system, making it the most complex red blood cell antigen system.

In routine blood typing and crossmatching tests, only one of these 50 antigens, the D antigen, also known as the Rh factor or $Rh_o[D]$, is tested for. If the D antigen is present, that person is Rh-positive; if the D antigen is absent, that person is Rh-negative.

Other important antigens in the Rh system are C, c, E, and e. These antigens are not usually tested for in routine blood typing tests. Testing for the presence of these antigens, however, is useful in paternity testing, and in cases in which a technologist screens blood to identify unexpected Rh antibodies or find matching blood for a person with antibodies to one or more of these antigens.

Unlike the ABO system, antibodies to Rh antigens don't develop naturally. They develop only as an immune response after a transfusion or during pregnancy. The incidence of the Rh blood types varies between racial groups, but not as widely as the ABO blood types: 85% of Caucasians and 90% of African Americans are Rh-positive; 15% of Caucasians and 10% of African Americans are Rh-negative.

The distribution of ABO and Rh blood groups in the overall United States population is as follows:

- O Rh-positive, 38%
- O Rh-negative, 7%
- A Rh-positive, 34%
- A Rh-negative, 6%
- B Rh-positive, 9%
- B Rh-negative, 2%
- AB Rh-positive, 3%
- AB Rh-negative, 1%

In transfusions, the Rh system is next in importance after the ABO system. Most Rh-negative people who receive Rh-positive blood will develop anti-D antibodies.

A later transfusion of Rh-positive blood may result in a severe or fatal transfusion reaction.

Rh incompatibility is the most common and severe cause of HDN. This incompatibility may occur when an Rh-negative mother and an Rh-positive father have an Rh-positive baby. Cells from the baby can cross the placenta and enter the mother's bloodstream, causing the mother to make anti-D antibodies. Unlike ABO antibodies, the structure of anti-D antibodies makes it likely that they will cross the placenta and enter the baby's bloodstream. There, they can destroy the baby's red blood cells, causing a severe or fatal anemia.

The first step in preventing HDN is to find out the Rh types of the expectant parents. If the mother is Rh-negative and the father is Rh-positive, the baby is at risk for developing HDN. The next step is performing an antibody screen of the mother's serum to make sure she doesn't already have anti-D antibodies from a previous pregnancy or transfusion. Finally, the Rh-negative mother is given an injection of Rh immunoglobulin (RhIg) at 28 weeks of gestation and again after delivery if the baby is Rh positive. The RhIg attaches to any Rh-positive cells from the baby in the mother's bloodstream, preventing them from triggering anti-D antibody production in the mother. An Rh-negative woman should also receive RhIg following a miscarriage, abortion, or ectopic pregnancy.

OTHER BLOOD GROUP SYSTEMS. Several other blood group systems may be involved in HDN and transfusion reactions, although they are much less common than ABO and Rh incompatibilities. Some of the other groups are the Duffy, Kell, Kidd, MNS, and P systems. Tests for antigens from these systems are not included in routine blood typing, but they are commonly used in paternity testing.

Like Rh antibodies, antibodies in these systems do not develop naturally, but as an immune response after transfusion or during pregnancy. An antibody screening test is done before a crossmatch to check for unexpected antibodies to antigens in these systems. A person's serum is mixed in a test tube with commercially prepared cells containing antigens from these systems. If hemagglutination, or clumping, occurs, the antibody is identified.

Antibody screening

Antibody screening is done to look for unexpected antibodies to other blood groups, such as certain Rh (e.g., E, e, C, c), Duffy, MNS, Kell, Kidd, and P system antigens. The recipient's serum is mixed with screening reagent red blood cells. The screening reagent red blood cells are cells with known antigens. This test is sometimes called an indirect antiglobulin or Coombs' test. If an antibody to an antigen is present, the mixture will cause agglutination (clumping) of the red blood cells or cause hemolysis (breaking of the red cell membrane). If an antibody to one of these antigens is found, only blood without that antigen will be compatible in a crossmatch. This sequence must be repeated before each transfusion a person receives.

Testing for infectious disease markers

Pretransfusion testing includes analyzing blood for the following infectious disease markers:

- Hepatitis B surface antigen (HBsAg). This test detects the outer envelope of the hepatitis B virus.
- Antibodies to the core of the hepatitis B virus (Anti-HBc). This test detects an antibody to the hepatitis B virus that is produced during and after an infection.
- Antibodies to the hepatitis C virus (Anti-HCV).
- Antibodies to human immunodeficiency virus, types 1 and 2 (Anti-HIV-1, -2).
- HIV-1 p24 antigen. This test screens for antigens of HIV-1. The advantage of this test is that it can detect HIV-1 infection a week earlier than the antibody test.
- Antibodies to human T-lymphotropic virus, types I and II (Anti-HTLV-I, -II). In the United States, HTLV infection is most common among intravenous drug users.
- Syphilis. This test is performed to detect evidence of infection with the spirochete *Treponema pallidum*.
- Nucleic acid amplification testing (NAT). NAT uses a new form of blood testing technology that directly detects the genetic material of the HCV and HIV viruses.
- Confirmatory tests. These are done to screen out false positives.

Crossmatching

Crossmatching is the final step in pretransfusion testing. It is commonly referred to as compatibility testing, or "type and cross." Before blood from a donor and the recipient are crossmatched, both are ABO and Rh typed. To begin the crossmatch, a unit of blood from a donor with the same ABO and Rh type as the recipient is selected. Serum from the patient is mixed with red blood cells from the donor. The crossmatch can be performed either as a short (5–10 min) incubation intended only to verify ABO compatibility, or as a long (45 min) incubation with an antihuman globulin test intended to verify compatibility for all other red cell antigens. If clumping occurs, the blood is not compatible; if clumping does not occur, the blood is compatible. If an unexpected antibody is found in either the patient or the donor, the blood bank does further testing to ensure that the blood is compatible.

In an emergency, when there is not enough time for blood typing and crossmatching, O red blood cells may be given, preferably Rh-negative. O-type blood is called the universal donor because it has no ABO antigens for a patient's antibodies to combine with. In contrast, AB blood type is called the universal recipient because it has no ABO antibodies to combine with the antigens on transfused red blood cells. If there is time for blood typing, red blood cells of the recipient type (type-specific cells) are given. In either case, the crossmatch is continued even though the transfusion has begun.

Autologous donation

The practice of collecting a patient's own blood prior to **elective surgery** for later transfusion is called autologous donation. Since the safest blood for transfusion is the patient's own, autologous donation is particularly useful for patients with rare blood types. Two to four units of blood are collected several weeks before surgery, and the patient is given iron supplements to build up his or her hemoglobin levels.

Preparation

To collect the 10 mL of blood needed for these tests, a healthcare worker ties a tourniquet above the patient's elbow, locates a vein near the inner elbow, cleans the skin overlying the vein, and inserts a needle into that vein. The blood is drawn through the needle into an attached vacuum tube. Collection of the sample takes only a few minutes.

Blood typing and screening must be done three days or less before a transfusion. A person does not need to change diet, medications, or activities before these tests. Patients should tell their health care provider if they have received a blood transfusion or a plasma substitute during the last three months, or have had a radiology procedure using intravenous contrast media. These can give false clumping reactions in both typing and crossmatching tests.

Aftercare

The possible side effects of any blood collection are discomfort, bruising, or excessive bleeding at the site where the needle punctured the skin, as well as dizziness or fainting. Bruising and bleeding is reduced if pressure is applied with a finger to the puncture site until the bleeding stops. Discomfort can be treated with warm packs to the puncture site.

Risks

Aside from the rare event of infection or bleeding, there are no risks from blood collection. Blood

KEY TERMS

ABO blood type—Blood type based on the presence or absence of the A and B antigens on the red blood cells. There are four types: A, B, AB, and O.

Acute hemolytic transfusion reaction (AHTR)—A severe transfusion reaction with abrupt onset, most often caused by ABO incompatibility. Symptoms include difficulty breathing, fever and chills, pain, and sometimes shock.

Antibody—A protein produced by B-lymphocytes that binds to an antigen, facilitating its removal by phagocytosis or lysis.

Antigen—Any substance that stimulates the production of antibodies and combines specifically with them.

Autologous donation—Donation of the patient's own blood, made several weeks before elective surgery.

Blood bank—A laboratory that specializes in blood typing, antibody identification, and transfusion services.

Blood type—Any of various classes into which human blood can be divided according to immunological compatibility based on the presence or absence of certain antigens on the red blood cells. Blood types are sometimes called blood groups.

Crossmatch—A laboratory test done to confirm that blood from a donor and blood from the recipient are compatible. Serum from each is mixed with red blood cells from the other and observed for hemagglutination.

Ectopic pregnancy—The implantation of a fertilized egg in a woman's fallopian tube instead of the uterus.

Gene—A piece of DNA, located on a chromosome, that determines how traits such as blood type are inherited and expressed.

Hemagglutination—The clumping of red blood cells due to blood type incompatibility.

Hematocrit—The proportion of the volume of a blood sample that consists of red blood cells. It is expressed as a percentage.

Indirect Coombs' test—A test used to screen for unexpected antibodies against red blood cells. The patient's serum is mixed with reagent red blood cells, incubated, washed, tested with antihuman globulin, and observed for clumping.

Lysis—Destruction or decomposition.

Pathologist—A doctor who specializes in the study of diseases. The ABO blood groups were discovered by an Austrian pathologist.

Rh blood type—In general, refers to the blood type based on the presence or absence of the D antigen on the red blood cells. There are, however, other antigens in the Rh system.

Serum (plural, sera)—The clear, pale yellow liquid that separates from a clot when blood coagulates.

Tourniquet—A thin piece of tubing or other device used to stop bleeding or control circulation by compressing the blood vessels in an arm or leg. Health care professionals apply a tourniquet before drawing blood.

Transfusion—The therapeutic introduction of blood or a blood component into a patient's bloodstream.

transfusions, however, always have the risk of an unexpected transfusion reaction. These complications may include an acute hemolytic transfusion reaction (AHTR), which is most commonly caused by ABO incompatibility. The patient may complain of pain, difficult breathing, fever and chills, facial flushing, and nausea. Signs of shock may appear, including a drop in blood pressure and a rapid but weak pulse. If AHTR is suspected, the transfusion should be stopped at once.

Other milder transfusion reactions include a delayed hemolytic transfusion reaction, which may occur one to two weeks after the transfusion. It consists of a slight fever and a falling **hematocrit**, and is usually self-limited. Patients may also have allergic reactions to unknown components in donor blood.

Results

The blood type is labeled as A+, A−, B+, B−, O+, O−, AB+, or AB−, based on both the ABO and Rh systems. If antibody screening is negative, only a crossmatch is necessary. If the antibody screen is positive, then blood that is negative for those antigens must be identified. The desired result of a crossmatch is that compatible donor blood is found. Compatibility testing procedures are designed to provide the safest blood product possible for the recipient, but a compatible crossmatch is no guarantee that an unexpected adverse reaction will not appear during the transfusion.

Except in an emergency, a person cannot receive a transfusion without a compatible crossmatch result.

In rare cases, the least incompatible blood has to be given.

Resources

BOOKS

Bope, E. T. *Conn's Current Therapy*. Philadelphia: Saunders/Elseier, 2013.

Ferri, Fred, ed. *Ferri's Clinical Advisor 2013*. Philadelphia: Mosby Elsevier, 2013.

Goldman, Lee, and Andrew I. Schafer. *Goldman's Cecil Medicine*. 24th ed. Philadelphia: Saunders/Elsevier, 2012.

Hoffman, R., et al. *Hematology: Basic Principles and Practice*. 6th ed. Philadelphia: Elsevier, 2012.

McPherson, Richard A., and Matthew R. Pincus, eds. *Henry's Clinical Diagnosis and Management by Laboratory Methods*. 22nd ed. Philadelphia: Saunders/Elsevier, 2011.

Rakel, R. *Textbook of Family Medicine*. 8th ed. Philadelphia: Saunders/Elsevier, 2011.

PERIODICALS

Reich, David, and Melissa S. Pessin. "Rational Preoperative Blood Type and Screen Testing Criteria." *Anesthesiology* 116, no. 4 (2012): 749–50.

WEBSITES

A.D.A.M. Medical Encyclopedia. "Blood Typing." MedlinePlus. http://www.nlm.nih.gov/medlineplus/ency/article/003345.htm (accessed August 1, 2013).

American Association for Clinical Chemistry. "Blood Typing." Lab Tests Online. http://labtestsonline.org/understanding/analytes/blood-typing (accessed August 1, 2013).

American Red Cross. "Blood Types." http://www.redcrossblood.org/learn-about-blood/blood-types (accessed August 1, 2013).

"The Blood Typing Game." Nobelprize.org. http://www.nobelprize.org/educational/medicine/bloodtypinggame (accessed August 1, 2013).

Women's Health Connecticut. "Routine Lab Tests." http://www.womenshealthct.com/your_health/pregnancy/routine_care_during_pregnancy/routine_lab_tests (accessed August 1, 2013).

ORGANIZATIONS

AABB (American Association of Blood Banks), 8101 Glenbrook Rd., Bethesda, MD 20814-2749, (301) 907-6977, Fax: (301) 907-6895, aabb@aabb.org, http://www.aabb.org.

American Congress of Obstetricians and Gynecologists, 409 12th St. SW, Washington, DC 20024-2188, (202) 638-5577, (800) 673-8444, resources@acog.org, http://www.acog.org.

American Red Cross, 2025 E St., Washington, DC 20006, (800) RED-CROSS (733-2767), http://www.redcross.org.

Mark A. Best

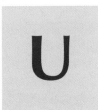

U

Ultrasound

Definition

Medical ultrasound imaging involves the use of high frequency sound waves to produce images of different parts of the inside of the body. This medical procedure is painless, safe, and noninvasive. Ultrasound imaging uses sound waves to visualize internal body structures, as opposed to techniques like x-ray, which uses radiation. Ultrasound images provide dynamic images in "real time" and not just a static picture taken at a single moment such as in x-ray. Therefore, ultrasound imaging can help to show movement inside of body organs as well as the structure of the organs. Most people are familiar with ultrasound imaging being used during pregnancy to look safely and carefully at the developing fetus. There are also many other uses in medicine for ultrasound imaging.

The following are some other uses for medical ultrasound imaging:

• Cardiac ultrasound is used to diagnose problems with the heart and major blood vessels surrounding the heart.

• Ultrasound imaging in gynecology is used to diagnose problems with the female reproductive tract including being used to diagnose problems associated with infertility. Ultrasound is also used to monitor infertility treatments.

• Ultrasound imaging is used to look for problems with other internal organs, such as the gallbladder, bladder, testicles, liver, spleen, kidneys, and pancreas.

• Ultrasound imaging is also used to look for problems with glands, such as the thyroid.

• Vascular ultrasound imaging is used to watch the blood flow in blood vessels or blood flow to tumors. Ultrasound doppler imaging and color flow mapping can show the flow of blood.

• Ultrasound imaging is also used during medical procedures such as needle biopsies or egg retrieval during in vitro fertilization.

Purpose

The purpose of ultrasound imaging in medicine is to help the physician diagnose, monitor and treat medical conditions.

Description

Ultrasound imaging is performed by using a transducer, which is a small device that the technician holds in his/her hand and is attached to a cord that connects to the ultrasound machine. The ultrasound machine has a keyboard, a computer, and a display screen. The patient is usually lying down on an examination table and clear gel (cold or warm) is applied to the area of the body that is to be imaged or scanned so that the transducer makes easy contact with the body and can easily be slid back and forth during the ultrasound. As the transducer is moved over that part of the body, it sends out high frequency sound waves, looks for the returning echo and instantly puts that image up onto the screen. An ultrasound examination is usually painless; however, on occasion, discomfort from the pressure being pressed on the body may occur, especially if the patient's bladder is full, or if the area being scanned is injured or tender. Sometimes ultrasound imaging is performed by using an ultrasound probe that is inserted into an area of the body, such as the vagina or the esophagus. Vaginal ultrasounds are used to scan for early pregnancy or to look carefully at the ovaries or guide the physician during procedures such as egg

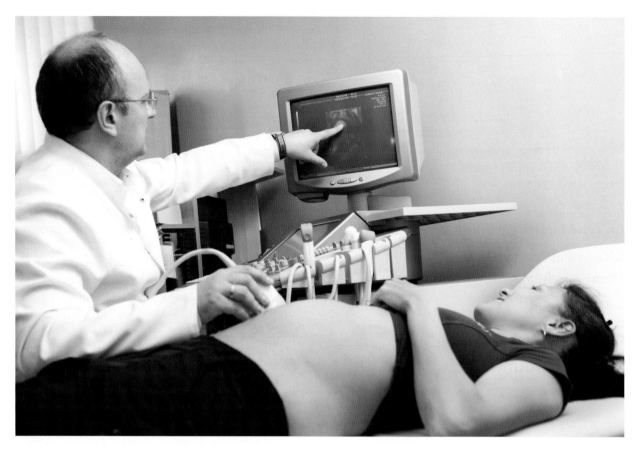

Pregnant woman receiving an ultrasound. *(Dmitry Kalinovsky/Shutterstock.com)*

retrieval for **in vitro fertilization**. This ultrasound is not usually painful, but to some may be uncomfortable. Transesophageal **echocardiography** involves inserting a narrow, flexible tube with a transducer in its tip into the throat. This allows the viewing of high-quality images of the heart, its valves and blood vessels, and the presence of any clots. Ultrasound may also be used to guide the placement of a needle when aspirating a tumor for a biopsy.

Precautions

The greatest precaution that should be taken when using ultrasound imaging to diagnose medical problems is the over and under diagnosing of problems by staff that is not properly trained, using poor equipment or not adequately supervised. This is especially true in the obstetrical setting where it is important to have properly trained ultrasound technicians (sonographers) to perform routine and advanced diagnostic ultrasounds on pregnant women. The Society of Diagnostic Medical Sonography and the American Institute for Ultrasound in Medicine are great resources for helping to find certified sonographers from accredited programs.

Preparation

Preparation for an ultrasound examination depends upon the area of the body that is to be scanned. For example, during pregnancy, a patient may be instructed to drink water and not to empty her bladder prior to the ultrasound examination to help with visualization during the ultrasound. Other procedures may require no eating or drinking prior to the ultrasound examination. Comfortable, loose clothing should be worn, although a gown may be provided to be worn for the ultrasound examination. It is important to ask for and follow the instructions that are given prior to the ultrasound examination so that the procedure does not need to be rescheduled.

Aftercare

After the ultrasound, the gel is wiped off and the patient is usually able to return to normal activity. Usually, after the examination, the technician has the images reviewed by the physician and the physician may then speak to the patient at that time. Otherwise, the results are called to the patient or discussed at a later visit. On occasion, especially during pregnancy, the technician or physician will discuss the results of the ultrasound while the ultrasound is being performed. If an ultrasound examination shows abnormal results, those results may need to be followed-up with other tests or consultations to discuss possible treatment.

Risks

For routine diagnostic ultrasound imaging, there are no known risks to humans and therefore, if necessary it is safe to repeat the procedure as often as needed to monitor a particular health concern or treatment. For over 30 years, diagnostic ultrasound imaging has been used on pregnant women. A multitude of studies on the effects of ultrasound use during pregnancy have been reported and although there have been a number of small studies citing possible hearing problems, low birthweight and left handedness, these studies have not been verified by larger studies. Overall, there has been no evidence that ultrasound is harmful to a developing fetus; however, the medical community should be diligent about preventing unnecessary use of ultrasound in pregnancy.

Resources

BOOKS

Mettler, Fred A. Jr. *Essentials of Radiology*. 3rd ed. Philadelphia: Saunders/Elsevier, 2014.

WEBSITES

MedlinePlus. "Ultrasound." U.S. National Library of Medicine, National Institutes of Health. http://www.nlm.nih.gov/medlineplus/ultrasound.html (accessed October 18, 2013).

Radiological Society of North America. "Ultrasound—General." http://www.radiologyinfo.org/en/info.cfm?pg=genus (accessed October 18, 2013).

ORGANIZATIONS

American Institute of Ultrasound in Medicine, 14750 Sweitzer Ln., Ste. 100, Laurel, MD 20707-5906, (301) 498-4100, (800) 638-5352, Fax: (301) 498-4450, http://www.aium.org.

Radiological Society of North America (RSNA), 820 Jorie Blvd., Oak Brook, IL 60523-2251, (630) 571-2670, (800) 381-6660, http://www.rsna.org.

Society of Diagnostic Medical Sonography, 2745 Dallas Pkwy., Ste. 350, Plano, TX 75093-8730, (214) 473-8057, (800) 229-9506, Fax: (214) 473-8563, http://www.sdms.org.

Renee Laux, MS

Umbilical hernia repair *see* **Hernia repair, umbilical**

Undescended testicle repair *see* **Orchiopexy**

Upper gastrointestinal exam

Definition

An upper gastrointestinal (GI) examination is a fluoroscopic examination (a type of x-ray imaging) of the upper gastrointestinal tract, including the pharynx (throat), esophagus, stomach, and upper small intestine (duodenum). An x-ray examination that evaluates only the pharynx and esophagus is called a barium swallow.

Purpose

An upper GI series is frequently requested when a patient experiences unexplained symptoms of abdominal pain, difficulty in swallowing (dysphagia), regurgitation (reflux), diarrhea, unexplained vomiting, blood in the stool, or unexplained weight loss. It is used to help diagnose disorders and diseases of, or related to, the upper gastrointestinal tract. Some of these conditions are: hiatal hernia, diverticula, tumors, obstruction, gastroesophageal reflux disease (GERD), pulmonary aspiration, and inflammation (e.g., ulcers, enteritis, and Crohn's disease).

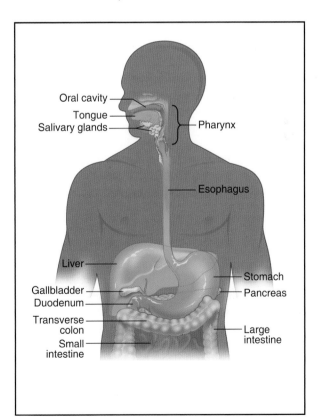

Gastrointestinal (GI) system. *(Illustration by Electronic Illustrators Group. Copyright © 2014 Cengage Learning®.)*

Glucagon, a medication sometimes given prior to an upper GI procedure, may cause nausea and dizziness. It is used to relax the natural movements of the stomach, which will enhance the overall study.

Description

An upper GI series takes place in a hospital or clinic setting, and is performed by an x-ray technologist and a radiologist. Before the test begins, the patient is sometimes given a glucagon injection, a medication that slows stomach and bowel activity, to provide the radiologist with a clear picture of the gastrointestinal tract. In order to further improve the upper GI picture clarity, the patient may be given a cup of fizzing baking soda crystals to swallow, which distends the esophagus and stomach by producing gas. This procedure is called a double-contrast or air-contrast upper GI.

Once these preparatory steps are complete, the patient stands against an upright x-ray table, and a fluoroscopic screen is placed in front of him or her. The patient will be asked to drink from a cup of flavored barium sulfate, a thick and chalky-tasting liquid, while the radiologist views the esophagus, stomach, and duodenum on the fluoroscopic screen. The patient will be asked to change positions frequently to coat the entire surface of the gastrointestinal tract with barium, move overlapping loops of bowel to isolate each segment, and provide multiple views of each segment. The technician or radiologist may press on the patient's abdomen to spread the barium throughout the folds within the lining of the stomach. The x-ray table will also be moved several times throughout the procedure. The radiologist will ask the patient to hold his or her breath periodically while exposures are taken. After the radiologist completes his or her portion of the exam, the technologist takes three to six additional films of the GI tract. The entire procedure takes approximately 15–30 minutes.

In addition to the standard upper GI series, a physician may request a detailed small bowel follow-through (SBFT), which is a timed series of films. After the preliminary upper GI series is complete, the patient will drink additional barium sulfate, and will be escorted to a waiting area while the barium moves through the small intestines. X-rays are initially taken at 15-minute intervals until the barium reaches the colon (the only way to be sure the terminal ileum is fully seen is to see the colon or ileocecal valve). The interval may be increased to 30 minutes, or even one hour if the barium passes slowly. Then the radiologist will obtain additional views of the terminal ileum (the most distal segment of the small bowel, just before the colon). This procedure can take from one to four hours.

KEY TERMS

Contrast medium—Any substance that is swallowed or injected in order to increase the visibility of body structures or fluids.

Crohn's disease—A chronic, inflammatory bowel disease usually affecting the ileum, colon, or both.

Diverticula (singular, diverticulum)—Pouch-like herniations through the muscular wall of an organ such as the stomach, small intestine, or colon.

Enteritis—Inflammation of the mucosal lining of the small intestine.

Gastroesophageal reflux disease (GERD)—A painful, chronic condition in which stomach acid flows back into the esophagus causing heartburn and, in time, erosion of the esophageal lining.

Hiatal hernia—Protrusion of the stomach up through the diaphragm.

Esophageal radiography, also called a barium esophagram or a barium swallow, is a study of the esophagus only, and is usually performed as part of the upper GI series (sometimes only a barium swallow is done). It is commonly used to diagnose the cause of difficulty in swallowing (dysphagia), and to detect a hiatal hernia. The patient drinks a barium sulfate liquid, and sometimes eats barium-coated food while the radiologist examines the swallowing mechanism on a fluoroscopic screen. The test takes approximately 30 minutes.

Preparation

Patients must not eat, drink, chew gum, or smoke for eight hours prior to undergoing an upper GI examination. Longer dietary restrictions may be required, depending on the type and diagnostic purpose of the test. Patients undergoing a small-bowel follow-through exam may be asked to take **laxatives** the day before the test. Patients are required to wear a hospital gown, or similar attire, and to remove all jewelry, to provide the camera with an unobstructed view of the abdomen.

Aftercare

No special aftercare treatment or regimen is required for an upper GI series. The patient may eat and drink as soon as the test is completed. The barium sulfate may make the patient's stool white for several days, and can cause constipation; therefore, patients are encouraged to drink plenty of water to eliminate it from their system.

Risks

Because the upper GI series is an x-ray procedure, it does involve minor exposure to ionizing radiation. Unless the patient is pregnant, or multiple radiological or fluoroscopic studies are required, the small dose of radiation incurred during a single procedure poses little risk. However, multiple studies requiring fluoroscopic exposure that are conducted in a short time period have been known, on very rare occasions, to cause skin death (necrosis) in some individuals. This risk can be minimized by careful monitoring and documentation of cumulative radiation doses.

Some patients find the barium liquid unpleasant to the taste or difficult to swallow. The radiologist may be able to provide a strawberry- or chocolate-flavored version. In addition, some patients feel gassy, bloated, or nauseated while they are being tilted on the examination table or having their abdomen pressed.

A few patients are allergic to barium and other contrast materials. Patients should inform the radiologist of any known allergies.

Results

A normal upper GI series shows a healthy, normally functioning, and unobstructed digestive tract. Hiatal hernia, obstructions, inflammation (including ulcers or polyps of the esophagus, stomach, or small intestine), or irregularities in the swallowing mechanism are just a few of the possible abnormalities that may appear on an upper GI series. Additionally, abnormal peristalsis, or digestive movements of the esophagus, stomach, and small intestine can often be visualized on the fluoroscopic part of the exam, and in the interpretation of the SBFT.

Resources

BOOKS

Brant, William E., and Clyde A. Helms. *Fundamentals of Diagnostic Radiology.* 4th ed. Philadelphia: Lippincott Williams & Wilkins, 2012.

PERIODICALS

Nandurkar, S., et al. "Rates of Endoscopy and Endoscopic Findings among People with Frequent Symptoms of Gastroesophageal Reflux in the Community." *American Journal of Gastroenterology* 100 (July 2005): 1459–65.

"Patient Page: Upper GI Series." *Radiologic Technology* 77 (May–June 2006): 415–16.

WEBSITES

American College of Gastroenterology. "Common GI Symptoms." http://patients.gi.org/topics/common-gi-symptoms (accessed October 14, 2013).

National Digestive Diseases Information Clearinghouse. "Upper GI Series." National Institute of Diabetes and Digestive and Kidney Diseases. http://digestive.niddk.nih.gov/ddiseases/pubs/uppergi (accessed October 14, 2013).

Radiological Society of North America. "X-ray (Radiography)—Upper GI Tract." RadiologyInfo.org. http://www.radiologyinfo.org/en/info.cfm?pg=uppergi&bhcp=1 (accessed October 14, 2013).

ORGANIZATIONS

American College of Gastroenterology, 6400 Goldsboro Rd., Ste. 200, Bethesda, MD 20817, (301) 263-9000, info@acg.gi.org, http://gi.org.

American College of Radiology, 1891 Preston White Dr., Reston, VA 20191, (703) 648-8900, info@acr.org, http://www.acr.org.

National Digestive Diseases Information Clearinghouse (NDDIC), 2 Information Way, Bethesda, MD 20892-3570, (800) 891-5389, (866) 569–1162, Fax: (703) 738–4929, nddic@info.niddk.nih.gov, http://www.digestive.niddk.nih.gov.

Radiological Society of North America (RSNA), 820 Jorie Blvd., Oak Brook, IL 60523-2251, (630) 571-2670, (800) 381-6660, http://www.rsna.org.

Debra Novograd, BS, RT(R)(M)
Lee A. Shratter, MD
Rebecca Frey, PhD

Ureteral stenting

Definition

A ureteral stent is a thin, flexible tube threaded into the ureter to help urine drain from the kidney to the bladder or to an external collection system.

Purpose

Urine is normally carried from the kidneys to the bladder via a pair of long, narrow tubes called ureters (each kidney is connected to one ureter). A ureter may become obstructed as a result of a number of conditions including kidney stones, tumors, blood clots, postsurgical swelling, or infection. A ureteral stent is placed in the ureter to restore the flow of urine to the bladder. Ureteral stents may be used in patients with active kidney infection or with diseased bladders (e.g., as a result of cancer or radiation therapy). Alternatively, ureteral stents may be used during or after urinary tract surgical procedures to provide a mold around which healing can occur, to divert the urinary flow away from areas of leakage, to manipulate kidney stones or prevent stone migration prior to treatment, or to make the ureters more easily identifiable during difficult surgical procedures. The stent may remain in place on a short-term (days to weeks) or long-term (weeks to months) basis.

Demographics

Chronic blockage of a ureter affects approximately five individuals out of every 1,000; acute blockage affects one out of every 1,000. Bilateral obstruction (blockage to both ureters) is more rare; chronic blockage affects one individual per 1,000 people, and acute blockage affects five per 10,000.

Description

The size, shape, and material of the ureteral stent to be used depends on the patient's anatomy and the reason why the stent is required. Most stents are 5–12 inches (12–30 cm) in length, and have a diameter of 0.06–0.2 inches (1.5–6 mm). One or both ends of the stent may be coiled (called a pigtail stent) to prevent it from moving out of place; an open-ended stent is better suited for patients who require temporary drainage. In some instances, one end of the stent has a thread attached to it that extends through the bladder and urethra to the outside of the body; this aids in stent removal. The stent material must be flexible, durable, non-reactive, and radiopaque (visible on an x-ray).

The patient is usually placed under **general anesthesia** for stent insertion; this ensures the physician that the patient will remain relaxed and will not move during the procedure. A cystoscope (a thin, telescope-like instrument) is inserted into the urethra to the bladder, and the opening to the ureter to be stented is identified. In some instances, a guide wire is inserted into the ureter under the aid of a fluoroscope (an imaging device that uses x-rays to visualize structures on a fluorescent screen). The guide wire provides a path for the placement of the stent, which is advanced over the wire. Once the stent is in place, the guide wire and cystoscope are removed. Patients who fail this method of ureteral stenting may have the stent placed percutaneously (through the skin), into the kidney, and subsequently into the ureter.

A stent that has an attached thread may be pulled out by a physician in an office setting. **Cystoscopy** may also be used to remove a stent.

Diagnosis

A number of different technologies aid in the diagnosis of ureteral obstruction. These include:

- cystoscopy (a procedure in which a thin, tubular instrument is used to visualize the interior of the bladder)

KEY TERMS

Acute—A condition that has a short but severe course.

Chronic—A condition that is persistent or recurs frequently.

Cystoscopy—Examination or treatment of the interior of the urinary bladder by looking through a special instrument with reflected light.

Kidney stones—Small, solid masses that form in the kidney.

Urethra—The tube through which urine travels from the bladder to the outside of the body.

- ultrasonography (an imaging technique that uses high-frequency sound waves to visualize structures inside the body)
- computed tomography (an imaging technique that uses x-rays to produce two-dimensional cross-sections on a viewing screen)
- pyelography (x-rays taken of the urinary tract after a contrast dye has been injected into a vein or into the kidney, ureter, or bladder)

Preparation

Prior to ureteral stenting, the procedure should be thoroughly explained by a medical professional. No food or drink is permitted after midnight the night before surgery. The patient wears a hospital gown during the procedure. If the stent insertion is performed with the aid of a cystoscope, the patient will assume a position that is typically used in a gynecological exam (lying on the back, with the legs flexed and supported by stirrups).

Aftercare

Stents must be periodically replaced to prevent fractures within the catheter wall or build-up of encrustation. Stent replacement is recommended approximately every six months; more often in patients who form stones.

Risks

Complications associated with ureteral stenting include:

- bleeding (usually minor and easily treated, but occasionally requiring transfusion)
- catheter migration or dislodgement (may require readjustment)

- coiling of the stent within the ureter (may cause lower abdominal pain or flank pain on urination, urinary frequency, or blood in the urine)

- introduction or worsening of infection

- penetration of adjacent organs (e.g., bowel, gallbladder, or lungs)

Results

Normally, a ureteral stent re-establishes the flow of urine from the kidney to the bladder. Postoperative urine flow will be monitored to ensure the stent has not been dislodged or obstructed.

Morbidity and mortality rates

Serious complications occur in approximately 4% of patients undergoing ureteral stenting, with minor complications in another 10%.

Alternatives

If a ureter is obstructed and ureteral stenting is not possible, a **nephrostomy** may be performed. During this procedure, a tube is placed through the skin on the patient's back, into the area of the kidney that collects urine. The tube may be connected to an external drainage bag. In other cases, the tube is connected directly from the kidney to the bladder.

Health care team roles

Ureteral stenting is typically performed in a hospital by an interventional radiologist (a physician who specializes in the treatment of medical disorders using specialized imaging techniques) or a urologist (a physician who specializes in the diagnosis and treatment of diseases of the urinary tract and genital organs).

Resources

BOOKS

Wein, Alan J., et al. *Campbell-Walsh Urology.* 10th ed. Philadelphia: Saunders/Elsevier, 2012.

PERIODICALS

Al-Aown, Abdulrahman, et al. "Ureteral Stents: New Ideas, New Designs." *Therapeutic Advances in Urology* 2, no. 2 (2013): 85–92. http://dx.doi.org/10.1177/1756287210370699 (accessed October 4, 2013).

Beraldo, S., et al. "The Prophylactic Use of a Ureteral Stent in Laparoscopic Colorectal Surgery." *Scandinavian Journal of Surgery* 102, no. 2 (2013): 87–89. http://dx.doi.org/10.1177/1457496913482247 (accessed October 4, 2013).

Divakaruni, Naveen, et al. "Forgotten Ureteral Stents: Who's at Risk?" *Journal of Endourology* 27, no. 8 (2013): 1051–54. http://dx.doi.org/10.1089/end.2012.0754 (accessed October 4, 2013).

OTHER

University of Michigan Health System. *Frequently Asked Questions about Ureteral Stents.* August 2007. http://www.med.umich.edu/1libr/urology/umureteral_stents.pdf (accessed October 4, 2013).

WEBSITES

Bristol Urological Institute. "Having a Ureteric Stent—What to Expect and How to Manage." http://bui.ac.uk/PatientInfo/ureterstent.html (accessed October 4, 2013).

Ohio State University Wexner Medical Center. "Ureteral Stents/FAQ." http://urology.osu.edu/22746.cfm (accessed October 4, 2013).

ORGANIZATIONS

Urology Care Foundation, 1000 Corporate Blvd., Linthicum, MD 21090, (410) 689-3700, (800) 828-7866, Fax: (410) 689-3998, info@urologycarefoundation.org, http://auafoundation.org.

Kathleen D. Wright, RN
Stephanie Dionne Sherk

Ureterocutaneostomy *see* **Ureterostomy, cutaneous**

Ureterosigmoidostomy

Definition

Ureterosigmoidostomy is a surgical procedure that treats urinary incontinence by joining the ureters to the lower colon, thereby allowing urine to evacuate through the rectum.

Ureterosigmoidostomy

Purpose

The surgery is indicated when there is resection (surgical removal), malformation, or injury to the bladder. The bladder disposes of wastes passed to it from the kidneys, which is the organ that does most of the blood filtering and retention of needed glucose, salts, and minerals.

Wastes from the kidneys drip through the ureters to the bladder, and on to the urethra where they are expelled via urination. Waste from the kidneys is slowed or impaired when the bladder is diseased because of ulcerative, inflammatory, or malignant conditions; is malformed; or if it has been removed. In these cases, the kidney is unable to get rid of the wastes, resulting in hydronephrosis (distention of the kidneys). Over time, this leads to kidney deterioration. Saving the kidneys by bladder diversion is as important as restoring urinary continence.

The surgical techniques for urinary and fecal diversion fall into two categories: continent diversion and conduit diversion. In continent diversion, an internal reservoir for urine or feces is created, allowing natural evacuation from the body. In urinary and fecal conduit diversion, a section of existing tissue is altered to serve as a passageway to an external reservoir or ostomy. Both continent and conduit diversions reproduce bladder or colon function that was impaired due to surgery, obstruction, or a neurogenically (nerve dysfunction) created condition. Both the continent and conduit diversion methods have been used for years, with advancements in minimally invasive surgical techniques and biochemical improvements in conduit materials and ostomy appliances.

Catheterization was the original solution for urinary incontinence, especially when major organ failure or removal was involved. But catheterization was found to have major residual back flow of urine into the kidneys over the long term. With the advent of surgical anastomosis—the grafting of vascularizing tissue for the repair and expansion of organ function—and with the ability to include flap-type valves to prevent back-up into the kidneys, major continent restoring procedures have become routine in **urologic surgery**. Catheterization has been replaced as a permanent remedy for persistent incontinence. Continent surgical procedures developed since the 1980s offer the possibility of safely retaining natural evacuation functions in both colonic (intestinal) and urinary systems.

Quality of life issues associated with urinary diversion are increasingly important to patients and, along with medical requirements, put an optimal threshold on the requirements for the surgical procedure.

KEY TERMS

Bladder exstrophy—One of many bladder and urinary congenital abnormalities. Occurs when the wall of the bladder fails to close in embryonic development and remains exposed to the abdominal wall.

Conduit diversion—A surgical procedure that restores urinary and fecal continence by diverting these functions through a constructed conduit leading to an external waste reservoir (ostomy).

Cystectomy—The surgical resection of part or all of the bladder.

Urinary continent diversion—A surgical procedure that restores urinary continence by diverting urinary function around the bladder and into the intestines, thereby allowing for natural evacuation through the rectum or an implanted artificial sphincter.

The bladder substitute or created reservoir must offer the following advantages:

• maintain continence

• maintain sterile urine

• empty completely

• protect the kidneys

• prevent absorption of waste products

• maintain quality of life

Ureterosigmoidostomy is one of the earliest continent diversions for a resected bladder, bladder abnormalities, and dysfunction. It is one of the more difficult surgeries, and has significant complications. Ureterosigmoidostomy does have a major benefit; it allows the natural expelling of wastes without the construction of a stoma—an artificial conduit—by using the rectum as a urinary reservoir. When evacuation occurs, the urine is passed along with the fecal matter.

Ureterosigmoidostomy is a single procedure, but there are additional refinements that allow rectal voiding of urine. A procedure known as the Mainz II pouch has undergone many refinements in attempts to lessen the complications that have traditionally accompanied ureterosigmoidostomy. This surgery is indicated for significant and serious conditions of the urinary tract, including:

• Cancer or ulceration of the bladder that necessitates a radical cystectomy or removal of the bladder, primarily occurring in adults, particularly those of advanced age.

- Various congenital abnormalities of the bladder in infants, especially eversion of part or all of the bladder. Eversion (or exstrophy) is a malformation of the bladder in which the wall adjacent to the abdomen fails to close. In some children, the bladder plate may be too small to fashion a closure.

Demographics

Bladder cancer affects over 50,000 people annually in the United States. The average age at diagnosis is 68 years. It accounts for approximately 10,000 deaths per year. Bladder cancer is the fifth leading cause of cancer deaths among men older than 75 years. Male bladder cancer is three times more prevalent than female bladder cancer.

In the United States, radical **cystectomy** (total removal of the bladder) is the standard treatment for muscle-invading bladder cancer. The operation usually involves removal of the bladder (with oncology staging) and pelvic lymph node, and prostate and seminal conduits with a form of urinary diversion. Ureterosigmoidostomy is one option that restores continence.

Pediatric ureterosigmoidostomy is performed primarily for bladder abnormalities occurring at birth. Classic bladder exstrophy occurs in 3.3 per 100,000 births, with a male to female ratio of 3 to 1 (6 to 1 in some studies).

Description

The most basic ureterosigmoidostomy modification is the Mainz II pouch. There is a 2.4 in. (6 cm) cut along antimesenteric border of the colon, both on the proximal and distal sides of the rectum/sigmoid colon junction. The ureters are drawn down into the colon. A special flap technique is applied by folding the colon to stop urine from refluxing back to the kidneys. After the colon is closed, the result is a small rectosigmoid reservoir that holds urine without refluxing it back to the upper urinary tract. Some variations of the Mainz II pouch include the construction of a valve, as in the Kock pouch, that confines urine to the distal segment of the colon.

Ureterosigmoidostomy is typically performed in patients with complex medical problems, often those who have had numerous surgeries. Ureterosigmoidostomy as a continent diversion technique relies heavily upon an intact and functional rectal sphincter. The treatment of pediatric urinary incontinence due to bladder eversion or other anatomical anomalies is a technical challenge, and is not always the first choice of **surgeons**. In Europe, early urinary diversion with ureterosigmoidostomy is used widely for most exstrophy patients.

Its main advantage is the possibility for spontaneous emptying by evacuation of urine and stool.

Diagnosis

A number of tests are performed as part of the pre-surgery diagnostic workup for bladder conditions such as cancer, ulcerative or inflammatory disease, or pediatric abnormalities. Tests may include:

- cystoscopy (bladder inspection with a laparoscope)
- CT scan
- liver function
- renal function
- rectal sphincter function evaluation (The rectal sphincter will be a critical factor in urination after the surgery, and it is important to determine its ability to function. Adult patients are often asked to have an oatmeal enema and sit upright for a period of time to test sphincter function.)

Preparation

In adult patients, a discussion of continent diversion is conducted early in the diagnostic process. Patients are asked to consider the possibility of a conduit urinary diversion if the ureterosigmoidostomy proves impossible to complete. Educational sessions on specific conduit alternatives take place prior to surgery. Topics include options for placement of a **stoma**, and appliances that may be a part of the daily voiding routine after surgery. Many doctors provide a stomal therapist to consult with the patient.

Aftercare

After surgery, patients may remain in the hospital for a few days to undergo blood, renal, and liver tests, and monitoring for fever or other surgical complications. In pediatric patients, a cast keeps the legs abducted (apart) and slightly elevated for three weeks. Bladder and kidneys are fully drained via multiple catheters during the first few weeks after surgery. **Antibiotics** are continued after surgery. Permanent follow-up with the urologist is essential for proper monitoring of kidney function.

Results

Good results have been reported, especially in children; however, ureterosigmoidostomy offers some severe morbid complications. Postsurgical bladder function and continence rates are very high. However, many newly created reservoirs do not function normally; some deteriorate over time, creating a need for more than one diversion surgery. Many patients have difficulty voiding after surgery. Five-year survival rates for bladder surgery patients are 50%–80%, depending on the grade, depth of bladder penetration, and nodal status.

Morbidity and mortality rates

The continence success rate with ureterosigmoidostomy and its variants is higher than 95% for exstrophy; however, long-term malignancy rates are quite high. Adenocarcinoma is the most common of these malignancies, and may be caused by chronic irritation and inflammation of exposed mucosa of the exstrophic bladder. In one series of studies, adenocarcinoma was reported in more than 10% of patients. However, the malignancy is actually higher in untreated patients whose bladders are left exposed for years before surgery.

Upper urinary tract deterioration is a potential complication, caused by reflux of urine back to the kidneys, resulting in febrile infections.

Alternatives

Other options include construction of a full neo-bladder in certain carefully defined circumstances, and bladder enhancement for congenitally shortened or abnormal bladders. Surgical bladder resection is often followed by continent operations using other parts of the colon, and by various conduit surgeries that utilize an external ostomy appliance.

Health care team roles

Ureterosigmoidostomy is usually performed by a urological surgeon with advanced training in urinary continent surgeries, often in consultation with a neonatologist (in newborn patients) or an oncological surgeon. The surgery takes place in a general hospital.

Resources

BOOKS

Wein, Alan J., et al. *Campbell-Walsh Urology.* 10th ed. Philadelphia: Saunders/Elsevier, 2012.

PERIODICALS

Pettersson, Louise, et al. "Half Century of Followup After Ureterosigmoidostomy Performed in Early Childhood." *The Journal of Urology* 189, no. 5 (2013): 1870–75. http://dx.doi.org/10.1016/j.juro.2012.11.179 (accessed October 4, 2013).

Tollefson, Matthew K., et al. "Long-Term Outcome of Ureterosigmoidostomy: An Analysis of Patients with >10 Years of Follow-Up." *BJU International* 105, no. 6 (2010): 860–63. http://dx.doi.org/10.1111/j.1464-410X.2009.08811.x (accessed October 4, 2013).

OTHER

University of North Carolina Health Care. *Living with Your Ureterosigmoidostomy: A Guide to Home Care.* http://www.unchealthcare.org/site/Nursing/servicelines/wocn/patient%20educational%20materials_new/LLWOCNWebEdUSig.pdf (accessed October 4, 2013).

WEBSITES

Ochsner. "Ureterosigmoidostomy." http://healthlibrary.ochsner.org/Library/HealthSheets/3,S,41095 (accessed October 4, 2013).

ORGANIZATIONS

National Institute of Diabetes and Digestive and Kidney Diseases (NIDDK), 31 Center Drive, MSC 2560, Bldg. 31, Rm. 9A06, Bethesda, MD 20892-2560, (301) 496-3583, http://www2.niddk.nih.gov.

Society for Pediatric Urology, 500 Cummings Ctr., Ste. 4550, Beverly, MA 01915, (978) 927-8330, Fax: (978) 524-8890, http://spuonline.org.

Urology Care Foundation, 1000 Corporate Blvd., Linthicum, MD 21090, (410) 689-3700, (800) 828-7866, Fax: (410) 689-3998, info@urologycarefoundation.org, http://auafoundation.org.

Nancy McKenzie, PhD

Ureterostomy, cutaneous

Definition

A cutaneous ureterostomy, also called ureterocutaneostomy, is a surgical procedure that detaches one or both ureters from the bladder, and brings them to the surface of the abdomen with the formation of an opening (**stoma**) to allow passage of urine.

Purpose

The bladder is the membranous pouch that serves as a reservoir for urine. Contraction of the bladder results in urination. A ureterostomy is performed to divert the flow of urine away from the bladder when the bladder is not functioning or has been removed. The following conditions may result in a need for ureterostomy.

- bladder cancer
- spinal cord injury
- malfunction of the bladder
- birth defects, such as spina bifida

Demographics

Bladder disorders afflict millions of people in the United States. According to the American Cancer Society (ACS), there were 72,570 new cases of bladder cancer in the United States in 2013, with approximately 15,210 deaths from the disease.

Description

Urostomy is the generic name for any surgical procedure that diverts the passage of urine by re-directing the ureters (fibromuscular tubes that carry the urine from the kidney to the bladder). There are two basic types of urostomies. The first features the creation of a passage called an "ileal conduit." In this procedure, the ureters are detached from the bladder and joined to a short length of the small intestine (ileum). The other type of urostomy is cutaneous ureterostomy. With this technique, the surgeon detaches the ureters from the bladder and brings one or both to the surface of the abdomen. The hole created in the abdomen is called a stoma, a reddish, moist abdominal protrusion. The stoma is not painful; it has no sensation. Since it has no muscles to regulate urination, urine collects in a bag.

There are four common types of ureterostomies:

- single ureterostomy—brings only one ureter to the surface of the abdomen
- bilateral ureterostomy—brings both ureters to the surface of the abdomen, one on each side
- double-barrel ureterostomy—brings both ureters to the same side of the abdominal surface
- transuretero ureterostomy (TUU)—brings both ureters to the same side of the abdomen, through the same stoma

Preparation

Ureterostomy patients may have the following tests and procedures as part of their diagnostic work-up:

- renal function tests, including blood, urea, nitrogen (BUN) and creatinine
- blood tests, including complete blood count (CBC) and electrolytes
- imaging studies of the ureters and renal pelvis

KEY TERMS

Anastomosis—An opening created by surgical, traumatic, or pathological means between two separate spaces or organs.

Cecum—The pouch-like start of the large intestine (colon) at the end of the small intestine.

Gastrointestinal (GI) tract—The entire length of the digestive tract, from the stomach to the rectum.

Ileum—The last portion of the small intestine that communicates with the large intestine.

Large intestine—Also called the colon, this structure has six major divisions: cecum, ascending colon, transverse colon, descending colon, sigmoid colon, and rectum.

Ostomy—General term meaning a surgical procedure in which an artificial opening is formed to either allow waste (stool or urine) to pass from the body, or to allow food into the GI tract. An ostomy can be permanent or temporary, as well as single-barreled, double-barreled, or a loop.

Small intestine—The small intestine consists of three sections: duodenum, jejunum, and ileum.

Spina bifida—A congenital defect in the spinal column, characterized by the absence of the vertebral arches through which the spinal membranes and spinal cord may protrude.

Stent—A tube made of metal or plastic that is inserted into a vessel or passage to keep it open and prevent closure.

Stoma—A surgically created opening in the abdominal wall.

Ureter—The fibromuscular tube that transports the urine from the kidney to the bladder.

The quality, character, and usable length of the ureters is usually assessed using any of the following tests:

- Intravenous pyelogram (IVP) is a special diagnostic test that follows the time course of excretion of a contrast dye through the kidneys, ureters, and bladder after it is injected into a vein.
- Retrograde and antegrade pyelograms are x-ray studies of the kidneys and urinary tract.
- Computed tomography (CT) is a special imaging technique that uses a computer to collect multiple x-ray images into a two-dimensional cross-sectional image.

• Magnetic resonance imaging (MRI) with intravenous gadolinium is a special technique used to image internal structures of the body, particularly the soft tissues. An MRI image is often superior to a routine x-ray image.

The presurgery evaluation also includes an assessment of overall patient stability. The surgery may take from two to six hours, depending on the health of the ureters, and the experience of the surgeon.

Aftercare

After surgery, the condition of the ureters is monitored by IVP testing, repeated postoperatively at six months, one year, and then yearly.

Following ureterostomy, urine needs to be collected in bags. Several designs are available. One popular type features an open bag fitted with an anti-reflux valve, which prevents the urine from flowing back toward the stoma. A urostomy bag connects to a night bag that may be attached to the bed at night. Urostomy bags are available as one- and two-piece bags:

• With one-piece bags, the adhesive and the bag are sealed together. The advantage of using a one-piece appliance is that it is easy to apply, and the bag is flexible and soft.

• For two-piece bags, the bag and the adhesive are two separate components. The adhesive does not need to be removed frequently from the skin, and can remain in place for several days while the bag is changed as required.

Risks

The complication rate associated with ureterostomy procedures is less than 5%–10%. Risks during surgery include heart problems, pulmonary (lung) complications, development of blood clots (thrombosis), blocking of arteries (embolism), and injury to adjacent structures, such as bowel or vascular entities. Inadequate ureteral length may also be encountered, leading to ureteral kinking and subsequent obstruction. If plastic tubes need inserting, their malposition can lead to obstruction and eventual breakdown of the opening (anastomosis). Anastomotic leak is the most frequently encountered complication.

Results

Normal results for a ureterostomy include the successful diversion of the urine pathway away from the bladder, and a tension-free, watertight opening to the abdomen that prevents urinary leakage.

Morbidity and mortality rates

The outcome and prognosis for ureterostomy patients depends on a number of factors. The highest rates of complications exist for those who have pelvic cancer or a history of radiation therapy.

In one study, a French medical team followed 69 patients for a minimum of one year (an average of six years) after TUU was performed. They reported one complication per four patients (6.3%), including a case requiring open drainage, prolonged urinary leakage, and common ureteral death (necrosis). Two complications occurred three and four years after surgery. The National Cancer Institute performed TUU for pelvic malignancy in 10 patients. Mean follow-up was 6.5 years. Complications include common ureteral narrowing (one patient); subsequent kidney removal, or **nephrectomy** (one patient); recurrence of disease with ureteral obstruction (one patient); and disease progression in a case of inflammation of blood vessels, or vasculitis (one patient). One patient died of sepsis (infection in the bloodstream) due to urine leakage at the anastomosis, one died after a heart attack, and three died from metastasis of their primary cancer.

Alternatives

There are several alternative surgical procedures available:

• In an ileal conduit urostomy, also known as "Bricker's loop," the two ureters that transport urine from the kidneys are detached from the bladder, and then attached so that they will empty through a piece of the ileum. One end of the ileum piece is sealed off and the other end is brought to the surface of the abdomen to form the stoma. It is the most common technique used for urinary diversion.

• With cystostomy, the flow of urine is diverted from the bladder to the abdominal wall. It features placement of a tube through the abdominal wall into the bladder, and is indicated in cases of blockage or stricture of the ureters. It can be temporary or permanent.

• An Indiana pouch refers to the construction of a pouch from the end part of the ileum and the first part of the large intestine (cecum). The remaining ileum is first attached to the large intestine to maintain normal digestive flow. A pouch is then created from the removed cecum, and the attached ileum is brought to the surface of the abdominal wall to create a stoma.

• Percutaneous nephrostomy diverts the flow of urine from the kidneys to the abdominal wall. Tubes are placed within the kidney to collect the urine as it is generated, and transport it to the abdominal wall. This procedure is usually temporary; however, it may be permanent for cancer patients.

Health care team roles

Ureterostomy is performed in a hospital setting by experienced **surgeons** trained in urology, the branch of medicine concerned with the diagnosis and treatment of diseases of the urinary tract and urogenital system. Specially trained nurses called wound ostomy continence nurses (WOCN) are commonly available for consultation in most major medical centers.

Resources

BOOKS

Door Mullen, Barbara, and Kerry Anne McGinn. *The Ostomy Book: Living Comfortably With Colostomies, Ileostomies, and Urostomies.* 3rd ed. Boulder, CO: Bull Publishing, 2008.

Graham, Sam D., and Thomas E. Keane, eds. *Glenn's Urologic Surgery.* Philadelphia: Wolters Kluwer/Lippincott Williams & Wilkins, 2010.

PERIODICALS

Rodríguez, Alejandro R., et al. "Cutaneous Ureterostomy Technique for Adults and Effects of Ureteral Stenting: An Alternative to the Ileal Conduit." *The Journal of Urology* 186, no. 5 (2011): 1939–43. http://dx.doi.org/10.1016/j.juro.2011.07.032 (accessed October 4, 2013).

Zilberman, D. E., et al. "Long-Term Urinary Bladder Function following Unilateral Refluxing Low Loop Cutaneous Ureterostomy." *Korean Journal of Urology* 53, no. 5 (2012): 355–59.

WEBSITES

American Cancer Society. "What Are the Key Statistics about Bladder Cancer?" http://www.cancer.org/cancer/bladder cancer/detailedguide/bladder-cancer-key-statistics (accessed October 14, 2013).

National Kidney and Urologic Diseases Information Clearinghouse. "Urostomy and Continent Urinary Diversion."
National Institute of Diabetes and Digestive and Kidney Diseases. http://www.kidney.niddk.nih.gov/kudiseases/pubs/urostomy (accessed October 4, 2013).

ORGANIZATIONS

National Institute of Diabetes and Digestive and Kidney Diseases (NIDDK), 31 Center Dr., MSC 2560, Bldg. 31, Rm. 9A06, Bethesda, MD 20892-2560, (301) 496-3583, http://www2.niddk.nih.gov.

United Ostomy Associations of America, Inc. (UOAA), PO Box 512, Northfield, MN 55057-0512, (800) 826-0826, info@ostomy.org, http://www.ostomy.org.

Urology Care Foundation, 1000 Corporate Blvd., Linthicum, MD 21090, (410) 689-3700, (800) 828-7866, Fax: (410) 689-3998, info@urologycarefoundation.org, http://auafoundation.org.

Monique Laberge, PhD

Uric acid tests *see* **Kidney function tests**

Urinalysis

Definition

A urinalysis is a group of manual and/or automated qualitative and semi-quantitative tests performed on a urine sample. It is also known as routine and microscopy (R&M). A routine urinalysis usually includes the following tests: color, transparency, specific gravity, pH, protein, glucose, ketones, blood, bilirubin, nitrite, urobilinogen, and leukocyte esterase. Some laboratories include a microscopic examination of urinary sediment with all routine urinalysis tests. If not, they customarily perform the microscopic exam if transparency, glucose, protein, blood, nitrite, or leukocyte esterase is abnormal.

Purpose

Routine urinalyses are performed for several reasons:

- general health screening to detect renal and metabolic diseases
- diagnosis of diseases or disorders of the kidneys or urinary tract
- monitoring of patients with diabetes

In addition, quantitative urinalysis tests may be performed to help diagnose many specific disorders, such as endocrine diseases, bladder cancer, osteoporosis, and porphyrias (a group of disorders caused by chemical imbalance). Quantitative analysis often requires the use of a timed urine sample. The urinary microalbumin test

KEY TERMS

Acidosis—A condition of the blood in which bicarbonate levels are below normal.

Alkalosis—A condition of the blood and other body fluids in which bicarbonate levels are higher than normal.

Bilirubin—A yellow bile pigment found as sodium (soluble) bilirubinate or as an insoluble calcium salt found in gallstones.

Biliverdin—A green bile pigment formed from the oxidation of heme, which is a bilin with a structure almost identical to that of bilirubin.

Cast—An insoluble gelled protein matrix that takes the form of the renal tubule in which it was deposited. Casts are washed out by normal urine flow.

Catheter—A thin flexible tube inserted through the urethra into the bladder to allow urine to flow out.

Clean-catch specimen—A urine specimen that is collected from the middle of the urine stream after the first part of the flow has been discarded.

Cystine—An amino acid normally reabsorbed by the kidney tubules. Cystinuria is an inherited disease in which cystine and some other amino acids are not reabsorbed by the body in normal amounts. Cystine crystals then form in the kidney, which leads to obstructive renal failure.

Epithelium—A general term for the layer of cells that lines blood vessels or small body cavities.

Ketones—Substances produced during the breakdown of fatty acids. They are produced in excessive amounts in diabetes and certain other abnormal conditions.

Meatus—A general term for an opening or passageway in the body. The urethral meatus should be cleansed before a urine sample is collected.

pH—A chemical symbol that denotes the acidity or alkalinity of a fluid, ranging from 1 (more acid) to 14 (more alkaline).

Porphyrias—A group of disorders involving heme biosynthesis, characterized by excessive excretion of porphyrins. The porphyrias may be either inherited or acquired (usually from the effects of certain chemical agents).

Trichomonads—Parasitic protozoa commonly found in the digestive and genital tracts of humans and other animals. Some species cause vaginal infections in women characterized by itching and a frothy discharge.

Turbidity—The degree of cloudiness of a urine sample (or other solution).

Urethra—The tube that carries urine from the bladder to the outside of the body.

Urinalysis (plural, urinalyses)—The diagnostic testing of a urine sample.

Voiding—The medical term for emptying the bladder or urinating.

---

measures the rate of albumin excretion in the urine using laboratory tests. This test is used to monitor kidney function of persons with diabetes mellitus. In diabetics, the excretion of greater than 200 μg/mL albumin is predictive of impending kidney disease.

Precautions

Voided specimens

All patients should avoid intense athletic training or heavy physical work before the test, as these activities may cause small amounts of blood to appear in the urine. Many urinary constituents are labile, and samples should be tested within one hour of collection or refrigerated. Samples may be stored at 36–46°F (2–8°C) for up to 24 hours for chemical urinalysis tests; however, the microscopic examination should be performed within four hours of collection, if possible. To minimize sample contamination, women who require a urinalysis during menstruation should insert a fresh tampon before providing a urine sample.

Over two dozen drugs are known to interfere with various chemical urinalysis tests. These include:

• ascorbic acid

• chlorpromazine

• L-dopa

• nitrofurantoin (Macrodantin, Furadantin)

• penicillin

• phenazopyridine (Pyridium)

• rifampin (Rifadin)

• tolbutamide

The preservatives that are used to prevent loss of glucose and cells may affect biochemical test results. The use of preservatives should be avoided whenever possible in urine tests.

Description

Routine urinalysis consists of three testing groups: physical characteristics, biochemical tests, and microscopic evaluation.

Physical tests

The physical tests measure the color, transparency (clarity), and specific gravity of a urine sample. In some cases, the volume (daily output) may be measured. Color and transparency are determined from visual observation of the sample.

COLOR. Normal urine is straw yellow to amber in color. Abnormal colors include bright yellow, brown, black (gray), red, and green. These pigments may result from medications, dietary sources, or diseases. For example, red urine may be caused by blood or hemoglobin, beets, medications, and some porphyrias. Black-gray urine may result from melanin (melanoma) or homogentisic acid (alkaptonuria, a rare metabolic disorder). Bright yellow urine may be caused by bilirubin (a bile pigment). Green urine may be caused by a bile pigment or certain medications. Orange urine may be caused by some medications or excessive urobilinogen (a chemical produced in the intestines). Brown urine may be caused by excessive amounts of porpholbilin or urobilin (chemical relatives of urobilinogen).

TRANSPARENCY. Normal urine is transparent. Turbid (cloudy) urine may be caused by either normal or abnormal processes. Normal conditions giving rise to turbid urine include precipitation of crystals, mucus, or vaginal discharge. Abnormal causes of turbidity include the presence of blood cells, yeast, and bacteria.

SPECIFIC GRAVITY. The specific gravity of urine is a measure of the concentration of dissolved solutes (substances in a solution), and it reflects the ability of the kidneys to concentrate the urine (conserve water). Specific gravity is usually measured by determining the refractive index of a urine sample (refractometry) or by chemical analysis. Specific gravity varies with fluid and solute intake. It will be increased (above 1.035) in persons with diabetes mellitus and persons taking large amounts of medication. It will also be increased after radiologic studies of the kidney owing to the excretion of x-ray contrast dye. Consistently low specific gravity (1.003 or less) is seen in persons with diabetes insipidus. In renal (kidney) failure, the specific gravity remains equal to that of blood plasma (1.008–1.010) regardless of changes in the patient's salt and water intake. Urine volume below 400 mL per day is considered oliguria

(low urine production) and may occur in persons who are dehydrated and those with some kidney diseases. A volume in excess of 2 liters (slightly more than 2 quarts) per day is considered polyuria (excessive urine production); it is common in persons with diabetes mellitus and diabetes insipidus.

Biochemical tests

Biochemical testing of urine is performed using dry reagent strips, often called dipsticks. A urine dipstick consists of a white plastic strip with absorbent microfiber cellulose pads attached to it. Each pad contains the dried reagents needed for a specific test. The person performing the test dips the strip into the urine, lets it sit for a specified amount of time, and compares the color change to a standard chart.

Additional tests are available for measuring the levels of bilirubin, protein, glucose, ketones, and urobilinogen in urine. In general, these individual tests provide greater sensitivity and permit detection of a lower concentration of the respective substance.

pH. A combination of pH indicators (methyl red and bromothymol blue) react with hydrogen ions (H^+) to produce a color change over a pH range of 5.0 to 8.5. The pH measurements are useful in determining metabolic or respiratory disturbances in acid-base balance. For example, kidney disease often results in retention of H^+ (reduced acid excretion). The pH varies with a person's diet, tending to be acidic in people who eat meat but more alkaline in vegetarians. The pH testing is also useful for the classification of urine crystals.

PROTEIN. Based upon a phenomenon called the "protein error of indicators," this test uses a pH indicator, such as tetrabromophenol blue, that changes color (at constant pH) when albumin is present in the urine. Albumin is important in determining the presence of glomerular damage. The glomerulus is the network of capillaries in the kidneys that filters low molecular weight solutes such as urea, glucose, and salts, but normally prevents passage of protein or cells from blood into filtrate. Albuminuria occurs when the glomerular membrane is damaged, a condition called glomerulonephritis.

GLUCOSE (SUGAR). The glucose test is used to monitor persons with diabetes. When blood glucose levels rise above 160 mg/dL, the glucose will be detected in urine. Consequently, glycosuria (glucose in the urine) may be the first indicator that diabetes or another hyperglycemic condition is present. The glucose test may be used to screen newborns for galactosuria and other disorders of carbohydrate metabolism that cause urinary excretion of a sugar other than glucose.

KETONES. Ketones are compounds resulting from the breakdown of fatty acids in the body. These ketones are produced in excess in disorders of carbohydrate metabolism, especially Type 1 diabetes mellitus. In diabetes, excess ketoacids in the blood may cause life-threatening acidosis and coma. These ketoacids and their salts spill into the urine, causing ketonuria. Ketones are also found in the urine in several other conditions, including fever; pregnancy; glycogen storage diseases; and weight loss produced by a carbohydrate-restricted diet.

BLOOD. Red cells and hemoglobin may enter the urine from the kidney or lower urinary tract. Testing for blood in the urine detects abnormal levels of either red cells or hemoglobin, which may be caused by excessive red cell destruction, glomerular disease, kidney or urinary tract infection, malignancy, or urinary tract injury.

BILIRUBIN. Bilirubin is a breakdown product of hemoglobin. Most of the bilirubin produced in humans is conjugated by the liver and excreted into the bile, but a very small amount of conjugated bilirubin is reabsorbed and reaches the general circulation to be excreted in the urine. The normal level of urinary bilirubin is below the detection limit of the test. Bilirubin in the urine is derived from the liver, and a positive test indicates hepatic disease or hepatobiliary obstruction.

SPECIFIC GRAVITY. Specific gravity is a measure of the ability of the kidneys to concentrate urine by conserving water.

NITRITE. Some disease bacteria, including the lactose-positive *Enterobacteriaceae*, *Staphylococcus*, *Proteus*, *Salmonella*, and *Pseudomonas*, are able to reduce nitrate in urine to nitrite. A positive test for nitrite indicates bacteriuria, or the presence of bacteria in the urine.

UROBILINOGEN. Urobilinogen is a substance formed in the gastrointestinal tract by the bacterial reduction of conjugated bilirubin. Increased urinary urobilinogen occurs in prehepatic jaundice (hemolytic anemia), hepatitis, and other forms of hepatic necrosis that impair the circulation of blood in the liver and surrounding organs. The urobilinogen test is helpful in differentiating these conditions from obstructive jaundice, which results in decreased production of urobilinogen.

LEUKOCYTES. The presence of white blood cells in the urine usually signifies a urinary tract infection, such as cystitis, or renal disease, such as pyelonephritis or glomerulonephritis.

Microscopic examination

A urine sample may contain cells that originated in the blood, the kidney, or the lower urinary tract. Microscopic examination of urinary sediment can provide valuable clues regarding many diseases and disorders involving these systems.

The presence of bacteria or yeast and white blood cells helps to distinguish between a urinary tract infection and a contaminated urine sample. White blood cells are not seen if the sample has been contaminated. The presence of cellular casts (casts containing RBCs, WBCs, or epithelial cells) identifies the kidneys, rather than the lower urinary tract, as the source of such cells. Cellular casts and renal epithelial (kidney lining) cells are signs of kidney disease.

The microscopic examination also identifies both normal and abnormal crystals in the sediment. Abnormal crystals are those formed as a result of an abnormal metabolic process and are always clinically significant. Normal crystals are formed from normal metabolic processes; however, they may lead to the formation of renal calculi, or kidney stones.

Preparation

A urine sample is collected in an unused disposable plastic cup with a tight-fitting lid. A randomly voided sample is suitable for routine urinalysis, although the urine that is first voided in the morning is preferable because it is the most concentrated. The best sample for analysis is collected in a sterile container after the external genitalia have been cleansed using the midstream void (clean-catch) method. This sample may be cultured if the laboratory findings indicate bacteriuria.

Specific methods for collecting a clean-catch sample vary based on the patient:

• Females should use a clean cotton ball moistened with lukewarm water (or antiseptic wipes provided with collection kits) to cleanse the external genital area before collecting a urine sample. To prevent contamination with menstrual blood, vaginal discharge, or germs from the external genitalia, they should release some urine before beginning to collect the sample.

• Males should use a piece of clean cotton moistened with lukewarm water or antiseptic wipes to cleanse the head of the penis and the urethral meatus (opening). Uncircumcised males should draw back the foreskin. After the area has been thoroughly cleansed, they should use the midstream void method to collect the sample.

• For infants, a parent or healthcare worker should cleanse the baby's outer genitalia and surrounding skin. A sterile collection bag should be attached to the child's genital area and left in place until he or she has urinated. It is important not to touch the inside of the bag and to remove it as soon as a specimen has been obtained.

Methenamine

People with certain medical conditions may have additional problems with this medicine; it may worsen liver or kidney disease.

Ciprofloxacin

Ciprofloxacin can worsen muscle weakness in people who have a nervous system disorder called myasthenia gravis and increase risk of tendinitis. The medication also makes the skin more sensitive to sunlight or other ultraviolet light.

Nitrofurantoin

Pregnant women should not take this medicine within two weeks of their delivery date and should not use it during labor and delivery, as this could cause problems in the baby.

Women who are breast-feeding should check with their physicians before using this medicine, as it passes into breast milk and could cause problems. This is especially true for babies with glucose-6-phosphate dehydrogenase (G6PD) deficiency. The medicine also should not be given directly to babies up to one month of age, as they are particularly sensitive to its effects.

Older people may be more likely to experience side effects when taking nitrofurantoin, because they are more sensitive to the drug's effects.

Taking nitrofurantoin may also cause problems for people with certain medical conditions. Side effects may be greater, for example, in people with lung disease or nerve damage. In people with kidney disease, the medicine may not work as well as it should and may cause more side effects. Those with glucose-6-phosphate dehydrogenase (G6PD) deficiency who take nitrofurantoin may develop anemia.

People with diabetes should be aware that this medicine may cause false results on some urine sugar tests. They should check with a physician before making any changes in diet or diabetes medicine based on the results of a urine test.

Levofloxacin

Levofloxacin is a quinolone antibiotic, so people who are allergic to quinolone antibiotics may experience a reaction. The medication can affect the heart's rhythm and cause serious problems by making a person's heart beat irregularly or too rapidly. Levofloxacin also can cause muscle weakness or tendinitis.

Symptoms should improve within a few days of starting to take a urinary anti-infective. If they do not, or if they become worse, check with a physician. Patients who need to take this medicine for long periods should see their physicians regularly, so that the physician can check their progress.

Anyone who has had unusual reactions to urinary anti-infectives in the past should let his or her physician know before taking the drugs again. The physician should also be told about any allergies to foods, dyes, preservatives, or other substances. Patients taking nalidixic acid should tell their physicians if they have ever had reactions to medicines such as cinoxacin (Cinobac), ciprofloxacin (Cipro), enoxacin (Penetrex), norfloxacin (Noroxin), or ofloxacin (Floxin), all of which are also used to treat or prevent infections. Anyone taking nitrofurantoin should let the physician know if he or she has had an unusual reaction to medicines such as furazolidone (Furoxone) or nitrofurazone (Furacin).

Side effects

While each drug is associated with known side effects, anyone who has unusual symptoms while taking a urinary anti-infective should contact his or her physician.

Methenamine

Nausea and vomiting are not common but may occur. These side effects do not need medical attention unless they are severe. Taking oral methenamine with food or milk can ease some of the nausea. One side effect that should be brought to a physician's attention immediately is a skin rash.

Ciprofloxacin

Taking ciprofloxacin can cause a patient to have nausea, vomiting, stomach pain, and diarrhea. Heartburn also can be a side effect, but people on ciprofloxacin should not take certain antacids immediately before taking the medication. Headache also has been reported. More serious side effects might indicate a serious reaction and should be reported immediately to a doctor. These include difficulty breathing or swallowing, hives, rashes, tingling or swelling of the face, and wheezing.

Nitrofurantoin

This medicine may make the urine turn reddish-yellow to brown, but it is nothing to worry about. Other possible side effects that do not need medical attention unless they become severe include pain in the stomach or abdomen, stomach upset, diarrhea, loss of appetite, and nausea or vomiting.

Anyone who has chest pain, breathing problems, fever, chills, or a cough while taking nitrofurantoin should consult their physician immediately.

Levofloxacin

Some side effects are minor, such as nausea, vomiting, stomach pain, constipation, and diarrhea. If diarrhea becomes severe, the person taking levofloxacin should notify the prescribing doctor. Other serious side effects include skin rashes, itching, fainting, rapid or irregular heartbeat, and unusual bruising or bleeding. Severe allergic reactions are rare but can occur; symptoms include a rash, itching, swelling around the mouth and throat, and dizziness.

Interactions

Patients should check with a physician or pharmacist before combining a urinary anti-infective with any other prescription or nonprescription (over-the-counter) medicine. Patients who are taking any kind of herbal preparation or other alternative medicine should give their doctor and pharmacist a list of all the compounds that they use on a regular basis. Most of these preparations are unlikely to interact with urinary anti-infectives, but there is much that is still unknown about possible interactions between standard prescription medications and alternative medicines.

Methenamine

Certain medicines may make methenamine less effective. These include thiazide **diuretics** (water pills) and medicines that make the urine less acidic, such as antacids, bicarbonate of soda, and the drugs acetazolamide (Diamox), dichlorphenamide (Daranide), and methazolamide (Neptazane), which are used to treat glaucoma, epilepsy, altitude sickness, and other conditions.

Ciprofloxacin

Several medications can interact with ciprofloxacin. Among them are tizanidine (Zanaflex) and warfarin (Coumadin, Jantoven). Several antidepressants and antipsychotic medicines can also cause an interaction, as can high levels of caffeine.

Nitrofurantoin

Patients should inform their physicians of any medications or herbal supplements they are taking before using nitrofurantoin. Antacids, antibiotics, and benztropine (Cogentin) are some of the medications or supplements that may cause reactions.

Levofloxacin

Several medications can interact with levofloxacin, including tizanidine (Zanaflex), warfarin (Coumadin,

---

KEY TERMS

Anticoagulant—A type of medication given to prevent the formation of blood clots. Anticoagulants are sometimes called blood thinners.

Bacteria—Microscopically small one-celled forms of life that cause many diseases and infections.

Glucose-6-phosphate dehydrogenase (G6PD) deficiency—An inherited disorder in which the body lacks an enzyme that normally protects red blood cells from toxic chemicals. Certain drugs can cause patients' red blood cells to break down, resulting in anemia. This may also happen when they have a fever or an infection. The condition usually occurs in males. About 10% of black males have it, as do a small percentage of people from the Mediterranean region.

Granule—A small grain or pellet. Medicines that come in granule form are usually mixed with liquids or sprinkled on food before they are taken.

pH—A measure of the acidity or alkalinity of a substance or compound. The pH scale ranges from 0 to 14. Values below 7 are acidic; values above 7 are alkaline.

Quinolones—A group of synthetic antibacterial drugs originally derived from quinine. Nalidixic acid is the first quinolone that was approved for clinical use.

Jantoven), and **nonsteroidal anti-inflammatory drugs**. Several antidepressants and antipsychotic medicines can also cause interactions.

Resources

BOOKS

Mandell, G. L., et al. *Principles and Practice of Infectious Diseases.* 6th ed. London: Churchill Livingstone, 2005.

Wein, A. J., et al. *Campbell-Walsh Urology.* 9th ed. Philadelphia: Saunders, 2007.

PERIODICALS

Chang, S. L. "Pediatric Urinary Tract Infections." *Pediatric Clinics of North America* 53 (June 2006): 379–400.

Emmerson, A. M., and A. M. Jones. "The Quinolones: Decades of Development and Use." *Journal of Antimicrobial Chemotherapy* 51 (May 2003): Supplement 1, 13–20.

Juthani-Mehta, M. "Asymptomatic Bacteriuria and Urinary Tract Infections in Older Adults." *Clinics of Geriatric Medicine* 23 (August 2007): 585–594.

WEBSITES

A.D.A.M. "Urinary Tract Infection—Treatment." University of Maryland Medical Center (UMMC). http://www.nlm.nih.gov/medlineplus/druginfo/meds/a697040.html (accessed June 4, 2013).

AHFS Consumer Medication Information. "Levofloxacin." AHFS Consumer Medication Information. Available from: http://www.nlm.nih.gov/medlineplus/druginfo/meds/a697040.html (accessed June 4, 2013).

ORGANIZATIONS

American Society of Health-System Pharmacists, 7272 Wisconsin Ave., Bethesda, MD 20814, (301) 664-8700, (866) 279-0681, custserv@ashp.org, http://www.ashp.org.

U.S. Food and Drug Administration, 10903 New Hampshire Ave., Silver Spring, MD 20993, (888) INFO-FDA (463-6332), http://www.fda.gov.

Nancy Ross-Flanigan
Sam Uretsky, PharmD
Teresa G. Odle

Urinary artificial sphincter *see* **Artificial sphincter insertion**

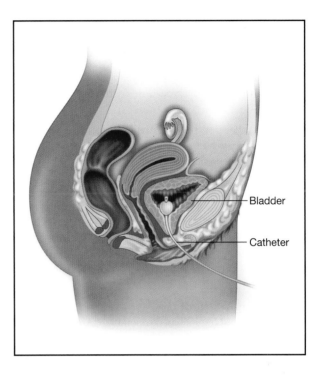

Female urinary catheterization. *(Illustration by Electronic Illustrators Group. Copyright © 2014 Cengage Learning®.)*

Urinary catheterization

Definition

Urinary catheterization is the insertion of a catheter through the urethra into the urinary bladder for withdrawal of urine. Straight catheters are used for intermittent drainage, while indwelling (Foley) catheters are inserted and retained in the bladder for continuous drainage of urine into a closed system.

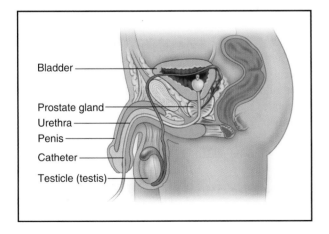

Male urinary catheterization. *(Illustration by Electronic Illustrators Group. Copyright © 2014 Cengage Learning®.)*

Purpose

Intermittent catheterization is used to:

• obtain a sterile urine specimen for diagnostic evaluation

• empty bladder contents when an individual is unable to void (urinate) due to urinary retention, bladder distention, or obstruction

• measure residual urine after urinating

• instill medication for a localized therapeutic effect in the bladder

• instill contrast material (dye) into the bladder for cystourethrography (x-ray study of the bladder and urethra)

• empty the bladder for increased space in the pelvic cavity to protect the bladder during labor and delivery or during pelvic and abdominal surgery

• monitor the urinary output and fluid balance of critically ill patients

Indwelling catheterization is used to:

• provide palliative care for incontinent persons who are terminally ill or severely impaired, and for whom bed and clothing changes are uncomfortable

• manage skin ulcerations caused or exacerbated by incontinence

• maintain a continuous outflow of urine for persons undergoing surgical procedures that cause a delay in bladder sensation, or for individuals with chronic neurological disorders that cause paralysis or loss of sensation in the perineal area

• keep with standard preoperative preparation for urologic surgery and procedures for bladder outlet obstruction

• provide relief for persons with an initial episode of acute urinary retention, allowing the bladder to regain its normal muscle tone

Description

The male urethral orifice (urinary meatus) is a vertical, slit-like opening, 0.15–0.2 in. (4–5 mm) long, located at the tip of the penis. The foreskin of the penis may conceal the opening. This must be retracted to be able to insert a catheter.

The female urethral orifice is a vertical, slit-like, or irregularly ovoid (egg-shaped) opening, 0.16–0.2 in. (4–5 mm) in diameter, located between the clitoris and the vagina. The urinary meatus (opening) is concealed between the labia minora, which are the small folds of tissue that need to be separated to view the opening and insert a catheter. Perineal care or cleansing may be required to ensure a clean procedural environment.

The male urethra is longer than the female urethra and has two curves in it as it passes through the penis to the bladder. Catheterization of the male patient is traditionally performed without the use of local anesthetic gel to facilitate catheter insertion. Glands along the urethra provide some natural lubrication. Older men may require lubrication; in such an instance, an anesthetic or antibacterial lubricant should be used.

Since there are no lubricating glands in the female urethra, the risk of trauma from a simple catheter insertion is increased. Therefore, an ample supply of an anesthetic or antibacterial lubricant should be used.

When inserting a urinary catheter, the healthcare provider will first wash the hands and put on gloves and clean the skin of the area around the urethra (in females) or the tip of the penis (in males). The catheter is threaded up the urethra and into the bladder until the urine starts to flow. Once the catheter is inserted, it is secured as appropriate for the catheter type. A straight catheter is typically secured with adhesive tape. An indwelling catheter is secured by inflating a bulb-like device inside of the bladder.

Catheter choices

TYPES. Silastic catheters have been recommended for short-term catheterization after surgery because they are known to decrease incidence of urethritis (inflammation of the urethra). However, due to lower cost and acceptable outcomes, latex is the catheter of choice for long-term catheterization. Silastic catheters should be reserved for individuals who are allergic to latex products.

Additional types of catheters include:

• PTFE (plastic)-coated latex indwelling (Foley) catheters

• hydrogel-coated latex indwelling catheters

• pure silicone indwelling catheters

• silicone-coated latex indwelling catheters

SIZE. The diameter of a catheter is measured in millimeters. Authorities recommend using the narrowest and softest tube that will serve the purpose of the catheterization. Rarely is a catheter larger than size 18 F(rench) required, and sizes 14 or 16 F are used more often. Catheters greater than size 16 F have been associated with patient discomfort and urine bypassing. A size 12 F catheter has been successfully used in children and in patients with urinary restriction.

DRAINAGE SYSTEM. The healthcare provider should discuss the design, capacity, and emptying mechanism of several urine drainage bags with the patient. For patients with normal bladder sensation, a catheter valve for intermittent drainage may be an acceptable option.

Preparation

Healthcare practitioners performing the catheterization should have a good understanding of the anatomy and physiology of the urinary system, be trained in antiseptic techniques, and have proficiency in catheter insertion and catheter care.

After determining the primary purpose for the catheterization, practitioners should give the patient and primary caregiver a detailed explanation. Patients requiring self-catheterization should be instructed and trained in the technique by a qualified health professional.

Sterile disposable catheterization sets are available in clinical settings and for home use. These sets contain most of the items needed for the procedure, such as antiseptic agent, perineal drapes, gloves, lubricant, specimen container, label, and tape. Anesthetic or antibacterial lubricant, catheter, and a drainage system may need to be added.

Aftercare

Patients using intermittent catheterization to manage incontinence may require a period of adjustment as they try to establish a catheterization schedule that is adequate for their normal fluid intake.

Antibiotics should not be prescribed as a preventative measure for patients at risk for urinary tract infection (UTI). Prophylactic use of antibacterial agents may lead to the development of drug-resistant bacteria. Patients who practice intermittent self-catheterization can reduce their risk for UTI by using antiseptic techniques for insertion and catheter care.

The extended portion of the catheter should be washed with a mild soap and warm water to keep it free of accumulated debris.

If the patient is sexually active, the practitioner must explain that intercourse can take place with the catheter in place. The patient and his or her partner can also be taught to remove the catheter before intercourse and replace it with a new one afterwards.

Risks

Complications that may occur from the catheterization procedure include:

• trauma or introduction of bacteria into the urinary system, leading to infection and, rarely, septicemia

• trauma to the urethra or bladder from incorrect insertion or attempting to remove the catheter with the balloon inflated; repeated trauma may cause scarring or stricture (narrowing) of the urethra

• passage of urine around the catheter; inserting a different size catheter can minimize this problem

Urinary catheterization should be avoided whenever possible. Clean intermittent catheterization, when practical, is preferable to long-term catheterization.

Catheters should not be routinely changed. Before the catheter is changed, each patient should be monitored for indication of obstruction, infection, or complications. Some patients require weekly catheter changes, while others may need one change in several weeks. Fewer catheter changes will reduce trauma to the urethra and reduce the incidence of UTI.

Because the urinary tract is normally a sterile system, catheterization presents the risk of causing a UTI. The presence of residual urine in the bladder due to incomplete voiding provides an ideal environment for bacterial growth. The catheterization procedure must be sterile, and the catheter must be free from bacteria.

Frequent intermittent catheterization and long-term use of indwelling catheterization predisposes a person to UTI. Care should be taken to avoid trauma to the urinary meatus or urothelium (urinary lining) with catheters that are too large or inserted with insufficient use of lubricant. Patients with an indwelling catheter must be reassessed

KEY TERMS

Catheter—A tube for evacuating or injecting fluid.

Foley catheter—A double-channel retention catheter; one channel provides for the inflow and outflow of bladder fluid, the second (smaller) channel is used to fill a balloon that holds the catheter in the bladder.

Incontinence—The inability to retain urine or control urine flow.

Intermittent catheterization—Periodic catheterization to facilitate urine flow.

Perineal area—The genital area between the vulva and anus in a woman.

Prophylactic—Intended to prevent or protect against disease.

Septicemia—An infection in the blood.

Urethra—The tube that allows passage of urine out of the urinary bladder.

Urethritis—Inflammation of the urinary bladder.

Urinary retention—The inability to void (urinate) or discharge urine.

periodically to determine if an alternative treatment will be more effective.

Males

Phimosis is constriction of the prepuce (foreskin) so that it cannot be drawn back over the glans penis. This may make it difficult to identify the external urethral meatus. Care should be taken when catheterizing men with phimosis to avoid trauma from forced retraction of the prepuce or by incorrect positioning of the catheter.

Females

Sexual activity and menopause can also compromise the sterility of the urinary tract. Irritation of the urethra during intercourse promotes the migration of perineal bacteria into the urethra and bladder, causing UTIs. Postmenopausal women may experience more UTIs than younger women.

Results

A catheterization program that includes correctly inserted catheters and is appropriately maintained will usually control urinary incontinence.

The patient and his or her caregiver should be taught to use **aseptic technique** for catheter care. Nursing interventions and patient education can make a difference in the incidence of UTIs in hospitals, **nursing homes**, and **home care** settings.

Morbidity and mortality rates

Injuries resulting from catheterization are infrequent. Deaths are extremely rare. Both complications are usually due to infections that result from improper catheter care.

Alternatives

An alternative to catheterization is to use a pad to absorb voided urine.

Health care team roles

Urinary catheterization can be performed by healthcare practitioners, by home caregivers, or by patients themselves in hospitals, long-term care facilities, or personal homes.

Resources

BOOKS

Perry, Anne Griffin, Patricia A. Potter, and Martha Keene Elkin. *Nursing Interventions & Clinical Skills*. 5th ed. St. Louis, MO: Mosby/Elsevier, 2012.

Taal, Maarten W., et al. *Brenner & Rector's The Kidney*. 9th ed. Philadelphia: Saunders/Elsevier, 2012.

Wein, Alan J., et al. *Campbell-Walsh Urology*. 10th ed. Philadelphia: Saunders/Elsevier, 2012.

PERIODICALS

Johnson, J. R. "Safety of Urinary Catheters." *Journal of the American Medical Association* 289, no. 3 (2003): 300–301.

Krien, Sarah L., et al. "Barriers to Reducing Urinary Catheter Use: A Qualitative Assessment of a Statewide Initiative." *JAMA Internal Medicine* 173, no. 10 (2013): 881–86. http://dx.doi.org/10.1001/jamainternmed.2013.105 (accessed October 23, 2013).

Magers, Tina L. "Using Evidence-Based Practice to Reduce Catheter-Associated Urinary Tract Infections." *American Journal of Nursing* 113, no. 6 (2013): 34–42. http://dx.doi.org/10.1097/01.NAJ.0000430923.07539.a7 (accessed October 23, 2013).

WEBSITES

A.D.A.M. Medical Encyclopedia. "Urinary Catheters." MedlinePlus. http://www.nlm.nih.gov/medlineplus/ency/article/003981.htm (accessed May 28, 2013).

NHS (UK National Health Service). "Urinary Catheterisation." http://www.nhs.uk/conditions/Urinary-catheterization/Pages/Introduction.aspx (accessed May 28, 2013).

ORGANIZATIONS

American Board of Urology, 600 Peter Jefferson Pkwy., Ste. 150, Charlottesville, VA 22911, (434) 979-0059, Fax: (434) 979-0266, http://www.abu.org.

National Kidney and Urologic Diseases Information Clearinghouse, 3 Information Way, Bethesda, MD 20892-3580, (800) 891-5390, (866) 569-1162, Fax: (703) 738–4929, nkudic@info.niddk.nih.gov, http://kidney.niddk.nih.gov.

Urology Care Foundation, 1000 Corporate Blvd., Linthicum, MD 21090, (410) 689-3700, (800) 828-7866, Fax: (410) 689-3998, info@urologycarefoundation.org, http://auafoundation.org.

L. Fleming Fallon, Jr, MD, DrPH

Urinary diversion *see* **Ureterostomy, cutaneous**

Urinary diversion surgery *see* **Ileal conduit surgery**

Urine culture

Definition

A urine culture is a diagnostic laboratory test performed to detect the presence of bacteria in the urine (bacteriuria).

Purpose

Culture of the urine is a method of diagnosis for urinary tract infection (UTI) that determines the number of microorganisms present in a given quantity of urine.

Description

There are several different methods for collection of a urine sample. The most common is the midstream clean-catch technique. Hands should be washed before beginning. For females, the external genitalia (sex organs) are washed two or three times with a cleansing agent and rinsed with water. In males, the external head of the penis is similarly cleansed and rinsed. The patient is then instructed to begin to urinate, and the urine is collected midstream into a sterile container. In infants, a urinary collection bag (plastic bag with an adhesive seal on one end) is attached over the labia in girls or the penis in boys to collect the specimen.

Another method is the catheterized urine specimen, in which a lubricated catheter (thin rubber tube) is inserted through the urethra and into the bladder. This avoids contamination from the urethra or external genitalia. If the patient already has a urinary catheter in place, the specimen may be collected by clamping the tubing below the collection port and using a sterile needle and syringe to obtain the urine sample; urine cannot be taken from the drainage bag, as it is not fresh and has had an opportunity to grow bacteria at room temperature. On rare occasions, the healthcare provider may collect a urine sample by inserting a needle directly into the bladder (suprapubic tap) and draining the urine; this method is used only when a sample is needed quickly.

Negative culture results showing no bacterial growth are available after 24 hours. Positive results require 24–72 hours to complete identification of the number and type of bacteria found.

Precautions

If delivery of the urine specimen to the laboratory within one hour of collection is not possible, it should be refrigerated. The healthcare provider should be informed of any **antibiotics** currently or recently taken.

Preparation

Drinking a glass of water 15–20 minutes before the test is helpful if there is no urge to urinate. There are no other special preparations or aftercare required for the test.

Aftercare

No aftercare is required for a urine culture.

Risks

There are no risks associated with the culture test itself. If insertion of a urinary catheter (thin rubber tube) is required to obtain the urine, there is a slight risk of introducing infection from the catheter.

Results

No growth of bacteria is considered the normal result, and this indicates absence of infection.

KEY TERMS

Bacteriuria—The presence of bacteria in the urine.

Urethra—The tube that carries urine from the bladder to outside the body. In females, the urethral opening is between the vagina and clitoris; in males, the urethra travels through the penis, opening at the tip.

Abnormal results

Abnormal results, or a positive test, where bacteria are found in the specimen, may indicate a UTI. Contamination of the specimen from hair, external genitalia, or the rectum may cause a false-positive result. Identification of the number and type of bacteria, with consideration of the method used in obtaining the specimen, is important for diagnosis.

Escherichia coli causes approximately 80% of infections in patients without catheters, abnormalities of the urinary tract, or calculi (stones). Other bacteria that account for a smaller portion of uncomplicated infections include *Proteus, Klebsiella*, and *Enterobacter*.

Resources

BOOKS

McGhee, M. *A Guide to Laboratory Investigations*. 5th ed. Oxford, England: Radcliffe Publishing Ltd, 2008.

Pagana, Kathleen Deska, and Timothy J. Pagana. *Mosby's Diagnostic and Laboratory Test Reference*. 11th ed. St. Louis, MO: Mosby/Elsevier, 2013.

Price, C. P. *Evidence-Based Laboratory Medicine: Principles, Practice, and Outcomes*. 2nd ed. Washington, DC: AACC Press, 2007.

Scott, M. G., A. M. Gronowski, and C. S. Eby. *Tietz's Applied Laboratory Medicine*. 2nd ed. New York: Wiley-Liss, 2007.

PERIODICALS

Giesen, Callen D., et al. "Performance of Flow Cytometry to Screen Urine for Bacteria and White Blood Cells Prior to Urine Culture." *Clinical Biochemistry* 46, no. 9 (2013): 810–13. http://dx.doi.org/10.1016/j.clinbiochem.2013.03.005 (accessed October 23, 2013).

WEBSITES

A.D.A.M. Medical Encyclopedia. "Urine Culture." MedlinePlus. http://www.nlm.nih.gov/medlineplus/ency/article/003751.htm (accessed May 22, 2013).

American Association for Clinical Chemistry. "Urine Culture." Lab Tests Online. http://labtestsonline.org/understanding/analytes/urine-culture (accessed May 28, 2013).

Urologic surgery

ORGANIZATIONS

American Society for Clinical Laboratory Science, 1861
International Dr., Ste. 200, McLean, VA 22102, (571)
748-3770, ascls@ascls.org, http://www.ascls.org.

American Society for Clinical Pathology (ASCP), 33 W.
Monroe St., Ste. 1600, Chicago, IL 60603, (312)
541-4999, (800) 267-2727, Fax: (312) 541-4998, http://
www.ascp.org.

College of American Pathologists, 325 Waukegan Rd.,
Northfield, IL 60093-2750, (847) 832-7000, (800)
323-4040, Fax: (847) 832-8000, http://www.cap.org.

L. Fleming Fallon, Jr, MD, DrPH

Urobilinogen test *see* **Urinalysis**

Urologic surgery

Definition

Urologic surgery is the integration of surgical activities for the pelvis—the colon, urogenital, and gynecological organs—primarily for the treatment of obstructions, dysfunction, malignancies, and inflammatory diseases. Common urologic operations include:

• renal (kidney) surgery

• kidney removal (nephrectomy)

• surgery of the ureters, including ureterolithotomy or removal of calculus (stones) in the ureters

• bladder surgery

• pelvic lymph node dissection

• prostatic surgery, removal of the prostate

• testicular (scrotal) surgery

• urethra surgery

• surgery to the penis

Purpose

Conditions that commonly dictate a need for urologic surgery include kidney stones, urologic cancers, neurogenic sources like spinal cord injury, injuries to the pelvic organs, urinary-voiding dysfunctions, and prostate enlargement and inflammation. There are many other common chronic and malignant diseases that can benefit from resection, surgical augmentation, or surgery to clear obstructions. These conditions impact the digestive, renal, and reproductive systems.

Most organs are susceptible to cancer in the form of tumors and invasion of the surrounding tissue. Urologic malignancies are on the rise. Other conditions that are seen more frequently include genitourinary anomalies in children and infections of the genitourinary tract.

Urologic surgery has been revolutionized by striking advances in urodynamic diagnostic systems. Changes in these areas have been particularly beneficial for urologic surgery: **laparoscopy**, endoscopic examination for colon cancer, robotic-assisted techniques, implantation procedures, and imaging techniques. These procedural and imaging advances have brought the field of urology to a highly active and innovative stage, with new surgical options evolving constantly.

Demographics

According to the National Kidney Foundation, kidney and urologic diseases affect at least 5% of the American population, and cause over 260,000 deaths. As the population ages, these conditions are expected to increase, especially among ethnic minorities who have a disproportionate share of urologic diseases. Major urologic surgery includes radical and partial resections for malignant and benign conditions, and diversion and transplantation surgeries.

Cancer

Prostate cancer is the most common cancer affecting males in the United States. One in six men will have the disease at some time in his life. It is, however, treated successfully with surgery or radiation therapy.

According to the Urological Foundation, more than 63,200 new cases of bladder cancer are detected each year. In the United States, bladder cancer is the fourth most common cancer in men and the eighth most common for women.

Kidney cancer occurs in 51,190 new patients per year, with almost 13,000 deaths. It is the eighth most common cancer in men and the tenth most common cancer in women. Renal cell carcinoma makes up 85% of all kidney tumors. In adults ages 50–70 years, kidney cancer occurs twice as often in men as women. At the time of diagnosis, metastasis is present in 25%–30% of patients with renal cell carcinoma.

Other conditions

Enlarged prostate (benign prostate hyperplasia, BPH) is very common and often treated with surgery. Interstitial cystitis (bladder infection of unknown origin) often affects women, and symptoms include severe pain and incontinence. The condition, like other forms of severe incontinence, may sometimes surgery.

Incontinence is increasingly diagnosed as a problem among the aging population in the United States, and is gaining recognition for its highly debilitating effects both in its fecal and urinary forms. According to the National Institute of Diabetes & Digestive & Kidney Diseases (NIDDK), more than 6.5 million Americans have fecal incontinence. Fecal incontinence affects people of all ages; many cases are never reported. Women are five times more likely than men to have fecal incontinence. This is primarily due to obstetric injury, especially with forceps delivery and anal sphincter laceration.

Urinary incontinence affects an estimated 38% of women aged 60 or older, and an estimated 17% of men aged 60 or older. According to one study published in the *American Journal of Gastroenterology*, only 34% of incontinent patients have ever mentioned their problem to a physician, even though 23% wear absorbent pads, 12% take medications, and 11% lead lives restricted by their incontinence.

Many surgical procedures are now available to correct incontinence. They include retropubic slings for urinary incontinence, artificial sphincter implants for urinary incontinence, and bladder diversion surgeries for restoration of voiding with an outside appliance (stoma) called a urostomy. Kidney surgery and transplantation account for a large segment of urologic surgery. Benign conditions include sexual dysfunction, kidney stones, and fertility issues.

Description

Until the late twentieth century, urological operations usually involved open abdominal surgery with full incision, lengthy hospital stays, and long recovery periods. Today, surgery is less traumatic, with shortened hospitalizations. Minimally invasive surgeries are the norm in many cases, with new laparoscopic procedures developed each year. Laparoscopic surgery is effective for many kidney tumors and kidney removal (**nephrectomy**), lymph node excision, prostate and ureteral cancers, as well as incontinence, urological reconstruction, kidney stones, and some cases of bladder dysfunction. Newer, robotic-assisted techniques allow for greater precision, and eliminate interference from even the slightest degree of imprecision that can be associated with a normal amount of operator hand tremor.

Preparation

Testing is often required to determine if a patient is better suited for open or laparoscopic surgery. Blood tests for some cancers, as well as function tests for the affected organs, will be required. Radiographic or **ultrasound** techniques are helpful in providing images of abnormalities.

KEY TERMS

Genitourinary reconstruction—Surgery that corrects birth defects or the results of disease that involve the genitals and urinary tract, including the kidneys, ureters, bladder, urethra, and the male and female genitals.

Nephrectomy—Surgical removal of a kidney.

Neurogenic bladder—Bladder dysfunction caused by neurological diseases that alter the brain's messages to the bladder.

Prostatectomy—Prostate cancer surgery that includes partial or complete removal of the prostate.

Cystoscopy is often used with bladder and urethra surgery. In this procedure, a thin telescope-like instrument is inserted directly into the bladder. Disorders of the colon may be studied with endoscopes, imaging instruments inserted directly into the colon. Urodynamic studies of the bladder and sphincter determine how the bladder fills and empties. Digital rectal exams diagnose prostatic disorders. In this procedure, the physician feels the prostate with a gloved, lubricated finger inserted into the rectum.

Aftercare

Hospital stays range from one day to one week, depending upon the level of organ involvement and type of urologic surgery (open versus laparoscopic). Major urologic surgeries may require stents (temporary diversion of urine or feces) and catheters that are removed after surgery. Some surgeries are staged in two parts to accommodate the removal of diseased tissue, and the augmentation or reconstruction to replace function. Laparoscopic surgery patients benefit from shorter hospital stays, more rapid recovery, and possibly lower morbidity rates than open surgery procedures. This is increasingly true for prostate cancer surgeries.

Risks

The risks of urologic surgery vary with the type of surgical procedure (open or laparoscopic), and the extent of organ involvement. According to one study of 2,407 urologic surgeries in four centers, the overall complication rate was 4.4%, with a mortality rate of 0.08%.

Open surgery poses the standard surgery and anesthetic risks associated with strain on the heart and lungs. Risks of infection at the wound site accompany all surgeries, open and laparoscopic. The risk of injury to adjacent organs is higher in laparoscopic surgery. Kidney removal and transplantation have many risks because of the extent of the surgery, as do surgeries of the colon, bladder, and prostate.

Significant gains have been made in prostate surgery. Urinary control issues following prostate surgery, especially radical **prostatectomy**, have improved. However, postoperative urinary incontinence remains a significant risk, with 27% of patients in one study reporting the need for some kind of leakage protection. In the same study, only 14.2% of previously potent men reported the ability to achieve and maintain a postoperative erection that is sufficient for sexual intercourse. Urologic **surgeons** are well versed in the risks and benefits of the surgeries they perform, and they expect to be asked questions related to these issues.

Results

The expected surgery result is a topic that the urologic surgeon and patient should address prior to surgery. It is important that the patient understands the issues of recovery, rehabilitation, training or retraining, and the limitations surgery may offer for basic daily functions and enjoyment. Results of urologic surgery are individual, and depend upon the health of the patient and his or her motivation to deal with postoperative recovery issues and changes to organ function brought about by the surgery.

Alternatives

Many urological diseases can be dealt with through diet, weight loss, and lifestyle changes. These modifications are especially significant in preventing and treating conditions of the urinary tract. Obesity and nutrition play a significant role in urologic diseases, and impact many urologic cancers, inflammatory and ulcerative conditions, incontinence, and sexual dysfunction.

Medical interventions are another form of treatment, particularly for infectious and inflammatory urologic conditions. They are particularly useful along with special adjunctive surgical procedures for the treatment of incontinence and painful bladder and kidney conditions. While many cancers must be treated surgically, prostate cancer is often treated with a "wait and see" approach due to its slow rate of growth. There is an increasing trend for men with slow-growing prostate cancers to have regular check-ups instead of immediate treatment.

Health care team roles

Urologic surgery is performed by surgeons who specialize in the treatment of urologic conditions.

QUESTIONS TO ASK YOUR DOCTOR

- How many procedures does my surgeon and this hospital perform compared to other facilities?
- What are the urination and sexual intercourse risks of this surgery?
- Are there alternatives to surgery?

Surgery is performed in a general hospital, regional center, or clinic, depending upon the type of procedure.

Resources

BOOKS

Wein, Alan J., et al. *Campbell-Walsh Urology*. 10th ed. Philadelphia: Saunders/Elsevier, 2012.

PERIODICALS

Kallingal, George J. S., and Dipen J Parekh. "Rise of Robotics in Urologic Surgery: Current Status and Future Directions." *Expert Review of Medical Devices* 10, no. 3 (2013): 287–89. http://dx.doi.org/10.1586/erd.13.15 (accessed September 19, 2013).

Nicolaides, A., R. D. Hull, and J. Fareed. "Urologic Surgery." *Clinical and Applied Thrombosis/Hemostatis* 19, no. 2 (2013): 133–34. http://dx.doi.org/10.1177/107602 9612474840d (accessed September 19, 2013).

Oh, Tae Hee. "Current Status of Laparoendoscopic Single-Site Surgery in Urologic Surgery." *Korean Journal of Urology* 53, no. 7 (2012): 443–50. http://dx.doi.org/10.4111/kju.2012.53.7.443 (accessed September 19, 2013).

van den Berg, Nynke S., Fijs W. B.van Leeuwen, and Henk G. van der Poel. "Fluorescence Guidance in Urologic Surgery." *Current Opinion in Urology* 22, no. 2 (2012): 109–20. http://dx.doi.org/10.1097/MOU.0b01 3e3283501869 (accessed September 19, 2013).

Wszolek, Matthew, et al. "Laparoscopy for the Detection and Treatment of Early Complications from Minimally Invasive Urologic Surgery." *Journal of Endourology* (June 26, 2012): e-pub ahead of print. http://dx.doi.org/10.1089/end.2012.0165 (accessed September 19, 2013).

WEBSITES

Urology Care Foundation. "Kidney And Ureteral Stones: Surgical Management." http://www.urologyhealth.org/urology/index.cfm?article=32&display=1 (accessed September 19, 2013).

Urology Care Foundation. "Prostate Cancer: Surgical Management." http://www.urologyhealth.org/urology/index.cfm?article=30&display=1 (accessed September 19, 2013).

ORGANIZATIONS

American Society of Nephrology, 1510 H St. NW, Ste. 800, Washington, DC 20005, (202) 640-4660, email @asn-online.org, http://asn-online.org.

National Institute of Diabetes and Digestive and Kidney Diseases (NIDDK), 31 Center Drive, MSC 2560, Bldg. 31, Rm. 9A06, Bethesda MD 20892-2560, (301) 496-3583, http://www2.niddk.nih.gov.

National Kidney and Urologic Diseases Information Clearinghouse, 3 Information Way, Bethesda, MD 20892-3580, (800) 891-5390, (866) 569-1162, Fax: (703) 738–4929, nkudic@info.niddk.nih.gov, http://kidney.niddk.nih.gov.

National Kidney Foundation, 30 E. 33rd St., New York, NY 10016, (212) 889-2210, (800) 622-9010, Fax: (212) 689-9261, http://www.kidney.org.

Urology Care Foundation, 1000 Corporate Blvd., Linthicum, MD 21090, (410) 689-3700, (800) 828-7866, Fax: (410) 689-3998, info@urologycarefoundation.org, http://auafoundation.org.

Nancy McKenzie, PhD

Uterine fibroid removal *see* **Myomectomy**

Uterus removal *see* **Hysterectomy**

Uvulopalatoplasty *see* **Snoring surgery**

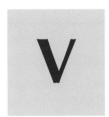

Vagal nerve stimulation *see* **Vagus nerve stimulation**

Vaginal wall repair *see* **Colporrhaphy**

Vaginotomy *see* **Colpotomy**

Vagotomy

Definition

Vagotomy is the surgical cutting of the vagus nerve to reduce acid secretion in the stomach.

Purpose

The vagus nerve trunk splits into branches that go to different parts of the stomach. Stimulation from these branches causes the stomach to produce acid. Too much stomach acid leads to ulcers that may eventually bleed and create an emergency situation.

A vagotomy is performed when acid production in the stomach can not be reduced by other means. The purpose of the procedure is to disable the acid-producing capacity of the stomach. It is used when ulcers in the stomach and duodenum do not respond to medication and changes in diet. It is an appropriate surgery when there are ulcer complications, such as obstruction of digestive flow, bleeding, or perforation. The frequency with which elective vagotomy is performed has decreased in the past 20 years as it has become clear that the primary cause of ulcers is an infection by a bacterium called *Helicobacter pylori*. Drugs have become increasingly effective in treating ulcers. However, the number of vagotomies performed in emergency situations has remained about the same.

A vagotomy procedure is often performed in conjunction with another gastrointestinal surgery, such as partial removal of the stomach (**antrectomy** or subtotal **gastrectomy**).

Demographics

Gastric (peptic) ulcers are included under the general heading of gastrointestinal (GI) diseases. GI disorders affect an estimated 25%–30% of the world's population. In the United States, 60 million adults experience gastrointestinal reflux at least once a month, and 25 million adults suffer daily from heartburn. Left untreated, these conditions often evolve into ulcers. Four million people have active peptic ulcers; about 350,000 new cases are diagnosed each year. Four times as many duodenal ulcers as gastric ulcers are diagnosed. The first-degree relatives of patients with duodenal ulcer have a two to three times greater risk of developing duodenal ulcer. Relatives of gastric ulcer patients have a similarly increased risk of developing a gastric ulcer.

Description

A vagotomy can be performed using closed (laparoscopic) or open surgical techniques. The indications for a laparoscopic vagotomy are the same as for open vagotomy.

There are four basic types of vagotomy procedures:

- In truncal or total abdominal vagotomy, the main vagal trunks are divided, and surgery is accompanied by a drainage procedure, such as pyloroplasty.

- With selective (total gastric) vagotomy, the main vagal trunks are dissected to the point where the branch leading to the biliary tree divides, and there is a cut at the section of vagus close to the hepatic branch. This procedure is rarely indicated or performed.

- Highly selective vagotomy (HSV) selectively deprives the parietal cells of vagal nerves and reduces their sensitivity to stimulation and the release of acid. It does not require a drainage procedure. The branches of Latarjet's nerve are divided from the esophagogastric

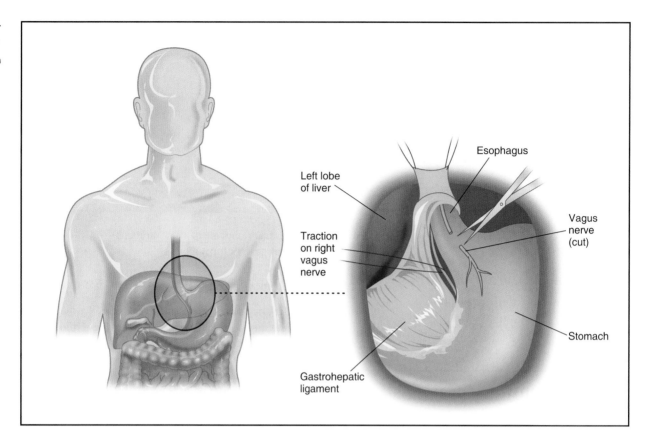

To perform a vagotomy, the surgeon makes an incision in the patient's abdomen. Once the stomach is located, the vagus nerves are cut. *(Illustration by Electronic Illustrators Group. Copyright © 2014 Cengage Learning®.)*

junction to the crow's foot along the lesser curvature of the stomach.

- Thoracoscopic vagotomy is performed through the third, sixth, and seventh left intercostal spaces. The posterior vagus trunk is isolated, clipped, and a segment excised.

A vagotomy is performed under **general anesthesia**. The surgeon makes an incision in the abdomen and locates the vagus nerve. Either the trunk or the branches leading to the stomach are cut. The abdominal muscles are sewn back together, and the skin is closed with sutures.

Often, other gastrointestinal surgery is performed (e.g., part of the stomach may be removed) at the same time. Vagotomy causes a decrease in peristalsis, and a change in the emptying patterns of the stomach. To ease this, a **pyloroplasty** is often performed to widen the outlet from the stomach to the small intestine.

Preparation

A gastroscopy and x-rays of the gastrointestinal system determine the position and condition of the ulcer. Standard preoperative blood and urine tests are done. The patient discusses with the anesthesiologist any medications or conditions that might affect the administration of anesthesia.

Aftercare

Patients who have had a vagotomy stay in the hospital for about seven days. Nasogastric suctioning is required for the first three or four days. A tube is inserted through the nose and into the stomach. The stomach contents are then suctioned out. Patients eat a clear liquid diet until the gastrointestinal tract regains function. When patients return to a regular diet, spicy and acidic foods should be avoided.

It takes about six weeks to fully recover from the surgery. The sutures that close the skin can be removed in seven to ten days. Patients are encouraged to move around soon after the operation to prevent the formation of deep vein blood clots. Pain medication, stool softeners, and **antibiotics** may be prescribed following the operation.

Risks

Standard surgical risks, such as excessive bleeding and infection, are potential complications. In addition,

KEY TERMS

Duodenum—The section of the small intestine closest to the stomach.

Gastric glands—Branched tubular glands located in the stomach.

Gastric ulcer—An ulcer of the stomach, duodenum, or other part of the gastrointestinal system. Also called a peptic ulcer.

Latarjet's nerve—Terminal branch of the anterior vagal trunk, which runs along the lesser curvature of the stomach.

Parietal cells—Cells of the gastric glands that secrete hydrochloric acid and intrinsic factor.

Peristalsis—The rhythmic contractions that move material through the bowel.

Pyloroplasty—Widening of the pyloric canal and any adjacent duodenal structure by means of a longitudinal incision.

QUESTIONS TO ASK YOUR DOCTOR

- What are the possible complications involved in vagotomy surgery?
- What surgical preparation is needed?
- What type of anesthesia will be used?
- How is the surgery performed?
- How long is the hospitalization?
- How many vagotomies does the surgeon perform in a year?

the emptying patterns of the stomach are changed. This can lead to dumping syndrome and diarrhea. Dumping syndrome is a condition in which the patient experiences palpitations, sweating, nausea, cramps, vomiting, and diarrhea shortly after eating.

The following complications are also associated with vagotomy surgery:

- Gastric or esophageal perforation may occur from an electrocautery injury or by clipping the branch of the nerve of Latarjet.
- Delayed gastric emptying is most common after truncal or selective vagotomy, particularly if a drainage procedure is not performed.

People who use alcohol excessively, smoke, are obese, and are very young or very old are at higher risk for complications.

Results

Normal recovery is expected for most patients. Ulcers recur in about 10% of those who have a vagotomy without stomach removal. Recurrent ulcers are also found in 2%–3% of patients who have some portion of their stomach removed.

Morbidity and mortality rates

In the United States, approximately 3,000 deaths per year are due to duodenal ulcers and 3,000 to gastric ulcers. There has been a marked decrease in reported hospitalization and mortality rates for gastric ulcers.

Alternatives

The preferred short-term treatment for gastric ulcers is drug therapy. A recent review surveying medical articles published from 1977 to 1994 concluded that drugs such as cimetidine, ranitidine, famotidine, H2 blockers, and sucralfate were efficient, with omeprazole considered the "gold standard" for active gastric ulcer treatment. Surgical intervention, however, is recommended for people who do not respond to medical therapy.

Health care team roles

Patients who receive vagotomies are most often seen in emergency situations where bleeding and perforated ulcers require immediate intervention. A vagotomy is usually performed by a board-certified surgeon, either a general surgeon who specializes in gastrointestinal surgery or a gastrointestinal endoscopic surgeon. The procedure is performed in a hospital setting.

Resources

BOOKS

Doherty, Gerard. *CURRENT Diagnosis and Treatment Surgery.* 13th ed. New York: McGraw-Hill, 2010.

Lawrence, Peter F., ed. *Essentials of General Surgery.* 5th ed. Philadelphia: Lippincott Williams & Wilkins, 2013.

PERIODICALS

Hunter, J., et al. "Effectiveness of Thoracoscopic Truncal Vagotomy in the Treatment of Marginal Ulcers after Laparoscopic Roux-en-Y Gastric Bypass." *The American Surgeon* 78, no. 6 (2012): 663–68.

Tait, Laura F., et al. "Resolution of Uncontrolled Type 2 Diabetes after Laparoscopic Truncal Vagotomy, Subtotal Gastrectomy, and Roux-en-Y Gastrojejunostomy for a

Patient with Intractable Gastric Ulcers." *Case Reports in Surgery* art. ID 102752 (November 3, 2012). http://dx.doi.org/10.1155/2012/102752 (accessed October 4, 2013).

WEBSITES

Draper, Richard. "Ulcer Surgery and Its Complications." Patient.co.uk. http://www.patient.co.uk/doctor/Ulcer-Surgery-and-its-Complications.htm (accessed October 4, 2013).

ORGANIZATIONS

American College of Surgeons, 633 N. Saint Clair St., Chicago, IL 60611-3211, (312) 202-5000, (800) 621-4111, Fax: (312) 202-5001, postmaster@facs.org, http://www.facs.org.

Society of American Gastrointestinal Endoscopic Surgeons (SAGES), 11300 West Olympic Blvd., Ste. 600, Los Angeles, CA 90064, (310) 437-0544, Fax: (310) 437-0585, webmaster@sages.org, http://www.sages.org.

Tish Davidson, AM
Monique Laberge, PhD

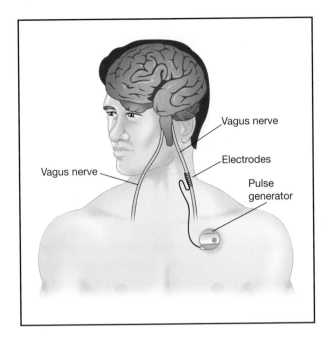

Vagus nerve stimulation. *(Illustration by Electronic Illustrators Group. Copyright © 2014 Cengage Learning®.)*

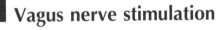

Vagus nerve stimulation

Definition

Vagus nerve stimulation, also referred to as vagal nerve stimulation, is a treatment for epilepsy in which an electrode is implanted in the neck to deliver electrical impulses to the vagus nerve. Newer uses of this technique involves the treatment of medication refractory depression. Research is being done to determine its efficacy in the treatment of other brain disorders, including multiple sclerosis, Alzheimer's disease, and severe migraine disease.

Purpose

Vagus nerve stimulation is an alternative to medication or surgical removal of brain tissue in controlling epileptic seizures. The seizures of epilepsy are caused by uncontrolled electrical discharges spreading through the brain. Antiseizure drugs interrupt this process by reducing the sensitivity of individual brain cells to stimulation. Brain surgery for epilepsy either removes the portion of the brain where seizures originate, or cuts nerve fibers to prevent the nerve impulses that occur during a seizure from spreading to other parts of the brain. Vagus nerve stimulation uses a different approach: It provides intermittent electrical stimulation to a nerve outside the brain—the vagus, or tenth cranial nerve, which influences certain patterns of brain activity.

This same vagus stimulation can be harnessed in the treatment of severe depression. Stimulation of the vagus seems to change metabolic activity in certain areas of the brain, leading to lessening of depressive symptoms some months after implantation.

The vagus nerve is a major connection between the brain and the rest of the body. It carries sensory information from the body to the brain, and motor commands from the brain to the body. The vagus is involved in complex control loops between these destinations; its precise pathways and mechanisms are still not fully understood. It is also not known how stimulation of the vagus nerve works to reduce seizure activity—it may stimulate inhibitory pathways that prevent the brain's electrical activity from getting out of control, interrupt some feedback loops that worsen seizures, or act in some other fashion.

Vagus nerve stimulation has been effective in reducing seizure frequency in patients whose seizures are not controlled by drugs, and who are either not candidates for other types of brain surgery or who have chosen not to undergo these procedures.

Demographics

About 2.2 million people in the United States have been diagnosed with epilepsy. While 50% of people given antiseizure medications will have a good response, almost 30% of people with epilepsy have seizures that are unresponsive to treatment. For these individuals, vagus nerve stimulation may provide relief. Vagus nerve stimulation was first performed in the United States in 1988 and received final approval by the United States Food and Drug Administration (FDA) in July 1997.

Almost 9.5% of people in the United States, or 18.8 million individuals, have clinically diagnosable depression at any given time. Of these, about 8% do not respond to antidepressant medications or experience intolerable side effects. Vagus nerve stimulation is an alternative for individuals with medication-resistant depression.

Description

The vagal nerve stimulator (VNS) has two parts: an electrode that wraps around the left vagus nerve in the neck, and a pulse generator, which is implanted under the skin below the collarbone. The two parts are connected by a wire. Stimulation is performed only on the left vagal nerve, as the right vagal nerve helps control the heartbeat.

Surgery to implant a VNS device takes about two hours. A neurosurgeon implants the electrode and generator while the patient is under **general anesthesia**. A vertical incision is made in the left side of the neck, and the helical electrode is attached to the nerve itself. A second incision is made on the left side of the chest below the collarbone, and the pulse generator (a disc about 2 in. [5 cm] in diameter) is implanted under the skin. The connecting wire is threaded around the muscles and bones to join the electrode and generator. The

generator makes a small bulge under the skin, but is hidden by clothing after the operation.

Before the neurosurgeon closes the incisions, he or she tests the VNS device to make sure it is working, and programs it to deliver the lowest amount of stimulation. The device is usually timed to stimulate the vagus nerve for 30 seconds every five minutes.

Preparation

A candidate for vagus nerve stimulation will have had many tests already to determine the focal point of seizure activity. Preoperative tests include neuroimaging, as well as psychological tests to determine the patient's cognitive (thinking) strengths and weaknesses.

The patient must be fully informed about VNS—how it works, its advantages and disadvantages, what will happen during surgery—before the operation is scheduled. A video as well as written material about VNS is available to view and discuss with the doctor.

Aftercare

Implantation of the stimulator in an adult may be performed as either an outpatient or inpatient procedure. In the latter case, the patient will remain in the hospital overnight for monitoring of heart function and other **vital signs**. Children who are receiving a VNS are usually scheduled for an overnight stay. Pain medication is given as needed.

The stimulation parameters are adjustable, and the neurologist may require several visits to find the right settings. Settings are adjusted with a magnetic wand that delivers commands to the stimulator's computer chip. The patient will be taught how to use a magnet to temporarily increase stimulation, to prevent a seizure, or to abort it once it begins.

The VNS generator is powered by a battery that lasts several years. It is replaced during an outpatient procedure under **local anesthesia**.

Risks

The most common adverse effects from vagus nerve stimulation are a hoarse voice, cough, headache, and ear pain. These side effects can be reduced by adjusting the stimulation settings, and may subside on their own over time. Infection and device malfunction are possible, though rare.

Patients who have had a VNS implanted must avoid strong magnets, which may affect the stimulator settings. Areas with warning signs posted regarding **pacemakers** should be avoided. The patient should consult with the neurologist and the neurosurgeon about other hazards.

Results

In patients with epilepsy, vagus nerve stimulation results in about one-third of patients enjoying a 50% reduction in their seizures. Another third enjoy some benefit, but not a 50% reduction in seizure activity. The last third notes no difference in seizure activity. Fewer than 5% of patients who undergo this procedure end up completely seizure-free. Most patients who continue to take antiseizure medications can reduce their dosage, however, which offers some relief from the side effects of these drugs.

Success rates for depression treatment with vagus nerve stimulation have not been completely clarified. Imaging reveals changes in brain metabolism some months before patients report an improvement in depressive symptoms.

Morbidity and mortality rates

Vagus nerve stimulation is a relatively safe procedure. Pilot studies of 300 patients that were done prior to FDA approval of VNS reported the following complication rates: hoarseness, 37% of patients; coughing, 14%; voice alteration, 13%; chest pain, 12%; and nausea, 2%. Lastly, patients contemplating the implantation of this device should be aware that the battery will require changing (and with that, a minor surgical procedure) between every three to every eight years.

Alternatives

Some individuals with epilepsy who are candidates for vagus nerve stimulation are also likely to be candidates for a **corpus callosotomy**, temporal lobectomy, or other surgical procedures. Individuals with depression may benefit from transcranial magnet stimulation or electroconvulsive therapy.

Health care team roles

The implanting of a VNS device is performed by a neurosurgeon in a hospital, in consultation with a neurologist.

Resources

BOOKS

Daroff, Robert B., et al. *Bradley's Neurology in Clinical Practice*. 6th ed. Philadelphia: Saunders/Elsevier, 2012.

PERIODICALS

Dugan, Patricia, & Orrin Devinsky. "Epilepsy: Guidelines on Vagus Nerve Stimulation for Epilepsy." *Nature Reviews Neurology* (October 15, 2013): e-pub ahead of print. http://dx.doi.org/10.1038/nrneurol.2013.211 (accessed October 18, 2013).

WEBSITES

American Association of Neurological Surgeons. "Vagus Nerve Stimulation." http://www.aans.org/Patient%20Information/Conditions%20and%20Treatments/Vagus%20Nerve%20Stimulation.aspx (accessed October 18, 2013).

Epilepsy Foundation. "VNS." http://www.epilepsyfoundation.org/aboutepilepsy/treatment/VNS (accessed October 18, 2013).

NYU Langone Medical Center, Comprehensive Epilepsy Center. "Vagus Nerve Stimulation (VNS)." http://epilepsy.med.nyu.edu/diagnosis-treatment/vagus-nerve-stimulation-vns (accessed October 18, 2013).

ORGANIZATIONS

American Academy of Neurology, 201 Chicago Ave., Minneapolis, MN 55415, (612) 928-6000, (800) 879-1960, Fax: (612) 454-2746, memberservices@aan.com, http://www.aan.com.

American Association of Neurological Surgeons, 5550 Meadowbrook Dr., Rolling Meadows, IL 60008-3852, (847) 378-0500, (888) 566-AANS (2267), Fax: (847) 378-0600, info@aans.org, http://aans.org.

Epilepsy Foundation, 8301 Professional Pl., Landover, MD 20785-2353, (800) 332-1000, (866) 748-8008 (Spanish), ContactUs@efa.org, http://www.epilepsyfoundation.org.

Richard Robinson

Valvuloplasty, balloon *see* **Balloon valvuloplasty**

Varicose vein sclerotherapy *see* **Sclerotherapy for varicose veins**

Vascular access devices

Definition

Vascular access devices (VADs) are thin, flexible plastic tubes—called catheters or access ports—that are inserted temporarily or permanently into a larger blood vessel for administering medications and/or nutrients, for frequent withdrawal of blood samples, or for hemodialysis.

Purpose

VADs are designed for long-term and/or more secure access to a blood vessel than can be achieved with a simple intravenous (IV) line. They allow ready access to a blood vessel without repeated puncture of the skin and vessel, thereby avoiding the inflammation and scarring from needle pricks and irritation and blood clots that can occur with IV lines. VADs reduce patient discomfort and anxiety. Furthermore, many fluids and medications cannot be administered through IV lines because of irritation or toxicity.

VADs are used for:

- chemotherapy for cancer treatment
- antibiotics or other drug treatments that last more than three to four weeks
- administration of certain heart medications in children
- transfusions of blood or blood products
- administration of fluids
- long-term feeding and total parenteral nutrition (TPN)
- repeated withdrawal of blood samples
- emergency access for managing cardiopulmonary arrest or trauma
- critical care monitoring
- hemodialysis for kidney failure
- patients for whom a simple IV line is not possible

Description

There are several different types of VADs available, including central, implantable, and other devices.

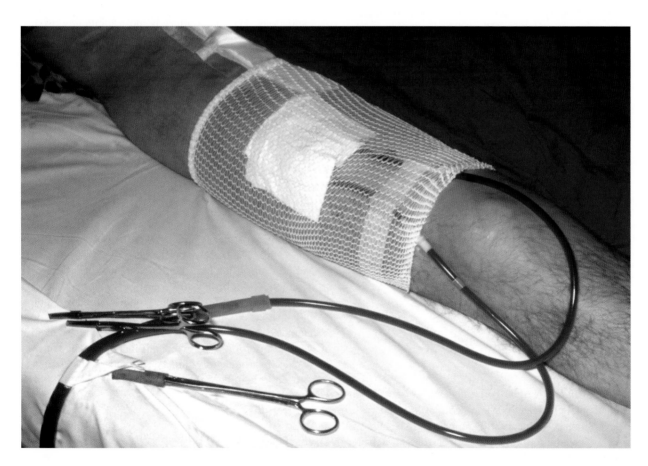

Vascular access devices are thin tubes that provide easy access to a patient's vein. (© Medical-on-Line/Alamy)

Central VADs

Central VADs are also called venous access catheters, venous access ports, or central venous catheters (CVCs). They are pencil-sized or smaller and may have a single cavity or lumen or multiple lumina that are used for different purposes. CVCs are inserted into a large vein that terminates near the heart, such as a vein in the neck, chest, arm, leg, or sometimes the groin. Non-tunneled catheters are fixed to the outside of the body at the insertion site. Tunneled catheters pass under the skin from the insertion site to an exit site, usually in the chest, so they are less visible. The catheter tip is most often placed within the superior vena cava. CVC placement usually takes 30–45 minutes. They may remain in place for weeks, months, or even years.

There are various types of CVCs:

• A peripherally inserted central catheter (PICC) is designed for short-to-medium-term use. It is a long catheter that extends from an arm or leg vein into the inferior or superior vena cava, the large veins near the heart. The tip of a midline catheter remains in a large vein but does not extend into the largest central vein. PICCs are commonly used for outpatient therapy and for many purposes. Some can be used for injecting contrast substances for CT scans.

• A percutaneous polyethylene catheter is for long-term use and is appropriate for most medications. It can be inserted into various veins, including the subclavian, internal jugular, and femoral. Like a PICC, it can be implanted in an emergency.

• Silicone CVCs are for long-term use, are safe for most medications, and are less likely than other types to cause clots or infection. They are more pliable and easier on veins than polyethylene catheters; however, they are expensive and require surgical insertion. A non-tunneled central catheter may have a larger diameter than a PICC and is placed in a large, central vein such as the jugular or the femoral vein in the groin. The exit point is close to the entry point of the vein. Tunneled silicone catheters are used for long-term treatment, such as total parenteral nutrition (TPN) or chemotherapy. An attached cuff is often impregnated with antibiotics. A CVC for hemodialysis may have a cuff that stimulates tissue growth to hold it in place.

Other VADs

Implantable VADs, port catheters, or subcutaneous implantable ports are for long-term or permanent use. They eliminate some of the problems associated with CVCs, including infection, frequent dressing changes, visibility, and restriction of daily activities such as showering or bathing. The injection port is made of a hard, durable protective shell, such as titanium, overlaid with a silicone diaphragm that is surgically implanted under the skin of the chest. The injection port is connected to a silicone catheter placed in the vein. The port is accessed by puncturing the diaphragm with a needle.

There are other VADs for specific purposes:

• Intraosseous devices are inserted into veins in the bone marrow that drain directly into the central venous circulation for emergency access, usually for resuscitation medications. They must be removed within 12–24 hours.

• Venous cutdown devices are used for emergency access but can remain in place long term. The saphenous vein of the lower leg is a usual site of insertion.

• The umbilical vein can be used for access in newborns. However, after the first few days of life, a surgical cutdown may be needed to access the vein. It can be used for monitoring central venous pressure as well as administering fluid and drugs and sampling blood. An artery in the umbilical stump can also be used for drugs and fluid, blood samples, and monitoring arterial blood pressure.

• Arterial vascular access is used to measure blood gases and continuously monitor blood pressure in critical-care situations. The radial artery is most commonly used.

Insertion

Ultrasound or x-rays and fluoroscopy are typically used to identify a suitable vein for catheter placement and for inserting the guide wire and catheter. A midline catheter and some PICC lines can be inserted through a vein near the elbow and threaded through a large vein in the upper arm at the patient's bedside without imaging. PICC insertion does not usually require sedation.

Other VAD procedures are usually performed in an interventional radiology suite or **operating room**. These procedures are often performed under a local anesthetic with mild sedation. A small needle is used to advance a guide wire. The catheter is advanced over the guide wire and positioned in a large central vein, and the guide wire is removed. A **chest x-ray** confirms the correct catheter position. The catheter is secured to the skin with a suture, and the insertion site is covered with a dressing. Tunneled catheters and subcutaneous ports require surgical insertion with two small incisions. The catheter is placed through the tunnel. The end of the tunnel is stitched to help hold the catheter in place.

Benefits

VADs have various benefits:

• There are a wide variety available for different circumstances.

- They can be used immediately after placement, some will function for a year or longer, and they are easily removed.
- They can provide a simple and pain-free means of drawing blood and administering TPN and drugs, sparing the patient stress and discomfort.
- For prolonged treatments such as chemotherapy, VADs avoid the need for repeatedly inserting an IV, which can result in badly scarred arm veins.
- PICCs are particularly useful for administering fluids or medicines that irritate vessel walls.
- VADs avoid other complications of IV lines, such as local tissue damage from leakage of toxic drugs.
- VADs are less likely to be dislodged.
- A VAD may be the only choice for hemodialysis.

Precautions

Most VADs eventually require replacement. The reservoir septa of implanted ports are useful for about 1,000 punctures, after which they must be replaced. PICCs may be difficult to position in a central vein and may occlude (close up).

Preparation

The careful selection of an appropriate VAD can have a profound effect on quality of life, and patient involvement in the choice of a VAD can improve outcomes. Blood tests may be performed before VAD insertion to assess kidney function and blood clotting. If the blood is too thin and not clotting properly, the patient may be given medication or blood products or the procedure may be postponed. Patients may have to discontinue **aspirin**, nonsteroidal anti-inflammatories, or blood thinners. **Informed consent** is required for the procedure. Patients may be told not to eat or drink for several hours before the procedure and will remove any clothing, jewelry, or other items that could interfere with x-ray imaging.

Heart rate and blood pressure monitors are attached to the patient. The insertion site—usually the arm for PICCs and the upper chest for tunneled catheters—is shaved, sterilized, covered with a surgical drape, and numbed with a local anesthetic. An IV line may be inserted, and the patient may be sedated.

Pediatric

Pediatric VADs are appropriately sized for children of different ages and may be inserted under **general anesthesia** using special equipment. X-ray doses are lower.

Pregnant or breast-feeding

Women should inform their physician and x-ray technician if there is any possibility that they are pregnant. Pregnancy may preclude the use of x-ray-guided insertion.

Aftercare

X-ray imaging confirms that the VAD is correctly positioned. Fluid is injected through the catheter to confirm that the device is functioning properly.

VAD procedures are often performed on an outpatient basis, but the patient must be driven home. The patient should rest for the remainder of the day and resume normal activities the following day, while avoiding heavy lifting. Pain medicine may be taken for any bruising, swelling, or tenderness in the chest, neck, or shoulder. The catheter site must be kept clean and dry for the first week. The physician may recommend cleaning the site with peroxide, applying an antibiotic ointment, and bandaging. Patients may shower after one week, with plastic wrap covering the catheter site, but the site cannot be immersed in water. Proper care of the incision can reduce the risk of infection. Patients may be told to flush the catheter with heparin to prevent clotting.

Removing PICCs and non-tunneled CVCs is similar to removing an IV and can be performed by nurses or technicians. Tunneled and port catheters are removed by a physician, with the skin numbed with **local anesthesia**. Removal takes about 15 minutes. The site must be kept dry until the incision has completely healed.

Risks

VAD complications can be serious or life threatening, and as many as 50% of VAD patients have complications. Approximately 10%–25% of hospital admissions are related to VAD complications, and patient morbidity is at least 10%.

The most common complications of peripheral catheters are displacement or clogging, which can cause fluids to extravasate into tissues outside the vein and requires removal of the catheter. Extravasation of hypertonic or irritating solutions can cause serious complications, including tissue death. PICC lines have an increased occlusion rate because their lumens are often small. Venous access sites that are exhausted from overuse can have serious implications for chronically ill patients.

The most common acute complication of central venous access is pneumothorax—a collection of air in the chest that causes a lung to collapse while a catheter or port is being positioned in the chest or neck. Pneumothorax occurs in up to 4% of VAD placements. Air embolism—the introduction of air into the vein—is another serious and often unrecognized risk. Other risks associated with VAD placement include:

• temporary disturbance of normal heart rhythm

• poor catheter placement

• hemothorax or bleeding into the chest due to blood vessel injury from the needle

• bruising or bleeding at the puncture site

• infection around the catheter or port

• bleeding, hemorrhaging, or nerve damage in surrounding tissue

• damage to the thoracic duct

• heart complications, such as irritation or perforation

• rarely, insertion of the catheter into an artery instead of a vein

The risk of long-term complications increases with the duration of catheterization. Infection is the most common complication. Any central venous line used for long-term access is prone to at least one infection. Thrombosis (blot clots), catheter occlusion, and catheter migration are also common. Delayed risks of a VAD include:

• infection at the insertion site

• sepsis—a life-threatening release of bacteria into the bloodstream, which can result from an infected VAD or non-sterile handling of the device

• catheter movement or dislodgement

• VAD malfunction

• a hole or break in the catheter resulting in leakage of fluid

• obstruction of the VAD by clotted blood or fibrin sheath

• occlusion of the catheterized vein, leading to swelling of the arm, shoulder, neck, or head

• deep-vein thrombosis (DVT)—a blood clot that causes swelling of the affected extremity and which can break off and travel to the lung, causing a life-threatening pulmonary embolism (PE)

• phlebitis (inflammation) of the vein

• superior vena cava syndrome

• air in the catheter that causes chest pain or shortness of breath—a medical emergency

• endocarditis from bacteria or fungi traveling from the VAD to the heart valves

• rarely, a skipped or irregular heartbeat related to catheter position

Pediatric

Infection rates from VADs are highest in newborns. Catheter removal usually eliminates infection in children.

KEY TERMS

Catheter—A hollow, flexible tube, such as a vascular access device, that is inserted into a body cavity, duct, or vessel for the passage of fluids.

Central venous catheter (CVC)—A vascular access device that is inserted into a central vein such as the jugular.

Deep-vein thrombosis (DVT)—A clot in a deep vein, as in the leg or pelvis.

Fluoroscopy—A technique for observing veins through shadows cast on a fluorescent screen by x-rays.

Hemodialysis—The process of removing blood from a kidney patient, purifying it by dialysis, and returning it to the body.

Heparin—A medication that prevents blood clotting.

Inferior vena cava—The largest vein in the body, which returns blood to the right atrium of the heart from the lower portion of the body.

Intravenous (IV)—Nutrition, fluids, or medications administered through a peripheral vein.

Peripherally inserted central catheter (PICC)—A vascular access device that is inserted through an arm or leg vein to the inferior or superior vena cava near the heart.

Pulmonary embolism (PE)—A blood clot that travels to the pulmonary artery, usually from a vein in the leg or pelvis.

Sepsis—Septicemia; a bacterial infection of the bloodstream.

Superior vena cava—The second largest vein in the body, which returns blood to the right atrium of the heart from the upper half of the body.

Thrombosis—The formation of a blood clot within a blood vessel.

Total parenteral nutrition (TPN)—Complete nutritional support that is provided outside of the intestines, as through a vascular access device.

Ultrasound—An imaging method in which high-frequency sound waves are used to outline internal body structures, such as veins.

Research and general acceptance

Because of the large number of variables, as well as insufficient research, the choice of a particular VAD for a given patient is not always clear. Several algorithms for selecting a VAD have been developed based on clinical variables. One study identified eight variables that were important to patients. These same variables, with the exception of "comfort," were identified by nurses as very important:

- safety, especially relative risk of infection

- pre-existing problems and treatment duration

- convenience for activities of daily living

- amount and type of care required

- availability of caregivers

- visibility

- comfort

- cost

Research has shown that patient education increases compliance and improves outcomes. However, the above study reported that 100% of African American and Hispanic patients and 60% of white patients said they had not received information on care and maintenance of their VAD, activity restrictions, and potential complications. A 2013 study found that both massage therapy and structured attention to patients were beneficial for relieving preoperative anxiety in cancer patients undergoing port placement.

Resources

BOOKS

Sansivero, Gail Egan, Gary Siskin, and David Singh. "Role of Ultrasound in Central Vascular Access Device Placement." In *Diagnostic Medical Sonography: The Vascular System*, edited by Ann Marie Kupinski. Philadelphia: Wolters Kluwer/Lippincott Williams & Wilkins, 2013.

PERIODICALS

Rosen, Jennifer, et al. "Massage for Perioperative Pain and Anxiety in Placement of Vascular Access Devices." *Advances in Mind-Body Medicine* 27, no. 1 (Winter 2013): 12–23.

WEBSITES

Larson, Shawn D. "Vascular Access Overview." Medscape Reference. http://emedicine.medscape.com/article/1018395-overview#showall (accessed September 25, 2013).

Macklin, Denise C. "Developing a Patient-Centered Approach to Vascular Access Device Selection." Medscape Reference. http://www.medscape.com/viewarticle/508093 (accessed September 25, 2013).

Radiological Society of North America. "Vascular Access Procedures." RadiologyInfo.org. http://www.radiology info.org/en/info.cfm?pg=vasc_access&bhcp=1&mobile bypass=1 (accessed September 25, 2013).

ORGANIZATIONS

American College of Radiology, 1891 Preston White Drive, Reston, VA 20191, (703) 648-8900, info@acr.org, http://www.acr.org.

Radiology Society of North America, 820 Jorie Boulevard, Oak Brook, IL 60523-2251, (630) 571-2670, Fax: (630) 571-7837, (800) 381-6660, http://www.rsna.org.

U.S. Food and Drug Administration, 10903 New Hampshire Avenue, Silver Spring, MD 20993-0002, (888) INFO-FDA (463-6332), http://www.fda.gov.

Margaret Alic, PhD

Vascular study *see* **Angiography**

Vascular surgery

Definition

Vascular surgery is the treatment of surgery on patients diagnosed with diseases of the arterial, venous, and lymphatic systems (excluding the intracranial and coronary arteries).

Purpose

Vascular surgery is indicated when a patient has vascular disease that cannot be treated by less invasive, nonsurgical treatments. The purpose of vascular surgery is to treat vascular diseases, which are diseases of the arteries and veins. Arterial disease is a condition in which blood clots, arteriosclerosis, and other vascular conditions occur in the arteries. Venous disease involves problems that occur in the veins. Some vascular conditions occur only in arteries, others occur only in the veins, and some affect both veins and arteries.

Demographics

As people age, vascular diseases are very common. Since they rarely cause symptoms in the early stages,

Abdominal aortic aneurysm—Occurs when an area in the aorta (the main artery of the heart) is weakened and bulges like a balloon. The abdominal section of the aorta supplies blood to the lower body.

Aneurysm—A weakening of the artery wall, due to atherosclerosis, causing a bulge that can rupture, and lead to thrombosis or embolism.

Angiography or angiogram—An x-ray exam of the arteries and veins (blood vessels) to diagnose blockages and other blood vessel problems.

Ankle-brachial index (ABI) test—A means of checking the blood pressure in the arms and ankles using a regular blood pressure cuff and a special ultrasound stethoscope (Doppler). The pressure in the ankle is compared to the pressure in the arm.

Aorta—A large, elastic artery beginning at the upper part of the left ventricle of the heart that becomes the main trunk of the arterial system.

Aortic aneurysms—Occurs when an area in the aorta (the main artery of the heart) is weakened and bulges like a balloon.

Arteriogram—An x-ray picture of an artery achieved by injecting an opaque dye with a needle or tube into the affected artery.

Artery—A blood vessel conveying blood in a direction away from the heart.

Atherosclerosis—A form of arteriosclerosis affecting the innermost area of the artery; a series of calcified deposits that can close down the vessel.

Bruit—A roaring sound created by a partially blocked artery.

Capillary—Smallest extremity of the arterial vessel, where oxygen and nutrients are released from the blood into the cells, and cellular waste is collected.

Carotid artery—Major artery leading to the brain, blockages of which can cause temporary or permanent strokes.

Carotid artery disease—A condition in which the arteries in the neck that supply blood to the brain become clogged, causing the danger of a stroke.

Carotid endarterectomy—A surgical technique for removing intra-arterial obstructions of the internal carotid artery.

Cerebral aneurysm—The dilation, bulging, or ballooning out of part of the wall of a vein or artery in the brain.

Cholesterol—An abundant fatty substance in animal tissues. High levels in the diet are a factor in the cause of atherosclerosis.

Claudication—Attacks of lameness or pain chiefly in the calf muscles, brought on by walking because of a lack of oxygen reaching the muscle.

Collaterals—Alternate pathways for arterial blood.

Computed tomography (CT) scan—An imaging technique that produces three-dimensional pictures of organs and structures inside the body using a 360° x-ray beam.

Coronary—Of or relating to the heart.

Doppler ultrasound—A diagnostic procedure that uses sound waves to evaluate blood flow through major arteries and veins.

many people do not realize that they suffer from these diseases. A large percentage of the 10 million people in the United States who may have peripheral vascular disease (PVD) or peripheral artery disease (PAD) are males. In the majority of cases, the blockage is caused by one or more blood clots that travel to the lungs from another part of the body. Factors that increase the chances of vascular disease include:

• increasing age (which results in a loss of elasticity in the veins and their valves)

• a family history of heart or vascular disease

• illness or injury

• pregnancy

• prolonged periods of inactivity sitting, standing, or bed rest

• smoking

• obesity

• hypertension, diabetes, high cholesterol, or other conditions that affect the health of the cardiovascular system

• lack of exercise

Description

Vascular surgery involves techniques relating to endovascular surgeries, including balloon **angioplasty** and/or stenting, aortic and peripheral vascular

Embolism—Obstruction or closure of a vessel by a transported clot of foreign matter.

Endovascular grafting—A procedure that involves the insertion of a delivery catheter through a groin artery into the abdominal aorta under fluoroscopic guidance.

Intracranial—Existing or occurring within the cranium; affecting or involving intracranial structures.

Lower extremity amputation—To cut a limb from the body.

Lymphangiography—Injection of dye into lymphatic vessels followed by x-rays of the area. It is a difficult procedure, as it requires surgical isolation of the lymph vessels to be injected.

Lymphoscintigraphy—A technique in which a radioactive substance that concentrates in the lymphatic vessels is injected into the affected tissue and mapped using a gamma camera, which images the location of the radioactive tracer.

Magnetic resonance imaging (MRI)—A noninvasive diagnostic technique that produces computerized images of internal body tissues and is based on nuclear magnetic resonance of atoms within the body induced by the application of radio waves.

Plethysmography—A test in which a patient sits inside a booth called a plethysmograph and breathes through a mouthpiece, while pressure and air flow measurements are collected to measure the total lung volume.

Pulmonary embolism—A blocked artery in the lung.

Renal artery aneurysm—An aneurysm relating to, involving, or located in the region of the kidneys.

Thoracic aortic aneurysm—Occurs when an area in the thoracic section of the aorta (the chest) is weakened and bulges like a balloon. The thoracic section supplies blood to the upper body.

Thrombolysis—A treatment that opens up blood flow and may prevent permanent damage to the blood vessels.

Thrombosis—The formation or presence of a blood clot within a blood vessel.

Thrombus—A blood clot that may form in a blood vessel or in one of the cavities of the heart.

Ulcer—A lesion or rough spot formed on the surface of an artery.

Ultrasound scan—The scan produces images of arteries on a screen and is used to evaluate the blood flow, locate blockages, and measure the size of the artery.

Varicose veins—Twisted, enlarged veins near the surface of the skin, which develop most commonly in the legs and ankles.

Vascular—Relating to the blood vessels.

Vasculogenic erectile dysfunction—The inability to attain or sustain an erection satisfactory for coitus, due to atherosclerotic disease of penile arteries, inadequate impedance of venous outflow (venous leaks), or a combination of both.

Venous stasis disease—A condition in which there is pooling of blood in the lower leg veins that may cause swelling and tissue damage, and lead to painful sores or ulcers.

endovascular stent/graft placement, thrombolysis, and other adjuncts for vascular reconstruction.

The vascular system is the network of blood vessels that circulate blood to and from the heart and lungs. The circulatory system (made up of the heart, arteries, veins, capillaries, and the circulating blood) provides nourishment to the body's cells and removes their waste. The arteries carry oxygenated blood from the heart to the cells. The veins return the blood from the cells back to the lungs for reoxygenation and recirculation by the heart. The aorta is the largest artery leaving the heart; it then subdivides into smaller arteries going to every part of the body. The arteries, as they narrow, are connected to smaller vessels called capillaries. In these capillaries, oxygen and nutrients are released from the blood into the cells, and cellular wastes are collected for the return trip. The capillaries then connect to veins, which return the blood back to the heart.

The aorta stems from the heart, arches upward, and then continues down through the chest (thorax) and the abdomen. The iliac arteries, which branch out from the aorta, provide blood to the pelvis and legs. The thoracic section of the aorta supplies blood to the upper body, as it continues through the chest. The abdominal section of the aorta, which supplies blood to the lower body, continues through the abdomen.

Vascular diseases are usually caused by conditions that clog or weaken blood vessels, or damage valves that control the flow of blood in and out of the veins, thus robbing them of vital blood nutrients and oxygen. A few common diseases affecting the arteries are peripheral vascular disease (PVD), carotid artery disease, and aortic aneurysms.

Surgery is used to treat specific diseased arteries, such as atherosclerosis, to help prevent strokes or heart attacks, improve or relieve angina or hypertension, remove aneurysms, improve claudication, and save legs that would otherwise have to be amputated. The choices involve repairing the artery, bypassing it, or replacing it.

As people age, atherosclerosis, commonly called hardening of the arteries, occurs with the constant passage of blood through the arteries. It can take on a number of forms, of which atherosclerosis (hardening of the innermost portion) is the most common. This occurs when fatty material containing cholesterol or calcium (plaque) is deposited on the innermost layer of the artery. This causes a narrowing of the inside diameter of the blood vessel. Eventually, the artery becomes so narrow that a blood clot (thrombus) forms, and blocks blood flow to an entire portion of the body. This condition is called PVD, or peripheral arterial disease. In another form of atherosclerosis, a rough area or ulcer forms in the diseased interior of the artery. Blood clots then tend to develop on this ulcer, break off, and travel further along, forming a blockage where the arteries get narrower. A blockage resulting from a clot formed elsewhere in the body is called an embolism.

People who have few areas affected by PVD may be treated with angioplasty by opening up the blood vessel with a balloon placed on the end of a catheter. A stent is often used with angioplasty to help keep the artery open. The type of surgery used to treat PVD is based upon the size and location of the damaged artery. The surgery techniques used for severe PVD include:

• Bypass surgery is preferred for people who have many areas of blockage or a long, continuous blockage.

• Aortobifemoral bypass is used for PVD affecting the major abdominal artery (aorta) and the large arteries that branch off of it.

• In a technique called thromboendarterectomy, the inner diseased layers of the artery are removed, leaving the relatively normal outer coats of the artery.

• Resection involves a technique to remove a diseased artery following an aneurysm; a bypass is created with a synthetic graft.

• In a bypass graft, a vein graft from another part of the body or a graft made from artificial material is used to create a detour around a blocked artery.

• Tibioperoneal bypass is used for PVD affecting the arteries in the lower leg or foot.

• Femoral-femoral bypass is a procedure to bypass occlusive disease in the unilateral common or external iliac artery.

• Femoropopliteal (fem-pop) bypass surgery is used for PVD affecting the arteries above and below the knee.

• Embolectomy is a technique in which an embolic clot on the wall of the artery is removed, using an inflatable balloon catheter.

• Thrombectomy is a technique in which a balloon catheter is inserted into the affected artery beyond a blood clot. The balloon is then inflated and pulled back, bringing the clot with it.

An aneurysm occurs when weakened blood vessels bulge like balloons as blood flows through them. Once they have grown to a certain size, there is a risk of rupture and life-threatening bleeding. There are two types of aortic aneurysms: abdominal aortic aneurysm (AAA) and thoracic aortic aneurysm. This classification is based on where the aneurysm occurs along the aorta. Aneurysms are more common in the abdominal section of the aorta than the thoracic section.

Most blood clots originate in the legs, but they can also form in the veins of arms, the right side of the heart, or even at the tip of a catheter placed in a vein. Venous disease conditions that usually occur in the veins of the legs include:

• varicose veins
• phlebitis
• venous stasis disease
• deep vein thrombosis (DVT)
• claudication
• blood clots

Carotid artery disease is a condition in which the arteries in the neck that supply blood to the brain become clogged; this condition can cause a stroke.

Lymphatic obstruction involves blockage of the lymph vessels, which drain fluid from tissues throughout the body and allow immune cells to travel where they are needed. Some of the causes of lymphatic obstruction (also known as swelling of the lymph passages), include infections such as chronic cellulitis, or parasitic infections such as filariasis, trauma, tumors, certain surgeries including **mastectomy**, and radiation therapy. There are rare forms of congenital lymphedema that probably result from abnormalities in the development of the lymphatic vessels. Most patients with lymphedema will not need surgery, as the symptoms are usually managed by other techniques. Surgical therapy for lymphedema includes removal of tissue containing abnormal lymphatics, and less commonly, transplant of tissue from areas with normal lymphatic tissues to areas with abnormal lymphatic drainage. In rare cases, bypass of abnormal lymphatic tissue is attempted, sometimes using vein grafts.

Other examples of vascular surgery include:

- cerebral aneurysm
- acute arterial and graft occlusion
- carotid endarterectomy
- endovascular grafting
- vasculogenic erectile dysfunction
- renal artery aneurysm
- surgery on varicose veins
- lower extremity amputation

Diagnosis

In order for a patient to be diagnosed with a vascular disease, he or she must be clinically evaluated by a vascular surgeon, which includes a history and **physical examination**. A vascular surgeon also treats vascular disorders by non-operative means, including drug therapy and risk factor management.

The symptoms produced by atherosclerosis, thrombosis, embolisms, or aneurysms depend on the particular artery affected. These conditions can sometimes cause pain, but often there are no symptoms at all.

A physician has many ways of feeling, hearing, measuring, and even seeing arterial blockages. Many arteries in the body can be felt or palpated. A doctor can feel for a pulse in an area he or she believes is afflicted. Usually, the more advanced the arteriosclerosis, the less pulse in a given area.

As the artery becomes blocked, it can cause a noise very much like water roaring over rocky rapids. The physician can listen to this noise (bruit) directly, or can use special amplification systems to hear the noise.

There are other tests that can be done to determine if arterial blood flow is normal, including:

- ankle-brachial index (ABI) test
- arteriogram
- segmental pressure test
- ultrasound scan
- magnetic resonance imaging (MRI)
- computed tomography (CT) scan
- angiography
- lymphangiography
- lymphoscintigraphy
- plethysmography
- duplex ultrasound scanning

There may be no symptoms of vascular disease caused by blood clots until the clot grows large enough to block the flow of blood through the vein. Symptoms that may come on suddenly include:

- pain
- sudden swelling in the affected limb
- reddish blue discoloration
- enlargement of the superficial veins
- skin that is warm to the touch

The physician will probably do an evaluation of all organ systems, including the heart, lungs, circulatory system, kidneys, and the gastrointestinal system. The decision whether to have surgery or not is based on the outcome of these evaluations.

Preparation

For high-risk patients undergoing vascular surgery, research has shown that taking oral beta-blockers one to two weeks before surgery and continuing for at least two weeks after the operation can significantly reduce the chance of dying or having a heart attack. Scientists suspect that the drug improves oxygen balance in the wall of the heart and stabilizes plaques in the arteries.

Aftercare

The length of time in intensive care and hospitalization will vary with each surgery, as will the recovery time, depending on numerous factors. Because surgery for an AAA is more serious, the patient can expect to be in intensive care for 24 hours, and in the hospital for five to 10 days, providing the patient was healthy and had a smooth operative and postoperative course. The hospital stay will likely increase if there are complications. It may take as long as six months to fully recover from surgery for an AAA.

Living a heart-healthy lifestyle is the best way of preventing and controlling vascular disease: quit smoking; eat nutritious foods low in fat; **exercise**; maintain a healthy weight; and control risk factors such as high blood pressure, high cholesterol, diabetes, hypertension, and other factors that contribute to vascular disease.

Medications that may be used to treat PVD include:

- aspirin and other antiplatelet medications to treat leg pain
- statins to lower cholesterol levels
- medications to control high blood pressure
- medications to control diabetes

• anticoagulants (these are rarely, but not generally, used to treat PVD unless the person is at an increased risk for forming blood clots)

Risks

All surgeries carry some risks. There is a risk of infection whenever incisions are required. Operations in the chest or those that involve major blood vessels carry a higher risk of complications. Patients that have high blood pressure, chronic lung or kidney disease, or other illnesses are at greater risk of complications during and after surgery. Other risks of vascular surgery include:

• bleeding

• failed or blocked grafts

• heart attack or stroke

• smoking

• leg swelling if a leg vein is used

• people over 65 years are at greater risk for brain impairment after major surgery

• the more damaged the circulatory system is before surgery, the higher susceptibility to mental decline after vascular surgery

• impotence

The patient should discuss risks with the surgeon after careful review of the patient's medical history and a physical examination.

Results

The success rate for vascular surgery varies depending on a number of factors that may influence the decision on whether to have surgery or not, as well as the results.

The chance that an aneurysm will rupture generally increases with the size of the aneurysm; AAAs smaller than 1.6 in. (4 cm) in diameter have up to a 2% risk of rupture, while ones larger than 2 in. (5 cm) in diameter have a 22% risk of rupture within two years.

Arterial bypass surgery and peripheral bypass surgery have very good success rates. Most of those who undergo AAA surgery recover well, except in the case of a rupture. Most patients who have a ruptured aortic aneurysm die due to excessive, rapid blood loss.

Surgical therapy for lymphedema has met with limited success, and requires significant experience and technical expertise.

Morbidity and mortality rates

Peripheral vascular disease affects 10 million people in the United States, including 5% of those over 50. Only

QUESTIONS TO ASK YOUR DOCTOR

• Can my vascular disease be controlled with lifestyle changes?

• If a procedure is required, am I a candidate for a less invasive, interventional radiology treatment?

• What are the risks and benefits of this operation?

• What are the normal results of this operation?

• What happens if this operation does not go as planned?

• What is the expected recovery time?

• How much discomfort can I expect in the short term? Over the long term?

• How many times have you performed this procedure?

• What tests or evaluation techniques will you perform to see if the procedure has been beneficial for me?

• What changes in my health can I expect to see after my procedure?

• Will I have any residual physical limitations after my procedure?

• What kind of changes can I expect to see with the medications you have prescribed for me?

• If I am to take some of these drugs long term, will I need regular blood tests or other tests to check for their effectiveness?

• What are the side effects associated with the medications you have prescribed for me?

• What symptoms or adverse effects are important enough that I should seek immediate treatment?

• Can you recommend an organization that will provide me with additional information about my condition?

a quarter of PVD sufferers are receiving treatment. More than two million people in the United States develop DVT each year. More than 650,000 Americans experience a pulmonary embolism every year. Of those, approximately 200,000 people die from the condition.

Alternatives

There a few alternatives to treating vascular disease, although extensive research has not been done. Acupuncture is used to aid in hypertension and chelation therapy is thought to stabilize the effects of vascular disease. The focus should be on maintaining a proper diet and being aware of a family history of vascular disease so as to catch it as early as possible.

Health care team roles

A vascular surgeon performs the procedure in a hospital **operating room**. Applicants for residency training in vascular surgery must have successfully completed a **general surgery** residency and be eligible for the board examination in general surgery. An individual must meet the standards set by the Vascular Surgery Board of the American Board of Surgery for cognitive knowledge and hypothetical case management. At the completion of a vascular surgery residency, both a written and oral examination must be completed before certification. A vascular surgeon is required to undergo periodic written reexamination.

Resources

BOOKS

Ascher, Enrico, ed. *Haimovici's Vascular Surgery.* 6th ed. New York: Wiley-Blackwell, 2012.

Berger, Zackary. *Talking to Your Doctor: A Patient's Guide to Communication in the Exam Room and Beyond.* Lanham, MD: Rowman & Littlefield Publishers, 2013.

Justesen, Sammie L. *The Smart Patient's Guide to Surgery.* Martinsville IN: NorLightsPress, 2009.

Mohler, Emile R. III, and Alan T. Hirsch. *100 Questions & Answers About Peripheral Artery Disease.* Sudbury, MA: Jones and Bartlett Publishers, 2010.

Schroeder, Juerrgen. *Peripheral Vascular Interventions: An Illustrated Manual.* New York: Thieme, 2013.

PERIODICALS

Sirignano, P., et al. "What is the Present Situation of Vascular Surgery? Considerations and Reflections Based on Real Practice." *Journal of Cardiovascular Surgery* 54, no. 5 (2013): 633–37. http://dx.doi.org/10.1136/jech-2013-203098.19 (accessed September 26, 2013).

van der Slegt, Jasper, et al. "Implementation of a Bundle of Care to Reduce Surgical Site Infections in Patients Undergoing Vascular Surgery." *PLoS ONE* 8, no. 8 (August 13, 2013). http://dx.doi.org/10.1371/journal.pone.0071566 (accessed September 26, 2013).

Vanniyasingam, Thuvaraha. "Predicting the Occurrence of Major Adverse Cardiac Events within 30 Days after a Patient's Vascular Surgery: An Individual Patient-Data Meta-Analysis." *Journal of Epidemiology & Community Health* 67, no. 10 (2013): e2. http://dx.doi.org/10.1136/jech-2013-203098.19 (accessed September 26, 2013).

WEBSITES

American Board of Surgery. "Specialty of Vascular Surgery Defined." http://www.absurgery.org/default.jsp?about vascularsurgerydefined (accessed September 26, 2013).

MedlinePlus. "Vascular Diseases." U.S. National Library of Medicine, National Institutes of Health. http://www.nlm.nih.gov/medlineplus/vasculardiseases.html (accessed September 26, 2013).

Society for Vascular Surgery. VascularWeb. http://www.vascularweb.org/Pages/default.aspx (accessed September 26, 2013).

ORGANIZATIONS

American Heart Association, 7272 Greenville Ave., Dallas, TX 75231, (800) AHA-USA-1 (242-8721), http://www.heart.org.

National Heart, Lung, and Blood Institute Information Center, PO Box 30105, Bethesda, MD 20824-0105, (301) 592-8573, Fax: (240) 629-3246, nhlbiinfo@nhlbi.nih.gov, http://www.nhlbi.nih.gov.

Society for Clinical Vascular Surgery (SCVS), 500 Cummings Ctr., Ste. 4550, Beverly, MA 01915, (978) 927-8330, Fax: (978) 524-8890, http://scvs.org.

Society for Vascular Surgery, 633 N. Saint Clair St., 22nd Fl., Chicago, IL 60611, (312) 334-2300, (800) 258-7188, vascular@vascularsociety.org, http://www.vascularweb.org.

Texas Heart Institute, 6770 Bertner Ave., Houston, TX 77030, (832) 355-4011, (800) 292-2221, hic@heart.thi.tmc.edu, http://www.texasheartinstitute.org.

World Heart Federation, 7, rue des Battoirs, 1211 Geneva, Switzerland, +41 22 807 03 20, info@worldheart.org, http://www.world-heart-federation.org.

Crystal H. Kaczkowski, MSc
Laura Jean Cataldo, RN, EdD

Vasectomy

Definition

A vasectomy is a surgical procedure performed on adult males in which the vasa deferentia (tubes that carry sperm from the testicles to the seminal vesicles) are cut, tied, cauterized (burned or seared), or otherwise interrupted. The semen no longer contains sperm after the tubes are cut, so conception cannot occur. The testicles continue to produce sperm, but the sperm die and are absorbed by the body.

Purpose

The purpose of the vasectomy is to provide reliable contraception. Research indicates that the level of effectiveness is 99.6%. Vasectomy is the most reliable method of contraception and has fewer complications and a faster recovery time than female sterilization

Vasectomy

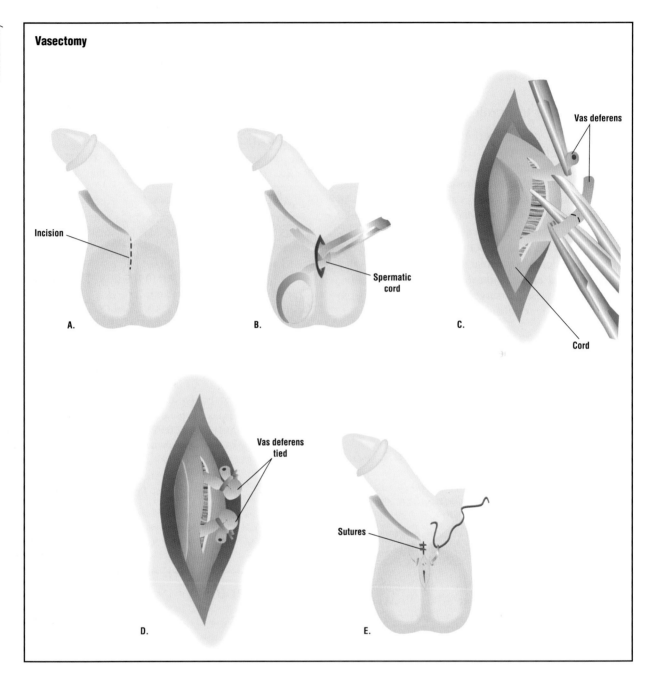

In a vasectomy, an incision is made in the man's scrotum (A). The spermatic cord is pulled out (B) and incised to expose the vas deferens, which is then severed (C). The ends may be cauterized or tied off (D). After the procedure is repeated on the opposite cord, the scrotal incision is closed (E). *(Illustration by GGS Information Services. Copyright © Cengage Learning®.)*

methods. Some insurance plans will cover the cost of the procedure.

Demographics

Approximately 500,000 vasectomies are performed annually in the United States. About one out of every six men over the age of 35 has had a vasectomy. Higher vasectomy rates are associated with higher levels of education and income.

Description

Vasectomies are usually performed in the doctor's office or an outpatient clinic using **local anesthesia**. The area around the patient's scrotum (the sac containing the

KEY TERMS

Ejaculation—The act of expelling the sperm through the penis during orgasm. The fluid that is released is called the ejaculate.

Epididymitis—Inflammation of the small tube that rests on top of the testicle and is part of the system that carries sperm from the testicle to the penis. The condition can be successfully treated with antibiotics, if necessary.

Scrotum—The sac that contains the testicles.

Sperm granuloma—A collection of fluid that leaks from an improperly sealed or tied vas deferens. The fluid usually disappears on its own, but can be drained, if necessary.

Testicles—The two egg-shaped organs found in the scrotum that produce sperm.

Tubal ligation—A female sterilization surgical procedure in which the fallopian tubes are tied in two places and cut between. This prevents eggs from moving from the ovary to the uterus.

Vas deferens (plural, vasa deferentia)—The Latin name for the duct that carries sperm from the testicle to the epididymis. In a vasectomy, a portion of each vas deferens is removed to prevent the sperm from entering the seminal fluid.

Vasovasostomy—A surgical procedure that is done to reverse a vasectomy by reconnecting the ends of the severed vasa deferentia.

testicles that produce sperm) is shaved and cleaned with an antiseptic solution to reduce the chance of infection. A small incision is made in the scrotum. Each vas deferens (one from each testicle) is tied in two places with nonabsorbable (permanent) sutures and the tube is severed between the ties. The ends may be cauterized (burned or seared) to decrease the chance that they will leak or grow back together.

"No-scalpel" vasectomies are gaining in popularity. Instead of an incision, a small puncture is made into the scrotum. The vasa deferentia are cut and sealed in a manner similar to that described above. No stitches are necessary and the patient has less pain. Other advantages include less damage to the tissues, less bleeding, less risk of infection, and less discomfort after the procedure. The no-scalpel method was developed in China in the mid-1970s and has been used in the United States since 1988. About one-third of vasectomies in the United States are performed with this technique.

The patient is not sterile immediately following the procedure. Men must use other methods of contraception until two consecutive semen analyses confirm that there are no sperm present in the ejaculate. It takes about four to six weeks, or 15–20 ejaculations, to clear all of the sperm from the tubes.

In some cases, vasectomies may be reversed by a procedure known as a **vasovasostomy**. In this procedure, the surgeon reconnects the ends of the severed vasa deferentia. A vasectomy should be considered permanent, however, as there is no guarantee of successful reversal. Vasovasostomies are successful in approximately 40%–50% of men, although the success rate varies considerably with the individual surgeon. In the mid 2000s between 6% and 12% of American men were requesting reversals of their vasectomies. The cost of the procedure in the United States can be considerable, ranging from $5,000–20,000.

Preparation

No special physical preparation is required for a vasectomy. The physician will first assess the patient's general health in order to identify any potential problems that could occur. The doctor will then explain the possible risks and side effects of the procedure. The patient is asked to sign a consent form that indicates that he understands the information he has received, and gives the doctor permission to perform the operation.

Aftercare

Following the surgery, ice packs are often applied to the scrotum to decrease pain and swelling. A dressing (or athletic supporter) that supports the scrotum can also reduce pain. Mild over-the-counter (OTC) pain medication such as **aspirin** or **acetaminophen** (Tylenol) should be able to control any discomfort. Activities may be restricted for one or two days, and no sexual intercourse for three or four days.

Risks

There are very few risks associated with vasectomy other than infection, bruising, epididymitis (inflammation of the tube that carries the sperm from the testicle to the penis), and sperm granulomas (collections of fluid that leaks from a poorly sealed or tied vas deferens). These complications are easily treated if they do occur. Patients do not experience difficulty achieving an erection, maintaining an erection, or ejaculating. There is no decrease in the production of the male hormone (testosterone), and the patient's sex drive and sexual performance are not altered. Vasectomy is safer and less expensive than **tubal ligation** (sterilization of a female by cutting the fallopian tubes to prevent conception).

According to both the World Health Organization (WHO) and the National Institutes of Health (NIH), there is no evidence that a vasectomy will increase a man's long-term risk of testicular cancer, prostate cancer, or heart disease.

Results

Vasectomies are more than 99% successful in preventing conception. As such, male sterilization is one of the most effective methods of contraception available.

Morbidity and mortality rates

Complications occur in approximately 5% of vasectomies. The rates of incidence of some of the more common complications include:

• mild bleeding into the scrotum: 1 in 400

• major bleeding into the scrotum: 1 in 1,000

• infection: 1 in 100

• epididymitis: 1 in 100

• sperm granuloma: 1 in 500

• persistent pain: 1 in 1,000

Fournier gangrene is a very rare but possible complication of vasectomy in which the lining of tissue underneath the skin of the scrotum becomes infected (a condition called fasciitis). Fournier gangrene progresses very rapidly and is treated with aggressive antibiotic therapy and surgery to remove necrotic (dead) tissue. Despite treatment, a mortality rate of 45% has been reported for this condition.

Alternatives

There are numerous options available to couples who are interested in preventing pregnancy. The most common methods are female sterilization, oral contraceptives, and the male condom. Female sterilization has a success rate of 99.5%; oral contraceptives, 95–99.5%; and the male condom, 86%–97%.

Health care team roles

Vasectomy is a minor procedure that can be performed in a clinic or doctor's office on an outpatient basis. The procedure is generally performed by a urologist, who is a medical doctor that has completed specialized training in the diagnosis and treatment of diseases of the urinary tract and genital organs.

QUESTIONS TO ASK YOUR DOCTOR

• How often do you perform vasectomies?
• What is your rate of complications?
• How long will the procedure take?
• What will the procedure cost?
• Will my insurance cover the cost?
• Do you perform vasectomy reversal? If so, what is your success rate?

Resources

PERIODICALS

"Male Factor Infertility: Vasectomy Guidelines Help Avoid Unnecessary Procedures." *Nature Reviews Urology* 10, no. 10 (2013): 556. http://dx.doi.org/10.1038/nrurol.2013.191 (accessed October 14, 2013).

WEBSITES

American Academy of Family Physicians. "Vasectomy: What to Expect." http://familydoctor.org/familydoctor/en/prevention-wellness/sex-birth-control/birth-control/vasectomy-what-to-expect.html (accessed October 14, 2013).

MedlinePlus. "Vasectomy." U.S. National Library of Medicine, National Institutes of Health. http://www.nlm.nih.gov/medlineplus/surgery.html (accessed October 14, 2013).

Planned Parenthood Federation of America. "Vasectomy." http://www.nlm.nih.gov/medlineplus/vasectomy.html (accessed October 14, 2013).

Urology Care Foundation. "Vasectomy." http://www.urologyhealth.org/urology/index.cfm?article=53 (accessed October 14, 2013).

ORGANIZATIONS

Guttmacher Institute, 1301 Connecticut Ave. NW, Ste. 700, Washington, DC 20036, (202) 296-4012, (877) 823-0262, Fax: (202) 223-5756, http://www.guttmacher.org.

Planned Parenthood Federation of America, 434 W. 33rd St., New York, NY 10001, (212) 541-7800, (800) 230-PLAN (7526), Fax: (212) 245-1845, http://www.plannedparenthood.org.

Donald G. Barstow, RN
Stephanie Dionne Sherk
Tish Davidson, AM

Vasectomy reversal *see* **Vasovasostomy**

Vasovasostomy

Definition

A vasovasostomy is a surgical procedure in which the effects of a **vasectomy** (male sterilization) are reversed. During a vasectomy, the vasa deferentia, which are ducts that carry sperm from the testicles to the seminal vesicles, are cut, tied, cauterized (burned or seared), or otherwise interrupted. A vasovasostomy creates an opening between the separated ends of each vas deferens so that the sperm may enter the semen before ejaculation.

Purpose

The purpose of a vasovasostomy is to restore a man's fertility, whereas a vasectomy, or male sterilization, is performed to provide reliable contraception (birth control). Research indicates that the level of effectiveness of vasectomies in preventing pregnancy is 99.6%. Vasectomy is the most reliable method of contraception for men and has less risk of complications and a faster recovery time than female sterilization methods.

In many cases, a vasectomy can be reversed. Vasectomy reversal does not, however, guarantee a successful pregnancy. The longer the time elapsed since a man has had a vasectomy, the more difficult the reversal and the lower the success rate. The rate of sperm return if a vasovasostomy is performed within three years of a vasectomy is 97%; this number decreases to 88% by 3–8 years after vasectomy, 79% at 9–14 years, and 71% after 15 years. In addition, other factors affect the success rate of vasectomy reversal, including the age of the female partner, her fertility potential, the method of reversal used, and the experience of the surgeon performing the procedure.

Vasovasostomies are also performed in men who are sterile because of genital tract obstructions rather than prior vasectomies. A vasovasostomy may be performed on occasion to relieve pain associated with post-vasectomy pain syndrome.

Demographics

An estimated 5% of men who have had a vasectomy later decide that they would like to have children. Some

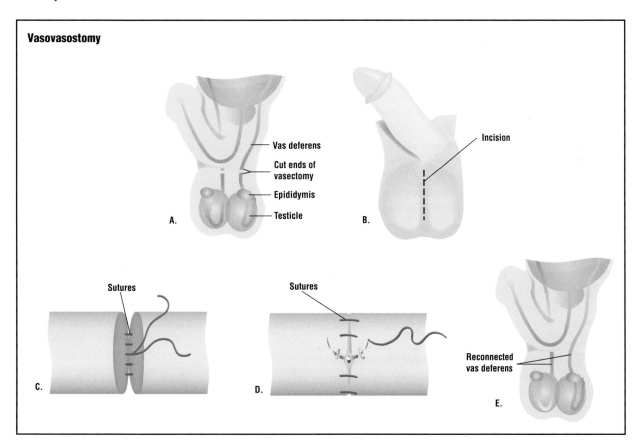

Vasovasostomy

Vas deferens
Cut ends of vasectomy
Epididymis
Testicle
A.

Incision
B.

Sutures
C.

Sutures
D.

Reconnected vas deferens
E.

In a vasovasostomy, or reverse vasectomy, the surgeon makes an incision in the scrotum at the site of the vasectomy scar (B). The spermatic cords are located, and the two vas deferens are reconnected with two layers of suture (C and D). *(Illustration by GGS Information Services. Copyright © Cengage Learning®.)*

reasons for wanting a vasectomy reversal include death of a child, death of a spouse, divorce, or experiencing a change in circumstances so that having more children is possible. One study found that divorce was the most commonly reported reason for a vasovasostomy and that the average age of men requesting a vasovasostomy was approximately 40 years.

About 7.4% of infertile men have primary genital tract obstructions caused by trauma, gonorrhea or other venereal infections, or congenital malformations of the vasa deferentia. Many of these men are good candidates for surgical treatment of their infertility.

Description

Most **surgeons** prefer to have the patient given either a continuous anesthetic block or **general anesthesia** because of the length of time required for the operation. A vasovasostomy generally takes two to three hours to perform, depending on the complexity of the surgery and the experience of the operating physician. More complex surgeries may take as long as five hours. The advantage of general anesthesia is that the patient remains unconscious for the duration of the surgery, which ensures that he remains comfortable. Regional anesthesia, such as a spinal block, allows the patient to remain awake during the procedure while blocking pain in the area of the surgery.

After an adequate level of anesthesia has been reached, the surgeon will make an incision from the top of one side of the scrotum, sometimes moving upward as far as several inches into the abdominal area. A similar incision will then be made on the other side of the scrotum. The vasa deferentia will be identified and isolated from surrounding tissue. Fluid will be removed from the testicular end of each vas deferens and analyzed for presence of sperm. If sperm are found, then a simpler procedure to connect the cut ends of the vasa deferentia will be performed. If no sperm are found, a more complex procedure called a vasoepididymostomy or epididymovasostomy (in which the vas deferens is attached to the epididymis, a structure in which the sperm mature and are stored) may be more successful in restoring sperm flow.

There are two techniques that may be used to reconnect the cut ends of the vasa deferentia. A single-layer closure involves stitching the outer layer of each cut end of the tube together with a very fine suture thread. This procedure takes less time but is often less successful in restoring sperm flow. A double-layer closure, however, involves stitching the inner layer of each cut end of the tube first, and then stitching the outer layer. After reconnection is established, the vasa deferentia are

KEY TERMS

Congenital—Present at birth.

Epididymis—A coiled cord-like structure at the upper border of the testis, in which sperm mature and are stored.

Hematoma—A localized collection of blood in an organ or tissue due to broken blood vessels.

In vitro fertilization (IVF)—A process in which sperm are incubated with a female egg under carefully controlled conditions, then transferred to the female uterus once fertilization has occurred.

Intracytoplasmic sperm injection (ICSI)—A process in which a single sperm is injected into a female egg.

Scrotum—The sac that contains the testicles.

Vas deferens (plural, vasa deferentia)—The Latin name for the duct that carries sperm from the testicle to the epididymis. In a vasectomy, a portion of each vas deferens is removed to prevent the sperm from entering the seminal fluid.

Vasoepididymostomy—A type of vasectomy reversal in which the vas deferens is attached to the epididymis, the structure where sperm matures and is stored.

returned to their anatomical place and the scrotal incisions closed.

Preparation

Before a vasovasostomy is performed, the patient will undergo a preoperative assessment, including a **physical examination** of the scrotum. This evaluation will allow the surgeon to determine what sort of vasectomy reversal should be performed and how extensive the surgery might be. A medical history will be taken. The physician will review the patient's medical records in order to determine how the patient's vasectomy was performed; if large portions of the vasa deferentia were removed during surgery, the vasectomy reversal will be more complicated and may have a lower chance of success. The patient's partner should also undergo a fertility assessment, including a gynecologic exam, to assess her reproductive health.

Some surgeons prefer to give the patient a broad-spectrum antibiotic about half an hour before surgery as well as a mild sedative.

Aftercare

After the procedure the patient will be transferred to a recovery room where he will remain for approximately three hours. The patient will be asked to void urine before discharge. Pain medication is prescribed and usually required for one to three days after the procedure. **Antibiotics** may be given after the procedure as well as beforehand to prevent infection. Ice packs applied to the scrotum will help to decrease swelling and discomfort. Heavy lifting, **exercise**, and sexual activity should be avoided for up to four weeks while the vasovasostomy heals.

Patients are usually allowed to return to work within three days. They may shower within two days after surgery, but should avoid soaking the incision (by taking a tub bath or going swimming) for about two weeks. The surgeon will schedule the patient for an incision check about a week after surgery and a semen analysis three months later.

Risks

The complications that most commonly occur after vasovasostomy include swelling, bruising, and symptoms associated with anesthesia (nausea, headache, etc.). There is a risk of low sperm count if the operation is done inadequately or if scarring partially blocks the channel inside the vasa deferentia. Less common complications are infection or severe hematoma (collection of blood under the skin). The most serious potential complication of a vasovasostomy is testicular atrophy (wasting away), which may result from damage to the spermatic artery during the procedure.

Results

If a successful vasectomy reversal has been performed, the average time to achieving pregnancy after the procedure is one year, with most pregnancies occurring within the first two years. A good sperm count usually returns within three to six months.

Morbidity and mortality rates

The chance that the vasa deferentia will become obstructed after a successful reversal is approximately 10%. Some doctors recommend that patients bank their sperm as a precautionary measure. Scrotal hematoma occurs in 1%–2% of patients after vasovasostomy, and infection in less than 1%.

Alternatives

A vasoepididymostomy may be performed if the physician determines that a vasovasostomy will be

---

QUESTIONS TO ASK YOUR DOCTOR

- How often do you perform vasectomy reversals?
- What is your success rate?
- What are the possible complications?
- What are my chances of success?
- What technique do you recommend for reestablishing sperm flow?
- How long will the procedure take?
- How much will my vasectomy reversal cost? Will my insurance cover the cost?

---

insufficient in restoring sperm flow. The determining factor is usually the absence of sperm or fluid in the testicular end of the cut vas deferens (which is found during surgery), although a swollen or blocked epididymis found during a preoperative scrotal examination may also indicate a vasoepididymostomy will be necessary.

There are some options available to men and their partners who are seeking to conceive after a vasectomy but wish to avoid vasectomy reversal. As sperm are no longer present in the man's ejaculate, they may be retrieved from the testicle or epididymis by extraction (removal of tissue) or aspiration (removed by a needle). The sperm may then be incubated with a female egg under carefully controlled conditions, then transferred to the female uterus once fertilization has occurred; this process is called **in vitro fertilization** (IVF). A process called intracytoplasmic sperm injection (ICSI) may be used to improve the success rate of IVF; in this procedure, a single sperm is injected into the female egg.

Health care team roles

A vasovasostomy can be performed in a hospital, clinic, or doctor's office on an outpatient basis. The procedure is generally performed by a urologist, a medical doctor who has completed specialized training in the diagnosis and treatment of diseases of the urinary tract and genital organs.

Resources

PERIODICALS

Schwarzer, J. Ullrich, and Heiko Steinfatt. "Current Status of Vasectomy Reversal." *Nature Reviews Urology* 10, no. 4 (2013): 195–205. http://dx.doi.org/10.1038/nrurol.2013.14 (accessed October 14, 2013).

WEBSITES

Mayo Clinic staff. "Vasectomy Reversal: Surgery to Undo a Vasectomy." http://www.mayoclinic.com/health/vasectomy-reversal/MY00326 (accessed October 14, 2013).

Ohio State University Wexner Medical Center. "Vasectomy Reversal (Vasovasostomy)." http://urology.osu.edu/19777.cfm (accessed October 14, 2013).

University of Wisconsin School of School of Medicine and Public Health. "Vasectomy Reversal (Vasovasostomy)." http://www.uwhealth.org/health/topic/surgicaldetail/vasectomy-reversal-vasovasostomy/hw227277.html (accessed October 14, 2013).

ORGANIZATIONS

American Board of Urology, 600 Peter Jefferson Pkwy., Ste. 150, Charlottesville, VA 22911, (434) 979-0059, Fax: (434) 979-0266, http://www.abu.org.

Stephanie Dionne Sherk

Vein ligation and stripping

Definition

Vein ligation and stripping is a surgical approach to the treatment of varicose veins. It is also sometimes called phlebectomy. Ligation refers to the surgical tying-off of a large vein in the leg called the greater saphenous vein, while stripping refers to the removal of this vein through incisions in the groin area or behind the knee. If some of the valves in the saphenous vein are healthy, the weak portion of the vein can be closed off by ligation. If the entire vein is weak, it is closed off and pulled downward and out through an incision made below it. Tying and removal of the greater saphenous vein are done to reduce the pressure of blood flowing backward through this large vein into the smaller veins that feed into it.

Phlebectomy is one of the oldest forms of treatment for varicose veins; the earliest description of it was written by Aulus Cornelius Celsus, a Roman historian of medicine, in 45 A.D. The first description of a phlebectomy hook comes from a textbook on surgery published in 1545. The modern technique of ambulatory (outpatient) phlebectomy was developed around 1956 by a Swiss dermatologist named Robert Muller. Surgical ligation and stripping of the saphenous vein are performed increasingly less frequently because of the introduction of less invasive forms of treatment.

Purpose

The purpose of vein ligation and stripping is to reduce the number and size of varicose veins that cannot be treated or closed by other measures. The reasons for **vascular surgery** in general include:

• improvement of the appearance of the legs

• relief from any pain, leg cramps, or fatigue that may be associated with varicose veins

• treatment of skin problems that may develop as complications of varicose veins, such as chronic eczema, skin ulceration, external bleeding, or abnormal pigmentation of the skin

• prevention of such disorders as thrombophlebitis and pulmonary blood clots

Demographics

The World Health Organization (WHO) estimates that about 25% of adults around the world have some type of venous disorder in the legs. The proportion of the general population with varicose veins is higher, however, in the developed countries. The American College of Phlebology (ACP), which is a group of dermatologists, plastic **surgeons**, gynecologists, and general surgeons with special training in the treatment of venous disorders, states that more than 80 million people in the United States suffer from varicose veins. In the past, the female-to-male ratio has been close to four to one, but this figure is changing due to the rapid rise in obesity among adult males in the past two decades.

Varicose veins are more common in middle-aged and elderly adults than in children or young adults. Although varicose veins tend to run in families, they do not appear to be associated with specific racial or ethnic groups.

Description

Causes of varicose veins

The venous part of the circulatory system returns blood to the heart to be pumped to the lungs for oxygenation, in contrast to the arterial system, which carries oxygenated blood away from the heart to be distributed throughout the body. Veins are more likely than arteries to expand or dilate if blood volume or pressure increases, because they consist of only one layer of tissue; this is in contrast to arteries, in which there are three layers.

There are three major categories of veins: superficial veins, deep veins, and perforating veins. All varicose veins are superficial veins; they lie between the skin and a layer of fibrous connective tissue called fascia, which

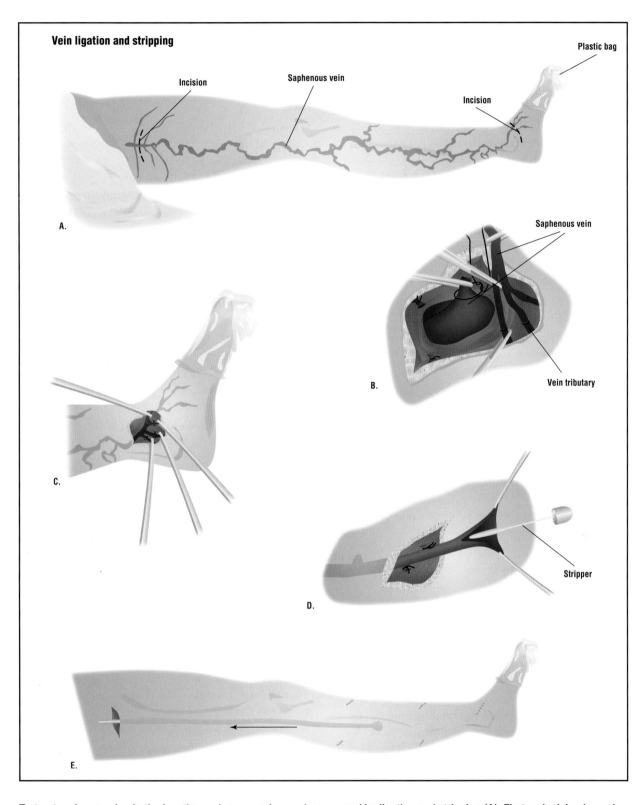

Vein ligation and stripping

To treat varicose veins in the leg, the saphenous vein may be removed by ligation and stripping (A). First an incision is made in the upper thigh, and the saphenous vein is separated from its tributaries (B). Another incision is made above the foot (C). The lower portion of the vein is cut, and a stripper is inserted into the vein (D). The stripper is pulled through the vein and out the incision in the upper thigh (E). *(Illustration by GGS Information Services. Copyright © Cengage Learning®.)*

KEY TERMS

Ablation—The destruction or removal of a body part. Saphenous ablation refers to several techniques for closing and destroying the greater saphenous vein without cutting or stripping.

Edema—The presence of abnormally large amounts of fluid in the soft tissues of the body.

Endovascular—Inside a blood vessel. Endovascular treatments of varicose veins are those that are performed inside the veins.

Incompetent—In a medical context, insufficient. An incompetent vein is one that is not performing its function of carrying blood back to the heart.

Ligation—The act of tying off a blood vessel.

Lumen—The channel or cavity inside a tube or hollow organ of the body.

Palpation—Examining by touch as part of the process of physical diagnosis.

Percussion—Thumping or tapping a part of the body with the fingers for diagnostic purposes.

Phlebectomy—Surgical removal of a vein or part of a vein.

Phlebology—The study of veins, their disorders, and their treatments. A phlebologist is a doctor who specializes in treating spider veins, varicose veins, and associated disorders.

Saphenous veins—Two large superficial veins in the leg that may be treated by ligation and stripping as therapy for varicose veins. The greater saphenous vein runs from the foot to the groin area, while the short saphenous vein runs from the ankle to the knee.

Sclerose—To harden or undergo hardening. Sclerosing agents are chemicals that are used in sclerotherapy to cause swollen veins to fill with fibrous tissue and close down.

Seroma—A collection of blood serum or lymphatic fluid in body tissues. It is an occasional complication of vascular surgery.

Telangiectasia—The medical term for the visible discolorations produced by permanently swollen capillaries and smaller veins.

Thrombophlebitis—The inflammation of a vein associated with the formation of blood clots.

Trendelenburg's test—A test that measures the speed at which the lower leg fills with blood after the leg has first been raised above the level of the heart. It is named for Friedrich Trendelenburg (1844–1924), a German surgeon.

Tumescent anesthesia—A type of local anesthesia originally developed for liposuction in which a large volume of diluted anesthetic is injected into the tissues around the vein until they become tumescent (firm and swollen).

Varicose—Abnormally enlarged and distended.

Varix (plural, varices)—The medical term for an enlarged blood vessel.

cover and support the muscles and the internal organs. The deep veins of the body lie within the muscle fascia. This distinction helps to explain why a superficial vein can be removed or closed without damage to the deep circulation in the legs. Perforating veins are veins that connect the superficial and deep veins.

Veins contain one-way valves that push blood inward and upward toward the heart against the force of gravity when they are functioning normally. The blood pressure in the superficial veins is usually low, but if it rises and remains at a higher level over a period of time, the valves in the veins begin to fail. The blood flows backward and collects in the lower veins, and the veins dilate, or expand. Veins that are not functioning properly are said to be incompetent. As the veins expand, they become more noticeable under the surface of the skin. Small veins, or capillaries, often appear as spider-shaped or tree-like networks of reddish or purplish lines under the skin. The medical term for these is telangiectasias, but they are commonly known as spider veins or thread veins. Larger veins that form flat, blue-green networks often found behind the knee are called reticular varicosities. True varicose veins are formed when the largest superficial veins become distorted and twisted by a long-term rise in blood pressure in the legs.

The most important veins in the lower leg are the two saphenous veins: the greater saphenous vein, which runs from the foot to the groin area, and the short saphenous vein, which runs from the ankle to the knee. It is thought that varicose veins develop when the valves at the top of the greater saphenous vein fail, allowing more blood to flow backward down the leg and increase the pressure on the valves in the smaller veins in turn. The practice of ligation and stripping of the greater saphenous vein is based on this hypothesis.

Some people are at increased risk for developing varicose veins. These risk factors include:

- Sex. Females in any age group are more likely than males to develop varicose veins. It is thought that female sex hormones contribute to the development of varicose veins by making the veins dilate more easily. Many women experience increased discomfort from varicose veins during their menstrual periods.
- Genetic factors. Some people have veins with abnormally weak walls or valves. They may develop varicose veins even without a rise in blood pressure in the superficial veins. This characteristic tends to run in families.
- Pregnancy. A woman's total blood volume increases during pregnancy, which increases the blood pressure in the venous system. In addition, the hormonal changes of pregnancy cause the walls and valves in the veins to soften.
- Using birth control pills.
- Obesity. Excess body weight increases the pressure on the veins.
- Occupational factors. People who have jobs that require standing or sitting for long periods of time—without the opportunity to walk or move around—are more likely to develop varicose veins.

Ambulatory phlebectomy

Ambulatory phlebectomy is the most common surgical procedure for treating medium-sized varicose veins. It is also known as stab avulsion or micro-extraction phlebectomy. An ambulatory phlebectomy is performed under **local anesthesia**. After the patient's leg has been anesthetized, the surgeon makes a series of very small vertical incisions 0.39–1.18 in. (1–3 mm) in length along the length of the affected vein. These incisions do not require stitches or tape closure afterward. Beginning with the more heavily involved areas of the leg, the surgeon inserts a phlebectomy hook through each micro-incision. The vein segment is drawn through the incision, held with a mosquito clamp, and pulled out through the incision. This technique requires the surgeon to be especially careful when removing varicose veins in the ankle, foot, or back of the knee. The procedure takes about 45–50 minutes.

After all the vein segments have been removed, the surgeon washes the patient's leg with hydrogen peroxide and covers the area with a foam wrap, several layers of cotton wrap, and an adhesive bandage. A compression stocking is then drawn up over the wrapping. The **bandages** are removed three to seven days after surgery, but the compression stocking must be worn for another two to four weeks to minimize bruising and swelling.

The patient is encouraged to walk around for 10 or so minutes before leaving the office; this mild activity helps to minimize the risk of a blood clot forming in the deep veins of the leg.

Transilluminated powered phlebectomy

Transilluminated powered phlebectomy (TIPP) is a newer technique that avoids the drawbacks of stab avulsion phlebectomy, which include long operating times, the risk of scar formation, and a relatively high risk of infection developing in the micro-incisions. Transilluminated powered phlebectomy is performed with an illuminator and a motorized resector. After the patient has been anesthetized with light **general anesthesia**, the surgeon makes only two small incisions: one for the illuminating device and the other for the resector. After making the first incision and introducing the illuminator, the surgeon uses a technique called tumescent anesthesia to plump up the tissues around the veins and make the veins easier to remove. Tumescent anesthesia was originally developed for **liposuction**. It involves the injection of large quantities of a dilute anesthetic into the tissues surrounding the veins until they become firm and swollen.

After the tumescent anesthesia has been completed, the surgeon makes a second incision to insert the resector, which draws the vein by suction toward an inner blade. The suction then removes the tiny pieces of venous tissue left by the blade. After all the clusters of varicose veins have been treated, the surgeon closes the two small incisions with a single stitch or Steri-Strips. The incisions are covered with a gauze dressing and the leg is wrapped in a sterile compression dressing.

Diagnosis

Vein ligation and stripping and ambulatory phlebectomies are considered elective cosmetic procedures; they are not performed on an emergency basis. For this reason, patients should check with their insurance provider to see whether these procedures are covered. Costs vary but generally run between $600 and $2,000 per leg for the surgeon's fee; anesthesia and hospitalization are extra.

The process of diagnosis may begin with the patient's complaints about the appearance of the legs or of pain and cramps, as well as with the physician's observations. It is important to note that there is no correlation between the size or number of a patient's varicose veins and the amount of pain that is experienced. Some people experience considerable discomfort from fairly small varices, while others may have no symptoms from clusters of extremely swollen varicose veins. If the patient mentions pain, burning sensations, or other physical symptoms, the doctor will need to rule out other possible causes, such as nerve root irritation, osteoarthritis, diabetic neuropathy, or problems in the arterial circulation. Relief of pain when the leg is elevated is the most significant diagnostic sign of varicose veins.

After taking the patient's medical history and a family history of venous disorders, the doctor examines the patient from the waist down to note the location of varicose veins and to palpate (touch with gentle pressure) for signs of other venous disorders. Palpation helps the doctor locate both normal and abnormal veins; further, some varicose veins can be detected by touch even though they cannot be seen through the skin. Ideally, the examiner will have a small raised platform for the patient to stand on during the **physical examination**. The doctor will ask the patient to turn slowly while standing, and will be looking for scars or other signs of trauma, bulges, and areas of discoloration in the skin, or other indications of chronic venous insufficiency. While palpating the legs, the doctor will note areas of unusual warmth or soreness, cysts, and edema (swelling of the soft tissues due to fluid retention). Next, the doctor will percuss (tap on) certain parts of the legs where the larger veins lie closer to the surface. By gently tapping or thumping on the skin over these areas, the doctor can feel if there are any fluid waves in the veins and determine whether further testing for venous insufficiency is required.

The next stage of the diagnostic examination is an evaluation of the valves in the patient's greater saphenous vein. The doctor places a tourniquet around the patient's upper thigh while the patient is lying on the examination table with the leg raised. The patient is then asked to stand on the floor. If the valves in this vein are working properly, the lower superficial veins should not fill up rapidly as long as the tourniquet remains tied. This test is known as Trendelenburg's test. It has, however, been largely replaced by the use of duplex Doppler **ultrasound**, which maps the location of the varicose veins in the patient's leg and provides information about the condition of the valves in the veins. Most insurance companies now also require a Doppler test before authorizing surgical treatment. The doctor's findings will determine whether the greater saphenous vein will require ligation and stripping or endovenous ablation before smaller varicose veins can be treated.

Some disorders or conditions are contraindications for vascular surgery, including:

• cellulitis and other infectious diseases of the skin

• severe edema associated with heart or kidney disease (these disorders should be brought under control before a phlebectomy is performed)

• uncontrolled diabetes

• disorders that affect the immune system, including HIV infection

• severe heart or lung disorders

Preparation

Patients preparing for vascular surgery are asked to discontinue **aspirin** or aspirin-related products for a week before the procedure. They should not eat or drink after midnight on the day of surgery. They should not apply any moisturizers, creams, tanning lotions, or sun block to the legs on the day of the procedure.

A patient scheduled for an ambulatory phlebectomy should arrive at the surgical center about an hour and a half before the procedure. All clothing must be removed before changing into a hospital gown. The patient is asked to walk up and down in the room or hallway for about 20 minutes to make the veins stand out. The surgeon marks the outlines of the veins with an indelible ink marker on the patient's legs while he or she is standing up. An ultrasound may be done at this point to verify the location and condition of the veins. The patient is then taken into the **operating room** for surgery.

Although patients are encouraged to walk around for a few minutes after an ambulatory phlebectomy, they should make arrangements for a friend or relative to drive them home from the surgical facility.

Aftercare

Surgical ligation and stripping of the greater saphenous vein usually requires an overnight stay in the hospital and two to eight weeks of **recovery at home** afterward.

Aftercare following surgical treatment of varicose veins includes wearing medical compression stockings that apply either 20–30 mm Hg or 30–40 mm Hg of pressure for two to six weeks after the procedure. Wearing compression stockings minimizes the risk of edema, discoloration, and pain. Fashion support stockings are a less acceptable alternative because they do not apply enough pressure to the legs.

The elastic surgical dressing applied at the end of an ambulatory phlebectomy should be left in place after returning home. Mild pain-killing medications may be taken for discomfort.

The patient is advised to watch for redness, swelling, pus, fever, and other signs of infection.

Patients are encouraged to walk, ride a bicycle, or participate in other low-impact forms of **exercise** (such as yoga and tai chi) to prevent the formation of blood clots in the deep veins of the legs. They should lie down with the legs elevated above heart level for 15 minutes at least twice a day, and use a foot stool when sitting to keep the legs raised.

Risks

Vein ligation and stripping carries the same risks as other surgical procedures under general anesthesia, such as bleeding, infection of the incision, and an adverse reaction to the anesthetic. Patients with leg ulcers or fungal infections of the foot are at increased risk of developing infections in the incisions following surgical treatment of varicose veins.

Specific risks associated with vascular surgery include:

- Deep venous thrombosis.

- Bruising. Bruising is the most common complication of phlebectomies, but heals itself in a few days or weeks.

- Scar formation. Phlebectomy has been found to produce permanent leg scars more frequently than sclerotherapy.

- Injury to the saphenous nerve. This complication results in numbness, tingling, or burning sensations in the area around the ankle. It usually goes away without further treatment within six to 12 months.

- Seromas. A seroma is a collection of uninfected blood serum or lymphatic fluid in the tissues. Seromas usually resolve without further treatment, but can be drained by the surgeon, if necessary.

- Injury to the arteries in the thigh and groin area. This complication is extremely rare, but it can have serious consequences. One example is amputation of the leg.

- Leg swelling. This complication is caused by disruption of the lymphatic system during surgery. This lasts about two to three weeks and can be managed by wearing compression stockings.

- Recurrence of smaller varicose veins.

Results

Normal results of vein ligation and stripping, or ambulatory phlebectomy, include reduction in the size and number of varicose veins in the leg. About 95% of patients also experience significant relief of pain.

Morbidity and mortality rates

The mortality rate following vein ligation and stripping has been reported to be one in 30,000. The incidence of deep venous thrombosis (DVT) following vascular surgery is estimated to be 0.6%.

Alternatives

Conservative treatments

Patients who are experiencing discomfort from varicose veins may be helped by any or several of the following approaches:

- Exercise. Walking or other forms of exercise that activate the muscles in the lower legs can relieve aching and cramping because these muscles keep the blood moving through the leg veins. One specific exercise that is often recommended is repeated flexing of the ankle joint. Flexing the ankles five to 10 times every few minutes and walking around for one to two minutes every half hour throughout the day helps to prevent the venous congestion that results from sitting or standing in one position for hours at a time.

- Avoiding high-heeled shoes. Shoes with high heels do not allow the ankle to flex fully when the patient is walking. This limitation of the range of motion of the ankle joint makes it more difficult for the leg muscles to contract and force venous blood upward toward the heart.

- Elevating the legs for 15–30 minutes once or twice a day. This change of position is frequently recommended for reducing edema of the feet and ankles.

- Wearing compression hosiery. Compression benefits the leg veins by reducing inflammation as well as improving venous outflow. Most manufacturers of medical compression stockings now sell some relatively sheer hosiery that looks attractive in addition to providing support.

- Medications. Drugs that have been used to treat the discomfort associated with varicose veins include nonsteroidal anti-inflammatory drugs (NSAIDs) and preparations of vitamins C and E. One prescription medication that is sometimes given to treat circulatory problems in the legs and feet is pentoxifylline, which improves blood flow in the smaller capillaries. Pentoxifylline is sold under the brand name Trendar.

If appearance is the patient's primary concern, varicose veins can be partially covered with specially formulated cosmetics that come in a wide variety of skin tones. Some of these preparations are available in waterproof formulations for use during swimming and other athletic activities.

Endovenous ablation

Endovenous ablation refers to two newer and less invasive methods for treating incompetent saphenous veins. In the Closure® method, which was approved by the U.S. Food and Drug Administration (FDA) in 1999, the surgeon passes a catheter into the lumen of the saphenous vein. The catheter is connected to a radio-frequency generator and delivers heat energy to the vein through an electrode in its tip. As the tissues in the wall of the vein are heated, they shrink and coagulate, which closes and seals the vein. The temperature inside the wall of the vein is limited to 185°F (85°C) to prevent heat damage to surrounding tissues. Radiofrequency ablation of the saphenous vein has been demonstrated to be safe and at least as effective as surgical stripping of the vein; in addition, patients can return to work the next day. About 95% of patients are satisfied with the procedure and would recommend it to others. The procedure produces good cosmetic results that last at least five years; the longer-term effectiveness of radiofrequency ablation, however, is not known. Its chief risk is loss of feeling in a patch of skin about the size of a quarter above the knee. This numbness usually resolves in about six months. One limitation of radiofrequency ablation is that present catheters cannot be used with extremely twisted or crooked veins. The most frequent complication reported with this procedure is deep vein thrombosis.

Endovenous laser treatment, or EVLT, uses a laser instead of a catheter with an electrode to heat the tissues in the wall of an incompetent vein in order to close the vein. Although EVLT appears to be as safe and effective as radiofrequency ablation, patients experience more discomfort and bruising afterward; most require two to three days of recovery at home after laser treatment. EVLT is reported to give as good results as surgery or laser ablation, with a low rate (less than 7%) of varicose vein recurrence after two years. As with radiofrequency ablation, EVLT cannot be used in extremely crooked veins. EVLT is not yet widely used; fewer than 10,000 cases worldwide had been reported as of 2007. The major side effect that has been described is skin burns.

Sclerotherapy

Sclerotherapy is a treatment method in which irritating chemicals in liquid or foam form are injected into spider veins or smaller reticular varicosities to close them off. The chemicals cause the vein to become inflamed, and lead to the formation of fibrous tissue and closing of the lumen, or central channel of the vein. Sclerotherapy is sometimes used in combination with other techniques to treat larger varicose veins.

Complementary and alternative (CAM) treatments

According to Dr. Kenneth Pelletier, former director of the program in complementary and alternative treatments at Stanford University School of Medicine, horse chestnut extract works as well as compression stockings when used as a conservative treatment for varicose veins. Horse chestnut (*Aesculus hippocastanum*)

QUESTIONS TO ASK YOUR DOCTOR

- Can my varicose veins be treated without ligation and stripping?
- Am I a candidate for treatment with EVLT or radiofrequency ablation?
- What specific technique(s) do you perform most frequently?
- Which treatment technique(s) do you recommend and why?
- What are the risks of these techniques?
- Are other patients satisfied with the results?

preparations have been used in Europe for some years to treat circulatory problems in the legs; most recent research has been carried out in Great Britain and Germany. The usual dosage is 75 mg twice a day, at meals. The most common side effect of oral preparations of horse chestnut is occasional indigestion in some patients.

Health care team roles

Surgical treatment of varicose veins is usually performed by general surgeons or by vascular surgeons, who are trained in the diagnosis and medical management of venous disorders as well as surgical treatment of them. Most vascular surgeons have completed five years of residency training in surgery after medical school, followed by one to two years of specialized fellowship training.

Phlebectomies and endovenous ablation treatments are performed in **ambulatory surgery centers** as outpatient procedures. Ligation and stripping of the greater saphenous vein, however, is more commonly performed in a hospital as an inpatient operation.

Resources

BOOKS

Bergan, John, and Nisha Bunke. *The Vein Book*. 2nd ed. Oxford, NY: Oxford University Press, 2014.

PERIODICALS

Jibiki, M., et al. "The Effect of Short Saphenous Vein Stripping in Patients with Deep Venous Reflux." *Annals of Vascular Diseases* 6, no. 3 (2013): 612–16.

WEBSITES

American College of Phlebology. "Treatment Options." http://www.phlebology.org/patientinfo/treatment.html (accessed October 17, 2013).

Healthwise. "Vein Ligation and Stripping." NorthShore University HealthSystem. http://www.uwhealth.org/healthfacts/B_EXTRANET_HEALTH_INFORMATION-FlexMember-Show_Public_HFFY_1126651684814.html (accessed October 17, 2013).

MedlinePlus. "Varicose Veins." U.S. National Library of Medicine, National Institutes of Health. http://www.nlm.nih.gov/medlineplus/varicoseveins.html (accessed October 17, 2013).

University of Wisconsin School of Medicine and Public Health. "Your Care at Home After Varicose Vein Ligation and Stripping and/or Radiofrequency Ablation." http://www.uwhealth.org/healthfacts/B_EXTRANET_HEALTH_INFORMATION-FlexMember-Show_Public_HFFY_1126651684814.html (accessed October 17, 2013).

ORGANIZATIONS

American Academy of Dermatology, 930 E. Woodfield Rd., Schaumburg, IL 60173, (847) 240-1280, (866) 503-SKIN (7546), http://www.aad.org.

American College of Phlebology, 101 Callan Ave., Ste. 210, San Leandro, CA 94577, (510) 346-6800, http://www.phlebology.org.

Peripheral Vascular Surgery Society (PVSS), 100 Cummings Ctr., Ste. 124A, Beverly, MA 01915, (978) 927-7800, Fax: (978) 927-7872, pvss@administrare.com, http://www.pvss.org.

Society for Vascular Surgery, 633 N. Saint Clair St., 22nd Fl., Chicago, IL 60611, (312) 334-2300, (800) 258-7188, vascular@vascularsociety.org, http://www.vascularweb.org.

Rebecca Frey, PhD

Venography *see* **Phlebography**

Venous thrombosis prevention

Definition

Venous thrombosis prevention is the use of medications, devices, and/or lifestyle changes to prevent blood clots (thrombi) from forming in veins.

Purpose

More than 200,000 people develop venous thrombosis every year in the United States. Deep-vein thrombosis (DVT)—the formation of blood clots in the deep veins of the legs and occasionally the arms—is a common medical problem. DVT in the lower leg affects one out of every 1,000 people. Although most cases of DVT resolve spontaneously, if the thrombus breaks loose and travels through the veins to the lungs, it can cause a pulmonary embolism (PE). Every year, about 100,000 people in the United States die within the first hour of a PE, making it the third most common cause of cardiovascular-related mortality. However, venous thrombosis is often preventable.

Description

Although blood clots can form in any vein in the body, DVT usually occurs in the leg or pelvis and occasionally in an arm. If the thrombus is large enough, it can block the blood flow within the vein, cutting off oxygen to the tissues. An embolus (a clot that breaks away from the wall of the blood vessel) can travel to the lung, the heart, or the brain causing a life-threatening PE, heart attack, or stroke. Some blood clots distend the walls of the blood vessel, creating a sac called an aneurysm. Sometimes the aneurysm bursts and leaks or hemorrhages blood. If this occurs within the brain, the heart, or the lungs, it can be fatal.

Classic symptoms of DVT include pain, swelling, and redness of the affected leg and dilation of the surface veins. The absence of these signs and symptoms, however, does not mean that the patient does not have DVT. Likewise, PE often occurs with little or no warning. Autopsies indicate that approximately 80% of all cases of DVT and PE are undiagnosed even when they are the immediate cause of death. About 90% of PE are a result of a clot from DVT in the leg or pelvis moving to the lung and blocking the pulmonary artery.

Risk factors

Prevention of venous thrombosis is closely related to risk factors for blood clots. Rudolf Virchow (1821–1902), a German physician and pathologist, first described the association between venous thrombosis in the legs and PE in 1846. He also described three factors integral to the development of venous thrombosis, which became known as Virchow's triad: slow or obstructed blood flow in the veins (venous stasis), blood thickness and coagulation, and vein damage. Anything that slows or obstructs the flow of venous blood can cause venous stasis, increased viscosity, and the formation of small thrombi that may enlarge. Long periods of immobilization from surgery, injury, or illness—even long airplane flights—can cause venous stasis. Coagulation can increase due to an imbalance of various factors in the blood. Damage to the lining of blood vessels can aggravate the formation of clots.

DVT is most common during recovery from surgery. Blood vessel disease, such as inflammation of the walls of veins (phlebitis), or hereditary blood clotting disorders can increase the chances of developing DVT. Heart disease, heart failure, stroke, or cancer can also cause venous thrombosis. Some drugs used in cancer chemotherapy increase the risk of DVT. Autoimmune disorders such as systemic lupus erythematosus increase the risk of DVT: about 9% of lupus patients develop spontaneous DVT. People who have had surgery to remove or close varicose veins have an increased risk of DVT. However, prolonged periods of bed rest or inactivity are particularly risky. Even the young and fit can die from travel-related DVT strokes. In 2003, NBC reporter David Bloom, who covered the war in Iraq embedded with the U.S. Army, died of PE from riding in a cramped position for long hours over several days.

The most common risk factors for DVT are a history of venous thromboembolism (VTE), which includes both DVT and PE, obesity, cancer, surgery, and immobility. Hospitalized and nursing home patients account for about half of all DVT cases. Other risk factors include:

- advanced age
- pregnancy and postpartum
- smoking
- major surgery in the previous four weeks
- automobile or airplane trips of more than four hours in the previous four weeks
- stroke
- heart attack
- congestive heart failure
- sepsis
- kidney disease
- Crohn's disease and ulcerative colitis
- multiple trauma
- central nervous system/spinal cord injury
- burns
- lower extremity fractures
- various inherited disorders
- intravenous drug use
- oral contraceptive use or estrogen therapy

Prevention

There are several methods for helping to prevent blood clots, including medications, mechanical means, behavioral changes, or a combination. However, regular activity and healthy living are the best preventive measures. Pregnant women with risk factors for venous thrombosis—a strong family history of clots or inherited thrombophilia or who require bed rest or are likely to have a cesarean delivery—may need medications or other preventive treatments.

LIFESTYLE. Regular **exercise**, maintaining a healthy weight, not smoking, and moving around as soon as

KEY TERMS

Aneurysm—A blood-filled stretching of a vessel, usually an artery.

Anticoagulant—Blood thinner; a medication such as heparin or warfarin that prevents coagulation or clotting of the blood.

Deep-vein thrombosis (DVT)—A clot in a deep vein, as in the leg or pelvis.

Embolus—A clot that breaks away from the wall of the blood vessel and travels through the body.

Inferior vena cava filter—A device implanted in the inferior vena cava—the largest vein in the body—to prevent clots or clot fragments from reaching the heart or lungs.

Phlebitis—Inflammation of the walls of a vein.

Prophylaxis—A measure for preserving health and/or preventing disease.

Pulmonary embolism (PE)—A blood clot that travels to the pulmonary artery, usually from a vein in the leg or pelvis.

Stent—A plastic mesh tube inserted in a blood vessel to hold it open and prevent clotting.

Stroke—A brain event caused by bleeding or oxygen deprivation in the brain, as from an aneurysm or clot.

Thrombophilia—An inherited or acquired tendency for thrombosis.

Thrombus—A clot that forms within a blood vessel and remains attached to its place of origin.

Venous thromboembolism (VTE)—The formation or presence of a thrombus or embolus in a vein, including deep-vein thrombosis and pulmonary embolism.

Virchow's triad—Three categories of factors that increase the risk of venous thrombosis: slowing of blood flow, increased blood coagulation, and injury to the lining of the veins.

possible after prolonged bed rest reduce the risk of DVT. Staying hydrated by drinking plenty of fluids can help prevent venous thrombosis. Other simple preventive measures include:

- occasionally raising the legs six in. (15 cm) above the heart
- raising the foot of the bed 4–6 in. (10–15 cm) with books or blocks

- avoiding sitting or standing for more than one hour at a time
- avoiding bumping or injuring the legs
- avoiding crossing the legs
- never using pillows under the knees
- reducing salt intake

Preventive measures when sitting for long periods or traveling for more than four hours include:

- exercising the legs while sitting, such as raising and lowering the toes with the heels on the floor and raising and lowering the heels with the toes on the floor, tightening and relaxing leg muscles, and performing ankle circles and leg lifts
- standing and walking every two to three hours
- wearing loose-fitting clothing, socks, and stockings
- drinking plenty of water
- avoiding alcohol and caffeine
- changing positions frequently

Prolonged travel increases the risk of VTE two–four-fold, especially in people with risk factors or traveling for more than four hours. In addition to walking around every one to two hours and wearing loose-fitting comfortable clothes, travelers should change positions frequently, flex and extend ankles and knees, and avoid crossing their legs. High-risk travelers should wear knee-high compression stockings or take blood thinners before traveling. Alcohol and sedatives or other medications that interfere with moving about should be avoided.

MEDICATIONS. Anticoagulants (blood thinners), such as warfarin (Coumadin) and heparin, are traditional prophylaxis for venous thrombosis. Newer oral anti-coagulants include dabigatran and rivaroxaban. These drugs decrease the clotting ability of the blood. One study indicated that anticoagulant prophylaxis prevented about 48% of potential DVT. Following an episode of DVT, patients generally take blood thinners for three to six months. By preventing the enlarging of existing clots and the formation of new clots, these drugs can free the body to dissolve any existing clots. However, blood thinners can interact with other medications and some dietary foods and lead to excessive bleeding. Although high-risk surgical patients, especially those undergoing bone, joint, or cancer surgery, may be given prophylactic anticoagulants, these should not be given to nonsurgical hospitalized patients unless the risk of VTE is greater than the risk of bleeding. Although the risk of venous thrombosis may persist after hospital discharge, clinical trials have failed to show a clear benefit from continued anticoagulant prophylaxis. Anticoagulants are also pre-scribed with caution to high-risk women during and following pregnancy.

Aspirin has traditionally been used to prevent arterial thrombosis—blood clots in arteries. As far back as 1977, 600 mg of aspirin twice daily were shown to reduce the risk of venous thrombosis after hip replacement. However, aspirin is not a mainstay of VTE prophylaxis, as there is not enough positive data from multiple studies. Patients with VTE are usually treated initially with heparin, followed by several months of warfarin treatment. Once anticoagulant treatment is suspended, the risk of VTE and other cardiovascular events increases again. However, recent studies have shown that subsequent low-dose (100 mg) daily aspirin reduces the risk of unprovoked VTE recurrence—as well as the risk of stroke, heart attack, or cardiovascular death—by one-third in patients without cancer or cardiovascular disease. Furthermore, the risk of bleeding while on aspirin therapy was low.

MECHANICAL. Mechanical stimulation of the calf muscles of the leg can help improve blood flow. Many hospitals require all surgical patients, especially those recovering from abdominal or cardiac surgery, to wear pneumatic compression stockings, also called leg pumps. These devices wrap around the lower leg from ankle to knee, with some reaching as high as the thigh. A pneumatic device pumps air into chambers within the stockings, gently tightening them around the legs for a few seconds and then releasing. This pulsing massage keeps the blood flowing and discourages venous thrombosis. The randomized CLOTS (Clots in Legs Or sTockings after Stroke) trial of almost 3,000 patients found that the use of leg pumps reduced DVT occurrence in immobile stroke patients, and there was a suggestion of mortality reduction. There have also been reports of successful DVT prevention by combining heparin administration and pneumatic compression stockings, particularly in patients undergoing colorectal or cardiac surgery. Mechanical devices are not recommended for preventing VTE in hospitalized nonsurgical patients.

Compression stockings, sometimes called graduated or medical compression stockings or support hose, are often recommended for preventing DVT and edema and for treating varicose veins and phlebitis. Graduated compression stockings apply more pressure at the ankle, gradually decreasing the pressure up to the knee. This pressure may help prevent backflow of blood and clot formation.

An inferior vena cava filter that blocks clots from traveling to the lungs is sometimes implanted in patients who cannot take anticoagulants because of bleeding or who have suffered a PE while taking anticoagulants. If blockage in a vein is believed to have caused DVT, the blockage may be opened with a balloon and stent to prevent recurrence.

QUESTIONS TO ASK YOUR DOCTOR

- Am I at risk for venous thrombosis?
- Should I take a prescription anticoagulant to prevent venous thrombosis?
- Should I take daily baby aspirin?
- What lifestyle changes would help prevent venous thrombosis?
- Do you recommend the use of compression stockings?

Preparation

Patients should discuss their risk of developing blood clots with their physician. If medication is prescribed, patients should be carefully instructed in its use and potential side effects. Special exercises should be described to the patient, as well as the benefits of a daily walk.

Results

There is no question that preventive measures can reduce the risk of venous thrombosis after surgery or during long periods of inactivity such as bed rest or travel. Travelers and sedentary workers may find that moving around and drinking fluids are the best methods for preventing blood clots. For patients recovering from surgery, however, a combination of methods, such as pneumatic compression pumps and anticoagulants, may be the best option.

Resources

BOOKS

Moliterno, David J., S. D. Kristensen, and R. De Caterina, eds. *Therapeutic Advances in Thrombosis*, 2nd ed. Hoboken, NJ: Wiley-Blackwell, 2012.

PERIODICALS

Ageno, Walter. "Do Medical Patients Need to Receive Pharmacologic Prophylaxis for the Prevention of Venous Thromboembolism?" *Internal and Emergency Medicine* Suppl. 7 (October 2012): S189–92.

Brighton, Timothy A., et al. "Low-Dose Aspirin for Preventing Recurrent Venous Thromboembolism." *New England Journal of Medicine* 367, no. 21 (November 22, 2012): 1979–87.

Hou, Li L., et al. "Preventive Effect of Electrical Acupoint Stimulation on Lower-Limb Thrombosis: A Prospective Study of Elderly Patients After Malignant Gastrointestinal Tumor Surgery." *Cancer Nursing* 36, no. 2 (March/April 2013): 139.

Larkin, Brenda G., Kimberly M. Mitchell, and Kathryn Petrie. "Translating Evidence to Practice for Mechanical Venous Thromboembolism Prophylaxis." *AORN Journal* 96, no. 5 (November 2012): 513–27.

Rusk, Matthew, and Robert K. Cato. "Aspirin Reduces the Risk for Recurrent VTE After an Initial Unprovoked Deep Venous Thrombosis or Pulmonary Embolism." *Annals of Internal Medicine* 158, no. 8 (April 16, 2013): 615.

Shah, Dhruvil, et al. "Nomograms to Predict Risk of In-Hospital and Post-Discharge Venous Thromboembolism after Abdominal and Thoracic Surgery: An American College of Surgeons National Surgical Quality Improvement Program Analysis." *Journal of Surgical Research* 183, no. 1 (2013): 462–71. http://dx.doi.org/10.1016/j.jss.2012.12.016 (accessed August 6, 2013).

Warkentin, Theodore E. "Aspirin for Dual Prevention of Venous and Arterial Thrombosis." *New England Journal of Medicine* 367, no. 21 (November 22, 2012): 2039–41.

OTHER

American College of Physicians. *Preventing Venous Thromboembolism in Hospitalized Patients: Recommendations From the American College of Physicians.* 2011. http://annals.org/data/Journals/AIM/20366/0000605-2011 11010-00002.pdf (accessed August 2, 2013).

WEBSITES

Agency for Healthcare Research and Quality. "Your Guide to Preventing and Treating Blood Clots." http://www.ahrq.gov/patients-consumers/prevention/disease/bloodclots.html (accessed August 2, 2013).

American Academy of Orthopaedic Surgeons. "Deep Vein Thrombosis." http://orthoinfo.aaos.org/topic.cfm?topic=a00219 (accessed August 5, 2013).

American College of Obstetricians and Gynecologists. "Preventing Deep Vein Thrombosis." Frequently Asked Questions. Women's Health. May 2011. http://www.acog.org/~/media/For%20Patients/faq174.pdf?dmc=1&ts=20130802T1949310234 (accessed August 2, 2013).

Centers for Disease Control and Prevention. "Are You at Risk for Deep Vein Thrombosis?" CDC Features. March 7, 2011. http://www.cdc.gov/Features/Thrombosis (accessed August 2, 2013).

CLOTS (Clots in Legs Or sTockings after Stroke) Trials Collaboration. "Effectiveness of Intermittent Pneumatic Compression in Reduction of Risk of Deep Vein Thrombosis in Patients Who Have Had a Stroke (CLOTS 3): A Mulicentre Randomised Controlled Trial." *Lancet.* May 31, 2013. http://www.thelancet.com/journals/lancet/article/PIIS0140-6736(13)61050-8/abstract (accessed August 3, 2013).

MedlinePlus. "Deep Vein Thrombosis." U.S. National Library of Medicine, National Institutes of Health. http://www.nlm.nih.gov/medlineplus/deepveinthrombosis.html (accessed August 2, 2013).

Office of the Surgeon General. "Fact Sheet: Deep Vein Thrombosis and Pulmonary Embolism." http://www.surgeongeneral.gov/library/calls/deepvein/fact sheetdvt_pe.html (accessed August 2, 2013).

Pai, Menaka, and James D. Douketis. "Patient Information: Deep Vein Thrombosis (DVT) (Beyond the Basics)." UpToDate. http://www.uptodate.com/contents/deep-vein-thrombosis-dvt-beyond-the-basics?view=print (accessed August 2, 2013).

Patel, Kaushal (Kevin). "Deep Venous Thrombosis." Medscape Reference. http://emedicine.medscape.com/article/1911303-overview#showall (accessed August 2, 2013).

Vascular Disease Foundation. "How Can I Prevent DVT?" This Is Serious. http://www.thisisserious.org/prevention (accessed August 3, 2013).

ORGANIZATIONS

American College of Phlebology, 101 Callan Avenue, Ste. 210, San Leandro, CA 94577, (510) 346-6800, Fax: (510) 346-6808, http://www.phlebology.org.

American Heart Association, 7272 Greenville Avenue, Dallas, TX 75231, (800) AHA-USA-1 (242-8721), http://www.heart.org.

Society for Clinical Vascular Surgery, 500 Cummings Center, Ste. 4550, Beverly, MA 01915, (978) 927-8330, Fax: (978) 524-8890, http://scvs.org.

U.S. Centers for Disease Control and Prevention, 1600 Clifton Rd., Atlanta, GA 30333, (800) CDC-INFO (232-4636), cdcinfo@cdc.gov, http://www.cdc.gov.

Vascular Disease Foundation, 550 M Ritchie Highway, PMB-281, Severna Park, MD 21146, (443) 261-5564, robert.greenberg@vdf.org, http://vasculardisease.org.

Janie Franz
Rebecca Frey, PhD
Margaret Alic, PhD

Ventilation *see* **Mechanical ventilation**

Ventral hernia repair *see* **Hernia repair, incisional**

Ventricular assist device

Definition

A ventricular assist device (VAD), also called a heart pump, is a battery-operated mechanical system with a blood pump and a control unit that is used to support blood circulation. It pumps blood out of a lower heart chamber—ventricle—to decrease the workload on a weakened heart and maintain adequate blood flow and blood pressure. Most VADs are left ventricular assist devices (LVADs) that pump blood from the left ventricle to the aorta and hence throughout the body. A right ventricular assist device (RVAD) pumps blood from the right ventricle to the pulmonary artery leading to the lungs. An LVAD and RVAD used together are known as a biventricular assist device (BVAD or BIVAD).

Purpose

A VAD is a life-sustaining device that can replace the left ventricle, the right ventricle, or both ventricles. It is used short-term when the heart muscle is damaged and requires rest to recover or heal, including:

• during and after heart surgery

• after a massive heart attack

• for heart failure when there is a delay in implementing a treatment plan

• when a patient cannot be weaned from a heart-lung bypass following treatment

• for an infection in the heart wall that does not respond to conventional treatments

• when patients are undergoing high-risk procedures to clear blockages in a coronary artery

For more than two decades, LVADs have been used as a lifesaving "bridge" for patients awaiting a heart transplant. However, the wait for a compatible heart can be so long that the LVAD pump may be implanted in the chest for the long term. An LVAD can maintain life and improve the quality of life for such patients. Other long-term uses of LVADs include severe heart conditions in which blood flow out of the heart is inadequate, such as with congestive heart failure, ventricular arrhythmia, or cardiogenic shock that cannot be controlled with medications, a pacemaker, or other treatments. LVADs are also used in patients whose bodies have rejected a transplanted heart. More recently, LVADs have come to be used as "destination therapy" for patients with end-stage heart failure who are not candidates for heart transplants.

Until recently, LVAD pumps were so large that they could only be implanted in adults with relatively large chest cavities. However, LVADs are now available for smaller women and children. Newer VADs are not only smaller, they are more reliable, and thus have become a treatment option for more patients, including those in earlier stages of heart failure. The new Excor pediatric VAD, called the Berlin Heart, can often keep children with heart failure alive until a heart becomes available for transplant.

Demographics

On any given day, there are about 3,000 people in the United States on the waiting list for a heart transplant, but only 2,000 donor hearts become available each year;

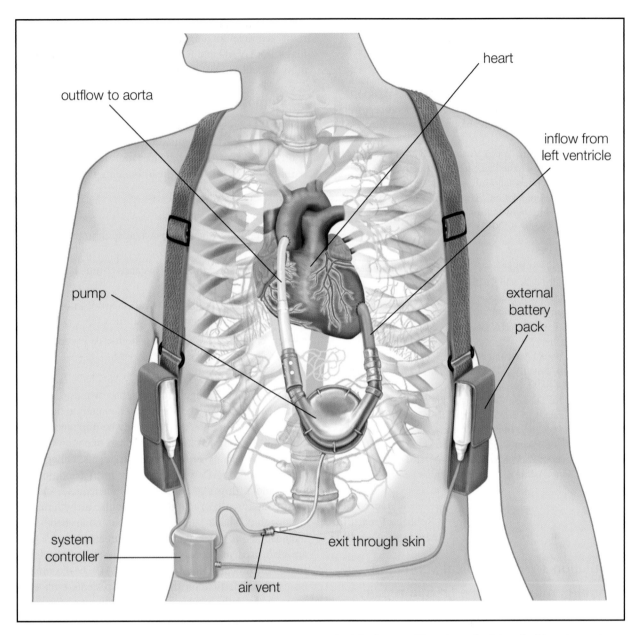

outflow to aorta

heart

inflow from left ventricle

pump

external battery pack

system controller

exit through skin

air vent

A ventricular assist device helps deliver oxygenated blood to the body's tissues. *(Encyclopaedia Britannica/Getty Images)*

thus, a large number of patients are using VADs while awaiting **heart transplantation**. The long-term use of VADs in patients that are not heart transplant candidates has also increased significantly in recent years.

Although approximately one in five people will eventually suffer left ventricular failure, only a relatively few of them are candidates for a VAD. To be considered for a VAD, patients must meet specific criteria with regard to blood flow, blood pressure, and general health. A VAD is contraindicated for patients with:

• irreversible kidney failure

• severe peripheral vascular disease

• irreversible brain damage

• cancer that has spread (metastasized)

• severe liver disease

• blood clotting disorders

• severe lung disease

• infections that do not respond to antibiotics

• advanced age

Description

A VAD helps the heart pump blood from a main pumping chamber, usually the left ventricle. The left

KEY TERMS

Anticoagulant—A medication for preventing the formation of blood clots in the circulatory system.

Aorta—The main artery arising from the left ventricle of the heart and carrying blood to the rest of the body.

Artery—A blood vessel that carries blood from the heart to other parts of the body.

Biventricular assist device (BVAD, BIVAD)—The combined use of left and right ventricular assist devices.

Coronary blood vessels—The arteries and veins that connect to the heart.

Echocardiogram—Ultrasound images of the heart.

Electrocardiogram (ECG, EKG)—A recording of the electrical impulses produced with each heartbeat.

Left ventricular assist device (LVAD)—The most common type of ventricular assist device, used to help the left ventricle pump blood to the rest of the body.

Palliative care—Care that focuses on relieving pain and suffering at the end of life.

Pulmonary artery—The major artery that carries blood from the right ventricle of the heart to the lungs.

Right ventricular assist device (RVAD)—A ventricular assist device that pumps blood from the right ventricle of the heart to the pulmonary artery that carries blood to the lungs.

Transcutaneous—Passing through the skin.

Ventilator—A mechanical breathing machine.

Ventricle—Either of the two lower chambers of the heart that receive blood from the atria and pump it into the major arteries.

ventricle pumps blood into the aorta—the main artery that carries oxygen-rich blood to the rest of the body. A VAD consists of a heart pump, a portable battery power source, a computerized control system, and tubes that attach it to the heart. The control unit has alarms to warn of low power or malfunction.

There are various types of VADs. The choice of a VAD depends on how long it will be needed, the patient's size, the amount of support (total or partial) required, and the type of flow desired (pulsatile or continuous). Different heart problems require different types of flow. Pulsatile VADs pump blood in pulses like the heart. Continuous-flow VADs supply the body with blood without maintaining a normal pulse. First-generation VADs were all pulsatile flow. Newer continuous-flow pumps are smaller and more durable.

A transcutaneous VAD is used for short-term support, such as during and after surgery. Both the pump and the power source are located outside of the body. The pump is connected to the heart by tubes running through small holes in the abdomen. RVADs are generally used only for short-term support of the right ventricle following heart surgery, including surgery to implant an LVAD.

With a typical implanted LVAD, a tube pulls blood from the left ventricle into the pump implanted into the upper part of the abdomen. The pump sends the blood to the aorta. A second tube from the pump comes out through the abdominal wall and attaches to the battery and control system. A VAD pump weighs from 1–2 pounds (460–900 grams). The battery pack is carried in a waistband or shoulder harness. Some fully implanted VADs require that a cord attached to the body be plugged into an electrical outlet at night.

A VAD is implanted under **general anesthesia** in a hospital **operating room**. A tube is guided down the throat to the lungs and connected to a ventilator so that the patient can breathe during the surgery. The surgeon makes an incision in the center of the chest, separates the breastbone, and opens the rib cage to reach the heart. A catheter is inserted into the jugular vein in the neck and threaded through the pulmonary artery, which carries blood from the right ventricle of the heart to the lungs. The catheter is used to measure the oxygen levels in the blood and to administer medications. A urinary catheter is inserted to measure the urine output. The surgeon sutures the catheters in place and attaches tubing to connect the catheters to the VAD pump. The pump is implanted beneath the skin and tissues in the upper part of the abdominal wall. Once the pump is turned on, blood flows out of the diseased ventricle, through the pump, and into the aorta. The patient's heart may be stopped so that the surgeon can operate on a still heart with the patient connected to a heart-lung bypass machine. After the LVAD has been implanted, the surgeon closes the incisions in the heart and the chest wall. The complete surgery usually takes four to six hours.

Preparation

VADs are used long-term in patients who have not benefited from other forms of treatment for heart disease, and most people who undergo VAD surgery are already in the hospital for heart failure. Some hospitals use palliative care specialists to help patients decide whether they want an LVAD, with all its incumbent risks and limitations. To evaluate patient eligibility for a VAD, **cardiac catheterization** is used to measure pressure in the heart chambers and demonstrate poor cardiac function. Monitoring of heart function also includes an electrocardiogram (EKG) and measurements of arterial and venous blood pressure. An echocardiogram uses sound waves to detail the size and shape of the heart and the functioning of the chambers and valves. The patient will probably also be given a **chest x-ray**. Blood samples are drawn to measure the levels of blood cells and electrolytes in the patient's circulation and to evaluate liver and kidney function The patient must be strong enough for the surgery. Sometimes, extra nutrition through a feeding tube is required prior to surgery.

Prior to surgery, patients and their caregivers will be taught how the VAD functions. They will be taught how to safely handle the device, how to wash and shower with it, how to travel with it, how to respond to its alarms, and how to handle an emergency such as loss of power.

Aftercare

Patients are gradually weaned from a short-term VAD. After VAD implants, patients are monitored in an **intensive care unit** (ICU) for up to five days and often remain hospitalized for much longer. Patients with severe heart disease may need to remain on a ventilator for breathing assistance for several days after surgery and may require intravenous fluids and nutrition. A tube in the bladder drains urine, and other tubes drain blood and fluid from the heart and chest. Anticoagulant (blood-thinning) medications, such as warfarin (Coumadin) and **aspirin**, are given to prevent the formation of blood clots. Anticoagulants are usually necessary as long as the VAD is in place. **Antibiotics** may be prescribed before and after surgery as a preventive measure, and patients are carefully watched for signs of infection.

The VAD lines penetrating the chest or abdominal cavity and connected to the control console must be cleansed and bandaged to prevent infection of the device. With appropriate training, the patient can continue treatment at home. VAD patients usually begin the process of hospital discharge by going home for a few hours and then returning, followed by going home for the day and returning to the hospital to sleep. Some patients go to a special care facility for up to two weeks. For the first month after hospital discharge, patients may have weekly outpatient visits, followed by visits every other week and then every other month.

VAD patients may undergo cardiac rehabilitation, including **exercise** training, education on "heart healthy" living, and counseling for stress and returning to a more active life. As patients improve, they begin a regular supervised exercise program. This is important because prior to VAD surgery, patients with weak hearts were unable to exercise and their muscles weakened. Recovery depends considerably on the patient's condition prior to surgery. Patients can usually resume most of their daily activities. They may be able to return to work, drive, and engage in sexual activity. Patients awaiting a heart transplant must stay within two hours of the hospital in case a heart becomes available.

Risks

VAD insertion carries risks of severe complications. Bleeding occurs in as many as 30%–50% of patients. Other complications include blood clots, partial paralysis of the diaphragm, respiratory failure, kidney failure, VAD failure, damage to coronary blood vessels, stroke, and infection. Blood clots in the legs may travel to the lungs or form in the VAD itself. A VAD also increases the risk of heart attack and bleeding from the gastrointestinal tract.

An additional risk is physical dependency on the device. With VADs in both ventricles, the heart may become so dependent that the patient cannot be weaned from ventricular support.

Many patients find that their emotions and cognitive functions are affected by the implantation procedure. Depression, mood swings, and memory loss are not unusual in VAD patients, many of whom find it difficult to be continuously plugged into a machine.

Results

Because VADs are used in the treatment of critically ill patients, outcomes vary widely according to the patient's condition before surgery. Signs of a successful implant include normal cardiac output with normal blood pressure and systemic and pulmonary vascular resistance. An LVAD can relieve symptoms such as shortness of breath and reduce the risk of death from end-stage heart failure by 50% at six and 12 months, extend life from 3.1 months to more than 10 months, and provide a better quality of life. VADs can enable patients to perform many daily activities that would otherwise be impossible.

Successful VAD implants can enable heart transplant candidates to remain at home and survive until a donor organ becomes available. In fact, as many as 5% of patients with implanted VADs recover an adequate level of heart muscle function to avoid the need for a heart transplant. Studies have found that children with heart failure who received the new pediatric VAD while

QUESTIONS TO ASK YOUR DOCTOR

- What factors should I consider when deciding whether to have a VAD?
- What are the benefits and risks of a VAD?
- What type of VAD will I receive?
- What is your success rate with VAD implants?
- Will a VAD extend my life and improve my quality of life?

awaiting a transplant had six-month outcomes similar to those of adults.

VADs are undergoing continual improvement. Newer continuous-flow VADs have yielded markedly better results compared with older pulsatile VADs. A newly developed continuous-flow pump is small enough to be partially implanted directly into the left ventricle, with the remainder of the device in the space around the heart. This device uses centrifugal flow, which may provide greater pulsatility and reduce arrhythmias. It may also reduce the occurrence of internal bleeding that is often associated with continuous-flow VADs.

Health care team roles

VADs are available at most heart transplant centers. A VAD is implanted by a cardiothoracic surgeon in a hospital that handles cardiopulmonary bypass procedures. The surgeon is trained in the specific techniques required to implant particular types of VADs. However, this special training and the cost of the materials limit the number of implant procedures that a hospital can perform.

Surgical nurses and anesthesiologists are part of the **surgical team**. If necessary, a perfusionist operates the heart-lung bypass machine during surgery. A team that includes the heart surgeon, cardiologist, critical care nurse, physical therapist, dietitian, and social worker help the VAD patient prepare for transition from hospital to home.

Resources

BOOKS

Deedwania, Prakash C. *Heart Failure*. Philadelphia: Saunders, 2012.

Joyce, David L., and Lyle D. Joyce. *Mechanical Circulatory Support: Principles and Clinical Applications*. New York: McGraw-Hill Professional, 2012.

PERIODICALS

Addonizio, Linda J. "Pediatric Ventricular Assist Devices—First Steps for Babies." *New England Journal of Medicine* 367, no. 6 (August 9, 2012): 567–68.

Fraser, Charles D., et al. "Prospective Trial of a Pediatric Ventricular Assist Device." *New England Journal of Medicine* 367, no. 6 (August 9, 2012): 532–41.

Gilotra, Nisha A., and Stuart D. Russell. "Patient Selection for Mechanical Circulatory Support." *Heart Failure Reviews* 18, no. 1 (January 2013): 27–34.

Kraemer, Felicitas. "Ontology or Phenomenology? How the LVAD Challenges the Euthanasia Debate." *Bioethics* 27, no. 3 (March 2013): 140–50.

Lee, Sangjin, et al. "Left Ventricular Assist Devices: From the Bench to the Clinic." *Cardiology* 125, no. 1 (May 2013): 1–12.

Milano, Carmelo A., and Alan A. Simeone. "Mechanical Circulatory Support: Devices, Outcomes and Complications." *Heart Failure Reviews* 18, no. 1 (January 2013): 35–53.

Raiten, Jesse M., and Mark D. Neuman. "'If I Had Only Known'—On Choice and Uncertainty in the ICU." *New England Journal of Medicine* 367, no. 19 (November 8, 2012): 1779–81.

WEBSITES

American Heart Association. "Implantable Medical Devices for Heart Failure." http://www.heart.org/HEARTORG/Conditions/HeartFailure/PreventionTreatmentofHeartFailure/Implantable-Medical-Devices-for-Heart-Failure_UCM_306354_Article.jsp (accessed September 8, 2013).

American Heart Association. "Recognizing Advanced Heart Failure and Knowing Your Options." http://www.heart.org/HEARTORG/Conditions/HeartFailure/Recognizing-Advanced-Heart-Failure-and-Knowing-Your-Options_UCM_441926_Article.jsp (accessed September 8, 2013).

Gordon, Serena. "Mechanical Device Helps Kids Waiting for Heart Transplant." *U.S. News & World Report*. August 8, 2012. http://health.usnews.com/health-news/news/articles/2012/08/08/mechanical-device-helps-kids-waiting-for-heart-transplant (accessed September 8, 2013).

MedlinePlus. "Ventricular Assist Device." National Institutes of Health. June 18, 2012. http://www.nlm.nih.gov/medlineplus/ency/article/007268.htm (accessed September 8, 2013).

National Heart, Lung, and Blood Institute. "What is a Ventricular Assist Device?" National Institutes of Health. March 31, 2012. http://www.nhlbi.nih.gov/health/health-topics/topics/vad (accessed September 8, 2013).

"New Pump to Treat Heart Failure in Waiting Transplant Patients Achieves Goal." American Heart Association. November 14, 2010. http://newsroom.heart.org/news/1188 (accessed September 8, 2013).

ORGANIZATIONS

American Heart Association, 7272 Greenville Ave., Dallas, TX 75231, (800) AHA-USA-1 (242-8721), http://www.heart.org.

National Heart, Lung, and Blood Institute, Health Information Center, PO Box 30105, Bethesda, MD 20824-0105, (301) 592-8573, Fax: (301) 592-8563, nhlbiinfo@nhlbi.nih.gov, http://www.nhlbi.nih.gov.

U.S. Food and Drug Administration, 10903 New Hampshire Ave., Silver Spring, MD 20993-0002, (888) INFO-FDA (463-6332), http://www.fda.gov.

Tish Davidson, AM
Allison J. Spiwak, MSBME
Margaret Alic, PhD

Ventricular shunt

Definition

A ventricular shunt is a tube that is surgically placed in one of the fluid-filled chambers inside the brain (ventricles). The fluid around the brain and the spinal column is called cerebrospinal fluid (CSF). When infection or disease causes an excess of CSF in the ventricles, the shunt is placed to drain it and thereby relieve excess pressure.

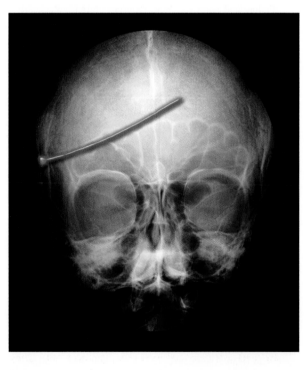

An x-ray of a skull with a ventricular shunt. *(Living Art Enterprises, LLC/Photo Researchers, Inc)*

Purpose

A ventricular shunt relieves hydrocephalus, a condition in which there is an increased volume of CSF within the ventricles. In hydrocephalus, pressure from the CSF usually increases. It may be caused by a tumor of the brain or of the membranes covering the brain (meninges), infection of or bleeding into the CSF, or inborn malformations of the brain. Symptoms of hydrocephalus may include headache, personality disturbances, loss of intellectual abilities (dementia), problems in walking, irritability, vomiting, abnormal eye movements, or a low level of consciousness.

Normal pressure hydrocephalus (a condition in which the volume of CSF increases without an increase in pressure) is associated with progressive dementia, problems walking, and loss of bladder control (urinary incontinence). Even though CSF is not thought to be under increased pressure in this condition, it may also be treated by ventricular shunting.

Demographics

The congenital form of hydrocephalus is believed to occur at an incidence of approximately one to four out of every 1,000 births. The incidence of acquired hydrocephalus is not exactly known. The peak ages for the development of hydrocephalus are in infancy, between four and eight years, and in early adulthood. Normal pressure hydrocephalus generally occurs in patients over the age of 60.

Description

The ventricular shunt tube is placed to drain fluid from the ventricular system in the brain to the cavity of the abdomen or to the large vein in the neck (jugular vein). Therefore, surgical procedures must be done both in the brain and at the drainage site. The tubing contains valves to ensure that fluid can only flow out of the brain and not back into it. The valve can be set at a desired pressure to allow CSF to escape whenever the pressure level is exceeded.

A small reservoir may be attached to the tubing and placed under the scalp. This reservoir allows samples of CSF to be removed with a syringe to check the pressure. Fluid from the reservoir can also be examined for bacteria, cancer cells, blood, or protein, depending on the cause of hydrocephalus. The reservoir may also be used to inject **antibiotics** for CSF infection or chemotherapy medication for meningeal tumors.

Precautions

As with any surgical procedure, the surgeon must know about any medications or health problems that may increase the patient's risk. Because infections are both common and serious, antibiotics are often given before and after surgery.

Diagnosis

The diagnosis of hydrocephalus should be confirmed by diagnostic imaging techniques, such as **computed tomography** scan (CT scan) or **magnetic resonance imaging** (MRI), before the shunting procedure is performed. These techniques will also show any associated brain abnormalities. CSF should be examined if infection or tumor of the meninges is suspected. Patients with dementia or intellectual disabilities should undergo neuropsychological testing to establish a baseline psychological profile before the shunting procedure.

Aftercare

To avoid infections at the shunt site, the area should be kept clean. CSF should be checked periodically by the doctor to be sure there is no infection or bleeding into the shunt. CSF pressure should be checked to be sure the shunt is operating properly. The eyes should be examined regularly because shunt failure may damage the nerve to the eyes (optic nerve). If not treated promptly, damage to the optic nerve causes irreversible loss of vision.

Risks

Serious and long-term complications of ventricular shunting are bleeding under the outermost covering of the brain (subdural hematoma), infection, stroke, and shunt failure. When a shunt drains to the abdomen (ventriculoperitoneal shunt), fluid may accumulate in the abdomen or abdominal organs may be injured. If CSF

QUESTIONS TO ASK YOUR DOCTOR

- Why is a ventricular shunt recommended in my case?
- What is the cause of the hydrocephalus?
- What diagnostic tests will be performed prior to the shunt being placed?
- Where will the shunt be placed?
- Are there any alternatives to a ventricular shunt?

---

pressure is lowered too much, patients may have severe headaches, often with nausea and vomiting, whenever they sit up or stand.

Results

After shunting, the ventricles get smaller within three or four days. This shrinkage occurs even when hydrocephalus has been present for a year or more. Clinically detectable signs of improvement occur within a few weeks. The cause of hydrocephalus, duration of hydrocephalus before shunting, and associated brain abnormalities affect the outcome.

Of patients with normal pressure hydrocephalus who are treated with shunting, 25%–80% experience long-term improvement. Normal pressure hydrocephalus is more likely to improve when it is caused by infection of or bleeding into the CSF than when it occurs without an underlying cause.

Morbidity and mortality rates

Complications of shunting occur in 30% of cases, but only 5% are serious. Infections occur in 5%–10% of patients, and as many as 80% of shunts develop a mechanical problem at some point and need to be replaced.

Alternatives

In some cases of hydrocephalus, certain drugs may be administered to temporarily decrease the amount of CSF until surgery can be performed. In patients with hydrocephalus caused by a tumor, removal of the tumor often cures the buildup of CSF. Approximately 25% of patients respond to therapies other than shunt placement.

Patients with normal pressure hydrocephalus may experience a temporary improvement in walking and mental abilities upon the temporary drainage of a moderate amount of CSF. This improvement may be an indication that shunting will improve their condition.

Health care team roles

Ventricular shunting is performed in a hospital **operating room** by a neurosurgeon, a surgeon who specializes in the treatment of diseases of the brain, spinal cord, and nerves.

Resources

BOOKS

Goetz, Christopher G. *Textbook of Clinical Neurology*. 3rd ed. Philadelphia: Saunders, 2007.

Townsend, Courtney M., et al. *Sabiston Textbook of Surgery*. 19th ed. Philadelphia: Saunders/Elsevier, 2012.

PERIODICALS

Bauer, David F., and James M. Markert. "Ventricular Shunt in Patients with Traumatic Brain Injury." *Neurosurgery* 68, no. 6 (2011): E1775–76. http://dx.doi.org/10.1227/NEU.0b013e31821815cc (accessed October 4, 2013).

Nigrovic, Lise E., et al. "The Prevalence of Traumatic Brain Injuries After Minor Blunt Head Trauma in Children With Ventricular Shunts." *Annals of Emergency Medicine* 61, no. 4 (2013): 389–93. http://dx.doi.org/10.1016/j.annemergmed.2012.08.030 (accessed October 4, 2013).

Rogers, Elisabeth Ashley, et al. "Predictors of Ventricular Shunt Infection among Children Presenting to a Pediatric Emergency Department." *Pediatric Emergency Care* 28, no. 5 (2012): 405–9. http://dx.doi.org/10.1097/PEC.0b013e318252c23c (accessed October 4, 2013).

WEBSITES

A.D.A.M. Medical Encyclopedia. "Ventriculoperitoneal Shunting." MedlinePlus. http://www.nlm.nih.gov/medlineplus/ency/article/003019.htm (accessed October 4, 2013).

Children's Hospital of the King's Daughters. "Hydrocephalus/Ventricular Shunts." http://www.chkd.org/healthlibrary/facts/content.aspx?pageid=0267 (accessed October 4, 2013).

Hydrocephalus Association. "Shunt Systems." http://www.hydroassoc.org/hydrocephalus-education-and-support/learning-about-hydrocephalus/shunts (accessed October 4, 2013).

ORGANIZATIONS

American Academy of Neurology, 201 Chicago Ave., Minneapolis, MN 55415, (612) 928-6000, (800) 879-1960, Fax: (612) 454-2746, memberservices@aan.com, http://www.aan.com.

Hydrocephalus Association, 4340 East West Hwy., Ste. 905, Bethesda, MD 20814, (301) 202-3811, (888) 598-3789, info@hydroassoc.org, http://www.hydroassoc.org.

Laurie Barclay, MD
Stephanie Dionne Sherk

Vertical banded gastroplasty

Definition

Vertical banded gastroplasty (VBG) is an elective surgical procedure in which the stomach is partitioned with staples and fitted with a plastic band to limit the amount of food that the stomach can hold at one time. Gastroplasty is a term that comes from two Greek words: *gaster*, or "stomach," and *plassein*, which means "to form or shape." Also known as stomach stapling, VBG is part of a surgical subspecialty called bariatric surgery. VBG is considered a restrictive bariatric procedure, since it controls the amount of food that the stomach can hold. Malabsorptive bariatric procedures, in contrast, reroute food within the digestive tract to prevent complete absorption of the nutrients.

Purpose

The purpose of VBG is the treatment of morbid obesity. It was one of the first successful procedures in bariatric surgery. VBG was developed in its present form in 1982 by Dr. Edward E. Mason, a professor of surgery at the University of Iowa.

Bariatric surgery in general has demonstrated long-term success in the majority of patients. Weight-reduction diets, **exercise** programs, and appetite-suppressant medications have had a low long-term success rate in managing morbid obesity. Most people who try to

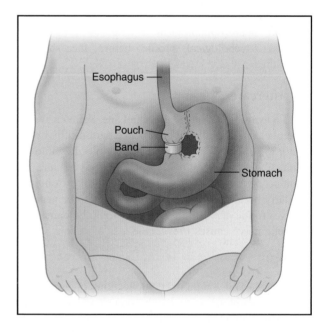

In vertical banded gastroplasty, a portion of the stomach is stapled shut, reducing its total size. *(Illustration by Electronic Illustrators Group. Copyright © 2014 Cengage Learning®.)*

lose weight on reduced-calorie diets regain two-thirds of the weight lost within one year; within five years, they have gained more weight in addition to all the weight they had lost previously. Appetite suppressants often have undesirable or harmful side effects, as well as having a low rate of long-term effectiveness; in 1997, the U.S. Food and Drug Administration (FDA) banned the sale of fenfluramine and phentermine ("fen-phen") when these substances were discovered to cause damage to heart valves.

Obesity is a major health problem not only because it is widespread in the American population—more than one-third of adults in the United States meet the National Institutes of Health (NIH) criteria for obesity—but because it greatly increases a person's risk of developing potentially life-threatening disorders. Obesity is associated with type 2 diabetes, hypertension, abnormal blood cholesterol levels, liver disease, coronary artery disease, sleep apnea syndrome, depression, urinary incontinence, and certain types of cancer. In addition to these disorders, obesity is a factor in what has been called lifestyle-limiting conditions. These conditions are not life-threatening, but they can have an enormous impact on people's day-to-day lives, particularly in their relationships and in the working world. Lifestyle-limiting conditions related to obesity include osteoarthritis and gout, urinary stress incontinence, heartburn, skin disorders caused by heavy perspiration accumulating in folds of skin, leg swelling and varicose veins, gallstones, and abdominal hernias. Women who are obese frequently suffer from irregular menstrual periods and infertility. Finally, societal prejudice against obesity may contribute to acute psychological distress. Surgical treatment of obesity has been demonstrated to relieve emotional pain as well as to reduce risks to the patient's physical health.

Demographics

Data from 2011 stated that more than one-third of U.S. adults (35.7%) were obese; however, VBG is performed only on patients who are severely or morbidly obese by NIH standards. Severe obesity is presently defined as a body mass index (BMI) of 35 or higher. BMI is a ratio of the weight and height calculated by a specific formula. Obesity is the epidemic with the greatest prevalence in the United States. In 2008, obesity among men was generally similar at all income levels, with a tendency to be slightly higher at higher income levels. Higher income women are less likely to be obese than low income women. According to a report from the U.S. Centers for Disease Control and Prevention, obesity may become a leading cause of mortality in the United States with an estimated 500,000 deaths per year. During the

past 20 years, there has been a dramatic increase in obesity in the United States. In 2008, medical costs associated with obesity were estimated at $147 billion. Non-Hispanic blacks have the highest age-adjusted rates of obesity (49.5%), compared with Mexican Americans (40.4%), all Hispanics (39.1%) and non-Hispanic whites (34.3%). In 2011, individual state data concluded that obesity prevalence ranged from 20.7% in Colorado to 34.9% in Mississippi. No individual state had a prevalence of obesity less than 20%. According to the American Society for Metabolic and Bariatric Surgery (ASMBS), formerly known as the American Society for Bariatric Surgery (ASBS), while the prevalence of obesity in the United States doubled between 1986 and 2000, the prevalence of morbid obesity quadrupled and the prevalence of super-obesity increased fivefold.

In the United States, the number of **gastric bypass** surgeries increased by more than 600% from 1993 to 2003. Between 2004 and 2006, more than 16,000 laparoscopic gastric bypass procedures and 6,000 gastric bypass procedures were performed. According to a recent study from the Agency for Healthcare Research and Quality (AHRQ), the mortality rate associated with bariatric surgery dropped by a staggering 78.7%, from 0.89% in 1998 to 0.19% in 2004. The mortality rate from morbid obesity was reduced by 89% after bariatric or metabolic surgery, according to a study published in the Annals of Surgery in 2004.

Description

There are two major types of VBG—open, which is the older of the two procedures; and laparoscopic, which is performed through very small incisions with the help of special instruments. Based on results of observational studies and small randomized controlled trials (RCTs), laparoscopic or minimally invasive techniques are thought to reduce potential complications and be safer for patients. Patients also have a faster recovery time with minimally invasive techniques.

Open vertical banded gastroplasty

The open VBG is done under **general anesthesia**. In most cases, it takes one to two hours to perform. The surgeon makes an incision several inches long in the patient's upper abdomen. After cutting through the layers of tissue over the stomach, the surgeon cuts a hole, or "window," into the upper part of the stomach a few inches below the esophagus. The second step involves placing a line of surgical staples from the window in the direction of the esophagus, which creates a small pouch at the upper end of the stomach. The surgeon must measure the size of this pouch very carefully; when completed, it is about 10% of the size of a

KEY TERMS

Appetite suppressant—A medication given to reduce the desire to eat.

Bariatrics—The branch of medicine that deals with the prevention and treatment of obesity and related disorders.

Body mass index (BMI)—A measurement that has replaced weight as the preferred determinant of obesity. The BMI can be calculated (in American units) as 703.1 times a person's weight in pounds divided by the square of the person's height in inches.

Comorbid—A term applied to a disease or disorder that occurs at the same time as another disease condition. There are a number of health problems that are comorbid with obesity.

Dehiscence—A separation or splitting apart. In a vertical banded gastroplasty, dehiscence refers to the coming apart of the line of staples used to form the stomach pouch.

Gastric pacing—An experimental form of obesity surgery in which electrodes are implanted in the muscle of the stomach wall. Electrical stimulation paces the timing of stomach contractions so that the patient feels full on less food.

Hernia—The protrusion of tissue or an organ through an incision, weakened area, or abnormal opening into other tissues or outside of a cavity. Incisional hernias sometimes occur after open VBGs.

Laparoscope—An instrument that allows a doctor to look inside the abdominal cavity. A less invasive form of VBG can be performed with the help of a laparoscope.

Malabsorptive—A type of bariatric surgery in which a part of the stomach is partitioned off and connected to a lower portion of the small intestine in order to reduce the amount of nutrients that the body absorbs from food.

Morbid—Unwholesome or bad for health. Morbid obesity is a condition in which the patient's weight is a very high risk to his or her health. The NIH (National Institutes of Health) prefers the term "severely obese" to "morbidly obese."

Obesity—Excessive weight gain due to accumulation of fat in the body, sometimes defined as a BMI (body mass index) of 30 or higher, or body weight greater than 30% above a person's desirable weight on standard height-weight tables.

Prevalence—The number of cases of a disease or disorder that are present in a given population at a specific time.

Restrictive—A type of bariatric surgery that works by limiting the amount of food that the stomach can hold. Vertical banded gastroplasty is a restrictive procedure.

Sleep apnea syndrome—A disorder in which the patient's breathing temporarily stops at intervals during the night due to obstruction of the upper airway. People with sleep apnea syndrome do not get enough oxygen in their blood and often develop heart problems.

Stricture—An abnormal narrowing of a body canal or opening. Sometimes strictures form near the plastic band in a VBG. A stricture may also be called an area of stenosis.

normal stomach and will hold about a tablespoon of solid food.

After forming the pouch and checking its size, the surgeon takes a band made out of polypropylene plastic and fits it through the window around the outlet of the stomach pouch. The vertical band is then stitched into place. Because the polypropylene does not stretch, it holds food in the stomach longer, which allows the patient to feel full on only a small amount of food.

Following the placement of the band, the surgeon will check to make sure that there is no leakage around the window and the line of surgical staples. The area of surgery will then be washed out with a sterile saline solution and the incision closed.

Laparoscopic vertical banded gastroplasty

A laparoscopic vertical banded gastroplasty, or LVBG, is performed with the help of a bariatric laparoscope. A laparoscope is a small tube, 0.39 in. (10 mm) in diameter, that holds a fiberoptic cable that allows the surgeon to view the inside of the abdominal cavity on a high-resolution video screen and record the operation on a video recorder. In a laparoscopic VBG, the surgeon makes three small incisions on the left side of the abdomen for inserting the laparoscope, and a fourth incision about 2.5 in. (14 cm) long on the right side. The formation of the stomach pouch and insertion of the plastic band are done through these small incisions. Because it is more difficult for the surgeon to maneuver the instruments through the small openings, an LVBG takes longer than an open VBG, about two to four hours.

A laparoscopic VBG requires that the surgeon spend more time training than with an open VBG. In the event of complications developing during a laparoscopic VBG, the surgeon usually completes the operation using the open procedure.

Diagnosis

Determination of obesity

The diagnosis of a patient who is considered to be eligible for bariatric surgery begins with measuring the degree of the patient's obesity. This measurement is crucial because the NIH and almost all health insurers have established specific limits for approval of bariatric procedures.

The obesity guidelines that are cited most often were drawn up by Milliman and Robertson, a nationally recognized company that establishes medical need for a wide variety of procedures for health insurers. The Milliman and Robertson criteria for weight-loss surgery specifies patients who:

- are at least 100 lb. (45 kg) over ideal weight, as defined by life insurance tables; have a BMI of 40 or higher; or have a BMI over 35 with a coexisting serious medical condition, such as diabetes or coronary artery disease

- demonstrate failure to lose weight or a tendency to regain weight despite having tried a multidisciplinary weight-control program

- have another cause of obesity, such as an endocrine disorder

- have attained full adult height

The patient must be treated not only by a doctor with special training in obesity surgery, but in a comprehensive program that includes: preoperative psychological screening and medical examination; nutritional counseling; exercise counseling; and participation in support groups.

There are several ways to measure obesity. Some are based on the relationship between a person's height and weight. The older measurements of this correlation are the so-called height-weight tables that listed desirable weights for a given height. The limitation of height-weight tables is that they do not distinguish between the weight of human fatty tissue and the weight of lean muscle tissue—many professional athletes and body-builders are overweight by the standards of these tables. A more accurate measurement of obesity is body mass index, or BMI. The BMI is an indirect measurement of body fat. The BMI is calculated in American

measurements by multiplying a person's weight in pounds by 703.1, then dividing that number by the person's height in inches squared. A BMI between 19 and 24 is considered normal; 25–29 is overweight; 30–34 is moderately obese; 35–39 is severely obese; 40 or higher is defined as morbidly obese; and 50 or higher is super-obese.

More direct methods of measuring body fat include measuring the thickness of the skinfold at the back of the upper arm, and bioelectrical impedance analysis (BIA). Bioelectrical impedance measures the total amount of water in the body, using a special instrument that calculates the different degrees of resistance to a mild electrical current in different types of body tissue. Fatty tissue has a higher resistance to the current than body tissues containing larger amounts of water. A higher percentage of body water indicates a greater amount of lean tissue.

Psychological evaluation

Psychiatric and psychological screening before a VBG is done to evaluate the patient's emotional stability and to ensure that weight loss expectations are not unrealistic. Because of social prejudice against obesity, some obese people who have felt isolated from others or suffered job discrimination come to think of weight loss surgery as a magical or quick solution to all the problems in their lives. In addition, the surgeon will want to make sure that the patient understands the long-term lifestyle adjustments that are necessary after surgery, and that the patient is committed to making those changes. A third reason for a psychological assessment before a VBG is to determine whether the patient's eating habits are compulsive. These would be characterized by the persistent and irresistible impulse to eat from unknown or unconscious purposes. Compulsive eating is not a reason for not having weight loss surgery, but it does mean that the psychological factors contributing to the patient's obesity will also require treatment.

Other tests and examinations

Patients must have a complete **physical examination** and blood tests before being considered for a VBG. Some bariatric **surgeons** will not accept patients with any of the following: histories of major psychiatric illness; alcohol or drug abuse; previous abdominal surgery; or collagen vascular diseases, which include systemic lupus erythematosus (SLE) and rheumatoid arthritis. Many will not accept patients younger than 16 or older than 55, although some surgeons report successful VBGs in patients over 70. In any event, patients will need to provide documentation of their physical condition, particularly comorbid diseases or disorders, to their insurance company.

Preparation

Preparation for bariatric surgery requires more attention to certain matters than most other forms of surgery requiring hospitalization.

Health insurance issues

Both bariatric surgeons and people who have had weight loss surgery report that obtaining preauthorization for a VBG from insurance companies is a lengthy, complicated, and frequently frustrating process. Insurance companies tend to reflect the prejudices against obese people that exist in the wider society. In addition, bariatric surgery is expensive—between $20,000 and $35,000 per procedure, according to the National Institutes of Health. Although this situation is slowly changing because of increasingly widespread recognition of the high costs of obesity-related diseases, people considering a VBG should contact their insurance provider early to secure approval for their operation.

Lifestyle changes

A VBG requires a period of **recovery at home** after **discharge from the hospital**. Since the patient's physical mobility will be limited, the following should be done before the operation:

- Arrange for leave from work, assistance at home, help with driving, and similar tasks and commitments.
- Obtain a handicapped parking permit.
- Check the house or apartment thoroughly for needed adjustments to furniture, appliances, lighting, and personal conveniences; specific recommendations include the purchase of a shower chair and toilet seat lift. People recovering from bariatric surgery must minimize bending, stooping, and any risk of falling.
- Stock up on prescription medications, nonperishable groceries, cleaning supplies, and similar items to minimize the need to go shopping. Food items should include plenty of clear liquids (juices, broth, soups) and soft foods (oatmeal and other cooked cereals, gelatin dessert mixes).
- Have a supply of easy-care clothing with elastic waistbands and simple fasteners. Shoes should be slip-ons or fastened with Velcro.
- Take "before" photographs prior to the operation, and make a written record of body measurements. These should include measurements of the neck, waist, wrist, widest part of the hips, bust or chest, knees, and ankles,

as well as shoe size. The pre-operation photographs and measurements help to document the rate and amount of weight lost. Patients who have had weight loss surgery also point out that these records serve to boost morale by allowing the patient to measure progress in losing weight after the surgery.

Pre-operation classes and support groups

In line with the Milliman and Robertson guidelines, most bariatric surgeons now have "pre-op" classes and ongoing support groups for patients scheduled for VBG and other types of bariatric surgery. Facilitators of these classes can answer questions regarding preparation for the operation and what to expect during recovery, particularly about changes in eating patterns. In addition, they provide opportunities for patients to share concerns and experiences. Patients who have attended group meetings for weight loss surgery often report that simply sharing accounts of the effects of severe obesity on their lives strengthened their resolve to have the operation. In addition, clinical studies indicate that patients who have attended pre-op classes are less anxious before surgery and generally recover more rapidly.

Medical preparation

Patients scheduled for a gastroplasty are advised to eat lightly the day before surgery. The surgeon will provide specific instructions about taking medications prescribed for other health conditions. The patient will be given pre-operation medications that usually include a laxative to clear the lower digestive tract, an antinausea drug, and an antibiotic to lower the risk of infection. Some surgeons ask patients to shower on the morning of their surgery with a special antiseptic skin cleanser.

Aftercare

Aftercare following a gastroplasty has long-term as well as short-term aspects.

Short-term aftercare

Patients who have had an open VBG usually remain in the hospital for four to five days after surgery; those who have had a laparoscopic VBG may return home after two to three days. Aftercare in the hospital typically includes:

- Pain medication. After returning from surgery, patients are given a patient-controlled anesthesia, or PCA device. The PCA is a small pump that delivers a dose of medication into the IV when the patient pushes a button.

- Clear fluids. Inpatient food is limited to a liquid diet following a VBG.

- Oxygen treatment and breathing exercises to get the patient's lungs back into shape. Patients are encouraged to get out of bed and walk around as soon as possible to prevent pneumonia.

- Regular change of surgical dressings. Patients may be given additional dressings for use at home, if needed.

Long-term aftercare

Long-term aftercare includes several adjustments to the patient's lifestyle:

- Slow progression from consuming liquids to eating a normal diet. For the first two weeks after surgery, the patient is limited to liquids and foods that have been pureed in a blender. The reintroduction of solid foods takes place gradually over several months. In addition, patients sometimes have unpredictable reactions to specific foods, although most of these resolve over time.

- Lifelong changes in eating habits. Patients who have had a VBG must learn to chew food thoroughly and to eat slowly to reduce the risk of nausea and vomiting. They must also be careful to avoid eating too many soft foods or sweets, to reduce the risk of regaining weight.

- A minimum of five years of follow-up visits to the surgeon to monitor weight maintenance and other health concerns. Patients considering bariatric surgery should choose a surgeon with whom they feel comfortable, as they are making a long-term commitment to aftercare with this professional.

- Ongoing support group meetings to deal with the physical and psychological aftereffects of surgery and weight loss.

- Beginning and maintaining an appropriate exercise program.

Risks

Patients who undergo a VBG are at risk for some of the same complications that may follow any major operation, including death, pulmonary embolism, the formation of blood clots in the deep veins of the leg, and infection of the surgical incision. These risks are increased for severely obese patients; for example, the risk of infection is about 10% for obese patients compared to 2% for patients of normal weight. With specific regard to VBGs, recent studies indicate that the risks of complications after surgery are about the same for open and laparoscopic VBGs. The ASMBS reported in 2005 that about 5% of VBGs result in complications, and that the mortality rate is 0.1%.

Specific risks of VBGs

Specific risks associated with vertical banded gastroplasty include:

- Incisional hernia. An incisional hernia is the protrusion of tissue through an incision. It results from the stress placed on the stitches holding the incision closed in extremely obese patients. Most can be repaired by resuturing the incision. Incisional hernias are more likely to occur with open VBGs than with laparoscopic procedures.

- Dehiscence. Dehiscence is the medical term for splitting open; it can occur in a VBG if the staples forming the pouch at the upper end of the stomach come loose.

- Nausea and vomiting. Nausea and vomiting usually result from eating more food than the stomach pouch can hold, or eating the food too quickly. In most cases, the vomiting disappears as the patient learns different eating habits.

- Formation of a stricture at the site of the plastic band. A stricture is an abnormal narrowing of a body canal or opening. It is also called a stenosis.

- Lodging of a food particle, pill, or capsule within the band or ring. If the object does not move further down the digestive tract within 24 hours, it must be removed by an endoscope.

- Damage to the spleen. The spleen lies very close to the stomach and can be injured in the process of bariatric surgery. In most cases, it can be repaired during the operation.

Long-term risks

The long-term risks of vertical banded gastroplasty include:

- Regaining weight. Patients who have had a VBG are more likely to regain lost weight than those who have had gastric bypass surgery. This is partly because the patient's digestive tract continues to absorb the nutrients in food in normal fashion. Because the stomach pouch in a VBG is small, many patients are tempted to eat ice cream and high-calorie liquids that pass quickly through the pouch. A 10-year follow-up study of 70 patients who had a VBG found that only 20% of the patients had lost and kept off the loss of 50% of their excess body weight.

- Ongoing vomiting and heartburn. About 20% of patients with VBGs report long-term digestive difficulties.

• Psychological problems. Some people have difficulty adjusting to the changes in their outward appearance and to others' changed reactions to them. Other patients experience feelings of depression, which are thought to be related to biochemical changes resulting from the weight loss.

Results

The most rapid weight loss following a VBG takes place in the first six months. It usually takes between 18 and 24 months after the operation for patients to lose 50% of their excess body weight, which is the measurement used to define success in bariatric surgery. At this point, most patients feel much better physically and psychologically; diabetes, high blood pressure, urinary stress incontinence, and other complications associated with severe obesity have either improved or completely resolved.

The primary drawback of VBG is its relatively high rate of failure in maintaining the patient's weight loss over a five-year period. The most common form of revision surgery for a failed VBG is the Roux-en-Y gastric bypass. For this reason, some bariatric surgeons recommend VBGs for patients at the lower end of the severe obesity spectrum; that is, those with BMIs between 35 and 40. The chief advantage of VBGs over malabsorptive types of weight loss surgery is that there is little risk of malnutrition or vitamin deficiencies.

Although bariatric surgeons advise patients to wait for two years after a VBG to have **plastic surgery** procedures, it is not unusual for patients to require operations to remove excess skin from the upper arms, abdomen, and other parts of the body that had large accumulations of fatty tissue.

Morbidity and mortality rates

According to the American Society of Bariatric Surgery, the rates of postsurgical complications are about 2% for leaks leading to infection and a need to reoperate; 1.5% for dehiscence; 1% for injury to the spleen; and 1% for pulmonary embolisms.

Alternatives

Established surgical alternatives

The primary restrictive alternative to a VBG is implanting a Lap-Band, which is an adjustable band that the surgeon positions around the upper end of the stomach to form the small pouch instead of using staples. The Lap-Band was approved by the U.S. Food and Drug Administration (FDA) for use in the United States in 2001. It can be implanted with the laparoscopic

technique. When the band is in place, it is inflated with saline solution. It can be tightened or loosened after the operation through a portal under the skin. Although the Lap-Band eliminates the risk of dehiscence, it produces such side effects as vomiting, heartburn, abdominal cramps, or enlargement of the stomach pouch due to the band slipping out of place. In one American study, 25% of patients eventually had the band removed.

The other major type of obesity surgery combines restriction of the size of the stomach with a malabsorptive approach. The combination surgery that is considered the safest and performed most frequently in the United States is the Roux-en-Y gastric bypass. In this procedure, the surgeon forms a stomach pouch and then divides the small intestine, connecting one part of it to the new pouch and reconnecting the other portion to the intestines at some distance from the stomach. The food bypasses the section of the stomach and the small intestine, where most nutrients are absorbed. The procedure takes its name from Cesar Roux, the Swiss surgeon who first performed it, and the "Y" shape formed by the reconnected intestines.

Experimental procedures

A newer technique in obesity surgery is known as gastric pacing or implantable gastric stimulation (IGS). In IGS, the surgeon implants electrodes in the muscle of the stomach wall that deliver a mild electrical current. These electrical impulses regulate the pace of stomach contractions so that the patient feels full on smaller amounts of food. Preliminary results from a team of Italian researchers on patients followed since 1995 indicate that gastric pacing is both safe and effective; studies in the United States have found similar results.

Another experimental surgical alternative in obesity surgery is staged surgery. This approach involves a first-stage less invasive procedure—usually a Lap-Band—that helps the patient reduce his or her weight to a safer level. Once the patient has lost some weight, the more complex Roux-en-Y gastric bypass is performed.

Health care team roles

A VBG is performed in a hospital regardless of whether the operation is an open or a laparoscopic gastroplasty. It is done by a bariatric surgeon, who is a medical doctor (MD) or doctor of osteopathy (DO) who has completed at least three years' training in **general surgery** after medical school and internship. Most bariatric surgeons have had additional training in gastrointestinal or biliary surgery before completing a fellowship in bariatric surgery with an experienced practitioner in this subspecialty.

QUESTIONS TO ASK YOUR DOCTOR

- Do I meet the eligibility criteria for bariatric surgery?
- Would you recommend a vertical banded gastroplasty (VBG) for me, a gastric bypass operation, IGS, or staged surgery?
- Am I a candidate for a laparoscopic VBG?
- How long have you been practicing bariatric surgery?
- How many VBGs do you perform each year?

In addition to demonstrating the technical skills necessary to perform a VBG, bariatric surgeons seeking hospital privileges must show that they are competent to provide the psychological and nutritional assessments and counseling included in weight loss surgery programs.

Resources

BOOKS

Cantor Goldberg, Merle, William Y. Marcus, and George Cowan, Jr. *Weight-Loss Surgery: Is It Right for You?* Garden City, NY: Square One Publishers, 2006.

Flancbaum, Louis, with Erica Manfred, and Deborah Biskin. *The Doctor's Guide to Weight Loss Surgery.* West Hurley, NY: Fredonia Communications, 2001.

Hochstrasser, April. *The Patient's Guide to Weight Loss Surgery: Everything You Need to Know about Gastric Bypass and Bariatric Surgery.* Long Island City, NY: Hatherleigh Press, 2004.

Thompson, Barbara. *Weight Loss Surgery: Finding the Thin Person Hiding Inside You.* 4th ed. Tarentum, PA: Word Association Publishers, 2008.

PERIODICALS

Buchwald, H. "Consensus Conference Statement. Bariatric Surgery for Morbid Obesity: Health Implications for Patients, Health Professionals, and Third-Party Payers." *Surgery for Obesity and Related Diseases* 1 (2005): 371–381.

Cigaina, V. "Gastric Pacing as Therapy for Morbid Obesity: Preliminary Results." *Obesity Surgery* 12 (April 2002), Supplement 1: 12S–16S.

Cummings, S., E. S. Parham, and G. W. Strain. "Position of the American Dietetic Association: Weight Management." *Journal of the American Dietetic Association* 102 (August 2002): 1145–1155.

Guisado, J. A., F. J. Vaz, J. Alarcon, et al. "Psychopathological Status and Interpersonal Functioning following Weight Loss in Morbidly Obese Patients Undergoing Bariatric Surgery." *Obesity Surgery* 12 (December 2002): 835–840.

Gumbs, A. A., A. Pomp, and M. Gagner. "Revisional Bariatric Surgery for Inadequate Weight Loss." *Obesity Surgery* 17 (September 2007): 1137–1145.

Magnusson, M., J. Freedman, E. Jonas, et al. "Five-Year Results of Laparoscopic Vertical Banded Gastroplasty in the Treatment of Massive Obesity." *Obesity Surgery* 12 (December 2002): 826–830.

Regan, J. P., et al. "Early Experience with Two-Stage Laparoscopic Roux-en-Y Gastric Bypass as an Alternative in the Super-Super Obese Patient." *Obesity Surgery* 13 (December 2003): 861–864.

Shai, I., Y. Henkin, S. Weitzman, and I. Levi. "Long-Term Dietary Changes After Vertical Banded Gastroplasty: Is the Trade-Off Favorable?" *Obesity Surgery* 12 (December 2002): 805–811.

Shikora, S. A. "'What Are the Yanks Doing?' The U.S. Experience with Implantable Gastric Stimulation (IGS) for the Treatment of Obesity—Update on the Ongoing Clinical Trials." *Obesity Surgery* 14 (September 2004): S40–S48.

Shikora, S. A., J. J. Kim, and M. E. Tarnoff. "Nutrition and Gastrointestinal Complications of Bariatric Surgery." *Nutrition in Clinical Practice* 22 (February 2007): 29–40.

Sugerman, H. J., E. L. Sugerman, E. J. DeMaria, et al. "Bariatric Surgery for Severely Obese Adolescents." *Journal of Gastrointestinal Surgery* 7 (January 2003): 102–108.

van Hout, G. C., J. J. Jakimowicz, F. A. Fortuin, et al. "Weight Loss and Eating Behavior Following Vertical Banded Gastroplasty." *Obesity Surgery* 17 (September 2007): 1226–1234.

WEBSITES

American Society for Metabolic and Bariatric Surgery. "Story of Obesity Surgery." http://asmbs.org/story-of-obesity-surgery (accessed September 26, 2013).

LeMont, Diane, Melodie Moorehead, Michael Parish, et al. "Suggestions for the Pre-Surgical Psychological Assessment of Bariatric Surgery Candidates." http://s3. amazonaws.com/publicASMBS/GuidelinesStatements/ Guidelines/PsychPreSurgicalAssessment.pdf (accessed September 26, 2013).

WebMD Health News. "FDA Approves Implanted Stomach Band to Treat Severe Obesity." http://www.webmd.com/ diet/news/20010605/fda-approves-stomach-band-fight-obesity (accessed September 26, 2013).

Weight-control Information Network. "Gastrointestinal Surgery for Severe Obesity." National Institute of Diabetes & Digestive & Kidney Diseases. http://win.niddk.nih.gov/ publications/gastric.htm (accessed September 26, 2013).

ORGANIZATIONS

American Society for Metabolic and Bariatric Surgery, 100 SW 75th St., Ste. 201, Gainesville, FL 32607, (352) 331-4900, Fax: (352) 331-4975, info@asmbs.org, http://asmbs.org.

American Society of Bariatric Physicians, 2821 S. Parker Rd., Ste. 625, Aurora, CO 80014, (303) 770-2526, Fax: (303) 779-4834, http://www.asbp.org.

Obesity Society, 8757 Georgia Ave., Ste. 1320, Silver Spring, MD 20910, (301) 563-6526, Fax: (301) 563-6595, http://www.obesity.org.

Weight-control Information Network (WIN), 1 WIN Way, Bethesda, MD 20892-3665, (877) 946-4627, win@info.niddk.nih.gov, http://www.win.niddk.nih.gov.

Rebecca Frey, PhD
Tammy Allhoff, CST/CSFA, AAS

Vital signs

Definition

Vital signs, or signs of life, include the following objective measures for a person: temperature, respiratory rate, heart beat (pulse), and blood pressure. When these values are not zero, they indicate that a person is alive. All of these vital signs can be observed, measured, and monitored. This will enable the assessment of the level at which an individual is functioning. Normal ranges of measurements of vital signs change with age and medical condition.

Purpose

The purpose of recording vital signs is to establish a baseline on admission to a hospital, clinic, professional office, or other encounter with a health care provider. Vital signs may be recorded by a nurse, physician, physician's assistant, or other health care professional. The health care professional has the responsibility of interpreting data and identifying any abnormalities from a person's normal state, and of establishing if current treatment or medications are having the desired effect.

Abnormalities of the heart are diagnosed by analyzing the heartbeat (or pulse) and blood pressure.

Normal vital sign averages

Blood pressure	90/60–120/80 mm/Hg
Pulse	60–100 beats per minute
Respiration	12–18 breaths per minute
Temperature	98.6 degrees F°

SOURCE: A.D.A.M. Medical Encyclopedia, "Vital Signs." Available online at: http://www.nlm.nih.gov/medlineplus/ency/article/002341.htm.

(Table by PreMediaGlobal. Copyright © 2014 Cengage Learning®.)

KEY TERMS

Auscultation—The process of listening to sounds that are produced in the body. Direct auscultation uses the ear alone, such as when listening to the grating of a moving joint. Indirect auscultation involves the use of a stethoscope to amplify sounds from within the body, such as those coming from the heart or intestines.

Blood pressure—The pressure exerted by arterial blood on the walls of arteries. This depends on the strength of the heart beat, elasticity of the arterial walls, and volume and viscosity (resistance to flow) of blood. The pressure of blood in the arteries is measured in millimeters of mercury by a sphygmomanometer or by an electronic device.

Hypothermia—An abnormally low body temperature.

Pyrexia—Fever or a febrile condition.

Respiration—The exchange of gases between red blood cells and the atmosphere.

Stethoscope—A Y-shaped instrument that amplifies body sounds such as heartbeat, breathing, and air in the intestine. Used in auscultation.

The rate, rhythm and regularity of the beat are assessed, as well as the strength and tension of the beat, against the arterial wall.

Vital signs are usually recorded from once hourly to four times hourly, as required by a person's condition.

The vital signs are recorded and compared with normal ranges for a person's age and medical condition. Based on these results, a decision is made regarding further actions to be taken.

All persons should be made comfortable and reassured that recording vital signs is normal part of health checks, and that it is necessary to ensure that the state of their health is being monitored correctly. Any abnormalities in vital signs should be reported to the health care professional in charge of care.

Description

Temperature

Temperature is recorded to check for fever (pyrexia or a febrile condition), or to monitor the degree of hypothermia.

Manufacturer guidelines should be followed when recording a temperature with an electronic **thermometer**.

The result displayed on the liquid crystal display (LCD) screen should be read, then recorded in a person's medical record. Electronic temperature monitors do not have to be cleaned after use. They have protective guards that are discarded after each use. This practice ensures that infections are not spread.

An alcohol or mercury thermometer can be used to monitor a temperature by three methods:

- Axillary, under the armpit. This method provides the least accurate results.

- Orally, under the tongue. This method is never used with infants or very young children because they may accidentally bite or break the thermometer. They also have difficulty holding oral thermometers under their tongues long enough for their temperatures to be accurately measured.

- Rectally, inserted into the rectum. This method provides the most accurate recording of recording the temperature. It is most often used for infants. A recent study reported that rectal thermometers were more accurate than ear thermometers in detecting high fevers. With the ability to detect low-grade fevers, rectal thermometers can be useful in discovering serious illnesses, such as meningitis or pneumonia. The tip of a rectal thermometer is usually blue, which distinguishes it from the silver tip of an oral, or axillary thermometer.

To record the temperature using an alcohol or mercury thermometer, one should shake down the thermometer by holding it firmly at the clear end and flicking it quickly a few times, with the silver end pointing downward. The health care provider who is taking the temperature should confirm that the alcohol or mercury is below a normal body temperature.

To record an axillary temperature, the silver tip of the thermometer should be placed under the right armpit. The arm clamps the thermometer into place, against the chest. The thermometer should stay in place for three to four minutes. After the appropriate time has elapsed, the thermometer should be removed and held at eye level. During the waiting period, the alcohol or mercury will have risen to a mark that indicates the temperature of a person.

To record an oral temperature, the axillary procedure should be followed, except that the silver tip of the thermometer should be placed beneath the tongue for three to four minutes, then read as described previously.

In both cases, the thermometer should be wiped clean with an antiseptic and stored in an appropriate container to prevent breakage.

To record a rectal temperature, a rectal thermometer should be shaken down, as described previously. A small amount of water-based lubricant should be placed on the colored tip of the thermometer. Infants must be placed on their stomachs and held securely in place. The tip of the thermometer is inserted into the rectum no more than 0.5 in. (1.3 cm) and held there for two to three minutes. The thermometer is removed, read as before, and wiped with an antibacterial wipe. It is then stored in an appropriate container to prevent breakage, because ingestion of mercury can be fatal.

Respiratory rate

An examiner's fingers should be placed on the person's wrist, while the number of breaths or respirations in one minute is recorded. Every effort should be made to prevent people from becoming aware that their breathing is being checked. Respiration results should be noted in the medical chart.

Heartbeat (pulse)

The pulse can be recorded anywhere that a surface artery runs over a bone. The radial artery in the wrist is the point most commonly used to measure a pulse. To measure a pulse, one should place the index, middle, and ring fingers over the radial artery. It is located above the wrist, on the anterior or front surface of the thumb side of the arm. Gentle pressure should be applied, taking care to avoid obstructing blood flow. The rate, rhythm, strength, and tension of the pulse should be noted. If there are no abnormalities detected, the pulsations can be counted for half a minute, and the result doubled. However, any irregularities discerned indicate that the pulse should be recorded for one minute. This will eliminate the possibility of error. Pulse results should be noted in the health chart.

Blood pressure

To record blood pressure, a person should be seated with one arm bent slightly, and the arm bare or with the sleeve loosely rolled up. With an aneroid or automatic unit, the cuff is placed level with the heart and wrapped around the upper arm, one inch above the elbow. Following the manufacturer's guidelines, the cuff is inflated and then deflated while an attendant records the reading.

If the blood pressure is monitored manually, a cuff is placed level with the heart and wrapped firmly but not tightly around the arm one inch above the elbow over the brachial artery. Wrinkles in the cuff should be smoothed out. Positioning a **stethoscope** over the brachial artery in front of the elbow with one hand and listening through the earpieces, the cuff is inflated well above normal levels (to about 200 mm Hg), or until no sound is heard.

Alternatively, the cuff should be inflated 10 mm Hg above the last sound heard. The valve in the pump is slowly opened. Air is allowed to escape no faster than 5 mm Hg per second to deflate the pressure in the cuff to the point where a clicking sound is heard over the brachial artery. The reading of the gauge at this point is recorded as the systolic pressure.

The sounds continue as the pressure in the cuff is released and the flow of blood through the artery is no longer blocked. At this point, the noises are no longer heard. The reading of the gauge at this point is noted as the diastolic pressure. "Lub-dub" is the sound produced by the normal heart as it beats. Every time this sound is detected, it means that the heart is contracting once. The noises are created when the heart valves click to close. When one hears "lub," the atrioventricular valves are closing. The "dub" sound is produced by the pulmonic and aortic valves.

With children, the clicking noise does not disappear but changes to a soft muffled sound. Because sounds continue to be heard as the cuff deflates to zero, the reading of the gauge at the point where the sounds change is recorded as the diastolic pressure.

Blood pressure readings are recorded with the systolic pressure first, then the diastolic pressure (e.g., 120/70).

Blood pressure should be measured using a cuff that is correctly sized for the person being evaluated. Cuffs that are too small are likely to yield readings that can be 10 to 50 millimeters (mm) Hg too high. Hypertension (high blood pressure) may be incorrectly diagnosed.

Preparation

As there may be no recorded knowledge of a person's previous vital signs for comparison, it is important that a health care professional be aware that there is a wide range of normal values that can apply to persons of different ages. The health care professional should obtain as detailed a medical history from the person as soon as possible. Any known medical or surgical history, prior measurements of vital signs, and details of current medications should be recorded, as well. Physical exertion prior to measurement of vital signs, such as climbing stairs, may affect the measurements. This should be avoided immediately before the measurement of blood pressure. Tobacco, caffeinated drinks, and alcohol should be avoided for 30 minutes prior to recording.

A person should be sitting down or lying comfortably to ensure that the readings are taken in a similar position each time. There should be little excitement, which can affect the results. The equipment required include a watch with a second hand, an electronic or other form of thermometer, an electronic or manual **sphygmomanometer** with an appropriate sized cuff, and a stethoscope.

Results

A normal body temperature taken orally is 98.6°F (37°C), with a range of 97.8–99.1°F (36.5–37.2°C). A fever is a temperature of 101°F (38.3°C) or higher in an infant younger than three months or above 102°F (38.9°C) for older children and adults. Hypothermia is recognized as a temperature below 96°F (35.5°C).

Respirations are quiet, slow, and shallow when the adult is asleep, and rapid, deeper, and noisier during and after activity.

Average respiration rates at rest are:

• infants: 34–40 per minute
• children five years of age: 25 per minute
• older children and adults: 16–20 per minute

Tachypnea is rapid respiration above 20 per minute.

The strength of a heart beat is raised during conditions such as fever and lowered by conditions such as shock or elevated intracranial pressure. The average heart rate for older children (aged 12 and older) and adults is approximately 72 beats per minute (BPM). Tachycardia is a pulse rate over 100 BPM, while bradycardia is a pulse rate of under 60 BPM.

Blood pressure is recorded for older children and adults. A normal adult blood pressure reading is 120/80.

Resources

BOOKS

Bickley, Lynn S. *Bates' Guide to Physical Examination and History Taking*. 10th ed. Philadelphia: Wolters Kluwer Health/Lippincott Williams & Wilkins, 2009.

Jarvis, Carolyn. *Physical Examination and Health Assessment*. 5th ed. St. Louis, MO: Saunders/Elsevier, 2008.

Seidel, Henry M., et al. *Mosby's Physical Examination Handbook*. 7th ed. St. Louis, MO: Mosby/Elsevier, 2011.

Swartz, Mark H. *Textbook of Physical Diagnosis: History and Examination*. 6th ed. Philadelphia: Saunders/Elsevier, 2010.

PERIODICALS

Ansermino, J. Mark. "Universal Access to Essential Vital Signs Monitoring." *Anesthesia & Analgesia* 117, no. 4 (2013): 883–90. http://dx.doi.org/10.1213/ANE.0b013e3182a1 f22f (accessed October 4, 2013).

Hyder, Joseph A, et al. "How to Improve the Performance of Intraoperative Risk Models: An Example with Vital

Signs Using the Surgical Apgar Score." *Anesthesia & Analgesia* (September 13, 2013): e-pub ahead of print. http://dx.doi.org/10.1213/ANE.0b013e3182a46d6d (accessed October 4, 2013).

WEBSITES

A.D.A.M. Medical Encyclopedia. "Vital Signs." MedlinePlus. http://www.nlm.nih.gov/medlineplus/ency/article/002341. htm (accessed October 4, 2013).

Ohio State University Wexner Medical Center. "Vital Signs (Body Temperature, Pulse Rate, Respiration Rate, Blood Pressure)." http://medicalcenter.osu.edu/patientcare/ healthcare_services/emergency_services/non_traumatic_ emergencies/vital_signs/Pages/index.aspx (accessed October 4, 2013).

ORGANIZATIONS

American Academy of Family Physicians (AAFP), 11400 Tomahawk Creek Pkwy., Leawood, KS 66211-2680, (913) 906-6000, (800) 274-2237, Fax: (913) 906-6075, http://www.aafp.org.

American Academy of Pediatrics, 141 Northwest Point Blvd., Elk Grove Village, IL 60007-1098, (847) 434-4000, (800) 433-9016, Fax: (847) 434-8000, http://www.aap.org.

American College of Physicians (ACP), 190 N. Independence Mall West, Philadelphia, PA 19106-1572, (215) 351-2400, (800) 523-1546, http://www.acponline.org.

L. Fleming Fallon, Jr., MD, DrPH

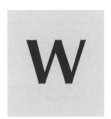

Water pills *see* **Diuretics**

Webbed finger or toe repair

Definition

Webbed finger or toe repair refers to corrective or **reconstructive surgery** performed to repair webbed fingers or toes, also called syndactyly. The long and ring fingers or the second and third toes are most often affected. Generally, syndactyly repairs are done between the ages of six months and two years.

Purpose

Webbing, or syndactyly, is a condition characterized by the incomplete separation or union of two or more fingers or toes, and usually only involves a skin connection between the two (simple syndactyly), but may—rarely—also include fusion of bones, nerves, blood vessels, and tendons in the affected digits (complex syndactyly). Webbing may extend partially up between the digits, frequently just to the first joint, or may extend the entire length of the digits. Polysyndactyly describes both webbing and the presence of an extra number of fingers or toes. The condition usually develops within six weeks after birth. Syndactyly can also occur in victims of fires, as the intense heat can melt the skin and fuse the epidermis and dermis of the phalanges, fingers, or toes. Burn victim syndactyly is always less invasive because bone fusion is not present in these cases. The purpose of repair surgery is to improve the appearance of the hand or foot and to prevent progressive deformity from developing as the child grows.

Demographics

In the United States, approximately one infant in every 2,000 births is born with webbed fingers or toes.

Both hands are involved in 50% of cases; the middle finger and ring finger in 41%; the ring finger and little finger in 27%; the index finger and middle finger in 23%; and the thumb and index finger in 9%.

Description

Polydactyly can be corrected by surgical removal of the extra digit or partial digit. Syndactyly can also be corrected surgically. This is usually accomplished with the addition of a skin graft from the groin.

There are several ways to perform this type of surgery; the design of the operation depends both on the features of the hand or foot and the surgeon's experience. The surgery is usually performed with zigzag cuts that cross back and forth across the fingers or toes so that the scars do not interfere with growth of the digits.

The procedure is performed under **general anesthesia**. The skin areas to be repaired are marked and the surgeon then proceeds to incise the skin, lifting small flaps at the sides of the fingers or toes and in the web. These flaps are sutured into position, leaving absent areas of skin. These areas may be filled in with full thickness skin grafts, usually taken from the skin in the groin area. The hand or foot is then immobilized with bulky **dressings**, or a cast. Webbed or toe repair surgery usually takes two to four hours.

Diagnosis

Syndactyly may be diagnosed during an examination of an infant or child, with the aid of x-rays. In its most common form, it is seen as webbing between the second and third toes. This form is often inherited. Syndactyly can also occur as part of a pattern of other congenital defects involving the skull, face, and bones.

An infant with webbed fingers or toes may have other symptoms that, when observed together, define a specific syndrome or medical condition. For example, syndactyly is a characteristic of Apert syndrome, Poland syndrome, Jarcho-Levin syndrome, oral-facial-digital

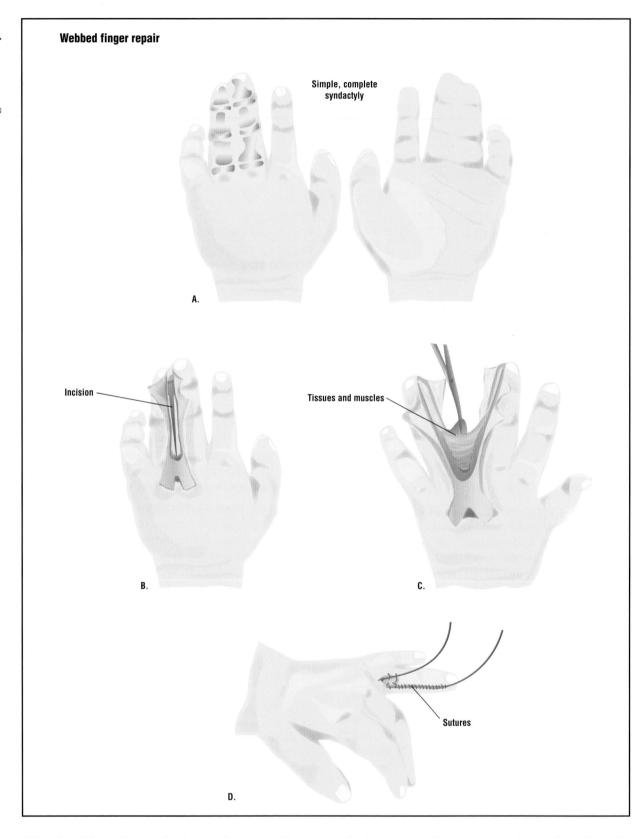

Webbed finger repair

Simple, complete syndactyly

A.

Incision

B.

Tissues and muscles

C.

Sutures

D.

This webbed finger shows a simple, complete syndactyly, meaning the bones for two fingers are complete, and only the soft tissues form the webbed section (A). To repair this, an incision is made in the skin of the webbing (B). Tissues and muscles are severed (C), and the two separated fingers are stitched (D). *(Illustration by GGS Information Services. Copyright © Cengage Learning®.)*

syndrome, Pfeiffer syndrome, and Edwards syndrome. Diagnosis of a syndrome is made on family history, medical history, and thorough physical evaluation. The medical history questions documenting the condition in detail usually include:

- Which fingers (toes) are involved?
- Are any other family members affected by the same condition?
- What other symptoms or abnormalities are also present?

Preparation

To prepare for surgery, seven to ten days before surgery, the child visits the family physician or pediatrician for a general **physical examination** and blood tests. The child cannot have solid food after midnight before surgery. Breast milk, formula, or milk (no pablum or other cereal may be added) up to six hours before the scheduled start of surgery is allowed, and then only clear fluids up to three hours before surgery. Thereafter, the child may not have anything else to eat or drink.

Aftercare

Hospital stays of one or two days are common for webbed finger or toe repair surgery. There is usually some swelling and bruising. Pain medications are given to alleviate any discomfort. The **bandages** must be kept clean and dry and must remain for two to three weeks for proper healing and protection. Skin grafts and the hand or foot may become very dry, so it is encouraged to dampen them with a good moisturizer such as Lubriderm or Nivea. Small children with hand syndactylies may have a cast put on that extends above the flexed elbow.

Sometimes, the cast extends beyond the fingers or toes. This protects the repaired areas from trauma.

The treating physician should be informed of any postoperative swelling, severe pain, fever, or fingers that tingle, are numb, or have a bluish discoloration.

Risks

Webbed finger or toe repair surgery carries the risks associated with any anesthesia, such as adverse reactions to medications, breathing problems, and sore throat from intubation. Risks associated with any surgery are excessive bleeding and infection.

Specific risks associated with the repair surgery include possible loss of skin graft and circulation damage from the cast or bandages.

Results

The results of webbed finger or toe repair depend on the degree of fusion of the digits and the repair is usually successful. When joined fingers share a single fingernail, the creation of two normal-looking nails is rarely possible. One nail will look more normal than the other. Some children may require a second surgery, depending on the type of syndactyly. If polydactyly or syndactyly are just cosmetic and not symptomatic of a condition or disorder, the outcome of surgery is usually very good. If it is symptomatic, the outcome will rely heavily on the management of the disorder.

Alternatives

Syndactyly does not generally pose any health risk, so it is not mandatory that the repair be performed. However, if the thumb is joined, or if the fingers are joined out toward their tips, they will grow in a progressively worsening bend over time.

Health care team roles

Webbed finger or toe repair surgery is usually performed in a children's hospital by a pediatric surgeon or orthopedic surgeon specializing in syndactyly surgery.

If prenatal screening indicates syndactyly in the fetus, arrangements are usually made so that the baby is delivered at a hospital with a pediatric surgeon on staff.

Resources

BOOKS

Jones, Kenneth Lyons, Marilyn C. Jones, and Miguel del Campo. *Smith's Recognizable Patterns of Human Malformation.* 7th ed. Philadelphia: Saunders/Elsevier, 2013.

Moore, Keith L., T. V. N. Persaud, and Mark G. Torchia. *Before We Are Born: Essentials of Embryology and Birth Defects.* 8th ed. Philadelphia: Saunders/Elsevier, 2013.

PERIODICALS

Chopra, K., et al. "Syndactyly Repair." *Eplasty* 13 (July 15, 2013): ic51.

"Polydactyly: A Review." *Bulletin of the Hospital for Joint Disease* 71, no. 1 (2013): 17–23.

WEBSITES

Detroit Medical Center. "Syndactyly: Infant Finger Separation." http://www.dmc.org/VideoLibrary/ShowVideo.aspx?Library=1&VideoID=155 (accessed October 4, 2013).

Yale School of Medicine. "Syndactyly." http://www.yalesurgery.org/plastics/care/hand/syndactyly.aspx (accessed October 4, 2013).

ORGANIZATIONS

American Academy of Orthopaedic Surgeons (AAOS), 6300 N. River Rd., Rosemont, IL 60018-4262, (847) 823-7186, Fax: (847) 823-8125, pemr@aaos.org, http://www.aaos.org.

American Society for Surgery of the Hand (ASSH), 822 W. Washington Blvd., Chicago, IL 60607, (312) 880-1900, Fax: (847) 384-1435, info@assh.org, http://www.assh.org.

Monique Laberge, PhD

Weight management

Definition

Weight management refers to a set of practices and behaviors that are necessary to keep weight at a healthful level. It is preferred to the term "dieting," because it involves more than regulation of food intake or treatment of overweight people. People diagnosed with eating disorders that are not obese or overweight still need to practice weight management. Some healthcare professionals use the term "nutritional disorders" to cover all disorders related to weight.

Purpose

The purpose of weight management is to help patients achieve and stay at the best weight possible for their overall health, occupation, and living situation. It may also be necessary for the prevention and treatment of diseases and disorders associated with obesity or with eating disorders. These disorders include depression and other psychiatric disturbances, in addition to the physical problems associated with nutritional disorders.

Demographics

Obesity has become a major public health concern in the last decade. Obesity ranks second only to smoking as a major cause of preventable deaths in the United States. It is estimated that 300,000 people die in the United States each year from weight-related causes. The proportion of overweight adults in the general population has continued to rise since the 1960s. According to a report published in 2010 by the National Health and Nutrition Examination Survey (NCHS), more than one-third of adults and almost 17% of youth were obese.

The prevalence of obesity in the United States varies somewhat according to sex, age, race, and socioeconomic status. Data from 2011 stated that more than one-third of U.S. adults (35.7%) are obese. The prevalence of obesity in men was virtually equal to that in women according to a report published in 2010 by the U.S. Department of Health and Human Services. In 2008, obesity among men was generally similar at all income levels with a tendency to be slightly higher at higher income levels. Higher income women are less likely to be obese than low income women. According to a report from the Centers for Disease Control and Prevention, obesity may become a leading cause of mortality in the United States with an estimated 500,000 deaths per year. During the past 20 years, there has been a dramatic increase in obesity in the United States. In 2008, medical costs associated with obesity were estimated at $147 billion. Non-Hispanic blacks have the highest age-adjusted rates of obesity (49.5 %) compared with Mexican Americans (40.4 %), all Hispanics (39.1%) and non-Hispanic whites (34.3%). In 2011, individual state data concludes that obesity prevalence ranges from 20.7 % in Colorado to 34.9 % in Mississippi.

Obesity may be responsible for:

• type 2 diabetes

• coronary heart disease

• gallstone attacks

KEY TERMS

Anorexia nervosa—An eating disorder marked by refusal to eat, intense fear of obesity, and distortions of body image.

Appetite suppressant—A medication given to reduce the desire to eat.

Bariatrics—The branch of medicine that deals with the prevention and treatment of obesity and related disorders.

Binge—A time-limited bout of excessive indulgence in eating; consuming a larger amount of food within a limited period of time than most people would eat in similar circumstances.

Binge eating disorder—An eating disorder in which the person binges, but does not try to get rid of the food afterward by vomiting, using laxatives, or exercising.

Body mass index (BMI)—A measurement that has replaced weight as the preferred determinant of obesity. The BMI can be calculated (in American units) as 703.1 times a person's weight in pounds divided by the square of the person's height in inches.

Bulimia nervosa—An eating disorder marked by episodes of binge eating followed by purging, over-exercising, or other behaviors intended to prevent weight gain.

Ephedra—A herb used in traditional Chinese medicine to treat asthma and hay fever. It should never be used for weight management.

Hoodia—A succulent African plant resembling a cactus said to contain a natural appetite suppressant.

Obesity—Excessive weight gain due to accumulation of fat in the body, sometimes defined as a BMI of 30 or higher, or body weight greater than 30% above a person's desirable weight on standard height-weight tables.

Prevalence—The number of cases of a disease or disorder that are present in a given population at a specific time.

Sedentary—Characterized by inactivity and lack of exercise. A sedentary lifestyle is a major risk factor for becoming overweight or obese.

• cases of hypertension

• breast cancers

• colon cancers

• pulmonary function impairment

• endocrine abnormalities

• obstetric complications

• trauma to weight-bearing joints

In addition, obesity intensifies the pain of osteoarthritis and gout, increases the risk of complications in pregnancy and childbirth, contributes to depression and other mental disorders, and makes a person a poor candidate for surgery. Many **surgeons** refuse to operate on patients who weigh more than 300 lb. (136 kg).

According to statistics for 2012 compiled by the National Association of Anorexia Nervosa and Associated Disorders (ANAD), almost 50% of people with eating disorders also meet the criteria for depression. Up to 24 million people of all ages and genders suffer from an eating disorder (anorexia, bulimia, and binge eating disorder) in the United States.

The long-term health consequences of eating disorders include gum disease and loss of teeth, irregular heart rhythm, disturbances in the chemical balance of the blood, and damage to the digestive tract. Eating disorders have the highest mortality rate of any mental illness. A study by the National Association of Anorexia Nervosa and Associated Disorders reported that 5%–10% of people with anorexia die within 10 years after contracting the disease, 18%–20% die within 20 years, and only 30%–40% fully recover. The mortality rate associated with anorexia nervosa is 12 times higher than the death rate of all causes of death for females 15–24 years old.

Description

The term "weight management" reflects a change in thinking about the treatment for obesity and being overweight during the past 20 years. Before 1980, treatment of overweight people focused on weight loss, with the goal of helping the patient reach an ideal weight as defined by standard life insurance height-weight charts. In recent years, however, researchers have discovered that most of the negative health consequences of obesity are improved or controlled by a relatively modest weight loss, perhaps as little as 10% of the patient's body weight. It is not necessary for the person to reach the ideal weight to benefit from weight management. Some nutritionists refer to this treatment goal as the

"10% solution." Second, the fact that most obese people who lose large amounts of weight from reduced-calorie diets regain it within five years has led nutrition experts to emphasize weight management rather than weight loss as an appropriate outcome of treatment.

Overweight and obese

Overweight and obese are not the same thing. People who are overweight weigh more than they should compared with set standards for their height. The excess weight may come from muscle tissue, bone, and body water, as well as from fat. A person who is obese has too much fat in comparison to other types of body tissue; hence, it is possible to be overweight without being obese.

There are several ways to determine whether someone is obese. Some measures are based on the relationship between the person's height and weight. The older measurements of this correlation are the so-called height-weight tables that list desirable weights for a given height. A more accurate measurement of obesity is body mass index, or BMI. The BMI is an indirect measurement of the amount of body fat. The BMI is calculated in American measurements by multiplying a person's weight in pounds by 703.1, and dividing that number by the person's height in inches squared. A BMI between 19 and 24 is considered normal; 25–29 is overweight; 30–34 is moderately obese; 35–39 is severely obese; and 40 or higher is defined as morbidly obese. More direct methods of measuring body fat include measuring the thickness of the skin fold at the back of the upper arm, and bioelectrical impedance analysis (BIA). Bioelectrical impedance analysis measures the total amount of water in the body by calculating the different degrees of resistance to an electrical current in different types of body tissue. Fatty tissue has a higher resistance to the current than body tissues containing larger amounts of water. A higher percentage of body water indicates a greater amount of lean tissue.

Eating disorders

Eating disorders are a group of psychiatric disturbances defined by unhealthy eating or weight management practices. Anorexia nervosa is an eating disorder in which people restrict their food intake severely, refuse to maintain a normal body weight, and express intense fear of becoming obese. Bulimia nervosa is a disorder marked by episodes of binge eating followed by attempts to avoid weight gain from the food by abusing **laxatives**, forcing vomiting, or over-exercising. A third type, binge eating disorder, is found in some obese people, as well as in people of normal weight. In binge eating disorder, the person has an eating binge but does not try to get rid of the food after eating it. Although most patients diagnosed with anorexia or bulimia are women, 40% of patients with binge eating disorder are men. An estimated 10%–15% of people with anorexia or bulimia are males.

To understand the goals and structure of nutritionally sound weight management programs, it is helpful to look first at the causes of being overweight, obesity, and eating disorders.

Causes of nutrition-related disorders

GENETIC/BIOLOGIC. Studies of twins separated at birth and research with genetically altered mice have shown that there is a genetic component to obesity. Some researchers think that there are also genetic factors involved in eating disorders.

LIFESTYLE-RELATED. The ready availability of relatively inexpensive, but high-caloric snacks and "junk food" is considered to contribute to the high rates of obesity in developed countries. In addition, the fast pace of modern life encourages people to select quick-cooking processed foods that are high in calories, rather than making meals that are more healthful but take longer to prepare. Lastly, changes in technology and transportation patterns mean that people today do not do as much walking or hard physical labor as earlier generations did. This sedentary or inactive lifestyle makes it easier for people to gain weight.

SOCIOCULTURAL. In recent years, many researchers have examined the role of advertising and the mass media in encouraging unhealthy eating patterns. On the one hand, advertisements for such items as fast food, soft drinks, and ice cream often convey the message that food can be used to relieve stress, reward or comfort oneself, or substitute for a fulfilling human relationship. On the other hand, the media also portray unrealistic images of human physical perfection. Their emphasis on slenderness as essential to beauty, particularly in women, is often cited as a major factor in the increase of eating disorders over the past three decades.

Another sociocultural factor that contributes to obesity among some Hispanic and Asian groups is the belief that children are not healthy unless they look plump. Overfeeding in infancy and early childhood, unfortunately, makes weight management in adolescence and adult life much more difficult. Eating disorders are one of the most common psychological problems facing women in Japan.

MEDICATIONS. Recent research has found that a number of prescription medications can contribute to weight gain. These drugs include steroid hormones, antidepressants, benzodiazepine tranquilizers, lithium, and antipsychotic medications.

Aspects of weight management

Since the late 1980s, nutritionists and healthcare professionals have come to recognize that successful weight management programs have three characteristics, including:

- They present weight management as a lifetime commitment to healthful patterns of eating and exercise, rather than emphasizing strict dieting alternating with carelessness about eating habits.
- They are tailored to each person's age, general health, living situation, and other individual characteristics.
- They recognize that the emotional, psychological, and spiritual dimensions of human life are as important to maintaining a healthy lifestyle as the medical and nutritional facets.

NUTRITION. The nutritional aspect of weight management programs includes education about healthful eating, as well as modifying the person's food intake.

DIETARY REGULATION. Most weight-management programs are based on a diet that supplies enough vitamins and minerals; 50–63 grams of protein each day; an adequate intake of carbohydrates (100 g) and dietary fiber (20–30 g); and no more than 30% of each day's calories from fat. Good weight-management diets are intended to teach people how to make wise food choices and to encourage gradual weight loss. Some diets are based on fixed menus, while others are based on food exchanges. In a food-exchange diet, a person can choose among several items within a particular food group when following a menu plan. For example, if a person's menu plan allows for two items from the vegetable group at lunch, they can have one raw and one cooked vegetable, or one serving of vegetable juice along with another vegetable.

NUTRITIONAL EDUCATION. Nutritional counseling is important to successful weight management because many people, particularly those with eating disorders, do not understand how the body uses food. They may also be trying to manage their weight in unhealthy ways. One recent study of adolescents found that 32% of the females and 17% of the males were using such potentially dangerous methods of weight control as smoking, fasting, over-the-counter (OTC) diet pills, or laxatives.

Exercise

Regular physical **exercise** is a major part of weight management because it increases the number of calories used by the body and because it helps the body to replace fat with lean muscle tissue. Exercise also serves to lower emotional stress levels and to promote a general sense of well-being. People should consult with a doctor before beginning an exercise program, however, to make sure that the activity that interests them is safe relative to any other health problems they may have. For example, people with osteoarthritis should avoid high-impact sports that are hard on the knee and ankle joints. Good choices for most people include swimming, walking, cycling, and yoga or other stretching exercises.

Psychological/psychiatric

Both obesity and eating disorders are associated with a variety of psychiatric disorders, most commonly major depression and substance abuse. Some obese people may feel harshly judged and criticized by others, and fear of obesity is a major factor in the development of both anorexia and bulimia. Many people find medications and/or psychotherapy to be a helpful part of a weight management program.

MEDICATIONS. In recent years, doctors have been cautious about prescribing appetite suppressants, which are drugs given to reduce the desire for food. In 1997, the U.S. Food and Drug Administration (FDA) banned the sale of two drugs: fenfluramine and phentermine (known as "fen-phen") when they were discovered to cause damage to heart valves. An appetite suppressant known as sibutramine (Meridia) was approved as safe in 1997, but it was removed from the market by the FDA in 2010 due to concerns over increased risk for stroke and other cardiovascular events. Another new drug that is sometimes prescribed for weight management is called orlistat (Xenical). It works by lowering the amount of dietary fat that is absorbed by the body. However, it can cause significant diarrhea or intestinal gas.

People with eating disorders are sometimes given antidepressant medications, most often fluoxetine (Prozac) or venlafaxine, to relieve the symptoms of depression or anxiety that often accompany eating disorders.

COGNITIVE-BEHAVIORAL THERAPY. Cognitive-behavioral therapy (CBT) is a form of psychotherapy that has been shown to be effective in reinforcing the changes in food selection and eating patterns that are necessary for successful weight management. In this form of therapy, usually offered in specialized clinics, patients learn to modify their eating habits by keeping diaries and records of what they eat, what events or feelings trigger overeating, and any other patterns that they notice about their choice of foods or eating habits. They also examine their attitudes toward food and weight management, and work to change any attitudes that are self-defeating or interfere with a healthy lifestyle. Most CBT programs also include nutritional education and counseling, but some researchers maintain that more work needs to be done on the use of CBT in real-world settings, not just university-related specialized clinics.

WEIGHT-MANAGEMENT GROUPS. Many doctors and nutritional counselors suggest that patients attend a weight-management group for social support. Social support is essential in weight management, especially for people who struggle with feelings of shame. Many people with obesity or an eating disorder may isolate themselves from others because they are afraid of being teased or criticized for their appearance. Such groups as Overeaters Anonymous (OA) or Take Off Pounds Sensibly (TOPS) help members in several ways: they help to reduce any levels of shame and anxiety that members feel; they teach strategies for coping with setbacks in weight management; they provide settings for making new friends; and they help people learn to handle problems in their workplace or in relationships with family members. Additional support groups and resources can be found by researching associations such as the National Association of Anorexia Nervosa or Associated Disorders, or The National Eating Disorders Association (NEDA).

ANTI-DISCRIMINATION GROUPS. Another approach to weight-related psychological issues is tackling public discrimination against overweight people, including educational and employment discrimination as well as verbal harassment and teasing. The two major groups in the United States are the Council on Size and Weight Discrimination (CSWD) and the National Association to Advance Fat Acceptance (NAAFA). The CWSD describes itself as "a not-for-profit group which works to change people's attitudes about weight. We act as consumer advocates for larger people, especially in the areas of medical treatment, job discrimination, and media images." NAAFA states its goals as "eliminat[ing] discrimination based on body size and provid[ing] fat people with the tools for self-empowerment through public education, advocacy, and member support."

Surgical

Bariatric surgery is the most successful approach to weight management for people who are morbidly obese (BMI of 40 or greater), or severely obese with additional health complications. Surgical treatment of obesity usually results in a large weight loss that is successfully maintained for longer than five years. The most common surgical procedures for weight management are **vertical banded gastroplasty** (VBG), sometimes referred to as "stomach stapling," and **gastric bypass**. Vertical banded gastroplasty works by limiting the amount of food the stomach can hold, while gastric bypass works by preventing normal absorption of the nutrients in the food.

Complementary and alternative medicine (CAM) approaches

Some forms of complementary and alternative medicine are beneficial additions to weight management programs.

MOVEMENT THERAPIES. Movement therapies include a number of forms of exercise, such as tai chi, yoga, dance therapy, Trager work, and the Feldenkrais method. Many of these approaches help people improve their posture and move their bodies more easily as well as keeping active. Tai chi and yoga, for example, are good for people who must avoid high-impact physical work-outs. Yoga can also be adapted to a person's individual needs or limitations with the help of a qualified teacher following a doctor's recommendations. Books and videos on yoga and weight management are available through most bookstores or the American Yoga Association.

SPIRITUAL AND RELIGIOUS PRACTICE. Prayer, meditation, and regular religious worship have been linked to reduced emotional stress in people struggling with weight issues. In addition, many people find that spiritual practice helps them to keep a healthy perspective on weight management, so that it does not crowd out other important interests and concerns in their lives.

HERBAL PREPARATIONS. The one type of alternative treatment that people should be extremely cautious about making part of a weight management program is over-the-counter herbal preparations advertised as "fat burners," muscle builders, or appetite suppressants. Within a two-week period in early 2003, the national media carried accounts of death or serious illness from taking these substances. One was ephedra, an herb used in traditional Chinese medicine that can cause strokes, heart attacks, seizures, and psychotic episodes. The other was usnic acid, a compound derived from lichens that can cause liver damage.

Another herbal preparation that has received considerable media attention since 2004 is hoodia (*Hoodia gordonii*), a succulent plant similar to a cactus that is native to South Africa and Namibia. Used for generations by the native inhabitants of these parts of Africa to treat indigestion, hoodia was studied by several pharmaceutical companies in the early 2000s as a natural appetite suppressant. In 2002, one such company stopped its research into hoodia on the grounds that it has potentially severe side effects on the liver. Nonetheless, hoodia has been featured on such popular television shows as *60 Minutes*, and is marketed in various diet products.

However, there is no scientific evidence that hoodia is effective in curbing appetite, and it is not recommended by any professional medical or nutrition society.

Results

Much more research needs to be done to improve the success of weight management programs. A position paper published by the Academy of Nutrition and Dietetics summarizes the present situation: "Although our knowledge base has greatly expanded regarding the complex causation of increased body fat, little progress has been made in long-term maintenance interventions, with the exception of surgery." A study published in the *Journal of the American Medical Association* showed that neither subjects randomly assigned to a commercial weight loss program nor those assigned to a self-help weight loss program lost more than a modest amount of weight and succeeded in keeping it off over a two-year period. Most adults in weight maintenance programs find it difficult to change eating patterns learned over a lifetime. Furthermore, their efforts are all too often undermined by friends or relatives, as well as by media messages that encourage overeating or the use of food as a mood-enhancing drug. More effective weight maintenance programs may well depend on broad-based changes in society.

Resources

BOOKS

American Psychiatric Association. "Eating Disorders." In *Diagnostic and Statistical Manual of Mental Disorders.* 5th ed. Arlington, VA: American Psychiatric Publishing, 2013.

Brownell, Kelly, ed. *Weight Bias: Nature, Consequences, and Remedies.* New York: Guilford Press, 2005.

Fairburn, Christopher, and Kelly Brownell. *Eating Disorders and Obesity: A Comprehensive Handbook.* 2nd ed. New York: Guilford Press, 2002.

Hornbacher, Marya. *Wasted: A Memoir of Anorexia and Bulimia.* New York: Harper Perennial Editions, 1999.

Murphy, Wendy. *Weight and Health.* Minneapolis, MN: Twenty First Century Books, 2008.

Pelletier, Kenneth R., "CAM Therapies for Specific Conditions: Obesity." In *The Best Alternative Medicine*, Part II. New York: Simon & Schuster, 2002.

Schauer, Philip. *Bariatric Surgery and Weight Management.* Cleveland, OH: Cleveland Clinic Press, 2008.

PERIODICALS

Bellafante, Ginia. "When Midlife Seems Just an Empty Plate." *New York Times*, March 9, 2003. http://query.nytimes.com/gst/fullpage.html?res=950DEED6103FF93AA35750C0A9659C8B63&scp=1&sq=When+Midlife+Seems+Just+an+Empty+Plate&st=nyt (accessed September 26, 2013).

Bindra, Jasjit S. "A Popular Pill's Hidden Dangers." *New York Times*, April 26, 2005. http://query.nytimes.com/gst/fullpage.html?res=9505E3D71231F935A15757C0A9639C8B63 (accessed September 26, 2013).

Chass, Murray. "Pitcher's Autopsy Points to Ephedra As One Factor." *New York Times*, March 14, 2003. http://www.nytimes.com/2003/03/14/sports/baseball/14BASE.html (accessed September 26, 2013).

Cummings, S., E. S. Parham, and G. W. Strain. "Position of the American Dietetic Association: Weight Management." *Journal of the American Dietetic Association* 102 (August 2002): 1145–1155.

Drohan, S. H. "Managing Early Childhood Obesity in the Primary Care Setting: A Behavior Modification Approach." *Pediatric Nursing* 28 (November–December 2002): 599–610.

Foster, Gary D., Angela P. Makris, and Brooke A. Bailer. "Behavioral Treatment of Obesity." *American Journal of Clinical Nutrition* 82 (July 2005): 230S–235S.

Heshka, Stanley, James W. Anderson, Richard L. Atkinson, et al. "Weight Loss with Self-help Compared with a Structured Commercial Program." *Journal of the American Medical Association* 289 (April 9, 2003): 1792–1798.

Holt, Richard I. G. "Obesity—An Epidemic of the Twenty-First Century: An Update for Psychiatrists." *Journal of Psychopharmacology* 19, no. 6 (2005): 6–15.

"Hoodia: Lose Weight Without Feeling Hungry?" *Consumer Reports* 71 (March 2006): 49.

James, W. Philip T. "The SCOUT Study: Risk-Benefit Profile of Sibutramine in Overweight High-Risk Cardiovascular Patients." *European Heart Journal* 7, suppl. (2005): L44–L48.

Lowry, R., D. A. Galuska, J. E. Fulton, et al. "Weight Management Goals and Practices Among U.S. High School Students: Associations with Physical Activity, Diet, and Smoking." *Journal of Adolescent Health* 31 (August 2002): 133–144.

WEBSITES

National Institute of Diabetes & Digestive & Kidney Diseases. "Choosing a Safe and Successful Weight-Loss Program." Weight-control Information Network. http://win.niddk.nih.gov/publications/choosing.htm (accessed September 26, 2013).

National Institute of Diabetes & Digestive & Kidney Diseases. "Do You Know the Health Risks of Being Overweight?" Weight-control Information Network. http://win.niddk.nih.gov/publications/health_risks.htm (accessed September 26, 2013).

National Institute of Diabetes & Digestive & Kidney Diseases. "Weight Loss for Life." Weight-control Information Network. http://win.niddk.nih.gov/publications/for_life.htm (accessed September 26, 2013).

ORGANIZATIONS

Academy of Nutrition and Dietetics, 120 S. Riverside Plz., Ste. 2000, Chicago, IL 60606-6995, (312) 899-0040, (800) 877-1600, http://www.eatright.org.

American Society for Metabolic and Bariatric Surgery, 100 SW 75th St., Ste. 201, Gainesville, FL 32607, (352) 331-4900, Fax: (352) 331-4975, info@asmbs.org, http://asmbs.org.

Obesity Society, 8757 Georgia Ave., Ste. 1320, Silver Spring, MD 20910, (301) 563-6526, Fax: (301) 563-6595, http://www.obesity.org.

Overeaters Anonymous, 6075 Zenith Ct. NE, Rio Rancho, NM 87144-6424, (505) 891-2664, http://www.oa.org.

Weight-control Information Network (WIN), 1 WIN Way, Bethesda, MD 20892-3665, (877) 946-4627, win@info. niddk.nih.gov, http://www.win.niddk.nih.gov.

Rebecca Frey, PhD
Tammy Allhoff, CST/CSFA, AAS

Weight-loss surgery *see* **Gastric bypass; Liposuction; Vertical banded gastroplasty**

Whipple procedure

Definition

A Whipple procedure, or pancreaticoduodenectomy, is a surgical procedure that generally removes the head of the pancreas, the majority of the duodenum (the first part of the small intestine), part or all of the common bile duct, and possibly the gallbladder. It sometimes includes removal of part of the stomach or the body of the pancreas. It is most often performed to treat pancreatic cancer.

Purpose

A Whipple procedure is the most common surgery for cancer of the pancreas. It may also be performed for cancer of the duodenum, cancer of the bile duct (cholangiocarcinoma), cancer of the ampulla (the area where the bile and pancreatic ducts enter the small intestine), and for chronic pancreatitis and benign (noncancerous) tumors involving the pancreatic head.

Demographics

The American Cancer Society estimates that 43,920 cases of pancreatic cancer were diagnosed in the United States in 2012, affecting approximately equal numbers of males and females. An estimated 34,290 people died of pancreatic cancer in 2012. The incidence of pancreatic cancer has been increasing at a rate 1.5% per year since 2004. Most people diagnosed with pancreatic cancer are over age 60.

Risk factors for the development of pancreatic cancer include smoking, a history of diabetes, a family

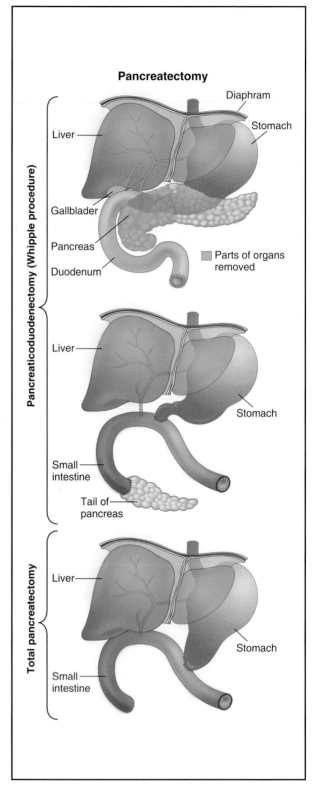

Pancreatectomy

Pancreaticoduodenectomy (Whipple procedure)

Liver — Diaphram — Stomach — Gallblader — Pancreas — Duodenum — ■ Parts of organs removed

Liver — Stomach — Small intestine — Tail of pancreas

Total pancreatectomy

Liver — Stomach — Small intestine

In a Whipple procedure, the gallbladder, duodenum, and pancreatic head are removed. The tail of the pancreas is attached to the remainder of the small intestine. *(Illustration by Electronic Illustrators Group. Copyright © Cengage Learning®.)*

history of pancreatic cancer, and a personal history of chronic pancreatitis. Environmental factors, such as certain workplace exposures or a high-fat diet, may also increase an individual's risk of pancreatic cancer.

Description

The pancreas is an organ located near the liver on the right side of the body. The exocrine pancreas produces digestive juices, and the endocrine pancreas produces hormones such as insulin, which is involved in the regulation of blood sugar and overall metabolism. Pancreatic cancer most often affects the exocrine pancreas, and the Whipple procedure is the most common surgery for removing tumors of the exocrine pancreas. It is also sometimes used to treat cancers of the endocrine pancreas.

Procedure

Although it was originally described by an Italian surgeon in 1898, the Whipple procedure is named after Dr. Alan O. Whipple, an American surgeon who developed an improved form of the surgery in 1935 and subsequently devised multiple refinements. It is a lengthy and complex operation, lasting between four and ten hours. It is only performed by experienced and skilled **surgeons**. **General anesthesia** is required.

A classic Whipple procedure requires a large abdominal incision. However, a minimally invasive laparoscopic Whipple procedure is now available. Laparoscopic surgery is performed through four small abdominal incisions, using a fiber-optic laparoscope and miniaturized **surgical instruments**, with or without robotic assistance.

There are several varieties of Whipple procedures. A standard Whipple procedure removes the head of the pancreas, the gallbladder, part of the duodenum, the small bottom portion of the stomach known as the pylorus (where the stomach empties into the duodenum), part of the common bile duct, and the lymph nodes near the head of the pancreas. Sometimes the body of the pancreas is also removed. A classic Whipple procedure removes 40% of the stomach as well. After the head of the pancreas has been removed, three important connections (anastomoses) must be made: the small intestine must be connected to the remains of the pancreas, to the remaining bile duct, and to the stomach. These anastomoses must be very carefully performed, so that pancreatic digestive enzymes, bile, and the contents of the stomach flow into the small intestine. Any leak may cause pancreatic juices to enter the abdomen, with the risk of severe complications. A pylorus-preserving Whipple leaves the pylorus intact. During a Whipple

procedure, a jejunostomy tube (j-tube) may be inserted temporarily into the digestive tract to maintain nutrition during recovery.

Precautions

A Whipple procedure is very complex surgery, and experienced surgeons and hospitals are associated with better outcomes. For the best outcome, patients are advised to choose a surgeon who has performed many such operations at a hospital that performs at least 20 Whipple procedures per year.

Potentially curative Whipple procedures usually treat cancers at the head of the pancreas. Since these cancers are near the bile duct, they may cause jaundice. If they are detected at an early enough stage to be completely removed by surgery, the cancer can be cured. Whipple procedures that involve other parts of the pancreas are generally only performed if all of the cancer can potentially be removed.

Preparation

Pancreatic cancer initially causes only vague symptoms and, thus, is often not diagnosed until later stages of the disease. Furthermore, pancreatic cancer spreads very quickly, so that the cancer has often widely metastasized by the time it is finally diagnosed. Symptoms of pancreatic cancer can include pain in the upper abdomen, often radiating to the back; jaundice (yellow eyes and skin); decreased appetite; weight loss; and depression.

A candidate for a Whipple procedure meets with the surgeon to discuss the details of the surgery and receive instructions on preoperative and **postoperative care**. Patients having their spleen removed during the procedure are often given certain vaccines prior to surgery, since their bodies will be less able to fight infection. Blood tests to evaluate bleeding time and an electrocardiogram (EKG) to evaluate heart function may be performed several days prior to the operation. Directly preceding surgery, an intravenous (IV) line is set to administer fluid and medications, and the patient is given a bowel prep to cleanse the bowel and prepare it for surgery.

Aftercare

Recuperation from a Whipple procedure may be slow and difficult. Depending on whether minimally invasive surgery or a traditional open incision is used, the hospital stay will range from 5 to 14 days. Because of the high likelihood of gastroparesis (slow gastric emptying), patients will remain on intravenous feeding for 5 or 6 days following the operation. A nasogastric tube may be required to remove excess stomach acid and juices that accumulate. The dietary advancement from clear liquids to full liquids, soft foods, and a regular diet is slow, with the timeframe depending on the patient's tolerance of each new step. Some patients take as long as four to six weeks for normal stomach emptying to return. A feeding tube that delivers a nutritional formula directly into the jejunum (the section of the small intestine below the duodenum) may be used if recovery is overly slow.

Following a Whipple procedure, the remaining portion of the pancreas often produces little or no digestive enzymes, and patients are prescribed pancreatic enzymes to be taken with all meals and snacks. Patients who have undergone surgery for pancreatic cancer usually must avoid large meals and fatty, greasy, or fried foods. Many patients must adhere to a low-fat diet containing 1.4–2.1 oz. (40–60 g) of fat per day for the long term. Small sips of fluids with meals can help prevent bloating, gas, abdominal cramping, and diarrhea. Patients should eat five or six small meals and snacks of nutrient-rich foods daily, with at least eight cups (237 mL) of fluids daily, taken an hour before or after meals. Nutrient beverages such as juices, smoothies, or food supplements may be taken with meals. Alcohol should be avoided. Vitamin supplements may be necessary.

A daily food journal is helpful. The amounts of specific foods, daily body weight, doses of pancreatic enzymes, bowel movements, and possibly blood glucose readings should be recorded. Such a journal can assist a physician or dietitian in making additional dietary recommendations.

Risks

Whipple procedures have a high risk of complications—30%–50%. Some of these complications may be fatal. Loss of 5%–10% of pre-surgical body weight is common. Digestive difficulties and other complications may be long term.

The most common complication of a Whipple procedure is delayed gastric emptying, in which the stomach takes too long to empty after meals, affecting approximately 19% of patients. Generally, the stomach begins to function properly after seven to ten days; however, if gastroparesis persists, a supplemental feeding tube may be necessary. The most serious potential complication of a Whipple procedure is leakage of pancreatic juices into the abdomen at the point where the pancreas connects with the intestine or other connections with the intestine. This occurs in approximately 10% of patients. Such leakage can cause infection or digestion of internal organs by the pancreatic enzymes: this can result in perforations (holes) in the intestine, stomach, or other nearby organs; abnormal connections between organs (fistulas); or necrosis (cell death) within an affected

---

KEY TERMS

Duodenum—The first portion of the small intestine, which connects with the bile and pancreatic ducts.

Fistula—An abnormal connection between two organs or between an organ and the outside of the body.

Gallbladder—The sac that stores bile from the liver.

Gastroparesis—Partial paralysis of the stomach, as can occur after a Whipple procedure.

Jaundice—A yellowish cast to the whites of the eyes and/or the skin, caused by excess bilirubin circulating in the bloodstream.

Jejunostomy tube—J-tube; a feeding tube that goes directly into the small intestine.

Laparoscopic surgery—Surgical procedures performed with a laparoscope through small incisions in the abdomen.

Pancreas—The organ beneath the stomach that produces digestive juices, insulin, and other hormones.

Pancreatitis—Inflammation of the pancreas.

Pylorus—The opening from the stomach into the small intestine.

Spleen—An abdominal organ that is involved in the filtration and storage of blood and the production of immune system cells.

---

organ. Whipple procedures can also result in complications due to general anesthesia or cause excessive bleeding or diabetes.

Results

Although recuperation times may be long, most patients return to their previous level of functioning and quality of life after a Whipple procedure. However, the risk of further advancement of the pancreatic cancer and death is very high, even though many patients receive chemotherapy and radiation treatments in addition to the surgery.

Morbidity and mortality

Whipple procedures have high rates of morbidity and mortality. When performed in cancer centers by experienced surgeons, less than 5% of patients die as a direct result of surgical complications; however, in small hospitals or with less experienced surgeons, fatality rates from the procedure may exceed 15%.

Only about 10% of pancreatic cancers appear to be contained entirely within the pancreas at the time of diagnosis, and once surgery has commenced, only about half of these contained cancers are truly resectable. Even when all of the cancer appears to have been removed, cancer cells have usually escaped from the pancreas and eventually affect other parts of the body. Nevertheless, surgery is the only curative option for exocrine pancreatic cancer. About 20% of all Whipple procedure patients survive for five years after their initial diagnosis of pancreatic cancer. Patients with no lymph node involvement at the time of surgery have a higher five-year survival rate of about 40%, compared with a five-year survival rate of only 5% with chemotherapy alone.

Certain conditions have better prognoses. Periampullary carcinoma that causes early obstructive jaundice, for example, has a Whipple procedure mortality rate of 3%–5%, a complete cancer removal rate of 70%, and a five-year survival rate of 20%–40%. Pancreatic neuroendocrine tumors are much more likely to be cured by a Whipple procedure than other types of pancreatic cancer. However, this treatment may involve removing the spleen, making patients more susceptible to infection.

Health care team roles

A Whipple procedure is performed in a hospital **operating room**. It is considered one of the most technically difficult operations and should be performed only by experienced, skilled surgeons who have successfully performed many such procedures. General surgeons, surgical gastroenterologists, and surgical oncologists usually perform Whipple procedures.

Resources

PERIODICALS

Fisher, William E., et al. "Assessment of the Learning Curve for Pancreaticoduodenectomy." *American Journal of Surgery* 206, no. 6 (June 2012): 684–90.

WEBSITES

American Cancer Society. "Surgery for Pancreatic Cancer." http://www.cancer.org/cancer/pancreaticcancer/detailed guide/pancreatic-cancer-treating-surgery (accessed April 5, 2013).

Pancreatic Cancer Action Network. "Nutrition After a Whipple Procedure." http://www.pancan.org/section_facing_pancreatic_cancer/learn_about_pan_cancer/diet_and_nutrition/After_Whipple_procedure.php (accessed April 5, 2013).

Pancreatic Cancer Action Network. "Whipple Procedure." http://www.pancan.org/section_facing_pancreatic_cancer/learn_about_pan_cancer/treatment/surgery/Whipple_procedure.php (accessed April 5, 2013).

Venugopal, Roshni L. "Pylorus-Preserving Pancreaticoduodenectomy (Whipple Procedure)." Medscape Reference. http://emedicine.medscape.com/article/1893199-overview (accessed April 5, 2013).

ORGANIZATIONS

American Cancer Society, 250 Williams St. NW, Atlanta, GA 30303, (800) 227-2345, http://www.cancer.org.

Pancreatic Cancer Action Network, 1500 Rosecrans Ave., Ste. 200, Manhattan Beach, CA 90226, (310) 725-0025, (877) 272-6226, Fax: (310) 725-0029, info@pancan.org, http://www.pancan.org.

Rosalyn Carson-DeWitt, MD
Margaret Alic, PhD

White blood cell count and differential

Definition

A white blood cell (WBC) count determines the concentration of white blood cells in the patient's blood. A differential determines the percentage of each of the five types of mature white blood cells.

Purpose

A WBC count is included in general health examinations and to help investigate a variety of illnesses. An elevated WBC count occurs in infection, allergy, systemic illness, inflammation, tissue injury, and leukemia. A low WBC count may occur in some viral

KEY TERMS

Band cell—An immature neutrophil at the stage just preceding a mature cell. The nucleus of a band cell is unsegmented.

Basophil—Segmented white blood cell with large dark blue-black granules that releases histamine in allergic reactions.

Cytoplasm—The part of a cell outside of the nucleus.

Differential—Blood test that determines the percentage of each type of white blood cell in a person's blood.

Eosinophil—Segmented white blood cell with large orange-red granules that increases in response to parasitic infections and allergic reactions.

Lymphocyte—Mononuclear white blood cell that is responsible for humoral (antibody mediated) and cell mediated immunity.

Monocyte—Mononuclear phagocytic white blood cell that removes debris and microorganisms by phagocytosis and processes antigens for recognition by immune lymphocytes.

Neutrophil—Segmented white blood cell normally comprising 50%–70% of the total. The cytoplasm contains both primary and secondary granules that take up both acidic and basic dyes of the Wright stain. Neutrophils remove and kill bacteria by phagocytosis.

Nucleus—The part of a cell that contains the DNA.

Phagocytosis—A process by which a white blood cell envelopes and digests debris and microorganisms to remove them from the blood.

infections, immunodeficiency states, and bone marrow failure. The WBC count provides clues about certain illnesses, and helps physicians monitor a patient's recovery from others. Abnormal counts that return to normal indicate that the condition is improving, while counts that become more abnormal indicate that the condition is worsening. The differential will reveal which WBC types are affected most. For example, an elevated WBC count with an absolute increase in lymphocytes having an atypical appearance is most often caused by infectious mononucleosis. The differential will also identify early WBCs, which may be reactive (e.g., a response to acute infection) or the result of a leukemia.

Description

White cell counts are usually performed using an automated instrument, but may be done manually using a microscope and a counting chamber, especially when counts are very low, or if the patient has a condition known to interfere with an automated WBC count.

An automated differential may be performed by an electronic cell counter or by an image analysis instrument. When the electronic WBC count is abnormal or a cell population is flagged, meaning that one or more of the results is atypical, a manual differential is performed. The WBC differential is performed manually by microscopic examination of a blood sample that is spread in a thin film on a glass slide. White blood cells are identified by their size, shape, and texture.

The manual WBC differential involves a thorough evaluation of a stained blood film. In addition to determining the percentage of each mature white blood cell, the following tests are preformed as part of the differential:

- An evaluation of RBC morphology includes grading of the variation in RBC size (anisocytosis) and shape (poikilocytosis); reporting the type and number of any abnormal or immature RBCs; and counting the number of nucleated RBCs per 100 WBCs.

- An estimate of the WBC count is made and compared with the automated or chamber WBC count. An estimate of the platelet count is made and compared with the automated or chamber platelet count. Abnormal platelets, such as clumped platelets or excessively large platelets, are noted on the report.

- Any immature WBCs are included in the differential count of 100 cells, and any inclusions or abnormalities of the WBCs are reported.

Precautions

Many medications affect the WBC count. Both prescription and non-prescription drugs, including herbal supplements, should be noted. Normal values for both the WBC count and differential are age-related.

Sources of error in manual WBC counting are due largely to variance in the dilution of the sample and the distribution of cells in the chamber, as well as the small number of WBCs that are counted. For electronic WBC counts and differentials, interference may be caused by small fibrin clots, nucleated red blood cells (RBCs), platelet clumping, and unlysed RBCs. Immature WBCs and nucleated RBCs may cause interference with the automated differential count. Automated cell counters may not be acceptable for counting WBCs in other body fluids, especially when the number of WBCs is less than

1,000 per microliter (μL) or when other nucleated cell types are present.

Preparation

This test requires a 3.5 mL sample of blood. Vein puncture with a needle is usually performed by a nurse or phlebotomist, a person trained to draw blood. There is no restriction on diet or physical activity.

Aftercare

Discomfort or bruising may occur at the puncture site. Pressure to the puncture site until the bleeding stops reduces bruising; warm packs relieve discomfort. Some people feel dizzy or faint after blood has been drawn and should be allowed to lie down and relax until they are stable.

Risks

Other than potential bruising at the puncture site, and/or dizziness, there are no complications associated with this test.

Results

Normal values vary with age. White blood cell counts are highest in children under one year of age, and then decrease somewhat until adulthood. The increase is largely in the lymphocyte population. Adult normal values include:

- WBC count: 4,500–11,000/μL
- polymorphonuclear neutrophils: 1800–7800/μL; (50%–70%)
- band neutrophils: 0–700/μL; (0%–10%)
- lymphocytes: 1,000–4,800/μL; (15%–45%)
- monocytes: 0–800/μL; (0%–10%)
- eosinophils: 0–450/μL; (0%–6%)
- basophils: 0–200/μL; (0%–2%)

Resources

BOOKS

Cohen, J., et al. *Infectious Diseases*. 3rd ed. St. Louis: Mosby/Elsevier, 2010.

Hoffman, Ronald, et al. *Hematology: Basic Principles and Practice*. 6th ed. Philadelphia: Saunders/Elsevier, 2013.

Long, Sarah S., Larry K. Pickering, and Charles G. Prober. *Principles and Practice of Pediatric Infectious Diseases*. 4th ed. New York: Churchill Livingstone, 2012.

McPherson, Richard A., and Matthew R. Pincus, eds. *Henry's Clinical Diagnosis and Management by Laboratory Methods*. 22nd ed. Philadelphia: Saunders/Elsevier, 2011.

WEBSITES

A.D.A.M. Medical Encyclopedia. "WBC Count." MedlinePlus. http://www.nlm.nih.gov/medlineplus/ency/article/003643.htm (accessed October 17, 2013).

American Association for Clinical Chemistry. "WBC Differential." Lab Tests Online. http://labtestsonline.org/understanding/analytes/differential (accessed October 17, 2013).

ORGANIZATIONS

American Association for Clinical Chemistry, 1850 K St. NW, Ste. 625, Washington, DC 20006, (800) 892-1400, Fax: (202) 887-5093, custserv@aacc.org, http://www.aacc.org.

Victoria E. DeMoranville
Mark A. Best
Rosalyn Carson-DeWitt, MD

Wound care

Definition

Wound care refers to the proper maintenance of a wound. A wound is a disruption in the continuity of cells—anything that causes cells that would normally be connected to become separated. Partial thickness injury is limited to the outermost layers of skin, with no damage to the dermal blood vessels. Healing occurs by regeneration of the outer layers of tissue. Full thickness injury involves loss of the dermis, extends to deeper tissue layers, and disrupts blood vessels.

Purpose

The purpose of wound care is to promote healing and prevent infection. If wounds are not properly cared for, they can result in severe consequences, including sympathetic stress response, hemorrhage and blood clotting, bacterial contamination, cell death, and immediate loss of all or part of organ functioning. The most important factor in minimizing these effects and promoting successful care is the prevention of infection, which can be accomplished by using sterile techniques when treating and dressing a wound.

Description

The first principle of wound care is the removal of nonviable tissue, including any dead tissue, slough, foreign debris, or residual material from **dressings**. Removal of nonviable tissue is referred to as **debridement**; removal of foreign matter is referred to as cleansing. Chronic wounds are usually colonized with bacteria, but are not necessarily infected. A wound is considered colonized when a limited number of bacteria are present in the wound, but are of no consequence in the healing process. A wound is considered infected when the bacterial burden overwhelms the immune response of the host, allowing the bacteria to grow unchecked. Clinical signs of infection include redness of the skin around the wound, purulent (pus-containing) drainage, foul odor, and edema (swelling).

The second principle of wound care is to provide a moist environment. This has been shown to promote skin growth and healing. Exposing wounds to air dries the surface and may impede the healing process. Gauze dressings that are kept moist in the wound—referred to as wet-to-dry dressings—help provide this environment. Generally, a saline-soaked gauze dressing is loosely placed into the wound and covered with a dry gauze dressing to prevent drying and contamination. It also supports autolytic debridement (the body's own capacity to dissolve dead tissue), absorbs exudate (thick layer of discharge), and traps bacteria, which are removed when the dressing is changed.

Preventing further injury is the third principle of wound care. This involves elimination or reduction of the condition that allowed the wound to develop. Factors that may contribute to the development of chronic wounds include losses in mobility, mental status changes, deficits of sensation, and circulatory deficits. Patients must be properly positioned to eliminate continued pressure on the chronic wound. Pressure-reducing devices, such as mattresses, cushions, supportive boots, foam wedges, and fitted shoes can be used to keep pressure off wounds.

Wound dressings

Dressings are applied to wounds to provide the proper environment for healing, absorb drainage, immobilize the wound, protect the wound and new tissue growth from mechanical injury and bacterial contamination, prevent bleeding, and provide mental and physical patient comfort. There are several types of dressings and most are designed to maintain a moist wound bed:

• Alginate is made of nonwoven fibers derived from seaweed and forms a gel as it absorbs exudate. It is used for wounds with moderate-to-heavy exudate or drainage and is changed every 12 hours to three days, depending on the amount of exudate.

• Composite dressings combine physically distinct components into a single dressing to provide bacterial protection, absorption, and adhesion. The frequency of dressing changes varies.

• Foam is used for wounds with moderate-to-heavy exudate or drainage. It is made from polyurethane and comes in various thicknesses having different absorption rates. Dressing changes occur every three to seven days.

• Gauze is available in a number of forms, including sponges, pads, ropes, strips, and rolls. It may be used with petroleum jelly, antimicrobials, or saline. Frequent changes are needed because gauze has limited moisture retention properties, and there is little protection from contamination. With removal of a dried dressing, there is a risk of wound damage to the healing skin surrounding the wound. Gauze dressings are changed two to three times a day.

• Hydrocolloid is made of gelatin or pectin and is available as a wafer, paste, or powder. While absorbing exudate, the dressing forms a gel. Hydrocolloid dressings are used for light-to-moderate exudate or drainage. Because it is almost totally occlusive, this type of dressing is not used for wounds with exposed tendon or bone; third-degree burns; or in the presence of bacterial, fungal, or viral infections or active cellulitis or vasculitis. Dressings are changed every three to seven days.

• Hydrogel is composed primarily of water and is used for wounds with minimal exudate. It is occasionally used with gauze or nonwoven sponge. Dressings are changed one to two times a day.

• Transparent film is an adhesive, waterproof membrane that keeps contaminants out while allowing oxygen and water vapor to cross through. It is used primarily for wounds with minimal exudate. It is also used as a secondary material to secure nonadhesive gauze. Dressings are changed every three to five days if the film is used as a primary dressing.

Cellular wound dressings

In cases where a wound is particularly severe, large, or a third-degree burn, cellular wound healing products may be used to close the wound and speed recovery. Cellular wound dressings help decrease the risk of infection, protect against fluid loss, lessen the need for skin grafts, and promote the healing process. These dressings provide a cover that keeps fluids from evaporating and prevents blood from oozing out once the dead skin has been removed. Some of these products grow in place and expand natural skin when it heals.

Cellular wound dressings may look and feel like skin, but they do not function exactly the same as skin because they are missing hair follicles, sweat glands, melanocytes, and Langerhans' cells. Some cellular wound dressings have a synthetic top layer structured like an epidermis. It peels away over time or is replaced with healthy skin through **skin grafting**. How these products are involved in wound repair is a subject of great scientific interest; it is known that they promote a higher rate of healing than standard wound care.

People with severe wounds, chronic wounds, burns, and ulcers can benefit from the use of cellular wound dressings:

- Apligraf is a two-layer wound dressing that contains live human skin cells combined with cow collagen. It delivers live cells from a different donor (circumcised infant foreskin). Thousands of pieces of Apligraf are produced in the laboratory from one small patch of cells from a single donor.

- Dermagraft is made from human cells placed on a dissolvable mesh material. The mesh material is gradually absorbed, and the human cells grow and replace the damaged skin after being placed on the wound or ulcer.

- Biobrane is used as a temporary dressing for a variety of wounds, including ulcers, lacerations, and full-thickness burns. It may also be used on wounds that develop on areas from which healthy skin is transplanted to cover damaged skin. It consists of an ultrathin silicone film and nylon fabric. The Biobrane is trimmed away as the wound heals, or until autografting becomes possible.

- TransCyte is used as a temporary covering over full-thickness and some partial-thickness burns until autografting is possible, as well as a temporary covering for some burn wounds that heal without autografting. It consists of human cells from circumcised infant foreskin and is grown on nylon mesh, combined with a synthetic epidermal layer. TransCyte starts with living cells, but these cells die when it is shipped in a frozen state to burn treatment facilities. The product is then thawed and stretched over a burn site. In one to two weeks, the TransCyte starts peeling off, and the surgeon trims it away as it peels.

- Integra Dermal Regeneration Template is used to treat full-thickness and some partial-thickness burns. Integra consists of two layers. The bottom layer, made of shark cartilage and collagen from cow tendons, acts as a matrix onto which a person's own cells migrate over two to three weeks. A new dermis is created as the cells gradually absorb the cartilage and collagen. The top layer is a protective silicone sheet that is peeled off after several weeks, while the bottom layer is a permanent cover. A very thin layer of the person's own skin is then grafted onto the neo-dermis.

- OrCel is also made from circumcised infant foreskin, grown on a cow collagen matrix, and used to treat donor sites in burn patients. It is also used to help treat epidermolysis bullosa, a rare skin condition in children.

Skin grafts

For burns, a skin graft will often be used. Although most **surgeons** prefer to use skin donated from another person (known as cadaver skin, or human allograft), skin donations are not always available. Surgeons must then rely on other available products, such as cellular wound dressings, for the treatment of burns. For skin grafting of full-thickness burn wounds, surgeons use healthy skin from another part of the person's own body (autografting) as a permanent treatment. Surgeons may use cellular wound dressings as a temporary covering when the skin damage is so extensive that there is not enough healthy skin available to graft initially. This helps prevent infection and fluid loss until autografting can be performed.

The survival rate for burn patients has increased considerably through the process of quickly removing dead tissue and immediately covering the wound. Burns covering half the body were routinely fatal 20 years ago, but today even people with extensive and severe burns have a good chance of survival, according to the American Burn Association.

Preparation

Effective wound care begins with an assessment of the entire patient. This includes obtaining a complete **health history** and a physical assessment. Assessing the patient assists in identifying causes and contributing factors of the wound. When examining the wound, it is important to document its size, location, appearance, and the surrounding skin. The healthcare professional should examine the wound for exudate, dead tissue, signs of infection, and drainage, and document how long the patient has had the wound. It is also important to know what treatment, if any, the patient has previously received for the wound.

The actual components of wound care include cleaning, dressing, determining frequency of dressing changes, and reevaluation. Dead tissue and debris can impede healing, and the goal of cleaning the wound is its removal. When cleaning the wound, protective goggles should be worn and sterile saline solution should be used. Povidone iodine, sodium hypochlorite, and hydrogen peroxide should never be used, as they are toxic to cells.

Gentle pressure should be used to clean the wound if there is no dead tissue. This can be accomplished by utilizing a syringe to apply the cleaning solution. If the wound has dead tissue, more pressure may be needed. Whirlpools can also be used for wounds that have a thick layer of discharge. Chemical or surgical debridement may be needed to remove excess debris.

KEY TERMS

Allograft skin—Skin donated from another person to treat burns.

Autograft skin—Use of a person's own skin to treat burns.

Dermis—The thick layer of skin below the epidermis.

Epidermis—The outermost layer of the skin.

Exudate—Fluid, cells, or other substances that are slowly discharged by tissue, especially due to injury or inflammation.

Hemostasis—Slowing down or stopping bleeding.

Langerhans' cells—Cells in the epidermis that help protect the body against infection.

Melanocytes—Cells within the epidermis that give skin its color.

Scar tissue—Scar tissue is the fibrous tissue that replaces normal tissue destroyed by injury or disease.

Aftercare

Once the wound has been treated, providing proper nutrition is the fourth principle of healing. Protein is especially essential for wound repair and cell regeneration. Amino acids also support the immune response. Adequate amounts of carbohydrates and fats are needed to prevent the amino acids from being oxidized for caloric needs. Glucose is also needed to meet the energy requirements of the cells involved in wound repair.

Risks

Various risks from wounds include:

• Hematoma. Dressings should be inspected for hemorrhage at intervals during the first 24 hours after surgery. A large amount of bleeding should be reported to a healthcare professional immediately. Concealed bleeding sometimes occurs in the wound, beneath the skin. If the clot formed is small, it will be absorbed by the body, but if large, the wound bulges and the clot must be removed for healing to continue.

• Infection. The second most frequent nosocomial (hospital-acquired) infection in hospitals is surgical wound infections with *Staphylococcus aureus*, *Escherichia coli*, and *Pseudomonas aeruginosa*. Prevention is accomplished with meticulous wound management. Cellulitis is a bacterial infection that spreads into tissue planes, and systemic antibiotics are usually prescribed

to treat it. If the infection is in an arm or leg, elevation of the limb reduces dependent edema and heat application promotes blood circulation. Abscess is a bacterial infection that is localized and characterized by pus. Treatment consists of surgical drainage or excision with the concurrent administration of antibiotics.

• Dehiscence (disruption of the surgical wound) and evisceration (protrusion of wound contents). This condition results from sutures giving way, infection, distention, and coughs. Dehiscence results in pain and the surgeon should be called immediately. Prophylactically, an abdominal binder may be utilized.

• Excessive growth of scar tissue (known as keloid scarring). Careful wound closure, hemostasis, and pressure support are used to ward off this complication.

Results

The desired result of wound care is successful wound healing and prevention of infection.

Resources

BOOKS

Baranoski, Sharon, and Elizabeth A. Ayello. *Wound Care Essentials: Practice Principles*. 3rd ed. Philadelphia: Lippincott Williams & Wilkins, 2012.

Dipietro, Luisa A., and Aime L. Burns, eds. *Wound Healing: Methods and Protocols*. Totowa, NJ: Humana Press, 2003.

Hess, Cathy Thomas. *Clinical Guide to Skin & Wound Care*. 7th ed. Philadelphia: Lippincott Williams & Wilkins, 2012.

Sheffield, Paul J., Adrianne P. S. Smith, and Caroline E. Fife, eds. *Wound Care Practice*. 2nd ed. Flagstaff, AZ: Best Pub Co., 2007.

PERIODICALS

Adkins, Carrie L. "Wound Care Dressings and Choices for Care of Wounds in the Home." *Home Healthcare Nurse* 31, no. 5 (2013): 259–67. http://dx.doi.org/10.1097/NHH.0b013e31828eb658 (accessed September 26, 2013).

Salcido, Richard. "Big Data and Disruptive Innovation in Wound Care." *Advances in Skin & Wound Care* 26, no. 8 (2013): 344. http://dx.doi.org/10.1097/01.ASW.0000432244.36301.fc (accessed September 26, 2013).

Vaienti, L., et al. "Limb Trauma: The Use of an Advanced Wound Care Device in the Treatment of Full-Thickness Wounds." *Strategies in Trauma and Limb Reconstruction* 8, no. 2 (2013): 111–15. http://dx.doi.org/10.1007/s11751-013-0165-8 (accessed September 26, 2013).

WEBSITES

MedlinePlus. "Wounds." U.S. National Library of Medicine, National Institutes of Health. http://www.nlm.nih.gov/medlineplus/wounds.html (accessed September 26, 2013).

ORGANIZATIONS

American Professional Wound Care Association, 406 W Street Rd., Feasterville, PA 19053, (215) 942-6095, wounds @apwca.org, http://www.apwca.org.

Wound Care Institute, 1100 NE 163rd St., Ste. #101, North Miami Beach, FL 33162, (305) 919-9192, FishmanTamara @hotmail.com, http://woundcare.org.

Wound Healing Society, 341 N. Maitland Ave., Ste. 130, Maitland, FL 32751, (407) 647-8839, info@woundheal. org, http://www.woundheal.org.

René A. Jackson, RN
Crystal H. Kaczkowski, MSc
Robert Bockstiegel

Wound culture

Definition

A wound culture is a diagnostic laboratory test in which microorganisms—such as bacteria or fungi from an infected wound, are grown in the laboratory on nutrient-enriched substance called media—then identified. Wound cultures always include an aerobic (with oxygen) culture, but Gram stain and anaerobic (without oxygen) cultures are not performed on every wound. These tests are performed when indicated or requested by the physician.

Purpose

The purpose of a wound culture is to isolate and identify bacteria or fungi causing an infection of the wound. Only then can **antibiotics** that will be effective in destroying the organism be identified.

Description

Wounds are injuries to body tissues caused by physical trauma or disease processes that may include surgery, diabetes, burns, punctures, gunshots, lacerations, bites, bed sores, and broken bones. Types of wounds may include:

- abrasions (caused by scraping)
- contusions (bruises or bleeding into tissue)
- incisions (formed by clean cuts)
- lacerations (tearing of skin or tissues caused by heavy pressure)
- perforations (wounds with an exit and an entry point, such as a gunshot)
- punctures (formed when something goes through the skin and into tissue)
- nonpenetrating or blunt trauma wounds (no disruption to the surface of the body; usually located in the thorax or abdomen)
- open wounds (tissues are exposed to air)
- penetrating wounds (disruption of the body surface and extension into the underlying tissue)

The chance of a wound becoming infected depends on the nature, size, and depth of the wound, its proximity to and involvement of nonsterile areas, such as the skin and gastrointestinal (GI) tract, the opportunity for organisms from the environment to enter the wound, and the immunologic, nutritional, and general health status of the person. In general, acute (sudden onset) wounds are more prone to infection than chronic (long-lasting) wounds. Wounds with a large loss of body surface, such as abrasions, are also easily infected. Puncture wounds can permit the growth of microorganisms because there is a break in the skin with minimal bleeding; they are also difficult to clean. Deep wounds, closed off from oxygen, are an ideal breeding environment for anaerobic infections. Foul-smelling odors, gas, or dead tissue at the infection site are signs of an infection caused by anaerobic bacteria. Surgical wounds can also cause infection by introducing bacteria from one body compartment into another.

Diagnosis

Diagnosing infection in a wound may be difficult. One of the chief signs the clinician looks for is slow healing. Within hours of injury, most wounds display a release of fluid, called exudate. This fluid contains compounds that aid in healing, and is normal. It should not be present 48–72 hours after injury. Exudate indicative of infection may be thicker than the initial exudate and may also be purulent (containing pus) and foul smelling. Clinicians will look at color, consistency, and the amount of exudate to monitor early infection. In addition, infected wounds may display skin discoloration, swelling, warmth to touch, and an increase in pain.

Wound infection prevents healing, and the bacteria or yeast can spread from wounds to other body parts, including the blood. Infection in the blood is termed septicemia and can be fatal. Symptoms of a systemic infection include a fever and rise in white blood cells (WBCs), along with confusion and mental status changes in the elderly. It is important to treat the infected wound early with a regimen of antibiotics to prevent further complications.

Wound infections often contain multiple organisms, including both aerobic and anaerobic gram-positive cocci and Gram-negative bacilli and yeast. The most common pathogens isolated from wounds are *Streptococcus* group A, *Staphylococcus aureus*, *Escherichia coli*, *Proteus*, *Klebsiella*, *Pseudomonas*, *Enterobacter*, *Enterococci*, *Bacteroides*, *Clostridium*, *Candida*, *Peptostreptococcus*, *Fusobacterium*, and *Aeromonas*.

The tissue used for the tests is obtained by three different methods: tissue biopsy, needle aspiration, or the swab technique. The biopsy method involves the removal of tissue from the wound using a cutting sheath. The swab technique is most commonly used, but contains the least amount of specimen.

Wound specimens are cultured on both nonselective enriched and selective media. Cultures are examined each day for growth and any colonies are Gram stained and subcultured (i.e., transferred) to appropriate media. The subcultured isolates are tested via appropriate biochemical identification panels to identify the species present. In some cases sensitivity testing will also be done. Sensitivity testing exposes the grown colonies to one or more antibiotics and monitors the response. This helps determine which antibiotics will be effective at treating the infection. The selection of antibiotics for testing depends on the organism isolated.

Preparation

A biopsy sample is usually preferred by clinicians, but this is a moderately invasive procedure and may not always be feasible. The health care professional prepares the patient by cleansing the affected area with a sterile solution, such as saline. **Antiseptics** such as ethyl alcohol are not recommended, because they kill bacteria and cause the culture results to be negative. The patient is given a local anesthetic and the tissue is removed by the practitioner, who uses a cutting sheath. Afterwards, pressure is applied to the wound to control bleeding.

Needle aspiration is less invasive and is a good technique to use in wounds where there is little loss of skin, such as in the case of puncture wounds. The skin around the wound is cleaned with an antiseptic to kill bacteria on the skin's surface, and a small needle is inserted. To obtain a sample of the fluid to be biopsied, the clinician pulls back on the plunger, then changes the angle of the needle two or three times to remove fluid from different areas of the wound. This procedure may be painful for the patient, so many initial cultures are done with the swab technique.

For a sample to be collected using the swab technique some of the wound must be exposed. A small sterile swab is inserted into the wound, or rubbed on top of the wound, rotated, and moved back and forth to collect as much fluid as possible from the wound. This is usually the least painful of the collection techniques, although it cannot be used with every type of wound. After completion of any of the three procedures, the wound should be cleaned thoroughly and bandaged.

Risks

The physician may choose to start the person on an antibiotic before the specimen is collected for culture. This may alter results, since antibiotics in the person's system may prevent microorganisms present in the wound from growing in culture. In some cases, the patient may begin antibiotic treatment after the specimen is collected. The antibiotic chosen may or may not be appropriate for one or more organisms recovered by culture.

Clinicians must be very careful when finishing a wound culture collection to ensure that the wound has been cleaned thoroughly and is bandaged properly. It is important to watch for bleeding and further infection from the procedure. In addition, patients may be in pain from the manipulation, so giving pain-killing drugs, such as **acetaminophen**, may be advised.

Results

The initial Gram-stain result is available the same day, or in less than an hour, if requested by the doctor. An early report, known as a preliminary report, is usually available after one day. After that, preliminary reports will be posted whenever an organism is identified. Cultures showing no growth are signed out after two to three days unless a slow-growing mycobacterium or fungus is found. These organisms take several weeks to grow and are held for four to six weeks. The final report includes complete identification, an estimate of the quantity of the microorganisms, and a list of the antibiotics to which each organism is sensitive and resistant.

Resources

BOOKS

Dealey, Carol and Janice Cameron. *Wound Management*. Malden, MA: Blackwell, 2008.

Krasner, Diane L., George T. Rodeheaver and R. Gary Sibbald, eds. *Chronic Wound Care: a Clinical Source Book for Healthcare Professionals*. 5th ed. Malvern, PA: HMP Communications, 2012.

Myers, Betsy A. *Wound Management: Principles and Practice*. 3rd ed. Upper Saddle River, NJ: Pearson/Prentice Hall, 2012.

PERIODICALS

Rushing, J. "Obtaining a Wound Culture Specimen." *Nursing* 37, no. 11 (2007): 18.

WEBSITES

American Association for Clinical Chemistry. "Bacterial Wound Culture." Lab Tests Online. http://labtestsonline.org/understanding/analytes/wound-culture (accessed October 17, 2013).

University of Rochester Medical Center. "Wound Culture." http://www.urmc.rochester.edu/encyclopedia/content.aspx?ContentTypeID=167&ContentID=wound_culture (accessed October 17, 2013).

ORGANIZATIONS

Wound Healing Society, 341 N. Maitland Ave., Ste. 130, Maitland, FL 32751, (407) 647-8839, info@woundheal.org, http://www.woundheal.org.

Jane E. Phillips, PhD
Mark A. Best, MD
Robert Bockstiegel

Wrist replacement

Definition

Wrist replacement surgery is performed to replace a wrist injured or damaged beyond repair. An artificial wrist joint replacement is implanted.

Purpose

Traumatic injuries or severe degenerative diseases affecting the wrist (such as osteoarthritis and rheumatoid arthritis with bony destruction) may require replacement of the painful wrist joint with an artificial wrist joint. The purpose of wrist replacement surgery is to restore wrist motion for activities of daily living and non-contact sports. A wrist replacement recovers lost strength by restoring length to the muscles and tendons of the fingers and wrist, and maintains a useful arc of motion and provides the stability required for an active life.

Description

Surgery to replace a wrist starts with an incision through the skin on the back of the wrist. The surgeon then moves the tendons extending over the back of the wrist out of the way to access the joint capsule on the back of the wrist joint, which is then opened to expose the wrist joint area. A portion of the carpal bones and the end of the radius and ulna are then removed from the wrist to allow room for the new artificial wrist joint. The bones of the hand and the radius bone of the forearm are prepared with the use of special instruments to form holes in the bones; the stems of the artificial joint components

can then fit in. Next, the components are inserted into the holes. After obtaining a proper fit, the surgeon verifies the range of motion of the joint to ensure that it moves correctly. Finally, the surgeon cements the two sides of the joint and replaces the tendons back into their proper position before closing the wound.

A total wrist replacement implant consists of the following components:

- An ellipsoid head that simulates the curvature of the natural wrist joint and allows for a functional range of motion. This ensures that the patient may flex and extend the wrist and move it side-to-side.

- An offset radial stem that anchors the implant in the forearm. The special shape of this component is designed to assist the function of the tendons used to extend the wrist and to ensure the stability of the implant.

- An elongated radial tray surface with a molded bearing usually made of polyethylene. This component is required to distribute forces over the entire surface of the artificial joint.

KEY TERMS

Arthritis—An inflammatory condition that affects joints.

Carpal bones—Eight wrist bones arranged in two rows that articulate proximally with the radius and indirectly with the ulna, and distally with the five metacarpal bones.

Metacarpal bones—Five cylindrical bones extending from the wrist to the fingers.

Osteoarthritis—Non-inflammatory degenerative joint disease occurring mostly in older persons accompanied by pain and stiffness, especially after prolonged activity.

Radius—One of the two forearm bones. The largest portion of the radius is at the wrist joint where it articulates with the carpal bones of the hand. Above, the radius articulates with the humerus at the elbow joint.

Rheumatoid arthritis—Chronic inflammatory disease in which there is destruction of joints.

Tendon—A fibrous, strong, connective tissue that connects muscle to bone.

Ulna—One of the two bones of the forearm. The largest section articulates with the humerus at the elbow joint and the smallest portion of the ulna articulates with the carpal bones in the wrist.

- A fixation stem that is secured to the patient's bone to add stability and eliminate rotation of the artificial joint within the bone.
- A curved metacarpal stem that secures the artificial wrist within the hand.

Preparation

The orthopedic surgeon who will perform the surgery will usually require a complete **physical examination** of the patient by the primary care physician to ensure that the patient will be in the best possible condition to undergo the surgery. The patient may also need to see the physical therapist responsible for managing rehabilitation after wrist replacement. The therapist prepares the patient before surgery to ensure readiness for rehabilitation post-surgery. The purpose of the preoperative examination is also for the physician to prerecord a baseline of information that will include measurements of the patient's current pain levels, functional wrist capacity, and the range of motion and strength of each hand.

Before surgery, patients are advised to take all of their normal medications, with the exception of blood thinners such as **aspirin**, ibuprofen, and other anti-inflammatory drugs that may cause greater blood loss during surgery. Patients may eat as they please the night before surgery, including solid food, until midnight. After midnight, patients should not eat or drink anything unless told otherwise by their doctor.

Aftercare

Following surgery, the patient's wrist, hand, and lower arm are placed into a bulky bandage and a splint. A small plastic tube may be inserted to drain any blood that gathers under the incision to prevent excessive swelling (hematoma). The tube is usually removed within 24 hours. Sutures may be removed 10–14 days after surgery.

Risks

Some of the most common risks associated with wrist replacement surgery are:

- Infection. Infection can be a very serious complication following wrist replacement surgery. Infection following wrist replacement occurs in approximately 1%–2% of cases. Some infections may appear before the patient leaves the hospital, while others may not become apparent for months, or even years, after surgery.
- Loosening. There is also a risk that the artificial joints may eventually fail, due to a loosening process where

---

QUESTIONS TO ASK YOUR DOCTOR

- Will the surgery restore my wrist flexibility?
- How long will rehabilitation require?
- What are the chances of infection?
- Is alternative treatment available?
- How many wrist replacement surgeries do you perform each year?
- What appearance will my wrist have after surgery?

---

the metal or cement meets the bone. There have been great advances in extending how long an artificial joint will last, but most will eventually loosen and require revision surgery. The risk of loosening is much greater in younger, more active people. A loose artificial wrist is a problem because of the resulting pain. Once the pain becomes unbearable, another operation is usually required to either revise the wrist replacement or perform a wrist fusion.

- Nerve injury. All of the nerves and blood vessels that go to the hand travel across the wrist joint. Wrist replacement surgery is performed very close to these structures, introducing a risk of injury either to the nerves or the blood vessels.

Results

Wrist replacement surgery often succeeds at restoring wrist function. On average, a wrist replacement is expected to last for 10–15 years.

Alternatives

An alternative to wrist replacement is wrist fusion (arthrodesis). Wrist fusion surgery eliminates pain by allowing the bones that make up the joint to grow together, or fuse, into one solid bone. The surgery reduces pain, but also reduces the patient's ability to move the wrist. Wrist fusions were very common before the invention of artificial joints, and they are still performed often.

Health care team roles

Wrist replacement surgery is performed by an orthopedic surgeon in an orthopedic hospital or in a specialized clinic.

Resources

BOOKS

Browner, Bruce D., et al. *Skeletal Trauma: Basic Science, Management, and Reconstruction.* 4th ed. Philadelphia: Saunders/Elsevier, 2009.

Canale, S. T., ed. *Campbell's Operative Orthopaedics.* 12th ed. St. Louis, MO: Mosby, 2012.

DeLee, Jesse, David Drez, and Mark D. Miller. *DeLee and Drez's Orthopaedic Sports Medicine: Principles and Practice.* 3rd ed. Philadelphia: Saunders/Elsevier, 2010.

PERIODICALS

Weiss, A. P., and E. Akelman. "Total Wrist Replacement." *Medicine and Health, Rhode Island* 95, no. 4 (2012): 117–19.

WEBSITES

American Academy of Orthopaedic Surgeons. "Preparing for Joint Replacement Surgery." OrthoInfo. http://orthoinfo.aaos.org/topic.cfm?topic=A00019 (accessed October 14, 2013).

American Academy of Orthopaedic Surgeons. "Wrist Joint Replacement (Wrist Arthroplasty)." OrthoInfo. http://orthoinfo.aaos.org/topic.cfm?topic=A00019 (accessed October 14, 2013).

ORGANIZATIONS

American Academy of Orthopaedic Surgeons (AAOS), 6300 N. River Rd., Rosemont, IL 60018-4262, (847) 823-7186, Fax: (847) 823-8125, pemr@aaos.org, http://www.aaos.org.

Monique Laberge, PhD

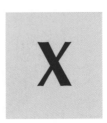

X

X-rays *see* **Bone x-rays; Skull x-rays**

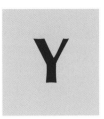

Y

YAG laser capsulotomy *see* **Laser posterior capsulotomy**

ORGANIZATIONS

The following is an alphabetical compilation of relevant organizations listed in the *Resources* sections of the main body entries. Although the list is comprehensive, it is by no means exhaustive. It is a starting point for gathering further information. Many of the organizations listed provide information for multiple disorders and have links to additional related websites. E-mail addresses and web addresses listed were provided by the associations; Gale, Cengage Learning is not responsible for the accuracy of the addresses or the contents of the websites.

A

AABB (formerly the American Association of Blood Banks)
8101 Glenbrook Rd.
Bethesda, MD 20814-2749
Phone: (301) 907-6977
Fax: (301) 907-6895
E-mail: aabb@aabb.org
Web site: http://www.aabb.org

AAGL (formerly the American Association of Gynecologic Laparoscopists)
6757 Katella Ave.
Cypress, CA 90630
Phone: (714) 503-6200
Toll free: (800) 554-2245
Web site: http://www.aagl.org

AARP (formerly the American Association of Retired Persons)
601 E. St. NW
Washington, DC 20049
Phone: (202) 434-3525
Toll free: (888) OUR-AARP (687-2277)
TTY: (877) 434-7598
Toll free: (877) 342-2277 (Spanish)
E-mail: member@aarp.org
Web site: http://www.aarp.org

ABCD (After Breast Cancer Diagnosis)
5775 N. Glen Park Rd., Ste. 201
Glendale, WI 53209
Phone: (414) 977-1780
Toll free: (800) 977-4121
Fax: (414) 977-1781
E-mail: abcdinc@abcdmentor.org
Web site: http://www.abcdbreastcancersupport.org

Academy of General Dentistry
560 W. Lake St., 6th Fl.
Chicago, IL 60611-1999
Phone: (888) AGD-DENT (243-3368)

Fax: (312) 335-3443
E-mail: membership@agd.org
Web site: http://www.agd.org

Academy of Nutrition and Dietetics
120 S. Riverside Plz., Ste. 2000
Chicago, IL 60606-6995
Phone: (312) 899-0040
Toll free: (800) 877-1600
Web site: http://www.eatright.org

Accreditation Association for Ambulatory Health Care (AAAHC)
5250 Old Orchard Rd., Ste. 200
Skokie, IL 60077
Phone: (847) 853-6060
Fax: (847) 853-9028
E-mail: info@aaahc.org
Web site: http://www.aaahc.org

Action on Smoking and Health
701 4th St. NW
Washington, DC 20001
Phone: (202) 659-4310
Fax: (202) 289-7166
E-mail: info@ash.org
Web site: http://ash.org

Administration for Community Living
One Massachusetts Ave. NW
Washington, DC 20001
Phone: (202) 619-0724
Toll free: (800) 677-1116 (Eldercare locator)
E-mail: aclinfo@acl.hhs.gov
Web site: http://acl.gov

Adult Congenital Heart Association (ACHA)
6757 Greene St., Ste. 335
Philadelphia, PA 19119-3508
Phone: (215) 849-1260
Toll free: (888) 921-ACHA (2242)
Fax: (215) 849-1261
E-mail: info@achaheart.org
Web site: http://www.achaheart.org

Agency for Healthcare Research and Quality
540 Gaither Rd.
Rockville, MD 20850
Phone: (301) 427-1104
Web site: http://www.ahrq.gov

AIDS Education and Training Centers (AETC) National Resource Center
School of Nursing, Rutgers, The State University of New Jersey, 65 Bergen St., 8th Fl.
Newark, NJ 07101
E-mail: info@aidsetc.org
Web site: http://www.aidsetc.org

AIDS*info*
PO Box 4780
Rockville, MD 20849-6303
Phone: (301) 315-2816
Toll free: (800) HIV-0440 (448-0440)
TTY: (888) 480-3739
E-mail: ContactUs@aidsinfo.nih.gov
Web site: http://aidsinfo.nih.gov

Alexander Graham Bell Association for the Deaf and Hard of Hearing
3417 Volta Pl. NW
Washington, DC 20007
Phone: (202) 337-5220
Fax: (202) 337-8314
E-mail: info@agbell.org
Web site: http://www.agbell.org

Alliance for the Prudent Use of Antibiotics
200 Harrison Ave., Posner 3 (Business)
Boston, MA 02111
Phone: (617) 636-0966
E-mail: apua@tufts.edu
Web site: http://www.tufts.edu/med/apua

Ambulatory Surgery Center Association (ASCA)
1012 Cameron St.
Alexandria, VA 22314-2427
Phone: (703) 836-8808
Fax: (703) 549-0976

E-mail: asc@ascassociation.org
Web site: http://www.ascassociation.org

American Academy for Pediatric Ophthalmology and Strabismus (AAPOS)
PO Box 193832
San Francisco, CA 94119-3832
Phone: (415) 561-8505
Fax: (415) 561-8531
E-mail: aapos@aao.org
Web site: http://www.aapos.org

American Academy of Allergy, Asthma & Immunology
555 E. Wells St., Ste. 1100
Milwaukee, WI 53202-3823
Phone: (414) 272-6071
E-mail: info@aaaai.org
Web site: http://www.aaaai.org

American Academy of Anesthesiologist Assistants (AAAA)
1231 Collier Rd. NW, Ste. J
Atlanta, GA 30318
Phone: (678) 222-4221
Fax: (404) 249-8831
E-mail: devon.bacon@politics.org
Web site: http://www.anesthetist.org

American Academy of Audiology
11480 Commerce Park Dr., Ste. 220
Reston, VA 20191
Phone: (703) 790-8466
Toll free: (800) AAA-2336 (222-2336)
Fax: (703) 790-8631
E-mail: infoaud@audiology.org
Web site: http://www.audiology.org

American Academy of Clinical Toxicology (AACT)
6728 Old McLean Village Dr.
McLean, VA 22101
Phone: (703) 556-9222
Fax: (703) 556-8729
E-mail: admin@clintox.org
Web site: http://www.clintox.org

American Academy of Cosmetic Surgery
737 N. Michigan Ave., Ste. 2100
Chicago, IL 60611-5641
Phone: (312) 981-6760
Fax: (312) 981-6787
E-mail: info@cosmeticsurgery.org
Web site: http://www.cosmeticsurgery.org

American Academy of Dermatology
930 E. Woodfield Rd.
Schaumburg, IL 60173
Phone: (847) 240-1280
Toll free: (866) 503-SKIN (7546)
Web site: http://www.aad.org

American Academy of Emergency Medicine
555 E. Wells St., Ste. 1100
Milwaukee, WI 53202-3823
Toll free: (800) 884-2236
Fax: (414) 276-3349
E-mail: info@aaem.org
Web site: http://www.aaem.org

American Academy of Facial Plastic and Reconstructive Surgery
310 S. Henry St.
Alexandria, VA 22314
Phone: (703) 299-9291
Fax: (703) 299-8898
E-mail: info@aafprs.org
Web site: http://www.aafprs.org

American Academy of Family Physicians (AAFP)
11400 Tomahawk Creek Pkwy.
Leawood, KS 66211-2680
Phone: (913) 906-6000
Toll free: (800) 274-2237
Fax: (913) 906-6075
E-mail: contactcenter@aafp.org
Web site: http://www.aafp.org

American Academy of Hospice and Palliative Medicine
8735 W. Higgins Rd., Ste. 300
Chicago, IL 60631
Phone: (847) 375-4712
Fax: (847) 375-6475
E-mail: info@aahpm.org
Web site: http://www.aahpm.org

American Academy of Implant Dentistry
211 E. Chicago Ave., Ste. 750
Chicago, IL 60611
Phone: (312) 335-1550
Toll free: (877) 335-AAID (2243)
E-mail: info@aaid.com
Web site: http://aaid.com

American Academy of Medical Acupuncture
1970 E. Grand Ave., Ste. 330
El Segundo, CA 90245
Phone: (310) 364-0193
E-mail: jdowden@prodigy.net
Web site: http://www.medicalacupuncture.org

American Academy of Neurological and Orthopaedic Surgeons
1516 N. Lakeshore Dr.
Chicago, IL 60610
Toll free: (800) 766-3427
Fax: (312) 787-9289
E-mail: nick@aanos.org
Web site: http://www.aanos.org

American Academy of Neurology
201 Chicago Ave.

Minneapolis, MN 55415
Phone: (612) 928-6000
Toll free: (800) 879-1960
Fax: (612) 454-2746
E-mail: memberservices@aan.com
Web site: http://www.aan.com

American Academy of Ophthalmology (AAO)
655 Beach St.
San Francisco, CA 94109
Phone: (415) 561-8500
Fax: (415) 561-8533
E-mail: patientinfo@aao.org
Web site: http://www.aao.org

American Academy of Orthopaedic Surgeons (AAOS)
6300 N. River Rd.
Rosemont, IL 60018-4262
Phone: (847) 823-7186
Fax: (847) 823-8125
E-mail: pemr@aaos.org
Web site: http://www.aaos.org

American Academy of Otolaryngology—Head and Neck Surgery
1650 Diagonal Rd.
Alexandria, VA 22314-2857
Phone: (703) 836-4444
Web site: http://www.entnet.org

American Academy of Pediatric Dentistry
211 E. Chicago Ave., Ste. 1700
Chicago, IL 60611-2637
Phone: (312) 337-2169
Fax: (312) 337-6329
Web site: http://www.aapd.org

American Academy of Pediatrics (AAP)
141 Northwest Point Blvd.
Elk Grove Village, IL 60007-1098
Phone: (847) 434-4000
Toll free: (800) 433-9016
Fax: (847) 434-8000
Web site: http://www.aap.org

American Academy of Sleep Medicine
2510 N. Frontage Rd.
Darien, IL 60561
Phone: (630) 737-9700
Fax: (630) 737-9790
E-mail: inquiries@aasmnet.org
Web site: http://www.aasmnet.org

American Association for Accreditation of Ambulatory Surgery Facilities (AAAASF)
PO Box 9500, 5101 Washington St., 2nd Fl.
Gurnee, IL 60031
Toll free: (888) 545-5222

Phone: (847) 775-1970
Fax: (847) 775-1985
E-mail: reception@aaaasf.org
Web site: http://www.aaaasf.org

American Association for Clinical Chemistry (AACC)
1850 K St. NW, Ste. 625
Washington, DC 20006
Toll free: (800) 892-1400
Fax: (202) 887-5093
E-mail: custserv@aacc.org
Web site: http://www.aacc.org

American Association for Hand Surgery
500 Cummings Ctr., Ste. 4550
Beverly, MA 01915
Phone: (978) 927-8330
Fax: (978) 524-8890
Web site: http://handsurgery.org

American Association for Long-Term Care Insurance (AALTCI)
3835 E. Thousand Oaks Blvd., Ste. 336
Westlake Village, CA 91362
Phone: (818) 597-3227
E-mail: info@aaltci.org
Web site: http://www.aaltci.org

American Association for Respiratory Care
9425 N. MacArthur Blvd. Ste. 100
Irving, TX 75063-4706
Phone: (972) 243-2272
E-mail: info@aarc.org
Web site: http://www.aarc.org

American Association for the Surgery of Trauma (AAST)
633 N. Saint Clair St., Ste. 2600
Chicago, IL 60611
Toll free: (800) 789-4006
Fax: (312) 202-5064
E-mail: aast@aast.org
Web site: http://www.aast.org

American Association for Thoracic Surgery (AATS)
500 Cummings Ctr., Ste. 4550
Beverly, MA 01915
Phone: (978) 927-8330
Fax: (978) 524-8890
Web site: http://www.aats.org

American Association of Cardiovascular and Pulmonary Rehabilitation (AACVPR)
330 N. Wabash Ave., Ste. 2000
Chicago, IL 60611
Phone: (312) 321-5146
Fax: (312) 673-6924
E-mail: aacvpr@aacvpr.org
Web site: https://www.aacvpr.org

American Association of Clinical Endocrinologists
245 Riverside Ave., Ste. 200
Jacksonville, FL 32202
Phone: (904) 353-7878
Fax: (904) 353-8185
Web site: https://www.aace.com

American Association of Critical-Care Nurses
101 Columbia
Aliso Viejo, CA 92656-4109
Toll free: (800) 899-AACN (2226)
Fax: (949) 362-2020
E-mail: info@aacn.org
Web site: http://www.aacn.org

American Association of Endocrine Surgeons
11300 W. Olympic Blvd., Ste. 600
Los Angeles, CA 90064
Phone: (310) 986-6452
Fax: (310) 437-0585
E-mail: information@endocrinesurgery.org
Web site: http://www.endocrinesurgery.org

American Association of Endodontists
211 E. Chicago Ave., Ste. 1100
Chicago, IL 60611-2691
Phone: (312) 266-7255
Toll free: (800) 872-3636
Fax: (312) 266-9867
E-mail: info@aae.org
Web site: http://www.aae.org

American Association of Hip and Knee Surgeons (AAHKS)
6300 N. River Rd., Ste. 615
Rosemont, IL 60018-4237
Phone: (847) 698-1200
Fax: (847) 698-0704
E-mail: helpdesk@aahks.org
Web site: http://www.aahks.org

American Association of Immunologists (AAI)
9650 Rockville Pike
Bethesda, MD 20814
Phone: (301) 634-7178
Fax: (301) 634-7887
E-mail: infoaai@aai.org
Web site: http://www.aai.org

American Association of Kidney Patients (AAKP)
2701 N. Rocky Point Dr., Ste. 150
Tampa, FL 33607
Phone: (813) 636-8100
Toll free: (800) 749-AAKP
Fax: (813) 636-8122
E-mail: info@aakp.org
Web site: http://www.aakp.org

American Association of Managed Care Nurses (AAMCN)
4435 Waterfront Dr., Ste. 101
Glen Allen, VA 23060
Phone: (804) 527-1905
Fax: (804) 747-5316
Web site: http://www.aamcn.org

American Association of Neurological Surgeons
5550 Meadowbrook Dr.
Rolling Meadows, IL 60008-3852
Phone: (847) 378-0500
Toll free: (888) 566-AANS (2267)
Fax: (847) 378-0600
E-mail: info@aans.org
Web site: http://aans.org

American Association of Neuromuscular & Electrodiagnostic Medicine (AANEM)
2621 Superior Dr. NW
Rochester, MN 55901
Phone: (507) 288-0100
E-mail: aanem@aanem.org
Web site: https://www.aanem.org

American Association of Nurse Anesthetists (AANA)
222 S. Prospect Ave.
Park Ridge, IL 60068-4001
Phone: (847) 692-7050
Toll free: (855) 526-2262
Fax: (847) 692-6968
E-mail: info@aana.com
Web site: http://www.aana.com

American Association of Nurse Practitioners (AANP)
PO Box 12846
Austin, TX 78711
Phone: (512) 442-4262
Fax: (512) 442-6469
E-mail: admin@aanp.org
Web site: http://www.aanp.org

American Association of Oral and Maxillofacial Surgeons (AAOMS)
9700 W. Bryn Mawr Ave.
Rosemont, IL 60018-5701
Phone: (847) 678-6200
Toll free: (800) 822-6637
Fax: (847) 678-6286
Web site: http://www.aaoms.org

American Association of Plastic Surgeons
500 Cummings Center, Ste. 4550
Beverly, MA 01915
Phone: (978) 927-8330
Fax: (978) 524-8890
Web site: http://www.aaps1921.org

American Association of Respiratory Care (AARC)
9425 N. MacArthur Blvd., Ste. 100
Irving, TX 75063-4706
Phone: (972) 243-2272
Fax: (972) 484-2720
E-mail: info@aarc.org
Web site: http://www.aarc.org

American Association of Tissue Banks
1320 Old Chain Bridge Rd., Ste. 450
McLean, VA 22101
Phone: (703) 827-9582
Fax: (703) 356-2198
E-mail: aatb@aatb.org
Web site: http://www.aatb.org

American Autoimmune Related Diseases Association (AARDA)
22100 Gratiot Ave.
Eastpointe, MI 48021
Phone: (586) 776-3900
Fax: (586) 776-3903
Web site: https://www.aarda.org

American Bar Association
321 N. Clark St.
Chicago, IL 60654
Phone: (312) 988-5000
Toll free: (800) 285-2221
Web site: http://www.americanbar.org

American Board of Anesthesiology
4208 Six Forks Rd., Ste. 1500
Raleigh, NC 27609-5765
Phone: (866) 999-7501
Fax: (866) 999-7503
Web site: http://www.theaba.org

American Board of Colon and Rectal Surgery
20600 Eureka Rd., Ste. 600
Taylor, MI 48180
Phone: (734) 282-9400
Fax: (734) 282-9402
E-mail: admin@abcrs.org
Web site: http://www.abcrs.org

American Board of Facial Plastic and Reconstructive Surgery (ABFPRS)
115C S. Saint Asaph St.
Alexandria, VA 22314
Phone: (703) 549-3223
Phone: (703) 549-3357
E-mail: lwirth@abfprs.org
Web site: http://www.abfprs.org

American Board of Medical Specialties
222 N. LaSalle St., Ste. 1500
Chicago, IL 60601
Phone: (312) 436-2600
Web site: http://www.abms.org

American Board of Neurological Surgery (ABNS)
245 Amity Road #208
Woodbridge, CT 06525
Phone: (203) 397-2267
Fax: (203) 392-0400
E-mail: abns@abns.org
Web site: http://www.abns.org

American Board of Obstetrics and Gynecology
2915 Vine St.
Dallas, TX 75204
Phone: (214) 871-1619
Fax: (214) 871-1943
Web site: http://www.abog.org

American Board of Ophthalmology
111 Presidential Blvd., Ste. 241
Bala Cynwyd, PA 19004-1075
Phone: (610) 664-1175
Fax: (610) 664-6503
E-mail: info@abop.org
Web site: http://abop.org

American Board of Plastic Surgery
1635 Market St., 7 Penn Ctr., Ste. 400
Philadelphia, PA 19103-2204
Phone: (215) 587-9322
E-mail: info@abplsurg.org
Web site: https://www.abplsurg.org

American Board of Registration of Electroencephalographic and Evoked Potential Technologists (ABRET)
2908 Greenbriar Dr., Ste. A
Springfield, IL 62704
Phone: (217) 726-7980
Fax: (217) 726-7989
E-mail: janice@abret.org
Web site: http://abret.org

American Board of Surgery
1617 John F. Kennedy Blvd., Ste. 860
Philadelphia, PA 19103-1847
Phone: (215) 568-4000
Fax: (215) 563-5718
Web site: http://www.absurgery.org

American Board of Urology
600 Peter Jefferson Pkwy., Ste. 150
Charlottesville, VA 22911
Phone: (434) 979-0059
Fax: (434) 979-0266
E-mail: denise@abu.org
Web site: http://www.abu.org

American Board of Wound Management
1155 15th St. NW, Ste. 500
Washington, DC 20005
Phone: (202) 457-8408
Fax: (202) 530-0659
E-mail: info@abwmcertified.org
Web site: http://www.abwmcertified.org

American Bone Health
1814 Franklin St., Ste. 620
Oakland, CA 94612
Phone: (510) 832-2663
Toll free: (888) 266-3015
Fax: (510) 208-7174
E-mail: info@americanbonehealth.org
Web site: http://www. americanbonehealth.org

American Brain Tumor Association (ABTA)
8550 W. Bryn Mawr Ave., Ste. 550
Chicago, IL 60631
Phone: (773) 577-8750
Toll free: (800) 886-2282
Fax: (773) 577-8738
E-mail: info@abta.org
Web site: http://www.abta.org

American Burn Association
311 S. Wacker Dr., Ste. 4150
Chicago, IL 60606
Phone: (312) 642-9260
Fax: (312) 642-9130
E-mail: info@ameriburn.org
Web site: http://www.ameriburn.org

American Cancer Society (ACS)
250 Williams St. NW
Atlanta, GA 30303
Toll free: (800) 227-2345
Web site: http://www.cancer.org

American Chiropractic Association
1701 Clarendon Blvd.
Arlington, VA 22209
Phone: (703) 276-8800
Fax: (703) 243-2593
E-mail: memberinfo@acatoday.org
Web site: http://www.acatoday.org

American Chronic Pain Association (ACPA)
PO Box 850
Rocklin, CA 95677
Toll free: (800) 533-3231
Fax: (916) 632-3208
E-mail: ACPA@theacpa.org
Web site: http://www.theacpa.org

American Cleft Palate-Craniofacial Association
1504 E. Franklin St., Ste. 102
Chapel Hill, NC 27514-2820
Phone: (919) 933-9044
Fax: (919) 933-9604
E-mail: info@acpa-cpf.org
Web site: http://www.acpa-cpf.org

American College of Allergy, Asthma & Immunology
85 W. Algonquin Rd., Ste. 550
Arlington Heights, IL 60005
Phone: (847) 427-1200
Fax: (847) 427-1294

E-mail: mail@acaai.org
Web site: http://www.acaai.org

American College of Cardiology
Heart House, 2400 N St. NW
Washington, DC 20037
Phone: (202) 375-6000, ext. 5603
Toll free: (800) 253-4636, ext. 5603
Fax: (202) 375-7000
E-mail: resource@acc.org
Web site: http://www.cardiosource.org

American College of Chest Physicians (ACCP)
3300 Dundee Rd.
Northbrook, IL 60062-2348
Phone: (847) 498-1400
Toll free: (800) 343-2227
Fax: (847) 498-5460
Web site: http://www.chestnet.org

American College of Clinical Pharmacy (ACCP)
13000 W. 87th Street Pkwy.
Lenexa, KS 66215-4530
Phone: (913) 492-3311
Fax: (913) 492-0088
E-mail: accp@accp.com
Web site: http://www.accp.com

American College of Emergency Physicians (ACEP)
1125 Executive Cir.
Irving, TX 75038-2522
Phone: (972) 550-0911
Toll free: (800) 798-1822
Fax: (972) 580-2816
Web site: http://www.acep.org

American College of Eye Surgeons/ American Board of Eye Surgery
334 E. Lake Rd., #135
Palm Harbor, FL 34685-2427
Phone: (727) 366-1487
Fax: (727) 836-9783
E-mail: quality@aces-abes.org
Web site: http://www.aces-abes.org

American College of Foot and Ankle Surgeons
8725 W. Higgins Rd., Ste. 555
Chicago, IL 60631-2724
Phone: (773) 693-9300
Toll free: (800) 421-2237
Fax: (773) 693-9304
E-mail: info@acfas.org
Web site: http://www.acfas.org

American College of Gastroenterology (ACG)
6400 Goldsboro Rd., Ste. 200
Bethesda, MD 20817
Phone: (301) 263-9000
E-mail: info@acg.gi.org
Web site: http://gi.org

American College of Healthcare Executives
One North Franklin St., Ste. 1700
Chicago, IL 60606-3529
Phone: (312) 424-2800
Fax: (312) 424-0023
E-mail: contact@ache.org
Web site: http://www.ache.org

American College of Medical Toxicology (ACMT)
10645 N. Tatum Blvd., Ste. 200-111
Phoenix, AZ 85028
Phone: (623) 533-6340
Fax: (623) 533-6520
E-mail: info@acmt.net
Web site: http://www.acmt.net

American College of Nurse-Midwives
8403 Colesville Rd., Ste. 1550
Silver Spring, MD 20910
Phone: (240) 485-1800
Fax: (240) 485-1818
Web site: http://www.midwife.org

American College of Phlebology
101 Callan Ave., Ste. 210
San Leandro, CA 94577
Phone: (510) 346-6800
Fax: (510) 346-6808
Web site: http://www.phlebology.org

American College of Physicians (ACP)
190 N. Independence Mall West
Philadelphia, PA 19106-1572
Phone: (215) 351-2400
Toll free: (800) 523-1546
Web site: http://www.acponline.org

American College of Radiology
1891 Preston White Dr.
Reston, VA 20191
Phone: (703) 648-8900
E-mail: info@acr.org
Web site: http://www.acr.org

American College of Sports Medicine (ACSM)
401 W. Michigan St.
Indianapolis, IN 46202-3233
Phone: (317) 637-9200
Fax: (317) 634-7817
E-mail: publicinfo@acsm.org
Web site: http://acsm.org

American College of Surgeons (ACS)
633 N. Saint Clair St.
Chicago, IL 60611-3211
Phone: (312) 202-5000
Toll free: (800) 621-4111
Fax: (312) 202-5001
E-mail: postmaster@facs.org
Web site: http://www.facs.org

American College of Surgeons Health Policy Research Institute
725 Martin Luther King Jr. Blvd., Campus Box 7590
University of North Carolina, Cecil G. Sheps Center for Health Services Research
Chapel Hill, NC 27599-7590
Phone: (919) 966-9425
E-mail: acs-hpri@facs.org
Web site: http://acshpri.org

American Congress of Obstetricians and Gynecologists (ACOG)
409 12th St. SW
Washington, DC 20024-2188
Phone: (202) 638-5577
Toll free: (800) 673-8444
Web site: http://www.acog.org

American Council on Exercise (ACE)
4851 Paramount Dr.
San Diego, CA 92123
Phone: (858) 279-8227
Toll free: (888) 825-3636
Fax: (858) 576-6564
E-mail: support@acefitness.org
Web site: http://www.acefitness.org

American Dental Association (ADA)
211 E. Chicago Ave.
Chicago, IL 60611
Phone: (312) 440-2500
Web site: http://www.ada.org

American Dental Education Association
1400 K St. NW, Ste. 1100
Washington, DC 20005
Phone: (202) 289-7201
Fax: (202) 289-7204
Web site: http://www.adea.org

American Dental Hygienists' Association
444 N. Michigan Ave., Ste. 3400
Chicago, IL 60611
Phone: (312) 440-8900
E-mail: member.services@adha.net
Web site: http://www.adha.org

American Diabetes Association
1701 N. Beauregard St.
Alexandria, VA 22311
Toll free: (800) DIABETES (342-2383)
E-mail: AskADA@diabetes.org
Web site: http://www.diabetes.org

American Fertility Association
315 Madison Ave., Ste. 901
New York, NY 10017
Toll free: (888) 917-3777
E-mail: Info@TheAFA.org
Web site: http://www.theafa.org

American Gastroenterological Association
4930 Del Ray Ave.
Bethesda, MD 20814
Phone: (301) 654-2055
Fax: (301) 654-5920
E-mail: member@gastro.org
Web site: http://www.gastro.org

American Geriatrics Society (AGS)
40 Fulton St., 18th Fl.
New York, NY 10038
Phone: (212) 308-1414
Fax: (212) 832-8646
E-mail: info.amger@americangeriatrics.
   org
Web site: http://www.
   americangeriatrics.org

American Health Lawyers Association
1620 Eye St. NW, 6th Fl.
Washington, DC 20006-4010
Phone: (202) 833-1100
Fax: (202) 833-1105
E-mail: MbrDept@healthlawyers.org
Web site: http://www.healthlawyers.org

American Hearing Research Foundation
310 W. Lake St., Ste. 111
Elmhurst, IL 60126
Phone: (630) 617-5079
Fax: (630) 563-9181
Web site: http://american-hearing.org

American Heart Association
7272 Greenville Ave.
Dallas, TX 75231
Phone: (214) 570-5978
Toll free: (800) AHA-USA-1 (242-8721)
Web site: http://www.heart.org

American Hospital Association
155 N. Wacker Dr.
Chicago, IL 60606
Phone: (312) 422-3000
Toll free: (800) 424-4301
Web site: http://www.aha.org

American Institute of Ultrasound in Medicine
14750 Sweitzer Ln., Ste. 100
Laurel, MD 20707-5906
Phone: (301) 498-4100
Toll free: (800) 638-5352
Fax: (301) 498-4450
Web site: http://www.aium.org

American Joint Committee on Cancer (AJCC)
633 N. Saint Clair St.
Chicago, IL 60611-3211
Phone: (312) 202-5205
Fax: (312) 202-5009
E-mail: ajcc@facs.org
Web site: http://www.cancerstaging.org

American Kidney Fund
11921 Rockville Pike, Ste. 300
Rockville, MD 20852
Toll free: (800) 638-8299
E-mail: patientservice@kidneyfund.org
Web site: http://www.kidneyfund.org

American Liver Foundation
39 Broadway, Ste. 2700
New York, NY 10006
Phone: (212) 668-1000
Toll free: (800) GO-LIVER (465-4837)
Fax: (212) 483-8179
Web site: http://www.liverfoundation.
   org

American Lung Association (ALA)
1301 Pennsylvania Ave. NW, Ste. 800
Washington, DC 20004
Phone: (202) 785-3355
Toll free: (800) LUNG-USA (586-
   4872)
Fax: (202) 452-1805
Web site: http://www.lung.org

American Medical Association
330 N. Wabash Ave.
Chicago, IL 60611
Toll free: (800) 621-8335
Web site: http://www.ama-assn.org

American Medical Informatics Association (AMIA)
4720 Montgomery Ln., Ste. 500
Bethesda, MD 20814
Phone: (301) 657-1291
Fax: (301) 657-1296
Web site: http://www.amia.org

American Nurses Association
8515 Georgia Ave., Ste. 400
Silver Spring, MD 20910-3492
Toll free: (800) 274-4ANA (4262)
Fax: (301) 628-5001
Web site: http://nursingworld.org

American Nystagmus Network
303-D Beltline Pl., #321
Decatur, AL 35603
Web site: http://nystagmus.org

American Optometric Association (AOA)
243 N. Lindbergh Blvd., 1 Fl.
St. Louis, MO 63141
Toll free: (800) 365-2219
Web site: http://www.aoa.org

American Orthopaedic Foot & Ankle Society
6300 N. River Rd., Ste. 510
Rosemont, IL 60018
Phone: (847) 698-4654
Toll free: (800) 235-4855
E-mail: aofasinfo@aofas.org
Web site: http://www.aofas.org

American Orthopaedic Society for Sports Medicine (AOSSM)
6300 N. River Rd., Ste. 500
Rosemont, IL 60018
Phone: (847) 292-4900
Toll free: (877) 321-3500
Fax: (847) 292-4905
E-mail: info@aossm.org
Web site: http://www.sportsmed.org

American Osteopathic Association (AOA)
142 E. Ontario St.
Chicago, IL 60611
Phone: (312) 202-8000
Toll free: (800) 621-1773
Fax: (312) 202-8200
E-mail: info@osteopathic.org
Web site: http://www.osteopathic.org

American Osteopathic Colleges of Ophthalmology and Otolaryngology—Head and Neck Surgery (AOCOO-HNS)
4764 Fishburg Rd., Ste. F
Huber Heights, OH 45424
Toll free: (800) 455-9404
Fax: (937) 233-5673
E-mail: info@aocoohns.org
Web site: http://www.aocoohns.org

American Pain Society
8735 W. Higgins Rd., Ste. 300
Glenview, IL 60631
Phone: (847) 375-4715
Fax: (866) 574-2654
E-mail: info@americanpainsociety.org
Web site: http://www.
   americanpainsociety.org

American Pediatric Surgical Association (APSA)
111 Deer Lake Rd., Ste. 100
Deerfield, IL 60015
Phone: (847) 480-9576
Fax: (847) 480-9282
E-mail: eapsa@eapsa.org
Web site: http://www.eapsa.org

American Physical Therapy Association
1111 N. Fairfax St.
Alexandria, VA 22314-1488
Phone: (703) 684-APTA (2782)
Toll free: (800) 999-APTA (2782)
TTY: (703) 683-6748
Fax: (703) 684-7343
E-mail: memberservices@apta.org
Web site: http://www.apta.org

American Podiatric Medical Association
9312 Old Georgetown Rd.
Bethesda, MD 20814-1621
Phone: (301) 581-9200
Web site: http://www.apma.org

American Pregnancy Association
1425 Greenway Dr., Ste. 440
Irving, TX 75038
E-mail: questions@americanpregnancy.
org
Web site: http://americanpregnancy.org

American Professional Wound Care Association
406 West Street Rd.
Feasterville, PA 19053
Phone: (215) 942-6095
Fax: (215) 942-6098
E-mail: wounds@apwca.org
Web site: http://www.apwca.org

American Prostate Society
10 E. Lee St., Ste. 1504
Baltimore, MD 21202
Phone: (410) 837-3735
Fax: (410) 837-8510
E-mail: info@americanprostatesociety.
com
Web site: http://
americanprostatesociety.com

American Psychiatric Association
1000 Wilson Blvd., Ste. 1825
Arlington, VA 22209
Phone: (703) 907-7300
Toll free: (888) 35-PSYCH (357-7924)
E-mail: apa@psych.org
Web site: http://www.psychiatry.org

American Psychological Association
750 First St. NE
Washington, DC 20002-4242
Phone: (202) 336-5500
Toll free: (800) 374-2721
TTY: (202) 336-6123
Web site: http://www.apa.org

American Red Cross
2025 E St. NW
Washington, DC 20006
Phone: (202) 303-4498
Toll free: (800) RED CROSS (733-2767)
Web site: http://www.redcross.org

American Registry of Diagnostic Medical Sonography (ARDMS)
1401 Rockville Pike, Ste. 600
Rockville, MD 20852-1402
Phone: (301) 738-8401
Toll free: (800) 541-9754
Fax: (301) 738-0312
Web site: http://www.ardms.org

American Sexual Health Association
PO Box 13827
Research Triangle Park, NC 27709
Phone: (919) 361-8400
Fax: (919) 361-8425
Web site: http://www.ashasexualhealth.
org

American Shoulder and Elbow Surgeons
6300 N. River Road, Ste. 727
Rosemont, IL 60018
Phone: (847) 698-1629
Fax: (847) 823-0536
E-mail: ases@aaos.org
Web site: http://www.ases-assn.org

American Sleep Apnea Association
6856 Eastern Ave. NW, Ste. 203
Washington, DC 20012
Toll free: (888) 293-3650
Web site: http://www.sleepapnea.org

American Social Health Association
PO Box 13827
Research Triangle Park, NC 27709-3827
Phone: (919) 361-8400
Toll free: (800) 227-8922
Fax: (919) 361-8425
Web site: http://www.ashastd.org

American Society for Aesthetic Plastic Surgery (ASAPS)
11262 Monarch St.
Garden Grove, CA 92841
Phone: (562) 799-2356
Toll free: (800) 364-2147
Fax: (562) 799-1098
E-mail: asaps@surgery.org
Web site: http://www.surgery.org

American Society for Blood and Marrow Transplantation (ASBMT)
85 W. Algonquin Rd., Ste. 550
Arlington Heights, IL 60005
Phone: (847) 427-0224
Fax: (847) 427-9656
E-mail: mail@asbmt.org
Web site: http://asbmt.org

American Society for Bone and Mineral Research (ASBMR)
2025 M St. NW, Ste. 800
Washington, DC 20036-3309
Phone: (202) 367-1161
Fax: (202) 367-2161
E-mail: asbmr@asbmr.org
Web site: http://www.asbmr.org

American Society for Clinical Laboratory Science
1861 International Dr., Ste. 200
McLean, VA 22102
Phone: (571) 748-3770
E-mail: ascls@ascls.org
Web site: http://www.ascls.org

American Society for Clinical Pathology (ASCP)
33 W. Monroe St., Ste. 1600
Chicago, IL 60603
Phone: (312) 541-4999
Toll free: (800) 267-2727

Fax: (312) 541-4998
Web site: http://www.ascp.org

American Society for Colposcopy and Cervical Pathology (ASCCP)
1530 Tilco Dr., Ste. C
Frederick, MD 21704
Phone: (301) 733-3640
Toll free: (800) 787-7227
Fax: (240) 575-9880
Web site: http://www.asccp.org

American Society for Dermatologic Surgery
5550 Meadowbrook Dr., Ste. 120
Rolling Meadows, IL 60008
Phone: (847) 956-0900
Fax: (847) 956-0999
Web site: http://www.asds.net

American Society for Gastrointestinal Endoscopy (ASGE)
3300 Woodcreek Dr.
Downers Grove, IL 60515
Phone: (630) 573-0600
Toll free: (866) 353-ASGE (2743)
Fax: (630) 963-8332
E-mail: info@asge.org
Web site: http://www.asge.org

American Society for Laser Medicine and Surgery
2100 Stewart Ave., Ste. 240
Wausau, WI 54401
Phone: (715) 845-9283
Toll free: (877) 258-6028
Fax: (715) 848-2493
E-mail: information@aslms.org
Web site: http://aslms.org

American Society for Metabolic and Bariatric Surgery
100 SW 75th St., Ste. 201
Gainesville, FL 32607
Phone: (352) 331-4900
Fax: (352) 331-4975
E-mail: info@asmbs.org
Web site: http://asmbs.org

American Society for Microbiology
1752 N St. NW
Washington, DC 20036-2904
Phone: (202) 737-3600
E-mail: service@asmusa.org
Web site: http://www.asm.org

American Society for Mohs Surgery
5901 Warner Ave., Box 391
Huntington Beach, CA 92649-4659
Phone: (714) 379-6262
Toll free: (800) 616-ASMS (2767)
Fax: (714) 379-6272
E-mail: info@mohssurgery.org
Web site: http://www.mohssurgery.org

American Society for Parenteral and Enteral Nutrition
8630 Fenton St., Ste. 412
Silver Spring, MD 20910
Phone: (301) 587-6315
Toll free: (800) 727-4567
Fax: (301) 587-2365
E-mail: aspen@nutr.org
Web site: https://www.nutritioncare.org

American Society for Reconstructive Microsurgery
20 N. Michigan Ave., Ste. 700
Chicago, IL 60602
Phone: (312) 456-9579
Fax: (312) 782-0553
E-mail: contact@microsurg.org
Web site: http://www.microsurg.org

American Society for Reproductive Medicine
1209 Montgomery Hwy.
Birmingham, AL 35216-2809
Phone: (205) 978-5000
Fax: (205) 978-5005
E-mail: asrm@asrm.org
Web site: http://www.asrm.org

American Society for Surgery of the Hand (ASSH)
822 W. Washington Blvd.
Chicago, IL 60607
Phone: (312) 880-1900
Fax: (847) 384-1435
E-mail: info@assh.org
Web site: http://www.assh.org

American Society of Anesthesiologists (ASA)
520 N. Northwest Hwy.
Park Ridge, IL 60068-2573
Phone: (847) 825-5586
Fax: (847) 825-1692
E-mail: communications@asahq.org
Web site: http://www.asahq.org

American Society of Bariatric Physicians
2821 S. Parker Rd., Ste. 625
Aurora, CO 80014
Phone: (303) 770-2526
Fax: (303) 779-4834
Web site: http://www.asbp.org

American Society of Cataract and Refractive Surgery (ASCRS)
4000 Legato Rd., Ste. 700
Fairfax, VA 22033
Phone: (703) 591-2220
Fax: (703) 591-0614
Web site: http://ascrs.org

American Society of Clinical Oncology (ASCO)
2318 Mill Rd., Ste. 800
Alexandria, VA 22314

Phone: (571) 483-1300
Toll free: (888) 282-2552
Web site: http://www.asco.org

American Society of Colon and Rectal Surgeons (ASCRS)
85 W. Algonquin Rd., Ste. 550
Arlington Heights, IL 60005
Phone: (847) 290-9184
Fax: (847) 290-9203
E-mail: ascrs@fascrs.org
Web site: http://www.fascrs.org

American Society of Cosmetic Breast Surgery (ASCBS)
1419 Superior Ave., Ste. 2
Newport Beach, CA 92663
Phone: (949) 645-6665
Fax: (949) 645-6784
E-mail: ascbs@mail.ascbs.org
Web site: http://www.ascbs.us

American Society of Echocardiography
2100 Gateway Centre Blvd., Ste. 310
Morrisville, NC 27560
Phone: (919) 861-5574
Fax: (919) 882-9900
Web site: http://www.asecho.org

American Society of Health-System Pharmacists
7272 Wisconsin Ave.
Bethesda, MD 20814
Phone: (301) 664-8700
Toll free: (866) 279-0681
E-mail: custserv@ashp.org
Web site: http://www.ashp.org

American Society of Hematology (ASH)
2021 L St. NW, Ste. 900
Washington, DC 20036
Phone: (202) 776-0544
Fax: (202) 776-0545
Web site: http://www.hematology.org

American Society of Nephrology (ASN)
1510 H St. NW, Ste. 800
Washington, DC 20005
Phone: (202) 640-4660
Fax: (202) 637-9793
E-mail: email@asn-online.org
Web site: http://asn-online.org

American Society of PeriAnesthesia Nurses
90 Frontage Rd.
Cherry Hill, NJ 08034-1424
Toll free: (877) 737-9696
Fax: (856) 616-9601
E-mail: aspan@aspan.org
Web site: http://www.aspan.org

American Society of Plastic Surgeons
444 E. Algonquin Rd.
Arlington Heights, IL 60005
Phone: (847) 228-9900
Web site: http://www.plasticsurgery.org

American Society of Radiologic Technologists (ASRT)
15000 Central Ave. SE
Albuquerque, NM 87123-3909
Phone: (505) 298-4500
Toll free: (800) 444-2778
Fax: (505) 298-5063
E-mail: memberservices@asrt.org
Web site: http://www.asrt.org

American Society of Transplant Surgeons (ASTS)
2461 South Clark St., Ste. 640
Arlington, VA 22202
Phone: (703) 414-7870
Fax: (703) 414-7874
E-mail: asts@asts.org
Web site: http://www.asts.org

American Society of Transplantation (AST)
15000 Commerce Pkwy., Ste. C
Mt. Laurel, NJ 08054
Phone: (856) 439-9986
Fax: (856) 439-9982
Web site: http://www.myast.org

American Speech-Language-Hearing Association (ASHA)
2200 Research Blvd.
Rockville, MD 20850-3289
Phone: (301) 296-5700
Toll free: (800) 638-8255
TTY: (301) 296-5650
Web site: http://www.asha.org

American Thoracic Society
25 Broadway, 18th Fl.
New York, NY 10004
Phone: (212) 315-8600
Fax: (212) 315-6498
E-mail: atsinfo@thoracic.org
Web site: http://www.thoracic.org

American Thyroid Association
6066 Leesburg Pike, Ste. 550
Falls Church, VA 22041
Phone: (703) 998-8890
Fax: (703) 998-8893
E-mail: thyroid@thyroid.org
Web site: http://www.thyroid.org

American Trauma Society (ATS)
201 Park Washington Ct.
Falls Church, VA 22046
Phone: (703) 538-3544
Toll free: (800) 556-7890
Fax: (703) 241-5603
E-mail: info@amtrauma.org
Web site: http://www.amtrauma.org

America's Blood Centers
725 15th St. NW, Ste. 700
Washington, DC 20005
Phone: (202) 393-5725
Fax: (202) 393-1282
E-mail: abc@americasblood.org
Web site: http://www.americasblood.org

America's Health Insurance Plans
601 Pennsylvania Ave. NW, S. Bldg., Ste. 500
Washington, DC 20004
Phone: (202) 778-3200
Fax: (202) 331-7487
E-mail: ahip@ahip.org
Web site: http://www.ahip.org

Amputee Coalition
9303 Center St., Ste. 100
Manassas, VA 20110
Toll free: (888) 267-5669
TTY: (865) 525-4512
Web site: https://www.amputee-coalition.org

Anesthesia Patient Safety Foundation (APSF)
8007 S. Meridian St., Bldg. 1, Ste. 2
Indianapolis, IN 46217-2922
E-mail: info@apsf.org
Web site: http://www.apsf.org

Arthritis Foundation
1300 W. Peachtree St., Ste. 100
Atlanta, GA 30309
Phone: (404) 872-7100
Web site: http://www.arthritis.org

ASET—The Neurodiagnostic Society
402 E. Bannister Rd., Ste. A
Kansas City, MO 64131-3019
Phone: (816) 931-1120
Fax: (816) 931-1145
E-mail: info@aset.org
Web site: http://www.aset.org

Association for Research in Otolaryngology (ARO)
19 Mantua Rd.
Mt. Royal, NJ 08061
Phone: (856) 423-0041
Fax: (856) 423-3420
E-mail: headquarters@aro.org
Web site: http://www.aro.org

Association of American Medical Colleges
2450 N. St. NW
Washington, DC 20037-1126
Phone: (202) 828-0400
Fax: (202) 828-1125
Web site: https://www.aamc.org

Association of periOperative Registered Nurses (AORN)
2170 S. Parker Rd., Ste. 400
Denver, CO 80231-5711
Phone: (303) 755-6300
Toll free: (800) 755-2676
Fax: (800) 847-0045
E-mail: custsvc@aorn.org
Web site: http://www.aorn.org

Association of Surgical Technologists
6 West Dry Creek Cir., Ste. 200
Littleton, CO 80120-8031
Phone: (303) 694-9130
Toll free: (800) 637-7433
Fax: (303) 694-9169
Web site: http://www.ast.org

Association of Women's Health, Obstetric, and Neonatal Nurses (AWHONN)
2000 L St. NW, Ste. 740
Washington, DC 20036
Phone: (202) 261-2400
Toll free: (800) 673-8499
Fax: (202) 728-0575
E-mail: customerservice@awhonn.org
Web site: http://www.awhonn.org

Asthma and Allergy Foundation of America
8201 Corporate Dr., Ste. 1000
Landover, MD 20785
Toll free: (800) 7-ASTHMA (727-8462)
E-mail: info@aafa.org
Web site: http://aafa.org

AVERT
4 Brighton Rd.
Horsham, West Sussex RH13 5BA
United Kingdom
Phone: +44 1403 210202
E-mail: info@avert.org
Web site: http://www.avert.org

B

Better Hearing Institute
1444 I St. NW, Ste. 700
Washington, DC 20005
Phone: (202) 449-1100
Fax: (202) 216-9646
E-mail: mail@betterhearing.org
Web site: http://betterhearing.org

Bladder & Bowel Foundation
SATRA Innovation Park, Rockingham Rd.
Kettering, Northants NN16 9JH
United Kingdom
Phone: +44 01536 533255
E-mail: info@bladderandbowel foundation.org
Web site: http://www.bladderandbowelfoundation.org

BMT InfoNet (Blood and Marrow Transplant Information Network)
2310 Skokie Valley Rd., Ste. 104
Highland Park, IL 60035
Phone: (847) 433-3313
Toll free: (888) 597-7674
Fax: (847) 433-4599
E-mail: help@bmtinfonet.org
Web site: http://www.bmtinfonet.org

Bone Marrow Donors Worldwide
Plesmanlaan 1-b
2333 BZ Leiden, The Netherlands
Phone: +31 71 5685300
Fax: +31 71 5210457
E-mail: BMDW@Europdonor.NL
Web site: http://www.bmdw.org

Brain Injury Association of America
1608 Spring Hill Rd., Ste. 110
Vienna, VA 22182
Phone: (703) 761-0750
Toll free: (800) 444-6443
Fax: (703) 761-0755
E-mail: info@biausa.org
Web site: http://www.biausa.org

Breastcancer.org
7 E. Lancaster Ave., 3rd Fl.
Ardmore, PA 19003
Phone: (610) 642-6550
Fax: (610) 642-6559
Web site: http://www.breastcancer.org

British Association of Oral and Maxillofacial Surgeons
Royal College of Surgeons of England, 35/43 Lincoln's Inn Fields
London, WC2A 3PE
United Kingdom
Phone: +44 207 405 8074
E-mail: office@baoms.org.uk
Web site: http://www.baoms.org.uk

British Heart Foundation
Greater London House, 180 Hampstead Rd.
London, NW1 7AW
United Kingdom
Phone: +44 0300 330 3322
Toll free: (800) 1 020 7554 0000
Web site: http://www.bhf.org.uk

C

Canadian Association of Gastroenterology
1540 Cornwall Rd., #224
Oakville, Ontario L6J 7W5
Canada
Phone: (905) 829-2504
Toll free: (888) 780-0007
Fax: (905) 829-0242
E-mail: general@cag-acg.org
Web site: http://www.cag-acg.org

Canadian Institute for Health Information (CIHI)
495 Richmond Rd., Ste. 600
Ottawa, Ontario K2A 4H6
Canada
Phone: (613) 241-5543
E-mail: communications@cihi.ca
Web site: http://www.cihi.ca

Canadian Ophthalmological Society
610-1525 Carling Ave.
Ottawa, Ontario K1Z 8R9
Canada
Phone: (613) 729-6779
Fax: (613) 729-7209
E-mail: cos@cos-sco.ca
Web site: http://www.eyesite.ca

Canadian Orthopaedic Foundation
PO Box 1036
Toronto, Ontario M5K 1P2
Canada
Phone: (416) 410-2341
Toll free: (800) 461-3639
E-mail: mailbox@canorth.org
Web site: http://www.canorth.org

The Canadian Society of Plastic Surgeons
1469 St. Joseph Blvd. E., #4
Montreal, Quebec H2J 1M6
Canada
Phone: (514) 843-5415
Fax: (514) 843-7005
Web site: http://www.plasticsurgery.ca

Cancer Research and Prevention Foundation
1600 Duke St., Ste. 500
Alexandria, VA 22314
Phone: (703) 836-4412
Toll free: (800) 227-2732
Fax: (703) 836-4413
E-mail: pcf@preventcancer.org
Web site: http://www.preventcancer.org

Cancer Research Institute
One Exchange Plz., 55 Broadway, Ste. 1802
New York, NY 10006
Phone: (212) 688-7515
Toll free: (800) 99-CANCER (992-2623)
Web site: http://cancerresearch.org

Cardiovascular and Interventional Radiological Society of Europe (CIRSE)
Neutorgasse 9/6
1010 Vienna, Austria
Phone: +43 1 904 2003
Fax: +43 1 904 2003 30
E-mail: info@cirse.org
Web site: http://www.cirse.org

CARES Foundation
2414 Morris Ave., Ste. 110
Union, NJ 07083
Toll free: (866) 227-3737
E-mail: contact@caresfoundation.org
Web site: http://www.caresfoundation.org

Caring Connections
Toll free: (800) 658-8898
Toll free: (877) 658-8896 (Multilingual)
E-mail: caringinfo@nhpco.org
Web site: http://www.caringinfo.org

Center for Emergency Medicine of Western Pennsylvania, Inc.
230 McKee Pl., Ste. 500
Pittsburgh, PA 15213
Phone: (412) 647-5300
Fax: (412) 647-4670
E-mail: kusmierekj@upmc.edu
Web site: http://centerem.org

Center for Medicare Advocacy
PO Box 350
Willimantic, CT 06226
Phone: (860) 456-7790
Fax: (860) 456-2614
Web site: http://www.medicareadvocacy.org

Center for Uterine Fibroids, Brigham and Women's Hospital
77 Ave. Louis Pasteur, New Research Building
Boston, MA 02115
Toll free: (800) 722-5520
Web site: http://fibroids.net/homepage.html

Center on Medical Record Rights and Privacy
Health Policy Institute, Georgetown University, Box 57144
Washington, DC 20057-1485
Phone: (202) 687-0880
Fax: (202) 687-3110
Web site: http://hpi.georgetown.edu/privacy

Centers for Disease Control and Prevention (CDC)
1600 Clifton Rd.
Atlanta, GA 30333
Toll free: (800) CDC-INFO (232-4636)
TTY: (888) 232-6348
E-mail: cdcinfo@cdc.gov
Web site: http://www.cdc.gov

Centers for Disease Control and Prevention, Division of Reproductive Health
1600 Clifton Rd.
Atlanta, GA 30333
Toll free: (800) CDC-INFO (232-4636)
TTY: (888) 232-6348
E-mail: cdcinfo@cdc.gov
Web site: http://www.cdc.gov/reproductivehealth

Centers for Disease Control and Prevention, National Center for Chronic Disease Prevention and Health Promotion (NCCDPHP)
4770 Buford Hwy. NE, MS F-76
Atlanta, GA 30341
Toll free: (800) CDC-INFO (232-4636)
TTY: (888) 232-6348
E-mail: cdcinfo@cdc.gov
Web site: http://www.cdc.gov/chronicdisease

Centers for Disease Control and Prevention, National Center for HIV, Viral Hepatitis, STD, and TB Prevention
1600 Clifton Rd.
Atlanta, GA 30333
Toll free: (800) CDC-INFO (232-4636)
E-mail: cdcinfo@cdc.gov
Web site: http://www.cdc.gov/nchhstp

Centers for Disease Control and Prevention, Office of Public Health Genomics
1600 Clifton Rd. NE, MS E61
Atlanta, GA 30333
Phone: (404) 498-0001
Toll free: (800) CDC-INFO (232-4636)
E-mail: genetics@cdc.gov
Web site: http://www.cdc.gov/genomics

Centers for Medicare & Medicaid Services
7500 Security Blvd.
Baltimore, MD 21244
Phone: (410) 786-3000
Toll free: (877) 267-2323
TTY: (866) 226-1819
Web site: http://www.cms.gov

Centre for Minimal Access Surgery (CMAS)
50 Charlton Ave. E.
Hamilton, Ontario L8N 4A6
Canada
Phone: (905) 522-1155, ext. 33185
Fax: (905) 521-6924
E-mail: info@cmas.ca
Web site: http://www.cmas.ca

Charles P. Felton National Tuberculosis Center
215 W. 125th St., 1st Fl., Ste. A.
New York, NY 10027
E-mail: tbcenter_info@columbia.edu

Children's Hospice International
1101 King St., Ste. 360
Alexandria, VA 22314
Phone: (703) 684-0330
E-mail: info@CHIonline.org
Web site: http://www.chionline.org

Children's Organ Transplant Association (COTA)
2501 W. COTA Dr.

Bloomington, IN 47403
Toll free: (800) 366-2682
Fax: (812) 336-8885
E-mail: cota@cota.org
Web site: http://www.cota.org

CIBMTR (Center for International Blood and Marrow Transplant Research)
Froedtert and the Medical College of Wisconsin Clinical Cancer Center, 9200 W. Wisconsin Ave., Ste. C5500
Milwaukee, WI 53226
Phone: (414) 805-0700
Fax: (414) 805-0714
E-mail: contactus@cibmtr.org
Web site: http://www.cibmtr.org

Clinical Islet Tranplantation (CIT) Consortium
Web site: http://www.citisletstudy.org

College of American Pathologists
325 Waukegan Rd.
Northfield, IL 60093-2750
Phone: (847) 832-7000
Toll free: (800) 323-4040
Fax: (847) 832-8000
Web site: http://www.cap.org

Colon Cancer Alliance
1025 Vermont Ave. NW, Ste. 1066
Washington, DC 20005
Phone: (202) 628-0123
Toll free: (877) 422-2030
Fax: (866) 304-9075
Web site: http://ccalliance.org

Colostomy Association
Enterprise House, 95 London St.
Reading, Berkshire RG1 4QA
United Kingdom
Phone: +44 118 939 1537
Toll free: (800) 328-4257
E-mail: cass@colostomyassociation. org.uk
Web site: http://www. colostomyassociation.org.uk

Congenital Heart Information Network (CHIN)
PO Box 3397
Margate City, NJ 08402-0397
Phone: (609) 823-4507
E-mail: mb@tchin.org
Web site: http://www.tchin.org

Congenital Heart Surgeons Society
500 Cummings Ctr., Ste. 4550
Beverly, MA 01915
Phone: (978) 927-8330
Fax: (978) 524-8890
Web site: http://chss.org

Crohn's & Colitis Foundation of America
733 Third Ave., Ste. 510
New York, NY 10017
Toll free: (800) 932-2423
E-mail: info@ccfa.org
Web site: http://www.ccfa.org

D

Delete Blood Cancer
100 Broadway, 6th Fl.
New York, NY 10005
Phone: (212) 209-6700
Fax: (212) 209-6710
E-mail: info@dkmsamericas.org
Web site: https://www. deletebloodcancer.org

DES Action USA
PO Box 7296
Jupiter, FL 33468
Toll free: (800) DES-9288 (337-9288)
E-mail: info@desaction.org
Web site: http://www.desaction.org

Donate Life America
701 E. Byrd St., 16th Fl.
Richmond, VA 23219
Toll free: (804) 377-3580
E-mail: donatelifeamerica@donatelife. net
Web site: http://donatelife.net

E

EA/TEF Family Support Connection
Web site: http://eatef.org

Electronic Privacy Information Center (EPIC)
1718 Connecticut Ave. NW, Ste. 200
Washington, DC 20009
Phone: (202) 483-1140
Fax: (202) 483-1248
Web site: http://epic.org

Endometriosis Association
8585 N. 76th Pl.
Milwaukee, WI 53223
Phone: (414) 355-2200
Fax: (414) 355-6065
Web site: http://endometriosisassn.org

Epilepsy Foundation
8301 Professional Pl.
Landover, MD 20785-2353
Toll free: (800) 332-1000; Spanish: (866) 748-8008
E-mail: ContactUs@efa.org
Web site: http://www. epilepsyfoundation.org

Epilepsy Society
Chesham Lane, Chalfont St. Peter
Buckinghamshire, SL9 0RJ
United Kingdom
Phone: +44 01494 601 300
Web site: http://www.epilepsysociety. org.uk

EuroGentest
Center for Human Genetics, University of Leuven, Herestraat 49 Box 602
Leuven, Belgium, 3000
Phone: +32 16 340321
Fax: +32 16 345997
E-mail: admin@eurogentest.org
Web site: http://www.eurogentest.org

European Institute of TeleSurgery (EITS)
Hôpitaux Universitaires 1, place de l'Hôpital
Strasbourg Cedex, France, 67091
Phone: +33 (0)3 88 11 90 00
Fax: +33 (0)3 88 11 90 99
E-mail: info@eits.fr
Web site: http://www.eits.fr

Extracorporeal Life Support Organization (ELSO)
2800 Plymouth Rd., Bldg. 300, Rm. 303
Ann Arbor, MI 48109-2800
Phone: (734) 998-6601
Fax: (734) 998-6602
Web site: http://elsonet.org

Eye Bank Association of America
1015 18th St. NW, Ste. 1010
Washington, DC 20036
Phone: (202) 775-4999
Web site: http://www.restoresight.org

Eye Cancer Network
115 E. 61st St., Ste. 5B
New York, NY 10065
Phone: (212) 832-8170
E-mail: contactus@eyecancer.com
Web site: http://www.eyecancer.com

F

FACES: The National Craniofacial Association
PO Box 11082
Chattanooga, TN 37401
Phone: (423) 266-1632
Toll free: (800) 3-FACES-3 (332-2373)
E-mail: faces@faces-cranio.org
Web site: http://www.faces-cranio.org

Federation of State Medical Boards
400 Fuller Wiser Rd., Ste. 300
Euless, TX 76039
Phone: (817) 868-4000
Fax: (817) 868-4099
Web site: http://www.fsmb.org

Fetal Hope Foundation
9786 S. Holland St.
Littleton, CO 80127
Toll free: (877) 789-HOPE (4673)
Phone: (303) 932-0553
Web site: http://www.fetalhope.org

Fetal Treatment Center, University of California, San Francisco
400 Parnassus Ave., A123
San Francisco, CA 94143-0570
Phone: (415) 353-8489
Toll free: (800) RX-FETUS (793-3887)
Fax: (415) 502-0660
E-mail: fetus@surgery.ucsf.edu
Web site: http://fetus.ucsfmedicalcenter.
   org

FORCE: Facing Our Risk of Cancer Empowered
16057 Tampa Palms Blvd. W, PMB #373
Tampa, FL 33647
Toll free: (866) 288-RISK (7475)
Fax: (954) 827-2200
E-mail: info@facingourrisk.org
Web site: http://www.facingourrisk.org

G

Gender Matters
The Mill House, 5b Bridgnorth Rd.
Wolverhampton, West Midlands WV6
   8AB
United Kingdom
Phone: +44 (0) 1902 744424
E-mail: info@gender-matters.org.uk
Web site: http://gender-matters.org.uk

The Glaucoma Foundation
80 Maiden Ln., Ste. 700
New York, NY 10038
Phone: (212) 285-0080
E-mail: info@glaucomafoundation.org
Web site: http://www.
   glaucomafoundation.org

Glaucoma Research Foundation
251 Post St., Ste. 600
San Francisco, CA 94108
Phone: (415) 986-3162
Toll free: (800) 826-6693
Fax: (415) 986-3763
E-mail: grf@glaucoma.org
Web site: http://www.glaucoma.org

Glaucoma Service Foundation to Prevent Blindness
Wills Eye Institute, 840 Walnut St., Ste.
   1130
Philadelphia, PA 19107-5598
Phone: (215) 928-3190
Fax: (215) 928-3194
Web site: http://willsglaucoma.org

Guttmacher Institute
1301 Connecticut Ave. NW, Ste. 700
Washington, DC 20036
Phone: (202) 296-4012
Toll free: (877) 823-0262
Fax: (202) 223-5756
Web site: http://www.guttmacher.org

H

Health Canada
Address Locator 0900C2
Ottawa, Ontario K1A 0K9
Canada
Phone: (613) 957-2991
Toll free: (866) 225-0709
Fax: (613) 941-5366
E-mail: Info@hc-sc.gc.ca
Web site: http://www.hc-sc.gc.ca

Health Care Without Harm
12355 Sunrise Valley Dr., Ste. 680
Reston, VA 20191
Phone: (703) 860-9790
Fax: (703) 860-9795
Web site: http://noharm.org

Hearing Link
27-28 The Waterfront
Eastbourne, East Sussex BN23 5UZ
United Kingdom
Phone: +44 1323 0300 111 1113
E-mail: enquiries@hearinglink.org
Web site: http://hearinglink.org

Heart Rhythm Society
1400 K St. NW, Ste. 500
Washington, DC 20005
Phone: (202) 464-3400
Fax: (202) 464-3401
E-mail: info@HRSonline.org
Web site: http://www.hrsonline.org

HelpHOPELive
Two Radnor Corporate Ctr., 100
   Matsonford Rd., Ste. 100
Radnor, PA 19087
Phone: (610) 727-0612
Toll free: (800) 642-8399
Fax: (610) 535-6106
Web site: http://www.helphopelive.org

Henry J. Kaiser Family Foundation
2400 Sand Hill Rd.
Menlo Park, CA 94025
Phone: (650) 854-9400
Fax: (650) 854-4800
Web site: http://www.kff.org

Hepatitis Foundation International
504 Blick Dr.
Silver Spring, MD 20904
Phone: (301) 879-6891

Toll free: (800) 891-0707
Fax: (301) 879-6890
E-mail: info@hepatitisfoundation.org
Web site: http://www.hepatitis
   foundation.org

Hospice Foundation of America
1710 Rhode Island Ave. NW, Ste. 400
Washington, DC 20036
Phone: (202) 457-5811
Toll free: (800) 854-3402
Fax: (202) 457-5815
E-mail: hfaoffice@hospicefoundation.
   org
Web site: http://www.hospice
   foundation.org

Hydrocephalus Association
4340 East West Hwy., Ste. 905
Bethesda, MD 20814
Phone: (301) 202-3811
Toll free: (888) 598-3789
Fax: (301) 202-3813
E-mail: info@hydroassoc.org
Web site: http://www.hydroassoc.org

Hyster Sisters
2436 S. I-35 E., Ste. 376-184
Denton, TX 76205
Web site: http://www.hystersisters.com

I

Immune Tolerance Network (ITN)
Benaroya Research Institute, 1201
   Ninth Ave.
Seattle, WA 98101-2795
Phone: (206) 342-6562
Fax: (206) 342-6588
Web site: http://www.immunetolerance.
   org

Infusion Nurses Society
315 Norwood Park S.
Norwood, MA 02062
Phone: (781) 440-9408
Fax: (781) 440-9409
E-mail: ins@ins1.org
Web site: http://www.ins1.org

Institute for Healthcare Improvement
20 University Rd., 7th Fl.
Cambridge, MA 02138
Phone: (617) 301-4800
Toll free: (866) 787-0831
Fax: (617) 301-4848
E-mail: info@ihi.org
Web site: http://www.ihi.org

Institute of Medicine, National Academy of Sciences
500 Fifth St. NW
Washington, DC 20001

Phone: (202) 334-2352
E-mail: iomwww@nas.edu
Web site: http://iom.edu

**Inter-Institutional Collaborating
Network on End-of-Life Care**
Phone: (415) 863-3045
Web site: http://www.growthhouse.org/
iicn.html

**International Association for the
Study of Pain (IASP)**
1510 H St. NW, Ste. 600
Washington, DC 20005-1020
Phone: (202) 524-5300
Fax: (202) 524-5301
E-mail: IASPdesk@iasp-pain.org
Web site: http://www.iasp-pain.org

**International Association for Trauma
Surgery and Intensive Care**
Secretariat IATSIC c/o ISS/SIC,
Seltisbergerstrasse 16
CH-4419 Lupsingen, Switzerland
Phone: +41 61 815 96 66
Fax: +41 61 811 47 75
E-mail: iatsic@iss-sic.ch
Web site: http://www.iatsic.org

**International Association of
Laryngectomees (IAL)**
925B Peachtree St. NE, Ste. 316
Atlanta, GA 30309
Toll free: (866) 425-3678
E-mail: webmaster@theial.com
Web site: http://www.theial.com

**International Association of Living
Organ Donors**
Web site: http://www.
livingdonorsonline.org

**International Cesarean Awareness
Network**
PO Box 31423
St. Louis, MO 63131
Toll free: (800) 686-ICAN (4226)
Web site: http://www.ican-online.org

**International Craniofacial
Institute**
Cleft Lip & Palate Treatment Center,
11970 N. Central Expy., Ste. 270
Dallas, TX 75243
Phone: (972) 331-1900
Toll free: (800) 344-4068
Fax: (972) 331-1909
E-mail: doctors@craniofacial.net
Web site: http://www.craniofacial.net

**International EECP Therapists
Association**
180 Linden Ave.
Westbury, NY 11590
Phone: (516) 997-4600
Toll free: (800) 455-EECP (3327)

Fax: (516) 997-2299
E-mail: info@eecp.com
Web site: http://www.eecp.com

**International Federation of
Gynecology and Obstetrics
(FIGO)**
FIGO House, Ste. 3, Waterloo Ct., 10
Theed St.
London SE1 8ST, United Kingdom
Phone: +44 20 7928 1166
Fax: +44 20 7928 7099
Web site: http://www.figo.org

**International Foundation for
Functional Gastrointestinal
Disorders (IFFGD)**
700 W. Virginia St., #201
Milwaukee, WI 53204
Phone: (414) 964-1799
Toll free: (888) 964-2001
Fax: (414) 964-7176
E-mail: iffgd@iffgd.org
Web site: http://www.iffgd.org

**International Myeloma Foundation
(IMF)**
12650 Riverside Dr., Ste. 206
North Hollywood, CA 91607
Phone: (818) 487-7455
Toll free: (800) 452-CURE (2873)
Fax: (818) 487-7454
E-mail: TheIMF@myeloma.org
Web site: http://www.myeloma.org

**International Osteoporosis
Foundation**
9, rue Juste-Olivier
CH-1260 Nyon, Switzerland, 1260
Phone: +41 22 994 0100
Fax: +41 22 994 0101
E-mail: info@iofbonehealth.org
Web site: http://www.iofbonehealth.org

**International Pancreas Transplant
Registry (IPTR)**
Division of Epidemiology Immunology
50 N. Brockway St., Ste. 304
Palatine, IL 60067
Phone: (847) 934-1918
E-mail: info@JCAAI.org
Web site: http://www.jcaai.org

K

Kaiser Family Foundation
2400 Sand Hill Rd.
Menlo Park, CA 94025
Phone: (650) 854-9400
Fax: (650) 854-4800
Web site: http://www.kff.org

L

**League Of Intravenous Therapy
Education Vascular Access
Network**
2400 Ardmore Blvd., Ste. 302
Pittsburgh, PA 15221
Phone: (412) 244-4338
Fax: (412) 243-5160
E-mail: info@lite.org
Web site: http://www.lite.org

The Leapfrog Group
1660 L St. NW, Ste. 308
Washington, DC 20036
Phone: (202) 292-6713
Fax: (202) 292-6813
E-mail: info@leapfroggroup.org
Web site: http://www.leapfroggroup.org

Leukemia & Lymphoma Society
1311 Mamaroneck Ave., Ste. 310
White Plains, NY 10605
Phone: (914) 949-5213
Toll free: (800) 955-4572
Fax: (914) 949-6691
E-mail: infocenter@lls.org
Web site: http://www.lls.org

**Life and Health Insurance
Foundation for Education (LIFE)**
1655 N. Fort Myer Dr., Ste. 610
Arlington, VA 22209
Toll free: (888) LIFE-777 (543-3777)
E-mail: info@lifehappens.org
Web site: http://www.lifehappens.org

Little Hearts
PO Box 171
Cromwell, CT 06416
Phone: (860) 635-0006
Toll free: (866) 435-HOPE (4673)
Web site: https://www.littlehearts.org

Lymphoma Research Foundation
115 Broadway, Ste. 1301
New York, NY 10006
Phone: (212) 349-2910
Toll free: (800) 500-9976
Fax: (212) 349-2886
E-mail: LRF@lymphoma.org
Web site: http://www.lymphoma.org

M

**Management of Myelomeningocele
Study (MOMS)**
GWU Biostatistics Center, 6110
Executive Blvd., Ste. 750
Rockville, MD 20852
Toll free: (866) ASK-MOMS (275-6667)
Fax: (866) 458-4621

E-mail: MOMS@biostat.bsc.gwu.edu
Web site: http://www.spinabifidamoms.
com

March of Dimes Foundation
1275 Mamaroneck Ave.
White Plains, NY 10605
Phone: (914) 997-4488
E-mail: askus@marchofdimes.com
Web site: http://www.marchofdimes.
com

Medicare Rights Center
520 Eighth Ave., N. Wing, 3rd Fl.
New York, NY 10018
Phone: (212) 869-3850
Toll free: (800) 333-4114
Fax: (212) 869-3532
E-mail: info@medicarerights.org
Web site: http://www.medicarerights.
org

Midwives Alliance of North America
1500 Sunday Dr., Ste. 102
Raleigh, NC 27607
Toll free: (888) 923-MANA (6262)
E-mail: info@mana.org
Web site: http://www.mana.org

Migraine Research Foundation
300 E. 75th St., Ste. 3K
New York, NY 10021
Phone: (212) 249-5402
Fax: (212) 249-5405
E-mail: info@migraineresearch
foundation.org
Web site: http://www.migraineresearch
foundation.org

**Miller Family Heart & Vascular
Institute at Cleveland Clinic**
9500 Euclid Ave.
Cleveland, OH 44195
Toll free: (800) 659-7822
TTY: (216) 444-0261
Web site: http://my.clevelandclinic.org/
heart/default.aspx

**Musculoskeletal Transplant
Foundation**
125 May St.
Edison, NJ 08837
Phone: (732) 661-0202
Toll free: (800) 946-9008
Fax: (732) 661-2298
Web site: http://www.mtf.org

N

National Abortion Federation
1660 L St. NW, Ste. 450
Washington, DC 20036
Phone: (202) 667-5881
Toll free: (800) 772-9100

Fax: (202) 667-5890
E-mail: naf@prochoice.org
Web site: http://www.prochoice.org

**National Alliance on Mental Illness
(NAMI)**
3803 N. Fairfax Dr., Ste. 100
Arlington, VA 22203
Phone: (703) 524-7600
Toll free: (800) 950-NAMI (6264)
Fax: (703) 524-9094
Web site: http://www.nami.org

National Amputation Foundation
40 Church St.
Malverne, NY 11565
Phone: (516) 887-3600
Fax: (516) 887-3667
E-mail: amps76@aol.com
Web site: http://www.
nationalamputation.org

**National Association for Continence
(NAFC)**
PO Box 1019
Charleston, SC 29402-1019
Phone: (843) 377-0900
Toll free: (800) BLADDER (252-3337)
Fax: (843) 377-0905
E-mail: memberservices@nafc.org
Web site: http://www.nafc.org

**National Association for Home Care
& Hospice**
228 Seventh St. SE
Washington, DC 20003
Phone: (202) 547-7424
Fax: (202) 547-3540
Web site: http://www.nahc.org

**National Association of Emergency
Medical Technicians**
132-A E. Northside Dr.
Clinton, MS 39056
Phone: (601) 924-7744
Toll free: (800) 34-NAEMT (346-2368)
Fax: (601) 924-7325
E-mail: info@naemt.org
Web site: http://www.naemt.org

**National Association of Neonatal
Nurses**
8735 W. Higgins Rd., Ste. 300
Chicago, IL 60631
Phone: (847) 375-3660
Toll free: (800) 451-3795
Fax: (866) 927-5321
E-mail: info@nann.org
Web site: http://www.nann.org

National Association of the Deaf
8630 Fenton St., Ste. 820
Silver Spring, MD 20910
Phone: (301) 587-1788
TTY: (301) 587-1789
Fax: (301) 587-1791

Web site: http://nad.org

**National Birth Defects Prevention
Network**
14781 Memorial Dr. #1561
Houston, TX 77079
E-mail: nbdpn@nbdpn.org
Web site: http://www.nbdpn.org

**National Bone Marrow Transplant
Link**
20411 W. 12 Mile Rd., Ste. 108
Southfield, MI 48076
Phone: (248) 358-1886
Toll free: (800) LINK-BMT (546-5268)
Fax: (248) 358-1889
E-mail: info@nbmtlink.org
Web site: http://nbmtlink.org

National Breast Cancer Coalition
1101 17th St. NW, Ste. 1300
Washington, DC 20036
Phone: (202) 296-7477
Toll free: (800) 622-2838
Fax: (202) 265-6854
Web site: http://www.
breastcancerdeadline2020.org

National Breast Cancer Foundation
2600 Network Blvd., Ste. 300
Frisco, TX 75034
Web site: http://www.nationalbreast
cancer.org

National Cancer Institute (NCI)
9609 Medical Center Dr.
Bethesda, MD 20892-9760
Toll free: (800) 4-CANCER (422-6237)
Web site: http://cancer.gov

National Caregivers Library
901 Moorefield Park Dr., Ste. 100
Richmond, VA 23236
Phone: (804) 327-1111
E-mail: info@caregiverslibrary.com
Web site: http://www.caregiverslibrary.
org

**National Center for Complementary
and Alternative Medicine
(NCCAM)**
9000 Rockville Pike
Bethesda, MD 20892
Toll free: (888) 644-6226
TTY: (866) 464-3615
Web site: http://nccam.nih.gov

**National Center on Sleep Disorders
Research**
6701 Rockledge Dr.
Bethesda, MD 20892
Phone: (301) 435-0199
Fax: (301) 480-3451
Web site: http://www.nhlbi.nih.gov/
about/ncsdr/index.htm

National Cervical Cancer Coalition (NCCC)
PO Box 13827
Research Triangle Park, NC 27709
Toll free: (800) 685-5531
Fax: (919) 361-8425
E-mail: nccc@ashastd.org
Web site: http://www.nccc-online.org

National Committee for Quality Assurance (NCQA)
1100 13th St. NW, Ste. 1000
Washington, DC 20005
Phone: (202) 955-3500
Toll free: (888) 275-7585
Fax: (202) 955-3599
E-mail: customersupport@ncqa.org
Web site: http://www.ncqa.org

National Comprehensive Cancer Network (NCCN)
275 Commerce Dr., Ste. 300
Fort Washington, PA 19034
Phone: (215) 690-0300
Fax: (215) 690-0280
Web site: http://www.nccn.org

National Consumer Voice for Quality Long-Term Care
1001 Connecticut Ave. NW, Ste. 425
Washington, DC 20036
Phone: (202) 332-2275
Fax: (866) 230-9789
E-mail: info@theconsumervoice.org
Web site: http://www.theconsumer
  voice.org

National Diabetes Information Clearinghouse (NDIC)
1 Information Way
Bethesda, MD 20892-3560
Toll free: (800) 860-8747
TTY: (866) 569-1162
Fax: (703) 738-4929
E-mail: ndic@info.niddk.nih.gov
Web site: http://diabetes.niddk.nih.gov

National Digestive Diseases Information Clearinghouse (NDDIC)
2 Information Way
Bethesda, MD 20892-3570
Toll free: (800) 891-5389
TTY: (866) 569-1162
Fax: (703) 738-4929
E-mail: nddic@info.niddk.nih.gov
Web site: http://www.digestive.niddk.
  nih.gov

National Down Syndrome Society (NDSS)
666 Broadway, 8th Fl.
New York, NY 10012
Toll free: (800) 221-4602
E-mail: info@ndss.org
Web site: http://www.ndss.org

National Endocrine and Metabolic Diseases Information Service
6 Information Way
Bethesda, MD 20892-3569
Toll free: (888) 828-0904
Fax: (703) 738-4929
E-mail: endoandmeta@info.niddk.nih.
  gov
Web site: http://www.endocrine.niddk.
  nih.gov

National Eye Institute (NEI)
NEI Information Office, 31 Center Dr.,
  MSC 2510
Bethesda, MD 20892-2510
Phone: (301) 496-5248
E-mail: 2020@nei.nih.gov
Web site: http://www.nei.nih.gov

National Foundation for Transplants
5350 Poplar Ave., Ste. 430
Memphis, TN 38119
Phone: (901) 684-1697
Toll free: (800) 489-3863
Fax: (901) 684-1128
E-mail: info@transplants.org
Web site: http://www.transplants.org

National Heart, Lung, and Blood Institute, Division of Blood Diseases and Resources
Two Rockledge Ctr., Ste. 9030, 6701
  Rockledge Dr., MSC 7950
Bethesda, MD 20892-7950
Phone: (301) 435-0080
Web site: http://www.nhlbi.nih.gov/
  about/dbdr/index.htm

National Heart, Lung, and Blood Institute Information Center
PO Box 30105
Bethesda, MD 20824-0105
Phone: (301) 592-8573
Fax: (301) 592-8563
E-mail: nhlbiinfo@nhlbi.nih.gov
Web site: http://www.nhlbi.nih.gov

National Highway Traffic Safety Administration (NHTSA)
1200 New Jersey Ave. SE, West Bldg.
Washington, DC 20590
Toll free: (888) 327-4236
TTY: (800) 424-9153
Web site: http://www.nhtsa.gov

National Hospice and Palliative Care Organization (NHPCO)
1731 King St., Ste. 100
Alexandria, VA 22314
Phone: (703) 837-1500
Toll free: (800) 646-6460
Fax: (703) 837-1233
E-mail: nhpco_info@nhpco.org
Web site: http://www.nhpco.org

National Human Genome Research Institute
National Institutes of Health, 9000
  Rockville Pike, Bldg. 31, Rm. 4B09,
  31 Center Dr., MSC 2152
Bethesda, MD 20892-2152
Phone: (301) 402-0911
Fax: (301) 402-2218
Web site: http://www.genome.gov

National Institute for Jewish Hospice
732 University St.
North Woodmere, NY 11581
Phone: (516) 791-9888
Toll free: (800) 446-4448
E-mail: shirlamm@nijh.org
Web site: http://www.nijh.org

National Institute of Allergy and Infectious Diseases (NIAID)
Office of Communications and
  Government Relations, 6610
  Rockledge Dr., MSC 6612
Bethesda, MD 20892-6612
Phone: (301) 496-5717
Toll free: (866) 284-4107
TTY: (800) 877-8339
Fax: (301) 402-3573
E-mail: ocpostoffice@niaid.nih.gov
Web site: http://www.niaid.nih.gov

National Institute of Arthritis and Musculoskeletal and Skin Diseases (NIAMS)
NIAMS Information Clearinghouse, 1
  AMS Cir.
Bethesda, MD 20892-3675
Phone: (301) 495-4484
Toll free: (877) 22-NIAMS (226-4267)
TTY: (301) 565-2966
Fax: (301) 718-6366
E-mail: NIAMSinfo@mail.nih.gov
Web site: http://www.niams.nih.gov

National Institute of Biomedical Imaging and Bioengineering
9000 Rockville Pike, Bldg. 31, Rm.
  1C14
Bethesda, MD 20892-8859
Phone: (301) 496-8859
E-mail: info@nibib.nih.gov
Web site: http://www.nibib.gov

National Institute of Dental and Craniofacial Research (NIDCR)
Toll free: (866) 232-4528
Fax: (301) 480-4098
E-mail: nidcrinfo@mail.nih.gov
Web site: http://www.nidcr.nih.gov

National Institute of Diabetes and Digestive and Kidney Diseases (NIDDK)
31 Center Dr., MSC 2560, Bldg. 31,
  Rm. 9A06
Bethesda, MD 20892-2560

Phone: (301) 496-3583
Web site: http://www2.niddk.nih.gov

National Institute of Environmental Health Sciences (NIEHS)
PO Box 12233, MD K3-16
Research Triangle Park, NC 27709
Phone: (919) 541-3345
Fax: (301) 480-2978
E-mail: webcenter@niehs.nih.gov
Web site: http://www.niehs.nih.gov

National Institute of Mental Health (NIMH)
6001 Executive Blvd., Rm. 6200, MSC 9663
Bethesda, MD 20892-9663
Phone: (301) 443-4513
Toll free: (866) 615-6464
TTY: (866) 415-8051
Fax: (301) 443-4279
E-mail: nimhinfo@nih.gov
Web site: http://www.nimh.nih.gov

National Institute of Neurological Disorders and Stroke (NINDS)
NIH Neurological Institute, PO Box 5801
Bethesda, MD 20824
Phone: (301) 496-5751
Toll free: (800) 352-9424
Web site: http://www.ninds.nih.gov

National Institute on Aging (NIA)
31 Center Dr., MSC 2292, Bldg. 31, Rm. 5C27
Bethesda, MD 20892
Toll free: (800) 222-2225
TTY: (800) 222-4225
E-mail: niaic@nia.nih.gov
Web site: http://www.nia.nih.gov

National Institute on Deafness and Other Communication Disorders (NIDCD)
NIDCD Office of Health Communication and Public Liaison, 31 Center Dr., MSC 2320
Bethesda, MD 20892-2320
Phone: (301) 496-7243
Toll free: (800) 241-1044
TTY: (800) 241-1055
Fax: (301) 402-0018
E-mail: nidcdinfo@nidcd.nih.gov
Web site: http://www.nidcd.nih.gov

National Institutes of Health (NIH)
9000 Rockville Pike
Bethesda, MD 20892
Phone: (301) 496-4000
TTY: (301) 402-9612
E-mail: NIHinfo@od.nih.gov
Web site: http://www.nih.gov

National Jewish Health's Lung Line
Toll free: (800) 222-LUNG (222-5864)

E-mail: lungline@njhealth.org
Web site: http://www.nationaljewish.org

National Kidney and Urologic Diseases Information Clearinghouse
3 Information Way
Bethesda, MD 20892-3580
Toll free: (800) 891-5390
TTY: (866) 569-1162
Fax: (703) 738-4929
E-mail: nkudic@info.niddk.nih.gov
Web site: http://kidney.niddk.nih.gov

National Kidney Foundation
30 E. 33rd St.
New York, NY 10016
Toll free: (800) 622-9010
Fax: (212) 689-9261
E-mail: info@kidney.org
Web site: http://www.kidney.org

National Lung Health Education Program
18000 W. 105th St.
Olathe, KS 66061
Phone: (913) 895-4631
E-mail: nlhep@goamp.com
Web site: http://www.nlhep.org

National Lymphedema Network
116 New Montgomery St., Ste. 235
San Francisco, CA 94105
Phone: (415) 908-3681
Toll free: (800) 541-3259
Fax: (415) 908-3813
E-mail: nln@lymphnet.org
Web site: http://lymphnet.org

National Marrow Donor Program (NMDP)
3001 Broadway St. NE, Ste. 100
Minneapolis, MN 55413-1753
Phone: (612) 627-5800
Toll free: (800) MARROW2 (627-7692)
E-mail: patientinfo@nmdp.org
Web site: http://bethematch.org

National Organization for Rare Disorders (NORD)
55 Kenosia Ave.
Danbury, CT 06810
Phone: (203) 744-0100
Toll free: (800) 999-6673
Fax: (203) 798-2291
Web site: http://rarediseases.org

National Osteoporosis Foundation
1150 17th St. NW, Ste. 850
Washington, DC 20036
Phone: (202) 223-2226
Toll free: (800) 231-4222
Fax: (202) 223-2237
E-mail: info@nof.org
Web site: http://www.nof.org

National Parkinson Foundation
1501 NW 9th Ave./Bob Hope Rd.
Miami, FL 33136-1494
Phone: (305) 243-6666
Toll free: (800) 4PD-INFO (473-4636)
Fax: (305) 243-6073
E-mail: contact@parkinson.org
Web site: http://www.parkinson.org

National Patient Advocate Foundation
725 15th St. NW, 10th Fl.
Washington, DC 20005
Phone: (202) 347-8009
Fax: (202) 347-5579
E-mail: action@npaf.org
Web site: http://www.npaf.org

National Patient Safety Foundation
268 Summer St., 6th Fl.
Boston, MA 02210
Phone: (617) 391-9900
Fax: (617) 391-9999
Web site: http://www.npsf.org

National Pressure Ulcer Advisory Panel
1025 Thomas Jefferson St. NW, Ste. 500 E.
Washington, DC 20007
Phone: (202) 521-6789
Fax: (202) 833-3636
Web site: http://www.npuap.org

National Prevention Information Network, Centers for Disease Control and Prevention (CDC NPIN)
PO Box 6003
Rockville, MD 20849-6003
E-mail: info@cdcnpin.org
Web site: http://www.cdcnpin.org

National Scoliosis Foundation
5 Cabot Pl.
Stoughton, MA 02072
Toll free: (800) NSF-MYBACK (673-6922)
E-mail: nsf@scoliosis.org
Web site: http://www.scoliosis.org

National Society of Genetic Counselors
330 N. Wabash Ave., Ste. 2000
Chicago, IL 60611
Phone: (312) 321-6834
Fax: (312) 673-6972
E-mail: nsgc@nsgc.org
Web site: http://www.nsgc.org

National Stroke Association
9707 E. Easter Ln., Ste. B
Centennial, CO 80112
Toll free: (800) STROKES (787-6537)
Fax: (303) 649-1328
E-mail: info@stroke.org
Web site: http://www.stroke.org

**National Women's Health Network
(NWHN)**
1413 K St. NW, 4th Fl.
Washington, DC 20005
Phone: (202) 682-2640
Fax: (202) 682-2648
E-mail: nwhn@nwhn.org
Web site: http://www.nwhn.org

Nemours Foundation
10140 Centurion Pkwy. N.
Jacksonville, FL 32256
Phone: (904) 697-4100
Web site: http://www.nemours.org

**New England Ophthalmological
Society**
PO Box 9165, 50 Staniford St., 7th Fl.
Boston, MA 02114
Phone: (617) 227-6484
Fax: (617) 367-4908
E-mail: neosjudy@aol.com
Web site: http://www.neos-eyes.org

**North American Society for Pediatric
Gastroenterology, Hepatology and
Nutrition**
PO Box 6
Flourtown, PA 19031
Phone: (215) 233-0808
Fax: (215) 233-3918
E-mail: naspghan@naspghan.org
Web site: http://www.naspghan.org

**North American Spine Society
(NASS)**
7075 Veterans Blvd.
Burr Ridge, IL 60527
Phone: (630) 230-3600
Toll free: (866) 960-6277
Fax: (630) 230-3700
Web site: http://www.spine.org

O

Obesity Society
8757 Georgia Ave., Ste. 1320
Silver Spring, MD 20910
Phone: (301) 563-6526
Toll free: (800) 974-3084
Fax: (301) 563-6595
Web site: http://www.obesity.org

**Occupational Safety and Health
Administration (OSHA)**
200 Constitution Ave.
Washington, DC 20210
Toll free: (800) 321-OSHA (6742)
TTY: (877) 889-5627
Web site: http://www.osha.gov

**Office of Cancer Complementary and
Alternative Medicine (OCCAM)**
9609 Medical Center Dr., Rm. 5-W-136

Rockville, MD 20850
Phone: (240) 276-6595
Fax: (240) 276-7888
E-mail: ncioccam1-r@mail.nih.gov
Web site: http://cam.cancer.gov

Office on Women's Health
U.S. Department of Health and Human
Services, 200 Independence Ave.
SW, Rm. 712E
Washington, DC 20201
Phone: (202) 690-7650
Toll free: (800) 994-9662
Fax: (202) 205-2631
Web site: http://womenshealth.gov

Oral Cancer Foundation
3419 Via Lido, #205
Newport Beach, CA 92663
Phone: (949) 646-8000
E-mail: info@oralcancerfoundation.org
Web site: http://oralcancerfoundation.
org

Oregon Health Study
5211 NE Glisan St.
Portland, OR 97213
Toll free: (877) 215-0686
E-mail: info@oregonhealthstudy.org
Web site: http://oregonhealthstudy.org

Orthopaedic Trauma Association
6300 N. River Rd., Ste. 727
Rosemont, IL 60018-4226
Phone: (847) 698-1631
Fax: (847) 823-0536
E-mail: OTA@aaos.org
Web site: http://www.ota.org

Overeaters Anonymous
6075 Zenith Ct. NE
Rio Rancho, NM 87144-6424
Phone: (505) 891-2664
Fax: (505) 891-4320
Web site: http://www.oa.org

P

**Pan Birmingham Cancer Research
Network**
Old Queen Elizabeth Hospital,
Mindelsohn Way
Birmingham B15 2SQ
United Kingdom
Phone: +44 0121 414 8283
E-mail: pbcrn@uhb.nhs.uk
Web site: http://www.
birminghamcancer.nhs.uk

Pancreatic Cancer Action Network
1500 Rosecrans Ave., Ste. 200
Manhattan Beach, CA 90226
Phone: (310) 725-0025

Toll free: (877) 272-6226
Fax: (310) 725-0029
E-mail: info@pancan.org
Web site: http://www.pancan.org

**Patient Safety Partnership/Safe Care
Campaign**
625 Aunt Lucy Ln., Ste. 20
Smyrna, GA 30082
Phone: (678) 309-9600
E-mail: vnahum@patientsafety
partnership.org; anahum@
patientsafetypartnership.org
Web site: http://www.patientsafety
partnership.org; http://www.safecare
campaign.org

**Peripheral Vascular Surgery Society
(PVSS)**
100 Cummings Ctr., Ste. 124A
Beverly, MA 01915
Phone: (978) 927-7800
Fax: (978) 927-7872
E-mail: pvss@administrare.com
Web site: http://www.pvss.org

**The Philadelphia Center For
Transgender Surgery**
19 Montgomery Ave.
Bala Cynwyd, PA 19004
Phone: (610) 667-1888
E-mail: DrShermanLeis@DrSherman
Leis.com
Web site: http://www.
thetransgendercenter.com

Pioneer Network
35 E. Wacker Dr., Ste. 850
Chicago, IL 60601
Phone: (312) 224-2574
Fax: (312) 644-8557
E-mail: info@pioneernetwork.net
Web site: http://www.pioneernetwork.
net

**Planned Parenthood Federation of
America**
434 W. 33rd St.
New York, NY 10001
Phone: (212) 541-7800
Toll free: (800) 230-PLAN (7526)
Fax: (212) 245-1845
Web site: http://www.planned
parenthood.org

Prevent Blindness America
211 W. Wacker Dr., Ste. 1700
Chicago, IL 60606
Toll free: (800) 331-2020
Web site: http://www.preventblindness.
org

Privacy Rights Clearinghouse
3108 Fifth Ave., Ste. A
San Diego, CA 92103

Phone: (619) 298-3396
Web site: https://www.privacyrights.org

Prostate Cancer Foundation
1250 Fourth St.
Santa Monica, CA 90401
Phone: (310) 570-4700
Toll free: (800) 757-CURE (2873)
Fax: (310) 570-4701
E-mail: info@pcf.org
Web site: http://www.pcf.org

Pulmonary Paper
PO Box 877
Ormond Beach, FL 32175-0877
Toll free: (800) 950-3698
E-mail: info@pulmonarypaper.org
Web site: https://www.pulmonarypaper.org

PULSE (Persons United Limiting Substandards and Errors in Health Care
Toll free: (800) 96-PULSE
E-mail: PULSE516@aol.com;
PULSEofFlorida@gmail.com
Web site: http://www.pulseamerica.org

Queensland Health
147-163 Charlotte St.
Brisbane, Queensland 4000
Australia
Phone: +61 7 3234 0111
Web site: http://www.health.qld.gov.au

R Adams Cowley Shock Trauma Center, University of Maryland Medical Center
22 S. Greene St.
Baltimore, MD 21201-1595
Toll free: (800) 492-5538
Web site: http://www.umm.edu/shocktrauma

Radiological Society of North America (RSNA)
820 Jorie Blvd.
Oak Brook, IL 60523-2251
Phone: (630) 571-2670
Toll free: (800) 381-6660
Fax: (630) 571-7837
Web site: http://www.rsna.org

RESOLVE: The National Infertility Association
1760 Old Meadow Rd., Ste. 500
McLean, VA 22102

Phone: (703) 556-7172
Fax: (703) 506-3266
Web site: http://www.resolve.org

Royal College of Surgeons of England
35-43 Lincoln's Inn Fields
London, WC2A 3PE
England
Phone: +44 20 7405 8074
E-mail: office@baoms.org.uk
Web site: http://www.baoms.org.uk

Rural Assistance Center
501 N. Columbia Rd., Stop 9037
Grand Forks, ND 58202-9037
Toll free: (800) 270-1898
Fax: (800) 270-1913
E-mail: info@raconline.org
Web site: http://www.raconline.org

S

Scientific Registry of Transplant Recipients (SRTR)
914 S. 8th St., Ste. S-4.100
Minneapolis, MN 55404
Phone: (877) 970-SRTR
Fax: (612) 347-5878
E-mail: srtr@srtr.org
Web site: http://srtr.org

Screening for Mental Health, Inc.
One Washington St., Ste. 304
Wellesley Hills, MA 02481
Phone: (781) 239-0071
Fax: (781) 431-7447
E-mail: smhinfo@mentalhealthscreening.org
Web site: http://www.mentalhealthscreening.org

Second Wind Lung Transplant Association
Toll free: (888) 855-9463
Web site: http://www.2ndwind.org

Simon Foundation for Continence
PO Box 815
Wilmette, IL 60091
Phone: (847) 864-3913
Toll free: (800) 23-SIMON (237-4666)
Fax: (847) 864-9758
E-mail: info@simonfoundation.org
Web site: http://simonfoundation.org

Sinai Center for Geriatric Surgery
Sinai Hospital, 2401 W. Belvedere Ave.
Baltimore, MD 21215
Phone: (410) 601-5719
E-mail: jocolema@lifebridgehealth.org
Web site: http://www.lifebridgehealth.org/GeriatricSurgery/GeriatricSurgery1.aspx

Skin Cancer Foundation
149 Madison Ave., Ste. 901
New York, NY 10016
Phone: (212) 725-5176
Web site: http://www.skincancer.org

Society for Clinical Vascular Surgery (SCVS)
500 Cummings Ctr., Ste. 4550
Beverly, MA 01915
Phone: (978) 927-8330
Fax: (978) 524-8890
Web site: http://scvs.org

Society for Gastroenterology Nurses and Associates
330 N. Wabash Ave., Ste. 2000
Chicago, IL 60611-7621
Phone: (312) 321-5165
Toll free: (800) 245-7462
Fax: (312) 673-6694
E-mail: sgna@smithbucklin.com
Web site: http://www.sgna.org

Society for Neuro-Oncology (SNO)
4617 Birch St.
Bellaire, TX 77401-5509
Phone: (281) 554-6589
Web site: http://www.soc-neuro-onc.org

Society for Pediatric Urology
500 Cummings Ctr., Ste. 4550
Beverly, MA 01915
Phone: (978) 927-8330
Fax: (978) 524-8890
Web site: http://spuonline.org

Society for Technology in Anesthesia
6737 W. Washington St., Ste. 1300
Milwaukee, WI 53214
Phone: (414) 389-8600
Fax: (414) 276-7704
E-mail: STAhq@STAhq.org
Web site: http://www.stahq.org

Society for the Advancement of Blood Management (SABM)
350 Engle St.
Englewood, NJ 07631
Phone: (434) 977-3716
Web site: http://www.sabm.org

Society for Vascular Surgery
633 N. Saint Clair St., 22nd Fl.
Chicago, IL 60611
Phone: (312) 334-2300
Toll free: (800) 258-7188
Fax: (312) 334-2320
E-mail: vascular@vascularsociety.org
Web site: http://www.vascularweb.org

Society of American Gastrointestinal Endoscopic Surgeons (SAGES)
11300 W. Olympic Blvd., Ste. 600
Los Angeles, CA 90064
Phone: (310) 437-0544

Fax: (310) 437-0585
E-mail: sagesweb@sages.org
Web site: http://www.sages.org

Society of Critical Care Medicine
500 Midway Dr.
Mount Prospect, IL 60056
Phone: (847) 827-6869
Fax: (847) 827-6886
E-mail: info@sccm.org
Web site: http://www.sccm.org

Society of Diagnostic Medical Sonography
2745 Dallas Pkwy., Ste. 350
Plano, TX 75093-8730
Phone: (214) 473-8057
Toll free: (800) 229-9506
Fax: (214) 473-8563
Web site: http://www.sdms.org

Society of Gynecologic Oncology (SGO)
230 W. Monroe St., Ste. 710
Chicago, IL 60606-4703
Phone: (312) 235-4060
Fax: (312) 235-4059
E-mail: sgo@sgo.org
Web site: https://www.sgo.org

Society of Hospital Medicine (SHM)
1500 Spring Garden, Ste. 501
Philadelphia, PA 19130
Toll free: (800) 843-3360
Fax: (267) 702-2690
E-mail: webmaster@hospitalmedicine.org
Web site: http://www.hospitalmedicine.org

Society of Interventional Radiology
3975 Fair Ridge Dr., Ste. 400 N.
Fairfax, VA 22033
Phone: (703) 691-1805
Toll free: (800) 488-7284
Fax: (703) 691-1855
Web site: http://www.sirweb.org

Society of Laparoendoscopic Surgeons
7330 SW 62nd Pl., Ste. 410
Miami, FL 33143-4825
Phone: (305) 665-9959
Fax: (305) 667-4123
E-mail: Info@SLS.org
Web site: http://www.sls.org

Society of NeuroInterventional Surgery
975 Fair Ridge Dr., Ste. 200 N.
Fairfax, VA 22033
Phone: (703) 691-2272
Fax: (703) 537-0650
Web site: http://www.snisonline.org

Society of Nuclear Medicine and Molecular Imaging
1850 Samuel Morse Dr.
Reston, VA 20190
Phone: (703) 708-9000
Fax: (703) 708-9015
E-mail: feedback@snm.org
Web site: http://www.snm.org

Society of Robotic Surgery
1100 E. Woodfield Rd., Ste. 350
Schaumburg, IL 60173
Phone: (847) 517-7225
E-mail: srs@wjweiser.com
Web site: http://www.srobotics.org

The Society of Thoracic Surgeons
633 N. Saint Clair St., Fl. 23
Chicago, IL 60611
Phone: (312) 202-5800
Fax: (312) 202-5801
Web site: http://sts.org

Society of Toxicology
1821 Michael Faraday Dr., Ste. 300
Reston, VA 20190
Phone: (703) 438-3115
Fax: (703) 438-3113
E-mail: sothq@toxicology.org
Web site: http://www.toxicology.org

Society of Urologic Nurses and Associates (SUNA)
E. Holly Ave., Box 56
Pitman, NJ 08071-0056
Toll free: (888) 827-7862
E-mail: suna@ajj.com
Web site: http://suna.org

Southern Thoracic Surgical Association
633 N. Saint Clair St., Fl. 23
Chicago, IL 60611-3658
Phone: (312) 202-5892
Toll free: (800) 685-7872
Fax: (773) 289-0871
E-mail: stsa@stsa.org
Web site: http://stsa.org

Spina Bifida Association of America
4590 MacArthur Blvd. NW, Ste. 250
Washington, DC 20007-4226
Phone: (202) 944-3285
Toll free: (800) 621-3141
Fax: (202) 944-3295
E-mail: sbaa@sbaa.org
Web site: http://www.spinabifidaassociation.org

T

Texas Heart Institute
6770 Bertner Ave.
Houston, TX 77030

Phone: (832) 355-4011
Toll free: (800) 292-2221
E-mail: hic@heart.thi.tmc.edu
Web site: http://www.texasheartinstitute.org

Transplant Foundation
701 SW 27th Ave., Ste. 705
Miami, FL 33135
Phone: (305) 817-5645
Toll free: (866) 900-3172
Fax: (305) 541-6500
E-mail: ecompton@med.miami.edu
Web site: http://transplantfoundation.org

Transplant Recipients International Organization (TRIO)
2100 M St. NW, #170-353
Washington, DC 20037-1233
Phone: (202) 293-0980
Toll free: (800) TRIO-386 (874-6386)
E-mail: info@trioweb.org
Web site: http://www.trioweb.org

TransWeb.org
University of Michigan Transplant Center, 3868 Taubman Ctr., 1500 E. Medical Center Dr., SPC 5391
Ann Arbor, MI 48109-5391
Phone: (734) 232-1113
E-mail: transweb@umich.edu
Web site: http://www.transweb.org

U

UCSF Cochlear Implant Center
University of California, San Francisco, Department of Otolaryngology, 2380 Sutter St., 1st Fl.
San Francisco, CA 94115
Phone: (415) 353-2464
Fax: (415) 353-2603
E-mail: cochlearimplant@ucsfmedctr.org
Web site: http://cochlear.ucsf.edu

UK Department of Health
Richmond House, 79 Whitehall
London, England, SW1A 2NS
Phone: +44 20 7210 4850
Fax: +44 20 7210 5952
Web site: https://www.gov.uk/dh

United Cerebral Palsy (UCP)
1825 K St. NW, Ste. 600
Washington, DC 20006
Phone: (202) 776-0406
Toll free: (800) 872-5827
Web site: http://www.ucp.org

United Hospital Fund
1411 Broadway, 12th Fl.
New York, NY 10018

Phone: (212) 494-0700
Fax: (212) 494-0800
Web site: http://www.uhfnyc.org

United Network for Organ Sharing (UNOS)
700 N. 4th St.
Richmond, VA 23219
Phone: (804) 782-4800
Toll free: (888) 894-6361
Web site: http://www.unos.org

United Ostomy Associations of America, Inc. (UOAA)
PO Box 512
Northfield, MN 55057-0512
Toll free: (800) 826-0826
E-mail: info@ostomy.org
Web site: http://www.ostomy.org

University of Arizona Center for Integrative Medicine
PO Box 245153
Tucson, AZ 85724-5153
Phone: (520) 626-6489
Web site: http://integrativemedicine.arizona.edu

University of California, San Francisco (UCSF) Center for HIV Information
4150 Clement St., Bldg. 16, VAMC 111V-UCSF
San Francisco, CA 94121
Phone: (415) 379-5601
Fax: (415) 379-5547
E-mail: chi@ucsf.edu
Web site: http://chi.ucsf.edu

University of Maryland School of Medicine, Center for Integrative Medicine
Kernan Hospital, 2200 Kernan Dr.
Baltimore, MD 21207
Phone: (410) 448-6361
Fax: (410) 448-1873
E-mail: clinic@compmed.umm.edu
Web site: http://www.compmed.umm.edu

University of Michigan Kellogg Eye Center
1000 Wall St.
Ann Arbor, MI 48105
Phone: (734) 763-8122
E-mail: contactkellogg@umich.edu
Web site: http://www.kellogg.umich.edu

Urology Care Foundation
1000 Corporate Blvd.
Linthicum, MD 21090
Phone: (410) 689-3700
Toll free: (800) 828-7866
Fax: (410) 689-3998

E-mail: info@urologycarefoundation.org
Web site: http://www.urologyhealth.org

U.S. Chemical Safety Board (CSB)
2175 K. St. NW, Ste. 400
Washington, DC 20037-1809
Phone: (202) 261-7600
Fax: (202) 261-7650
E-mail: public@csb.gov
Web site: http://www.csb.gov

U.S. Department of Health and Human Services
200 Independence Ave. SW
Washington, DC 20201
Toll free: (877) 696-6775
Web site: http://www.hhs.gov

U.S. Environmental Protection Agency
1200 Pennsylvania Ave. NW
Washington, DC 20460
Phone: (202) 272-0167
TTY: (202) 272-0165
Web site: http://www.epa.gov

U.S. Food and Drug Administration (FDA)
10903 New Hampshire Ave.
Silver Spring, MD 20993
Toll free: (888) INFO-FDA (463-6332)
Web site: http://www.fda.gov

U.S. Food and Drug Administration (FDA), National Center for Toxicological Research (NCTR)
3900 NCTR Rd.
Jefferson, AR 72079
Phone: (870) 543-7000
E-mail: NCTRinformation@fda.hhs.gov
Web site: http://www.fda.gov/AboutFDA/CentersOffices/OC/OfficeofScientificandMedical Programs/NCTR/default.htm

U.S. Living Will Registry
523 Westfield Ave., PO Box 2789
Westfield, NJ 07091-2789
Toll free: (800) LIV-WILL (548-9455)
Fax: (908) 654-1919
E-mail: admin@uslivingwillregistry.com
Web site: http://www.uslivingwillregistry.com

U.S. Pharmacopeial Convention (USP)
12601 Twinbrook Pkwy.
Rockville, MD 20852-1790
Phone: (301) 881-0666
Toll free: (800) 227-8772
Web site: http://www.usp.org

U.S. Renal Data System (USRDS)
701 Park Ave., Ste. S2.100
Minneapolis, MN 55415
Phone: (612) 347-7776
Toll free: (888) 99-USRDS (998-7737)
Fax: (612) 347-5878
E-mail: usrds@usrds.org
Web site: http://www.usrds.org

V

Vascular Birthmarks Foundation
PO Box 106
Latham, NY 12110
Toll free: (877) VBF-4646 (823-4646)
E-mail: hvbf@aol.com
Web site: http://birthmark.org

Vascular Disease Foundation
550 M Ritchie Hwy., PMB-281
Severna Park, MD 21146
Phone: (443) 261-5564
E-mail: robert.greenberg@vdf.org
Web site: http://vasculardisease.org

Vestibular Disorders Association (VEDA)
5018 NE 15th Ave.
Portland, OR 97211
Toll free: (800) VESTIBU (837-8428)
E-mail: info@vestibular.org
Web site: http://vestibular.org

VNAA (Visiting Nurse Associations of America)
601 Thirteenth St. NW, Ste. 610N
Washington, DC 20005
Phone: (202) 384-1420
Toll free: (888) 866-8773
E-mail: vnaa@vnaa.org
Web site: http://vnaa.org

W

Washington Home Center for Palliative Care Studies
4200 Wisconsin Ave. NW, 4th Fl.
Washington, DC 20016
Phone: (202) 895-2625
Fax: (202) 966-5410
E-mail: info@medicaring.org
Web site: http://medicaring.org

Weight-control Information Network (WIN)
1 WIN Way
Bethesda, MD 20892-3665
Toll free: (877) 946-4627
Fax: (202) 828-1028
E-mail: win@info.niddk.nih.gov
Web site: http://www.win.niddk.nih.gov

Wills Eye Institute
840 Walnut St.
Philadelphia, PA 19107
Toll free: (877) AT-WILLS (289-4557)
Web site: http://www.willseye.org

World Health Organization
Avenue Appia 20
1211 Geneva 27, Switzerland
Phone: +41 22 791 21 11
Fax: +41 22 791 31 11
Web site: http://www.who.int

World Heart Federation
7, rue des Battoirs
1211 Geneva, Switzerland
Phone: +41 22 807 03 20
E-mail: info@worldheart.org
Web site: http://www.world-heart-
     federation.org

**World Professional Association for
     Transgender Health**
1300 S. Second St., Ste. 180
Minneapolis, MN 55454
E-mail: wpath@wpath.org
Web site: http://www.wpath.org

Wound Care Institute, Inc.
1100 NE 163rd St., Ste. 101
North Miami Beach, FL 33162
Phone: (305) 919-9192
E-mail: FishmanTamara@hotmail.com
Web site: http://woundcare.org

Wound Healing Society
9650 Rockville Pike
Bethesda, MD 20814
Phone: (301) 634-7600
E-mail: info@woundheal.org
Web site: http://www.woundheal.org

**Wound Ostomy and Continence
     Nurses Society (WOCN)**
15000 Commerce Pkwy., Ste. C
Mount Laurel, NJ 08054
Toll free: (888) 224-9626
Fax: (856) 439-0525
E-mail: wocn_info@wocn.org
Web site: http://www.wocn.org

Z

Zen Hospice Project
273 Page St.
San Francisco, CA 94102
Phone: (415) 913-7682
Fax: (415) 374-7458
E-mail: guesthouse@zenhospice.org
Web site: http://www.zenhospice.org

GLOSSARY

The glossary is an alphabetical compilation of terms and definitions listed in the *Key Terms* sections of the main body entries. Although the list is comprehensive, it is by no means exhaustive.

A

ABCDE. A survey standard used by emergency responders to do an initial assessment of patients in a non-healthcare setting; stands for Airway, Breathing, Circulation, Disability, and Exposure.

ABDOMEN. The portion of the body that lies between the thorax and the pelvis.

ABDOMINAL ANEURYSM. Aneurysm that involves the descending aorta, from the diaphragm to the point at which it separates into two iliac arteries.

ABDOMINAL AORTIC ANEURYSM. Occurs when an area in the aorta (the main artery of the heart) is weakened and bulges like a balloon. The abdominal section of the aorta supplies blood to the lower body.

ABDOMINAL DISTENSION. Swelling of the abdominal cavity, which creates painful pressure on the internal organs.

ABDOMINAL HERNIA. A defect in the abdominal wall through which the abdominal organs protrude.

ABLATION. Removal or destruction of tissue, such as by burning or cutting.

ABLATION THERAPY. A procedure used to treat arrhythmias, especially atrial fibrillation. During the procedure, a catheter (small flexible tube) is inserted in a vein and threaded to the heart. High-frequency electrical energy is delivered through the catheter to disconnect the pathway in the heart that is causing the abnormal rhythm.

ABO ANTIGEN. Protein molecules located on the surfaces of red blood cells that determine a person's blood type: A, B, or O.

ABO BLOOD GROUPS. A system in which human blood is classified according to the A and B antigens found in red blood cells. Type A blood has the A antigen, type B has the B antigen, type AB has both, and type O has neither.

ABO BLOOD TYPE. Blood type based on the presence or absence of the A and B antigens on the red blood cells. There are four types: A, B, AB, and O.

ABSCESS. A localized collection of pus at the site of an infection.

ACCESS SITE. The point where a needle or catheter is inserted for dialysis.

ACCESSORY ORGAN. A lump of tissue adjacent to an organ that is similar to the organ but serves no important purpose (if it functions at all). While not necessarily harmful, such organs can cause problems if they are confused with a mass or, in rare cases, if they grow too large or become cancerous.

ACETABULAR DYSPLASIA. A type of arthritis resulting in a shallow hip socket.

ACETABULUM. The socket-shaped part of the pelvis that forms part of the hip joint.

ACETAMINOPHEN. A common pain reliever (e.g., Tylenol).

ACETIC ACID. The acid in vinegar.

ACHALASIA. Failure of the lower end of the esophagus (or another tubular valve) to open, resulting in obstruction.

ACID. Any chemical or compound that lowers the pH of a solution below 7.0, meaning that there is a surplus of hydrogen ions dissociated within that solution.

ACIDOSIS. Increased acidity of the blood, usually defined as a pH below 7.35 in arterial blood.

ACL RECONSTRUCTION. Repairing a tear of the anterior cruciate ligament (ACL) of the knee using arthroscopy and/or open surgery.

ACOUSTIC NERVE. Nerve within the inner ear that supplies hearing and assists with balance.

ACOUSTIC WINDOW. Area through which ultrasound waves move freely.

ACQUIRED IMMUNODEFICIENCY SYNDROME (AIDS). A disease syndrome in which the patient's immune cells are destroyed by HIV virus, leaving the patient open to opportunistic infections that a healthy immune system could keep at bay.

ACROMIOCLAVICULAR (AC) JOINT. The shoulder joint.

ACROMIOCLAVICULAR DISLOCATION. Disruption of the normal articulation between the acromion and the collarbone. The acromioclavicular joint (AC joint) is normally stabilized by several ligaments that can be torn in the process of dislocating the AC joint.

ACROMION. The triangular projection of the spine of the shoulder blade that forms the point of the shoulder and articulates with the collarbone.

ACTINIC KERATOSIS (AK). A crusty, scaly precancerous skin lesion caused by damage from the sun; also known as solar keratosis.

ACTIVATED PARTIAL THROMBOPLASTIN TIME (APTT). A lab test that detects coagulation defects in the intrinsic clotting cascade; used to regulate heparin dosing.

ACTIVITIES OF DAILY LIVING (ADLS). Self-care activities performed during the course of a normal day, such as eating, bathing, dressing, etc.

ACUITY. Sharpness or clarity of vision.

ACUPUNCTURE. The insertion of tiny needles into the skin at specific spots on the body for curative purposes.

ACUTE. Referring to a condition that has a short but severe course.

ACUTE CARE SURGERY (ACS). A newer medical specialty that encompasses trauma, emergency, and critical care surgery.

ACUTE HEMOLYTIC TRANSFUSION REACTION (AHTR). A severe transfusion reaction with abrupt onset, most often caused by blood type incompatibility. Symptoms include difficulty breathing, fever and chills, pain, and sometimes shock.

ACUTE OTITIS MEDIA. Inflammation of the middle ear with signs of infection lasting less than three months.

ACUTE PAIN. Pain that is usually temporary and results from something specific, such as a surgery, an injury, or an infection.

ACUTE RENAL FAILURE. Also known as acute kidney failure, the rapid loss of the kidney's ability to function due to kidney damage. Acute renal failure decreases the kidney's ability to filter waste products from the blood for excretion in the urine.

ACUTE TUBULAR NECROSIS. A kidney disease involving damage to the portion of the kidney known as the tubules that causes kidney failure.

ADAPTIVE IMMUNE SYSTEM. The part of the immune system that develops responses to specific antigens and maintains immunological memory. It is also known as the acquired immune system.

ADDICTION. Compulsive, overwhelming involvement with a specific activity, such as smoking, gambling, alcohol, or drug use.

ADDISONIAN CRISIS. A medical emergency resulting from severe adrenal insufficiency. It can be caused by sudden withdrawal from oral glucocorticoid medications, as well as from damage to the adrenal gland itself. Untreated Addisonian crisis can be fatal.

ADDISON'S DISEASE. A disease involving decreased functioning of the adrenal glands, caused by either a problem in the adrenal glands or in the pituitary gland (which secretes a hormone that affects the adrenal glands).

ADENOCARCINOMA. A cancer originating in glandular cells.

ADENOIDS. Small lumps of lymphoid tissue near the tonsils on the walls of the upper throat behind the nose.

ADENOMA. A benign tumor that develops out of glandular tissue.

ADHESION. A fibrous band of tissue that forms an abnormal connection between two adjacent organs or other structures; may form after surgery or trauma.

ADJUVANT THERAPY. In cancer treatment, a secondary therapy used after surgery to help kill any remaining cancer cells or to keep the cancer in remission. Examples include chemotherapy and radiation therapy.

ADRENERGIC. Activated by adrenaline (norepinephrine); loosely applied to the sympathetic nervous system responses.

ADSORB. To attract and hold another substance on the surface of a solid material.

ADVANCE DIRECTIVES. Documents prepared in advance of medical care that reflect a patient's wishes toward specific medical procedures (for or against), to be used in the event that the patient becomes incapacitated and unable to make those decisions.

ADVERSE EVENT. An undesirable or unintended result of a medical treatment or intervention.

AEROBIC BACTERIA. Bacteria that grow freely in oxygen-rich environments.

AEROBIC EXERCISE. Any type of exercise that is intended to increase the body's oxygen consumption and improve the functioning of the cardiovascular and respiratory systems.

AESTHETIC. Pertaining to beauty or appearance. Plastic surgery done to improve a patient's appearance is sometimes called aesthetic surgery.

AFFECT. The external manifestation of a mood or state of mind. Affect is usually observed in facial expression or other body language.

AFFERENT NERVE FIBER. A nerve fiber in a receptor or a sense organ that carries nerve impulses toward the central nervous system.

AFFORDABLE CARE ACT (ACA). Patient Protection and Affordable Care Act (PPACA); signed into law by President Barack Obama in March of 2010, the ACA overhauled the U.S. healthcare system.

AGAINST MEDICAL ADVICE (AMA). Treatment refusal by leaving a hospital or other medical facility without being discharged.

AGENESIS. The absence of an organ or body part due to developmental failure.

AIDS. Acquired immunodeficiency syndrome. A disease caused by infection with the human immunodeficiency virus (HIV). The disease causes the immune system to break down, increasing the risk of other infections and some types of cancer.

AIRBORNE PATHOGEN. A disease-causing organism that is transmitted through air.

AIRWAY. The passageway through the mouth, nose, and throat that allows air to enter and leave the lungs; the term can also refer to a tube or other artificial device used to create an air passageway into and out of the lungs when a patient is under general anesthesia or unable to breathe properly.

ALDOSTERONE. A hormone secreted by the adrenal glands that prompts the kidneys to hold onto sodium.

ALGORITHM. A procedure or formula for solving a problem. It is often used to refer to a sequence of steps used to program a computer to solve a specific problem.

ALKALINE. Any chemical or compound that raises the pH of a solution above 7.0, meaning that there is a relative shortage of hydrogen ions dissociated within that solution.

ALKALOSIS. A pathological state in which there is a relative excess of hydroxide ions in the arterial blood.

ALLELE. Types of genes that occupy the same site on a chromosome.

ALLERGEN. A substance that provokes an allergic response.

ALLOGENEIC. Referring to the transplantation of blood, bone marrow, or stem cells from one person to another person.

ALLOGRAFT. Tissue that is taken from one person's body and grafted to another person.

ALLOPLAST. An implant made of an inert foreign material such as silicone or hydroxyapatite.

ALOPECIA. Hair loss or baldness.

ALPHA 1-ANTITRYPSIN DEFICIENCY. A genetic disorder characterized by insufficient production of alpha 1-antitrypsin (A1AT), a substance that protects the elasticity of lung tissue. Patients with insufficient A1AT are at high risk of developing emphysema, particularly if they are smokers.

ALPHA-FETOPROTEIN (AFP). A substance produced by a fetus's liver that can be found in the amniotic fluid and in the mother's blood. Abnormally high levels suggest there may be defects in the fetal neural tube, the structure that develops into the brain and spinal cord. Abnormally low levels suggest the possibility of Down syndrome.

ALPHA-FETOPROTEIN SCREEN. A test that measures the level of alpha-fetoprotein (AFP) in the mother's blood.

ALTERNATIVE MEDICINE. Any nonconventional treatment or substance that is used in place of mainstream medical or surgical treatment.

ALTERNATIVES TO SURGERY. Other treatments for a condition or illness that do not involve surgery; these are usually tried before surgery is an option.

ALVEOLAR ARCH. An arch formed by the ridge of the alveolar process of the mandible (jawbone) or maxilla.

ALVEOLAR PART OF THE MAXILLA. The part of the bony upper jaw that contains teeth (the upper gum).

ALVEOLAR PROCESS. A ridge of bone on the lower surface of the maxilla (upper jaw) and the upper surface of the mandible (lower jaw) that contains the tooth sockets. It is also known as the alveolar bone.

ALVEOLUS (PLURAL, ALVEOLI). One of the tiny air sacs in the lungs where carbon dioxide in the blood is exchanged for oxygen from the air.

ALZHEIMER'S DISEASE. A disease involving progressive cognitive deterioration. Symptoms include loss of memory, judgment, and intellect; disorientation; confusion; and a general inability to mentally function in social situations. The disease may begin as early as late mid-life and results in eventual death. It is associated with specific physical changes to the brain that can be visualized using medical imaging techniques.

AMBLYOPIA. Lazy eye; poor vision in one eye with no apparent structural cause.

AMBULATE. To move from place to place (walk).

AMBULATORY. Able to move; not bedridden.

AMBULATORY CARE FACILITY. A facility in which patients undergo invasive procedures but are typically released within 24 hours following the procedure; also referred to as an outpatient facility.

AMBULATORY MONITORING. Electrocardiograph (ECG) recording over a prolonged period during which the patient can move around.

AMBULATORY MONITORS. Small portable electrocardiograph machines that record the heart's rhythm; e.g., the Holter monitor, loop recorder, and trans-telephonic transmitter.

AMBULATORY SURGERY. Surgery done on an outpatient basis, meaning the patient goes home the same day.

AMBULATORY SURGERY CENTER. An outpatient facility with at least two operating rooms, either connected or not connected to a hospital.

AMINE. A chemical compound that contains NH_3 (a nitrogen-hydrogen combination) as part of its structure.

AMNIOCENTESIS. A procedure where a needle is inserted through a pregnant woman's abdomen and into the uterus to withdraw a sample of amniotic fluid surrounding the fetus.

AMNIOTIC FLUID. The watery fluid within the amniotic membrane that surrounds the fetus.

AMNIOTIC MEMBRANE. A thin membrane that contains the fetus and the protective amniotic fluid surrounding the fetus.

AMOEBA. A type of protozoa (one-celled animal) that can move or change its shape by extending projections of its cytoplasm.

AMYOTROPHIC LATERAL SCLEROSIS (ALS). A progressive neurodegenerative disease affecting nerve cells in the brain and the spinal cord; often referred to as Lou Gehrig's disease.

ANAEROBIC. An organism that lives without oxygen. Anaerobic bacteria are commonly found in the mouth and the intestines.

ANALGESIA. Relief from pain.

ANALGESIC. A medication given to relieve pain.

ANALYTE. A material or chemical substance subjected to analysis.

ANAPHYLACTIC. A serious allergic reaction to a foreign protein or other material.

ANAPHYLACTIC SHOCK. A potentially fatal allergic reaction that causes a severe drop in blood pressure, swelling of the respiratory tract, rash, and possible convulsions.

ANAPHYLAXIS. Increased sensitivity caused by previous exposure to an allergen that can result in blood vessel dilation (swelling) and smooth muscle contraction. Anaphylaxis can result in sharp blood pressure drops and difficulty breathing.

ANAPLASIA. The loss of distinctive cell features, which is a distinct characteristic of malignant neoplasms, or tumors.

ANASTOMOSIS. The surgical connection of two structures, such as blood vessels or sections of the intestine.

ANDROGENS. A class of chemical compounds (hormones) that stimulate the development of male secondary sexual characteristics.

ANEMIA. A disorder marked by low hemoglobin levels in red blood cells, which leads to a deficiency of oxygen in the blood.

ANENCEPHALY. A hereditary defect resulting in the partial to complete absence of a brain and spinal cord. It is fatal.

ANEROID MONITOR. A monitor that works without fluids (mercury free).

ANESTHESIA. Use of drugs that produce sedation, amnesia, analgesia, and immobility in order to accomplish surgical and other invasive procedures with minimal discomfort to the patient.

ANESTHESIOLOGIST. A physician who has special training and expertise in administering anesthesia.

ANESTHESIOLOGY. The branch of medicine that specializes in the study of anesthetic agents, their effects on patients, and their proper use and administration.

ANESTHETIC. A drug that causes unconsciousness or loss of sensation.

ANESTHETIST. A nurse trained in anesthesiology who assists the anesthesiologist in administering anesthesia during surgery and monitors the patient after surgery.

ANEURYSM. A potentially life-threatening enlargement or bulge in an artery, caused by a weakening of the artery wall above or below an area of blockage.

ANGINA. Also called angina pectoris, chest pain or discomfort that occurs when diseased blood vessels restrict blood flow to the heart.

ANGIOEDEMA. An allergic skin disease characterized by patches of circumscribed swelling involving the skin and its subcutaneous layers, the mucous membranes, and sometimes the viscera—also called angioneurotic edema, giant urticaria, Quincke's disease, or Quincke's edema.

ANGIOGRAM. X-ray of a blood vessel after a special x-ray dye has been injected into it.

ANGIOGRAPHY. A technique for visualizing blood vessels that involves injecting dye into the arteries so they show up on an x-ray.

ANGIOMA. A benign skin tumor consisting primarily of blood vessels.

ANGIOPLASTY. The surgical repair of a blood vessel.

ANGIOTENSIN-CONVERTING ENZYME (ACE) INHIBITOR. A drug that lowers blood pressure by interfering with the breakdown of a protein-like substance involved in blood pressure regulation.

ANGLE. The open point in the anterior chamber of the eye at which the iris meets the cornea.

ANGLE CLOSURE. A blockage of the angle of the eye, causing an increase in pressure in the eye and possible glaucoma.

ANKLE-BRACHIAL INDEX (ABI) TEST. A means of checking the blood pressure in the arms and ankles using a regular blood pressure cuff and a special ultrasound stethoscope (Doppler). The pressure in the ankle is compared to the pressure in the arm.

ANKYLOSING SPONDYLITIS. A form of inflammatory arthritis in which the bones in the spine and pelvis gradually fuse when inflamed connective tissue is replaced by bone.

ANNULUS. A ring-shaped structure.

ANOMALY. A marked deviation from normal structure or function.

ANOREXIA NERVOSA. A serious eating disorder that can lead to severe weight loss, malnutrition, and death.

ANTACID. A substance that counteracts or neutralizes acidity, usually of the stomach. Antacids have a rapid onset of action compared to histamine H-2 receptor blockers and proton pump inhibitors, but they have a short duration of action and require frequent dosing.

ANTERIOR CERVICAL DISKECTOMY AND FUSION (ACDF). Disc removal and spinal fusion performed through the front of the neck.

ANTERIOR CHAMBER. The fluid-filled space at the front of the eye between the iris and the inner surface of the cornea.

ANTERIOR CRUCIATE LIGAMENT (ACL). A crossing ligament that attaches the femur to the tibia and stabilizes the knee against forward motion of the tibia.

ANTERIOR LUMBAR INTERBODY FUSION (ALIF). Spinal fusion performed through the left side of the abdomen following disk removal.

ANTERIOR MEDIASTINOTOMY. A surgical procedure to look at the organs and tissues between the lungs and between the breastbone and spine for abnormal areas. An incision (cut) is made next to the breastbone and a thin, lighted tube is inserted into the chest. Tissue and lymph node samples may be taken for biopsy.

ANTIARRHYTHMIC. Medication used to treat abnormal heart rhythms.

ANTIBIOTIC. A medicine used to treat infections.

ANTIBODY. A protein that the body produces in response to a foreign invader, such as a virus, bacteria, fungus, or allergen. The production of each antibody is triggered by a specific antigen.

ANTICHOLINERGICS. Drugs that inhibit secretion of bodily fluids (e.g., saliva, perspiration, stomach acid).

ANTICOAGULANT. Medication given to prevent the formation of blood clots; also called blood thinners.

ANTICONVULSANT. A medication used to prevent or control seizures.

ANTIDIURETIC HORMONE (ADH). Also called vasopressin; a hormone produced by the hypothalamus and stored in and excreted by the pituitary gland. ADH acts on the kidneys to reduce the flow of urine, increasing total body fluid.

ANTIEMETIC. A type of drug given to prevent or relieve nausea and vomiting.

ANTIGEN. A molecule, usually a protein, that elicits the production of a specific antibody or immune response.

ANTIHISTAMINE. Medicine that prevents or relieves allergy symptoms.

ANTIMETABOLITE. An immunosuppressive drug that works by interfering with a cell's use of a metabolite (a byproduct of normal metabolism). Antimetabolites thus inhibit the growth and division of cells.

ANTIMICROBIAL. A substance or action that kills or inhibits the growth of microorganisms.

ANTINUCLEAR ANTIBODIES. Autoantibodies that attack substances found in the center, or nucleus, of all cells.

ANTIPLATELET DRUG. Drug that inhibits platelets from aggregating to form a plug.

ANTIPYRETIC. A medication that lowers fever.

ANTISEPTIC. A substance that inhibits the growth of harmful bacteria and other organisms.

ANTITHROMBOTIC. Preventing clot formation.

ANTITRYPSIN. A substance that inhibits the action of trypsin, a digestive enzyme.

ANTRECTOMY. A surgical procedure for ulcer disease in which the antrum, a portion of the stomach, is removed.

ANTROSTOMY. The opening of a body cavity, usually for drainage purposes.

ANTRUM. The lower part of the stomach that lies between the pylorus and the body of the stomach. It is also called the gastric antrum or antrum pyloricum.

ANUS. The terminal orifice of the bowel.

ANXIETY. A psychological state characterized by strong feelings of worry, nervousness, apprehension, or agitation; may also be accompanied by physical symptoms, including sweating, tension, and increased pulse.

ANXIETY ATTACK. A disorder in which sudden feelings of dread, fear, and apprehension enter a person's mind in an overwhelming manner. Attacks may lead to a state of hyperventilation.

ANXIOLYTICS. Medications given to reduce anxiety; also known as tranquilizers.

AORTA. The largest artery in the body; carries oxygenated blood from the heart to the rest of the body.

AORTIC ANEURYSM. Occurs when an area in the aorta (the main artery of the heart) is weakened and bulges like a balloon.

AORTIC DISSECTION. A situation in which a tear in the interior lining of the wall of the aorta causes bleeding between the layers of that major artery.

AORTIC VALVE. The valve between the heart's left ventricle and ascending aorta that prevents regurgitation of blood back into the left ventricle.

APERT SYNDROME. A congenital disorder characterized by malformations of the skull, face, hands, and feet, including a peaked shape to the head. Named for the French physician who first described it in 1906, Apert syndrome affects about one in every 65,000 live births.

APFEL SCORE. A score that predicts a patient's risk of postoperative nausea and vomiting, based on four risk factors (female gender, nonsmoker, history of motion sickness, and opioid pain relievers planned for postoperative administration). Each factor counts one point.

APHAKIC. Referring to an eye without a lens.

APHERESIS. A procedure in which whole blood is withdrawn from a donor, a specific blood component is separated and collected, and the remainder is reinfused into the patient.

APICAL. Rounded end of the root of a tooth that is embedded in hard tissue (bone); toward the apex of the root.

APICOECTOMY. Also called root resectioning, a procedure in which the root tip of a tooth is accessed in the bone and a small amount is shaved away. The diseased tissue is removed and a filling is placed to reseal the canal.

APLASTIC ANEMIA. A disorder in which the body produces inadequate amounts of red blood cells and hemoglobin due to underdeveloped or missing bone marrow.

APNEA. Cessation of breathing.

APPENDECTOMY. Removal of the appendix.

APPENDIX. A pouch-shaped organ that is attached to the upper part of the large intestine.

APPETITE SUPPRESSANT. A medication given to reduce the desire to eat.

APPLANATION TONOMETRY. A type of tonometry that involves flattening a portion of the patient's cornea to obtain a reading of intraocular pressure. The two most widely used applanation tonometers are the Goldmann tonometer and the Perkins tonometer.

APROTININ. A protein derived from cows' lungs included in some fibrin sealants to prevent the fibrin clot from dissolving.

AQUEOUS HUMOR. The clear, watery fluid between the cornea and the crystalline lens of the eye.

AREA POSTREMA. A small tongue-shaped structure that lies on the floor of the fourth ventricle of the brain.

AREFLEXIA. A condition in which the body's normal reflexes are absent.

AREOLA. The pigmented ring around the nipple.

ARGON. A colorless, odorless gas.

AROMATASE INHIBITOR. A medication for preventing or treating breast cancer in postmenopausal women by inhibiting the body's production of estrogen.

ARREST. A sudden stopping of the function of a body organ, such as breathing (respiratory arrest) or the beating of the heart (cardiac arrest).

ARRHYTHMIA. An abnormal heart rhythm.

ARTERIAL BLOOD. Blood from the arteries, the blood vessels that carry oxygen from the lungs to supply the body tissues.

ARTERIAL BLOOD GAS (ABG). A type of blood laboratory test done to check the blood for imbalances in pH or gases that affect pH.

ARTERIAL EMBOLISM. A blood clot arising from another location that blocks an artery.

ARTERIAL LINE. A catheter inserted into an artery and connected to a physiologic monitoring system to allow direct measurement of oxygen, carbon dioxide, and invasive blood pressure.

ARTERIES. Blood vessels that carry blood away from the heart to the cells, tissues, and organs of the body.

ARTERIOGRAM. A diagnostic test that involves viewing the arteries and/or attached organs by injecting a contrast medium, or dye, into the artery and taking an x-ray.

ARTERIOLAR BED. An area in which arterioles cluster between arteries and capillaries.

ARTERIOLES. The smallest branches of arteries.

ARTERIOSCLEROSIS. A chronic condition characterized by thickening and hardening of the arteries and the build-up of plaque on the arterial walls; also called atherosclerosis.

ARTERIOTOMY. An incision made into a blood vessel.

ARTERIOVENOUS FISTULA. An abnormal channel or passage between an artery and a vein that results in a disruption of normal blood flow patterns. It can be acquired or congenital.

ARTERIOVENOUS MALFORMATION. Abnormal, direct connection between the arteries and veins. Arteriovenous malformations can range from very small to large.

ARTERY. Blood vessel that carries blood away from the heart to the body.

ARTHRITIS. A painful inflammatory condition that affects joints.

ARTHRODESIS. Surgery that joins (or fuses) two bones together so that the joint can no longer move; it may be done on joints such as the fingers, knees, ankles, or vertebrae of the spine.

ARTHROGRAPHY. Visualization of a joint by radiographic means following injection of a contrast dye into the joint space.

ARTHROPLASTY. The surgical repair of a joint.

ARTHROSCOPE. An instrument that contains a miniature camera and light source mounted on a flexible tube, allowing a surgeon to see the inside of a joint or bone during surgery.

ARTHROSCOPY. A minimally invasive procedure in which a specialized endoscope called an arthroscope is inserted into a joint to examine the joint and make small repairs.

ARTHROSIS. A disease of a joint.

ARTIFACT. Extra electrical activity typically caused by interference.

ARTIFICIAL SPHINCTER. An implanted device that functions to control the opening and closing of the urethral or anal canal for the expelling of urine or feces, respectively.

ASCITES. An abnormal collection of fluid within the abdomen.

ASCITIC FLUID. The fluid that accumulates in the peritoneal cavity in ascites.

ASEPTIC. Free from infection or diseased material; sterile.

ASEPTIC TECHNIQUE. Practices performed before, during, and after a clinical procedure to prevent or reduce contamination and postprocedural infection.

ASHERMAN'S SYNDROME. The cessation of menstruation and/or infertility caused by intrauterine adhesions.

ASPIRATE. Remove fluids by suction, often through a needle; also, to take into the lungs by breathing.

ASPIRATION. The process of removing fluids or gases from the body by suction.

ASPIRIN. Also medically referred to as acetylsalicylic acid, a drug in the family of salicylates that is often used to relieve aches and pain.

ASSAY. An analysis of the chemical composition or strength of a substance.

ASTHMA. An inflammatory respiratory disorder in which the airway becomes obstructed and breathing is difficult.

ASTIGMATISM. A condition in which one or both eyes cannot filter light properly and images appear blurred and indistinct.

ATELECTASIS. Partial or complete collapse of the lung, usually due to a blockage of the air passages with fluid, mucus, or infection.

ATHERECTOMY. A nonsurgical technique for treating diseased arteries with a rotating device that cuts or shaves away obstructing material inside the artery.

ATHEROMA. An accumulation of plaque blocking a portion of an artery.

ATHEROSCLEROSIS. A disease characterized by the buildup of fatty deposits (plaque) on the insides of artery walls, which results in the clogging, narrowing, and hardening of the arteries; also known as arteriosclerosis.

ATKINS DIET. A diet that involves eating high amounts of protein and fat with low amounts of carbohydrates.

ATONIC SEIZURE. Also called a drop seizure or a drop attack, this is a seizure in which an individual loses muscle tone and falls down. These seizures carry a high risk of accidental injury.

ATRESIA. Absence of a normal opening.

ATRIA (SINGULAR, ATRIUM). The right and left upper chambers of the heart.

ATRIAL FIBRILLATION. A dangerous, rapid, irregular heartbeat.

ATRIAL FLUTTER. A rapid pulsation of the upper chambers of the heart that interferes with normal heart function. Atrial flutter is usually more organized and regular than atrial fibrillation, but often converts to atrial fibrillation.

ATRIOVENTRICULAR. Referring to the valves regulating blood flow from the upper chambers of the heart (atria) to the lower chambers (ventricles). There are two such valves, one connecting the right atrium and ventricle and one connecting the left atrium and ventricle.

ATROPHY. Wasting of body tissues.

ATTENTION DEFICIT HYPERACTIVITY DISORDER (ADHD). A disorder involving a developmentally inappropriate degree of inattention and impulsivity. Hyperactivity may or may not be a component. This disorder usually appears in childhood and manifests itself as difficulty at home or school. It sometimes persists into adulthood where it may affect work, relationships, and other social situations.

AUDIOGRAM. A test of hearing at a range of sound frequencies.

AUDIOLOGIST. A health care professional who performs diagnostic testing of impaired hearing.

AUDITORY NERVE. The nerve that carries electrical signals from the cochlea to the brain.

AURICLE. The portion of the external ear that is not contained inside the head. It is also called the pinna.

AUSCULTATION. The process of listening to sounds that are produced in the body. Direct auscultation uses the ear alone, such as when listening to the grating of a moving joint. Indirect auscultation involves the use of a stethoscope to amplify the sounds from within the body, such as the heartbeat.

AUTISM. A childhood disorder that manifests as an inability to communicate with or relate to others, or interact in social situations in a healthy, normal manner. Autism may range from mild to severe and includes repetitive behaviors, the inability to cope with changes from routine activities, and obsessions with specific objects. Autism is sometimes associated with below-normal intelligence or anxiety.

AUTOANTIBODY. An antibody formed by a person's immune system against one of its own proteins.

AUTOCLAVE. A heavy vessel that uses pressurized steam for disinfecting and sterilizing surgical instruments.

AUTOGENOUS TISSUE. Tissue or skin taken from any part of a person's body to graft onto another part of the body that needs repairing; laid on as a patch.

AUTOGRAFT. Tissue that is taken from one part of a person's body and transplanted to a different part of the same person.

AUTOIMMUNE DISORDER. A condition in which the body makes antibodies against its own cells or tissues.

AUTOLOGOUS. From the same person; e.g., in an autologous blood transfusion, blood is removed from and then transfused back to the same person at a later time.

AUTOLOGOUS BLOOD DONATION. The patient's own blood is drawn and set aside before surgery for use in case a transfusion is needed.

AUTONOMIC NERVOUS SYSTEM. The part of the nervous system that regulates the activity of the heart muscle, smooth muscle, and glands.

AUTOSOMAL DISEASE. A disease caused by a gene mutation located on a chromosome other than a sex chromosome.

AUTOTRANSFUSION. Also known as blood salvage, a technique for recovering blood during surgery, separating and concentrating the red blood cells, and reinfusing them in the patient.

AUXILIARY HOSPITAL SERVICES. A term used broadly to designate such nonmedical services as financial services, birthing classes, support groups, etc., that are instituted in response to consumer demand.

AVASCULAR NECROSIS. A disorder in which bone tissue dies and collapses following the temporary or permanent loss of its blood supply; also known as osteonecrosis.

AVULSION. A type of injury caused by ripping or tearing.

AXILLA. Armpit.

AXILLARY. Pertaining to the armpit.

AXILLARY LYMPH NODES. Lymph nodes located under the arm.

AXILLARY VEIN. A blood vessel that takes blood from tissues back to the heart to receive oxygenated blood.

AYURVEDA. The traditional medical system of India.

B

B CELL. A type of white blood cell derived from bone marrow. B cells are sometimes called B lymphocytes; they secrete antibodies and have a number of other complex functions within the human immune system.

B LYMPHOCYTE. A type of blood cell that is active in immune response.

BACTERIA. Microscopic, one-celled forms of life that cause many diseases and infections.

BACTERICIDAL. An agent that kills bacteria.

BACTERIOSTATIC. An agent that stops the multiplication of bacteria.

BACTERIURIA. The presence of bacteria in the urine.

BALANCED ANESTHESIA. The use of a combination of inhalation and intravenous anesthetics, often with opioids for pain relief and neuromuscular blockers for muscle paralysis.

BALLOON ANGIOPLASTY. X-ray-guided insertion of a balloon catheter into a blocked blood vessel to remove plaque and open the vessel for better blood flow.

BAND CELL. An immature neutrophil at the stage just preceding a mature cell. The nucleus of a band cell is unsegmented.

BARIATRIC SURGERY. Weight-loss surgery, such as gastric banding or gastric bypass.

BARIATRICS. The branch of medicine that deals with the prevention and treatment of obesity and related disorders.

BARIUM. A metallic element used in its sulfate form as a contrast medium for x-ray studies of the digestive tract.

BARIUM ENEMA. An x-ray test of the bowel performed after giving the patient an enema of barium to outline the colon and the rectum.

BARIUM SULFATE. A barium compound used during a barium enema to block the passage of x-rays during the exam.

BARIUM SWALLOW. A diagnostic test that uses barium to coat the upper digestive tract, allowing it to be better visualized on an x-ray.

BAROTRAUMA. Ear pain caused by unequal air pressure on the inside and outside of the eardrum; also called barotitis media.

BARRETT'S ESOPHAGUS. A potentially precancerous change in the type of cells that line the esophagus, caused by acid reflux disease.

BARTTER SYNDROME. An inherited disorder that affects a number of body processes, including the functioning of the part of the kidney that regulates potassium excretion and absorption. People with Bartter syndrome have abnormally low blood potassium levels (hypokalemia).

BASAL CELL CARCINOMA (BCC). The most common malignant tumor and the most common type of skin cancer.

BASELINE FUNCTIONING. A term used in medicine to describe the initial set of measurements taken of a patient's vital functions in order to have a basis for comparison with later observations.

BASOPHIL. Segmented white blood cell with large dark blue-black granules that releases histamine in allergic reactions.

BELL. The cup-shaped portion of the head of a stethoscope, useful for detecting low-pitched sounds.

BELL'S PALSY. One-sided paralysis of the face that may be due to damage to the facial nerve.

BENIGN. Noncancerous.

BENIGN PROSTATIC HYPERPLASIA (BPH). A noncancerous condition of the prostate that causes overgrowth of the prostate tissue; also called benign prostatic enlargement (BPE).

BENIGN TUMOR. An abnormal growth that is not cancerous and does not spread to other areas of the body.

BETA BLOCKER. An antihypertensive drug that limits the activity of epinephrine, a hormone that increases blood pressure.

BETA CELL. The specific type of cell within the islets of Langerhans in the pancreas that produces insulin.

BEVEL. The slanted opening on one side of the tip of a needle.

BEZOAR. A collection of foreign material, usually hair or vegetable fibers or a mixture of both, that may occasionally occur in the stomach or intestines and block the passage of food.

BILATERAL. Occurring on both the right and left sides.

BILATERAL CLEFT LIP. Cleft that occurs on both sides of the lip.

BILE. A bitter yellowish-brown fluid secreted by the liver that contains bile salts, bile pigments, cholesterol, and other substances. It helps the body to digest and absorb fats.

BILE DUCTS. Tubes carrying bile from the liver to the intestines.

BILEVEL POSITIVE AIRWAY PRESSURE (BIPAP). A type of mechanical ventilator that delivers a higher pressure on inhalation and low pressure on exhalation.

BILIARY. Relating to bile.

BILIARY ATRESIA. A disease in which the ducts that carry bile out of the liver are missing or damaged.

BILIARY SYSTEM. The system of ducts that carries the bile flow through the liver and gallbladder to the duodenum (first portion of the small intestine).

BILIARY TRACT. The passages that allow the flow of bile from the gallbladder to the intestines.

BILIRUBIN. A yellow bile pigment, found as sodium (soluble) bilirubinate or as an insoluble calcium salt found in gallstones.

BILIVERDIN. A green bile pigment formed from the oxidation of heme, with a structure almost identical to that of bilirubin.

BINGE. A time-limited bout of excessive indulgence; consuming a larger amount of food within a limited period of time than most people would eat in similar circumstances.

BINGE EATING DISORDER. An eating disorder in which a person binges but does not try to get rid of the food afterward by vomiting, using laxatives, or exercising excessively.

BIOLOGICAL TISSUE VALVE. A replacement heart valve that is harvested from the patient (autograft); a human cadaver (homograft or allograft); or an animal, such as a pig (heterograft).

BIOMECHANICS. The application of mechanical laws to the structures in the human body, such as measuring the force and direction of stresses on a joint.

BIOPSY. The removal and microscopic examination of a small sample of tissue to determine if cancerous or other abnormal cells are present.

BISMUTH. A substance used in medicines to treat diarrhea, nausea, and indigestion.

BIVENTRICULAR ASSIST DEVICE (BVAD, BIVAD). The combined use of left and right ventricular assist devices.

BLADDER. A membranous sac that serves as a reservoir for urine. Contraction of the bladder results in urination.

BLADDER EXSTROPHY. One of many bladder and urinary congenital abnormalities; occurs when the wall of the bladder fails to close in embryonic development and remains exposed to the abdominal wall.

BLADDER IRRIGATION. To flush or rinse the bladder with a stream of liquid (as in removing a foreign body or medicating).

BLADDER MUCOSA. Mucous coat of the bladder.

BLADDER TUMOR MARKER STUDIES. Tests to detect specific substances released by bladder cancer cells into the urine.

BLADDER WASHING. A procedure in which bladder washing samples are taken by placing a salt solution into the bladder through a catheter (tube) and then removing the solution for microscopic testing.

BLAST PHASE. Stage of chronic myelogenous leukemia where large quantities of immature cells are produced by the marrow and are not responsive to treatment.

BLEB. A thin-walled auxiliary drain created on the outside of the eyeball during filtering surgery for glaucoma. It is sometimes called a filtering bleb.

BLEEDING DISORDER. A problem related to the clotting mechanism of the blood.

BLEEDING TIME TEST. A test done to evaluate platelet function and blood clotting ability. It involves the use of a blood pressure cuff and the making of two small cuts on the patient's forearm rather than venipuncture.

BLEPHAROPLASTY. Surgical reshaping of the eyelid.

BLOOD BANK. A laboratory that specializes in blood typing, antibody identification, and transfusion services.

BLOOD PRESSURE. The pressure exerted by arterial blood on the walls of arteries, measured in millimeters of mercury (mm Hg) by a sphygmomanometer (blood pressure cuff) or an electronic device.

BLOOD TYPE. Any of various classes into which human blood can be divided according to immunological compatibility based on the presence or absence of certain antigens on the red blood cells. Blood types are sometimes called blood groups; they include A, B, AB, and O.

BLOOD UREA NITROGEN (BUN). The nitrogen portion of urea in the bloodstream. Urea is a waste product of protein metabolism in the body.

BODY DYSMORPHIC DISORDER (BDD). A psychiatric condition marked by excessive preoccupation with an imaginary or minor defect in a facial feature or localized part of the body. Many people with BDD seek cosmetic surgery as a treatment for their perceived flaw.

BODY MASS INDEX (BMI). A weight-to-height ratio that is used by some as a determinant of obesity. BMI is calculated (in English units) as 703.1 times a person's weight in pounds divided by the square of the person's height in inches. The metric formula is weight in kilograms divided by the square of height in meters.

BODY PLETHYSMOGRAPHY. A very sensitive test given to measure damage to the lungs that might be missed by routine pulmonary function tests. The patient sits within a so-called airtight body box while various devices measure both the air pressure in the patient's alveoli and the airflow through the respiratory system.

BOLUS. A mass of food ready to be swallowed, or a preparation of medicine to be given by mouth or intravenously all at once rather than gradually.

BONE DENSITOMETRY TEST. A test that measures bone density.

BONE MARROW. Soft tissue that fills the hollow centers of bones. Blood cells and platelets (disk-shaped bodies in the blood that are important in clotting) are produced in the bone marrow.

BONE MARROW BIOPSY. A test involving the insertion of a thin needle into the breastbone or, more commonly, the hip, in order to aspirate (remove) a sample of the marrow. A small piece of cortical bone may also be obtained for biopsy.

BONE MORPHOGENETIC PROTEINS. A family of substances in human bones and blood that encourage the process of osteoinduction.

BONE SPUR. A calcified growth on a bone.

BONY LABYRINTH. A series of cavities contained in a capsule inside the temporal bone of the skull. The endolymph-filled membranous labyrinth is suspended in a fluid inside the bony labyrinth.

BORBORYGMI. Sounds created by the passage of food, gas, or fecal material in the stomach or intestines.

BOTULINUM TOXIN. A toxin produced by the spores and growing cells of *Clostridium botulinum*. It causes muscle paralysis and is used in plastic surgery to reduce frown lines by temporarily paralyzing the muscles in the face that contract when a person frowns or squints.

BOUGIE. A slender, flexible tube or rod inserted into the urethra in order to dilate it.

BOWEL LUMEN. The space within the intestine.

BRACHIAL. Referring to the arm; the brachial artery is an artery that runs from the shoulder to the elbow.

BRACHYTHERAPY. The use of radiation during angioplasty to prevent the artery from narrowing again (a process called restenosis).

BRADYCARDIA. Slow heartbeat, usually under 60 beats per minute.

BRAIN DEATH. Irreversible cessation of brain function. Patients with brain death have no potential capacity for survival or for recovery of any brain function.

BRAIN LESION. Physical damage done to a specific part or location of the brain.

BRCA1, BRCA2. Breast cancer susceptibility genes; specific mutations in these genes greatly increase the risk of breast and ovarian cancers.

BREAST AUGMENTATION. A surgery to increase the size of the breasts.

BREAST BIOPSY. A procedure where suspicious tissue is removed and examined by a pathologist for cancer or other disease. The breast tissue may be obtained by open surgery, or through a needle.

BREAST-CONSERVING SURGERY. Breast cancer treatment, such as a lumpectomy or partial mastectomy, that removes only the cancerous tissue rather than the entire breast.

BREATHING RATE. The number of breaths per minute.

BREECH PRESENTATION. A baby entering the birth canal buttocks or feet first rather than head first; also known as breech position.

BRONCHI. The network of tubular passages that carries air to and from the lungs.

BRONCHIECTASIS. Persistent and progressive dilation of bronchi or bronchioles as a consequence of inflammatory disease such as lung infections, obstructions, tumors, or congenital abnormalities.

BRONCHIOLES. Small airways extending from the bronchi into the lobes of the lungs.

BRONCHITIS. Inflammation of the air passages of the lungs.

BRONCHOALVEOLAR LAVAGE. Washing cells from the air sacs at the end of the bronchioles.

BRONCHODILATOR. A drug that relaxes the bronchial muscles, resulting in expansion of the bronchial air passages.

BRONCHOPLEURAL FISTULA. An abnormal connection between an air passage and the membrane that covers the lungs.

BRONCHOSCOPE. A tubular illuminated instrument used for inspecting or passing instruments into the bronchi.

BRONCHOSCOPY. A medical test that enables the physician to see the breathing passages and the lungs through a hollow, lighted tube.

BRONCHOSPASM. A spasmodic contraction of the muscles that line the two branches of the trachea that lead into the lungs, causing difficulty in breathing.

BRUCELLOSIS. An infectious disease transmitted to humans from farm animals, most commonly goats, sheep, cattle, and dogs. It is marked by high fever, pains in the muscles and joints, heavy sweating, headaches, and depression.

BRUIT. A roaring sound created by a partially blocked artery.

BRUNESCENT. Developing a brownish or amber color over time.

BUCCAL. The interior surface of the cheek.

BUCCAL SULCUS. Groove in the upper part of the upper jaw (where there are teeth).

BUERGER'S DISEASE. An episodic disease that causes inflammation and blockage of the veins and arteries of the limbs. It tends to be present almost exclusively in men under age 40 who smoke, and may require amputation of the hand or foot.

BULIMIA NERVOSA. An eating disorder marked by episodes of binge eating followed by purging, over-exercising, or other behaviors intended to prevent weight gain.

BUNION. A swelling or deformity of the big toe, characterized by the formation of a bursa and a sideways displacement of the toe.

BURCH PROCEDURE. A surgical procedure, also called retropubic colposuspension, in which the neck of the bladder is suspended from nearby ligaments with sutures. It is performed to treat urinary incontinence.

BURSA (PLURAL, BURSAE). A fluid-filled sac found in connective tissue that reduces friction between tendon and bone.

BURSITIS. Inflammation of a bursa.

BYWATERS' SYNDROME. Another name for crush syndrome, derived from the name of the British physician who first described it during World War II.

C

CADAVER. A dead body.

CADAVER ORGAN. A pancreas, kidney, or other organ from a deceased organ donor.

CADAVERIC DONOR. An organ donor who has recently died of causes not affecting the organ intended for transplant.

CALCITONIN. A hormone made by the thyroid gland. Calcitonin is involved in regulating levels of calcium and phosphorus in the blood.

CALCIUM. A mineral that helps build bone. After menopause, when women start making less of the bone-protecting hormone estrogen, they may need to increase their intake of calcium.

CALCIUM CHANNEL BLOCKER. A drug that lowers blood pressure by regulating calcium-related electrical activity in the heart.

CALCULUS (PLURAL, CALCULI). A term for plaque buildup on the teeth that has crystallized; also, a kidney or gallbladder stone.

CALDWELL-LUC PROCEDURE. A surgical procedure in which the surgeon enters the maxillary sinus by making an opening under the upper lip above the teeth.

CALLUS. A localized thickening of the outer layer of skin cells, caused by friction or pressure from shoes or other articles of clothing.

CANCER. A disease caused by uncontrolled growth of the body's cells.

CANCER STAGING. A surgical procedure to determine the extent of a cancer and how far it has spread.

CANCER SURGERY. Surgery in which the goal is to remove a tumor and any surrounding tissue found to be malignant.

CANINE TOOTH. In humans, the tooth located in the mouth next to the second incisor. The canine tooth has a pointed crown and the longest root of all the teeth.

CANKER SORE. A painful sore inside the mouth.

CANNULA (PLURAL, CANNULAE). A small, flexible tube.

CAPILLARIES. Tiny blood vessels that aid in the exchange of oxygen and carbon dioxide.

CAPILLARITY. The capability of suture material to harbor bacteria and transmit fluid along the length of the strand.

CAPILLARY. Smallest extremity of the arterial vessel, where oxygen and nutrients are released from the blood into the cells, and cellular waste is collected.

CAPSULAR CONTRACTURE. Thick scar tissue around a breast implant, which may tighten and cause discomfort and/or firmness.

CAPSULE. A general medical term for a structure that encloses another structure or body part.

CAPSULORHEXIS. The creation of a continuous circular tear in the front portion of the lens capsule during cataract surgery to allow for removal of the lens nucleus.

CAPSULOTOMY. A procedure that is sometimes needed after extra capsular cataract extraction (ECCE) to open a lens capsule in the eye that has become cloudy.

CARBOHYDRATE. A nutrient that the body uses as an energy source. Carbohydrates provide four calories of energy per gram.

CARBON DIOXIDE. Abbreviated CO_2, a heavy, colorless gas that dissolves in water.

CARBON MONOXIDE DIFFUSING TEST. Also called the transfer factor test, this test measures the ability of a patient's lungs to transfer blood gases.

CARCINOMA. A cancerous growth that arises from epithelium, found in skin or, more commonly, the lining of body organs.

CARCINOMA IN SITU. Malignant cells that have not yet spread.

CARDIAC. Of or relating to the heart.

CARDIAC ANGIOGRAPHY. A procedure used to visualize blood vessels of the heart.

CARDIAC ARREST. Abrupt cessation of the heartbeat.

CARDIAC ARRHYTHMIA. An irregular heart rate (frequency of heartbeats) or rhythm (the pattern of heartbeats).

CARDIAC CATHETER. Long, thin, flexible tube that is threaded into the heart through a blood vessel.

CARDIAC CATHETERIZATION. A minimally invasive technique that runs a catheter through veins into the heart to evaluate heart function.

CARDIAC MARKER. A substance in the blood that rises following a myocardial infarction (heart attack).

CARDIAC OUTPUT. The liter-per-minute blood flow generated by contraction of the heart.

CARDIAC PULMONARY BYPASS. A procedure where heart blood is diverted into an inserted pump in order to maintain appropriate blood flow.

CARDIAC REHABILITATION. A structured program of education and activity offered by hospitals and other organizations.

CARDIAC SURGERY. Surgery performed on the heart.

Glossary

GALE ENCYCLOPEDIA OF SURGERY AND MEDICAL TESTS, 3RD EDITION

2079

CARDIAC TAMPONADE. A condition in which the sac around the heart fills with blood, preventing the heart from functioning properly.

CARDIOLOGIST. A physician who specializes in problems of the heart.

CARDIOMYOPATHIES. Diseases of the heart muscle; usually refers to a disease of obscure etiology.

CARDIOPLEGIC ARREST. Halting the electrical activity of the heart by delivery of a high potassium solution to the coronary arteries. The arrested heart provides a superior surgical field for operation.

CARDIOPULMONARY. Involving both heart and lungs.

CARDIOPULMONARY BYPASS. Uses a heart-lung machine to maintain blood circulation while bypassing the heart and lungs.

CARDIOPULMONARY RESUSCITATION (CPR). An emergency procedure for restoring breathing and circulation.

CARDIOTHORACIC SURGERY. Surgery involving the chest body cavity known as the thoracic cavity.

CARDIOVASCULAR SYSTEM. The physiological system including the heart and the blood vessels.

CARDIOVERSION. A procedure used to restore the heart's normal rhythm by applying a controlled electric shock to the exterior of the chest.

CARDIOVERTER. A device to apply electric shock to the chest to convert an abnormal heartbeat into a normal heartbeat.

CAROTID ARTERY. Major artery in the neck that leads to the brain; blockages can cause temporary or permanent strokes.

CAROTID ARTERY DISEASE. A condition in which the arteries in the neck that supply blood to the brain become clogged, causing the danger of a stroke.

CAROTID ENDARTERECTOMY. A surgical technique for removing intra-arterial obstructions of the internal carotid artery.

CARPAL BONES. Wrist bones.

CARRIER. A person who harbors an infectious agent or a defective gene without showing any clinical signs but can transmit the infection to others or the defective gene to his/her children.

CARTILAGE. A tough, elastic connective tissue found in the joints, outer ear, nose, larynx, and other parts of the body.

CASE MANAGER. A healthcare professional who can provide assistance with a patient's needs beyond the hospital.

CAST. An insoluble gelled protein matrix that takes the form of the renal tubule in which it was deposited. Casts are washed out by normal urine flow.

CASTRATION. Removal or destruction by radiation of both testicles (in a male) or both ovaries (in a female), making the individual incapable of reproducing.

CATARACT. A clouding of the lens of the eye, leading to poor vision or blindness.

CATEGORICALLY NEEDY. Groups of people who qualify for the basic mandatory Medicaid benefits and that state Medicaid programs are either required to cover or have the option of covering.

CATGUT. A tough, natural suture material made from the dried intestines of sheep or horses.

CATHARTIC. An agent that stimulates defecation.

CATHARTIC COLON. A poorly functioning colon, resulting from the chronic abuse of stimulant cathartics.

CATHETER. A flexible tube inserted into the body to allow passage of fluids.

CATHETER-DRIVEN THROMBOLYSIS. A procedure performed in conjunction with or in place of thrombectomy that delivers a thrombolytic directly into a blood clot.

CATHETERIZATION. The use of or insertion of a catheter.

CAUDA EQUINA. A bundle of nerve roots in the lower (lumbar) region of the spinal canal that controls the leg muscles and functioning of the bladder, intestines, and genitals.

CAUDA EQUINA SYNDROME (CES). A group of symptoms characterized by numbness or pain in the legs and/or loss of bladder and bowel control, caused by compression and paralysis of the nerve roots in the cauda equina. CES is a medical emergency.

CAUSALGIA. A severe burning sensation sometimes accompanied by redness and inflammation of the skin. Causalgia is caused by injury to a nerve outside the spinal cord.

CAUTERIZE. To use heat or chemicals to stop bleeding, prevent the spread of infection, or destroy tissue.

CAUTERY. The burning, searing, or destroying of tissue.

CD4. A type of protein molecule in human blood that is present on the surface of 65% of human T cells. CD4 is a receptor for the HIV virus. When the HIV virus infects cells with CD4 surface proteins, it depletes the number of T cells, B cells, natural killer cells, and monocytes in the patient's blood. Most of the damage to an AIDS patient's immune system is done by the virus' destruction of CD4+ lymphocytes. CD4 is sometimes called the T4 antigen.

CECUM. The beginning of the large intestine and the place where the appendix attaches to the intestinal tract.

CELLULITE. Dimpled skin that is caused by uneven fat deposits beneath the surface.

CENTERS FOR MEDICARE & MEDICAID SERVICES (CMS). The division within the U.S. Department of Health and Human Services that administers Medicare and Medicaid.

CENTRAL LINE. A catheter passed through a vein into large blood vessels of the chest or the heart, used in various medical procedures.

CENTRAL NERVOUS SYSTEM (CNS). The part of the nervous system that includes the brain and the spinal cord.

CENTRAL VENOUS CATHETER (CVC). A vascular access device that is inserted into a central vein such as the jugular.

CENTRAL VENOUS LINE. A catheter inserted into a vein and connected to a physiologic monitoring system to directly measure venous blood pressure.

CEPHALOPELVIC DISPROPORTION (CPD). A condition in which the baby's head is too large to fit through the mother's pelvis.

CEREBRAL ANEURYSM. The dilation, bulging, or ballooning out of part of the wall of a vein or artery in the brain.

CEREBRAL CORTEX. The outer portion of the brain, consisting of layers of nerve cells and their connections. The cerebral cortex is the part of the brain in which thought processes take place.

CEREBRAL PALSY. Group of disorders characterized by loss of movement or loss of other nerve functions. These disorders are caused by injuries to the brain that occur during fetal development or near the time of birth.

CEREBROSPINAL FLUID (CSF). A clear fluid that fills the hollow cavity inside the brain and spinal cord.

CEREBROVASCULAR ACCIDENT. Brain hemorrhage, also known as a stroke.

CERTIFIED REGISTERED NURSE ANESTHETIST (CRNA). A registered nurse who has completed specialized education and training in the administration of anesthesia.

CERVICAL CRYOTHERAPY. Surgery performed after a biopsy has confirmed abnormal cervical cells (dysplasia).

CERVICAL INTRAEPITHELIAL NEOPLASIA (CIN). A term used to categorize degrees of dysplasia arising in the epithelium, or outer layer, of the cervix.

CERVIX. The neck-shaped opening at the lower part of the uterus.

CESAREAN DELIVERY ON MATERNAL REQUEST (CDMR). The choice to have a cesarean delivery when it is not medically necessary.

CESAREAN SECTION. Childbirth performed through surgical incisions in the abdominal and uterine wall; also referred to as cesarean delivery or c-section.

CHARCOT-MARIE-TOOTH DISEASE. An inherited neurological disorder that affects the peripheral nerves.

CHARCOT'S ARTHROPATHY. Also called neuropathic arthropathy, a condition in which the shoulder joint is destroyed following loss of its nerve supply.

CHARTING BY EXCEPTION (CBE). Medical charting that includes only significant or unusual findings.

CHELATION THERAPY. A method for removing lead from the body by administering an agent that binds lead ions in the body, allowing the body to excrete the lead through the urine. The agent most often used is dimercaptosuccinic acid (DMSA), also known as succimer.

CHEMICAL PEEL. A skin treatment that uses the application of chemicals, such as phenol or trichloroacetic acid (TCA), to remove the uppermost layer of skin.

CHEMICAL TOXICITY. State of physical illness induced by poisoning with toxic chemicals. Chemical toxicities may affect a person's behavior or mental function.

CHEMOPREVENTION. The use of drugs, vitamins, or other substances to reduce the risk of developing cancer or of a cancer returning.

CHEMORECEPTOR TRIGGER ZONE (CTZ). An area within the area postrema of the brain that is sensitive to drugs and neurotransmitters; it communicates with other nearby brain structures to trigger vomiting.

CHEMOTHERAPY. Cancer treatment that uses drugs to stop the growth of cancer cells, either by killing the cells or by stopping them from dividing.

CHEST SHELL. A type of mechanical ventilator that fits around the chest, creating a vacuum between the shell and the chest wall that causes the chest to expand and suck in air.

CHEST TUBE. A tube inserted into the chest to drain fluid and air from around the lungs.

CHEST X-RAY. A diagnostic procedure in which a small amount of radiation is used to produce an image of the structures of the chest (heart, lungs, and bones) on film.

CHILD LIFE SPECIALIST. A person who has had specific training in the care of children, including understanding growth and development specific to each age range and how to talk to children of different ages.

CHILDREN'S HEALTH INSURANCE PROGRAM (CHIP). Children's Medicaid; a federal program administered by the states that provides low-cost or free health insurance to children from families with incomes that have traditionally been too high to qualify for Medicaid.

CHIROPRACTIC. A form of manipulative therapy that emphasizes the adjustment and realignment of joints and muscles. Chiropractic is most often used as an alternative treatment for low back pain.

CHOLANGITIS. A bacterial infection of the biliary system.

CHOLECYSTECTOMY. Surgical removal of the gall-bladder.

CHOLECYSTITIS. Infection and inflammation of the gallbladder, causing severe pain and rigidity in the upper right abdomen.

CHOLELITHIASIS. Also known as gallstones, these hard masses are formed in the gallbladder or passages and can cause severe upper right abdominal pain as a result of blocked bile flow.

CHOLELITHOTOMY. Surgical incision into the gall-bladder to remove stones.

CHOLESTASIS. A blockage in the flow of bile.

CHOLESTEATOMA. A destructive and expanding sac that develops in the middle ear or mastoid process.

CHOLESTEROL. A waxy substance made by the liver that circulates in the bloodstream; it is also acquired through diet. Cholesterol is essential to the human body, but too much can increase the risk of cardiovascular disease and other conditions.

CHORDAE TENDINEAE. The strands of connective tissue that connect the mitral valve to the papillary muscle of the heart's left ventricle.

CHORDEE. A condition associated with hypospadias in which the penis bends downward during erections.

CHORIOAMNIONITIS. Infection of the amniotic sac.

CHORIONIC VILLUS SAMPLING (CVS). A procedure where a needle is inserted into the placenta to withdraw a sample of the placenta's inner wall cells surrounding the fetus.

CHORIORETINAL. Relating to the choroid coat of the eye and retina.

CHOROID. Middle layer of the eye, between the retina and sclera.

CHROMOSOMES. Strands of genetic material in a cell. Normal human cells contain 23 chromosome pairs—one in each pair inherited from the mother, and one from the father. Every human cell contains the exact same set of chromosomes.

CHRONIC. Long term.

CHRONIC ILLNESS. A condition that lasts a year or longer, limits activity, and may require ongoing care.

CHRONIC MYELOGENOUS LEUKEMIA (CML). Also called chronic myelocytic leukemia, a malignant disorder that involves abnormal accumulation of white cells in the marrow and bloodstream.

CHRONIC OTITIS MEDIA. Inflammation of the middle ear with signs of infection lasting three months or longer.

CHRONIC PAIN. Pain that lasts more than three months and threatens to disrupt daily life.

CHRONIC RENAL (KIDNEY) FAILURE. Progressive loss of kidney function over several years that can result in permanent kidney failure requiring dialysis.

CILIA. Short hairlike projections that are capable of a lashing movement.

CILIARY BODY. The part of the eye, located behind the iris, that makes the intraocular aqueous fluid.

CIRCULATION. The passage of blood and delivery of oxygen through the veins and arteries of the body.

CIRCUMCISION. The removal of the foreskin of the penis.

CIRRHOSIS. A type of chronic, progressive liver disease in which liver cells are replaced by scar tissue.

CLASSICAL INCISION. A vertical incision of the uterus during cesarean delivery.

CLATHRATES. Substances in which a molecule from one compound fills a space within the crystal lattice of another compound.

CLAUDICATION. Cramping or pain in the leg caused by poor blood circulation, frequently caused by hardening of the arteries (atherosclerosis). Intermittent claudication occurs only at certain times, usually after exercise, and is relieved by rest.

CLEAN-CATCH SPECIMEN. A urine specimen that is collected from the middle of the urine stream after the first part of the flow has been discarded.

CLEARANCE. The process of removing a substance or obstruction from the body.

CLEFT. Split or opening, which can occur in the lip or palate or both.

CLEFT PALATE. A birth defect in which the roof of the mouth is open because the two sides of the palate failed to join together during fetal development.

CLINICAL BREAST EXAM. An examination of the breast and surrounding tissue by a physician, who is feeling for lumps and other signs of abnormality.

CLINICAL NURSE SPECIALIST. A nurse with advanced training as well as a master's degree.

CLONIC SEIZURE. A seizure in which the body jerks uncontrollably.

CLOSTRIDIUM DIFFICILE. A bacterium that causes diarrhea and other serious intestinal illness and is commonly contracted during hospital stays.

CLOT. A soft, semi-solid mass that forms when blood gels.

CLOTTING FACTORS. Substances in the blood that act in sequence to stop bleeding by forming a clot.

COAGULATION. Blood clotting.

COAGULATION CASCADE. The sequence of biochemical activities, involving clotting factors, that stop bleeding by forming a clot.

COAGULATION FACTORS. Proteins produced in the liver and found in blood plasma that are necessary for the formation of blood clots to stop excessive bleeding.

COAGULOPATHY. A defect in the blood-clotting mechanism.

COARCTATION OF THE AORTA. A congenital defect in which severe narrowing or constriction of the aorta obstructs the flow of blood.

COATS' DISEASE. Also called exudative retinitis, a chronic abnormality characterized by the deposition of cholesterol on the outer retinal layers.

COBRA. Consolidated Omnibus Budget Reconciliation Act; a provision of the Health Insurance Portability and Accountability Act of 1996 that enables people who lose their health insurance to purchase coverage from their previous employer-based plan for a limited time period.

COCHLEA. The hearing part of the inner ear. This snail-shaped structure contains fluid and thousands of microscopic hair cells tuned to various frequencies, in addition to the organ of Corti (the receptor for hearing).

COGNITION. The mental activity of thinking, learning, and memory.

COLD SORE. A small blister on the lips or face, caused by a virus; also called a fever blister.

COLECTOMY. The surgical removal of the colon or part of the colon.

COLITIS. Inflammation of the colon (large bowel).

COLLAGEN. A type of protein found in connective tissue that gives it strength and flexibility.

COLLATERAL VESSEL. A side branch or network of side branches of a large blood vessel.

COLLATERALS. Alternate pathways for arterial blood.

COLON. The portion of the large intestine where stool is formed.

COLONOSCOPE. A thin, flexible, hollow, lighted tube that is used to view the inside of the large intestine.

COLONOSCOPY. An examination of the rectum and colon performed by inserting a colonoscope through the anus.

COLORECTAL. Pertaining to the large intestine and the rectum.

COLORECTAL CANCER. Cancer of the large intestine, or colon, including the rectum.

COLOSTOMY. The surgical construction of an artificial anus between the colon and the surface of the abdomen.

COLPORRHAPHY. A surgical procedure in which the vagina is sutured.

COLPOSCOPY. Examination of the cervix through a magnifying device to detect abnormal cells.

COLUMELLA. The strip of skin running from the tip of the nose to the upper lip, which separates the nostrils.

COMA. A state of unconsciousness from which a person cannot be aroused, even by strong or painful stimuli.

COMBINATION THERAPY. The use of two or more drugs to treat or manage a medical condition.

COMMISSURES. The normal separations between the valve leaflets in the heart.

COMMON BILE DUCT. The branching passage through which bile—a necessary digestive enzyme—travels from the liver and gallbladder into the small intestine. Digestive enzymes from the pancreas also enter the intestines through the common bile duct.

COMMON PATHWAY. In the coagulation cascade, the pathway that results from the merging of the extrinsic and intrinsic pathways. The common pathway includes the final steps before a clot is formed.

COMORBID. A term applied to a disease or disorder that occurs simultaneously with another condition in a patient.

COMPARTMENT SYNDROME. A condition in which tissue pressure within a closed muscle compartment is greater than perfusion pressure, resulting in the loss of blood supply to muscles and nerves.

COMPATIBLE DONOR. A person whose tissue and blood type are the same as the recipient's.

COMPLEMENTARY MEDICINE. A nonconventional therapy that is used together with or alongside mainstream treatment. Complementary medicine is not intended to treat a disease but instead is used to alleviate associated symptoms, such as pain or stress.

COMPLETE BLOOD COUNT (CBC). A blood test that checks the numbers of red blood cells, white blood cells, and platelets in the blood.

COMPOSITE TISSUE ALLOTRANSPLANTATION (CTA). Transplantation of a functional unit made up of different tissues, such as a hand or face.

COMPOUND FRACTURE. A fracture in which the broken end or ends of the bone have penetrated through the skin; also known as an open fracture.

COMPULSION. The uncontrollable impulse to perform a specific act. In mental health disorders, compulsions are often repetitive and carried out in response to anxiety.

COMPUTED TOMOGRAPHY (CT). An imaging technique that uses x-rays to produce detailed pictures (scans) of anatomical structures inside the body.

CONCHA. The hollow shell-shaped portion of the external ear.

CONDITIONING. Process of preparing a patient to receive a marrow donation, often through the use of chemotherapy and radiation therapy.

CONDUCTIVE HEARING LOSS. A type of medically treatable hearing loss in which the inner ear is usually normal, but there are specific problems in the middle or outer ears that prevent sound from getting to the inner ear.

CONDUIT DIVERSION. A surgical procedure that restores urinary and fecal continence by diverting these functions through a constructed conduit leading to an external waste reservoir (ostomy).

CONFIRMATORY TYPING. Repeat tissue typing to confirm the compatibility of a donor and patient before transplant.

CONGENITAL. Present at birth.

CONGENITAL CYSTIC ADENOMATOID MALFORMATION (CCAM). A condition in which one or more lobes of the fetal lungs develop into fluid-filled sacs called cysts.

CONGENITAL DEFECT. A defect present at birth.

CONGENITAL DIAPHRAGMATIC HERNIA (CDH). A condition in which the fetal diaphragm—the muscle dividing the chest and abdominal cavity—does not close completely.

CONGENITAL HEART DEFECTS. Congenital (conditions that are present at birth) heart disease includes a variety of defects that occur during fetal development.

CONGESTIVE HEART FAILURE. A serious condition caused by disease or damage to the heart that weakens the heart's ability to pump a sufficient amount of blood to the body tissues.

CONJUNCTIVA. The mucous membrane that lines the visible part of the eye and the inner eyelid.

CONJUNCTIVITIS. Inflammation of the conjunctiva, the membrane on the inner part of the eyelids and the covering of the white of the eye.

CONNECTIVE TISSUE. Cells such as fibroblasts, and material such as collagen and reticulin, that unite one part of the body with another.

CONSCIOUS SEDATION. A level of sedation during which the patient remains awake but very relaxed.

CONSENT. Permission or agreement.

CONSERVATION SURGERY. Surgery that preserves the aesthetics of the area undergoing an operation.

CONSERVATOR. Legal guardian.

CONSTIPATION. A condition in which there is difficulty in emptying the bowels, usually associated with hardened feces.

CONSTRICT. To squeeze tightly; compress; draw together.

CONSUMER OPERATED AND ORIENTED PLANS (CO-OPS). Independent, nonprofit, member-owned, and member-operated health insurance companies established under the Patient Protection and Affordable Care Act (PPACA).

CONTAMINATION. A breach in the preservation of a clean or sterile object or environment.

CONTINENT. Able to control the release of the contents of the bladder or bowel. A continent surgical procedure is one that allows the patient to keep waste products inside the body rather than collecting them in an external bag attached to a stoma.

CONTINUOUS POSITIVE AIRWAY PRESSURE (CPAP). A ventilation device that blows a gentle stream of air into the nose during sleep to keep the airway open; used in patients with sleep apnea.

CONTRACEPTION. The prevention of the union of the male's sperm with the female's egg.

CONTRACTURE. An abnormal persistent shortening of a muscle or the overlying skin at a joint, usually caused by the formation of scar tissue following an injury.

CONTRAST MEDIUM. A substance that is swallowed or injected into the body to increase the visibility of body structures or fluids on x-rays; also referred to as a contrast agent.

CONVULSION. Involuntary contractions of body muscles that accompany a seizure episode.

CO-PAYMENT. The amount that an insured individual pays out-of-pocket for healthcare services.

COR PULMONALE. Enlargement of the right ventricle of the heart caused by pulmonary hypertension that may result from emphysema or bronchiectasis; eventually, the condition leads to congestive heart failure.

CORACOID PROCESS. A long curved projection from the scapula overhanging the glenoid cavity; it provides attachment to muscles and ligaments of the shoulder and back region.

CORE NEEDLE BIOPSY (CNB). A procedure using a larger diameter needle to remove a core of tissue from the breast.

CORECTOMY. Another term for iridectomy.

CORN. A horny thickening of the skin on a toe, caused by friction and pressure from poorly fitted shoes or stockings.

CORNEA. The transparent layer of tissue at the very front of the eye that admits light.

CORNEAL TOPOGRAPHY. Mapping the cornea's surface with a specialized computer that illustrates corneal elevations.

CORONARY. Of or relating to the heart.

CORONARY ARTERY BYPASS GRAFT SURGERY (CABG). A surgical procedure where arteries or veins from elsewhere in the patient's body are grafted into the arteries of the heart as a way to bypass damaged or narrowed heart blood vessels.

CORONARY ARTERY DISEASE. A build-up of fatty matter and debris in the coronary artery wall that causes narrowing of the artery; also called atherosclerosis.

CORONARY BLOOD VESSELS. The arteries and veins that connect to the heart.

CORONARY BYPASS SURGERY. A surgical procedure that places a shunt to allow blood to travel from the aorta to a branch of the coronary artery at a point below an obstruction.

CORONARY OCCLUSION. Obstruction of an artery that supplies the heart. When the artery is completely blocked, a myocardial infarction (heart attack) results; an incomplete blockage may result in angina.

CORONARY STENT. An artificial support device used to keep a coronary vessel open.

CORONARY VASCULAR DISEASE. Cardiovascular disease; disease of the heart or blood vessels, such as atherosclerosis (hardening of the arteries).

CORTICOSTEROID. A type of synthetic hormone used to treat inflammatory conditions.

CORTISOL. A corticosteroid hormone produced by the adrenal gland.

CORTISONE. A steroid compound used to treat autoimmune diseases and inflammatory conditions.

COSMETIC SURGERY. Surgery that is intended to improve a patient's appearance; it is also called aesthetic surgery.

COUCHING. The oldest form of cataract surgery, in which the lens is dislocated and pushed backward into the vitreous body with a lance.

COX-2 SELECTIVE INHIBITOR. A type of nonsteroidal anti-inflammatory drug (NSAID) that targets the enzyme cyclooxygenase-2 (COX-2), which is responsible for pain and inflammation within the body.

CRANIOCAUDAL. Literally, "head to tail"; refers to an x-ray beam placed directly overhead the part being examined.

CRANIOFACIAL SURGERY. Surgery of the facial tissue and skull.

CRANIOPHARYNGEAL ACHALASIA. A swallowing disorder of the throat.

CRANIOSYNOSTOSIS. Premature closure of the skull, resulting in skull deformities and increased pressure on the brain.

CRANIOTOMY. A surgical procedure in which a piece of the skull is removed temporarily to provide access to the brain.

CRANIUM. The large, rounded upper part of the skull that encloses the brain.

CREATINE. A substance produced from protein and stored in the muscles. Creatine is a source for energy, allowing muscle contraction to take place.

CREATININE. A byproduct of creatine. Creatinine enters the bloodstream and goes to the kidneys. Healthy kidneys filter out this waste material from the blood and it leaves the body in urine.

CREATININE CLEARANCE RATE. The clearance of creatinine from the blood compared to its appearance in the urine. Since there is no reabsorption of creatinine, this measurement can help evaluate kidney function.

CREMASTERIC REFLEX. A reflex in which the cremaster muscle, which covers the testes and the spermatic cord, pulls the testicles back into the scrotum. It is important for a doctor to distinguish between an undescended testicle and a hyperactive cremasteric reflex in small children.

CRETINISM. Severe hypothyroidism that is present at birth and characterized by severe intellectual disability.

CRICOID CARTILAGE. A ring-shaped piece of cartilage that forms the lower and rear parts of the voice box or larynx; it is sometimes called the annular cartilage because of its shape.

CRICOTHYROID MEMBRANE. The piece of connective tissue that lies between the thyroid and cricoid cartilage.

CRICOTHYROIDOTOMY. An emergency tracheotomy that consists of a cut through the cricothyroid membrane to open the patient's airway as fast as possible.

CRITICAL CARE. Multidisciplinary healthcare specialty that provides care to patients with acute, life-threatening illness or injury.

CROHN'S DISEASE. Chronic inflammatory bowel disease that most commonly affects the last part of the small intestine (ileum) and/or the large intestine (colon and rectum).

CROSSMATCH. A test to determine whether patient and donor blood or tissues are compatible.

CROUZON SYNDROME. A genetic disorder caused by a mutation of a growth factor receptor on chromosome 10, characterized by early fusion of an infant's skull and facial bones.

CROWN. The natural crown of a tooth is that part of the tooth covered by enamel. A restorative crown is a protective shell that fits over a tooth.

CRUSH INJURY. Any injury caused when part of the body is trapped or caught between two objects forced together by pressure. Crush injuries range from minor household accidents to potentially life-threatening situations.

CRUSH SYNDROME. A potentially fatal condition in which localized crush injury leads to such systemic complications as metabolic abnormalities and acute kidney failure.

CRYOANESTHESIA. The use of the numbing effects of cold as a surgical anesthetic.

CRYOGEN. A substance with a very low boiling point, such as liquid nitrogen, used in cryotherapy treatment.

CRYOPEXY. Reattachment of a detached retina by freezing the tissue behind the tear with nitrous oxide.

CRYOPROSTATECTOMY. Freezing of the prostate through the use of liquid nitrogen probes guided by transrectal ultrasound of the prostate.

CRYOSURGERY. Freezing and destroying abnormal cells.

CRYOTHERAPY. The therapeutic use of cold to reduce discomfort or remove abnormal tissue.

CRYPTORCHIDISM. A developmental disorder in which one or both testes fail to descend from the abdomen into the scrotum before birth.

CRYPTOSPORIDIUM. A type of parasitic protozoa.

CUL-DE-SAC. The closed end of a pouch.

CULTURE. A laboratory test done from a sample of body fluid to identify microorganisms causing infection.

CUPID'S BOW. Double curve of the upper lip.

CURETTE. A spoon-shaped instrument used to remove tissue from the inner lining of the uterus.

CUSHING'S DISEASE. A condition resulting from excess cortisol in the body, characterized by high blood pressure, a round face, excessive sweating, thinning of the skin and easy bruising, and the growth of fat pads around the shoulders and back of the neck.

CUTANEOUS SQUAMOUS CELL CARCINOMA (SCC). A malignant (cancerous) skin tumor.

CYANOACRYLATE. The chemical name of liquid surgical adhesive.

CYANOSIS. Blue, gray, or dark purple discoloration of the skin caused by a loss of oxygen.

CYANOTIC. Inadequate oxygen in the systemic arterial circulation.

CYCLOCRYOTHERAPY. The use of subfreezing temperatures to treat glaucoma.

CYST. An abnormal saclike growth in the body that contains liquid or a semisolid material.

CYSTECTOMY. The surgical resection of part or all of the bladder.

CYSTIC ARTERY. An artery that brings oxygenated blood to the gallbladder.

CYSTIC FIBROSIS. A generalized disorder of infants, children, and young adults characterized by widespread dysfunction of the exocrine glands, and chronic pulmonary disease due to excess mucus production in the respiratory tract.

CYSTINE. An amino acid found in protein molecules that may form kidney stones when excreted in excessive amounts in the urine.

CYSTINURIA. A hereditary condition characterized by chronic excessive excretion of cystine and three other amino acids.

CYSTOPLASTY. Reconstructive surgery of the urinary bladder.

CYSTOSCOPE. A specialized endoscope (thin tube fixed with a lens and light) used to examine the urinary bladder and urethra.

CYSTOSCOPY. Examination of the bladder using a cystoscope.

CYSTOTOMY. An incision in the bladder.

CYTOKINE. Any of a group of signaling molecules, including interleukin, interferon, and tumor necrosis factor, that influence the functioning of the immune system and may have either pro- or anti-inflammatory effects.

CYTOLOGIST. A medical technologist who specializes in cytology.

CYTOLOGY. The field of medicine that focuses on the examination of biopsy specimens and cell specimens for changes that may indicate precancerous conditions or a specific stage of cancer.

CYTOPATHOLOGY. Another name for cytology; the study of cells or cell types.

CYTOPLASM. The part of a cell outside of the nucleus.

CYTOREDUCTION. Another term for debulking surgery; surgical removal of a tumor.

CYTOSTATIC DRUG. Any drug that inhibits or prevents cell division and proliferation.

D

DACRON GRAFT. A synthetic material used in the repair or replacement of blood vessels.

D-DIMER. A small protein fragment that is present in the blood after the fibrin in a blood clot has been broken down. The D-dimer level can be measured to evaluate a patient for thrombosis (inappropriate clot formation) or disseminated intravascular coagulation.

DEBRIDEMENT. Surgical removal of foreign material and dead or damaged tissue.

DEBULKING. Surgical removal of a major portion of a tumor so that there is less of the cancer left for later treatment by chemotherapy or radiation.

DECLOTTING. A procedure used to remove a blood clot.

DECOMPRESSION. Any surgical procedure done to relieve pressure on a nerve or other part of the body.

DEDUCTIBLE. The amount that an insured person is required to pay on each claim or over the course of a year.

DEEP VEIN THROMBOSIS. The development or presence of a blood clot in a vein deep within the leg.

DEFECATION. The act of passing a bowel movement.

DEFIBRILLATION. An electronic process that helps reestablish a normal heart rhythm.

DEFIBRILLATOR. A device that delivers an electric shock to the heart muscle through the chest wall in order to restore a normal heart rate.

DEFLAGRATION. The combustion of gas or other flammable material at speeds below the speed of sound, driven by heat transfer.

DEGENERATIVE ARTHRITIS. A non-inflammatory type of arthritis that usually occurs in older adults, characterized by degeneration of cartilage, enlargement of the margins of the bones, and changes in the membranes in the joints; also known as osteoarthritis.

DEGLOVING. Separating the skin of the penis from the shaft temporarily in order to correct chordee.

DEHISCENCE. Separation or splitting open of the different layers of tissue in a surgical incision. Dehiscence may be partial, involving only a few layers of surface tissue, or complete, reopening all the layers of the incision.

DEHYDRATION. A decreased amount of water in the tissues, caused by an excessive loss of bodily fluid or lack of adequate hydration.

DELIRIUM. An altered state of consciousness that includes confusion, disorientation, incoherence, agitation, and defective perception (such as hallucinations).

DELTOID MUSCLE. Muscle that covers the prominence of the shoulder.

DELUSION. Conviction of a false belief or wrong judgment despite obvious evidence to the contrary.

DEMENTIA. Disorder characterized by the progressive loss of cognitive and intellectual function.

DEMYELINATION. The loss of myelin, a protective cover that surrounds nerve cells, with preservation of the axons or fiber tracts. Central demyelination occurs within the central nervous system, and peripheral demyelination affects the peripheral nervous system.

DENTAL OCCLUSION. The medical term for the contact between the teeth in the upper and lower jaws. Misalignment of the jaws and teeth is called malocclusion.

DEOXYHEMOGLOBIN. Hemoglobin with oxygen removed.

DEPENDENCE. A state in which a person requires a steady concentration of a particular substance in order to avoid withdrawal symptoms.

DEPRESSANT. A drug or other substance that soothes or lessens tension of the muscles or nerves.

DERMABRASION. A technique for removing the upper layers of skin with planing wheels powered by compressed air.

DERMATITIS. A skin disorder that causes inflammation (redness, swelling, heat, and pain).

DERMATOLOGIST. A doctor who specializes in skin care and treatment.

DERMATOME. A surgical instrument used to cut thin slices of skin for grafts.

DERMATOSIS. A noninflammatory skin disorder.

DERMIS. The underlayer of skin, containing blood vessels, nerves, hair follicles, and oil and sweat glands.

DESICCATION. Tissue death.

DETONATION. A chemical reaction that propagates from reacted to unreacted material faster than the speed of sound, such that the heat of the explosion is preceded by a shock wave.

DETOXIFICATION. The process of removing a poison or toxin or the effect of a harmful substance.

DETRUSOR MUSCLE. The medical name for the layer of muscle tissue covering the urinary bladder. When the detrusor muscle contracts, the bladder expels urine.

DEVELOPMENTAL DISORDER. A disorder or disability that occurs because of prenatal or early childhood events that affect cognition, language, motor, or social skills.

DEVIATED SEPTUM. An abnormal configuration of the cartilage that divides the two sides of the nose. It can cause breathing problems if left uncorrected.

DEXA BONE DENSITY SCAN. A bone density scan that uses a rotating x-ray beam to measure the strength of an individual's bones and his or her fracture risk.

DIABETES MELLITUS. A disease in which a person cannot effectively use glucose to meet the needs of the body, caused by a lack of the hormone insulin.

DIABETIC NEPHROPATHY. A progressive kidney disease associated with diabetes that interferes with the kidney's ability to filter waste products from the blood.

DIABETIC RETINOPATHY. Degeneration of the retina related to diabetes; both type 1 and type 2 diabetes can lead to diabetic retinopathy.

DIAGNOSTIC WINDOW. A cardiac marker's timeline for rising, peaking, and returning to normal after a heart attack.

DIALYSATE. A chemical bath used in dialysis to draw fluids and toxins out of the bloodstream and supply electrolytes and other chemicals to the bloodstream.

DIALYSIS. A blood filtration therapy that replaces the function of the kidneys, filtering fluids and waste products out of the bloodstream. There are two types of dialysis treatment: hemodialysis, which uses an artificial kidney, or dialyzer, as a blood filter; and peritoneal dialysis, which uses the patient's abdominal cavity (peritoneum) as a blood filter.

DIALYSIS PRESCRIPTION. The general parameters of dialysis treatment that vary according to each patient's individual needs. Treatment length, type of dialyzer and dialysate used, and rate of ultrafiltration are all part of the dialysis prescription.

DIALYZER. An artificial kidney, usually composed of hollow fiber, that is used in hemodialysis to eliminate waste products from the blood and remove excess fluids from the bloodstream.

DIAPHRAGM. The large flat muscle that runs horizontally across the bottom of the chest cavity and aids in breathing; alternately, the flat-shaped portion of the head of a stethoscope.

DIAPHYSIS. The shaft of a long bone.

DIASTOLE. Period between contractions of the heart.

DIASTOLIC. Minimum arterial blood pressure during ventricular rest.

DIATHERMY. Also called electrocautery, this is a procedure that heats and destroys abnormal cells.

DIETHYLSTILBESTROL (DES). A synthetic form of estrogen that was widely prescribed to women from 1940 to 1970 to prevent complications during pregnancy, later linked to several serious birth defects and disorders of the reproductive system in daughters of women who took DES.

DIFFERENTIAL. Blood test that determines the percentage of each type of white blood cell in a person's blood.

DIFFUSE ESOPHAGEAL SPASM (DES). An uncommon condition characterized by abnormal simultaneous contractions of the esophagus.

DIFFUSION TENSOR IMAGING (DTI). A refinement of magnetic resonance imaging (MRI) that allows the doctor to measure the flow of water and track the pathways of white matter in the brain. DTI is able to detect abnormalities in the brain that do not show up on standard MRI scans.

DIGESTIVE TRACT. The stomach, intestines, and other parts of the body through which food passes.

DIGITAL RECTAL EXAM (DRE). Procedure in which the physician inserts a gloved finger (digit) into the rectum to examine the rectum and the prostate gland for signs of cancer.

DIGITS. Fingers or toes.

DILATE. To expand or open.

DILATION AND CURETTAGE (D&C). A surgical procedure that expands the cervical canal (dilation) so that the lining of the uterus can be scraped (curettage).

DIRECTED DONATION. Blood donated by a patient's family member or friend, to be used by the patient.

DISCHARGE PLANNER. A healthcare professional who helps patients arrange for health and home care needs after they go home from the hospital.

DISEASE-MODIFYING ANTIRHEUMATIC DRUGS (DMARDS). A group of medications that can be given to slow or stop the progression of rheumatoid arthritis. DMARDs include such drugs as oral or injectable methotrexate, leflunomide, and penicillamine.

DISINFECT. To remove most microorganisms.

DISKECTOMY. The surgical removal of a portion or all of an intervertebral disk in the spine.

DISSEMINATED INTRAVASCULAR COAGULATION (DIC). A potentially fatal condition in which blood clots form within blood vessels throughout the body, disrupting normal blood flow to vital organs and eventually resulting in uncontrolled bleeding from the respiratory and gastrointestinal tracts. DIC can result from traumatic injuries as well as from cancer and certain infectious diseases.

DISSEMINATED INTRAVASCULAR DISSEMINATION. A condition in which the clotting factors in the blood are rapidly used up, resulting in a severe deficit in clotting factors and a very high risk of severe, uncontrollable bleeding.

DIURETIC. A type of medication that increases the amount of urine produced and relieves excess fluid buildup in body tissues. Diuretics may be used in treating high blood pressure, lung disease, premenstrual syndrome, and other conditions.

DIVERTICULA (SINGULAR, DIVERTICULUM). Sacs or pouches in the colon wall. They are usually asymptomatic (without symptoms) but may cause difficulty if they become inflamed.

DIVERTICULITIS. Inflammation or infection of diverticula.

DIVERTICULOSIS. The development of diverticula.

DNA. Deoxyribonucleic acid; the substance within the nucleus of all human cells in which genetic information is stored.

DO NOT RESUSCITATE (DNR) ORDER. Instructions for medical personnel that a patient is not to be resuscitated in the event of cardiac or respiratory arrest.

DOMINANT. Referring to a genetic trait that is expressed when only one copy of the gene is present.

DOMINANT HAND. The hand that an individual prefers to use for most activities, especially writing.

DON. To put on.

DONOR. A person who supplies organ(s), tissue, or blood to another person for transplantation or transfusion.

DOPPLER. The Doppler effect refers to the apparent change in frequency of sound-wave echoes returning to a stationary source from a moving target. If the object is moving toward the source, the frequency increases; if the object is moving away, the frequency decreases. The size of this frequency shift can be used to compute the object's speed—be it a car on the road or blood in an artery.

DOPPLER ECHOCARDIOGRAPHY. A testing technique that uses Doppler ultrasound technology to evaluate the pattern and direction of blood flow in the heart.

DOPPLER ULTRASONOGRAPHY. A diagnostic ultrasound procedure that uses reflected sound waves to evaluate blood flow through major arteries and veins; also referred to as Doppler ultrasound.

DORSAL. Referring to a position closer to the back than to the stomach. The laminae in the spinal column are located on the dorsal side of each vertebra.

DOSE LIMITING. Circumstance in which the side effects of a drug prevent an increase in dose.

DOWN SYNDROME. The most prevalent of a class of genetic defects known as trisomies, in which cells contain three copies of certain chromosomes rather than the usual two. Down syndrome, or trisomy 21, usually results from three copies of chromosome 21 and is characterized by intellectual disability and risk of heart defects.

DRAINAGE. The withdrawal or removal of blood and other fluid matter from an incision or wound. An incision that is oozing blood or tissue fluids is said to be draining.

DRESSING. A bandage, gauze pad, or other material placed over a wound or incision to cover and protect it.

DRY EYE. Corneal dryness due to insufficient tear production.

DRY SOCKET. A painful condition following tooth extraction in which a blood clot does not properly fill the empty socket. Dry socket leaves the underlying bone exposed to air and food particles.

DUAL ELIGIBLES. Low-income elderly and people with physical or mental disabilities who are eligible for both Medicaid and Medicare.

DUANE SYNDROME. A hereditary congenital syndrome in which the affected eye shows a limited capacity to move and is deficient in convergence with the other eye.

DUCTUS ARTERIOSUS. A fetal blood vessel that connects the aorta and pulmonary artery.

DUMPING SYNDROME. A complex physical reaction to food passing too quickly from the stomach into the small intestine, characterized by sweating, nausea, abdominal cramps, dizziness, and other symptoms.

DUODENECTOMY. Excision of the duodenum.

DUODENUM. The section of the small intestine closest to the stomach.

DURA MATER. The outermost and strongest of the three membranes that cover the brain and spinal cord.

DURABLE MEDICAL POWER OF ATTORNEY. A legal document that empowers a person to make medical decisions for a patient, should the patient become incapacitated.

DYSMENORRHEA. Painful menstruation.

DYSMOTILITY. A lack of normal muscle movement (motility), especially in the esophagus, stomach, or intestines.

DYSPHAGIA. Difficulty or discomfort in swallowing.

DYSPLASIA. Abnormal development of or changes in cells.

DYSPNEA. Difficulty breathing.

DYSTOCIA. Failure to progress in labor, either because the cervix will not dilate (expand) further or (after full dilation) the baby's head does not descend through the mother's pelvis.

DYSVASCULAR AMPUTATION. Amputation due to vascular disease.

E

EALES DISEASE. A disorder marked by recurrent hemorrhages into the retina and vitreous body of the eye. It occurs most often in males between the ages of 10 and 25.

EAR MOLDING. A nonsurgical method for treating ear deformities shortly after birth with the application of a mold held in place by tape and surgical glue.

EARLY AND PERIODIC SCREENING, DIAGNOSIS, AND TREATMENT (EPSDT). Children's services that Medicaid programs are required to cover.

ECG. Abbreviation for electrocardiogram or electrocardiography.

ECHOCARDIOGRAM. Ultrasound image of the heart.

ECHOCARDIOGRAPHY. An imaging procedure that uses high-frequency sound waves to create a picture of the heart's movement, valves, and chambers.

ECLAMPSIA. A serious, life-threatening complication of pregnancy, in which high blood pressure results in a variety of problems, including seizures.

ECTOPIC. Located in an abnormal site or tissue.

ECTOPIC BEAT. Abnormal heartbeat arising elsewhere than from the sinoatrial node.

ECTOPIC PARATHYROID TISSUE. Parathyroid tissue located in an abnormal place.

ECTOPIC PREGNANCY. A pregnancy that occurs outside of the uterus, most often in the fallopian tubes.

ECTROPION. A complication of blepharoplasty, in which the lower lid is pulled downward, exposing the inner surface.

EDEMA. Swelling of body tissues caused by excess fluid.

EFFUSION. The escape of fluid from blood vessels or the lymphatic system and its collection in a cavity.

EGOBRONCHOPHONY. Increased intensity of the spoken voice.

EJACULATION. The act of expelling the sperm through the penis during orgasm. The fluid that is released is called the ejaculate.

EJECTION FRACTION. The amount of blood pumped out at each heartbeat, usually expressed as a percentage.

EKG. Abbreviation for electrocardiogram or electrocardiography.

ELECTIVE SURGERY. Surgery that is chosen by the patient (or a guardian); an elective operation may be beneficial to the patient but is not urgently needed.

ELECTROCARDIOGRAM. A graphic tracing of the electrical activity of the heart.

ELECTROCARDIOGRAPHY. A test that measures electrical impulses in the heart using small electrode patches attached to the skin.

ELECTROCAUTERY. The cauterization of tissue using an electric current to generate heat.

ELECTROCOAGULATION. The coagulation or destruction of tissue through the application of a high-frequency electrical current; also referred to as diathermy.

ELECTRODE. A medium for conducting an electrical current.

ELECTRODESICCATION. A method of treating spider veins or drying up tissue by passing a small electric current through a fine needle into the affected area; also referred to as electrofulguration.

ELECTROENCEPHALOGRAM (EEG). A diagnostic test that measures the electrical activity of the brain (brain waves) using highly sensitive recording equipment attached to the scalp by electrodes.

ELECTROLYTES. Ions in the body that participate in metabolic reactions. The major human electrolytes are sodium (Na^+), potassium (K^+), calcium (Ca^{2+}), magnesium (Mg^{2+}), chloride (Cl^-), phosphate (HPO_4^{2-}), bicarbonate (HCO_3^-), and sulfate (SO_4^{2-}).

ELECTROMYOGRAPHY. A test that measures muscle response to nerve stimulation. It is used to evaluate muscle weakness and to determine if the weakness is related to the muscles themselves or to a problem with the nerves that supply the muscles.

ELECTRONIC HEALTH RECORD (EHR). An electronic version of a patient's complete medical history.

ELECTRONYSTAGMOGRAM. A test that involves the graphic recording of eye movements.

ELECTROPHORESIS. A method of separating complex protein molecules suspended in a gel by running an electric current through the gel.

ELECTROPHYSIOLOGICAL STUDY (EPS). A test that monitors the electrical activity of the heart in order to diagnose arrhythmia. An electrophysiological study measures electrical signals through a cardiac catheter that is inserted into an artery in the leg and guided up into the atrium and ventricle of the heart.

ELECTROPHYSIOLOGY. Study of how electrical signals in the body relate to physiologic function.

ELECTROSECTION. Electrosurgical cutting out of tissues.

ELECTROSURGICAL DEVICE. A medical device that uses electrical current to cauterize or coagulate tissue during surgical procedures.

ELECTROTHERAPY. The treatment of body tissues by passing electrical currents through them, stimulating the nerves and muscles.

EMASCULATION. Another term for castration of a male.

EMBALMING. Process of treating a dead body with chemicals to preserve it from decay.

EMBOLISM. A blood clot, air bubble, or clot of foreign material that travels and blocks the flow of blood in an artery. When blood supply to a tissue or organ is blocked by an embolism, infarction (death of the tissue the artery feeds) occurs. Without immediate and appropriate treatment, an embolism can be fatal.

EMBOLIZATION. The purposeful introduction of a substance into a blood vessel to stop blood flow.

EMBOLUS (PLURAL, EMBOLI). A gas or air bubble, bit of tissue, blood clot, or foreign object that circulates in the bloodstream until it lodges in a vessel. A large embolus can narrow or block the vessel, which leads to decreased blood flow in the organ supplied by that vessel.

EMBRYO. A developing human from the time of conception to the end of the eighth week after conception.

EMESIS. The medical term for vomiting.

EMESIS BASIN. A basin used to collect sputum or vomit.

EMPHYSEMA. A disease in which the small air sacs in the lungs become damaged, causing shortness of breath. In severe cases it can lead to respiratory or heart failure.

EMPYEMA. An accumulation of pus in the lung cavity, usually as a result of infection.

ENCEPHALITIS. An inflammation or infection of the brain and spinal cord caused by a virus or as a complication of another infection.

ENCEPHALOCELES. Protrusion of the brain through a defect in the skull.

ENDARTERECTOMY. Endarterectomy is the surgical removal of plaque buildup from an artery.

ENDEMIC. Present in a specific population or geographical area at all times.

ENDOCARDITIS. An infection of the inner membrane lining of the heart.

ENDOCRINE. A type of organ or gland that secretes hormones or other products into the bloodstream or the lymphatic system.

ENDOCRINE SYSTEM. Group of glands and parts of glands that control metabolic activity. The pituitary, thyroid, adrenals, ovaries, and testes are all part of the endocrine system.

ENDOCRINOLOGIST. A physician who specializes in treating persons with diseases of the thyroid, parathyroid, adrenal glands, and the pancreas.

ENDODONTIC. Pertaining to the inside structures of the tooth, including the dental pulp and tooth root, and the periapical tissue surrounding the root.

ENDODONTIST. A dentist who specializes in the diagnosis and treatment of disorders affecting the inside structures of teeth.

ENDOLYMPH. The watery fluid contained in the membranous labyrinth of the inner ear.

ENDOLYMPHATIC SAC. The pouch at the end of the endolymphatic duct that connects to the membranous labyrinth of the inner ear.

ENDOMETRIAL POLYPS. Growths in the lining of the uterus (endometrium) that may cause bleeding and can develop into cancer.

ENDOMETRIOSIS. A condition in which the endometrial tissue that lines the uterus (endometrium) spreads to other parts of the body.

ENDOMETRIOSIS ABLATION. Procedure of removing endometrial tissue from deposition on structures within the abdominal cavity.

ENDOMETRIUM. The lining of the uterus.

ENDOMYOCARDIAL BIOPSY. Removal of a small sample of heart tissue to check it for signs of damage caused by organ rejection.

ENDOPHTHALMITIS. An infection on the inside of the eye that can result in vision loss.

ENDORPHINS. Any of a group of proteins with analgesic (pain-relieving) properties that occur naturally in the brain.

ENDOSCOPE. A narrow, flexible tube with a fiber-optic light that is used to see inside body cavities.

ENDOSCOPIC. Of, relating to, or performed by means of an endoscope or endoscopy.

ENDOSCOPIC RETROGRADE CHOLANGIOPANCREA-TOGRAPHY (ERCP). A procedure to x-ray the ducts (tubes) that carry bile from the liver to the gallbladder and from the gallbladder to the small intestine.

ENDOSCOPIC ULTRASOUND. An imaging procedure that uses high-frequency sound waves to visualize the esophagus via a lighted telescopic instrument (endoscope) and a monitor.

ENDOSCOPIST. A physician or other medical professional highly trained in the use of the endoscope and related diagnostic and therapeutic procedures.

ENDOSCOPY. The visual inspection of any cavity of the body using an endoscope.

ENDOSTEAL IMPLANTS. Dental implants that are placed within the bone.

ENDOTRACHEAL. Located inside the trachea.

ENDOTRACHEAL INTUBATION. A procedure in which a tube is inserted into the trachea in order to administer anesthesia or ventilate the patient.

ENDOTRACHEAL TUBE. A tube inserted into the trachea (windpipe) through the nose or mouth to deliver air to the lungs.

ENDOVASCULAR. Within the walls of a blood vessel.

ENDOVASCULAR COILING. Interventional or endo-vascular neuroradiology; a nonsurgical procedure for repairing cerebral aneurysms.

ENDOVASCULAR GRAFTING. A procedure that involves the insertion of a delivery catheter through a groin artery into the abdominal aorta under fluoroscopic guidance.

END-STAGE HEART FAILURE. Severe heart disease that does not respond adequately to medical or surgical treatment.

END-STAGE LUNG FAILURE. Severe lung disease that does not respond adequately to medical or surgical treatment.

END-STAGE RENAL DISEASE. Chronic or permanent kidney failure.

ENEMA. The injection of liquid into the rectum through the anus for cleansing, for stimulating evacuation of the bowels, or for other therapeutic or diagnostic purposes.

ENGRAFTMENT. The process of transplanted stem cells reproducing new cells.

ENHANCEMENT. In ocular surgery, a secondary refractive procedure performed in an attempt to achieve better visual acuity.

ENOPHTHALMOS. A condition in which the eye falls back into the socket and inhibits proper eyelid function.

ENTERAL NUTRITIONAL SUPPORT. Nutrition utilizing an intact gastrointestinal tract, but bypassing another organ such as the stomach or esophagus.

ENTERIC. Pertaining to the intestine.

ENTERIC COAT. A coating put on some tablets or capsules to prevent their disintegration in the stomach. The contents of coated tablets or capsules will be released only when the dose reaches the intestine. This may be done to protect the drug from stomach acid, to protect the stomach from drug irritation, or to delay the onset of action of the drug.

ENTERITIS. Inflammation of the mucosal lining of the small intestine.

ENTEROSTOMAL THERAPIST. A healthcare provider who specializes in the care of patients with enterostomies (e.g., ileostomies or colostomies).

ENTEROTOXIGENIC. Refers to an organism that produces toxins in the gastrointestinal tract that cause such things as vomiting, diarrhea, and other symptoms of food poisoning.

ENUCLEATION. Surgical removal of the eyeball.

ENZYME. A protein that changes the rate of a chemical reaction within the body without being depleted in the reaction.

ENZYME-LINKED IMMUNOSORBENT ASSAY (ELISA). A diagnostic blood test used to screen patients for AIDS or other viruses.

EOSINOPHIL. Segmented white blood cell with large orange-red granules that increases in response to parasitic infections and allergic reactions.

EPHEDRA. An herb used in traditional Chinese medicine to treat asthma and hay fever. It should never be used for weight management.

EPICONDYLES. The two rounded knuckle-like knobs on the lower end of the humerus bone. The epicondyle closer to the outside of the elbow is called the lateral epicondyle; the other (and larger) epicondyle is called the medial epicondyle.

EPIDERMIS. The outermost layer of the skin.

EPIDIDYMIS. A coiled, cord-like structure within the scrotum, in which sperm mature and are stored.

EPIDIDYMITIS. Inflammation of the epididymis.

EPIDURAL. Between the vertebrae and the dura mater of the spinal cord.

EPIDURAL ANESTHESIA. A type of anesthesia that is injected into the epidural space of the spinal cord to numb the nerves leading to the lower half of the body.

EPIDURAL CATHETER. A thin plastic tube, through which pain medication is delivered, inserted into the patient's back before surgery.

EPIDURAL SPACE. The space surrounding the spinal fluid sac.

EPIGLOTTIS. A leaf-shaped piece of cartilage lying at the root of the tongue that protects the respiratory tract from aspiration during the swallowing reflex.

EPIKERATOPHAKIA. A procedure in which the donor cornea is attached directly onto the host cornea.

EPILEPSY. A neurological disorder characterized by recurrent seizures with or without a loss of consciousness.

EPINEPHRINE. A substance that occurs naturally in the body and causes blood vessels to constrict or narrow. As a drug, it is used to reduce bleeding.

EPIPHYSIODESIS. A surgical procedure that partially or totally destroys an epiphysis and may incorporate a bone graft to produce fusion of the epiphysis or premature cessation of its growth; usually performed to equalize leg length.

EPIPHYSIS. A part of a long bone where bone growth occurs.

EPITHELIAL CELLS. Cells that form a thin surface coating on the outside of a body structure.

EPITHELIUM. A general term for the layer of cells that lines blood vessels or small body cavities.

ERBIUM:YAG. A crystal made of erbium, yttrium, aluminum, and garnet that produces light that is well absorbed by the skin; used for skin resurfacing treatments.

EROSION. A gradual breakdown or ulceration of the uppermost layer of tissue lining the esophagus or stomach.

ERUPTION. The emergence of a tooth through the gum tissue.

ERYTHROBLASTOSIS FETALIS. A condition in which the incompatibility between a mother's Rh-negative blood type and a baby's Rh-positive blood type results in destruction of the baby's red blood cells by maternal antibodies.

ERYTHROPOIETIN. A hormone produced by the kidneys that stimulates the production of red blood cells.

ESCHAR. A hardened dry crust that forms on skin exposed to burns or corrosive agents.

ESOPHAGEAL SPHINCTER. Muscle at the opening to the stomach that keeps the stomach contents from traveling into the esophagus.

ESOPHAGEAL VARICES. Varicose veins at the lowermost portion of the esophagus. Esophageal varices are easily injured, and bleeding from them is often difficult to stop.

ESOPHAGECTOMY. Surgical removal of the esophagus.

ESOPHAGITIS. Inflammation of the esophagus.

ESOPHAGUS. The muscular passageway between the throat and the stomach.

ESRD. End-stage renal disease.

ESSENTIAL HEALTH BENEFITS (EHB). Minimum services that must be provided by health insurance plans under the Patient Protection and Affordable Care Act (PPACA).

ESTATE PLANNING. Preparation of a plan of administration and disposition of a person's property before or after death, including will, trusts, gifts, and power of attorney.

ESTROGENS. A class of chemical compounds (hormones) that stimulate the development of female secondary sexual characteristics.

ETHMOID SINUSES. Paired labyrinth of air cells between the nose and eyes.

ETHYLENE OXIDE. A colorless gas used to sterilize surgical sutures, bandages, and most other surgical materials or implements.

EUSTACHIAN TUBE. A canal that extends from the middle ear to the pharynx.

EUTHANASIA. To bring about the death of another person who has an incurable disease or condition.

EVENT RECORDER. A small machine worn by a patient to record his or her heart activity when an abnormal symptom is detected.

EVIDENCE-BASED PRACTICE. The process by which healthcare providers incorporate the best research or evidence into clinical practice in combination with clinical expertise and within the context of patient values.

EX UTERO INTRAPARTUM TREATMENT (EXIT). A cesarean section in which the infant is removed from the uterus but the umbilical cord is not cut until after surgery; treats congenital defects that block an air passage.

EXCHANGES. American Health Benefit Exchanges; state systems through which individuals can compare and purchase health insurance under the Patient Projection and Affordable Care Act (PPACA).

EXCIMER LASER. An instrument that is used to vaporize tissue.

EXCISION. Removal by cutting.

EXCISIONAL BIOPSY. Procedure in which a surgeon removes all of a lump or suspicious area and an area of healthy tissue around the edges. The tissue is then examined under a microscope to check for cancer cells.

EXCLUSIVE PROVIDER ORGANIZATION (EPO). A managed care plan that only covers services provided by doctors, specialists, and hospitals within the plan's network.

EXOPHTHALMOS. A condition in which the eyes bulge out of their sockets and inhibit proper eyelid function.

EXOTHERMIC REACTION. A chemical reaction that releases energy in the form of light or heat.

EXTRACAPSULAR SURGERY. A cataract surgical procedure in which an incision is made in the cornea to remove the hard center of the lens. The natural lens is then replaced with an intraocular lens (IOL).

EXTRACORPOREAL. Outside of the body.

EXTRACORPOREAL CIRCUIT (ECC). The path a hemodialysis patient's blood takes outside of the body. It typically consists of plastic tubing, a hemodialysis machine, and a dialyzer.

EXTRACORPOREAL SHOCK WAVE LITHOTRIPSY (ESWL). The use of focused shock waves, generated outside the body, to fragment kidney stones.

EXTRACTION. In the context of oral surgery, the surgical removal of a tooth from its socket in a bone.

EXTRACTION SITE. In the context of oral surgery, the empty tooth socket following removal of a tooth.

EXTRAOCULAR MUSCLES. The muscles (lateral rectus, medial rectus, inferior rectus, superior rectus, superior oblique, and inferior oblique) that move the eyeball.

EXTRINSIC PATHWAY. One of three pathways in the coagulation cascade (blood-clotting process).

EXTRUSION. Pushing out or expulsion.

EXUDATE. Fluid, cells, or other substances that are slowly discharged by tissue, especially due to injury or inflammation.

EXUDATIVE. Pertaining to exudate.

EXUDATIVE RETINAL DETACHMENT. A type of retinal detachment caused by the accumulation of tissue fluid underneath the retina.

F

FACE LIFT. Plastic surgery performed to remove sagging skin and wrinkles from an individual's face.

FACTOR XIII. A substance found in blood that forms cross-links between strands of fibrin during the process of blood coagulation. Factor XIII is an ingredient in some types of fibrin sealants. It is also known as fibrin stabilizing factor.

FAILURE TO RESCUE. Patient death after a major surgical complication.

FALLOPIAN TUBES. Tubes that extend from either end of the uterus and convey the egg from the ovary to the uterus during each monthly cycle.

FALSE NEGATIVE. Test results showing no problem when one exists.

FALSE POSITIVE. Test results showing a problem when one does not exist.

FASCIA (PLURAL, FASCIAE). Thin connective tissue that separates and supports organs and other structures in the body.

FASCIOTOMY. Surgical cutting or removal of a fascia or fasciae to relieve the loss of circulation in muscle tissue; it is sometimes called fasciectomy.

FAST FOURIER TRANSFORM (FFT). A mathematical process used in electroencephalogram (EEG) analysis to investigate the composition of an EEG signal.

FAST-TRACK. A protocol for postoperative patients with projected shorter recovery times. Fast-tracking patients means that they will either bypass the post-anesthesia care unit (PACU) completely, or spend a shorter time there with less intensive staff intervention and monitoring.

FATIGUE. Physical or mental weariness.

FECAL INCONTINENCE. Inability to control bowel movements.

FECES. Material excreted by the intestines.

FEDERAL POVERTY LEVEL (FPL). The U.S. government's definition of poverty for families of a given size, adjusted annually for inflation and used as the reference point for determining Medicaid eligibility.

FELLOWSHIP TRAINING. Additional specialty training that follows completion of medical residency training; fellowships are typically one to two years in length.

FELON. A very painful abscess on the lower surface of the fingertip, resulting from infection in the closed space surrounding the bone in the fingertip. It is also known as whitlow.

FEMALE STERILIZATION. The process of permanently ending a woman's ability to conceive by tying off or cutting apart the fallopian tubes.

FEMORAL. Pertaining to the thigh region.

FEMORAL ARTERY. An artery located in the groin area.

FEMORAL HEAD. The upper end of the femur.

FEMUR. The medical name for the thighbone.

FERRITIN. A protein found in the liver, spleen, and bone marrow that stores iron.

FETOSCOPE. A fiber-optic instrument for viewing the fetus inside the uterus.

FETUS. The stage in human development from the second month of pregnancy until birth.

FIBER. Carbohydrate material in food that cannot be digested.

FIBER OPTICS. In medicine, fiber optics refers to the use of glass or plastic fibers to transmit light through a specially designed tube inserted into organs or body cavities, where it transmits a magnified image of the internal body structures.

FIBRILLATION. Rapid, uncoordinated contractions of the upper or the lower chambers of the heart.

FIBRIN. The protein formed as the end product of the blood clotting process when fibrinogen interacts with thrombin.

FIBRINOGEN. Also known as factor I, a soluble clotting factor in the blood that is converted into the insoluble fibrin by the action of thrombin.

FIBROBLAST. A type of cell found in connective tissue that is involved in collagen production as well as tendon formation and healing.

FIBROID. A benign tumor of the uterus.

FIBROSIS. A condition characterized by the presence of scar tissue, or reticulin and collagen proliferation in tissues to the extent that it replaces normal tissues.

FIBROUS CONNECTIVE TISSUE. Dense tissue found in various parts of the body containing very few living cells.

FIBULA. The smaller of the two bones in the lower leg.

FINE-NEEDLE ASPIRATION. Use of a very thin type of needle to withdraw cells and body fluid for examination.

FINGER STICK. A technique for collecting a very small amount of blood from the fingertip area.

FIRST RESPONDER. The first medically trained responder to arrive at the scene of an emergency, accident, natural or human-made disaster, or similar event. First responders may be police officers, fire fighters, emergency medical services personnel, or bystanders with some training in first aid.

FIRST-LINE DRUG. A drug (or class of drugs) regarded as the medication of choice to treat a given condition.

FISTULA (PLURAL, FISTULAE). An abnormal opening between two organs or an abnormal opening leading to the outside of the body.

FISTULA TEST. Compression or rarefaction of the air in the external auditory canal.

FIXATIVE. A chemical that preserves tissue without destroying or altering the structure of the cells.

FIXATOR. A device providing rigid immobilization through external skeletal fixation by means of rods attached to pins that are placed in or through the bone.

FIXED. A term used to describe chemically preserved tissue. Fixed tissue is dead so it does not bleed or sense pain.

FLAGELLATE. A microorganism that uses flagella (hair-like projections) to move.

FLAIL CHEST. Occurs when a section of the thoracic wall such as the rib cage separates from the rest of the chest wall.

FLAP. A section of tissue moved from one area of the body to another.

FLIGHT OF IDEAS. A psychiatric term describing a thought disorder where streams of unrelated words or ideas enter a patient's mind too quickly to be properly vocalized despite the rushed and rapid rate of the patient's speech.

FLOATERS. Spots in the field of vision.

FLORA. Refers to normal bacteria found in a healthy person.

FLOW METER. Device for measuring the rate of a gas (especially oxygen) or liquid.

Glossary

FLUORESCEIN DYE. An orange dye used to illuminate the blood vessels of the retina in fluorescein angiography.

FLUOROSCOPE. An imaging device used to display real-time x-rays of the body.

FLUOROSCOPY. A diagnostic imaging procedure that uses x-rays and contrast agents to visualize anatomy and motion in real time.

FOLEY CATHETER. A thin tube that is inserted into the urethra (the tube that runs from the bladder to the outside of the body) to allow the drainage of urine.

FOLIC ACID. A water-soluble vitamin belonging to the B-complex group of vitamins.

FOOTPLATE. A flat oval plate of bone that fits into the oval window on the wall of the inner ear; the base of the stapes.

FORAMEN (PLURAL, FORAMINA). The medical term for a natural opening or passage. The foramina of the spinal column are openings between the vertebrae for the spinal nerves to branch off from the spinal cord.

FORAMINOTOMY. Surgery to take pressure off nerves in a foramen; often combined with disk removal.

FORCED EXPIRATORY VOLUME (FEV). The maximum volume of air expelled during a set time (usually 0.5, 1, 2, and 3 seconds).

FORCED VITAL CAPACITY (FVC). A measurement of the volume of air that a patient can exhale from the lungs after taking a deep breath. To measure the FVC, the patient is asked to take the deepest breath they can and then exhale into a sensor as hard as possible for as long as possible.

FORCEPS. An instrument for grasping, holding firmly, or exerting traction upon objects.

FORENSIC. Referring to the application of scientific methods in matters related to civil or criminal law.

FORESKIN. A covering fold of skin over the tip of the penis.

FORMALIN. A clear solution of diluted formaldehyde that is used to preserve biopsy specimens until they can be examined in the laboratory.

FRACTIONATED RADIOSURGERY. Radiosurgery in which the radiation is delivered in several smaller doses over a period of time rather than the full amount in a single treatment.

FRACTIONATION. The process of separating the various components of whole blood.

FREE FLAP. A section of tissue is detached from its blood supply, moved to another part of the body, and reattached by microsurgery to a new blood supply.

FREE FLAP FACIAL SURGERY. Facial reconstruction using skin obtained from another part of the patient's body.

FREQUENCY. Sound, whether traveling through air or the human body, produces vibrations—molecules bouncing into each other—as the shock wave travels along. The frequency of a sound is the number of vibrations per second. Within the audible range, frequency means pitch: the higher the frequency, the higher a sound's pitch.

FRONTAL BONE. The part of the skull that lies behind the forehead.

FRONTAL LOBE EPILEPSY (FLE). The second most common type of epilepsy, characterized by brief, recurring seizures, often while an individual is sleeping.

FUCHS' DYSTROPHY. A hereditary disease of the inner layer of the cornea.

FUNCTIONAL RESERVE. The degree to which a vital organ can tolerate a workload higher than its usual level.

FUNCTIONAL RESIDUAL CAPACITY (FRC). The volume of air left in the lungs at the end of passive expiration (breathing out).

FUNDOPLICATION. Surgery in which the upper portion of the stomach is wrapped around the lower portion of the esophagus and sutured in place to prevent gastroesophageal reflux. Developed by the Swiss surgeon Rudolph Nissen, it is also referred to as Nissen fundoplication.

FUNGAL. Caused by a fungus, a member of a group of simple organisms that are related to yeast and molds.

FUSION. A union or joining together of materials.

G

GADOLINIUM. A very rare metallic element useful for its sensitivity to electromagnetic resonance, among other things. Traces of it can be injected into the body to enhance magnetic resonance imaging (MRI) scans.

GAIT. A person's habitual manner or style of walking.

GALLBLADDER. The sac that stores bile from the liver.

GAMETE INTRAFALLOPIAN TUBE TRANSFER (GIFT). An assisted reproductive technique where eggs are taken from a woman's ovaries, mixed with sperm, and then deposited into the woman's fallopian tube.

GAMMA CAMERA. A camera used to photograph internal organs after the patient has been injected with a radioactive material.

GAMMA RAYS. Extremely short-wavelength electromagnetic radiation released during the process of radioactive decay.

GANGLION. A knot or knot-like mass; it can refer either to groups of nerve cells outside the central nervous system or to cysts that form on the sheath of a tendon.

GANGLIONECTOMY. Surgery to excise a ganglion cyst.

GANGRENE. The death of tissue, usually associated with loss of blood supply and followed by bacterial infection.

GANGRENOUS. Referring to tissue that is dead.

GANTRY. A name for the portion of a computed tomography (CT) scanner that houses the x-ray tube and detector array used to capture image information and send it to the computer.

GAS CHROMATOGRAPHY. A method for separating the various chemicals in a test sample by vaporizing a portion of a sample, mixing it with a carrier gas (usually nitrogen), and passing the mixture through a long column of adsorbent material. The different chemicals in the sample will pass through the column at different rates of speed and can then be identified.

GAS GANGRENE. A severe form of gangrene caused by *Clostridium* infection.

GASTRECTOMY. A surgical procedure in which all or a portion of the stomach is removed.

GASTRIC (OR PEPTIC) ULCER. An ulcer (sore or hole) in the stomach lining, duodenum, or other part of the gastrointestinal system.

GASTRIC ANTRAL VASCULAR ECTASIA (GAVE). A type of arteriovenous malformation (AVM) that develops in the antrum. The dilated blood vessels in the AVM resemble the stripes of a watermelon, so GAVE is also referred to as watermelon stomach.

GASTRIC GLANDS. Branched tubular glands located in the stomach.

GASTRIC PACING. An experimental form of obesity surgery in which electrodes are implanted in the muscle of the stomach wall. Electrical stimulation paces the timing of stomach contractions so that the patient feels full on less food.

GASTRIC ULCER. An ulcer of the stomach, duodenum, or other part of the gastrointestinal system; also called a peptic ulcer.

GASTRIN. A hormone produced by cells in the antrum of the stomach that stimulates the production of gastric acid.

GASTRODUODENOSTOMY. A surgical procedure that creates a new connection between the stomach and the duodenum (upper portion of the small intestine).

GASTROENTEROLOGIST. A physician who specializes in digestive disorders and diseases of the organs of the digestive tract, including the esophagus, stomach, and intestines.

GASTROENTEROLOGY. The branch of medicine that specializes in the diagnosis and treatment of disorders affecting the stomach and intestines.

GASTROESOPHAGEAL REFLUX DISEASE (GERD). A condition in which the contents of the stomach flow backward into the esophagus.

GASTROINTESTINAL (GI). Pertaining to the digestive tract.

GASTROINTESTINAL DISEASES. Diseases that affect the digestive system.

GASTROINTESTINAL TRACT. A group of organs and related structures that includes the esophagus, stomach, liver, gallbladder, pancreas, small intestine, large intestine, rectum, and anus.

GASTROINTESTINAL TUBE. A tube surgically inserted into the stomach for feeding a patient who is unable to eat by mouth.

GASTROJEJUNOSTOMY. A surgical procedure in which the stomach is surgically connected to the jejunum (middle portion of the small intestine).

GASTROPARESIS. Partial paralysis of the stomach, as can occur after a Whipple procedure.

GASTROSCHISIS. A defect of the abdominal wall caused by rupture of the amniotic membrane or by the delayed closure of the umbilical ring. It is usually accompanied by the protrusion of internal organs in the abdomen.

GBS. Group B streptococci.

GENDER IDENTITY DISORDER (GID). A condition in which a person strongly identifies with the opposite sex and feels uncomfortable with his or her biological sex.

GENDER REASSIGNMENT SURGERY. The surgical alteration and reconstruction of a person's sex organs to resemble those of the other sex as closely as possible; it is sometimes called sex reassignment surgery.

GENE. A piece of DNA, located on a chromosome, that determines how traits such as blood type are inherited and expressed.

GENERAL ANESTHESIA. Method used to sedate a patient and stop pain from being felt during an operation. General anesthesia is generally used only for major operations such as brain, neck, chest, abdomen, and pelvis surgery.

GENERAL SURGERY. General surgery includes procedures on the abdominal cavity organs and other body areas such as the breast and thyroid. It also includes procedures on various other body regions that may be associated with multiple specialties.

GENERALIZED INFECTION. An infection that has entered the bloodstream and has general systemic symptoms such as fever, chills, and low blood pressure.

GENETIC. Referring to genes.

GENIOPLASTY. Another word for mentoplasty, or chin augmentation surgery.

GENITAL. Sexual organ.

GENITOURINARY RECONSTRUCTION. Surgery that corrects defects of the genitals and urinary tract, including the kidneys, ureters, bladder, urethra, and the male and female genitals.

GENTIAN VIOLET. An antibacterial, antifungal dye that is commonly applied to the skin during dermabrasion.

GENUINE STRESS INCONTINENCE (GSI). A specific term for a type of incontinence that has to do with the instability of the urethra due to weakened support muscles.

GERIATRICIAN. A physician who specializes in the health care of the elderly. Geriatrics is considered a subspecialty of internal medicine and family practice.

GERMINOMA. A tumor of germ cells (ovum and sperm cells that participate in production of the developing embryo).

GESTATIONAL AGE. The length of time of growth and development of the young in the mother's womb.

GESTATIONAL DIABETES. A type of diabetes that occurs during pregnancy. Untreated, it can cause severe complications for the mother and the baby. However, it usually does not lead to long-term diabetes in either the mother or the child.

GIGANTISM. A condition in which an individual grows to an abnormally large size. Mental development may or may not be affected.

GINGIVITIS. Inflammation of the gingiva or gums caused by bacterial buildup in plague on the teeth.

GLANS. The cap-shaped structure at the end of the penis.

GLAUCOMA. Eye disease characterized by increased pressure within the eye, which can damage eye tissue and structures and, if untreated, result in blindness.

GLENOHUMERAL JOINT. A ball-and-socket synovial joint between the head of the humerus and the glenoid cavity of the scapula; also called the glenohumeral articulation or shoulder joint.

GLENOID CAVITY. The hollow cavity in the head of the shoulder blade that receives the head of the humerus to make the glenohumeral or shoulder joint.

GLOBIN. The protein component of hemoglobin. Newer fecal occult blood tests screen for the presence of globin in the stool rather than heme.

GLOMERULONEPHRITIS. A disease of the kidney that causes inflammation and scarring and impairs the kidney's ability to filter waste products from the blood.

GLOTTIS. The vocal part of the larynx, consisting of the vocal cords and the opening between them.

GLUCAGON. A hormone produced in the pancreas that is responsible for elevating blood glucose when it falls below a safe level for the body's organs and tissues.

GLUCOSE. A simple sugar that is the product of carbohydrate metabolism. It is the major source of energy for all of the organs and tissues of the body.

GLUCOSE-6-PHOSPHATE DEHYDROGENASE (G6PD) DEFICIENCY. An inherited disorder in which the body lacks an enzyme that normally protects red blood cells from toxic chemicals. Certain drugs or infections can cause patients' red blood cells to break down, resulting in anemia.

GLYCATED HEMOGLOBIN. A test that measures the amount of hemoglobin bound to glucose. It is a measure of how much glucose has been in the blood during a two to three month period beginning approximately one month prior to sample collection.

GLYCOGEN. The form in which glucose is stored in the body.

GLYCOPROTEIN. Any of a group of complex proteins that consist of a carbohydrate combined with a simple protein. Some tumor markers are glycoproteins.

GLYCYLCYCLINES. A subgroup of tetracyclines derived from minocycline, a semi-synthetic tetracycline.

GOITER. Chronic enlargement of the thyroid gland.

GONADOTROPINS. Hormones that stimulate the activity of the ovaries in females and testes in males.

GONIOSCOPY. A technique for examining the angle between the iris and the cornea with the use of a special mirrored lens applied to the cornea.

GONORRHEA. A sexually transmitted disease (STD) that causes infection in the genital organs and may cause disease in other parts of the body.

GRAFT. Replacement of a diseased or damaged part of the body with a compatible substitute that can be artificial (metal or other substance) or taken from the body itself, such as a piece of skin, healthy tissue, or bone.

GRAFT VERSUS HOST DISEASE. A life-threatening complication of bone marrow transplants in which the donated marrow causes an immune reaction against the recipient's body.

GRAM STAINING. Use of a purple dye to identify pathogens, usually bacteria.

GRANULE. A small grain or pellet. Medicines that come in granule form are usually mixed with liquids or sprinkled on food before they are taken.

GRANULOCYTES. White blood cells.

GRAVEL. The debris that is formed from a fragmented kidney stone.

GRAVES' DISEASE. The most common form of hyperthyroidism, characterized by bulging eyes, rapid heart rate, and other symptoms.

GROUP B STREPTOCOCCI. A type of bacteria that, if passed to an infant, can affect the brain, spinal cord, blood, or lungs. In some cases, it can result in infant death.

GUAIAC. A compound derived from the wood resin of guaiacum trees. Guaiac reacts with blood in the stool to produce a blue-colored reaction when peroxide is added to the sample.

GUGLIELMI DETACHABLE COIL (GDC). A platinum or titanium coil inserted to repair a cerebral aneurysm.

GUIDE WIRE. A wire that is inserted into an artery to guide a catheter to a certain location in the body.

GUIDED IMAGERY. A form of focused relaxation that coaches patients to visualize calm, peaceful images.

GUILLAIN-BARRÉ SYNDROME. A demyelinating disease involving nerves that affect the extremities, resulting in weakness and motor and sensory dysfunction.

GUILLOTINE AMPUTATION. An amputation in which the severed part is cut off cleanly by a blade or other sharp-edged object.

GUTTA-PERCHA. An inert, latex-like substance used for filling root canals.

GYNECOLOGIC SURGERY. Surgery on the female reproductive system.

GYNECOMASTIA. Overly developed or enlarged breasts in a male.

H

HAIR CELLS. Sensory receptors in the inner ear that transform sound vibrations into messages that travel to the brain.

HAIR FOLLICLE. A tube-like indentation in the skin from which a single hair grows.

HALLUCINATION. The perception of a person, object, event, or sensory stimulus that is not truly there. Hallucinations can be visual (seen), auditory (heard), olfactory (smelled), tactile (felt), gustatory (tasted), or a combination thereof.

HARMONIC SCALPEL. A scalpel that uses ultrasound technology to seal tissues while it is cutting.

HARVESTING. The process of removing tissues or organs from a donor and preserving them for transplantation.

HEAD-UPRIGHT TILT TABLE TEST. A test used to determine the cause of fainting spells. The patient is tilted at different angles on a special table for a period of time while heart rhythm, blood pressure, and other measurements are evaluated.

HEALTH CARE AGENT. A person who has the power of attorney to carry out a patient's wishes if the patient becomes incapacitated; also known as a surrogate or patient representative.

HEALTH INSURANCE PORTABILITY AND ACCOUNTABILITY ACT (HIPAA). A 1996 U.S. federal law that governs the privacy and security of personal health information.

HEALTH MAINTENANCE ORGANIZATION (HMO). A comprehensive private insurance plan that provides primary care physicians who control referrals to specialists and other services within the HMO's network.

HEALTHCARE PROXY. Healthcare power of attorney; a document that appoints a particular person to make medical decisions in the event that the person designating the proxy becomes incapable of expressing his or her own preferences.

HEALTHCARE-ACQUIRED INFECTION (HAI). An infection acquired in a hospital or other healthcare setting while receiving treatment for another condition; also referred to as a healthcare-associated infection or hospital-acquired infection.

HEART MONITOR LEADS. Sticky pads placed on the chest to monitor the electrical activity of the heart. The pads are connected to an electrocardiogram machine.

HEART VALVE REPLACEMENT SURGERY. Surgery performed to repair or replace the valves in the heart that control blood flow through the heart and are responsible for the audible heartbeat.

HEARTBURN. A sensation of warmth or burning behind the breastbone, rising upward toward the neck. It is often caused by stomach acid flowing backward from the stomach into the esophagus.

HEART-LUNG MACHINE. A machine that temporarily takes over the function of the heart and lungs during surgical procedures in order to maintain blood circulation and delivery of oxygen to body tissues while the heart is being repaired.

HELICAL. Having a spiral shape.

HELICOBACTER PYLORI. A spiral-shaped bacterium that was discovered in 1982 to be the underlying cause of most ulcers in the stomach and duodenum (upper portion of the small intestine).

HEMAGGLUTINATION. The clumping of red blood cells due to blood type incompatibility.

HEMATEMESIS. Vomiting blood.

HEMATOCRIT. The proportion of the volume of a blood sample that consists of red blood cells, expressed as a percentage.

HEMATOLOGIST. A specialist who treats diseases and disorders of the blood and blood-forming organs.

HEMATOMA. An accumulation of blood, often clotted, in a body tissue or organ, usually caused by a break or tear in a blood vessel.

HEME. The iron-containing pigment found in hemoglobin.

HEMIFACIAL MICROSOMIA (HFM). A term used to describe a group of complex birth defects characterized by underdevelopment of one side of the face.

HEMOCHROMATOSIS. A disorder of iron absorption characterized by bronze-colored skin. It can cause painful joints, diabetes, and liver damage if the iron concentration is not lowered.

HEMODIALYSIS. The process of removing blood from a kidney patient, purifying it by dialysis, and returning it to the body.

HEMODILUTION. A technique in which the fluid content of the blood is increased without increasing the number of red blood cells.

HEMODYNAMIC. Relating to the flow of blood through the circulatory system.

HEMODYNAMICS. Measurement of the movements involved in the circulation of the blood; it usually includes blood pressure and heart rate.

HEMOGLOBIN. The iron-containing protein found in blood that carries oxygen from the lungs to the rest of the body.

HEMOGLOBIN A1C (HBA1C). Glycated hemoglobin; glucose bound to hemoglobin A in the blood, which can be used to determine the average blood glucose levels for the previous two to three months.

HEMOLYSIS. Separation of hemoglobin from the red blood cells.

HEMOPTYSIS. The spitting up of blood or of blood-containing sputum.

HEMORRHAGE. Heavy bleeding.

HEMORRHAGIC SHOCK. Shock resulting from loss of blood.

HEMORRHAGIC STROKE. A disruption of the blood supply to the brain caused by bleeding into the brain.

HEMOSIDERIN. A form of iron that is stored inside tissue cells.

HEMOSIDEROSIS. An overload of iron in the body resulting from repeated blood transfusions.

HEMOSTASIS. Slowing down or stopping bleeding.

HEMOSTAT. A small surgical clamp used to hold a blood vessel closed.

HEMOSTATIC. Relating to blood clotting and coagulation.

HEMOTHORAX. A condition in which blood accumulates in the pleural cavity, commonly as a result of traumatic injury.

HEPARIN. A medication that prevents blood clots.

HEPATIC ARTERY. The blood vessel supplying arterial blood to the liver.

HEPATIC DUCT. A duct that carries bile from the liver.

HEPATITIS. Disease characterized by inflammation of the liver.

HEPATOCELLULAR CARCINOMA. The most common type of liver tumor.

HEPATOCYTES. Liver cells.

HEPATOMA. A liver tumor.

HEREDITARY. Something that is inherited or passed down from parents to offspring. In biology and medicine, the word pertains to inherited genetic characteristics.

HEREDITARY SPHEROCYTOSIS. A hereditary disorder that leads to a chronic form of anemia (too few red blood cells) due to an abnormality in the red blood cell membrane.

HERNIA. The protrusion of a loop or section of an organ or tissue through an abnormal opening.

HERNIATED DISK. A blister-like bulging or protrusion of the contents of an intervertebral disk; also called a prolapsed, slipped, displaced, or ruptured disk.

HERNIORRHAPHY. The surgical repair of any type of hernia.

HETEROTOPIC BONE. Bone that develops as an excess growth around a joint following surgery.

HETEROTROPHIC TRANSPLANTATION. The addition of a donor liver at another site, while the diseased liver is left intact.

HIATAL HERNIA. A condition in which part of the stomach pushes up through the diaphragm.

HIGH TIBIAL OSTEOTOMY (HTO). Surgical procedure in which the tibial bone is cut to redistribute weight on the knee for varus alignment deformities or injuries.

HIP DYSPLASIA. Abnormal development of the hip joint.

HIRSUTISM. Excessive or increased growth of facial or body hair in women resembling the male pattern of hair distribution.

HISTAMINE. A chemical released by mast cells that activates pain receptors and causes cells to become leaky.

HISTOCOMPATIBILITY ANTIGENS. Proteins scattered throughout body tissues that are unique for almost every individual.

HISTOCOMPATIBILITY TESTING. Testing of genotypes of a recipient and potential donor to determine the risk of rejection prior to organ or bone marrow transplantation.

HIV INFECTION. Human immunodeficiency virus; an infectious disease that impairs the immune system. If left untreated, it progresses to acquired immune deficiency syndrome (AIDS).

HODGKIN'S DISEASE. A type of cancer involving the lymph nodes and potentially affecting non-lymphatic organs in the later stage.

HOLISTIC. Pertaining to all aspects of the patient, including biological, psychosocial, and cultural factors.

HOLTER MONITOR. A small machine worn by a patient, usually for 24 hours, that continuously records the electrical activity of the patient's heart.

HOME HEALTH AIDE. An employee of a home care agency who provides the same services to a patient in the home as nurses aides perform in hospitals and nursing homes.

HOMEOPATHY. A system of alternative medicine that arose in Germany in the late eighteenth century that emphasizes treating the symptoms of a given disease with highly diluted remedies made from substances that cause the symptoms of the disease in healthy people.

HOMEOSTASIS. The process of maintaining balance in the normal vital life functions of a living organism.

HOMOCYSTEINE. An amino acid normally found in small amounts in the blood.

HOODIA. A succulent African plant resembling a cactus said to contain a natural appetite suppressant.

HORMONE. A chemical messenger produced by the body that is involved in regulating specific bodily functions such as growth, development, reproduction, metabolism, and mood.

HOSPICE. An approach for providing compassionate, palliative care to terminally ill patients and counseling or assistance for their families. The term may also refer to a hospital unit or freestanding facility devoted to the care of terminally ill patients.

HOSPITAL-ACQUIRED INFECTION (HAI). Also referred to as a healthcare-associated infection or nosocomial infection; an infection that is contracted while in the hospital.

HOSPITAL-ACQUIRED PNEUMONIA (HAP). Pneumonia acquired while in the hospital.

HOST. A living organism that harbors or potentially harbors infection.

HUMAN CHORIONIC GONADOTROPIN (HCG). A hormone produced by the placenta during pregnancy; used to detect pregnancy.

HUMAN IMMUNODEFICIENCY VIRUS (HIV). A transmissible retrovirus that causes AIDS in humans. Two forms of HIV are now recognized: HIV-1, which causes most cases of AIDS in Europe, North and South America, and most parts of Africa; and HIV-2, which is chiefly found in West African patients. HIV-2, discovered in 1986, appears to be less virulent than HIV-1, but may also have a longer latency period.

HUMAN IMMUNODEFICIENCY VIRUS (HIV) GROUPS. HIV classification has evolved into several groups; specific lineages are now termed as groups M, N, O, and P. M is considered the pandemic strain and comprises the vast majority of strains of HIV. Viruses from the M group are further divided into subtypes, of which there are currently 10 identified (A to J). Subtypes are also known as clades; the most common clade in the United States and Europe is HIV clade B, and HIV testing was originally developed to identify HIV clade B.

HUMAN LEUKOCYTE ANTIGEN (HLA). The major histocompatibility complex that is used to match donor organs with transplant recipients.

HUMAN PAPILLOMAVIRUS (HPV). A family of viruses that causes common warts of the hands and feet, as well as lesions in the genital and vaginal area. More than 50 types of HPV have been identified, some of which are linked to cancerous and precancerous conditions.

HUMERUS. The long bone of the upper arm that runs from the shoulder blade to the elbow joint.

HYDRAMNIOS. The excessive production of amniotic fluid due to either fetal or maternal conditions.

HYDROCELE. An accumulation of fluid in the membrane that surrounds the testes.

HYDROCEPHALUS. Abnormal accumulation of cerebrospinal fluid within the cavities inside the brain.

HYDROGEL. A gel that contains water, used as a dressing after laser skin resurfacing.

HYDROGEN. The simplest, most common element known in the universe. It is composed of a single electron (negatively charged particle) circling a nucleus consisting of a single proton (positively charged particle).

HYDROGEN IONS. Ions that contain one hydrogen atom with a positive charge.

HYDRONEPHROSIS. Severe swelling of the kidney due to backup of urine. It may occur because of an obstruction, calculi, tumor, or other pathological condition.

HYDROSALPINX. A condition in which a fallopian tube becomes blocked and filled with fluid.

HYDROXIDE IONS. Ions that contain one oxygen and one hydrogen atom, with a negative charge.

HYDROXYAPATITE. A calcium phosphate complex that is the primary mineral component of bone.

HYPERALDOSTERONISM. A disorder characterized by excessive secretion of the hormone aldosterone.

HYPERBARIC OXYGEN THERAPY (HBOT). Treatment in which a pressure chamber is used to deliver 100% oxygen to the patient at a level higher than atmospheric pressure.

HYPERCALCEMIA. Abnormally high levels of calcium in the blood.

HYPERCARBIA. An excess of carbon dioxide in the blood.

HYPERCHLOREMIA. Elevated serum (blood) chloride levels.

HYPERGLYCEMIA. Abnormally high blood glucose levels.

HYPERHIDROSIS. Excessive sweating. Hyperhidrosis can be caused by heat, overactive thyroid glands, strong emotion, menopause, or infection.

HYPERKALEMIA. An abnormally high concentration of potassium in the blood.

HYPERMOBILE URETHRA. A term that denotes the movement of the urethra that allows for leakage or spillage of urine.

HYPERNATREMIA. Elevated blood sodium levels.

HYPEROPIA. The inability to see near objects as clearly as distant objects; also known as farsightedness.

HYPEROSMOTIC. Hypertonic; containing a higher concentration of salts or other dissolved materials than normal tissues.

HYPEROSMOTIC AGENTS. Substances that cause abnormally rapid osmosis.

HYPERPARATHYROIDISM. Abnormal over-functioning of the parathyroid glands.

HYPERPHOSPHATEMIA. Elevated blood phosphate levels.

HYPERPIGMENTATION. Excessive pigmentation or color on part of the skin.

HYPERREFLEXIA. A condition in which the detrusor muscle of the bladder contracts too frequently, leading to an inability to hold urine.

HYPERRESONANCE ON PERCUSSION. Occurrence of a highly resonating sound when the physician taps gently on a patient's back; this is not a normal finding and should be investigated with an x-ray.

HYPERTENSION. High blood pressure.

HYPERTHYROIDISM. Disease of the thyroid gland involving overproduction of thyroid hormones.

HYPERTROPHY. The overgrowth of muscle.

HYPERVENTILATION. The act of breathing more rapidly or more deeply than normal, resulting in a lowered level of carbon dioxide in the blood, a raised pH level, and the risk of respiratory alkalosis.

HYPHEMA. Bleeding inside the anterior chamber of the eye.

HYPNOSIS. A specific verbal technique for refocusing a person's attention in order to change their perceptions, judgment, control of movements, and memory. A hypnotic medication is one that induces sleep.

HYPOALBUMINEMIA. An abnormally low concentration of albumin in the blood.

HYPOCALCEMIA. An abnormally low concentration of calcium in the blood.

HYPOCHLOREMIA. Low serum chloride levels.

HYPOCHROMIC. A descriptive term applied to a red blood cell with a decreased concentration of hemoglobin.

HYPODERMIC. Applied or administered beneath the skin. The modern hypodermic needle was invented to deliver medications below the skin surface.

HYPODERMOCLYSIS. A technique for restoring the body's fluid balance by injecting a solution of salt and water into the tissues beneath the skin rather than directly into a vein.

HYPOGLYCEMIA. Abnormally low blood glucose levels.

HYPOKALEMIA. An abnormally low concentration of potassium in the blood.

HYPONATREMIA. Low blood sodium levels.

HYPOPARATHYROIDISM. Insufficient production of parathyroid hormone (PTH) by the parathyroid glands.

HYPOPHARYNX. The last part of the throat or the pharynx.

HYPOPHOSPHATEMIA. Low blood phosphate levels.

HYPOPIGMENTATION. Decreased pigmentation or color on a portion of the skin.

HYPOPITUITARISM. A medical condition where the pituitary gland produces lower than normal levels of its hormones.

HYPOSPADIAS. A congenital deformity of the penis where the urinary tract opening is not at the tip of the glans.

HYPOTENSION. Low blood pressure. Hypotension is sometimes caused deliberately during surgery to decrease blood loss.

HYPOTHERMIA. Abnormally low body temperature, typically 95°F (35°C) or less.

HYPOTHYROIDISM. Disease of the thyroid gland involving underproduction of thyroid hormones.

HYPOTONY. Intraocular fluid pressure that is too low.

HYPOVOLEMIA. An abnormally low amount of blood in the body.

HYPOVOLEMIC SHOCK. Shock caused by a lack of circulating blood.

HYPOXEMIA. Oxygen deficiency, defined as an oxygen level less than 60 mm Hg (millimeters of mercury) or arterial oxygen saturation of less than 90%. Different values are used for infants and for patients with certain lung diseases.

HYPOXIA. A decreased amount of oxygen in the tissues.

HYSTERECTOMY. The surgical removal of the uterus.

HYSTEROSALPINGOGRAPHY (HSG). X-raying of the uterus and fallopian tubes following the injection of a contrast dye.

HYSTEROSCOPE. A specialized endoscope used to examine the uterus.

HYSTEROSCOPY. A procedure in which an endoscope is inserted through the cervix to view the cervix and uterus.

HYSTEROSONOGRAPHY. The use of a thin catheter to inject sterile saline into a woman's uterus to allow examination of the interior of the uterus with an ultrasound probe. It is a less invasive technique than hysteroscopy.

HYSTEROTOMY. A surgical incision of the uterus.

I

IATROGENIC. Resulting from the activity of the physician.

ICU (INTENSIVE CARE UNIT) PSYCHOSIS. Psychosis that develops from being confined in a hospital intensive care unit, possibly on mechanical ventilation.

IDIOPATHIC. Having an unknown cause or arising spontaneously.

IDIOPATHIC THROMBOCYTOPENIA PURPURA (ITP). A rare autoimmune disorder characterized by an acute shortage of platelets with resultant bruising and spontaneous bleeding.

ILEECTOMY. Excision (removal) of the ileum.

ILEOANAL RESERVOIR. A colon-like pouch created from the last few inches of the ileum to collect stool and allow for normal bowel movements after removal of the large intestine; also known as ileoanal anastomosis or ileoanal pull through.

ILEOSTOMY. Surgical connection of the ileum to an opening in the abdominal wall to create an artificial anus.

ILEUM. The final section of the small intestine before it joins the large intestine. The ileum in humans is between 6 and 12 feet long.

ILEUS. Obstruction in or immobility of the intestines. Symptoms include nausea and vomiting, absent bowel sounds, abdominal pain, and abdominal distension.

ILIAC ARTERY. Large blood vessel in the pelvis that leads into the leg.

ILIZAROV METHOD. A bone-fixation technique using an external fixator for lengthening limbs, correcting deformities, and assisting in the healing of fractures and infections. The method was designed by the Russian orthopedic surgeon Gavriil Abramovich Ilizarov (1921–1992).

IMMUNE RESPONSE. The body's natural defense against disease and infection.

IMMUNE SYSTEM. The network of organs, tissues, and cells that protects the body against foreign invaders, such as bacteria, viruses, and fungi.

IMMUNOASSAY. A laboratory method for detecting the presence of a substance by using an antibody that reacts with it.

IMMUNOCOMPROMISED. Lacking or deficient in defenses provided by the immune system, usually due to a disease or as a side effect of treatment.

IMMUNODEFICIENCY. A disorder in which the immune system is ineffective or disabled due either to acquired or inherited disease.

IMMUNOFLUORESCENCE ASSAY (IFA). A blood test sometimes used to confirm enzyme-linked immunosorbent assay (ELISA) results instead of using Western blotting. In an IFA test, HIV antigen is mixed with a fluorescent compound and then with a sample of the patient's blood. If HIV antibody is present, the mixture will fluoresce when examined under ultraviolet light.

IMMUNOGLOBULIN. An antibody.

IMMUNOGLOBULIN E (IGE). A type of protein in blood plasma that acts as an antibody to activate allergic reactions. About 50% of patients with allergic disorders have increased IgE levels in their blood serum.

IMMUNOSUPPRESSED. The impaired or nonfunctioning state of the immune system.

IMMUNOSUPPRESSION. A condition where the immune response is reduced or absent; may be caused by disease or by certain medications.

IMMUNOSUPPRESSIVE. Relating to the weakening or reducing of the immune system's responses to foreign material.

IMMUNOSUPPRESSIVE DRUGS. Medications that suppress the immune system to prevent rejection of transplanted tissue.

IMMUNOTHERAPY. A method of treating allergies in which small doses of substances that a person is allergic to are injected under the skin.

IMPACTED TOOTH. A tooth that is growing against another tooth, bone, or soft tissue.

IMPACTION GRAFTING. The use of crushed bone from a donor to fill in the central canal of the femur during joint revision surgery.

IMPLANT. In dentistry, a metal (usually titanium) screw placed within the bone of the upper or lower jaw that supports a prosthetic tooth or group of teeth.

IMPLANTABLE CARDIOVERTER-DEFIBRILLATOR (ICD). An electronic device that is surgically placed to constantly monitor the patient's heart rate and rhythm. If a very fast abnormal heart rate is detected, the device delivers electrical energy to the heart to beat in a normal rhythm again.

IN VITRO FERTILIZATION (IVF). An assisted reproductive technology in which sperm are incubated with a female egg under carefully controlled conditions, then transferred to the female uterus once fertilization has occurred.

INCARCERATED HERNIA. An inguinal hernia that is trapped in place and cannot slip back into the abdominal cavity, often causing intestinal obstruction.

INCARCERATED INTESTINE. Intestines trapped in the weakened area of a hernia that cannot slip back into the abdominal cavity.

INCARCERATION. The abnormal confinement of a section of the intestine or other body tissues. Hernia may lead to incarceration of part of the intestine.

INCENTIVE SPIROMETER. Device that is used postoperatively to prevent lung collapse and promote maximum inspiration. The patient inhales until a preset volume is reached, then sustains the volume by holding his or her breath for three to five seconds.

INCISION. A cut, usually referring to the cut made by a surgeon during a surgical procedure.

INCISIONAL BIOPSY. A procedure in which a surgeon cuts out a sample of a lump or suspicious area for further examination.

INCISIONAL HERNIA. Hernia occurring at the site of a prior surgery.

INCOMPETENT. Insufficient.

INCONTINENCE. The inability to control defecation (fecal incontinence) or urination (urinary incontinence).

INCUS. The middle of the three bones of the middle ear, also known as the anvil.

INDEMNITY. Protection, as by insurance, against damage or loss.

INDEPENDENT PRACTICE ASSOCIATION (IPA). A managed care plan that contracts with private physicians to treat plan participants.

INDICATED TEST. A test that is given for a specific clinical reason.

INDIRECT COOMBS' TEST. A test used to screen for unexpected antibodies against red blood cells. The patient's serum is mixed with reagent red blood cells, incubated, washed, tested with antihuman globulin, and observed for clumping.

INERT. Amount of tissue reaction.

INFARCTION. Tissue death resulting from a lack of oxygen to the area.

INFECTION CALCULI. Another name for struvite calculi.

INFECTIOUS DISEASE TEAM. A team of physicians who help control the hospital environment to protect patients against harmful sources of infection.

INFERIOR TURBINATE. Bony projections on each side of the nose.

INFERIOR VENA CAVA. The biggest vein in the body, returning blood to the heart from the lower half of the body.

INFERIOR VENA CAVA FILTER. A device implanted in the inferior vena cava—the largest vein in the body—to prevent clots or clot fragments from reaching the heart or lungs.

INFERTILITY. The inability to become pregnant or carry a pregnancy to term.

INFLAMMATION. A condition characterized by pain, redness, swelling, and warmth, often in response to an injury or infection.

INFLAMMATORY ARTHRITIS. An inflammatory condition that affects joints.

INFLAMMATORY BOWEL DISEASE (IBD). A chronic condition characterized by periods of diarrhea, bloating, abdominal cramps, and pain, sometimes accompanied by weight loss and malnutrition because of the inability to absorb nutrients. Crohn's disease and ulcerative colitis are the two types of IBD.

INFORMED. From full knowledge; not coerced.

INFORMED CONSENT. Patient consent to undergo a medical treatment or procedure after being informed of the details of the procedure and the potential risks and benefits.

INFRARED. A type of energy wave given off as heat.

INFUSION. Introduction of a substance directly into a vein or tissue by gravity flow.

INGUINAL. Referring to the groin area.

INGUINAL HERNIA. A weak spot in the lower abdominal muscles of the groin through which body organs, usually the large intestine, can push through as a result of abdominal pressure.

INHALATION CHALLENGE TEST. A test given to diagnose asthma by asking the patient to breathe cold air, methacholine, histamine, or another airway irritant and measuring the decline (if any) in the forced expiratory volume (FEV1).

INJECTION. Forcing a fluid into the body with a needle and syringe.

INJECTION SNOREPLASTY. A technique for reducing snoring by injecting a chemical that forms scar tissue near the base of the uvula, helping to anchor it and reduce its fluttering or vibrating during sleep.

INNATE IMMUNE SYSTEM. The part of the immune system that responds to infectious organisms in a nonspecific manner.

INNER EAR. The interior section of the ear, where sound vibrations and information about balance are translated into nerve impulses.

INNERVATE. To carry nerve impulses to a particular body part.

INPATIENT. A patient that has been admitted to the hospital.

INPATIENT SURGERY. Surgery that requires an overnight stay of one or more days in the hospital.

INSIDIOUS. Developing in a stealthy and inconspicuous way.

INSPECTION. The visual examination of the body using the eyes and a lighted instrument if needed. The sense of smell may also be used.

INSPIRATION. Inhalation; the flow of air taken into an organism through breathing.

INSTRUMENTAL ACTIVITIES OF DAILY LIVING (IADLS). Daily tasks that enable a person to live independently.

INSTRUMENTS. In medicine, tools or devices that perform such functions as cutting, dissecting, grasping, holding, retracting, or suturing.

INSUFFLATION. Inflation of the abdominal cavity using carbon dioxide, performed prior to laparoscopic procedures to give the surgeon space to maneuver surgical equipment; alternately, blowing air into the ear as a test for the presence of fluid in the middle ear.

INSULIN. A protein hormone synthesized in the pancreas that is required for the metabolism of carbohydrates, lipids, and proteins, and that regulates blood sugar levels.

INSULINOMA. A tumor within the pancreas that produces insulin, potentially causing the serum glucose level to drop to dangerously low levels.

INTEGRATED DELIVERY SYSTEM (IDS). An organization that provides a continuum of healthcare services. Some IDSs include a health maintenance organization (HMO), while others are a network of physicians and hospitals or of physicians only.

INTEGRATIVE MEDICINE. An approach to medicine that combines appropriate mainstream and alternative therapies, neither rejecting mainstream medicine nor accepting alternative treatments uncritically.

INTEGUMENT. A covering; in medicine, the skin as a covering for the body. The skin is also called the integumentary system.

INTENSIVE CARE UNIT (ICU). A specialized hospital unit for the constant monitoring and support of critically ill patients.

INTENSIVIST. A physician who specializes in caring for patients in intensive care units.

INTERCOSTAL ARTERY. Referring to an artery that runs from the aorta.

INTERLEUKIN. Any of a group of cytokines that were first found to be expressed by white blood cells and that help to regulate the responses of the immune system.

INTERLEUKIN-2 (IL-2). A cytokine derived from T helper lymphocytes that causes proliferation of T lymphocytes and activated B lymphocytes.

INTERMITTENT CATHETERIZATION. Periodic catheterization to facilitate urine flow.

INTERMITTENT CLAUDICATION. Pain that occurs on walking and is relieved on rest.

INTERNATIONAL NORMALIZED RATIO (INR) TEST. A version of the prothrombin time (PT) test (a test that evaluates blood-clotting ability) in which the results are standardized so that results from different laboratories can be understood in the same way. Normal INR results are 0.8–1.1.

INTERNIST. A physician who specializes in internal medicine.

INTERNSHIP. The first year of residency training.

INTERSTITIAL CYSTITIS. A chronic inflammatory condition of the bladder involving bladder pain, frequent urination, and burning during urination.

INTERSTITIAL LUNG DISEASE. A category of lung disease that can lead to breathing or heart failure; injury or foreign substances in the lungs (such as asbestos fibers), infections, cancers, or inherited disorders may cause one of the 180 conditions classified as interstitial lung disease.

INTERSTITIAL RADIATION THERAPY. The process of placing radioactive sources directly into a tumor. These radioactive sources may be temporary (removed after the proper dose is reached) or permanent.

INTERVERTEBRAL DISK. The cylindrical elastic-like gel pad that connects and separates each pair of vertebrae in the spine.

INTESTINAL ILEUS. Mechanical or dynamic obstruction of the bowel causing pain, abdominal distention, vomiting, and often fever.

INTESTINAL PERFORATION. A hole in the intestinal wall.

INTESTINE. Commonly called the bowels, divided into the small and large intestine. They extend from the stomach to the anus. The small intestine is about 20 ft. (6 m) long. The large intestine is about 5 ft. (1.5 m) long.

INTRA-ABDOMINAL PRESSURE. Pressure that occurs within the abdominal cavity.

INTRA-AORTIC BALLOON PUMP. A temporary device inserted into the femoral artery in the leg and guided up to the aorta. The small balloon helps strengthen heart contractions by maintaining improved blood pressure.

INTRACRANIAL. Existing or occurring within the cranium; affecting or involving intracranial structures.

INTRACYTOPLASMIC SPERM INJECTION (ICSI). A fertility procedure in which a single sperm is injected into a female egg.

INTRAOCULAR LENS (IOL) IMPLANT. A small, plastic device (IOL) that is usually implanted in the lens capsule of the eye to correct vision after the lens of the eye is removed. This is the implant used in cataract surgery.

INTRAOCULAR MELANOMA. A rare form of cancer in which malignant cells are found in the part of the eye called the uvea.

INTRAOCULAR PRESSURE (IOP). A measurement of the degree of pressure exerted by the aqueous fluid in the eye.

INTRAOPERATIVE. During surgery.

INTRAORAL. Inside the mouth.

INTRAPERITONEAL FLUID. Liquid that is produced in the abdominal cavity to lubricate tissue surfaces.

INTRAUTERINE DEVICE (IUD). A small flexible device that is inserted into the uterus to prevent pregnancy.

INTRAVENOUS (IV). Into or within a vein.

INTRAVENOUS PYELOGRAM (IVP). An x-ray of the urinary system after injecting a contrast solution that enables the doctor to see images of the kidneys, ureters, and bladder.

INTRAVENOUS SEDATION. A method of injecting a fluid sedative into the blood through the vein.

INTRAVENTRICULAR HEMORRHAGE. Hemorrhage in the ventricles of the brain.

INTRINSIC PATHWAY. One of three pathways in the coagulation cascade (blood-clotting process).

INTRINSIC SPHINCTER DEFICIENCY (ISD). A type of incontinence caused by the inability of the sphincter muscles to keep the bladder closed.

INTUBATION. The insertion of an endotracheal tube to supply oxygen to the lungs and heart.

INTUSSUSCEPTION. The telescoping of one part of the intestine inside an immediately adjoining part.

INVASIVE. Involving entry into the body.

INVASIVE SURGERY. A form of surgery that involves making an incision in the patient's body and inserting instruments or other medical devices into it.

INVASIVENESS. A term that refers to the extent of surgical intrusion into the body or a part of the body. An invasive procedure is one that requires the insertion of a needle, catheter, or surgical instrument.

INVOLUTION. The slow healing and resolution stage of a hemangioma (noncancerous tumor).

IONIZING RADIATION. A type of radiation that can damage living tissue by disrupting and destroying individual cells at the molecular level. All types of nuclear radiation, including x-rays, gamma rays, and beta rays, are potentially ionizing.

IOP. Intraocular pressure.

IRIDECTOMY. Removal of a portion of the iris.

IRIDO CORNEAL ENDOTHELIAL SYNDROME (ICE). A type of glaucoma in which cells from the back of the cornea spread over the surface of the iris and tissue that drains the eye, forming adhesions that bind the iris to the cornea.

IRIDOPLASTY. Surgery to alter the iris.

IRIDOTOMY. A procedure in which a laser is used to make a small hole in the iris to relieve fluid pressure in the eye.

IRIS. Pigmented tissue behind the cornea that gives color to the eye and varies the size of the pupil to control the amount of light entering the eye.

IRON LUNG. A mechanical ventilator that rhythmically oscillates the air pressure in the chamber surrounding the patient's chest to force air in and out of the lungs; previously used for polio patients.

IRON POISONING. A potentially fatal condition caused by swallowing large amounts of iron dietary supplements. Most cases occur in children who have taken adult-strength iron formulas. The symptoms of iron poisoning include vomiting, bloody diarrhea, convulsions, low blood pressure, and turning blue.

ISCHEMIA. Inadequate blood supply to an organ or area of tissue due to obstruction of a blood vessel.

ISCHEMIC. Characterized by ischemia.

ISCHEMIC STROKE. A stroke caused by the obstruction of blood to the brain, as from a clot.

ISLETS OF LANGERHANS. Groups of endocrine cells in the pancreas that secrete insulin.

ISOENZYMES. Enzymes that bring about the same reactions on the same chemicals but are different in their physical properties.

ISOSPORA BELLI. A type of parasitic protozoa.

J

JAMSHIDI NEEDLE. Special needle used to obtain a sample of bone marrow tissue.

JAUNDICE. Yellowing of the skin and eyes caused by a buildup of bile or excessive breakdown of red blood cells.

JEJUNECTOMY. Excision of all or a part of the jejunum (middle portion of the small intestine).

JEJUNOSTOMY TUBE. A feeding tube that goes directly into the small intestine; also called a J-tube.

JOINT COMMISSION. The accrediting organization that evaluates virtually all U.S. healthcare facilities and programs. Accreditation is maintained with on-site surveys every three years; laboratories are surveyed every two years.

JUGULAR VEIN. Major vein of the neck that returns blood from the head to the heart.

K

KARYOTYPE. A photomicrograph (picture taken through a microscope) of a person's 46 chromosomes, lined up in 23 pairs, that is used to identify some types of genetic disorders.

KEGEL EXERCISES. A series of contractions and relaxations of the muscles in the perineal area. These exercises are thought to strengthen the pelvic floor and may help prevent urinary incontinence in women.

KELOID. An abnormal type of scarring that involves progressive enlargement, elevated edges, and irregular shapes because of excessive collagen formation during healing.

KERATINOCYTES. Dead cells at the outer surface of the epidermis that form a tough protective layer for the skin. The cells underneath divide to replenish the supply.

KERATOCONUS. An eye condition in which the cornea bulges outward, interfering with normal vision; usually both eyes are affected.

KERATOMETER. A device that measures the curvature of the cornea. It is used to determine the correct power for an intraocular lens prior to cataract surgery.

KETOACIDOSIS. A potentially life-threatening condition in which abnormally high blood glucose levels result in the blood becoming too acidic.

KETONES. Substances produced during the breakdown of fatty acids. They are produced in excessive amounts in diabetes and certain other abnormal conditions.

KETOSIS. Abnormally elevated concentration of ketones in body tissues.

KIDNEY STONES. Small solid masses composed primarily of calcium that form in the kidney, causing pain, bleeding, obstruction, and infection.

KILOGRAM. Metric unit of weight, abbreviated as kg.

KNEE SURGERY. Refers primarily to repair, replacement, or revision of parts of the knee; includes both arthroscopic and open surgeries.

L

LABIAL. Of or pertaining to the lips.

LACERATION. A type of wound with rough, torn, or ragged edges.

LAMINA (SINGULAR, LAMINAE). The broad plates of bone on the upper surface of the vertebrae that fuse together at the midline to form a bony covering over the spinal canal.

LAMINECTOMY. Surgical removal of the lamina to reach and remove a herniated disk.

LAMINOTOMY. A less invasive alternative to a laminectomy in which a hole is drilled through the lamina.

LANGERHANS' CELLS. Cells in the epidermis that help protect the body against infection.

LAPAROSCOPE. An instrument equipped with a camera that allows a surgeon to see inside the abdominal cavity.

LAPAROSCOPIC CHOLECYSTECTOMY. Removal of the gallbladder using a laparoscope.

LAPAROSCOPIC PROCEDURES. Procedures performed using a laparoscope.

LAPAROSCOPIC SURGERY. Surgery performed using a laparoscope and surgical instruments inserted through small incisions; also referred to as keyhole surgery.

LAPAROSCOPY. Visual examination of the inside of the abdomen with a laparoscope.

LAPAROTOMY. A surgical procedure in which the surgeon makes a large incision through the wall of the abdomen in order to gain access to the organs inside the abdominal cavity.

LARGE INTESTINE. Also called the colon, this structure has six major divisions: cecum, ascending colon, transverse colon, descending colon, sigmoid colon, and rectum.

LARYNGECTOMY. Surgical removal of the larynx.

LARYNGOPHARYNGECTOMY. Surgical removal of both the larynx and the pharynx.

LARYNGOSCOPE. An endoscope equipped for viewing a patient's larynx through the mouth.

LARYNGOSCOPY. The visualization of the larynx and vocal cords. This may be done directly with a fiber-optic scope (laryngoscope) or indirectly with mirrors.

LARYNGOSPASM. Spasmodic closure of the larynx.

LARYNX. Also known as the voice box, the larynx is composed of cartilage that contains the apparatus for voice production. This includes the vocal cords and the muscles and ligaments that move the cords.

LASER. A device that emits electromagnetic radiation at specific wavelengths, usually in the ultraviolet, visible, or infrared regions of the spectrum.

LASER IRIDOTOMY. A procedure, using either the Nd: YAG laser or the argon laser, done to penetrate the iris so that fluid in the eye can drain.

LASER SKIN RESURFACING. The use of laser light to remove the uppermost layer of skin. Two types of lasers commonly used are CO_2 and erbium.

LASER THERAPY. A cancer treatment that uses a laser beam (a narrow beam of intense light) to kill cancer cells.

LASER-ASSISTED IN SITU KERATOMILEUSIS (LASIK). A type of refractive eye surgery that uses an excimer laser to reshape the cornea of the eye in order to correct a patient's vision.

LATARJET'S NERVE. Terminal branch of the anterior vagal trunk, which runs along the lesser curvature of the stomach.

LATERAL. Of or pertaining to a side (opposite of medial).

LATERAL EPICONDYLITIS. The medical term for tennis elbow.

LATERAL RELEASE SURGERY. Release of tissues in the knee that keep the kneecap from tracking properly in its groove (sulcus) in the femur; by realigning or tightening tendons, the kneecap can be forced to track properly.

LATEX. A milky white fluid, or sap, from certain plants that makes up certain rubber products.

LATISSIMUS DORSI. A large fan-shaped muscle that covers a wide area of the back; in Latin, this muscle literally means "widest of the back."

LAVAGE. Washing out.

LAXATIVE. An agent that stimulates defecation.

LE FORT FRACTURE. A term that refers to a system for classifying fractures of the facial bones into three groups according to the region affected.

LEAD POINT. A well-defined abnormality in the area where intussusception (telescoping of the bowel) begins.

LEADS. Color-coded wires that connect electrodes to monitor cables.

LEFT VENTRICULAR ASSIST DEVICE (LVAD). The most common type of ventricular assist device, used to help the left ventricle of the heart pump blood to the rest of the body.

LEGG-CALVE-PERTHES DISEASE (LCP). A disorder in which the femoral head deteriorates within the hip joint as a result of insufficient blood supply.

LEGIONNAIRES' DISEASE. A lung disease caused by *Legionella* bacteria.

LEIOMYOSARCOMA. Cancer that grows in the smooth muscle lining of certain organs.

LENS. A transparent structure in the eye that focuses light onto the retina.

LENS CAPSULE. A clear elastic membrane-like structure that covers the lens of the eye.

LENTICONUS. A rare, usually congenital condition in which the surface of the lens of the eye is conical.

LENTICULAR. Lens-shaped.

LESION. An area of abnormal or injured skin.

LEUKEMIA. A type of cancer that affects leukocytes, a type of white blood cell.

LEUKOCORIA. A pupil reflex that is white instead of red or that has white spots.

LEUKOCYTE. A general term for the various types of white blood cells in the immune system that protect the body against infectious disease agents and foreign substances.

LEVONORGESTREL. A synthetic female hormone used in some intrauterine devices (IUDs) to prevent conception by inhibiting the movement of sperm and reducing the formation of the endometrial tissue lining the walls of the uterus.

LICENSED PRACTICAL NURSE (LPN). A person who is licensed to provide basic nursing care under the supervision of a physician or a registered nurse.

LIFE SUPPORT. Methods of replacing or supporting a failing bodily function, such as using mechanical ventilation to support breathing. In treatable or curable conditions, life support is used temporarily to aid healing until the body can resume normal functioning.

LIGAMENT. A band of fibrous tissue that connects bones to other bones or holds internal organs in place.

LIGAMENTA FLAVA (SINGULAR, LIGAMENTUM FLAVUM). A series of bands of tissue that are attached to the vertebrae in the spinal column. They help to hold the spine straight and to close the spaces between the laminar arches. The Latin name means "yellow band(s)."

LIGATION. The act of tying off a blood vessel.

LIPID. Any organic compound that is greasy and insoluble in water but soluble in alcohol. Fats, waxes, and oils are examples of lipids.

LIPOMA. A type of benign tumor that develops within adipose or fatty tissue.

LIPOPROTEINS. Substances that carry fat through the blood vessels for use or storage in other parts of the body.

LIPOSHAVING. Method of removing fat that lies closer to the surface of the skin by using a needle-like instrument that contains a sharp-edged shaving device.

LIPOSUCTION. A surgical technique for removing fat from under the skin by vacuum suctioning.

LITHOTOMY POSITION. The position most often used in Western medicine for examinations and surgical procedures involving the lower abdomen and pelvis. The patient lies on the back with the genital area at the edge of the examination table, the knees bent and positioned above the hips, and the feet placed in stirrups to keep the knees spread apart.

LITHOTRIPSY. A technique for breaking up kidney stones within the urinary tract, followed by flushing out the fragments.

LITTRE'S HERNIA. A Meckel's diverticulum trapped in an inguinal hernia.

LIVING WILL. A document that states end-of-life decisions concerning medical treatment.

LOBECTOMY. Removal of a section of the lung.

LOBULAR CARCINOMA-IN-SITU (LCIS). Breast cancer that is confined to the milk-producing glands.

LOCAL ANESTHESIA. Anesthesia that numbs a localized area of the body, with the patient remaining conscious.

LOCALIZED INFECTION. An infection that is limited to a specific part of the body.

LOCKOUT TIME. The minimum amount of time (usually expressed in minutes) allowed between doses of pain medication.

LONG QT SYNDROME. A rare inherited heart condition in which a disorder of the heart rhythm results in rapid, chaotic heartbeats that can lead to a fainting spell or even sudden death. Certain medications can also trigger the condition. The phrase "long QT" refers to the pattern of this abnormal heartbeat as it appears on an electrocardiogram.

LONG-TERM CARE (LTC). Residential care over a period of time, such as a nursing home that offers nursing care and assistance with daily living.

LONG-TERM CARE (LTC) INSURANCE. Private insurance intended to cover the cost of long-term nursing home or home health care.

LOOP ELECTROSURGICAL EXCISION PROCEDURE (LEEP). A procedure that uses a thin wire loop that emits a low-voltage high-frequency radio wave to excise abnormal cervical tissue.

LOOSENESS OF ASSOCIATION. A psychiatric term describing a thought disorder where a patient makes irrelevant connections between seemingly unrelated topics. In a mental health assessment, the patient's responses may not seem to correspond to the question asked by the health care provider.

LOUPE. A convex lens used to magnify small objects at very close range. It may be held on the hand, mounted on eyeglasses, or attached to a headband.

LOW TRANSVERSE INCISION. An incision made horizontally across the lower end of the uterus in cesarean delivery.

LOWER ESOPHAGEAL SPHINCTER (LES). A ring of muscle in the lower esophagus that prevents stomach acid from refluxing back into the esophagus.

LOWER EXTREMITY AMPUTATION. Surgical removal of one of the lower limbs of the body.

LUMBAR. Pertaining to the part of the back between the chest and the pelvis.

LUMBAR VERTEBRAE. The vertebrae of the lower back below the level of the ribs.

LUMEN. The cavity or channel inside a blood vessel or tube-shaped organ.

LUMPECTOMY. Excision of a breast tumor and some surrounding tissue.

LUNG ALLOCATION SCORE (LAS). A numerical value from 0 to 100 calculated to determine a patient's priority of receiving a donor lung within the United States. The LAS system has been used by the United Network for Organ Sharing (UNOS) since 2005.

LUPUS. A chronic inflammatory disease that is caused by autoimmunity. Patients with lupus have antibodies that target their own body tissues. Lupus can cause disease of the skin, heart, lungs, kidneys, joints, and nervous system. Lupus is a hereditary condition, but the specific cause is unknown.

LUPUS ERYTHEMATOSUS. A chronic autoimmune disease that affects the skin, joints, and certain internal organs.

LUXATE. To loosen or dislocate a tooth from its socket.

LYMPH. An almost colorless fluid that bathes body tissues. Lymph is found in the lymphatic vessels and carries lymphocytes that have entered the lymph glands from the blood.

LYMPH GLANDS. Another name for lymph nodes.

LYMPH NODE BIOPSY. The removal of all or part of a lymph node to view under a microscope for cancer cells.

LYMPH NODE DISSECTION. The removal of underarm lymph nodes to check for the spread of cancer.

LYMPH NODES. Small masses of tissue that are located throughout the body and contain clusters of cells called lymphocytes. They filter out and destroy bacteria, foreign particles, and cancerous cells from the blood.

LYMPHANGIOGRAPHY. Injection of dye into lymphatic vessels followed by x-rays of the area. It is a difficult procedure, as it requires surgical isolation of the lymph vessels to be injected.

LYMPHATIC SYSTEM. The tissues and organs (including the bone marrow, spleen, thymus, and lymph nodes) that produce and store cells that fight infection, together with the network of vessels that carry lymph throughout the body.

LYMPHEDEMA. Swelling due to retention of lymph fluid.

LYMPHOCYTES. Type of white blood cells that are part of the immune system. The lymphocytes are composed of three main cell lines: B lymphocytes, T lymphocytes, and natural killer (NK) cells.

LYMPHOID TISSUE. Tissue that contains white blood cells of the immune system.

LYMPHOMA. A type of cancer that affects lymph cells and tissues, including certain white blood cells (T cells and B cells), lymph nodes, bone marrow, and the spleen.

LYMPHOPROLIFERATIVE. An increase in the number of lymphocytes.

LYMPHOSCINTIGRAPHY. A technique for detecting the presence of cancer cells in lymph nodes by using a radioactive tracer.

LYSIS. Destruction or decomposition; in medicine, the process of removing adhesions from an organ.

M

MACROCYTIC. A descriptive term applied to a larger than normal red blood cell.

MACROMASTIA. Excessive size of the breasts.

MACROPHAGE. A large white blood cell, found primarily in the bloodstream and connective tissue, that helps the body fight off infections by ingesting the disease organism.

MACROSOMIA. The term used to describe a newborn baby with an abnormally high birth weight.

MACULA. A small, yellowish depressed area on the retina that absorbs the shorter wavelengths of visible light and is responsible for fine detailed vision.

MACULAR DEGENERATION. A condition usually associated with age in which the macula becomes impaired due to hardening of the arteries (arteriosclerosis), interfering with vision.

MAGNETIC FIELD. The three-dimensional area surrounding a magnet, in which its force is active.

MAGNETIC RESONANCE IMAGING (MRI). An imaging technique that uses magnetic fields and radio waves to create detailed images of internal body organs and structures.

MALABSORPTION. Defective or inadequate absorption of nutrients from the intestinal tract.

MALABSORPTIVE. Referring to a type of bariatric surgery in which a part of the stomach is partitioned off and connected to a lower portion of the small intestine in order to reduce the amount of nutrients that the body absorbs from food.

MALIGNANCY. Conditions that are cancerous, meaning that they produce abnormal cells capable of invading and destroying other local and distant tissues.

MALIGNANT. Cancerous.

MALIGNANT GLAUCOMA. Glaucoma that gets worse even after iridectomy (surgical removal of part of the iris).

MALIGNANT HYPERTHERMIA. A type of reaction (probably with a genetic basis) that can occur during general anesthesia in which a patient experiences a high fever, muscle rigidity, and fluctuations in heart rate and blood pressure.

MALIGNANT TUMOR. A cancerous growth that has the potential to spread to other parts of the body.

MALLEUS. One of the three bones of the middle ear, also known as the "hammer."

MALOCCLUSION. Malpositioning and defective contact between opposing teeth in the upper and lower jaws.

MALPRACTICE. A doctor's or lawyer's failure in his or her professional duties through ignorance, negligence, or criminal intent.

MAMMARY ARTERY. A chest wall artery that descends from the aorta and is commonly used for bypass grafts.

MAMMARY HYPERPLASIA. Increased size of the breast.

MAMMOGRAM. A set of x-rays taken of the front and side of the breast, used to help diagnose various breast abnormalities.

MAMMOGRAPHY. A procedure during which x-rays are taken of the breast.

MAMMOPLASTY. Surgery performed to change the size or shape of breasts.

MANAGED CARE. The integration of financing and delivery of health care.

MANDIBLE. The horseshoe-shaped bone that forms the lower jaw (jawbone).

MANNITOL. A type of diuretic (drug that increases urine output).

MARFAN SYNDROME. A hereditary disorder that affects the connective tissues of the body, the lens of the eye, and the cardiovascular system.

MARGIN OF RESECTION. The area between the cancerous tumor and the edges of the removed tissue.

MASS CASUALTY INCIDENT (MCI). Any event involving multiple human casualties that overwhelms first responders and other resources by the number and severity of injuries. It is also known as a mass casualty event (MCE).

MASS SPECTROMETRY. A method of analyzing a test sample by converting a portion of the sample into charged ions and measuring the electric current produced when the charged ions strike a detector. Mass spectrometry can be used to measure the quantity as well as the identity of a substance in the test sample.

MAST CELLS. A type of immune system cell found in the lining of the nasal passages and eyelids. It displays immunoglobulin type E (IgE) on its cell surface and participates in the allergic response by releasing histamine from intracellular granules.

MASTECTOMY. Removal of all or a portion of breast tissue.

MASTOID. A large bony process at the base of the skull behind the ear. It contains air spaces that connect with the cavity of the middle ear.

MASTOID AIR CELLS. Numerous small intercommunicating cavities in the mastoid process of the temporal bone that empty into the mastoid antrum.

MASTOID ANTRUM. A cavity in the temporal bone of the skull, communicating with the mastoid cells and with the middle ear.

MASTOID BONE. The prominent bone behind the ear that projects from the temporal bone of the skull.

MASTOID PROCESS. The nipple-like projection of part of the temporal bone (the large irregular bone situated in the base and side of the skull).

MASTOIDECTOMY. Hollowing out of the mastoid process by curetting, gouging, drilling, or otherwise removing the bony partitions forming the mastoid cells.

MASTOIDITIS. An inflammation of the bone behind the ear (the mastoid bone) caused by an infection spreading from the middle ear to the cavity in the mastoid bone.

MASTOPEXY. Surgical procedure to lift up a breast; may be used on opposite breast to achieve symmetrical appearance with a reconstructed breast.

MATERNAL BLOOD SCREENING. A test done early in pregnancy to screen for a variety of conditions. Abnormal amounts of certain proteins in a pregnant woman's blood raise the probability of fetal defects. Amniocentesis is recommended if such a probability occurs.

MATERNITY. Refers to the mother.

MAXILLA. The facial bone that forms the upper jaw and holds the upper teeth.

MAXILLARY SINUSES. Sinuses located in the cheek under the eye next to the ethmoid sinus.

MAZE PROCEDURE. A surgical procedure used to treat atrial fibrillation (abnormal heartbeat). During the procedure, precise incisions are made in the right and left atria to interrupt the conduction of abnormal impulses. When the heart heals, scar tissue forms and the abnormal electrical impulses are blocked from traveling through the heart.

MEAN CORPUSCULAR HEMOGLOBIN (MCH). A calculation of the average weight of hemoglobin in a red blood cell.

MEAN CORPUSCULAR HEMOGLOBIN CONCENTRATION (MCHC). A calculation of the average concentration of hemoglobin in a red blood cell.

MEAN CORPUSCULAR VOLUME (MCV). A measure of the average volume of a red blood cell.

MEATUS. A general term for an opening or passageway in the body.

MECHANICAL VALVE. An artificial device used to replace a patient's heart valve. They include three types: ball, disk, and bileaflet.

MECKEL'S DIVERTICULUM. Tissue faults in the lining of the intestines that are the result of a congenital abnormality originating in the umbilical duct's failure to close. Largely asymptomatic, the diverticula in some cases can become infected or obstructed.

MEDIAL. Toward the middle or center (e.g., the chest is medial to the arm).

MEDIAL (OR LATERAL) NASAL PROMINENCE. The medial (toward the middle) or lateral (toward the sides) are anatomical structures that form and merge the nose of a developing embryo during weeks six to nine in utero.

MEDIASTINOSCOPE. A thin hollow tube for performing mediastinoscopy.

MEDIASTINOSCOPY. A surgical procedure to look at the organs, tissues, and lymph nodes between the lungs for abnormal areas. An incision (cut) is made at the top of the breastbone and a thin, lighted tube (mediastinoscope) is inserted into the chest. Tissue and lymph node samples may be taken for biopsy.

MEDIASTINOTOMY. Surgical incision into the mediastinum.

MEDIASTINUM. The space in the chest between the lungs that contains the heart and its vessels, lymph nodes, the trachea, esophagus, and thymus.

MEDICAID. Federally funded program in the United States that provides medical assistance to permanently disabled patients and to low-income households. It is administered by the individual states.

MEDICAL AGENT. A designated patient representative who is legally empowered to carry out the patient's wishes with respect to medial care.

MEDICAL DIRECTIVES. Legal documents that include the declaration of a person's wishes pertaining to medical treatment (living will) and the stipulation of a proxy decision maker (power of attorney).

MEDICAL SURROGATE. Another name for a medical agent, or person legally designated to represent a patient in regards to medical treatment.

MEDICALLY NEEDY. Defined as people with high medical expenses whose incomes are above the eligibility limits for Medicaid but whom states have the option of covering.

MEDICARE. U.S. government health insurance system for people age 65 and older.

MEDICARE ADVANTAGE PLANS. Medicare Part C; private managed care plans that include all Medicare Part A and Part B benefits and usually some additional benefits.

MEDICARE PART A. Original Medicare; hospitalization insurance that is provided for free to most Americans aged 65 and older.

MEDICARE PART B. Health insurance that pays for some services not covered by Medicare Part A and that requires recipients to pay a monthly premium.

MEDICARE PART C. Also known as Medicare Advantage Plans; private healthcare plans that include all Medicare Part A and Part B benefits and usually some additional benefits.

MEDICARE PART D. An optional, subsidized, outpatient prescription drug benefit provided through a private insurer.

MEDIGAP. Supplemental healthcare insurance policies that cover services not included in Medicare.

MEDIONECROSIS. Death of the tunica, which is the middle layer of tissues in a vessel.

MEDULLA OBLONGATA. The lower part of the brain stem in humans, which controls such involuntary functions as breathing, blood pressure, and heart rate.

MEDULLARY CAVITY. The marrow cavity in the shaft of a long bone.

MEGACOLON. Abnormally large colon associated with some chronic intestine disorders.

MELANOCYTES. Cells within the epidermis that give skin its color.

MELANOMA. The most dangerous form of skin cancer.

MELENA. The passing of blackish-colored stools containing blood pigments or partially digested blood.

MEMBRANOUS LABYRINTH. A complex arrangement of communicating membranous canals and sacs, filled with endolymph and suspended within the cavity of the bony labyrinth.

MENGHINI NEEDLE. Special needle used to obtain a sample of liver tissue.

MÉNIÈRE'S DISEASE. Also known as idiopathic endolymphatic hydrops, Ménière's disease is a disorder of the inner ear. It is named for Prosper Ménière (1799–1862), a French physician.

MENINGES. Membranes that cover the brain.

MENINGITIS. An infection of the membranes that cover the brain and spinal cord.

MENISCUS. The fibrous cartilage within the knee joint that covers the surfaces of the femur and the tibia as they join the patella.

MEPERIDINE. A type of narcotic pain killer that may be used after surgical procedures.

MERIDIANS. The channels or paths in the human body that carry qi (life force), according to traditional Chinese medicine.

MESENCHYMAL CELLS. Embryonic cells that develop into many structures, including the soft tissues in the lip.

MESENTERY. The membranes, or one of the membranes (consisting of a fold of the peritoneum and enclosed tissues), that connect the intestines and their appendages with the dorsal wall of the abdominal cavity.

MESOTHELIOMA. A rare form of cancer that develops in mesothelial tissue, which lines the lungs, thorax, and perineum; it is most often associated with exposure to asbestos.

METABOLIC. Pertaining to metabolism, the physical and chemical processes of living things that produce energy.

METABOLIC ACIDOSIS. A condition in which either too much acid or too little bicarbonate in the body results in a drop in the blood pH (toward acidity).

METABOLIC ALKALOSIS. A condition in which either too little acid or too much bicarbonate in the body results in an elevation in the blood pH (toward alkalinity).

METABOLIC DISTURBANCE. A disturbance in the general function of the body's basic life processes, such as energy production. The body's inability to provide the brain with appropriate nourishment can affect the mental status of the individual.

METABOLIC SYNDROME. The presence of three or more factors that increase a person's risk of developing type 2 diabetes and cardiovascular disease. Factors include high blood pressure, abdominal obesity, high triglyceride levels, low HDL cholesterol levels, and high fasting blood sugar.

METABOLISM. The sum of all the physical and chemical processes required to maintain life, including the transformation by which energy is made available for use by the body.

METABOLITES. Chemicals produced during the breakdown of nutrients, drugs, enzymes, or other materials in the body.

METABOLIZE. To break down or convert food or other substances into a form that is useable by the body.

METACARPAL BONES. Five cylindrical bones extending from the wrist to the fingers.

METAPHYSIS. The widened end of the shaft of a long tubular bone such as the femur.

METASTASIS. The spread of cancer cells from one part of the body to another.

METASTASIZE. Spread; used to refer to the growth of cancer cells from the original site to other parts of the body.

METASTATIC. Referring to the spread of cancer from one site in the body to another.

METASTATIC CANCER. Secondary cancer, or cancer that has spread from one body organ or tissue to another.

METATARSAL JOINT. The joints in the bones located between the heel and the toes.

METHICILLIN-RESISTANT STAPHYLOCOCCUS AUREUS (MRSA). A strain of Staph bacteria that is resistant to treatment with the antibiotic methicillin and is therefore difficult to control or kill.

METHOTREXATE. A drug that targets rapidly dividing fetal cells, preventing a fetus from developing further.

MICROCYTIC. A descriptive term applied to a smaller than normal red blood cell.

MICRODISKECTOMY. Minimally invasive spinal surgery (MISS) for disk removal; also known as microdecompression.

MICROGENIA. An extremely small chin. It is the most common deformity of the chin.

MICROKERATOME. A precision surgical instrument that can slice an extremely thin layer of tissue from the surface of the cornea.

MICROORGANISM. An independent unit of life that is too small to be seen with the naked eye.

MICROSPORIDA. A type of parasitic protozoa.

MICROSURGERY. Surgery on small body structures or cells performed with the aid of a microscope and other specialized instruments.

MICROTIA. The partial or complete absence of the auricle of the ear.

MIDDLE EAR. The cavity or space between the eardrum and the inner ear. It includes the eardrum; the three little bones (hammer, anvil, and stirrup) that transmit sound to the inner ear; and the Eustachian tube, which connects the inner ear to the nasopharynx (the back of the nose).

MIDDLE MEATUS. A curved passage in each nasal cavity located below the middle nasal concha and extending along the entire superior border of the inferior nasal concha.

MIDDLE TURBINATE. The lower of two thin bony processes on the ethmoid bone on the lateral wall of each nasal fossa that separates the superior and middle meatus of the nose.

MILIA. Small bumps on the skin that occur when sweat glands are clogged.

MILIARY TUMOR. A very small tumor, sometimes described as the size of a small seed or grain of sand. The English word "miliary" comes from the Latin word for millet seed.

MINIGRAFT OR MICROGRAFT. Transplantation of a small number (as few as one to three) of hair follicles.

MINIMALLY INVASIVE SURGERY. Surgery performed using surgical instruments and tiny video cameras inserted into several small incisions instead of one large incision.

MIOTICS. Medications that cause the pupil of the eye to contract.

MITOTIC. Relating to mitosis, or the process by which a cell divides into two cells, each with identical sets of chromosomes.

MITRAL VALVE. The bicuspid valve that connects the left atrium and left ventricle of the heart.

MIXED DENTITION. A mix of both "baby teeth" and permanent teeth.

MODIFIED RADICAL MASTECTOMY. Total mastectomy with axillary lymph node dissection, but with preservation of the chest muscles.

MOHS EXCISION. Referring to the excision of one layer of tissue during Mohs surgery.

MONOCHORIONIC PREGNANCY. A pregnancy in which twin fetuses share a placenta.

MONOCHORIONIC TWINS. Twins that share a single placenta.

MONOCLONAL ANTIBODY. A type of antibody produced by identical immune cells derived by cloning a unique parent cell. The generic names on monoclonal antibody drugs all end in –mab.

MONOCYTE. A large white blood cell that is formed in the bone marrow and spleen. About 4% of the white blood cells in normal adults are monocytes.

MONOFILAMENT. A single untwisted strand of suture material.

MONSEL'S SOLUTION. A solution used to stop bleeding.

MORBID. Unwholesome or bad for health.

MORBIDITY. The presence of illness; a statistic that provides the rate at which an illness or abnormality occurs.

MORBIDLY OBESE. A term used to describe individuals either 100 lb. (45 kg) or more than 50% overweight and/or who have a body mass index above 40.

MORCELLATION. The division of tissue or tumors into smaller pieces for easier removal.

MORPHOLOGY. The study of form. In medicine, morphology refers to the size, shape, and structure of a given organ rather than its function.

MORTALITY. The occurrence of death or a statistic representing death rate (i.e., the number of deaths per unit of population in any specific region, age group, disease, or other classification, usually expressed as deaths per 1,000, 10,000, or 1,000,000).

MOTILITY. Ability to move freely or spontaneously.

MOUTH GUARD. A plastic device that protects the upper teeth from injury.

MUCOCILIARY. Involving the cilia of the mucous membranes of the respiratory system.

MUCOUS MEMBRANE. The thin lining of certain body passages, such as the nose, that protects the passage and secretes mucus, the fluid-like substance that moistens and protects the lining.

MUCUS. A viscous, slippery secretion that is produced by the mucous membranes it moistens and protects.

MULTIFILAMENT. A braided strand of suture material. Multifilament sutures are generally thicker than monofilament and are used in such specialties as orthopedic surgery.

MULTIFOCAL MOTOR NEUROPATHY. A rare condition in which the muscles in the body become progressively weaker over time.

MULTIMODAL MANAGEMENT. The use of more than one method of treatment.

MULTIPLE MYELOMA. An uncommon disease that occurs more often in men than in women and is associated with anemia, hemorrhage, recurrent infections, and weakness. It is regarded as a malignant neoplasm that originates in bone marrow and involves mainly the skeleton.

MULTIPLE SCLEROSIS. A disease that destroys the covering (myelin sheath) of nerve fibers of the brain and spinal cord.

MURMUR. The sound made as blood moves through the heart when there is turbulence in the flow of blood through a blood vessel, or if a valve does not completely close.

MUSCULAR DYSTROPHY. A genetic muscle disease that causes progressive muscle weakness along with the breakdown and death of muscle tissue.

MYCOBACTERIUM. Any of a genus of nonmotile, aerobic, acid-fast bacteria, including numerous saprophytes and the pathogens that cause tuberculosis and leprosy.

MYDRIATIC. Causing dilation or widening of the pupil of the eye.

MYDRIATICS. A class of drugs administered to dilate the pupil of the eye.

MYELODYSPLASIA. A condition in which the bone marrow does not function normally, which can affect the various types of blood cells produced in the bone marrow. It is often referred to as myelodysplastic syndrome or preleukemia and may progress to acute leukemia.

MYELOFIBROSIS. An anemic condition in which bone marrow cells are abnormal or defective and become fibrotic.

MYELOGRAM. Image(s) of the spine produced with x-rays or computed tomography scans and a special dye.

MYELOMA. A tumor of plasma cells that originates in bone marrow and usually spreads to more than one bone.

MYELOMENINGOCELE (MMC). A protrusion in the vertebral column containing the spinal cord and meninges.

MYOCARDIAL. Referring to the heart muscle.

MYOCARDIAL INFARCTION. Commonly known as a heart attack; occurs when some of the heart's blood supply is severely cut off or restricted, causing the heart muscle to suffer and die from lack of oxygen.

MYOCARDITIS. Inflammation of the muscles of the walls of the heart due to a viral infection.

MYOCARDIUM. The medical term for the specialized involuntary muscle tissue found in the walls of the heart.

MYOGLOBIN. A protein that is the primary iron-carrying pigment in muscle tissue. Myoglobin is found in the bloodstream only after injury to muscle tissue.

MYOMA. A tumor consisting of muscle tissue.

MYOPIA. A refractive error that causes distant objects to appear blurry. Myopia results when light does not focus properly on the retina; it is also known as nearsightedness.

MYOSITIS. Inflammation of muscle tissue.

MYRINGOPLASTY. Surgical restoration of a perforated eardrum by grafting.

MYRINGOTOMY. A procedure that involves making a small incision in the eardrum to release pressure caused by excess fluid accumulation.

MYXEDEMA. Hypothyroidism; underactive thyroid function characterized by thick, puffy features; an enlarged tongue; and lack of emotion.

N

NARCOTIC. A drug derived from opium or compounds similar to opium. Narcotics are potent pain relievers but can affect mood and behavior, and long-term use can lead to dependence and tolerance.

NASAL CANNULA. A piece of flexible plastic tubing with two small clamps that fit into the nostrils and provide supplemental oxygen flow.

NASAL CONCHA. Any of three thin bony plates on the lateral wall of each side of the nasal cavity (fossa).

NASAL SEPTUM. The cartilage that divides the right and left airways of the nose. A deviated nasal septum is one that is significantly off center.

NASOGASTRIC TUBE. A tube inserted through the nose and throat and into the stomach for direct feeding of the patient.

NATRIURETIC PEPTIDES. Peptides (compounds comprised of two or more amino acids) that prompt the kidneys to excrete sodium into the urine and out of the body.

NATURAL KILLER (NK) CELL. A large-celled lymphocyte that functions as part of the innate immune system to respond to cells infected by viruses and tumor cells.

NATUROPATHY. A type of alternative medicine that maintains that humans have an innate vital force that can be fostered by noninvasive treatments, encouragement of natural healing, and minimal use of surgery and drugs.

NEARSIGHTEDNESS. A condition in which one or both eyes cannot focus normally, causing objects at a distance to appear blurred and indistinct; also called myopia.

NECROSIS. Cellular or tissue death.

NECROTIC. Referring to the death of tissue as a result of disease or trauma.

NEEDLE BIOPSY. The procedure of using a large hollow needle to obtain a sample of intact tissue for further examination.

NEOADJUVANT CHEMOTHERAPY. Chemotherapy that is given before the main or primary treatment, usually surgery.

NEOBLADDER. A term that refers to the creation of a reservoir for urine made from intestinal tissue that allows for evacuation.

NEONATAL INTENSIVE CARE UNIT (NICU). A level III hospital nursery that is equipped to handle newborn emergency care.

NEONATAL JAUNDICE. A disorder in newborns where the liver is too premature to conjugate bilirubin, which builds up in the blood.

NEONATE. A newborn baby.

NEOPLASIA. Abnormal growth of cells, which may lead to a neoplasm, or tumor.

NEOPLASM. An uncontrolled growth of new tissue.

NEOVASCULAR GLAUCOMA. A form of glaucoma that results from uncontrolled diabetes or hypertension.

NEPHELOMETRY. A method for measuring the light-scattering properties of a sample.

NEPHRECTOMY. Surgical removal of a kidney.

NEPHROLITHOTOMY. The removal of renal calculi by an incision through the kidney. The term by itself usually refers to the standard open procedure for the surgical removal of kidney stones.

NEPHROLOGIST. A doctor specializing in kidney disease.

NEPHROPATHY. An abnormality or disease of the kidney.

NEPHROSCOPE. An instrument used to view the inside of the kidney during percutaneous nephrolithotomy (PCNL). A nephroscope has channels for a fiberoptic light, a telescope, and an irrigation system for washing out the affected part of the kidney.

NEPHROTIC SYNDROME. A kidney disorder that causes a cluster of symptoms, including low serum protein, loss of protein in the urine, and body swelling.

NEPHROTOXIC. Destructive to kidney cells.

NEPHROTOXICITY. Buildup of poisons in the kidneys.

NEUROFIBROMATOSIS. A rare hereditary disease that involves the growth of lesions that may affect the spinal cord.

NEUROGENIC BLADDER. Bladder dysfunction caused by neurological diseases that alter the brain's messages to the bladder.

NEUROLOGICAL. Pertaining to the nervous system: peripheral nervous system, brain, and spinal cord.

NEUROLOGIST. A physician who specializes in diagnosing and treating disorders of the nervous system.

NEUROMODULATION. Electrical stimulation of a nerve for relief of pain.

NEUROPATHY. A usually degenerative disorder of the nerves or nervous system.

NEUROSURGEON. A surgeon who specializes in the nervous system, including the brain.

NEUROSURGERY. Surgery performed on the brain.

NEUROTOXIN. Any substance that affects the functioning of the human nervous system, such as lead, ethanol (beverage alcohol), nitric oxide, tetanus toxin, and botulinum toxin.

NEUROTRANSMITTER. One of a group of chemicals secreted by a nerve cell (neuron) to carry a chemical message to another nerve cell, often as a way of transmitting a nerve impulse. Examples of neurotransmitters include acetylcholine, dopamine, serotonin, and norepinephrine.

NEUTRALIZE. The way the body addresses acidity or alkalinity: adding acid to an alkaline environment to arrive at a neutral pH value, or adding bicarbonate to an acidic environment to arrive at a neutral pH value.

NEUTROPHIL. A type of white blood cell involved in acute inflammation. Neutrophils remove and kill bacteria by phagocytosis.

NICOTINE. A colorless, oily chemical found in tobacco that makes people physically dependent on smoking. It is poisonous in large doses.

NITROUS OXIDE. A colorless, sweet-smelling gas used by dentists for mild anesthesia. It is sometimes called laughing gas because it makes some people feel giddy or silly.

NOCICEPTOR. A nerve cell that is capable of sensing pain and transmitting a pain signal.

NOCTURNIST. A hospitalist who works only at night.

NODULAR GOITER. An enlargement of the thyroid (goiter) caused when groups of cells collect to form nodules.

NOMOGRAMS. Surgical adjustments of an excimer laser to fine-tune results.

NONINVASIVE. A procedure that does not penetrate the body.

NONINVASIVE TUMORS. Tumors that have not penetrated the muscle wall and/or spread to other parts of the body.

NONMYELOABLATIVE ALLOGENEIC BONE MARROW TRANSPLANT. A type of bone marrow transplant that involves receiving low doses of chemotherapy and radiation therapy, followed by the infusion of a donor's bone marrow or peripheral stem cells. The goal is to suppress the patient's own bone marrow with low-dose chemotherapy and radiation therapy to allow the donor's cells to engraft. It is also called a "mini" bone marrow transplant.

NONPALPABLE. Unable to be detected through the sense of touch.

NONPHARMACOLOGICAL. Referring to therapy that does not involve drugs.

NONPROFIT HOSPITALS. Hospitals that combine a teaching function with providing for uninsured patients within large, complex networks technically designated as nonprofit institutions. However, while the institution may be nonprofit, its services are allowed to make a profit.

NONSTEROIDAL ANTI-INFLAMMATORY DRUGS (NSAIDS). Drugs that relieve pain and reduce inflammation but are not related chemically to cortisone. Common drugs in this class include aspirin, ibuprofen (Advil, Motrin), and naproxen (Aleve, Naprosyn).

NONUNION. Referring to a bone fracture or defect induced by disease, trauma, or surgery that fails to heal within a reasonable time span.

NOREPINEPHRINE. A naturally occurring hormone that acts as a neurotransmitter and affects both alpha- and beta-adrenergic receptors. It is also known as noradrenaline.

NORMOCHROMIC. A descriptive term applied to a red blood cell with a normal concentration of hemoglobin.

NORMOCYTIC. A descriptive term applied to a red blood cell of normal size.

NOSOCOMIAL. Originating or taking place in a hospital or clinical setting.

NOSOCOMIAL INFECTION. An infection acquired in the hospital.

NPO. A term that means "nothing by mouth." NPO refers to the time after which a patient is not allowed to eat or drink prior to a procedure or treatment.

NSAIDS. Nonsteroidal anti-inflammatory drugs.

NUCLEAR IMAGING. Method of producing images by detecting radiation in different parts of the body after a radioactive tracer material is administered.

NUCLEAR MEDICINE. A branch of medicine that makes use of radioisotopes (also called radionuclides) to evaluate the rate of radioactive decay in diagnosing and treating various diseases.

NUCLEOTIDES. Small molecules that form the building blocks of DNA and RNA, play important roles in cell metabolism, and participate in cell signaling.

NUCLEUS. The part of a cell that contains the DNA.

NUCLEUS TRACTUS SOLITARIUS (NTS). A group of nerve cells in the medulla (lower brainstem) that receives sensory information from the digestive tract (as well as the cardiovascular and respiratory systems) and conveys it to the vagus and facial nerves.

NULLIPAROUS. Referring to a woman who has never given birth.

NURSE ANESTHETIST. A registered nurse who has obtained advanced training in anesthesia delivery and perioperative patient care.

NURSE MANAGER. The nurse responsible for managing the nursing care on the nursing unit and who also supervises all of the other personnel working on the nursing unit.

NURSING UNIT. The floor or section of the hospital where patient rooms are located.

NYHA HEART FAILURE CLASSIFICATION. A classification system for heart failure developed by the New York Heart Association (NYHA). It includes the following four categories: I, symptoms with more than ordinary activity; II, symptoms with ordinary activity; III, symptoms with minimal activity; IV, symptoms at rest.

NYSTAGMUS. An involuntary, rapid, rhythmic movement of the eyeball, which may be horizontal, vertical, rotatory, or mixed.

O

OBESITY. Excessive weight gain due to accumulation of fat in the body, sometimes defined as a BMI (body mass index) of 30 or higher, or body weight greater than 30% above a person's desirable weight on standard height-weight tables.

OBESITY PARADOX. The observation that, although obesity is usually linked to risk factors for various diseases and surgical complications, it sometimes appears to have a protective effect.

OBSESSION. A recurrent and persistent idea, thought, or impulse that an individual cannot repress.

OBSTRUCTIVE SLEEP APNEA. Recurrent interruption of breathing during sleep due to obstruction of the upper airway.

OBTURATOR. Any structure that occludes an opening.

OCCIPITAL BONE. Bone that forms the back part of the skull.

OCCLUSION. An obstruction or blockage; also, the bringing together of the upper and lower jaw.

OCCULT. Hidden; not easily detected.

OCULAR FUNDUS. The part of the eye opposite the pupil.

OCULAR HYPERTENSION. A condition in which fluid pressure inside the eye is higher than normal but without visual field loss or damage to the optic nerve.

OCULAR MELANOMA. A malignant tumor that arises within the structures of the eye. It is the most common eye tumor in adults.

OCULAR ORBIT. Bony cavity containing the eyeball.

OINTMENT. A thick spreadable substance that contains medicine and is meant to be used on the outside of the body.

OLECRANON. The bony hook-shaped tip at the upper end of the ulna (one of the two forearm bones).

OLIGURIA. Decreased urine production.

OMBUDSMAN. A patient representative who investigates patient complaints and problems related to hospital service or treatment. He or she may act as a mediator between the patient, the family, and the hospital.

OMENTECTOMY. Surgical removal of the omentum.

OMENTUM. A layer of fatty tissue that covers the contents of the abdomen. Surgical removal of the omentum is called an omentectomy.

OMPHALOCELE. A congenital hernia in which a small portion of the fetal abdominal contents, covered by a membrane sac, protrudes into the base of the umbilical cord.

ONCOGENE. A gene that is capable under certain conditions of triggering the conversion of normal cells into cancer cells.

ONCOLOGIST. A physician who specializes in the development, diagnosis, treatment, and prevention of tumors.

ONCOLOGY. The branch of medicine that deals with the diagnosis and treatment of cancer.

OOPHORECTOMY. Surgical removal of the ovaries.

OPACITY. An opaque spot in a normally transparent structure, such as the lens of the eye.

OPEN SURGERY. Surgery using a large incision to lay open an area for examination or treatment.

OPEN-ANGLE GLAUCOMA. A form of glaucoma in which fluid pressure builds up inside the eye even though the angle of the anterior chamber is open and looks normal when the eye is examined. Most cases of glaucoma are open-angle.

OPERATIVE NURSE. A nurse specially trained to assist surgeons and work in all areas of patient surgical care.

OPHTHALMOLOGIST. A physician who specializes in treating diseases and disorders of the eye. Ophthalmologists are qualified to practice eye surgery and prescribe medicines for eye disorders.

OPHTHALMOLOGY. The branch of medicine that deals with the diagnosis and treatment of eye disorders.

OPHTHALMOSCOPE. Lighted device for studying the interior of the eyeball.

OPIOID. A synthetic painkiller, such as morphine, that has narcotic properties similar to opiates but may or may not be derived from opium.

OPPORTUNISTIC INFECTION. An infection that develops only when a person's immune system is weakened.

OPTIC DISC. A visually inactive portion of the retina from which the optic nerve and blood vessels emerge.

OPTIC NERVE. A large nerve found in the posterior part of the eye, through which all the visual nerve fibers leave the eye on their way to the brain.

OPTOMETRIST. A health care professional who is trained to prescribe and fit corrective lenses to improve vision and to diagnose and treat various eye diseases.

ORAL. Pertaining to the mouth.

ORAL SURGEON. A dentist who specializes in surgical procedures of the mouth.

ORBICULARIS ORIS. Concentrically shaped muscle that surrounds the upper and lower lips.

ORBIT. The bony cavity in the skull that contains the eyeball.

ORCHIECTOMY. Surgical removal of one or both testicles in a male; also called an orchidectomy.

ORGAN PROCUREMENT. Includes the process of donor screening and the evaluation, removal, preservation, and distribution of organs for transplantation.

OROPHARYNX. The part of the throat at the back of the mouth.

ORTHODONTIC TREATMENT. The process of realigning and straightening teeth to correct their appearance and function.

ORTHOGNATHIC SURGERY. Surgery that corrects deformities or malpositioning of the bones in the jaw.

ORTHOPEDIC. Related to the musculoskeletal system, including the bones, joints, muscles, ligaments, and tendons.

ORTHOPEDIC SURGERY. Surgery performed on the bones.

ORTHOPEDICS. The branch of medicine that deals with bones and joints; also referred to as orthopaedics.

ORTHOTIC. A device designed to be inserted into a shoe to help keep the foot in proper alignment, stabilize the heel, support the arch, and distribute body weight more evenly over the foot.

ORTHOTOPIC TRANSPLANTATION. The replacement of a whole diseased liver with a healthy donor liver.

OSMOLALITY. A measurement of urine concentration that depends on the number of particles dissolved in it. Values are expressed as milliosmols per kilogram (mOsm/kg) of water.

OSMOSIS. Passage of a solvent through a membrane from an area of greater concentration to an area of lesser concentration.

OSMOTIC PRESSURE. The pressure in a liquid exerted by chemicals dissolved in it. It forces a balancing of water in proportion to the amount of dissolved chemicals in two compartments separated by a semipermeable membrane.

OSSICLES. The three small bones of the middle ear: the malleus (hammer), the incus (anvil), and the stapes (stirrup). These bones help carry sound from the eardrum to the inner ear.

OSSICULOPLASTY. Surgical insertion of an implant to replace one or more of the ear ossicles; also called ossicular replacement.

OSTEOARTHRITIS. A form of arthritis that occurs mainly in older people and involves the gradual degeneration of the cartilage of the joints.

OSTEOBLASTS. Bone cells that build new bone tissue.

OSTEOCLASTS. Bone cells that break down and remove bone tissue.

OSTEOCONDUCTION. Provision of a scaffold (structure) for the growth of new bone.

OSTEOCYTES. Bone cells that maintain bone tissue.

OSTEOGENESIS. Growth of new bone.

OSTEOINDUCTION. Acceleration of new bone formation by chemical means; also refers to the process of building, healing, and remodeling bone in humans.

OSTEOLYSIS. Dissolution and loss of bone resulting from inflammation.

OSTEOMALACIA. A softening of bones caused by a lack of vitamin D and/or calcium in the diet.

OSTEONECROSIS. Condition resulting from poor blood supply to an area of a bone and causing bone death.

OSTEOPATHY. A system of medicine that uses standard medical and surgical methods of diagnosis and treatment while emphasizing the importance of proper body alignment and manipulative treatment of musculoskeletal disorders.

OSTEOPOROSIS. A condition in which bones decrease in density and become fragile and more likely to break.

OSTEOTOMY. The surgical cutting of bone.

OSTEOTOMY OF THE KNEE. Realignment of the knee, using bone cutting to shift weight bearing from damaged cartilage to healthier cartilage.

OSTIA. A mouth-like opening in a body part.

OSTOMY. A surgical procedure that creates an opening from the inside of the body to the outside, usually to remove body wastes (feces or urine).

OTITIS. Inflammation of the ear, which may be marked by pain, fever, abnormalities of hearing, hearing loss, tinnitus and vertigo.

OTOLARYNGOLOGIST. A doctor who specializes in treating disorders of the ears, nose, and throat.

OTOLOGY. The branch of medicine that deals with the diagnosis and treatment of ear disorders.

OTOSCLEROSIS. Formation of spongy bone around the footplate of the stapes, resulting in conductive hearing loss.

OTOSCOPE. An instrument with a light for examining the internal ear.

OTOSCOPY. Examination of the ear with an otoscope, an instrument designed to evaluate the condition of the ear.

OUTCOMES. Results or consequences of care or treatment.

OUTPATIENT. A patient who has not been admitted to a hospital.

OUTPATIENT PROCEDURE. A procedure (or surgery) that does not require a hospital stay; also known as ambulatory surgery.

OVA. Eggs.

OVARIAN CYST. A fluid-filled cavity on the surface of the ovary; may be malignant (cancerous) or benign.

OVARIES. The reproductive organs of women that are located in the pelvis; egg cells are developed and stored there, and female sex hormones estrogen and progesterone are produced there.

OVEREXPRESSION. Production in abnormally high amounts.

OVULATION. A process in which a mature female egg is released from one of the ovaries (egg-shaped structures located to each side of the uterus) every 28 days.

OXIMETRY. Measuring the degree of oxygen saturation of circulating blood.

OXYGENATION. Saturation with oxygen.

OXYHEMOGLOBIN. Hemoglobin combined with oxygen.

P

PACEMAKER. A surgically implanted electronic device that sends out electrical impulses to regulate a slow or erratic heartbeat.

PACHYMETRY. A test performed to measure the thickness of the cornea. It may be done as part of glaucoma screening or prior to LASIK surgery.

PACU. Post-anesthesia care unit; where the patient is cared for after surgery.

PAIN DISORDER. A psychiatric disorder in which pain in one or more parts of the body is caused or made worse by psychological factors. The lower back is one of the most common sites for pain related to this disorder.

PALATE. The roof of the mouth.

PALLIATIVE. Offering relief of symptoms, but not a cure.

PALLIATIVE CARE. Care that focuses on relieving pain and suffering when recovery is not an option.

PALPATE. To examine by means of touch.

PALPATION. Examination of the body using the sense of touch.

PALPEBRAL FISSURE. Eyelid opening.

PALPITATIONS. Forcible pulsation or pounding of the heart that is perceptible to the patient.

PANCREAS. The organ beneath the stomach that produces digestive juices, insulin, and other hormones.

PANCREAS-AFTER-KIDNEY (PAK) TRANSPLANT. Pancreas transplantation in a recipient who has already had a kidney transplant.

PANCREATICODUODENECTOMY. Removal of all or part of the pancreas along with the duodenum; also known as Whipple's procedure.

PANCREATITIS. Inflammation of the pancreas, either acute (sudden and episodic) or chronic, usually caused by excessive alcohol intake or gallbladder disease.

PANIC DISORDER. An disorder in which people have sudden and intense attacks of anxiety in certain situations.

PAP TEST. The common term for the Papanicolaou test, a simple smear method of removing cervical cells to screen for abnormalities that may indicate cancer or precancerous conditions; also referred to as a Pap smear.

PARACENTESIS. Surgical puncture of the abdominal cavity for the aspiration of peritoneal fluid.

PARALYTIC ILEUS. Disruption of normal muscle contraction within the intestines.

PARAQUAT. A highly toxic restricted-use pesticide. Death following ingestion usually results from multiple organ failure.

PARASITE. An organism that lives on or inside another living organism (host), causing damage to the host.

PARASTOMAL HERNIA. A condition in which a portion of the intestine bulges through a weak area in the abdominal wall near a stoma situated in the digestive tract. Parastomal hernias affect almost 30% of all patients with intestinal ostomies.

PARASYMPATHETIC NERVOUS SYSTEM. The division of the autonomic (involuntary) nervous system that slows heart rate, increases digestive and glandular activity, and relaxes the sphincter muscles that close off body organs.

PARATHYROID GLANDS. Two pairs of smaller glands that lie close to the lower surface of the thyroid gland. They secrete parathyroid hormone, which regulates the body's use of calcium and phosphorus.

PARATHYROID HORMONE (PTH). A hormone that is secreted by the parathyroid glands. Parathyroid hormone is involved in the regulation of calcium levels in the blood.

PARATHYROIDECTOMY. A surgical procedure in which one or more parathyroid glands are removed.

PARENCHYMA. The essential elements of an organ; used as a general term to designate the functional elements of an organ, as opposed to its framework.

PARENTERAL NUTRITIONAL SUPPORT. Intravenous nutrition that bypasses the intestines.

PARESTHESIA. An abnormal touch sensation, such as a prickling or burning feeling, often in the absence of an external cause.

PARIETAL CELLS. Cells of the gastric glands that secrete hydrochloric acid and intrinsic factor.

PARIETAL PERICARDIUM. External or outer layer of the pericardial cavity (part of the membrane that surrounds the heart).

PARKINSON'S DISEASE. A neurological disorder caused by deficiency of dopamine, a neurotransmitter, which is a chemical that assists in transmitting messages between the nerves within the brain. It is characterized by muscle tremor or palsy and rigid movements.

PARONYCHIA. Inflammation of the folds of tissue surrounding the nail.

PARTIAL MASTECTOMY. Segmental mastectomy; removal of only the cancerous breast tissue and some of the surrounding normal tissue.

PARTIAL THROMBOPLASTIN TIME (PTT). A blood test that measures the activity of blood clotting factors, performed to detect disorders of blood clotting or to monitor the effects of anticoagulant therapy; also known as the activated partial thromboplastin time test (aPTT or APTT).

PATELLA. Kneecap; a triangular bone located at the front of the knee.

PATELLECTOMY. Surgical removal of the patella, or kneecap removal.

PATENCY. The state of being open or unblocked.

PATENT. Open.

PATENT DUCTUS ARTERIOSUS. A congenital defect in which the temporary blood vessel connecting the left pulmonary artery to the aorta in the fetus fails to close.

PATERNITY. Refers to the father.

PATHOGEN. A disease-causing organism.

PATHOGENIC. Disease-causing.

PATHOLOGIC. Characterized by disease or the structural and functional changes due to disease.

PATHOLOGIST. A doctor who specializes in the study and diagnosis of disease.

PATIENT SELF-DETERMINATION ACT (PSDA). Federal law that ensures that medical providers offer the option of medical directives to patients and include the documents in their medical records.

PATIENT-CONTROLLED ANALGESIA (PCA). An approach to pain management that allows patients to control the timing of intravenous doses of analgesic drugs. The dose is administered by pressing a button on a pump, which delivers the medication through a tube attached to either an IV or an epidural catheter.

PATIENT-CONTROLLED ANALGESIA PUMP. A pump used to self-administer medication to control pain.

PEAK EXPIRATORY FLOW RATE (PEFR). A test used to measure how fast air can be exhaled from the lungs. PEFR is measured by a small handheld device called a peak flow meter.

PEAK FLOW. Another name for peak expiratory flow rate.

PECTORALIS MINOR. A triangular-shaped muscle in front of (anterior) the axilla.

PECTUS CARINATUM. A chest wall deformity characterized by a protrusion of the sternum.

PECTUS EXCAVATUM. A chest wall deformity in which the chest wall appears sunken.

PEDIATRIC-AGED PATIENT. The pediatric-aged patient encompasses several periods during development. The first four weeks after birth are called the neonatal period. The first year after birth is called infancy, and childhood is from 13 months until puberty (between the ages of 12 and 15 years in girls and 13 and 16 years in boys).

PEDIATRICS. The medical specialty of caring for children.

PEDICLE FLAP. A section of tissue, with its blood supply intact, that is maneuvered to another part of the body; also called an attached flap.

PEDUNCULATED. Referring to a polyp attached to its mucous membrane by a narrow stalk.

PELVIC. Located near the pelvis, the skeletal structure comprised of four bones that encloses the pelvic cavity.

PELVIC INFLAMMATORY DISEASE (PID). Inflammation of the female reproductive organs and associated structures.

PELVIC ORGANS. The organs inside of the body that are located within the confines of the pelvis. These include the bladder and rectum in both sexes, and the uterus, ovaries, and fallopian tubes in females.

PERCUSSION. The thumping or tapping of a part of the body with the fingers for diagnostic purposes.

PERCUTANEOUS. Performed through the skin.

PERCUTANEOUS BIOPSY. A biopsy in which the needle is inserted and the sample removed through the skin.

PERCUTANEOUS TRANSLUMINAL CORONARY ANGIOPLASTY (PTCA). A cardiac intervention in which an artery blocked by plaque is dilated, using a balloon catheter to flatten the plaque and open the vessel; it is also called balloon angioplasty.

PERFORATION. An opening or hole; used in medicine to refer to the rupture or penetration of an organ or other tissue.

PERFUSION. In medicine, the passage of fluid through the lymphatic system or blood vessels to an organ or tissue.

PERFUSION SCAN. A lung scan in which a tracer is injected into a vein in the arm. It travels through the bloodstream and into the lungs to show areas of the lungs that are not receiving enough air or that retain too much air.

PERFUSIONIST. A specially trained team member that operates the extracorporeal circulatory and respiratory equipment known as the cardiopulmonary machine during any medical procedure requiring artificial support of the patient's circulatory or respiratory functions.

PERIAPICAL. Referring to the tissue surrounding the apex of a tooth's root.

PERICARDIAL FRICTION RUB. A crackly, grating, low-pitched sound that is heard when breathing in (inspiration) and out (expiration).

PERICARDIAL TAMPONADE. The collection of blood in the sac surrounding the heart that causes compression.

PERINEAL AREA. The genital area between the vulva and anus in a woman.

PERINEUM. Area between the anus and genitals.

PERIODONTITIS. Generalized disease of the gums in which unremoved calculus has separated the gingiva or gum tissue from the teeth and threatens support ligaments of the teeth and bone.

PERIOPERATIVE. Includes all phases of surgery: preoperative, intraoperative, and postoperative.

PERIPHERAL ARTERIAL DISEASE (PAD). Damage to the arteries outside of the heart, especially narrowing or obstruction of an artery supplying a leg.

PERIPHERAL ARTERIES. Arteries other than those of the heart and brain, especially those that supply the lower body organs and limbs.

PERIPHERAL ENDARTERECTOMY. The surgical removal of fatty deposits, called plaque, from the walls of arteries other than those of the heart and brain.

PERIPHERAL NERVES. The nerves outside of the brain and spinal cord.

PERIPHERAL NERVOUS SYSTEM (PNS). The part of the nervous system that consists of the nerves outside of the brain and spinal cord.

PERIPHERAL STEM CELLS. Stem cells that are taken directly from circulating blood and used for transplantation. Stem cells are more concentrated in the bone marrow, but they can also be extracted from the bloodstream.

PERIPHERAL VISION. The outer portion of the visual field.

PERIPHERALLY INSERTED CENTRAL CATHETER (PICC). A vascular access device that is inserted through an arm or leg vein to the inferior or superior vena cava near the heart.

PERISTALSIS. The rhythmic contractions that move material through the digestive system.

PERITONEAL. Abdominal.

PERITONEAL CAVITY. The space enclosed by the peritoneum.

PERITONEUM. The membrane lining the walls of the abdominal and pelvic cavities and enclosing their organs.

PERITONITIS. Inflammation of the membrane lining the abdominal cavity. It causes abdominal pain and tenderness, constipation, vomiting, and fever.

PERIURETHRAL. Surrounding the urethra.

PERSONAL CARE ATTENDANT. An employee hired either through a healthcare facility, home care agency, or private agency to assist a patient in performing activities of daily living (ADLs).

PERSONAL HEALTH RECORD (PHR). A commercial online system for creating a personal medical history.

PERSONAL PROTECTIVE EQUIPMENT (PPE). Protective equipment such as goggles, masks, shields, waterproof aprons, gowns, and gloves.

PERSONALITY DISORDER. Group of behavioral disorders characterized by maladaptive patterns of behavior, social interactions, or lifestyles that deviate from the healthy normal. Personality disorders are distinct from psychotic disorders.

PH. A value that indicates the balance between acid and base in a given substance.

PHACOEMULSIFICATION. A method of extracapsular cataract extraction in which the lens is broken apart by ultrasound energy and the fragments are removed by suction.

PHACOLYTIC GLAUCOMA. Type of glaucoma causing dissolution of the lens.

PHAGOCYTOSIS. A process by which a white blood cell envelopes and digests debris and microorganisms to remove them from the blood.

PHARMACOLOGIC CARDIOVERSION. The use of medications to restore normal heart rhythm; also called chemical cardioversion.

PHARMACOLOGICAL. Referring to therapy that relies on drugs.

PHARMACOLOGIST. A specialist who studies the effects of drugs and other substances.

PHARYNX. The cavity at the back of the mouth that opens into the esophagus.

PHENOTYPE. A trait produced by a gene.

PHENYLKETONURIA (PKU). A genetic disorder in which the body lacks an important enzyme. If untreated, the disorder can lead to brain damage and intellectual disability.

PHEOCHROMOCYTOMA. A tumor of specialized cells of the adrenal gland.

PHILTRAL DIMPLE. The skin or depression below the nose, extending to the upper lip in the midline.

PHILTRAL UNITS. A collection of anatomical landmarks, including the philtral dimple (the skin or depression below the nose extending to the upper lip in the midline), philtral columns (the skin columns on the right and left side of the philtral dimple), philtral tubercle (in the midline of the upper lip), white roll (a linear tissue prominence that joins the upper lip portion of the philtral dimple and vermilion—the dark pink tissue that makes up the lip), and nasal columella (the outer portion of the nose that divides the nostrils).

PHIMOSIS. A tightening of the foreskin that may close the opening of the penis.

PHLEBECTOMY. Surgical removal of a vein or part of a vein.

PHLEBITIS. Inflammation of a vein.

PHLEBOLOGIST. A doctor who specializes in treating spider veins, varicose veins, and associated disorders.

PHLEBOLOGY. The study of veins, their disorders, and their treatments. A phlebologist is a doctor who specializes in treating spider veins, varicose veins, and associated disorders.

PHLEBOTOMIST. A healthcare professional trained to obtain samples of blood.

PHLEGMASIA CERULEA DOLENS (PCD). A rare, very severe complication of a blood clot.

PHOBIA. An intense, abnormal, or illogical fear of something specific, such as heights or open spaces.

PHOTOCOAGULATION. Condensation of material by laser.

PHOTODYNAMIC THERAPY. A cancer treatment that uses a drug that is activated by exposure to light. When the drug is exposed to light, the cancer cells are killed.

PHOTOMULTIPLIER. A device that is designed to be extremely sensitive to electromagnetic radiation, especially within the ultraviolet, visible, and near-infrared ranges of the electromagnetic spectrum.

PHYSICAL ACTIVITY. Any activity that involves moving the body and that burns calories. Baseline physical activity refers to activities performed in daily life (e.g., walking, standing, and lifting everyday objects), while health-enhancing physical activity refers to any additional activity beyond everyday tasks (e.g., running, cycling, swimming, yoga).

PHYSICAL FITNESS. The combination of muscle strength and cardiovascular health usually attributed to regular exercise and good nutrition.

PHYSIOLOGICAL. Pertaining to the normal vital life functions of a living organism.

PHYSIOLOGICAL STATE. The status of the normal vital life functions of a living organism.

PILES. Another name for hemorrhoids.

PILOCARPINE. Drug used to treat glaucoma.

PINNA. Another name for the auricle, the visible portion of the external ear.

PISTON. The plunger that slides up and down inside the barrel of a syringe.

PITUITARY GLAND. A small, oval-shaped endocrine gland situated at the base of the brain in the fossa (depression) of the sphenoid bone. Its overall role is to regulate growth and metabolism. The gland is divided into the posterior and anterior pituitary, each responsible for the production of its own unique hormones.

PITUITARY TUMORS. Tumors found in the pituitary gland. Most pituitary tumors are benign, meaning that they grow very slowly and do not spread to other parts of the body.

PLACEBO EFFECT. A term used to describe a patient's response to a treatment (whether conventional or alternative) that is affected by the patient's expectations (whether positive or negative).

PLACENTA. The organ that provides oxygen and nutrition from the mother to the fetus during pregnancy. The placenta is attached to the wall of the uterus and leads to the fetus via the umbilical cord.

PLACENTA PREVIA. A placenta that partially or totally covers the cervix, preventing vaginal delivery.

PLACENTAL ABRUPTION. Separation of the placenta from the uterine wall, cutting off blood flow to the fetus.

PLANTAR FASCIITIS. An inflammation of the fascia on the bottom of the foot.

PLAQUE. A collection of wax-like fatty deposits on the insides of artery walls; alternately, a sticky film of saliva, food particles, and bacteria that attaches to the tooth surface and causes decay.

PLASMA. The fluid portion of blood, as distinguished from blood cells. Plasma constitutes about 55% of blood volume.

PLASMA CELLS. White blood cells in the blood and bone marrow that are formed from B lymphocytes and that produce antibodies.

PLASMAPHERESIS. A procedure in which blood is withdrawn from a patient's circulation, the plasma is separated from the blood cells, and the cells are returned to the patient's bloodstream. It may be used alongside immunosuppressive drugs in the treatment of autoimmune disorders.

PLATELETS. Disk-shaped structures found in blood that play an active role in blood clotting; also known as thrombocytes.

PLETHYSMOGRAPHY. A test in which a patient sits inside a booth called a plethysmograph and breathes through a mouthpiece, while pressure and air flow measurements are collected to measure the total lung volume.

PLEURA. The membrane that covers the outer layer of the lungs and adjoining structures and the inner chest wall.

PLEURAL CAVITY. The space between the lungs and the chest wall.

PLEURAL SPACE. The space between the layers of the pleura—the membrane lining the lungs and chest wall.

PLUMBISM. Another word for lead poisoning; it is derived from *plumbum*, the Latin word for lead.

PNEUMATIC RETINOPEXY. Reattachment of a detached retina using an injected gas bubble to hold the retina against the back of the eye.

PNEUMOBELT. A mechanical ventilator that applies oscillating pressure to the chest to force air in and out of the lungs.

PNEUMOCYSTIS CARINII PNEUMONIA (PCP). A lung infection that affects people with weakened immune systems.

PNEUMONIA. A disease in which the lungs become inflamed. Pneumonia may be caused by bacteria, viruses, or other organisms, or by physical or chemical irritants.

PNEUMOPERITONEUM. The presence of air or gas in a cavity.

PNEUMOTHORAX. A collection of air or gas in the chest cavity that can cause lung collapse.

PODIATRIST. A physician who specializes in the care and treatment of the foot.

POINT-OF-SERVICE (POS) PLAN. A managed care plan that includes aspects of both health maintenance organizations and preferred provider organizations.

POLAND SYNDROME. A condition associated with chest wall deformities in which varying degrees of underdevelopment of one side of the chest and arm may occur.

POLARITY THERAPY. A form of energy therapy developed in the United States that uses a combination of gentle touch, bodywork, and dietary recommendations to correct imbalances or remove blockages in the client's energy field.

POLIOMYELITIS. Disorder caused by a viral infection (poliovirus) that can affect the whole body, including muscles and nerves.

POLYCYSTIC KIDNEY DISEASE. A hereditary kidney disease that causes fluid- or blood-filled pouches of tissue called cysts to form on the tubules of the kidneys. These cysts impair normal kidney function.

POLYCYTHEMIA. A condition in which the amount of red blood cells are increased in the blood.

POLYCYTHEMIA VERA. A disease in which the bone marrow makes too many blood cells.

POLYDACTYLY. A developmental abnormality characterized by an extra digit on the hand or foot.

POLYGLYCOLIC ACID (PGA). A polyester compound used to make bioabsorbable sutures and staples. It is also used in tissue engineering.

POLYMERASE CHAIN REACTION (PCR). A test performed to evaluate false-negative results to the ELISA and Western blot tests. In PCR testing, numerous copies of a gene are made by separating the two strands of DNA containing the gene segment, marking its location, using DNA polymerase to make a copy, and then continuously replicating the copies. The amplification of gene sequences that are associated with HIV allows for detection of the virus by this method.

POLYMYALGIA RHEUMATICA. A condition with symptoms of achiness and stiffness, primarily striking older adults.

POLYP. Any mass of tissue that grows out of a mucous membrane in the digestive tract, uterus, or elsewhere in the body.

POLYPECTOMY. The removal of polyps in the colon, usually during colonoscopy or flexible sigmoidoscopy.

POLYPECTOMY SNARE. A wire loop device that is slipped over a polyp and cuts through the stalk of the polyp when the loop is closed.

POLYPHARMACY. The use of five or more prescription medications on a regular basis, which includes about 40% of adults over 65. The term is sometimes used to refer to the use of unnecessary medications.

POLYPOSIS. A condition in which numerous polyps form on a hollow internal organ, most often in the intestines.

POLYSOMNOGRAPHY. A test administered in a sleep laboratory to analyze heart rate, blood circulation, muscle movement, brain waves, and breathing patterns during sleep.

POLYSYNDACTYLY. Condition involving both webbing and the presence of an extra number of fingers or toes.

POLYTRAUMA. Traumatic injury to multiple organs or organ systems.

PORPHYRIAS. A group of disorders involving heme biosynthesis, characterized by excessive excretion of porphyrins. The porphyrias may be either inherited or acquired (usually from the effects of certain chemical agents).

PORTABLE CHEST X-RAY. An x-ray procedure taken with equipment that can be brought to the patient. The resulting radiographs may not be as high in quality as stationary x-ray radiographs, but they allow a technologist to come to the patient.

PORTAL. An entrance or a means of entrance.

PORTAL HYPERTENSION. Abnormally high pressure within the portal vein.

PORTAL VEIN. The main vessel that carries blood to the liver.

PORTAL VEIN THROMBOSIS. The development of a blood clot in the vein that brings blood into the liver. Untreated portal vein thrombosis causes portal hypertension.

POSITRON. A positively charged particle; also called an "antielectron," the antimatter counterpart of the electron.

POSITRON EMISSION TOMOGRAPHY (PET). A method of medical imaging capable of displaying the metabolic activity of organs; often used to find cancerous cells, which are more active than normal cells.

POSTERIOR CAPSULE OPACIFICATION (PCO). This refers to the opacities that form on the back of the lens capsule after cataract removal or extraction. It is synonymous with a secondary cataract.

POSTERIOR CHAMBER. The part of the eye located behind the lens that includes the retina, where the photoreceptors are located.

POSTMORTEM. After death.

POSTOPERATIVE. After surgery.

POSTOPERATIVE CARE. Medical care and support required after surgery to promote healing and recovery.

POSTOPERATIVE COGNITIVE DYSFUNCTION (POCD). A condition in which the patient has long-term problems with loss of memory, learning, and the ability to concentrate after surgery.

POSTOPERATIVE DELIRIUM. A condition in which some elderly patients become confused and disoriented for up to a week after surgery.

POST-THROMBOTIC SYNDROME (PTS). Leg swelling, discoloration, and ulcers resulting from deep-vein thrombosis.

POST-TRAUMATIC STRESS DISORDER (PTSD). A psychological response to a highly stressful event; typically characterized by depression, anxiety, flashbacks, nightmares, and avoidance of reminders of the traumatic experience.

POTASSIUM. A mineral found in whole grains, meat, legumes, and some fruits and vegetables. Potassium is important for many body processes, including proper functioning of nerves and muscles.

POUCHING SYSTEM. A medical device consisting of a pouch or bag for the collection of digestive wastes or urine that is held against the skin surrounding a stoma by an adhesive skin barrier.

PREECLAMPSIA. A pregnancy-related condition that causes high blood pressure and swelling.

PREFERRED PROVIDER ORGANIZATIONS (PPOS). Private health insurance plans that require beneficiaries to select healthcare providers from a list approved by the insurance company.

PREGNANCY CATEGORY. A system of classifying drugs according to their established risks for use during pregnancy.

PREGNANCY CATEGORY A. Controlled human studies have demonstrated no fetal risk.

PREGNANCY CATEGORY B. Animal studies indicate no fetal risk but there are no human studies, or adverse effects occur in animals but not in well-controlled human studies.

PREGNANCY CATEGORY C. No adequate human or animal studies exist, or adverse fetal effects occur in animal studies but there is no available human data.

PREGNANCY CATEGORY D. Evidence of fetal risk, but benefits outweigh risks.

PREGNANCY CATEGORY X. Evidence of fetal risk, and risks outweigh any benefits.

PREMIUM. The amount paid by an insurance policyholder for insurance coverage, usually on a monthly basis.

PREOPERATIVE. Before surgery.

PREPUCE. A fold like the foreskin that covers the clitoris; another name for foreskin.

PRESBYOPIA. A condition affecting people over the age of 40 where it becomes difficult to focus on near objects due to age-related hardening of the lens of the eye.

PRESCRIPTION DRUG "DONUT HOLE." The coverage gap in Medicare Part D that requires participants to pay all of their annual prescription drug costs, which fall between approximately $3,000 and $5,000 annually.

PRESSURE ULCER. Also known as a decubitus ulcer, pressure ulcers are open wounds that form whenever prolonged pressure is applied to skin covering bony outcrops of the body. Patients who are bedridden are at risk of developing pressure ulcers, commonly known as bedsores.

PREVALENCE. The number of cases of a disease or disorder that are present in a given population at a specific time.

PRIMARY CARE CASE MANAGEMENT (PCCM). A fee-for-service managed care plan in which Medicaid contracts with primary care providers to coordinate and monitor patient care.

PRIMARY CARE PHYSICIAN (PCP). A family practitioner, pediatrician, internist, or gynecologist who takes care of a patient's routine medical needs and refers him or her to a surgeon or other specialist when necessary.

PRIMARY SNORING. Simple snoring; snoring that is not interrupted by episodes of breathing cessation.

PRIMARY TEETH. A child's first set of teeth, sometimes called baby teeth.

PROBLEM-INTERVENTION-EVALUATION (PIE). A type of medical chart that focuses on a specific problem and its treatments.

PROCTOSIGMOIDOSCOPY. A visual examination of the rectum and sigmoid colon using a sigmoidoscope; also known as sigmoidoscopy.

PROLAPSE. A condition in which an organ falls or slips out of place.

PROLAPSED CORD. Pushing of the umbilical cord into the vagina ahead of the baby, cutting off its blood flow.

PROLAPSED UTERUS. A uterus that has slipped out of place, sometimes protruding down through the vagina.

PROLIFERATION. The rapid growth stage of a hemangioma.

PROLOTHERAPY. A technique for stimulating collagen growth in injured tissues by the injection of glycerin or dextrose.

PRONATION. The nature of the foot to turn in toward the center of the body when walking or running.

PROPHYLACTIC. Intended to prevent or protect against disease.

PROPHYLACTIC ANTIEMESIS. The administration of an antiemetic (antinausea drug) prior to recovery from anesthesia in order to prevent postoperative nausea and vomiting. The antiemetic may be administered before surgery, during surgery, or shortly before the patient awakens from anesthesia.

PROPHYLACTIC MASTECTOMY. Removal of a healthy breast to prevent future breast cancer.

PROPHYLAXIS. A measure designed to preserve health and/or prevent the spread of disease.

PROPRIETARY HOSPITALS. Hospitals owned by private entities (mostly corporations) that are intended to make a profit as well as provide medical services. Most hospitals in health maintenance organizations and health networks are proprietary institutions.

PROSTAGLANDINS. Compounds derived from fatty acids and produced in the body that are involved in a number of body functions, including the regulation of inflammation, contraction or relaxation of smooth muscle tissues, and contraction of uterine muscle tissue.

PROSTATE GLAND. A gland in the male that surrounds the neck of the bladder and urethra. The prostate contributes to the seminal fluid.

PROSTATECTOMY. Partial or complete removal of the prostate.

PROSTATITIS. Inflammation of the prostate gland that may be accompanied by discomfort, pain, frequent urination, infrequent urination, and sometimes fever.

PROSTHESIS. An artificial device to replace a missing body part.

PROSTHETIC. A custom-built artificial limb or other body part.

PROSTHETIC TOOTH. An artificial tooth.

PROTECTED HEALTH INFORMATION (PHI). Information that is protected by law that relates to an individual's past, present, or future physical or mental health, as well as conditions, treatments, services, and payments that can be traced to an identifiable individual.

PROTEIN. A polypeptide chain or a chain of amino acids linked together.

PROTHROMBIN. A protein in blood plasma that is converted to thrombin during the clotting process.

PROTHROMBIN TEST. A common test to measure the amount of time it takes for a patient's blood to clot, measured in seconds.

PROTHROMBIN TIME (PT). A blood test performed to measure the clotting tendency of blood.

PROTOCOL. A set of guidelines; a treatment plan.

PROTOZOA (SINGULAR, PROTOZOAN). Single-celled eukaryotic organisms, some of which cause disease in humans.

PROXY. A person authorized or empowered to act on behalf of another; also, the document or written authorization appointing that person.

PRUNE BELLY SYNDROME (PBS). A genetic disorder associated with abnormalities of human chromosomes 18 and 21. Male infants with PBS often have cryptorchidism (undescended testes) along with other defects of the genitals and urinary tract. PBS is also known as triad syndrome and Eagle-Barrett syndrome.

PSEUDOANEURYSM. A dilation of a blood vessel that resembles an aneurysm.

PSEUDOPHAKIC BULLOUS KERATOPATHY (PBK). Painful swelling of the cornea occasionally occurring after surgery to implant an artificial lens in place of a lens affected by cataracts.

PSORIASIS. A skin disease characterized by itchy, scaly, red patches on the skin.

PSYCHIATRIC NURSING. The nursing specialty concerned with the prevention and treatment of mental disorders and their consequences.

PSYCHIATRIST. A medical doctor (MD) who specializes in the treatment of mental health problems and can prescribe medication.

PSYCHOACTIVE. Affecting the mind or behavior.

PSYCHOLOGIST. A health care professional (PsyD or PhD) who is not a medical doctor but can evaluate or provide counseling for patients with mental health issues.

PSYCHOSIS. A general psychiatric term for a condition in which the patient loses touch with reality; symptoms include hallucinations, delusions, personality changes, and disordered thinking. Psychosis is usually one feature of an overarching disorder, not a disorder in itself.

PSYLLIUM. The seeds of the fleawort plant, taken with water to produce a bland, jelly-like bulk that helps to move waste products through the digestive tract and prevent constipation.

PSYLLIUM HYDROPHILIC MUCILLOID. A plant material contained in some laxatives.

PTOSIS. The medical term for drooping of the upper eyelid.

PUBIS. The front portion of the pelvis located in the anterior abdomen.

PUBOCERVICAL FASCIA. Fibrous tissue that separates the vagina and the bladder.

PUBOVAGINAL SLING. A general term for a procedure that places a sling around the urethra without the use of tension between the sling and the urethra; often referred to as the Tension-Free Vaginal Tape (TVT) procedure.

PULMONARY. Referring to the respiratory system.

PULMONARY ARTERY. The major artery that carries blood from the right ventricle of the heart to the lungs.

PULMONARY DISEASE. Any disease involving the lungs.

PULMONARY EMBOLISM. Potentially life-threatening blockage of a pulmonary artery by fat, air, or a blood clot that originated elsewhere in the body. Symptoms include acute shortness of breath and sudden chest pain.

PULMONARY FIBROSIS. Chronic inflammation and progressive formation of fibrous tissue in the pulmonary alveolar walls with steadily progressive shortness of breath, resulting in death from lack of oxygen or heart failure.

PULMONARY FUNCTION TESTS. A series of tests that measures how well air is moving in and out of the lungs and the blood's ability to carry oxygen.

PULMONARY HYGIENE. A set of methods used to clear secretions from the airway and lungs or to prevent their buildup.

PULMONARY HYPERTENSION. Increased blood pressure in the blood vessels of the lungs.

PULMONARY HYPOPLASIA. Underdeveloped lungs.

PULMONARY NODULE. A lesion surrounded by normal lung tissue. Nodules may be caused by bacteria, fungi, or a tumor (benign or cancerous).

PULMONARY REHABILITATION. A program that helps patients learn how to breathe easier and improve their quality of life. Pulmonary rehabilitation includes treatment, exercise training, education, and counseling.

PULMONARY VALVE. The heart valve that separates the right ventricle and the opening into the pulmonary artery.

PULMONARY VEIN ISOLATION. A surgical procedure used to treat atrial fibrillation (irregular heartbeat). During the procedure, a radio frequency probe, microwave probe, or cryoprobe is inserted and used to create lesion lines in the heart to interrupt the conduction of abnormal impulses.

PULMONOLOGIST. A physician who specializes in caring for people with lung diseases and breathing problems.

PULP. The soft, innermost part of a tooth, containing blood and lymph vessels and nerves.

PULP CHAMBER. The area within the tooth occupied by dental pulp.

PULPITIS. Inflammation of the pulp of a tooth involving the blood vessels and nerves.

PULSE OXIMETRY. A noninvasive test in which a device that clips onto the finger measures the oxygen level in the blood.

PULSUS PARADOXUS. A variation of the systolic pressure with respiration (diminished systolic pressure with inspiration and increased pressure with expiration).

PUNCH GRAFTING. A method of treating a deep scar involving excision of the damaged area, followed by the suturing of a similarly shaped punch of skin that is often taken from behind the ear.

PUPIL. The black circular opening at the center of the iris that regulates the amount of light that enters the eye.

PURSE-STRING CLOSURE. A technique used to close circular or irregularly shaped wounds that involves threading the suture through the edges of the wound and pulling it taut, bringing the edges together.

PURULENT. Containing pus.

PYLORIC SPHINCTER. A broad band of muscle in the pylorus valve at the bottom end of the stomach.

PYLOROPLASTY. Widening of the pyloric canal and any adjacent duodenal structure by means of a longitudinal incision.

PYLORUS. The area that controls food passage from the stomach to the first part of the small intestine (duodenum).

PYODERMA. A pus-containing bacterial skin infection.

PYREXIA. A temperature of 101°F (38.3°C) or higher in an infant younger than three months or above 102°F (38.9°C) for older children and adults.

Q

QI. In traditional Chinese medicine, the life force or energy flow within all living creatures.

QIGONG. A traditional Chinese practice that combines breathing exercises, movement, and focused awareness. It is sometimes classified as a martial art.

QRST COMPLEX. The combined waves of an electrocardiogram for monitoring the heart.

Q-SWITCHED LASER (QSL). The type of laser generally used for tattoo removal.

QUADRANTECTOMY. Removal of a quadrant, or about a quarter, of the breast.

QUADRICEPS MUSCLES. A set of four muscles on each leg located at the front of the thigh. The quadriceps straighten the knee and are used every time a person takes a step.

QUALITY MEASURES. Occurrences that are used to determine hospital quality scores, such as patient injuries, medication errors, and complication rates.

QUINOLONES. A group of synthetic antibacterial drugs originally derived from quinine.

R

RADIAL. Star-shaped or radiating out from a central point; used in medicine to describe the scar-folds that results from a purse-string closure, and also to refer to the lower arm.

RADIAL ARTERY. An artery located in the arm and used for bypass grafts.

RADIATION THERAPY. A cancer treatment that uses high-energy x-rays or other types of radiation to kill cancer cells.

RADICAL MASTECTOMY. Removal of the breast, chest muscles, axillary lymph nodes, and associated skin and subcutaneous tissue.

RADIO WAVES. Electromagnetic energy of the frequency range corresponding to that used in radio communications, usually 10,000–300,000,000,000 cycles per second. Radio waves are the same as visible light, x-rays, and all other types of electromagnetic radiation, but are of a higher frequency.

RADIOACTIVE. Relating to radiation emitted by certain substances.

RADIOFREQUENCY ABLATION. A procedure in which radiofrequency waves are used to destroy blood vessels and tissues.

RADIOGRAPH. The actual picture or film produced by an x-ray study.

RADIOGRAPHICALLY DENSE. An abundance of glandular tissue that results in diminished anatomic detail on a mammogram.

RADIOIMAGING. The process of using a radioactively labeled compound to visualize specific types of body tissue.

RADIOIMMUNOASSAY. A method that uses a radio-isotope label in an immunoassay.

RADIOISOTOPE. A radioactive, or radiation-emitting, form of an element.

RADIOLOGIC EXAMS. The use of radiation or other imaging methods to find signs of cancer.

RADIOLOGIST. A medical doctor specially trained in radiology (x-ray) interpretation and its use in the diagnosis of diseases and injuries.

RADIONUCLIDE. An atom with an unstable nucleus that emits gamma rays during the process of its radioactive decay.

RADIOPHARMACEUTICAL. A radioactive drug.

RADIOSURGERY. Surgery that uses ionizing radiation to destroy tissue rather than a surgical incision.

RADIOTHERAPY. The treatment of disease with high-energy radiation, such as x-rays or gamma rays.

RADIUS. The bone of the forearm that extends from the lateral side of the elbow to the thumb side of the wrist. It is the shorter of the two bones in the forearm.

RANGE OF MOTION. The normal extent of movement (flexion and extension) of a joint.

RASMUSSEN SYNDROME. A progressive neurological disease in children that manifests as seizures, language impairment, and intellectual disability. Researchers believe Rasmussen syndrome is an autoimmune disease.

RAYNAUD'S DISEASE. A disease found mainly in young women that causes decreased circulation to the hands and feet.

REAL-TIME ULTRASOUND. A type of ultrasound that takes multiple images over time in order to record movement, allowing observations during the scan (rather than having to wait until after the procedure to look at films).

RECEPTOR. A sensory nerve ending that responds to chemical or other stimuli of various kinds.

RECESSIVE. Referring to a genetic trait expressed only when present on both members of a pair of chromosomes, one inherited from each parent.

RECIPIENT. The person on the receiving end of a transplant or blood transfusion.

RECTAL. Pertaining to the rectum.

RECTUM. The last part of the large intestine (colon) that connects to the anus.

RECTUS MUSCLES. The muscles responsible for movement of the eye.

RECURRENT LARYNGEAL NERVE. A nerve that lies very near the parathyroid glands and serves the larynx or voice box.

RECURRENT ULCER. Stomach ulcers that return after apparently complete healing. These ulcers appear to be caused by *Helicobacter pylori* infections and can generally be successfully treated with a combination of antibiotics and gastric acid reducing compounds, particularly the proton pump inhibitors.

RED BLOOD CELLS. Cells that carry hemoglobin (the molecule that transports oxygen) and help remove wastes from tissues throughout the body; also known as erythrocytes.

RED CELL DISTRIBUTION WIDTH (RDW). A measure of the variation in the size of red blood cells.

REDUCTION. The correction of a hernia, fracture, or dislocation.

REFERRAL. The process of directing a patient to a specialist for further diagnostic evaluation or treatment.

REFLEX. An automatic response to a stimulus.

REFLUX. Backflow; also called regurgitation.

REFRACTION. The bending of light rays as they pass from one medium through another. Used to describe the action of the cornea and lens on light rays as they enter they eye; also used to describe the determination and measurement of the eye's focusing system by an optometrist or ophthalmologist.

REFRACTIVE ERROR. The inability of the eye to properly focus light due to an irregularly shaped cornea, resulting in blurry vision, nearsightedness, farsightedness, or astigmatism.

REGENERATIVE MEDICINE. A new branch of medicine that investigates ways to restore damaged tissues or organs by replacing them with new ones derived from stem cells or by stimulating the body's own repair mechanisms to heal damaged organs.

REGIONAL ANESTHESIA. Blocking of specific nerve pathways through the injection of an anesthetic agent into a specific area of the body. Under regional anesthesia, the patient remains awake.

REGISTERED NURSE. A graduate nurse who has passed a state nursing board examination and been registered and licensed to practice nursing.

REIKI. A spiritual practice that developed in Japan in the 1920s that is considered a form of energy therapy.

Reiki practitioners believe that they can convey healing energy to others through stylized hand positions that can be placed on or near the patient.

REJECTION. An immune response that occurs when a transplanted organ or other type of tissue is viewed as a foreign substance by the body. If left untreated, rejection can lead to organ failure and even death.

REMISSION. Disappearance of the signs and symptoms of a disease. A remission can be temporary or permanent.

RENAL ARTERY ANEURYSM. An aneurysm relating to, involving, or located in the region of the kidneys.

RENAL CELL CARCINOMA. Cancer of the kidney.

REOPERATION. Repeat of a surgical procedure; may be required for a variety of reasons, such as surgical failure, replacement of failed component parts, or treatment of progressive disease.

REPERFUSION INJURY. Damage to tissues and organs caused when blood flow returns to a body part after a period of ischemia (lack of blood flow).

REPERFUSION THERAPY. Restoration of blood flow to an organ or tissue.

REPLANTATION. The medical term for the reattachment of an amputated digit.

RESCUE ANTIEMESIS. The administration of an antiemetic (antinausea) drug after a patient develops postoperative nausea and vomiting.

RESECTABLE. Referring to part or all of an organ that can be removed by surgery.

RESECTION. Surgical removal of all or part of an organ or tissue.

RESIDENCY TRAINING. A five-year period of additional training that follows completion of medical school.

RESIDUAL VOLUME. The volume of air remaining in the lungs, measured after a maximum expiration.

RESISTANT INFECTIONS. Infections that are not cured by standard antibiotic treatment.

RESISTANT ORGANISMS. Organisms that are difficult to eradicate with antibiotics.

RESORBED. Absorbed by the body after lack of function.

RESPIRATION. The exchange of gases between red blood cells and the atmosphere; breathing.

RESPIRATOR. Ventilator; a device for maintaining artificial respiration.

RESPIRATORY. Referring to breathing in and breathing out, and the function of the lungs.

RESPIRATORY ACIDOSIS. A condition in which an abnormal exchange of oxygen and carbon dioxide in the lungs results in too much carbon dioxide being accumulated, with a resultant drop in the blood pH (toward acidity).

RESPIRATORY ALKALOSIS. A condition in which an abnormal exchange of oxygen and carbon dioxide in the lungs results in the exhalation of too much carbon dioxide and a resultant rise in the blood pH (toward alkalinity).

RESPIRATORY ARREST. Cessation of breathing due to failure of the lungs to contract.

RESPIRATORY DEPRESSION. Decreased breathing rate (number of breaths per minute) and depth (how much air is inhaled with each breath).

RESPIRATORY FAILURE. The sudden inability of the lungs to provide normal oxygen delivery or normal carbon dioxide removal.

RESPIRATORY FUNCTION. The ability of the breathing structures of the body, including the lungs, to function.

RESPIRATORY INFECTIONS. Infections that relate to or affect respiration or breathing.

RESPIRATORY THERAPIST. A healthcare professional who specializes in assessing, treating, and educating people with lung diseases.

RESPIRATORY THERAPY. The department of any healthcare facility or agency that provides treatment to patients to maintain or improve their breathing function.

RESTENOSIS. The repeated narrowing of blood vessels.

RESTRAINT. A physical device or medication designed to restrict a person's movement.

RESTRICTIVE SURGERY. A type of bariatric surgery that works by limiting the amount of food that the stomach can hold.

RESUSCITATION. Revival after apparent death.

RETINA. The light-sensing tissue within the eye that sends signals to the brain in order to generate a visual image.

RETINAL DETACHMENT (RD). A serious vision disorder in which the light-detecting layer of cells inside the eye (retina) is separated from its normal support tissue and no longer functions properly.

RETINOBLASTOMA. Malignant (cancerous) tumor of the retina.

RETINOPATHY. Disease or damage to the retina of the eye.

RETINOPATHY OF PREMATURITY (ROP). A disorder that occurs in premature infants in which blood vessels in the eye continue to grow in an abnormal pattern after delivery. It can lead to retinal detachment and blindness. ROP is also known as retrolental fibroplasia.

RETINOSCOPE. An instrument for determining the state of refraction of the eye by illuminating the retina with a mirror.

RETRACTION. A condition in which a stoma sinks inward to become level with the skin surface or falls completely below the surface.

RETRACTOR. An instrument used during surgery to hold an incision open and pull back underlying layers of tissue.

RETROBULBAR HEMATOMA. A rare complication of blepharoplasty (eyelid surgery), in which a pocket of blood forms behind the eyeball.

RETROGRADE PYELOGRAM. X-ray of the kidneys, ureters, and bladder, obtained via retrograde pyelography.

RETROGRADE PYELOGRAPHY. A test in which dye is injected through a catheter into the ureter to make the lining of the bladder, ureters, and kidneys easier to see on x-rays.

RETROPUBIC URETHROPEXY. A generic term for the Burch procedure and its variants, which treat mild stress incontinence by stabilizing the urethra with retropubic surgery.

RETROVIRUS. A virus that contains a unique enzyme called reverse transcriptase that allows it to replicate within new host cells.

REVASCULARIZATION. Restoring normal blood flow (circulation) in the body's vascular (veins and arteries) system.

REYE'S SYNDROME. A life-threatening disease that affects the liver and the brain and sometimes occurs after a viral infection, such as flu or chickenpox. Children or teenagers who are given aspirin for flu or chickenpox are at increased risk of developing Reye's syndrome.

RH (RHESUS) FACTOR. An antigen present in the red blood cells of 85% of humans. A person with Rh factor is Rh positive (Rh+); a person without it is Rh negative

(Rh-). The Rh factor was first identified in the blood of a rhesus monkey.

RH BLOOD TYPE. Blood type based on the presence or absence of the D antigen on the red blood cells. There are, however, other antigens in the Rh system.

RH IMMUNE GLOBULIN (RHOGAM). A vaccine that must be given to a woman after an abortion, miscarriage, or prenatal tests during which she may have been exposed to blood from the fetus, in order to prevent sensitization to the Rh factor. If a woman has been sensitized to the Rh factor, subsequent pregnancies may result in significant complications in the developing fetus.

RH NEGATIVE. A condition in which the red blood cells do not possess the Rh factor, which consists of genetically determined antigens in red blood cells that produce immune responses. If an Rh-negative woman is pregnant with an Rh-positive fetus, her body will produce antibodies against the fetus's blood, causing a disease known as Rh disease.

RHABDOMYOLYSIS. The rapid breakdown of muscle tissue.

RHEUMATIC CARDITIS. Inflammation of the heart muscle associated with acute rheumatic fever.

RHEUMATIC FEVER. An inflammatory disease that arises as a complication of untreated or inadequately treated strep throat infection. Rheumatic fever can seriously damage the heart valves.

RHEUMATOID ARTHRITIS. A chronic autoimmune disease characterized by inflammation of multiple joints and crippling pain and stiffness.

RHINITIS. Inflammation of the membranes inside the nose.

RHINOPLASTY. Surgery performed to change the shape of the nose.

RHYTIDECTOMY. Wrinkle excision; it is an older, alternative term for a face lift.

RHYTIDES. Very fine wrinkles, often of the face.

RIGHT VENTRICULAR ASSIST DEVICE (RVAD). A ventricular assist device that pumps blood from the right ventricle of the heart to the pulmonary artery, which carries blood to the lungs.

ROOT CANAL. The space within a tooth that runs from the pulp chamber to the tip of the root.

ROOT CANAL TREATMENT. The process of removing diseased or damaged pulp from a tooth, then filling and sealing the pulp chamber and root canals.

ROSACEA. A chronic inflammatory skin condition primarily affecting the skin of the nose, forehead, and cheeks, marked by flushing and reddening of the affected areas.

ROTOBLATION. A nonsurgical technique for treating diseased arteries in which a special catheter with a diamond-coated tip is guided to the point of narrowing in the artery. The catheter tip spins at high speed and grinds away the blockage or plaque on the artery walls.

ROUTINE TEST. A medical test performed on all patients without regard to specific medical conditions.

RUPTURE. The bursting of a blood vessel or organ.

S

SACCADIC. Refers to rapid, irregular eye movement as the eye changes focus from one point to another point.

SACRAL NERVE. The nerve in the lower back region of the spine that controls the need to urinate.

SACROCOCCYGEAL TERATOMA (SCT). A tumor occurring at the base of a fetus's tailbone.

SALICYLATES. A group of drugs that includes aspirin and related compounds, used to relieve pain, reduce inflammation, and lower fever.

SALIVARY GLANDS. Three pairs of glands that secrete into the mouth and aid digestion.

SALPINGECTOMY. The surgical removal of a fallopian tube.

SANITIZE. To reduce the number of microorganisms to safe levels.

SAPHENOUS VEINS. Two large superficial veins in the leg. The greater saphenous vein runs from the foot to the groin area; the short saphenous vein runs from the ankle to the knee.

SARCOIDOSIS. A chronic disease characterized by nodules (small masses of tissue) in the lungs, skin, lymph nodes, and bones, although any tissue or organ in the body may be affected.

SARCOMA. A form of cancer that arises in supportive tissues such as bone, cartilage, fat, or muscle.

SCALING AND ROOT PLANING. A dental procedure to treat gingivitis (gum disease) in which the teeth are scraped inside the gum area and the root of the tooth is planed to dislodge bacterial deposits.

SCAPULA. The shoulder blade; a large, flat, triangular bone that forms the back portion of the shoulder. It articulates with the clavicle (at the acromion process) and the humerus (at the glenoid).

SCAR TISSUE. Scar tissue is the fibrous tissue that replaces normal tissue destroyed by injury or disease.

SCHLEMM'S CANAL. A circular channel located at the point where the sclera of the eye meets the cornea. Schlemm's canal is the primary pathway for aqueous humor to leave the eye.

SCIATICA. Pain in the lower back, buttock, or leg along the course of the sciatic nerve.

SCINTILLATOR. A material that exhibits the property of luminescence (also called "scintillation") when it is excited by ionizing radiation.

SCLERA. The tough white fibrous membrane that forms the outermost covering of the eyeball.

SCLEROSANT. An irritating solution that stops bleeding by hardening the blood or vein it is injected into.

SCLEROSE. To harden or undergo hardening.

SCLEROSING AGENT. A chemical used in sclerotherapy that causes swollen veins to fill with fibrous tissue and close down.

SCLEROTHERAPY. A technique for shrinking hemorrhoids by injecting an irritating chemical into the blood vessels.

SCREEN. In medicine, any test or technique used to detect patients with a high likelihood of having a specific disease, or to detect one or more substances in body fluids or tissues.

SCROTUM. The pouch of skin on the outside of the male body that holds the testes and part of the spermatic cord.

SEBORRHEIC KERATOSIS. A benign skin tumor, usually light to dark brown or black with a warty texture.

SEDATION. A condition of calm or relaxation, brought about by the use of a drug or medication.

SEDATIVE. A type of medication given to calm or relax patients before surgery.

SEDENTARY. Characterized by inactivity and lack of exercise. A sedentary lifestyle is a major risk factor for becoming overweight or obese.

SEIZURE. A sudden attack, spasm, or convulsion.

SENSITIVITY TEST. A test that determines which antibiotics will kill specific bacteria.

SENSORINEURAL DEAFNESS. Hearing loss due to the inability to convert sound from vibration to electrical signals; often involves defects in the function of cochlear hair cells.

SENTINEL LYMPH NODE. The first lymph node or group of nodes to which cancer cells are likely to spread from a primary tumor; also referred to as the sentinel node.

SEPARATION ANXIETY. A fear of being separated from a parent or loved one.

SEPSIS. Refers to both a systemic bacterial infection and the body's inflammatory response to infection.

SEPTAL DEFECTS. Openings in the cardiac septum, the muscular wall separating the right and left sides of the heart. Atrial septal defects are openings between the two upper heart chambers and ventricular septal defects are openings between the two lower heart chambers.

SEPTAL MUCOSA. Mucous membrane of a septum.

SEPTIC ARTHRITIS. A pus-forming bacterial infection of a joint.

SEPTICEMIA. Systemic disease associated with the presence of pathogenic microorganisms or their toxins in the blood.

SEPTUM. A dividing barrier within organs or between tissue (e.g., nasal septum).

SEQUESTRATION. A process in which the spleen withdraws blood cells from the circulation and stores them.

SERIAL X-RAYS. A number of x-rays performed at set times during disease progression or treatment intervals. The radiographs are compared to one another to track changes.

SEROCONVERSION. The change from HIV- negative to HIV-positive status during blood testing.

SEROLOGY. The analysis of the contents and properties of blood serum.

SEROMA. An internal collection of fluid at a surgical site.

SERTOLI CELLS. Cells in the seminiferous tubules of the male testis that nourish the developing spermatozoa; they are named for the Italian physiologist who first described them in 1865.

SERUM. The clear, pale yellow liquid that separates from a clot when blood coagulates.

SERUM SICKNESS. An inflammatory reaction in humans to proteins in serum derived from animal sources that contain polyclonal antibodies. It develops within four to ten days after exposure and is characterized by fever, joint pain, itching, rashes, low blood pressure, an enlarged spleen, and protein and blood in the urine.

SESSILE. Referring to a polyp that lacks a stalk.

SESTAMIBI. A type of radioimaging pharmaceutical compound that has been deemed medically safe to use in the human body; tests done using sestamibi are called sestamibi scans.

SETBACK OTOPLASTY. A surgical procedure done to reduce the size or improve the appearance of large or protruding ears; it is also known as pinback otoplasty.

SETON TUBE. An implant placed in the eye that provides an alternative route for aqueous fluid drainage.

SEX-LINKED GENETIC DISORDER. A disease or disorder caused by a gene mutation located on the X (female) or Y (male) chromosome.

SEXUALLY TRANSMITTED DISEASE (STD). A disease that is passed from one person to another through sexual intercourse or other intimate sexual contact.

SHARPS. Surgical implements with thin cutting edges or a fine point. Sharps include suture needles, scalpel blades, and hypodermic needles.

SHIATSU. A form of massage therapy developed in Japan that emphasizes finger pressure placed on specific body locations rather than stroking or kneading motions. It is based on the concept of qi and the system of meridians found in traditional Chinese medicine.

SHINGLES. A disease caused by the Herpes zoster virus—the same virus that causes chickenpox. Symptoms of shingles include pain and blisters along one nerve, usually on the face, chest, stomach, or back.

SHOCK. A serious condition in which the body's blood circulation and metabolism is severely impaired by injury, pain, blood loss, or certain diseases. The symptoms of shock include a pale complexion, very low blood pressure, and a weak pulse.

SHORT BOWEL SYNDROME. A condition in which digestion and absorption in the small intestine are impaired.

SHOULDER RESECTION ARTHROPLASTY. Surgery performed to repair a shoulder acromioclavicular (AC) joint. The procedure is most commonly recommended for AC joint problems resulting from osteoarthritis or injury.

SHRAPNEL. Fragmentation, shards, or splinters of material thrown out by an explosion.

SHUNT. A passageway that diverts flow of blood or other fluids from one main route to another; often used to drain excess fluid.

SICKLE CELL ANEMIA. An inherited disorder in which red blood cells contain an abnormal form of hemoglobin, the protein that carries oxygen.

SIDEROPHILIN. Another name for transferrin.

SIGMOID COLON. The last third of the intestinal tract that is attached to the rectum.

SIGMOID SINUS. An S-shaped cavity on the inner side of the skull behind the mastoid process.

SIGMOIDOSCOPY. Examination of the rectum and lower colon with a flexible instrument passed through the anus.

SILICOSIS. A progressive disease that results in impairment of lung function and is caused by inhalation of dust containing silica.

SIMPLE OBSTRUCTION. A blockage in the intestine that does not affect the flow of blood to the area.

SIMULATION SCANS. Scans done to help plan a course of treatment; may include computed tomography scans, magnetic resonance imaging, positron emission tomography, and ultrasound. In stereotactic radiosurgery, the scan is done with the patient's head fitted in a stereotactic frame, as it would be during surgery.

SINUS. A narrow hollow in the body extending from an infected area to the surface of the skin.

SINUSITIS. Inflammation of a sinus.

SITZ BATH. A shallow tub or bowl, sometimes mounted above a toilet, that allows the perineum and buttocks to be immersed in circulating water.

SJÖGREN'S SYNDROME. A disease in which the immune system damages and destroys exocrine glands, such as those that produce tears and saliva. Dry eyes and mouth are the usual initial symptoms of this disorder, but other organ systems can also be severely affected over time, including the skin, pancreas, liver, lungs, brain, and kidneys.

SKELETAL TRACTION. Traction in which pins, screws, or wires are surgically connected to bone, to which weights or pulleys are attached to exert force.

SKILLED NURSING FACILITY (SNF). A facility equipped to handle individuals with 24-hour nursing, postoperative recuperation, or complex medical care needs, as well as chronically ill individuals who can no longer live independently. These facilities must be licensed by the state in which they operate to meet standards of safety, staffing, and care procedures.

SKIN FLAP. A piece of skin with underlying tissue that is used in grafting to cover a defect and that receives its blood supply from a source other than the tissue on which it is laid.

SKIN TRACTION. Traction in which weights or other devices are attached to the skin.

SKIN-SPARING MASTECTOMY. Removal of the breast tissue, leaving the skin intact for breast reconstruction.

SLEEP APNEA SYNDROME. A disorder in which a person's breathing temporarily stops at intervals during the night due to obstruction of the upper airway. People with sleep apnea syndrome do not get enough oxygen in their blood and often develop heart problems.

SLIDING GENIOPLASTY. A complex plastic surgery procedure in which the patient's jawbone is cut, moved forward or backward, and repositioned with metal plates and screws.

SLIT LAMP. An instrument that combines a binocular microscope with a high-powered light source that can be focused to shine a thin sheet (slit) of light into the eye.

SMALL BOWEL OBSTRUCTION (SBO). An obstruction of the small intestine that prevents the free passage of material; sometimes caused by postoperative adhesions.

SMALL BUSINESS HEALTH OPTIONS PROGRAM (SHOP). State systems under the Patient Projection and Affordable Care Act (PPACA) through which small businesses can compare and purchase health insurance for their employees.

SMALL INTESTINE. The small intestine consists of three sections: duodenum, jejunum and ileum, all of which are involved in the absorption of nutrients. The total length of the small intestine is approximately 22 ft. (6.5 m).

SOAP NOTES. Subjective, Objective, Assessment, Plan; a common medical chart format that includes subjective statements followed by a key objective statement regarding the patient's status, a clinical assessment, and a plan for addressing specific problems or concerns.

SOCIAL SECURITY DISABILITY INSURANCE (SSDI). A federal program that pays benefits and provides Medicare to disabled workers under age 65.

SOCIAL WORKER. A healthcare provider who can provide support to patients and families, including assistance with a patient's psychosocial adjustment needs and referrals for community support.

SOFT TISSUE. Layers of cells that form the skin.

SOMATIZATION DISORDER. A chronic condition in which psychological stresses are converted into physical symptoms that interfere with work and relationships. Lower back pain is a frequent complaint of patients with somatization disorder.

SOMNOPLASTY. A technique that uses radiofrequency signals to heat a thin needle inserted into the tissues of the soft palate. The heat from the needle shrinks the tissues, thus enlarging the patient's airway. Somnoplasty is also known as radiofrequency volumetric tissue reduction (RFVTR).

SONOGRAM. Image, or picture, obtained when using a machine called an ultrasound to look inside the uterus when the mother is pregnant. Ultrasound is a painless procedure that uses sound waves to display an image on a monitor.

SONOGRAPHER. A technologist or physician who uses an ultrasound unit to take sonograms.

SORBENT. A material used to adsorb toxic or waste substances from the blood in a process known as hemoperfusion. Most hemoperfusion systems use resin or activated carbon as sorbents.

SPASM. Sudden, involuntary tensing of a muscle or a group of muscles.

SPECIFIC GRAVITY. The ratio of the weight of a body fluid when compared with water.

SPECULUM. An instrument for enlarging the opening of any canal or cavity in order to facilitate inspection of its interior.

SPEECH-LANGUAGE PATHOLOGY. Formerly known as speech therapy, it includes the study and treatment of human communication—its development and disorders.

SPERM GRANULOMA. A collection of fluid that leaks from an improperly sealed or tied vas deferens. The fluid usually disappears on its own but can be drained if necessary.

SPERMATIC CORD. A tube-like structure that extends from the testicle to the groin area. It contains blood vessels, nerves, and a duct to carry spermatic fluid.

SPHENOIDAL ELECTRODES. Fine wire electrodes that are implanted under the cheek bones to measure temporal seizures.

SPHINCTER. A circular band of muscle fibers that constricts or closes a passageway in the body.

SPHINCTER DEFICIENCY. A term related both to urinary and fecal incontinence in which the inability of the sphincter to keep the reservoir closed is a source of severe incontinence.

SPIDER NEVUS (PLURAL, NEVI). A reddish lesion that consists of a central arteriole with smaller branches radiating outward. Spider nevi are also called spider angiomas; they are most common in small children and pregnant women.

SPIDER VEINS. Telangiectasias; swollen blood vessels that appear on the surface of the legs, characterized by a reddish central point with smaller veins branching out like the legs of a spider.

SPINA BIFIDA. Myelomeningocele; a congenital defect in which the fetal backbone and spinal canal do not close completely, allowing the spinal cord and its surrounding membranes to protrude.

SPINAL ANESTHESIA. Regional anesthesia produced by injecting the anesthetic agent into an area directly around the spinal cord.

SPINAL CANAL. The cavity or hollow space within the spine that contains the spinal cord and the cerebrospinal fluid.

SPINAL FUSION. An operation in which the bones of the spine are permanently joined together using a bone graft (usually from the hip).

SPINAL STENOSIS. Narrowing of the canals in the vertebrae or around the nerve roots, causing pressure on the spinal cord and nerves.

SPIRAL CT. A method of computed tomography (CT) scanning that allows for continuous 360-degree X-ray image capture; also referred to as helical CT.

SPIROMETER. A device used to measure the volume of air inhaled and exhaled by a patient's lungs. It can also be used to measure the rate at which the air is breathed in and out over a specified period of time.

SPLEEN. An abdominal organ that is involved in the filtration and storage of blood and the production of immune system cells.

SPLENECTOMY. Surgical removal of the spleen.

SPLENOMEGALY. Enlargement of the spleen.

SPLINT. A piece of rigid material that is used to hold structures in place during healing.

SPONGES. Pieces of absorbent material, usually cotton gauze, used to absorb fluids, protect tissue, or apply pressure and traction.

SPORADIC. Occurring on random occasions or irregular intervals; having no pattern in order or timing.

SPURS. Sharp horny outgrowths of the skin.

SPUTUM. A mucus-rich secretion that is coughed up from the bronchial tubes and the lungs.

SPUTUM CYTOLOGY. A lab test in which a microscope is used to check for cancer cells in the sputum.

SQUAMOUS CELL CARCINOMA. A type of cancer that develops in the cells in the top layer of tissue.

SQUAMOUS CELLS. Thin, flat cells in the surfaces of the skin and cervix and the linings of various organs.

SQUAMOUS INTRAEPITHELIAL LESION (SIL). A term used to categorize the severity of abnormal changes arising in the squamous, or outermost, layer of the cervix.

STABILIZER. A device used to provide a still, motionless field for suturing.

STAGHORN CALCULUS. A kidney stone that develops a branched shape resembling the antlers of a stag. Staghorn calculi are composed of struvite.

STAGING. The classification of cancers according to the extent of the tumor.

STAHL'S DEFORMITY. A congenital deformity of the ear characterized by a flattened rim and pointed upper edge caused by a fold in the cartilage; it is also known colloquially as Vulcan ear or Spock ear.

STAPEDOTOMY. A procedure in which a small hole is cut in the footplate of the stapes (a bone in the ear).

STAPHYLOCOCCAL INFECTION. An infection caused by any of several pathogenic species of Staphylococcus, commonly characterized by the formation of abscesses in the skin or other organs; also known as a Staph infection.

STEATORRHEA. An excess of fat in the stool.

STEM CELLS. Unspecialized cells, or "immature" blood cells, that serve as the precursors of white blood cells, red blood cells, and platelets.

STENOSIS. Narrowing or constriction of a blood vessel, valve, or other opening or passageway in the body.

STENOTIC. Abnormally narrowed.

STENT. A specially designed wire-mesh device that is placed inside a blood vessel to open or support it.

STENTING. The insertion of a plastic mesh or metal tube into an artery to hold it open.

STEREOTACTIC. Characterized by precise positioning in space. When applied to radiosurgery, stereotactic refers to a system of three-dimensional coordinates for locating a target site (e.g., tumor).

STERILE. Completely free of pathogens; alternately, referring to an inability to reproduce.

STERILIZATION. To make sterile.

STERNOTOMY. A surgical opening into the thoracic cavity through the sternum (breastbone).

STERNOXIPHOID JUNCTION. The lower junction of the sternum or breastbone.

STERNUM. The long flat bone in the middle of the chest; the breastbone.

STEROIDS. A class of hormones and drugs that includes sex and stress hormones, anti-inflammatory medications, contraceptives, and growth-promoting substances.

STETHOSCOPE. A rubber Y-shaped device used to listen to sounds produced by the human body.

STEVENS-JOHNSON SYNDROME. A severe inflammatory reaction that is sometimes triggered by sulfa medications. It is characterized by blisters and eroded areas in the mouth, nose, eyes, and anus; it may also involve the lungs, heart, and digestive tract. Stevens-Johnson syndrome is also known as erythema multiforme.

STIMULANT. A drug or other substance that increases the rate of activity of a body system.

STIMULUS. A factor capable of eliciting a response.

STOCKINETTE. A soft elastic material used for bandages and clothing for infants.

STOMA. A surgically created opening in the abdominal wall.

STOOL. The solid waste that is left after food is digested. Stool forms in the intestines and passes out of the body through the anus.

STRABISMUS. A condition in which the muscles of the eye do not work together, often causing double vision.

STRANGULATED HERNIA. A twisted piece of herniated intestine that can block blood flow to the intestines.

STRANGULATION. A condition in which a vessel, section of the intestine, or other body part is compressed or constricted to the point that blood cannot circulate.

STRANGULATION OBSTRUCTION. A blockage in the intestine that closes off the flow of blood to the area.

STREP THROAT. A sore throat caused by infection with *Streptococcus* bacteria. Symptoms include sore throat, chills, fever, and swollen lymph nodes in the neck.

STREPTOCOCCAL INFECTION. An infection caused by a pathogenic bacterium of one of several species of the genus *Streptococcus* or their toxins. Almost any organ in the body may be involved.

STRESS INCONTINENCE. Involuntary loss of urine that occurs during physical activity such as coughing, sneezing, laughing, or exercise.

STRESS TEST. A test used to determine how the heart responds to stress. It usually involves walking on a treadmill or riding a stationary bike at increasing levels of difficulty while heart activity and blood pressure are monitored. If the patient is unable to walk on a treadmill or ride a stationary bike, medications may be used to produce similar results.

STRESS ULCERS. Stomach ulcers that occur in connection with some types of physical injury, including burns and invasive surgical procedures.

STRICTURE. An abnormal narrowing of a duct or canal.

STRICTUREPLASTY. A procedure that shortens and widens strictures in the intestine without removing sections of the intestine; used to treat Crohn's disease.

STROKE. An event that impairs the circulation of the brain. Ischemic stroke is caused by a blood clot in the brain, while hemorrhagic stroke is caused by bleeding into the brain.

STROMA. The thickest part of the cornea between Bowman's membrane and Decemet's membrane.

STRUVITE. A crystalline form of magnesium ammonium phosphate. Kidney stones made of struvite form in urine with a pH above 7.2.

STURGE-WEBER SYNDROME. A birth defect that results in abnormal blood vessels on the surface of (usually) one side of the brain, causing seizures, skin abnormalities, and intellectual disabilities.

SUBARACHNOID. The space underneath the arachnoid membrane, a thin membrane enclosing the brain and spinal cord.

SUBARACHNOID HEMORRHAGE (SAH). Bleeding from a ruptured blood vessel in the subarachnoid space between the membranes covering the brain.

SUBARACHNOID SPACE. The space surrounding the spinal cord that is filled with cerebrospinal fluid.

SUBCAPSULAR. Inside the outer tissue covering of the testicle.

SUBCAPSULAR ORCHIECTOMY. A procedure in which the surgeon removes the inner glandular tissue of the testicle while leaving the outer capsule intact.

SUBCUTANEOUS. Under the skin.

SUBCUTANEOUS EMPHYSEMA. A pathologic accumulation of air underneath the skin resulting from improper insufflation technique.

SUBDURAL ELECTRODES. Strip electrodes that are placed under dura mater (the outermost, toughest, and most fibrous of the three membranes [meninges] covering the brain and spinal cord). They are used to locate foci of epileptic seizures prior to epilepsy surgery.

SUBFERTILE. Referring to the decreased ability to become pregnant.

SUBGLOTTIC STENOSIS. An abnormal narrowing of the trachea below the level of the vocal cords.

SUBJECTIVE. Influenced by the perspective of the information provider; potentially biased.

SUBLINGUAL. Under the tongue.

SUBMENTAL. Underneath the chin.

SUBSTRATE. A substance acted upon by an enzyme.

SUMMARY OF BENEFITS AND COVERAGE (SBC). A standard form that health insurance companies and plans must use to explain their plans and allow for easy comparisons of plans.

SUPERIOR VENA CAVA. The second largest vein in the body, which returns blood to the right atrium of the heart from the upper half of the body.

SUPINE. A position in which the patient lies on the back with the face upward, usually with the legs straight and the arms at the sides or folded over the abdomen.

SUPPLEMENTAL SECURITY INCOME (SSI). A federal program that provides cash assistance to low-income blind, disabled, and elderly people; in most states, people receiving SSI benefits are eligible for Medicaid.

SUPRAVENTRICULAR TACHYCARDIA (SVT). A fast heartbeat that originates above the ventricles.

SURGEON. A physician that has completed surgical residency training, passed all examinations, and is a Fellow of the American College of Surgeons.

SURGICAL ALTERNATIVES. A range of surgical procedures that may be used to treat a specific condition.

SURGICAL CLIPPING. Surgical repair of a cerebral aneurysm.

SURGICAL ONCOLOGY. The branch of surgery that specializes in the surgical management of cancer.

SURGICAL REVISION. The failure of a procedure, which requires additional surgery to improve the result.

SURGICAL SITE INFECTION (SSI). An infection that originates at a site in the body that was operated upon.

SURGICENTER. Another term for ambulatory surgical center (an outpatient facility).

SURROGATE. A person who represents the wishes of a patient, chosen by the patient and stipulated by a legal document as power of attorney.

SUSTAINED MAXIMAL INSPIRATION (SMI). Another term for incentive spirometry, a respiratory therapy done to improve breathing and prevent respiratory complications after surgery.

SUTURE. A loop of material used to draw together and align the edges of a wound or incision. Sutures may be either absorbable or nonabsorbable.

SWAGED NEEDLE. An eyeless surgical needle with the suture material preattached by the manufacturer.

SWAN-GANZ CATHETER. A type of catheter inserted into a large vessel in the neck or chest that is used to measure the amount of fluid in the heart and to determine how well the heart is functioning; also called a pulmonary artery catheter.

SYMPATHETIC NERVOUS SYSTEM. The part of the nervous system that regulates involuntary reactions to stress, such as changes in the heartbeat and breathing rate, sweating, and changes in digestive secretions.

SYMPATHOMIMETIC DRUGS. Another name for adrenergic drugs.

SYNCHRONIZED ELECTRICAL CARDIOVERSION. The term used to describe cardioversion by the application of a controlled electric shock to the patient's chest.

SYNCOPE. A fainting episode.

SYNDACTYLY. Union or webbing of two or more fingers or toes, which usually only involves a skin connection between the two.

SYNDROME. A set of signs or a series of events occurring together that often point to a single disease or condition as the cause.

SYNOVIAL FLUID. A fluid that lubricates the joints, facilitates motion, and helps prevent wearing of the bones.

SYNOVITIS. Inflammation of the synovium, a thin membrane that lines joints.

SYSTEMIC CIRCULATION. Blood vessels not involved in carrying blood to and from the lungs between the right and left sides of the heart.

SYSTEMS ANALYSIS. An approach to medical errors and other management issues that looks for problems in the work process rather than singling out individuals as incompetent.

SYSTOLE. Period while the heart is contracting.

SYSTOLIC. Referring to maximum arterial blood pressure during ventricular contraction.

T

T CELL. A type of small-cell lymphocyte that is part of the adaptive immune system. There are several types of T cells with different functions, including to assist other lymphocytes, destroy tumor cells, provide the immune system with "memory" of past infections, and protect against autoimmune disease.

TACHYCARDIA. Rapid heartbeat, generally over 100 beats per minute.

TACTILE FREMITUS. A tremor or vibration in any part of the body detected by palpation (gently feeling or pressing with hands).

TAMOXIFEN. A drug that blocks the activity of estrogen; used to prevent or treat breast cancer.

TARDIVE DYSKINESIA. A disorder brought on by certain medications that is characterized by uncontrollable muscle spasms.

TATTOOING. In a surgical context, refers to marking the location of a large or unusual-looking colonic polyp removed for biopsy by injecting a small amount of India ink or carbon black. Tattooing is done to allow the surgeon to identify the location of the polyp for future surgery or follow-up surveillance.

TAY-SACHS DISEASE. An inherited disease prevalent among the Ashkenazi Jewish population of the United States. Infants with the disease are unable to process a certain type of fat that accumulates in nerve and brain cells, causing mental and physical disabilities and death by age four.

TEACHING HOSPITALS. Hospitals whose primary mission is training medical personnel in collaboration with (or ownership by) a medical school or research center.

TEAR FILM. The coating of fluid on the surface of the cornea that serves to lubricate the eye and remove bacteria from the cornea. The tear film consists of three layers: a mucous layer, a liquid layer, and an oily or lipid layer. It is also called the precorneal film.

TELANGIECTASIA. The medical term for the visible discolorations produced by permanently swollen capillaries and smaller veins.

TEMPLATING. A term that refers to the surgeon's use of x-ray images of an old prosthesis as a template or pattern guide for a new implant.

TEMPORAL ARTERITIS. A condition in which inflammation of the blood vessels that supply the head and neck result in severe, chronic headache, particularly over one temple, as well as fever, weight loss, and severe fatigue.

TEMPORAL LOBE EPILEPSY (TLE). The most common type of epilepsy, with elaborate and multiple sensory, motor, and psychic symptoms. A common feature is the loss of consciousness and amnesia during seizures. Other manifestations may include more complex behaviors like bursts of anger, emotional outbursts, fear, or automatisms.

TEMPOROMANDIBULAR JOINTS (TMJ). The two joints, one on either side of the skull, where the human mandible articulates with the two temporal bones of the skull. Twenty percent of all facial injuries involve a fracture of the mandible.

TENACULUM. A surgical instrument consisting of a slender hook attached to a handle; used to hold tissue during surgical operations or other procedures.

TENDINITIS. Inflammation of a tendon.

TENDON. Connective tissue that attaches muscle to bone.

TESTICLES. The two egg-shaped organs found in the scrotum that produce sperm.

TESTICULAR TORSION. Twisting of the testicle around the spermatic cord, cutting off the blood supply to the testicle. It is considered a urologic emergency.

TESTIS (PLURAL, TESTES). The medical term for a testicle.

TESTOSTERONE. The major male sex hormone, produced in the testes.

TETANUS. An acute infectious disease caused by a toxin produced by the bacterium *Clostridium tetani* and usually introduced into the body through a wound.

TETANY. Inappropriately sustained muscle spasms.

TETRALOGY OF FALLOT. A cyanotic defect in which the blood pumped through the body has too little oxygen.

Tetralogy of Fallot includes four defects: a ventricular septal defect, narrowing at or beneath the pulmonary valve, infundibular pulmonary stenosis (obstruction of blood flow out of the right ventricle through the pulmonary valve), and overriding aorta (the aorta crosses the ventricular septal defect into the right ventricle).

THALASSEMIA. A group of inherited disorders that affect hemoglobin production. Because hemoglobin production is impaired, a person with this disorder may suffer mild to severe anemia. Certain types of thalassemia can be fatal.

THERAPEUTIC INDEX. The range of acceptable levels of a drug in the bloodstream; generally, the ratio of the highest dose producing no toxic symptoms to the lowest effective dose. It is also known as the therapeutic window.

THORACENTESIS. Removal of fluid from the pleural cavity.

THORACIC. Pertaining to the chest cavity, including the lungs and the area around the lungs.

THORACIC ANEURYSM. Aneurysm that involves the ascending, arch, or descending thoracic aorta using the diaphragm as a landmark for transition to abdominal aorta.

THORACIC AORTIC ANEURYSM. Occurs when an area in the thoracic section of the aorta (the chest) is weakened and bulges like a balloon. The thoracic section supplies blood to the upper body.

THORACIC VERTEBRAE. The vertebrae in the chest region to which the ribs attach.

THORACOSCOPY. Examination of the chest through a tiny incision using a thin, lighted tube-like instrument (thoracoscope).

THORACOTOMY. An open surgical procedure performed through an incision in the chest.

THORAX. The chest area, which runs between the abdomen and neck and is encased in the ribs.

THROMBIN. An enzyme in blood plasma that plays an important role in the blood-clotting process.

THROMBIN INHIBITOR. One type of anticoagulant medication used to help prevent formation of harmful blood clots in the body by blocking the activity of thrombin.

THROMBOCYTOPENIA. A disorder characterized by a drop in the number of platelets in the blood.

THROMBOCYTOSIS. A vascular condition characterized by high blood platelet counts.

THROMBOEMBOLISM. A blood clot that breaks free and blocks a blood vessel elsewhere in the body.

THROMBOLYSIS. The dissolving of a blood clot.

THROMBOLYTIC. A medication that dissolves blood clots.

THROMBOPHILIA. An inherited or acquired tendency for thrombosis.

THROMBOPHLEBITIS. Inflammation of veins, associated with the formation of blood clots.

THROMBOPLASTIN. A protein in blood that converts prothrombin to thrombin.

THROMBOSED. Affected by the formation of a blood clot, or thrombus, along the wall of a blood vessel.

THROMBOSIS. The formation or presence of a blood clot within a blood vessel.

THROMBOTIC. Relating to, caused by, or characterized by thrombosis.

THROMBUS. A blood clot that is blocking a blood vessel.

THYMUS. An organ near the base of the neck that produces cells that fight infection.

THYROID CARTILAGE. The largest cartilage in the human larynx, or voice box. It is sometimes called the Adam's apple.

THYROID DYSFUNCTION. A physical state that involves the failure of the thyroid gland to function properly. Thyroid dysfunction not only affects a person's physical state, but may have secondary effects on their mental state as well.

THYROID GLAND. A butterfly-shaped gland in front and to the sides of the upper part of the windpipe. The thyroid gland produces thyroid hormone, which influences body processes like growth, development, reproduction, and metabolism.

THYROID STORM. An unusual complication of thyroid function that is sometimes triggered by the stress of thyroid surgery. It is a medical emergency.

THYROIDITIS. Inflammation of the thyroid gland.

THYROTOXICOSIS. A condition resulting from high levels of thyroid hormones in the blood.

TIBIA. The larger of two leg bones that lie beneath the knee. The tibia is sometimes called the shin bone.

TIDAL VOLUME. The volume of air inhaled or exhaled with each breath.

TIME OUT. A surgical safety procedure done before the first incision to ensure that the patient, surgical site, and planned procedure are correct and that all required equipment, instruments, and imaging are in place.

TINNITUS. A buzzing or ringing sensation in the ear.

TISSUE PLASMINOGEN ACTIVATOR (TPA). A genetically engineered form of a natural human thrombolytic.

TISSUE-FLAP SURGERY. Breast reconstruction using tissues from elsewhere in the body.

TITER. A dilution of a substance with an exact known amount of fluid; for example, one part of serum diluted with four parts of saline is a titer of 1:4.

TNM. A system used for cancer staging. **T** stands for tumor, **N** refers to spread to lymph nodes, and **M** stands for metastasis.

TOCOLYTIC. A medication that inhibits uterine contractions to stop or delay labor.

TOLERANCE. A decrease in sensitivity to a drug. When tolerance occurs, a person must take more of the drug to get the same effect.

TONIC SEIZURE. A seizure in which the complete body becomes rigid.

TONIC-CLONIC SEIZURE. A two-phase epileptic seizure in which the body first becomes rigid and then jerks uncontrollably.

TONOMETRY. Measurement of the fluid pressure inside the eye.

TONSILLECTOMY. Surgical removal of the tonsils.

TONSILLITIS. Inflammation of a tonsil.

TONSILS. Two lumps of lymphoid tissue located on either side of the back of the throat.

TOPICAL. Applied to the surface; not ingested.

TOTAL LUNG CAPACITY. The volume of air in the lungs at the end of a deep breath. The normal value in adults is between 4 and 6 quarts.

TOTAL LUNG CAPACITY TEST. A test that measures the amount of air in the lungs after a person has breathed in as much as possible.

TOTAL MASTECTOMY. Removal of the breast tissue, nipple, and a small portion of the overlying skin; also known as a simple mastectomy.

TOTAL PARENTERAL NUTRITION (TPN). Intravenous administration of a solution containing all of the nutrients required by the body, such as protein, fat, calories, vitamins, and minerals. TPN provides a complete and balanced source of nutrients for patients who cannot consume a normal diet.

TOURNIQUET. A thin piece of tubing or other device used to stop bleeding or control circulation by compressing the blood vessels.

TOXIC THYROID ADENOMA. Self-contained concentrations of thyroid tissue that may produce excessive amounts of thyroid hormone.

TOXICOLOGY. The branch of science that deals with the study of drugs, poisons, and other chemicals, and their effects on human and animal bodies.

TOXIN. A poison; usually refers to protein poisons produced by bacteria, animals, and some plants.

TRABECULAR MESHWORK. The main drainage passageway for fluid to leave the anterior chamber of the eye.

TRABECULOPLASTY. Laser surgery that creates perforations in the trabecular meshwork to drain built-up fluid and relieve pressure.

TRACER. A substance containing a radioisotope that is injected into the body and tracked in order to obtain information about various metabolic processes in the body.

TRACHEA. Tube of cartilage that carries air into and out of the lungs; the windpipe.

TRACHEOBRONCHIAL. Pertaining both to the tracheal and bronchial tubes or to their junction.

TRACHEOSTOMY. A surgical opening through the neck into the trachea (windpipe) to allow the passage of air through a tracheostomy tube.

TRACHEOSTOMY TUBE. A breathing tube inserted in the neck, used when assisted breathing is needed for a long period of time.

TRACHEOTOMY. A surgical procedure in which an artificial opening is made in the trachea (windpipe) to allow air into the lungs.

TRADITIONAL CHINESE MEDICINE (TCM). The medical system of mainland China that combines herbal medicines, dietary treatments, massage, acupuncture, and physical exercise (qigong and tai chi).

TRANSCONJUCTIVAL BLEPHAROPLASTY. A type of blepharoplasty (eyelid surgery) in which the surgeon makes no incision on the surface of the eyelid and instead enters from behind to tease out the fat deposits.

TRANSCUTANEOUS. Passing through the skin.

TRANSDUCER. An instrument that sends sound waves into organs of the body in order to produce ultrasound images.

TRANSESOPHAGEAL ECHOCARDIOGRAM (TEE). An invasive imaging procedure used to create a picture of the heart's movement, valves, and chambers. The test uses high-frequency sound waves that come from a small transducer passed down the patient's throat.

TRANSFERRIN. A protein in blood plasma that carries iron derived from food intake to the liver, spleen, and bone marrow.

TRANSFUSION. The therapeutic introduction of blood or a blood component into a patient's bloodstream.

TRANSFUSION CONTAINER. An administration bag made of polyvinyl chloride or other latex-free polymer for collection of blood products for administration to the patient.

TRANSILLUMINATION. A technique in which the doctor shines a strong light through body tissues in order to examine an organ or structure.

TRANSLOCATION. The rearrangement or exchange of segments of chromosomes that does not alter the total number of chromosomes, but sometimes results in a genetic disorder or disease.

TRANSPLANTATION. The removal of tissue from one part of the body for implantation to another part of the body, or the removal of tissue or an organ from one individual and its implantation into another individual by surgery.

TRANSPOSITION OF THE GREAT VESSELS. A cyanotic defect in which the blood pumped through the body has too little oxygen because the pulmonary artery and aorta are reversed.

TRANSSEXUAL. Person desiring to acquire the external appearance of a member of the opposite gender.

TRANSTRACHEAL JET VENTILATION (TTJV). A technique for ventilating a patient that involves passing oxygen under pressure through a catheter that has been passed through the patient's cricothyroid membrane.

TRANSURETHRAL SURGERY. Surgery in which instruments are entered through the urethra and no external incision is needed.

TRANSVERSE PRESENTATION. Refers to a baby laying sideways across the cervix rather than head first.

TRAUMA CENTERS. Specialized hospital facilities that are equipped to deal with emergency life-threatening conditions.

TRAUMA SURGERY. Surgery performed as a result of injury.

TRAUMATIC BRAIN INJURY (TBI). Traumatic injury to the brain. Injury may occur either as a closed head injury, such as the head hitting a car's windshield, or as a penetrating head injury, as when a bullet pierces the skull. Both may cause damage that ranges from mild to profound. Very severe injury can be fatal because of profound brain damage.

TREACHER COLLINS SYNDROME. A disorder that affects facial development and hearing, thought to be caused by a gene mutation on human chromosome 5; sometimes called mandibulofacial dysostosis.

TREMOR. A trembling, quivering, or shaking.

TRENDELENBURG. Position in which the head is low and the body and legs are on an inclined plane.

TRENDELENBURG'S TEST. A test that measures the speed at which the lower leg fills with blood after the leg has first been raised above the level of the heart. It is named for Friedrich Trendelenburg (1844–1924), a German surgeon.

TREPHINE. A small surgical instrument that is rotated to cut a circular incision.

TREPONEME. A term used to refer to any member of the genus *Treponema*, which is an anaerobic bacteria consisting of cells 3–8 m in length, with acute, regular, or irregular spirals and no obvious protoplasmic structure.

TRIAGE. A method for determining the priority of patient treatment during a disaster or mass casualty event according to the severity of the injuries, likelihood of survival, and available resources.

TRIAL OF LABOR (TOL). A purposeful attempt to deliver vaginally after a previous cesarean delivery.

TRICHOMONADS. Parasitic protozoa commonly found in the digestive and genital tracts of humans and other animals. Some species cause vaginal infections in women characterized by itching and a frothy discharge.

TRICUSPID VALVE. The heart valve connecting the right atrium and right ventricle.

TRIGLYCERIDE. A substance formed in the body from the breakdown of fat in the diet. Triglycerides are the main fatty materials in the blood. Triglyceride levels are important in the diagnosis and treatment of many diseases, including high blood pressure, diabetes, and heart disease.

TROCAR. A surgical tool shaped as a hollow cylinder that is sometimes used to make an initial incision into a body cavity and through which other surgical tools are then passed.

TUBAL LIGATION. A female sterilization surgical procedure in which the fallopian tubes are tied in two places and cut between. This prevents eggs from moving from the ovary to the uterus.

TUBE FEEDING. Feeding or nutrition through a tube placed into the body through the esophagus, nose, stomach, intestines, or via a surgically constructed artificial orifice called a stoma.

TUBERCULOSIS. An infectious disease that usually affects the lungs but may also affect other parts of the body. Its symptoms include fever, weight loss, and coughing up blood.

TUBULE. Small tubular part of an animal.

TUMESCENT ANESTHESIA. A type of local anesthesia originally developed for liposuction in which a large volume of diluted anesthetic is injected into the tissues around the vein until they become tumescent (firm and swollen).

TUMOR. An uncontrolled mass of body cells that may be benign or malignant.

TUMOR MARKER. A circulating biochemical compound that indicates the presence of cancer. Tumor markers can be used in diagnosis and in monitoring the effectiveness of treatment.

TUMOR STAGING. The method used by oncologists to determine the risk from a cancerous tumor. A number—ranging from 1A–4B—is assigned to predict the level of invasion by a tumor, and offer a prognosis for morbidity and mortality.

TUNICA (PLURAL, TUNICAE). The medical term for a membrane or piece of tissue that covers or lines a body part.

TUNICA VAGINALIS. A sac-like membrane covering the outer surface of the testes.

TURBIDITY. The degree of cloudiness of a urine sample (or other solution).

TURBINATE. Relating to a nasal concha.

TWILIGHT ANESTHESIA. An intravenous mixture of sedatives and other medications that decrease a person's awareness of the procedure being performed.

TWIN REVERSED ARTERIAL PERFUSION (TRAP) SEQUENCE. A condition in which one fetus lacks a heart and the other fetus pumps the blood for both.

TWIN-TO-TWIN TRANSFUSION SYNDROME (TTTS). A condition in monochorionic twins where the connection between the two circulatory systems is such that the donor twin pumps the blood to the recipient twin without the return of blood to the donor.

TYMPANIC MEMBRANE. The eardrum; a thin disc of tissue that separates the outer ear from the middle ear.

TYMPANOPLASTY. Procedure to reconstruct the tympanic membrane (eardrum) and/or middle ear bone as the result of infection or trauma.

TYMPANOSTOMY TUBE. Ear tube. A small tube made of metal or plastic that is inserted during myringotomy to ventilate the middle ear.

U

ULCER. A lesion or rough spot formed on the surface of an artery.

ULCERATION. Death of tissue cells in a specific area, such as skin.

ULCERATIVE COLITIS. A chronic condition in which recurrent ulcers are found in the colon. It is manifested clinically by abdominal cramping and rectal bleeding.

ULNA. The longer of the two bones in the forearm, extending from the medial side of the elbow joint to the side of the wrist closest to the little finger.

ULNAR COLLATERAL LIGAMENT (UCL) RECONSTRUCTION. The medical name for Tommy John surgery.

ULTRASONOGRAM. Images of areas inside the body, created by ultrasonography.

ULTRASONOGRAPHY. A procedure where high-frequency sound waves that cannot be heard by human ears are bounced off internal organs and tissues. These sound waves produce a pattern of echoes that are then used by a computer to create images.

ULTRASOUND. A technique that uses high-frequency sound waves to create a visual image (a sonogram) of soft tissues. The technique is routinely used in prenatal care and diagnosis.

UMBILICAL RING. An opening through which the umbilical vessels pass to the fetus; it is closed after birth and its site is indicated by the navel.

UMBILICUS. The area where the umbilical cord was attached; also known as the navel or belly button.

UNCINATE PROCESS. A downwardly and backwardly directed process of each lateral mass of the ethmoid bone that joins with the inferior nasal conchae.

UNILATERAL CLEFT LIP. A cleft that occurs on either the right or left side of the lip.

UNITED STATES PHARMACOPOEIA (USP). An authoritative book, updated annually, that contains lists of medicines, dietary supplements, and surgical supplies. It defines doses or other units of measurement and sets quality standards for their production and proper use. The USP is used by 130 countries around the world in addition to the United States.

UREA. A by-product of protein metabolism that is formed in the liver. Because urea contains ammonia, which is toxic to the body, it must be quickly filtered from the blood by the kidneys and excreted in the urine.

URETER. The tube that carries urine from each kidney to the bladder.

URETEROSCOPE. A special type of endoscope that allows a surgeon to remove kidney stones from the lower urinary tract without the need for an incision.

URETHRA. The tube that carries urine from the bladder to outside the body. In females, the urethral opening is between the vagina and clitoris; in males, the urethra travels through the penis, opening at the tip.

URETHRA HYPERMOBILITY. Main factor in stress urinary incontinence, with severity based upon how far the urethra has descended into the pelvic floor through herniation or cystocele.

URETHRAL FASCIAL SLING. A support and compression aid to urethral function using auxiliary material made of patient or donor tissue.

URETHRITIS. Inflammation of the urinary bladder.

URGENCY. A sudden compelling need to urinate.

URIC ACID. A product of purine breakdown that is excreted by the kidney. High levels of uric acid, caused by various diseases, can cause the formation of kidney stones.

URINALYSIS. The diagnostic testing of a urine sample.

URINARY CONDUIT DIVERSION. A type of urinary diversion or rerouting that uses a conduit made from an intestinal segment to channel urine to an outside collection pouch.

URINARY CONTINENT DIVERSION. A surgical procedure that restores urinary continence by diverting urinary function around the bladder and into the intestines, thereby allowing for natural evacuation through the rectum or an implanted artificial sphincter.

URINARY INCONTINENCE. Inability to control urination.

URINARY RETENTION. The inability to void (urinate) or discharge urine.

URINARY STRESS INCONTINENCE. The involuntary release of urine due to pressure on the abdominal muscles during exercise, laughing, or coughing.

URINARY TRACT. The passage through which urine flows from the kidneys to the outside of the body.

URINE. A fluid containing water and dissolved substances excreted by the kidney.

URINE CREATININE LEVEL. A value obtained by testing a 24-hour collection of urine for the amount of creatinine present.

URINE CULTURE. A test that examines urine samples in the lab to see if bacteria are present.

URINE CYTOLOGY. The examination of urine under a microscope to look for cancerous or precancerous cells.

UROGENITAL. Also called genitourinary, the organ systems that are involved in reproduction and excretion.

UROGYNECOLOGIST. A physician that specializes in female medical conditions concerning the urinary and reproductive systems.

UROLITHIASIS. The medical term for the formation of kidney stones. It is also used to refer to disease conditions related to kidney stones.

UROLOGIST. A physician who specializes in problems of the urinary system.

UROLOGY. The branch of medicine that deals with disorders of the urinary tract in both males and females, and with the genital organs in males.

URORADIOLOGIST. A radiologist that specializes in diagnostic imaging of the urinary tract and kidneys.

UTERINE FIBROID. A noncancerous tumor of the uterus. Small fibroids require no treatment, but those causing serious symptoms may need to be removed.

UTERINE PROLAPSE. A condition in which the uterus descends into or beyond the vagina.

UTERINE SOUND. An instrument used to probe and measure the length and direction of a woman's cervix and uterus prior to inserting an intrauterine device (IUD). The sound is inserted into the uterus through the cervix.

UTERINE SUSPENSION. Procedure that places a sling under the uterus and holds it in place.

UTERUS. The womb; the hollow, muscular female organ that supports the development and nourishment of the unborn baby during pregnancy.

UVEA. The middle of the three coats of tissue surrounding the eye: the choroid, iris, and ciliary body. The uvea is pigmented and well supplied with blood vessels.

UVEITIS. Inflammation of any part of the uvea.

UVULA. A triangular piece of tissue that hangs from the roof of the mouth above the back of the tongue.

UVULOPALATOPHARYNGOPLASTY (UPPP). An operation to remove the tonsils and other excess tissue at the back of the throat to prevent it from closing the airway during sleep. This procedure may also be performed with a laser.

V

VACUTAINER. A tube with a rubber top from which air has been removed.

VAGINA. A canal in the female body that leads from the cervix to the external orifice opening to the outside of the body.

VAGINAL BIRTH AFTER CESAREAN (VBAC). The option of having subsequent vaginal deliveries after a cesarean delivery.

VAGINAL SPECULUM. An instrument that is inserted into the vagina that expands and allows for examination of the vagina and cervix.

VAGOTOMY. A surgical procedure in which the nerves that stimulate stomach acid production and gastric motility (movement) are cut.

VAGUS NERVE. The tenth of the twelve pairs of cranial nerves, which receives sensory information from the lungs and the digestive tract and is also involved in vomiting.

VALGUS. A deformity in which a body part is angled away from the midline of the body.

VALGUS ALIGNMENT. Alignment of the knee that angles outward due to injury or deformity.

VALVE. Flaps (leaflets) of tissue in the passageways between the heart's upper and lower chambers.

VAPORIZE. To dissolve solid material or convert it into smoke or gas.

VARICES. Swollen or enlarged veins.

VARICOSE. Abnormally enlarged and distended.

VARICOSE VEINS. The permanent enlargement and twisting of veins, usually in the legs. They are most often seen in people with occupations requiring long periods of standing, and in pregnant women.

VARIX (PLURAL, VARICES). The medical term for an enlarged blood vessel.

VARUS. A deformity in which a body part is angled toward the midline of the body.

VARUS ALIGNMENT. Alignment of the knee that angles inward due to injury or deformity.

VAS DEFERENS (PLURAL, VASA DEFERENTIA). The Latin name for the duct that carries sperm from the testicle to the epididymis.

VASCULAR. Pertaining to the veins, arteries, and organs in the body's circulatory system.

VASCULAR SURGERY. A branch of medicine that deals with the surgical repair of disorders of or injuries to the blood vessels.

VASCULOGENIC ERECTILE DYSFUNCTION. The inability to attain or sustain an erection satisfactory for coitus, due to atherosclerotic disease of penile arteries, inadequate impedance of venous outflow (venous leaks), or a combination of both.

VASECTOMY. Surgical sterilization of the male, done by removing a portion of the tube that carries sperm to the urethra.

VASOCONSTRICTION. Narrowing of blood vessels.

VASOEPIDIDYMOSTOMY. A type of vasectomy reversal in which the vas deferens is attached to the epididymis, the structure where sperm matures and is stored.

VASOSPASM. Alternating contraction and relaxation of the muscle coating of blood vessels.

VASOVAGAL REACTION. A collection of symptoms that includes dizziness, fainting, profuse sweating, hyperventilation, and/or low blood pressure that occurs in a small percentage of individuals who donate blood.

VASOVAGAL RESPONSE. A short-lived response of the vascular and nervous system mediated by the vagus nerve, usually triggered by fear or pain. The patient typically experiences bradycardia (slowed heart rate), heavy sweating, paleness of the face, dizziness or feeling faint, and a rapid drop in arterial blood pressure. The vasovagal response is also known as a vagal attack or a vasovagal episode.

VASOVASOSTOMY. A surgical procedure that is done to reverse a vasectomy by reconnecting the ends of the severed vasa deferentia.

VEIN. A blood vessel that returns oxygen-depleted blood from various parts of the body to the heart.

VENA CAVA. The large vein that drains directly into the heart after gathering incoming blood from the entire body.

VENIPUNCTURE. Puncture of a vein with a needle for the purpose of withdrawing a blood sample for analysis.

VENOGRAPHY. X-ray visualization of veins after the injection of a radiopaque contrast dye.

VENOUS BLOOD. Blood that carries carbon dioxide from the tissues to the heart and then the lungs to be oxygenated.

VENOUS GRAFT. Transfer of living vein tissue within the same host (from one place of the body to another in the same person).

VENOUS STASIS DISEASE. A condition in which there is pooling of blood in the lower leg veins that may cause swelling and tissue damage and lead to painful sores or ulcers.

VENOUS SYSTEM. Circulation system that carries blood that has passed through the capillaries of various tissues (except the lungs) and is found in the veins, the right chambers of the heart, and the pulmonary arteries.

VENOUS THROMBOEMBOLISM (VTE). The formation or presence of a thrombus or embolus in a vein, including deep-vein thrombosis and pulmonary embolism.

VENOUS VALVES. Folds on the inner lining of the veins that prevent the backflow of blood.

VENTILATE. To assist a patient's breathing by use of a mechanical device or surgical procedure.

VENTILATION SCAN. A lung scan in which a tracer gas is inhaled into the lungs to show the quantity of air that different areas of the lungs are receiving.

VENTILATOR. Respirator; a mechanical device that helps patients breathe.

VENTRICLES. A lower pumping chamber of the heart. There are two ventricles, right and left. The right ventricle pumps oxygen-poor blood to the lungs to be re-oxygenated; the left ventricle pumps oxygen-rich blood to the body.

VENTRICULAR DRAIN. Used to measure the pressure inside the head or to relieve a blockage of the flow of the cerebrospinal fluid.

VENTRICULAR FIBRILLATION. An erratic, disorganized firing of impulses from the ventricles, the lower chambers of the heart. The ventricles quiver instead of pumping in an organized way, preventing blood from pumping through the body. Ventricular fibrillation is a medical emergency.

VENTRICULAR SHUNT. A tube that is placed in one of the fluid-filled chambers inside the brain (ventricles) to drain excess fluid and relieve pressure.

VENTRICULAR TACHYCARDIA. A rapid heartbeat, usually over 100 beats per minute.

VERMILION. The dark pink tissue that makes up the lip.

VERTEBRA (PLURAL, VERTEBRAE). One of the bones of the spinal column. There are 33 vertebrae in the human spine.

VERTEBRAL RECONSTRUCTION. Procedure for reconstruction and support of the vertebrae of the skeletal system.

VERTIGO. A feeling of dizziness together with a sensation of movement and a feeling of rotating in space.

VESTIBULAR. Relating to the middle cavity of the inner ear.

VIDEOSCOPE. A surgical camera.

VIRAL LOAD TEST. A blood test for monitoring the speed of human immunodeficiency virus (HIV) replication in patients with acquired immune deficiency syndrome (AIDS).

VIRCHOW'S TRIAD. Three categories of factors that increase the risk of venous thrombosis: slowing of blood flow, increased blood coagulation, and injury to the lining of the veins.

VIRTUAL COLONOSCOPY. Technique that provides views of the colon to screen for colon polyps and cancer. The images are produced by computerized manipulations rather than direct observation through the colonoscope; one technique uses the x-ray images from a computed tomography (CT) scan, and the other uses magnetic images from a magnetic resonance imaging (MRI) scan.

VIRUS. A tiny, disease-causing structure that can reproduce only in living cells and that causes a variety of infectious diseases.

VISCERAL PERICARDIUM. Single layer of cells that lines both the internal surface of the heart with the parietal pericardium and the external surface of the heart.

VISUAL FIELD. The total area in which a person can see objects within his or her peripheral vision while the eyes are focused on a central point.

VITAL CAPACITY (VC). Maximal breathing capacity; the amount of air that can be expired after maximum inspiration.

VITAL SIGNS. A person's essential body functions, usually defined as pulse, body temperature, and breathing rate.

VITAMIN K. A group of structurally related fat-soluble vitamins needed in humans and other animals to make blood clotting factors. Vitamin K_1 is the form of the vitamin found in plants; vitamin K_2 is the form found in animals.

VITRECTOMY. Surgical removal and replacement of part or all of the vitreous body.

VITREOUS BODY. The transparent gel that fills the inner portion of the eyeball between the lens and the retina. It is also called the vitreous humor or crystalline humor.

VOIDING. The medical term for emptying the bladder or urinating.

VOLAR. Pertaining to the palm of the hand or the sole of the foot.

VOLATILE ANESTHETIC. An anesthetic administered as a gas through an anesthesia mask. Volatile anesthetics are also called inhalational anesthetics.

VOLUMETRIC. Relating to or involving the measurement of volume.

VOLVULUS. An intestinal obstruction caused by a knotting or twisting of the bowel.

V/Q SCAN. A test in which both a perfusion scan and ventilation scan are done (separately or together) to show the quantity of air that different areas of the lungs are receiving.

VULVA. The external portion of the female genital organs.

W

WARFARIN. An anticoagulant that is commonly used to treat various heart conditions and blood clots; sold under the brand name Coumadin.

WATCHFUL WAITING. Monitoring a patient's disease state carefully to see if the condition worsens before trying surgery or another therapy.

WEGENER'S GRANULOMATOSIS. A rare condition that consists of lesions within the respiratory tract.

WEIGHT TRACTION. Sometimes used interchangeably with skin traction (traction in which weights or other devices are attached to the skin).

WESTERN BLOT. A technique to determine the presence of HIV antibody that is used to confirm enzyme-linked immunosorbent assay (ELISA) results.

WHITE BLOOD CELL (WBC) DIFFERENTIAL. A white blood cell count in which the technician classifies the different white blood cells by type as well as calculating the number of each type.

WHITE BLOOD CELLS. Cells that protect the body against infection; also known as leukocytes.

WILSON'S DISEASE. A genetic disorder characterized by accumulation of copper in the liver and brain.

WITHDRAWAL. End of administration or use of a drug.

WITHDRAWAL SYMPTOMS. A group of physical or mental symptoms that may occur when a person suddenly stops using a drug to which he or she has become dependent.

WOLFF-PARKINSON-WHITE SYNDROME. An abnormal rapid heart rhythm, due to an extra pathway for the electrical impulses to travel from the atria to the ventricles.

WRONG-SITE SURGERY. Performance of the wrong surgery or surgery performed on the wrong body part or the wrong person.

X

XENOGRAFT. A tissue or organ transplanted from a member of one animal species to a member of a different species (e.g., pigs to humans).

X-RAY. A form of electromagnetic radiation with shorter wavelengths than normal light. X-rays can penetrate most structures.

Z

ZINC PROTOPORPHYRIN (ZPP) TEST. A blood test that can be performed to screen for high blood lead levels by measuring the levels of a compound called zinc protoporphyrin.

ZOLLINGER-ELLISON SYNDROME. A condition marked by stomach ulcers, with excess secretion of stomach acid and tumors of the pancreas.

Z-TRACK INJECTION. A special technique for injecting a drug into muscle tissue so that the drug does not leak (track) into the layers of tissue just beneath the skin.

ZYGOMA. The cheekbone in the front of the face below the eye socket, connected to the frontal bone of the forehead and the maxilla (upper jaw). It is sometimes called the os zygomaticum or zygomatic bone.

ZYGOMATIC ARCH. Cheekbone; quadrilateral bone forming the prominence of the cheek. It articulates (touches or moves) with the frontal, sphenoid, maxillary, and temporal bones.

ZYGOTE INTRAFALLOPIAN TUBE TRANSFER (ZIFT). An artificial reproductive technique where a woman's eggs are fertilized in a laboratory dish and then placed in her fallopian tube.

INDEX

The index is alphabetized using a word-by-word system. References to individual volumes are listed before colons; numbers following a colon refer to specific page numbers within that particular volume. **Boldface** references indicate main topical essays. Photographs and illustration references are highlighted with an italicized page number. Tables and figures are indicated with the page number followed by a lowercase, italicized *t* or *f*, respectively.

A

Abdomen
   muscles of, 1:*6*
   paracentesis, 3:1347–1348
   second-look surgery, 4:1619
Abdominal adhesions, 1:26, 27
Abdominal aortic aneurysm
   aortic aneurysm repair, 1:122–123
   endovascular stent surgery, 2:574–577
   vascular surgery, 4:1976–1978
Abdominal cerclage, 1:325
Abdominal cystocele repair, 1:476, 477
Abdominal hernia, 2:694
Abdominal hysterectomy, 2:873, 874
Abdominal pain
   abdominal ultrasound, 1:1
   gallstones, 2:677
   laparotomy, exploratory, 3:1015
Abdominal stoma, 4:1733–1734, 1736
Abdominal surgery
   complications, 4:1547
   incisional hernias, 2:800–804
   laparoscopy, 3:1004–1009
   laparotomy, exploratory, 3:1013–1016
   surgical risks, 4:1770
   trocar injury, 4:1897
   See also specific types
Abdominal ultrasound, 1:**1–5**, *2*
Abdominal wall defect repair, 1:**5–8**, 3:1383
Abdominoplasty, 1:**8–13**, *9*
Ablative pain management procedures, 3:1330–1331
ABO blood group, 4:1564, 1867, 1927–1928
Abortifacient drugs. *See* Medical abortions
Abortion, induced, 1:**13–18**
   dilatation and curettage, 2:512

   intrauterine device insertion following, 2:936
   obstetric and gynecologic surgery, 3:1273
Abscess drainage, 1:**18–20**
Absorptive disorders, 4:1739–1740
Academy of Nutrition and Dietetics, 4:2025
Acardiac twins, 2:649
Access to health care, 3:1369
Accident-only insurance policies, 3:1509
Accidents, automobile. *See* Traffic accidents
Accreditation
   ambulatory surgery centers, 1:49
   hospitals, 1:351
Accreditation Council for Graduate Medical Education, 2:853
ACE inhibitors. *See* Angiotensin-converting enzyme inhibitors
Acetaminophen, 1:**20–22**, 3:1077
Acetazolamide, 3:1023
Achalasia, 2:607, 775–776
Acidosis
   arterial blood gas tests, 1:134
   crush syndrome, 1:455
   pH monitoring, 3:1408, 1410
Acquired immune deficiency syndrome. *See* HIV/AIDS
Acromegaly, 4:1690
Acromioclavicular joint. *See* Shoulder joint
ACTH, 1:435, 436
Actinic keratosis, 1:464–467
Activated clotting time tests, 1:369, 372
Activities of daily living
   home care, 2:837
   nursing homes, 3:1261
   surgery and the elderly, 4:1755
Acupressure
   pain management, 3:1330

   postoperative antiemetics alternatives, 3:1464
Acupuncture
   hypertension, 4:1978
   with myringotomy, 3:1231
   pain management, 3:1330
   postoperative antiemetics alternatives, 3:1464
   smoking cessation, 4:1696
   snoring surgery alternatives, 4:1704
Acute appendicitis, 3:1384
Acute care
   physiologic monitoring system, 2:926, 3:1283
   pressure ulcers, 3:1497
Acute hemolytic transfusion reaction, 4:1869, 1930
Acute ischemic stroke, 4:1826
Acute knee injuries, 2:972–977, 978
Acute normo-volemic hemodilution, 1:165
Acute renal failure, 1:273
Acute stress disorder, 1:196
Acute surgical emergencies, 2:560
Adaptive equipment, 4:1543
Addiction. *See* Substance abuse and addiction
Addison's disease, 2:551
Adenocarcinoma, 4:1942
Adenoidectomy, 1:**22–25**, *23*, 2:531
Adenoids and snoring, 4:1701
Adenosine diphosphate, 1:448
Adhesions, 1:**25–29**
   intestinal obstruction repair, 2:929, 930
   intussusception reduction, 2:944
   second-look surgery, 4:1619
Adhesives
   fibrin sealants, 2:652–654
   incision care, 2:919
Adjustable gastric band restrictive surgery, 2:695

Attached flap surgery, 1:262

Augmentation cystoplasty. *See* Bladder augmentation

Auscultation, 4:1730–1732

Australia, 2:627

Autografts, 1:221, 4:1686

Autoimmune disorders
  antibody tests, 1:100
  antinuclear antibody tests, 1:112–113
  breast implants, 1:263
  immunosuppressant drugs, 2:897
  immunosuppression, 2:902–903
  liver function tests, 3:1074
  rheumatoid factor testing, 4:1566–1568
  thoracentesis, 4:1814

Autoimmune hemolytic disorders, 4:1717

Autologous blood donation, 1:**164–167**
  blood donation and registry, 1:205
  blood salvage, 1:211–212
  hip replacement, 2:821
  knee replacement, 2:985
  laparoscopy, 3:1006
  planning a hospital stay, 3:1437
  preparing for surgery, 3:1493
  presurgical preparations, 3:1504
  spinal fusion, 4:1709
  transfusions, 4:1868
  transplant surgery, 4:1874
  type and screen, 4:1929

Autologous bone marrow transplantation, 1:230, 231, 234

Autologous breast reconstruction, 1:262, 263

Autologous islet cell transplantation, 2:954

Autologous stem cell transplantation, 4:1725

Autolytic debridement, 2:486

Automated endoscope reprocessing system, 1:270

Automobile accidents. *See* Traffic accidents

Autonomic nervous system, 4:1783–1785

Autonomy
  do not resuscitate orders, 2:525
  patient rights, 3:1373

Autosomal disease, 2:720

Avascular necrosis, 2:819

Avulsion, tooth, 4:1848–1850

Avulsion injuries, 3:1315

Awareness during surgery, 1:72, 187

Axillary dissection, 1:**167–170**, *168*, 4:1629

Axillary temperature measurement, 4:1800, 1811–1812, 2013

Ayurveda
  integrative medicine, 1:405
  peptic ulcer disease, 1:120
  philosophy and practice, 1:403–404

Azathioprine, 2:896, 897, 899

B

Baby boomers, 3:1176

Bacille Calmette-Guerin therapy, 1:474

Back pain, 3:997–1003, 4:1709

Back surgery
  disk removal, 2:517–522
  spinal fusion, 4:1707–1711
  spinal instrumentation, 4:1711–1713

Bacteremia, 1:202–204

Bacterial infections
  abscess drainage, 1:18–20
  anaerobic bacteria cultures, 1:58–60
  antibiotic prophylaxis, 1:90–92
  antibiotics, 1:92–96
  antiseptics, 1:114–115
  blood cultures, 1:202–204
  cephalosporin, 1:313–315
  cerebral fluid analysis, 1:320–323
  drug-resistant organisms, 2:527–528
  ear infections, 3:1231
  erythromycin, 2:595–596
  gingivectomy, 2:725
  H. pylori, 3:1530–1533
  pneumonia, 4:1817
  sexually transmitted disease, 4:1661, 1683, 1684
  stool cultures, 4:1738–1739
  surgical risks, 4:1768
  topical antibiotics, 1:97–99
  urinalysis, 4:1948
  urine cultures, 4:1957
  wound cultures, 4:2035–2036

Baerveldt implants, 4:1905

Balance issues, 2:555–557, 4:1925

Balanced anesthesiology, 1:187

Baldness, 2:741–743

Balfour, William, 2:658

Balloon angioplasty, 1:427, 428, 431

Balloon atrial septostomy, 2:759

Balloon dilation, 4:1886

Balloon valvotomy, 1:127

Balloon valvuloplasty, 1:**171–174**, 2:759

Bandages and dressings, 1:**174–177**
  incision care, 2:919

tendon repair, 4:1803
  wound care, 4:2032–2033

Bankart procedure, 1:**177–180**, *178*

Bariatric surgery
  gastric bypass, 2:691–696
  weight management, 4:2024
  See also Vertical banded gastroplasty

Barium enemas, 1:*181*, **181–183**
  colorectal surgery, 1:387
  rectal resection, 4:1548
  sigmoidoscopy alternatives, 4:1673

Barium esophagography
  esophageal resection, 2:609–610
  gastric cancer, 2:698
  gastroesophageal reflux scans, 2:705–707
  upper gastrointestinal examinations, 4:1936–1937

Barotrauma, 1:195–196, 3:1230

Barrett's esophagus
  esophageal resection, 2:607
  gastroesophageal reflux surgery, 2:711
  Heller myotomy, 2:775
  nonsurgical management of, 2:610–611

Basal cell carcinomas, 1:464–467, 3:1219

Basic life support, 1:457

Basiliximab, 2:897, 898

Bathing and showering, 2:920

Batteries, pacemaker, 3:1325

Bed rest
  cervical cerclage alternatives, 1:326
  prenatal surgery, 3:1481–1482

Bedsores. *See* Pressure ulcers

Behavioral therapy. *See* Cognitive-behavioral therapy

Belladonna, 4:1614

Bell's palsy, 4:1790

Benign prostatic hyperplasia
  prostatectomy, 3:1513–1519
  transurethral resection of the prostate, 4:1882, 1884–1887
  tumor marker tests, 4:1912
  urologic surgery, 4:1958

Benzalkonium chloride, 1:114

Benzodiazepine, 1:88, 89, 90

Bernstein test, 2:603–604

Best interests of patients, 3:1373

Beta waves, 2:548–549

Beta$_2$-microglobulin tests, 2:835

Beta-adrenergic blockers, 1:108

Beta-blockers, 4:1977

Bicarbonate, 1:134, 2:552

Blood flow and circulation (*continued*)
enhanced external counterpulsation, 2:578–583
heart-lung machines, 2:768–771
horse chestnut, 4:1613, 1992
magnetic resonance angiography, 3:1115–1117
smoking cessation, 4:1695
vascular surgery, 4:1973–1979
ventricular assist devices, 4:1997–2001

Blood gas tests. *See* Arterial blood gas tests

Blood glucose levels, 2:731, 3:1295–1298

Blood pressure
hypotensive transfusion reaction, 4:1869
sphygmomanometers, 4:1705–1707
vital signs, 4:2013–2014

Blood pressure measurement, 1:**208–211**, 209*t*, *210*

Blood salvage, 1:165, **211–213**

Blood substitutes, 1:166, 4:1870

Blood sugar tests. *See* Glucose tests

Blood tests
complete blood count, 1:408–410
creatine phosphokinase tests, 1:447–449
electrolyte tests, 2:550–552
Epstein-Barr virus test, 2:594–595
HDL cholesterol tests, 2:752
hematocrit, 2:779–780
hemoglobin tests, 2:783–785
hepatitis virus tests, 2:794–796
HIV/AIDS tests, 2:830–836
human chorionic gonadotropin pregnancy tests, 2:855–857
human leukocyte antigen tests, 2:857–859
immunoassay tests, 2:889–891
iron tests, 2:950–952
kidney function tests, 2:964–966
latex allergies, 3:1043
LDL cholesterol test, 3:1046–1047
lipid profiles, 3:1060–1061
liver biopsy alternatives, 3:1071
lung transplantation, 3:1107
partial thromboplastin time, 3:1358–1359
peripheral endarterectomy, 3:1398
phlebotomy, 3:1420–1421
protein components test, 3:1520–1521
red blood cell indices, 4:1551–1553
Rh blood typing, 4:1564–1566

rheumatoid factor testing, 4:1566–1568
sedimentation rate, 4:1622–1624
serum calcium levels, 4:1635–1637
serum carbon dioxide levels, 4:1637–1638
serum chloride levels, 4:1639–1640
serum creatinine levels, 4:1640–1642
serum glucose levels, 4:1643–1645
serum lead levels, 4:1645–1649
serum phosphate levels, 4:1650–1651
serum potassium levels, 4:1651–1653
serum sodium levels, 4:1654–1656
thyroid function tests, 4:1830–1833
toxicology screens, 4:1853
tumor marker tests, 4:1910–1914
type and screen, 4:1926–1931
white blood cell count and differential, 4:2029–2031

Blood thinners. *See* Anticoagulant and antiplatelet drugs

Blood toxicity, 2:785–786

Blood transfusions. *See* Transfusions

Blood type. *See* Type and screen

Blood urea nitrogen tests, 1:**213–215**, 335, 2:965, 966

Blood urea nitrogen-creatinine ratio, 1:**271–275**

Blood vessel hemorrhages, 4:1897

Blood vessels, 1:120–124, 3:1195–1196

Blood-borne disease, 1:215

Bloodborne infections, 4:1787–1788

Bloodless surgery, 1:166, **215–218**, 4:1870

Bloodstream infections. *See* Sepsis

Bloom-Richardson-Elston tumor grading system, 4:1909

Blunt-force trauma, 1:196

Board certification, 2:655

Body dysmorphic disorder, 2:666

Body fluid glucose tests, 2:732

Body imaging, 3:1119

Body mass index
gastric bypass, 2:691, 693
obesity, 3:1267, 4:2022
postoperative nausea risk factors, 3:1462
vertical banded gastroplasty, 4:2007

Body plethysmography, 3:1527, 1528

Body scans, 1:411, 413, 3:1118

Body temperature, 4:1798–1800, 1810–1812, 2012–2014

Body-based therapies

complementary medicine and surgery, 1:404
knee revision surgery alternatives, 2:992
pain management, 3:1330
scar revision surgery alternatives, 4:1595

Bombings, 4:1888–1889

Bone cancer, 3:1057–1059

Bone cement, 4:1807, 1808

Bone density tests, 1:**218–220**, *219*, 2:821, 3:1107

Bone grafting, 1:**220–225**, *221*, 2:500

Bone marrow aspiration and biopsy, 1:*225*, **225–229**

Bone marrow disorders, 4:1725–1726

Bone marrow genetic testing, 2:722, 723

Bone marrow transplantation, 1:**229–237**, *230*
stem cell transplantation compared to, 4:1725

Bone morphogenetic proteins, 1:224

Bone scans, 1:**237–239**, 3:1260

Bone spurs, 3:1000

Bone tumors, 3:1057

Bone x-rays, 1:**239–241**, *240*

Bones, hand, 2:748

Boston Marathon bombings, 4:1888–1889

Botanical therapies. *See* Herbal medicine

Botox
face lift alternatives, 2:638
forehead lift alternatives, 1:68
migraines, effect on, 3:1198

Bowel disorders and spina bifida, 3:1185

Bowel diversion, 1:386

Bowel injuries and trocar use, 4:1897–1898

Bowel obstruction repair. *See* Intestinal obstruction repair

Bowel preparation, 1:**241–242**
barium enemas, 1:182
bowel resection, 1:245
bowel resection, small intestine, 1:250
colonoscopy, 1:382
colorectal surgery, 1:387
colostomy, 1:391
defecography, 2:496
preoperative care, 3:1489
rectal resection, 4:1548
sigmoidoscopy, 4:1672

Bowel resection, 1:**242–247**, *243*, 2:800

Bowel resection, small intestine, 1:**247–252**, *248*

Bowel strangulation, 2:931, 944

Cancer (continued)

bone marrow aspiration and biopsy, 1:225–228

bone scans, 1:237

bowel resection, 1:244, 246

bowel resection, small intestine, 1:249, 251

breast biopsy, 1:252–255

breast cancer demographics, 4:1586–1587

chest x-rays, 1:340, 341

circumcision, 1:354

colonic stents, 1:379–380

colony-stimulating factors, 2:893

comorbidity, 3:1169

complementary and alternative medicine, 1:404–405

cone biopsy, 1:414–416

craniofacial reconstruction, 1:440, 442, 444

cryotherapy, 1:460, 461

cystectomy, 1:472–474

debulking surgery, 2:488–492

dilatation and curettage, 2:512

elbow surgery, 2:540

endoscopic retrograde cholangiopancreatography, 2:566

esophageal resection, 2:605–611

exenteration, 2:618–622

eye enucleation, 2:583–585

gastrectomy, 2:685–687

gastric cancer, 1:116–117

genetic testing, 2:721

glossectomy, 2:729–731

hepatectomy, 2:790–793

hypophysectomy, 2:863–866

hypospadias repair, 2:868

ileal conduit surgery, 2:880

immunosuppressant drugs, 2:899–900, 904

intestinal obstruction repair, 2:929

iridectomy, 2:947, 948, 949

laparoscopy, 3:1006

laparotomy, exploratory, 3:1013, 1015

laryngectomy, 3:1017–1019

limb salvage, 3:1057–1059

lobectomy, pulmonary, 3:1087–1091

lumpectomy, 3:1095–1099

lung biopsy, 3:1099–1103

lymph node biopsy, 3:1108–1110

mammography, 3:1124–1127

mastectomy, 3:1133–1137

mediastinoscopy, 3:1156–1159

modified radical mastectomy, 3:1213–1216

Mohs surgery, 3:1217–1219

myelography, 3:1221–1222

nephrostomy, 3:1249, 1250

obesity, 3:1269

obstetric and gynecologic surgery, 3:1273–1274

oral and maxillofacial surgery, 3:1290–1294

orchiectomy, 3:1298–1303

otoplasty, 3:1313

pancreatectomy, 3:1340–1343

pancreatic and gallbladder cancer, 2:566–567

Pap tests, 3:1343–1346

paracentesis, 3:1347

parotidectomy, 3:1356–1357

pharyngectomy, 3:1415–1418

pneumonectomy, 3:1444–1448

polypectomy, 3:1449–1453

positron emission tomography, 3:1457–1458

pressure ulcers, 3:1498

prostate and testicular cancers, 3:1298–1299

prostate biopsy, 3:1509–1512

quadrantectomy, 4:1535

radical neck dissection, 4:1539–1542

rectal resection, 4:1548

reoperation, 4:1557

second opinions, 4:1616

second-look surgery, 4:1618–1619

segmentectomy, 4:1624–1628

sentinel lymph node biopsy, 4:1629

simple mastectomy, 4:1674–1678

skin biopsy, 4:1681–1682

splenectomy, 4:1717

stereotactic radiosurgery, 4:1727–1729

surgical oncology, 4:1762–1765

thoracentesis, 4:1814

thoracoscopy, 4:1819

thoracotomy, 4:1821, 1822

transplant surgery, 4:1875

tube enterostomy, 4:1903

tumor grading, 4:1908–1910

tumor marker tests, 4:1910–1914

tumor removal, 4:1914–1917

tumor staging, 4:1917–1922

ureterosigmoidostomy, 4:1940–1941, 1942

ureterostomy, cutaneous, 4:1943–1945

urologic surgery, 4:1958

Whipple procedure, 4:2026–2029

See also Bone marrow transplantation; specific types

Cancer recurrence, 3:1357, 4:1678

Capacity. See Competence

Capsular contraction, 1:264

Capsulotomy, 2:744

Car accidents. See Traffic accidents

Carbon dioxide, 1:133, 4:1637–1638

Carbon dioxide lasers, 3:1032

Carbon monoxide diffusing tests, 3:1526

Carbonic anhydrase inhibitors, 2:522

Carcinoembryonic antigens, 4:1912

Cardiac blood pool studies. See Multiple-gated acquisition scans

Cardiac catheterization, 1:**281–286**, *282*, 428–429, 2:757–758

Cardiac complications, 4:1756, 1769–1770

Cardiac event monitors, 1:**286–289**, *287*

Cardiac marker tests, 1:**289–292**

Cardiac monitors, 1:286–289, **292–294**, *293*

Cardiac rehabilitation, 4:2000

Cardiac stress tests. See Stress tests

Cardiac surgery. See Heart surgery

Cardiac tamponade, 3:1393–1395

Cardiac transplantation. See Heart transplantation

Cardiopulmonary resuscitation, 1:**294–298**, *295*

defibrillation, 2:497, 498

DNR orders, 3:1495

powers of attorney, 3:1475

Cardiothoracic surgery, 4:1773

Cardiovascular surgeons, 4:1750

Cardioversion, 1:298, **298–303**, 3:1145

Caregivers, 2:839, 3:1499, 1501

Carotid artery disease, 4:1976

Carotid endarterectomy, 1:**303–308**, *304*, 2:575

Carpal tunnel release, 1:**309–313**, *310*

Carpal tunnel syndrome, 1:309–313, 2:749

Carrier testing, 2:720

Cartilage transplantation, 2:988

Case management, 2:839, 3:1130

Castration. See Orchiectomy

Casts, 1:367, 4:1806

CAT scan. See Computed tomography

Cataracts, 1:**462–464**

extracapsular cataract extraction, 2:625–631

goniotomy, 2:737

iridectomy complications, 3:1025

Index

Cirrhosis
  aspartate aminotransferase tests, 1:160
  demographics, 3:1405
  liver transplantation, 3:1076
  peritoneovenous shunts, 3:1406
  portal vein bypass, 3:1454–1456
  thoracentesis, 4:1813
Cis-retinoic acid, 2:506
Cisternal puncture, 1:320
Claustrophobia, 3:1116, 1123
Claw toe surgery. *See* Hammer, claw, and mallet toe surgery
Cleft lip and palate repair, 1:**357–361**, *358*, 438
Cleveland Clinic, 1:307, 2:639–640
Clinical chemists, 4:1855–1856
Clinical interviews, 2:754–756
Clinical trials
  carotid endarterectomy, 1:305, 307
  drug-coated coronary stents, 1:429
  lung cancer, 3:1103
  traction, 4:1865
  transplant surgery alternatives, 4:1877
Clinical *vs.* pathological tumor stage, 4:1920–1921
Closed-angle glaucoma, 2:945–949, 3:1020–1025
Closed-fist injuries, 2:749
Clostridium difficile, 4:1738, 1739
Closures, 1:**362–366**, 2:918–921, 3:995–996
Clot-dissolving drugs. *See* Thrombolytic therapy
Clotting. *See* Blood clotting
ClozeX, 1:365
Club foot repair, 1:**366–368**
Coagulation and clotting tests, 1:**368–373**
Coats' disease, 4:1558, 1559
Cochlear implants, 1:*373*, **373–377**
Cochrane database review, 3:1464
Cognition and mental health assessment, 3:1187
  gastric bypass alternatives, 2:696
  sacral nerve stimulation alternatives, 4:1585
  smoking cessation, 4:1696
  weight management, 4:2023–2024
Cognitive impairment, 2:495, 4:1754
Cognitive-behavioral therapy, 4:1696, 2024–2025
Coherent ultrapulse carbon dioxide laser treatment, 2:639
Cold sores, 2:506
Cold-knife conization, 1:414

Colds, 2:601
Colectomy. *See* Bowel resection
Collaborative Corneal Transplantation Study, 1:419
Collagen dressings, 1:174, 175
Collagen periurethral injections, 1:**377–378**
Colon polyps, 3:1449–1453
Colonic stents, 1:**379–381**
Colonoscopy, 1:**381–385**, *382*
  barium enema alternatives, 1:181
  colonic stents, 1:379–380
  colorectal surgery, 1:385–386, 387
  polypectomy, 3:1449–1453
  rectal resection, 4:1548
  after sigmoidoscopy, 4:1673
Colony-stimulating factors, 1:233, 2:893, 895
Colorectal cancer
  colonic stents, 1:379–380
  colonoscopy, 1:383–384
  colorectal surgery, 1:385–386, 389
  fecal occult blood tests, 2:646, 647
  obesity, 3:1269
  rectal resection, 4:1548
  sigmoidoscopy, 4:1670–1674
Colorectal surgery, 1:**385–389**
  bowel section, 1:242, 247
  gastroenterologic surgery risks, 2:703
Colostomy, 1:*390*, **390–394**
  colorectal surgery, 1:386, 387
  gastroenterologic surgery, 2:701
  intestinal obstruction repair, 2:930
  stoma, 4:1733–1734
ColoSure, 2:646
Colpocentesis, 3:1347
Colporrhaphy, 1:**394–396**, 475, 477, 3:1273
Colposcopy, 1:*397*, **397–400**, 415, 3:1273, 1343, 1345–1346
Colpotomy, 1:**400–402**, 3:1273
Coma, 3:1149
Combat casualties, 4:1889
Commercialization of health care, 1:49
Commissurotomy, 3:1207
Committee on Obstetric Practice, ACOG, 1:331
Communication
  errors, 3:1171
  laryngectomy, 3:1019
  talking to the health care provider, 4:1789–1790
Community hospitals, 2:845
Community-based health care

Medicaid, 3:1161
Patient Protection and Affordable Care Act, 3:1369
Comorbidity, 3:**1167–1170**
  diabetes, 2:508
  esophageal atresia, 2:599
  minimally invasive heart surgery, 3:1202
  surgery and the elderly, 4:1756
Compartment syndrome, 1:455–457
Competence, 2:922, 3:1373
  See also Mental capacity
Complementary and alternative medicine, 1:**402–408**
  atherosclerosis prevention, 3:1399, 1404
  benign prostatic hyperplasia, 4:1886–1887
  bladder cancer, 4:1881
  cancer treatment, 1:235–236
  with hip replacement, 2:823
  with hip revision surgery, 2:829
  kidney stone prevention, 3:1248
  knee replacement alternatives, 2:988
  knee revision surgery, 2:991
  laminectomy alternatives, 3:1003
  pain management, 3:1330
  peptic ulcer disease, 1:120
  planning a hospital stay, 3:1435
  postoperative antiemetics alternatives, 3:1464–1465
  postoperative pain management, 3:1472–1473
  preparing for surgery, 3:1493
  pressure ulcers, 3:1500
  sclerostomy alternatives, 4:1604
  sclerotherapy for varicose veins alternatives, 4:1613
  smoking cessation, 4:1696
  with transplant surgery, 4:1877
  vein ligation and stripping alternatives, 4:1992
  weight management, 4:2024–2025
Complete blood counts, 1:**408–410**, 2:834, 4:1551–1553
Complete debulking, 2:489
Complete splenectomy, 4:1718–1719
Compliance. *See* Patient compliance
Complications. *See* specific procedures
Composite dressings, 1:174, 175, 4:2032
Composite skin grafts, 4:1687
Composite tissue allotransplantation, 2:639
Compressed oxygen, 3:1320
Compresses, 2:593, 3:1500
Compression injuries, 2:643

2164   GALE ENCYCLOPEDIA OF SURGERY AND MEDICAL TESTS, 3ᴿᴰ EDITION

Cultures
anaerobic bacteria culture, 1:58–60
sexually transmitted disease cultures, 4:1660–1663
skin cultures, 4:1682–1684
stool cultures, 4:1737–1739
urine cultures, 4:1956–1957
wound cultures, 4:2035–2036
Curettage, dental cleaning, 2:726
Curettage and electrosurgery, 1:**464–468**
Cushing's syndrome, 2:863
Custom LASIK, 3:1038
Cutaneous ureterostomy. *See* Ureterostomy, cutaneous
Cutting trocars, 4:1896
Cyanoacrylates, 1:364, 2:652, 919
Cyclocryotherapy, 1:*468*, **468–471**, 2:738
Cyclodestruction, 2:738, 4:1907
Cyclophotocoagulation, 1:470–471
Cyclosporine
diuretics interactions, 2:524–525
immunosuppressant drugs, 2:896, 897, 899
liver transplantation, 3:1079
Cystectomy, 1:**471–474**, 4:1941
Cystic fibrosis, 2:720
Cystine calculi, 3:1245
Cystocele repair, 1:**475–478**
Cystoceles, 1:394, *476*, 3:1236
Cystoid macular edema, 2:629–630
Cystoscopy, 1:*478*, **478–481**
polypectomy, 3:1449–1453
prostate biopsy, 3:1510–1511
before prostatectomy, 3:1515
ureteral stenting, 4:1938
urologic surgery, 4:1959
Cystostomy, 4:1944
Cytology, 1:**481–482**, 2:615
Cytoreduction. *See* Debulking surgery
Cytostatic drugs, 2:902
Cytotoxic drugs, 2:611

D

Da Vinci surgical system, 3:1516, 4:*1573*, 1574–1575
Daclizumab, 2:897
Dacron patches, 2:760
Damus-Kaye-Stansel procedures, 2:759
Darrow, Marc, 2:988
Databases and patient confidentiality, 3:1364
Daviel, Jacques, 2:625

Day care, 3:1232
D-dimer tests, 1:369–370, 372
Deafness. *See* Hearing impairment
Death and dying, 2:**483–486**, 841–843
DeBakey, Michael, 1:303
Debridement, 2:**486–488**
dental cleaning, 2:726
knee arthroscopic surgery, 2:975, 976
knee osteotomy, 2:979
knee replacement alternatives, 2:988
Debulking surgery, 2:**488–493**, 4:1915, 1916
Decentered ablation, 3:1039
Decision making, 3:1373
Decompression, spinal, 2:519–520
Decontamination, 1:197
Deductibles, insurance, 3:1506
Deep brain stimulation, 2:*493*, **493–496**, 3:1335
Deep vein thrombosis
cesarean section, 1:333
hip replacement, 2:822
knee replacement, 2:986, 987
phlebography, 3:1418–1419
prevention, 4:1993–1996
surgical risks, 4:1770
thrombectomy, 4:1823–1826
vein ligation and stripping, 4:1991
Defecography, 2:**496–497**
Defibrillation, 2:*497*, **497–499**
electrophysiology study of the heart, 2:559
implantable cardioverter defibrillators, 2:907–910
mitral valve repair alternatives, 3:1208
Deflagration, 1:194
Deformities
hammer, claw, and mallet toe surgery, 2:743–746
hip osteotomy, 2:815–817
knee osteotomy, 2:978, 979
leg lengthening or shortening, 3:1047–1052
mentoplasty, 3:1190–1193
oral and maxillofacial surgery, 3:1290, 1291
otoplasty, 3:1312–1316
pectus excavatum, 3:1377–1379
penile prostheses, 3:1390–1392
snoring surgery, 4:1701
See also Congenital abnormalities
Degenerative conditions
kneecap removal, 2:993

neurosurgery, 3:1255–1256
shoulder resection arthroplasty risks, 4:1669
wrist replacement, 4:2037
Dehiscence
incision care, 2:920–921
vertical banded gastroplasty, 4:2009
wounds, 4:2034
Dehydration
intravenous rehydration, 2:940–941
kidney stone risk factors, 3:1245
nursing homes, 3:1265
Delayed breast reconstruction, 1:261
Delayed gastric emptying
gastroesophageal reflux scans, 2:705
pancreatectomy, 3:1342
vagotomy, 4:1965
Whipple procedure, 4:2028
Delayed hemolytic transfusion reaction, 4:1869
Delirium, 3:1056, 4:1754, 1756, 1768–1769
Delta waves, 2:548–549
Demand inspiratory flow systems, 3:1321
Dementia
single photon emission computed tomography, 4:1679
surgery and the elderly, 4:1754, 1756
surgical risks, 4:1769
Demographics. *See* Age; Gender; Race/ethnicity
Dendritic ulcers, 4:1791
Dental assistants and hygienists, 2:504
Dental bridges, 2:501
Dental exams, 1:233
Dental implants and restoration, 2:*499*, **499–502**, 4:1578
Dental procedures and oral surgery
anesthesia, local, 1:75, 76
gingivectomy, 2:725–728
hip replacement precautions, 2:821
knee replacement precautions, 2:985, 986
root canal treatment, 4:1576–1578
tooth extraction, 4:1845–1848
tooth replantation, 4:1848–1850
Dental x-rays, 2:*502*, **502–505**
Dentoalveolar surgery, 3:1291
Dentures, 2:501
Denver shunts, 3:1405
Department of Health and Human Services, U.S., 3:1094
Depression
craniofacial reconstruction, 1:443

Diethylstilbestrol, 2:869, 3:1299

Dieting, 4:2004–2005, 2020, 2023

Dietitians, 3:1436

Diffusion tensor imaging, 3:1119

Digestive disorders
stool fat tests, 4:1739–1740
Whipple procedure, 4:2028

Digestive system, 2:879, 4:1935–1937

Digital rectal examinations, 4:1884

Digital subtraction angiography, 1:306

Digital thermometers, 4:1800, 1811, 1812

Digital tonometry, 4:1841

Digitalis, 2:525

Dilatation and curettage, 2:512–515, 513
abortion, 1:15
hysteroscopy, 2:876
obstetric and gynecologic surgery, 3:1273
uterine polypectomy, 3:1450

Dilatation and evacuation, 1:15–16

Dilatation and extraction, 1:16

Direct DNA tests, 2:719, 721

Directed donor blood, 1:205, 4:1868

Disability
Medicaid, 3:1160, 1161
Medicare, 3:1176
nursing homes, 3:1261, 1262
premature birth, 1:326
stroke, 1:305–306

Disasters
emergency surgery, 2:561
mass trauma, 4:1888–1889
triage, 4:1781

Discharge, hospital, 2:515–517, 847

Disk degeneration, 4:1709, 1710

Disk removal, 2:517–522, 518

Diskectomy. See Disk removal

Dislocations
Bankart procedure, 1:177–180
hand surgery, 2:750
hip prostheses, 2:822
knee arthroscopic surgery, 2:974
kneecap removal, 2:993

Displaced flaps, 3:1040

Disposable catheterization sets, 4:1954

Disposable intensive care unit equipment, 2:928

Disposable operating room equipment, 3:1283

Disposable thermometers, 4:1800

Distant metastases, 4:1764

Diuretics, 2:522–525
antihypertensive drugs, 1:109–110

endolymphatic shunt alternatives, 2:565
peritoneovenous shunt alternatives, 3:1406

Diverticulitis, 1:244, 246, 3:1153–1155

Diverticulosis, 1:386

Dizziness, 2:555–557, 4:1925

Do not intubate orders, 4:1894

Do not resuscitate orders, 2:525–527
death and dying, 2:484
planning a hospital stay, 3:1439
powers of attorney, 3:1475
preparing for surgery, 3:1495
presurgical preparations, 3:1504
treatment refusal, 4:1894

Dobutamine, 1:35

DocInfo, 2:656

Docusate, 3:1045, 1046

Dog bites, 1:454, 455

Domiciliary care. see Home care

Donor Deferral Register, 1:205

Dopamine, 1:35, 3:1334

Dopamine antagonists, 3:1464

Doppler echocardiography, 2:535

Doppler ultrasound
abdominal ultrasound, 1:3
pelvic ultrasound, 3:1388
peripheral endarterectomy, 3:1398
stenosis in the carotid artery, 1:306

Dorsal rhizotomy. See Rhizotomy

Dosage
medication monitoring, 3:1180–1183
sedation, conscious, 4:1621
See also specific substances

Double-barrel colostomy, 1:391

Double-contrast barium studies, 1:117, 181

Down syndrome
alpha-fetoprotein tests, 1:46
amniocentesis, 1:51–52, 54
craniofacial reconstruction, 1:438, 442
genetic testing, 2:721
heart surgery for congenital defects, 2:757
prenatal testing, 3:1486

Drainage and drains
chest tube insertion, 1:336–339
endolymphatic shunts, 2:562–565
functional endoscopic sinus surgery, 2:672–675
gastrostomy, 2:713
incision care, 2:919
mastoidectomy, 3:1139
pharyngectomy, 3:1417

pneumonectomy, 3:1446
radical neck dissection, 4:1540
simple mastectomy, 4:1677
urinary catheterization, 4:1954
ventricular shunts, 4:2002–2004

Dressings. See Bandages and dressings

Driving, 4:1543, 1852, 1853

Driving under the influence, 4:1852, 1854

Drop attacks. See Epilepsy

Drug tests. See Toxicology screens

Drug-coated coronary stents, 1:429

Drug-resistant organisms, 2:527–529
antibiotic overuse, 1:95
fluoroquinolone, 2:662–663
hospital-acquired infections, 2:850–851
nursing homes, 3:1264
topical antibiotics, 1:98
urinary tract infections, 4:1955

Drugs, pharmaceutical. See Pharmaceutical drugs

Dry eye, 3:1040, 1287

Dry socket, 4:1846–1847

Dual eligibles, 3:1130, 1367

Dual Energy X-ray Absorptiometry (DEXA), 1:219

Duane syndrome, 2:633

Duchenne muscular dystrophy, 4:1709

Ductal carcinoma in situ, 3:1215

Duke Treadmill Score, 4:1744–1745

Dumping syndrome
antrectomy, 1:118
gastrectomy, 2:687
gastric bypass, 2:693, 694
gastroduodenostomy risks, 2:699
vagotomy, 4:1965

Duodenal ulcers, 4:1963, 1965

Duodenogastric reflux, 2:699

Durable powers of attorney. See Powers of attorney

Dye allergies. See Allergies

Dysmenorrhea, 1:400

Dysphagia
esophageal atresia repair, 2:601
esophageal cancer, 4:1816
esophageal resection alternatives, 2:611
pharyngectomy, 3:1417

Dysplasia, 3:1343, 1345, 1346

Dysrhythmias, 2:544–546

Dystocia, 1:329

Dystonia, 2:493, 494

E

E. coli, 4:1738, 1957

Ear, nose, and throat surgery, 2:**531–534**, *532*, 672–675

Ear infections, 3:1138–1140, 1229–1232

Ear molding, 3:1316

Ear temperature measurement, 4:1800, 1811

Ear tubes, 3:*1229*, **1229–1233**

Eardrum repair. *See* Tympanoplasty

Ears, 2:562–565, 3:1312–1316

Eastern cultures, 2:842

Eastern traditional medicine, 1:403–404

Eating disorders, 4:2020–2024

Echocardiography, 2:*534*, **534–536**, 3:1107, 4:1742–1744

Ectopic pregnancy
  in vitro fertilization, 2:913
  intrauterine devices, 2:938
  obstetric and gynecologic surgery, 3:1274
  salpingostomy, 4:1589–1592
  tubal ligation, 4:1901

Education, patient. *See* Patient education

Education and training, professional
  anesthesiologists, 1:78–79
  cardiopulmonary resuscitation, 1:297
  choosing a surgeon, 3:1491
  dental x-ray certification, 2:504
  finding a surgeon, 2:654–655
  general surgery, 2:716
  hospitalists, 2:853
  intensive care unit equipment, 2:928
  microsurgery, 3:1195
  oral and maxillofacial surgeons, 3:1291–1292
  orthopedic surgeons, 3:1310
  surgeons, 4:1751–1752
  surgical training, 4:1776–1778
  syringes and needles use, 4:1787–1788

EEG. *See* Electroencephalography

Egg retrieval, 3:1273

80/20 rule, 3:1368

Ejection fraction tests, 1:286

Elbow surgery, 2:**537–541**

Eldercare, 2:840

Elderly persons. *See* Aging and the aged; Surgery and the elderly

Elective surgery, 2:**541–543**
  bloodless surgery, 1:216
  cesarean section, 1:329–330, 331

extracapsular cataract extraction, 2:629
  finding a surgeon, 2:654–657
  gastric bypass, 2:691–696
  health insurance coverage, 2:617
  hernia repair, umbilical, 2:810–813
  laser-assisted in situ keratomileusis, 3:1035–1041
  Maze procedure for atrial fibrillation, 3:1141
  obesity, 3:1271
  oral and maxillofacial surgery, 3:1291
  photorefractive keratectomy, 3:1427
  plastic, reconstructive, and cosmetic surgery, 3:1441–1444
  preparing for, 3:1491–1496
  presurgical testing, 3:1502–1504
  vein ligation and stripping, 4:1986–1992

Electrocardiography, 2:*544*, **544–546**
  cardiac monitors, 1:292
  electrophysiology study of the heart, 2:557–559
  enhanced external counterpulsation, 1:426, 431–432
  lung transplantation, 3:1106–1107

Electrocoagulation, 2:565

Electroconvulsive therapy, 4:1968

Electrodesiccation, 1:465, 4:1613

Electroencephalography, 1:188–189, 433, 2:**546-550**, *547*

Electrofulguration, 1:465

Electrolyte tests, 2:**550–553**, 550*t*
  chemistry screens, 1:335–336
  serum carbon dioxide levels, 4:1637
  serum chloride levels, 4:1639
  serum creatinine levels, 4:1641
  serum glucose levels, 4:1643
  serum phosphate levels, 4:1650, 1652
  serum sodium levels, 4:1654

Electromyography, 1:153, 2:**553–555**, *554*

Electronic digital thermometers, 4:1800, 1811, 1812

Electronic health records
  medical charts, 3:1164, 1165–1166
  medical errors, 3:1173
  patient confidentiality, 3:1364

Electronic indentation tonometry, 4:1838

Electronystagmography, 2:**555–557**, *556*

Electrophysiologists, 2:910

Electrophysiology study of the heart, 2:**557–560**

Electrosection, 1:465

Electrosurgery. *See* Curettage and electrosurgery

Electrotherapy with debridement, 2:487

Eligibility
  Medicaid, 3:1369
  private insurance plans, 3:1507

Elschnig's pearls, 3:1026, 1028

Emasculation. *See* Orchiectomy

Embalming, 4:1896

Embolectomy, 4:1976

Embolisms
  hip replacement, 2:822
  knee replacement, 2:986
  mortality, 4:1978
  peripheral arterial disease, 3:1397
  peripheral endarterectomy, 3:1398
  phlebography, 3:1418–1419
  plastic, reconstructive, and cosmetic surgery, 3:1443
  prevention, 4:1993–1996
  sclerotherapy for varicose veins, 4:1612
  thoracentesis, 4:1813, 1814
  thrombectomy, 4:1823

Embolization *vs.* hysterectomy, 2:874

Embryonic stem cells, 4:1726

Emergencies and emergency care
  blast injuries, 1:196–197
  cardiopulmonary resuscitation, 1:294–297
  defibrillation, 2:497–499
  do not resuscitate orders, 2:525–526
  intensive care unit equipment, 2:927–928
  mass trauma, 4:1888–1889
  Patient Protection and Affordable Care Act, 3:1366, 1369, 1372
  pediatric concerns, 3:1380
  sclerotherapy for esophageal varices, 4:1606
  surgical triage, 4:1779–1780
  thyroid storm, 4:1836
  type and screen, 4:1929
  See also Emergency surgery

Emergency Laparotomy Network, 3:1014

Emergency physicians, 4:1855

Emergency resuscitation equipment, 3:1282

Emergency rooms, 2:769

Emergency Severity Index, 4:1780

Emergency surgery, 2:**560–562**
  chest tube insertion, 1:337–339
  cricothyroidotomy, 1:450–454

F

Hospitals, choosing, 1:**349–353**, 349*t*
 medical errors, avoiding, 3:1174
 pediatric concerns, 3:1381
 planning a stay, 3:1435
 preparing for surgery, 3:1492
 surgery centers, 3:1284
Hospitals, discharge from. *See* Discharge, hospital
Hospitals and hospitalization, 2:844*f*
 ambulatory surgery centers *vs.*, 1:50
 blast injuries, 1:196–197
 blood banks, 1:205
 crush injuries, 1:457
 do not resuscitate orders, 2:526
 hospice, 2:642
 hospitalists, 2:852–855
 intensive care unit equipment, 2:926–928
 intensive care units, 2:923–926
 length of stay, 3:1053–1057
 against medical advice, 4:1894
 operating rooms, 3:1281–1284
 outpatient surgery, 3:1317–1318
 ownership, 2:844*f*
 pediatric concerns, 3:1379–1381
 post-anesthesia care units, 3:1459–1460
 pressure ulcers, 3:1497–1498
 surgery risks and surgery volume, 4:1765, 1775
 surgical triage, 4:1779–1783
House, William, 2:563
Household safety, 1:458
HPV. *See* Human papillomavirus
Human bites, 2:749, 3:1314, 1315
Human chorionic gonadotropin tests, 2:**855–857**, 889, 4:1912–1913
Human error. *See* Medical errors
Human immunodeficiency virus. *See* HIV/AIDS
Human leukocyte antigen tests, 2:**857–859**
Human leukocyte antigens, 1:231, 232
Human papillomavirus (HPV)
 circumcision, 1:354
 curettage and electrosurgery, 1:465
 oral cancers, 2:729
 sexually transmitted disease cultures, 4:1662
Huntington's disease, 2:720–721
Hutchinson v. United States, 2:922–923
Hybrid Capture II test, 4:1662
Hyde shunts, 3:1405
Hydration, 3:1247

Hydrocelectomy, 2:**859–863**, *860*, 3:1385
Hydrocephalus, 4:2002–2004
Hydrocolloid dressings, 1:174, 175, 4:2032
Hydrocortisone, 1:435
Hydrofibers, 1:174, 175
Hydrogels, 1:174, 175, 4:2032
Hydrogen peroxide, 1:114
Hydropolymers, 1:174, 175
Hydrosalpinx, 4:1591
Hygiene
 circumcision, 1:354
 incision care, 2:920
 preoperative care, 3:1489
 pressure ulcer prevention, 3:1500
Hyperbaric oxygen therapy, 1:217, 457, 3:1319
Hyperglycemia, 2:687, 733
Hyperhidrosis, 4:1784, 1785
Hyperkalemia, 2:551
Hypernatremia, 2:550–551
Hyperosmotic agents, 3:1023–1024
Hyperosmotic laxatives, 3:1045
Hyperparathyroidism
 parathyroid hormone tests, 3:1349–1350
 parathyroidectomy, 3:1351–1353
 postoperative, 2:934
 sestamibi scans, 4:1656–1657
Hypersplenism, 4:1717
Hypertension
 acupuncture, 4:1978
 antihypertensive drugs, 1:107–110
 blood pressure measurement, 1:210
 carotid endarterectomy, 1:303, 305
 kidney dialysis, 2:959
Hypertrichosis, 4:1612
Hypertrophic scars, 1:360
Hyphema
 extracapsular cataract extraction, 2:629
 sclerostomy, 4:1604
 tube-shunt surgery, 4:1907
Hypnosis, 3:1293, 1330
Hypocalcemia, 2:933
Hypodermic needles. *See* Syringes and needles
Hypoglycemia, 2:699, 732, 733
Hypoparathyroidism, 2:933, 3:1353
Hypopharyngeal carcinomas, 3:1415, 1417–1418
Hypophysectomy, 2:*863*, **863–866**
Hypophysis. *See* Hypophysectomy
Hypopituitarism, 2:864

Hypoplastic left heart syndrome, 3:1480, 1481
Hypospadias repair, 2:**866–871**, *867*
Hypotension
 blood pressure measurement, 1:210
 bloodless surgery, 1:216–217
 kidney dialysis, 2:961–962
Hypotensive transfusion reaction, 4:1869
Hypothyroidism, 4:1836
Hypotony, 2:737, 4:1604
Hypoxemia, 3:1319–1322
Hysterectomy, 2:**871–875**, *872*
 colpotomy, 1:400, 402
 cone biopsy alternatives, 1:416
 dilatation and curettage alternatives, 2:514
 laparoscopy for endometriosis alternatives, 3:1012
 myomectomy alternatives, 3:1228
 obstetric and gynecologic surgery, 3:1273
 oophorectomy compared to, 3:1280
 postoperative pain, 3:1472
 salpingo-oophorectomy, 4:1586, 1588
Hysterosalpingography, 4:1591
Hysteroscopy, 2:**875–878**, *876*
 adhesions, 1:27
 dilatation and curettage alternatives, 2:514
 second-look surgery, 4:1620
Hysterosonography, 3:1389
Hysterotomy, 1:16

I

ICU. *See* Intensive care units
ICU psychosis, 3:1152
Idaho Radiation Network, 2:504
Ileal conduit surgery, 2:**879–882**, 4:1944
Ileoanal anastomosis, 1:386, 2:**882–886**, *883*, 888, 4:1736
Ileoanal reservoir surgery, 2:701
Ileostomy, 1:386, 2:**886–889**, *887*
 gastroenterologic surgery, 2:701
 ileoanal anastomosis *vs.*, 2:882, 884
 intestinal obstruction repair, 2:930
 stoma, 4:1733–1734
 stoma alternatives, 4:1736
Imaging studies
 adhesions, 1:27
 adrenalectomy, 1:33
 aortic aneurysms, 1:123

Infections

abscess drainage, 1:18–20
anaerobic bacteria cultures, 1:58–60
antibiotic prophylaxis, 1:90–92
antibiotics, 1:92–96
antibody tests, 1:101
appendectomy, 1:130–131
artificial sphincter insertion, 1:154
aseptic technique, 1:155–158
blood cultures, 1:202–204
bone scans, 1:237–238
bronchoscopy, 1:270
cephalosporin, 1:313–315
cerebral fluid analysis, 1:320–323
Chagas disease, 2:775
cryotherapy, 1:461
disk removal, 2:521
drug-resistant organisms, 2:527–528
extracapsular cataract extraction, 2:629
fetoscopy, 2:651
glaucoma, 4:1857
H. pylori, 3:1530–1533
hand surgery, 2:749
heart transplantation, 2:766
hepatitis virus tests, 2:794–796
hip replacement, 2:822–823
hospital-acquired infections, 2:848–851
hydrocelectomy, 2:862
hypophysectomy, 2:865
immunosuppressant drugs, 2:899–900, 904
incision care, 2:920–921
integrative medicine, 1:405–406
intrauterine device complications, 2:938
kidney dialysis, 2:962
knee replacement, 2:986, 987
laceration repair, 3:996
laser surgery risks, 3:1034
laser-assisted in situ keratomileusis risks, 3:1040
leg lengthening or shortening, 3:1050
limb salvage, 3:1058–1059
liver transplantation, 3:1081
lung transplantation, 4:1817
mechanical ventilation, 3:1152
mediastinoscopy, 3:1158
mitral valve repair, 3:1206
nephrolithotomy, percutaneous, 3:1247
neurosurgery, 3:1256
nursing homes, 3:1264
oral surgery, 2:727

paracentesis, 3:1347
phacoemulsification for cataracts, 3:1414
pharyngectomy, 3:1417
plastic, reconstructive, and cosmetic surgery, 3:1443
postoperative infections, 3:1468–1470
prenatal testing, 3:1486
pressure ulcers, 3:1497–1501
prostate biopsy, 3:1511
recovery at home, 4:1543
Robinson catheterization, 4:1949
sclerostomy, 4:1603
sexually transmitted disease cultures, 4:1660–1663
simple mastectomy, 4:1677
skin cultures, 4:1682–1684
skin grafts, 4:1687
skull x-rays, 4:1690
spinal instrumentation, 4:1713
splenectomy, 4:1720
stapedectomy, 4:1723
stem cell transplantation, 4:1726
stool cultures, 4:1737–1739
sulfonamides, 4:1745–1748
surgical risks, 4:1767–1768
syringes and needles use, 4:1787–1788
tendon repair, 4:1804
tooth extraction, 4:1845, 1846–1847
total parenteral nutrition, 4:1851
transplant surgery, 4:1876
tube enterostomy, 4:1904
urinary anti-infectives, 4:1949–1952
urinary catheterization, 4:1956
urologic surgery, 4:1959–1960
vascular access devices, 4:1972
white blood cell count and differential, 4:2029–2031
wound cultures, 4:2035–2036
wounds, 4:2034
wrist replacement, 4:2038
Infectious diseases
in vitro fertilization, 2:911–913
kidney dialysis, 2:962
negative pressure rooms, 3:1238–1239
prenatal testing, 3:1486–1487
sexually transmitted disease cultures, 4:1660–1663
transfusions, 4:1869
tuberculosis, 3:1132–1133
type and screen, 4:1929
Inferior vena cava filters, 4:1995

Infertility
genetic testing, 2:722
salpingostomy, 4:1589–1592
Inflammation
hip replacement, 2:823
laser iridotomy, 3:1024
sclerotherapy for varicose veins, 4:1612
sedimentation rate, 4:1622–1624
Inflammatory bowel disease, 3:1384–1385
Information disclosure and informed consent, 2:922–923
Information resources, 2:656, 3:1174
Informed consent, 2:**921–923**
anesthesia, 1:71
do not resuscitate orders, 2:525
enhanced external counterpulsation, 2:581
genetic testing, 2:722
goniotomy, 2:736
hip replacement, 2:821
hospital services, 2:846
knee replacement, 2:985
laparoscopy, 3:1006
lung biopsy, 3:1101
planning a hospital stay, 3:1438–1439
preoperative care, 3:1489–1490
preparing for surgery, 3:1494–1495
presurgical preparations, 3:1504
transplant surgery, 4:1874
treatment refusal, 4:1892
tube-shunt surgery, 4:1906
Infrared coagulation, 2:787
Infrared ear thermometers, 4:1800
INFUSE Bone Grafts, 1:224
Infusion pumps, 2:927, 3:1282
Inguinal hernia repair, 2:**805–809**, *806*, 3:1385
Inguinal orchiectomy, 3:1300
Inhalation anesthetics, 1:70
Inhalation challenge tests, 3:1527, 1528
Inhalation testing, 1:44, 45
Injectable local anesthetics, 1:74, 75
Injection snoreplasty, 4:1701
Injuries
blast injuries, 1:193–198
bowel resection, small intestine, 1:249
cataracts, 2:628
craniofacial reconstruction, 1:438, 440
crush injuries, 1:454–458
eye injuries, 2:584

Intravenous anesthetics, 1:70–71

Intravenous pain medications, 3:1472

Intravenous rehydration, 1:457, 2:*940*, **940–942**

Intravesical Bacille Calmette-Guerin therapy, 1:474

Intravesical medications, 4:1585

Intrinsic sphincter deficiency

    needle bladder neck suspension, 3:1236

    retropubic suspension, 4:1561, 1563

    sling procedure, 3:1237, 4:1692–1694

Intuitive Surgical, 4:1574

Intussusception reduction, 2:*942*, **942–945**, 3:1383

Invasive ventilation, 3:1150

Iodine, 1:114, 115, 141

Iridectomy, 2:**945–950**, 3:1025

Irido corneal endothelial syndrome, 1:25–26

Iridotomy. *See* Laser iridotomy

Iron lungs, 3:1151

Iron tests, 2:**950–952**

Irregular heartbeat. *See* Arrhythmia

Ischemia, 1:455

Islam, 1:353

Islet cell transplantation, 2:**952–955**, 3:1337

Isoflurane, 1:70

Isolation units, 1:158–159

Isometric exercises, 2:638

Isoproterenol, 1:36

J

Jacobson, Jules, 3:1193

Jaundice, 3:1385

Jehovah's Witnesses, 1:211

Joint Commission

    ambulatory surgery centers, 1:49

    evaluating a hospital, 3:1435

    finding a surgeon, 2:655

    hospital accreditation, 1:351

    medical errors, 3:1171

    preparing for surgery, 3:1492

    surgery risks and surgery volume, 4:1775

Joint fluid analysis, 2:**957–958**

Joint radiography. *See* Arthrography

Joint replacement surgery. *See* specific joints

Joint resection. *See* Arthroplasty

Joints

    arthrography, 1:140–142

    arthroplasty, 1:142–146

    arthroscopic surgery, 1:146–150

    joint fluid analysis, 2:957–958

    magnetic resonance imaging, 3:1119

    See also specific joints

J-pouch surgery. *See* Ileoanal anastomosis

Judaism, 1:353, 356, 2:843

Juvenile-onset open angle glaucoma, 2:735, 736

K

Kamami, Yves-Victor, 4:1700–1701

Karyotype tests, 2:720

Kegel exercises

    colporrhaphy alternatives, 1:396

    cystocele repair alternatives, 1:477

    retropubic suspension alternatives, 4:1564

Kelman, Charles, 3:1411

Keloids

    cleft lip and palate repair, 1:360

    dermabrasion, 2:507

    scar revision surgery, 4:1593, 1595, 1596

Keratoacanthoma, 1:464

Ketones, 4:1948

Ketorolac, 3:1473

Keyhole surgery, 1:28

Kidney angiography, 1:81–82

Kidney cancer

    nephrectomy, 3:1240–1241, 1242

    pediatric surgery, 3:1386

    urologic surgery, 4:1958

Kidney defects with esophageal atresia, 2:599

Kidney dialysis, 1:135–140, 2:**959–964**, *960*

Kidney disease

    abdominal ultrasound, 1:2

    anesthesia complications, 3:1478

    arteriovenous fistula creation, 1:135–140

    blood urea nitrogen-creatinine ratio, 1:272–274

    diabetes, 2:508

    diuretics, 2:524

    paracentesis, 3:1347

Kidney failure

    crush injuries, 1:457

    diabetes, 2:511

kidney dialysis, 2:959–963

Kidney function tests, 2:**964–967**

    albumin tests, 1:41

    blood urea nitrogen tests, 1:213–214

    chemistry screens, 1:335

    kidney dialysis, 2:962

    kidney transplantation, 2:970

    serum creatinine levels, 4:1641–1642

Kidney removal. *See* Nephrectomy

Kidney stones

    lithotripsy, 3:1065–1067

    nephrostomy, 3:1249–1250

    percutaneous nephrolithotomy, 3:1243–1248

    second-look surgery, 4:1620

Kidney transplantation, 2:**967–971**

    diabetes, 2:510–511

    donors, 4:1873

    kidney dialysis alternatives, 2:963

    nephrectomy, 3:1241, 1242

    obesity, 3:1269

Kidney-pancreas transplantation, 3:1338–1339

Klinefelter syndrome, 2:721

Knee arthroscopic surgery, 2:**972–977**, *973*

Knee osteotomy, 2:**977–980**

Knee replacement, 2:**980–989**, *981*

    after knee osteotomy, 2:979

    knee revision surgery, 2:989–992

    smoking cessation, 4:1695

Knee revision surgery, 2:**989–992**

Kneecap removal, 2:**993–994**

Kock pouch, 1:386, 2:886, 888

Komatsu, Shigeo, 2:659

Krupin implants, 4:1905, 1907

Kübler-Ross, Elisabeth, 2:841

L

Labor and delivery

    anesthesiologists, 1:78

    cesarean section, 1:328–333

    colpotomy, 1:400

    dilatation and curettage, 2:512

    epidural therapy, 2:588–590

    episiotomy, 2:590–593

    hospitals, choosing, 1:351–352

    intrauterine device insertion, 2:936

    length of hospital stay, 3:1054

    obstetric and gynecologic surgery, 3:1273

    Patient Protection and Affordable Care Act, 3:1366, 1372

M

Meniscus injuries, 2:975

Menopause, 4:1588

Mental capacity, 2:922, 3:1373

See also Competence

Mental disorders

comorbidity, 3:1168–1169

mental health assessment, 3:1186–1189

treatment refusal, 4:1891

Mental health assessment, 3:**1186–1190**

Mental health care, 3:1369, 1373

Mental status examinations, 3:1186–1187

Mentoplasty, 3:**1190–1193**

Mentoring, 4:1798

Mercury thermometers, 4:1800, 1811

Mesothelioma, 2:490, 492

Metabolic acidosis/alkalosis, 1:134

Metabolic imbalance, 3:1245, 4:1851

Metabolic panels, 4:1641, 1643

Metabolic syndrome, 3:1267

Metaraminol, 1:36

Metastases, cancer

bladder cancer, 4:1880

esophageal resection, 2:610

lymphadenectomy, 3:1111

neurosurgery, 3:1255

surgical oncology, 4:1764

tumor staging, 4:1919

Methenamine, 4:1950–1952

Methotrexate

abortion, induced, 1:14–15

ectopic pregnancies, 4:1591–1592

Methyl tert-butyl ether, 2:679

Meyer-Overton theory, 1:69–70

Microdermabrasion, 2:506, *506*, 4:1596

Microdiscectomy, 2:519–520, 3:1003

Microlaparoscopy, 3:1005, 1006

Microorganisms and pathogens

antiseptics, 1:114

drug-resistant organisms, 2:527–528

negative pressure rooms, 3:1238–1239

skin cultures, 4:1682–1684

stool cultures, 4:1737–1739

urine cultures, 4:1956–1957

wound cultures, 4:2035–2036

See also Bacterial infections; Fungal infections; Viral infections

Microscopy, 3:1194

Microsurgery, 1:27, 3:**1193–1197**, *1194*

Microtia, 3:1312–1316

Microvascular surgery, 3:1193

Midazolam, 4:1621

Middle ear

mastoidectomy, 3:1138–1140

myringotomy and ear tubes, 3:1229–1232

stapedectomy, 4:1721–1724

Mifepristone, 1:15

Migraine headaches

glaucoma, 4:1603

postoperative nausea risk factors, 3:1462

Migraine surgery, 3:**1198–1199**

Mild electrical stimulation, 4:1564

Military

blast injuries, 1:194

craniofacial reconstruction, 1:441

telesurgery, 4:1797

Millard rotation, 1:359–360

Milliman and Robertson guidelines, 4:2007, 2008

Mind/body therapies, 1:404, 405

Mindfulness-based stress reduction, 1:405

Mineral oil, 3:1045, 1046

Mineralocorticoids, 1:435

Mini-laparotomy, 4:1900

Minimally invasive heart surgery, 3:**1199–1204**, *1200*

Minimally invasive surgery

hip replacement, 2:820

laminotomy, 3:1003

mitral valve repair, 3:1206

obesity, 3:1271

operating rooms, 3:1283

spine surgery, 2:519–520

surgery and the elderly, 4:1757

surgical teams, 4:1773, 1774

See also Laparoscopy

Mini-percutaneous nephrolithotomy, 3:1246, 1248

Minor crush injuries, 1:457

Minoxidil, 2:742

Mirena intrauterine devices, 2:935

Miscarriage

amniocentesis, 3:1487

dilatation and curettage, 2:512

genetic testing, 2:723

Mismatched blood transfusions, 4:1869

Mistakes. *See* Medical errors

Mitotane, 2:865–866

Mitral commissurotomy, 3:1204–1205

Mitral valve repair, 3:**1204–1209**, *1205*, 1212

Mitral valve replacement, 3:1208, *1209*, **1209–1213**

Mixed incontinence, 4:1562

Mobile cardiovascular telemetry, 1:288

Model of End-Stage Liver Disease score, 3:1078

Modified radical mastectomy, 3:1135, **1213–1217**, *1214*, 4:1676

Modified radical mastoidectomy, 3:1139, 1140

Mohs, Frederick E., 4:1916

Mohs surgery, 1:467, 3:**1217–1220**, 4:1916

Molecular neurosurgery, 3:1256

Molteno implants, 4:1905

Monitoring. *See* Patient monitoring

Monitoring equipment, 3:1281, 1283

Monoclonal antibodies, 2:897

Monoclonal antibody therapy, 2:953

Mood and affect, 3:1187

Morbid obesity, 2:691–696

See also Vertical banded gastroplasty

Morbidity. *See* specific conditions; specific procedures

Morphine, 1:65

Mortality

abdominal aortic aneurysms, 1:123

abortion, induced, 1:17

anesthesia, general, 1:73

antrectomy, 1:118

aortic valve replacement, 1:127

appendicitis, 1:131

bariatric surgery, 4:2005

bladder cancer, 4:1943

blast injuries, 1:198

bone marrow transplantation, 1:234–235

bowel resection, small intestine, 1:251

breast cancer, 1:169, 3:1098, 1214, 1216, 4:1677–1678

bronchoscopy, 1:271

burns, 4:1688, 2033

cancer, 4:1917

cardiac catheterization, 1:285

carotid endarterectomy, 1:307

cerebral aneurysm repair, 1:319

cervical cancer, 1:399

cholecystectomy, 1:345

colorectal cancer, 1:383–384, 4:1670

colorectal surgery, 1:389

colostomy, 1:393

comorbidity, 3:1168

coronary artery bypass graft surgery, 1:425, 4:1557

cricothyroidotomy alternatives, 1:453

cystectomy, 1:474

dehydration, 2:941

diabetes, 2:511

N

Paracentesis, 3:*1347*, **1347–1348**, 1406–1407

Paralysis
anesthesia, local, 1:76
eyelids, 4:1790–1791
spinal instrumentation, 4:1712

Parasites, 2:775, 4:1738, 1740–1742

Parastomal hernia, 1:388–389, 393, 4:1735

Parathyroid hormone tests, 3:**1348–1350**
electrolyte tests, 2:551
intraoperative parathyroid hormone measurement, 2:932–934
serum calcium levels, 4:1635

Parathyroid scans, 3:**1350–1351**

Parathyroidectomy, 2:932–934, 3:**1351–1354**, *1352*

Paravaginal surgery. *See* Needle bladder neck suspension

Paré, Ambroise, 1:365, 3:1290

Parentage testing, 2:857, 3:**1354–1356**, 4:1927–1928

Parenteral nutrition. *See* Total parenteral nutrition

Parents and treatment refusal, 4:1892

Parkinson's disease, 2:493–495, 3:1333–1335

Parotidectomy, 3:*1356*, **1356–1358**

Partial cystectomy, 1:472

Partial dentures, 4:1578

Partial mastectomy, 3:1133, 4:1676
See also Quadrantectomy

Partial meniscectomy, 2:976

Partial pancreas transplantation, 3:1337

Partial splenectomy, 4:1719

Partial thromboplastin time, 1:369, 371, 372, 3:1102, **1358–1360**

Particle immunoassays, 2:890

Partnership to Improve Dementia Care, 3:1264

Passive smoking, 3:1232

Pastoral care, 3:1436

Patches, pain management, 3:1330

Patella-femoral syndrome, 2:974, 975

Patella-tracking surgery, 2:976

Patellectomy. *See* Kneecap removal

Patent ductus arteriosus, 2:760

Patent urachus repair, 3:**1360–1362**, *1361*

Paternal age, 1:357

Paternity testing. *See* Parentage testing

Pathogens. *See* Microorganisms and pathogens

Patient compliance
glaucoma medications, 4:1858–1859
tendon repair, 4:1804

toxicology screens, 4:1852

Patient confidentiality, 3:**1362–1365**, 1372
See also Privacy

Patient education
analgesics, opioid, 1:67
enhanced external counterpulsation, 2:581
gastrostomy, 2:714
immunosuppressant drugs, 2:903
kidney disorders, 2:966
patient-controlled analgesia, 3:1376
planning a hospital stay, 3:1436
plastic, reconstructive, and cosmetic surgery, 3:1442
postoperative care, 3:1467
postoperative pain, 3:1472–1473, 1474
preoperative care, 3:1490
preparing for surgery, 3:1496
stoma, 4:1734
transplant surgery, 4:1874
urinary catheterization, 4:1955–1956
vascular access devices, 4:1973
ventricular assist devices, 4:2000
vertical banded gastroplasty, 4:2008

Patient history, 3:1186, 1477

Patient monitoring, 2:926–927, 928, 4:1621–1622

Patient Protection and Affordable Care Act, 3:**1365–1370**, 1366*t*
managed care plans, 3:1131
Medicaid, 3:1159–1162
Medicare, 3:1177–1179
nursing homes, 3:1262
patient rights, 3:1372–1373
physical examinations, 3:1431
private insurance plans, 3:1507–1508, 1509

Patient rights, 3:**1370–1374**

Patient Self-Determination Act, 3:1082, 1372

Patient State Analyzer, 1:190

Patient-based surgical risks, 4:1767–1771

Patient-centered care, 4:1755

Patient-Centered Outcomes Research Institute, 3:1369

Patient-controlled analgesia, 3:*1374*, **1374–1377**
analgesics, opioid, 1:66
hospice, 2:843
medication monitoring, 3:1182
pain and pain management, 3:1330
postoperative pain, 3:1472, 1473
preoperative care, 3:1490

Patients and medical error prevention, 3:1172–1173

Patients' rights
confidentiality, 3:1362–1365
nursing homes, 3:1262–1263
planning a hospital stay, 3:1436
treatment refusal, 4:1891–1894

Pauling, Linus, 1:70

Pectus excavatum repair, 3:*1377*, **1377–1379**

Pediatric concerns, 3:**1379–1381**

Pediatric services, hospital, 3:1436

Pediatric surgery, 3:**1381–1387**, 4:1750, 1773

Pediatric ventricular assist devices, 4:2000–2001

Pedicle screws, 4:1712

Pelletier, Kenneth, 3:1232, 4:1992

Pelvic adhesions, 1:25, 26, 27

Pelvic cancer, 3:1249, 1250

Pelvic cysts, 1:400

Pelvic disease and second-look surgery, 4:1619

Pelvic exenteration, 2:*618*, 618–621

Pelvic infections, 2:938

Pelvic inflammatory disease, 4:1586

Pelvic osteotomy, 2:816

Pelvic pain, 1:25, 26

Pelvic prolapse, 1:475–477

Pelvic ultrasound, 3:**1387–1390**

Penetrating keratoplasty, 1:417–418

Penetrating wounds, 1:116, 196

Penicillin, 1:93–94, 95

Penile cancer, 1:354

Penile prostheses, 3:**1390–1392**, *1391*, 4:1557

Peptic ulcers
antrectomy, 1:116–118, 120
gastrectomy, 2:686
pyloroplasty, 3:1530–1533
vagotomy, 4:1963–1965

Percutaneous balloon angioplasty, 3:1203

Percutaneous balloon valvuloplasty. *See* Balloon valvuloplasty

Percutaneous catheter drainage, 1:19

Percutaneous heart procedures, 3:1271

Percutaneous mechanical thrombectomy, 4:1824

Percutaneous nephrolithotomy. *See* Nephrolithotomy, percutaneous

Percutaneous polyethylene catheters, 4:1970

Percutaneous thrombectomy, 4:1824

Percutaneous transhepatic cholangiography, 1:185, 2:568

Q

R

Index

W

Wages. *See* Salaries

Wait and see approach. *See* Watchful waiting

Waiting lists, transplantation

    heart transplantation, 2:764, 4:1997–1998

    islet cell transplantation, 2:953

    kidney transplantation, 2:967–969, 971

    mortality, 4:1876

    by organ type, 4:1871*t*

    pancreas transplantation, 3:1336

    United Network for Organ Sharing process, 4:1874

Walking. *See* Ambulation

Walter Reed Hospital, 4:1701

War

    craniofacial reconstruction, 1:441

    telesurgery, 4:1797

    trauma surgery, 4:1889

Warfarin

    medication monitoring, 3:1182

    prothrombin time, 3:1522–1523

    thrombectomy alternatives, 4:1826

Warnings, fluoroquinolone, 2:663

Warts, cryotherapy for, 1:459–460

Washington University School of Medicine, 3:1005

Watchful waiting

    cataracts, 2:631

    cryptorchidism, 3:1304–1305

    ectopic pregnancies, 4:1591

    hemangioma excision alternatives, 2:778–779

    melanoma of the iris, 2:949

    orchiectomy alternatives, 3:1303

    parotidectomy alternatives, 3:1357

    percutaneous nephrolithotomy alternatives, 3:1247

    polypectomy alternatives, 3:1452–1453

    prostate cancer, 4:1960

    stapedectomy alternatives, 4:1723

    umbilical hernias, 2:810

Water pills. *See* Diuretics

Water-induced thermotherapy, 4:1886

Watermelon stomach. *See* Gastric antral vascular ectasia syndrome

Webbed finger or toe repair, 4:**2017–2020**, *2018*

Weber's test, 4:1722–1723

Weight management, 4:**2020–2026**

    abdominoplasty, 1:8, 9

coronary artery bypass graft surgery, 1:424

coronary stenting, 1:430

heart disease management, 2:581

incisional hernia prevention, 2:803, 804

inguinal hernias prevention, 2:808

knee osteotomy alternatives, 2:979

knee replacement, 2:985, 987

laminectomy alternatives, 3:1001

Maze procedure for atrial fibrillation, 3:1144

plaque formation reduction, 2:577

Weight regain after vertical banded gastroplasty, 4:2009

Wellness programs, 3:1369

Western alternative medicine, 1:404

Western blot test, 2:831, 836, 4:1662

Whipple, Alan O., 4:2027

Whipple procedure, 3:1340, 4:*2026*, **2026–2029**

White blood cell count and differential, 4:**2029–2031**

White blood cells

    cerebrospinal fluid analysis, 1:322, 323

    cholecystitis, 1:344

    complete blood count, 1:409

    human leukocyte antigen tests, 2:857–859

    immunosuppression, 2:901

    transfusions, 4:1866

    urinalysis, 4:1948

Whole blood glucose tests, 2:732

Whole blood transfusions, 4:1866

Whole-brain radiation treatment, 4:1729

Wigs, 2:742

Wills Eye Institute, 2:633

Wilms' tumor, 3:1386

Withdrawal, smoking, 4:1697

Wolters Kluwer Health Clinical Solutions, 2:516

Women

    abortion, induced, 1:13–17

    cervical cerclage, 1:324–326

    collagen periurethral injections, 1:377–378

    colporrhaphy, 1:394–396

    colposcopy, 1:397–399

    cone biopsy, 1:414–416

    cystocele repair, 1:475–477

    debulking surgery, 2:488–492

    dilatation and curettage, 2:512–515

    hip revision surgery, 2:827

    hysterectomy, 2:871–875

    hysteroscopy, 2:875–878

    in vitro fertilization, 2:911–913

    intrauterine adhesions, 1:25

    intrauterine device insertion and removal, 2:934–939

    laparoscopy for endometriosis, 3:1010–1012

    laryngectomy, 3:1019

    lumpectomy, 3:1095–1099

    mammography, 3:1124–1127

    modified radical mastectomy, 3:1213–1216

    myomectomy, 3:1226–1228

    needle bladder neck suspension, 3:1236–1238

    oophorectomy, 3:1277–1280

    Pap tests, 3:1343–1346

    Patient Protection and Affordable Care Act, 3:1366, 1368, 1372

    pelvic adhesions, 1:26

    pelvic ultrasound, 3:1387–1389

    quadrantectomy, 4:1535–1537

    salpingo-oophorectomy, 4:1586–1589

    sentinel lymph node biopsy, 4:1629–1631

    simple mastectomy, 4:1674–1678

    tendon juries, 4:1801

    tubal ligation, 4:1898–1901

    uterine polypectomy, 3:1450

Wood, Alexander, 4:1786

Work hours, surgical residents', 3:1171, 4:1751–1752

Work settings

    hospitalists, 2:853–854

    orthopedic surgeons, 3:1310

    surgeons, 4:1752

Workers' compensation, 3:999

World Health Organization

    cataracts, 2:627

    pain management guidelines, 3:1329

    stomach cancer, 2:685

    venous disorders, 4:1986

World Heart Federation, 3:1204

World War I, 1:441

Wound care, 4:1687, **2031–2035**

Wound cultures, 4:**2035–2037**

Wound dehiscence, 2:870

Wound fillers, 1:175, 176

Wound pouches, 1:175, 176

Wounds

    bandages and dressings, 1:174–176

    closures, 1:362–366

    debridement, 2:486–488

    incision care, 2:918–921

X

Y

Z